Continued

Contents—cont'd

Mosby's
ONCOLOGY NURSING ADVISOR

A Comprehensive
Guide to Clinical Practice

Mosby's ONCOLOGY NURSING ADVISOR

A Comprehensive Guide to Clinical Practice

Susan Newton, RN, MS, AOCN®, AOCNS®
Oncology Advanced Practice Nurse
Project Leader, Innovex
Dayton, Ohio

Margaret Hickey, RN, MSN, MS, OCN®, CORLN
Associate Director
Novartis Oncology
Florham Park, New Jersey

Joyce Marrs, RN, MS, CNP, FNP-BC, AOCNP®
Oncology Nurse Practitioner
Dayton Physicians, Hematology and Oncology
Dayton, Ohio

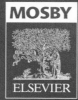

MOSBY

ELSEVIER

11830 Westline Industrial Drive
St. Louis, Missouri 63146

MOSBY'S ONCOLOGY NURSING ADVISOR: ISBN: 978-0-323-04597-1
A COMPREHENSIVE GUIDE TO CLINICAL PRACTICE
Copyright © 2009 by Mosby, Inc., an affiliate of Elsevier Inc.

Notice

Knowledge and best practice in this field are constantly changing. As new research and experience broaden our knowledge, changes in practice, treatment and drug therapy may become necessary or appropriate. Readers are advised to check the most current information provided (i) on procedures featured or (ii) by the manufacturer of each product to be administered, to verify the recommended dose or formula, the method and duration of administration, and contraindications. It is the responsibility of the practitioner, relying on their own experience and knowledge of the patient, to make diagnoses, to determine dosages and the best treatment for each individual patient, and to take all appropriate safety precautions. To the fullest extent of the law, neither the Publisher nor the Editors assumes any liability for any injury and/or damage to persons or property arising out or related to any use of the material contained in this book.

The Publisher

Library of Congress Control Number: 2007943782

Senior Acquisitions Editor: Sandra E. Clark
Senior Developmental Editor: Cindi Anderson
Book Production Manager: Gayle May
Project Manager: Tracey Schriefer
Design Direction: Julia Dummitt

Printed in Canada
Last digit is the print number: 9 8 7 6 5 4 3 2 1

Acknowledgment

To my loving husband Jack, who cheered me on through numerous deadlines and late nights. It is through his support and encouragement that I was able to take on this task while not missing out on the joy of raising three boys together. Thanks also to Alex, Casey, and Jackson, who have been understanding and patient while Mom was writing.

Susie

I had a "ghost" editor living in my home. He listened to me read out loud, encouraged me, and was supportive of the time I spent locked away in the office. I want to thank the love of my life, Kenny, for his role in making this book happen and for making my life complete.

Margie

I would like to thank Susie for giving me this opportunity. My gratitude goes to Cindi Anderson, Sandra Clark, and Tracey Schriefer at Elsevier for their help and guidance during the process. And most importantly, thanks to my family, friends, and co-workers, who have provided the support and encouragement throughout this time. This book would not have been possible without your support. Finally, to you the reader, may this book help you to provide excellent patient care.

Joyce

Contributors

Brooke M. Aghajani, MSN
Clinical Trainer
Genentech Incorporated
South San Francisco, California

Barbara Baum, RN, BSN, OCN®
Rockwall, Texas

Laura M. Benson, RN, MS, ANP, AOCN®
Senior Director, Medical Communications
OSI Pharmaceuticals
Melville, New York

Carol S. Blecher, MS, APN, C, AOCN®, CSB
Advanced Practice Nurse/Clinical Educator
Trinitas Comprehensive Cancer Center
Elizabeth, New Jersey

Christa Braun-Inglis, MS, APRN, FNP-BC, AOCNP®
Oncology Nurse Practitioner
OnCare Hawaii, INC
Honolulu, Hawaii

Patty Woods Bunch, RN, BSN, OCN®
Research Nurse Manager
University of Alabama at Birmingham
Birmingham, Alabama

Kristin A. Cawley, RN, MSN, OCN®
Nurse Leader
Ambulatory Care Services
Memorial Sloan-Kettering Cancer Center
New York, New York

Mary Collins, RN, MSN, OCN®
Carle Clinic Cancer Center
Urbana, Illinois

Dorothy Lynn Crider, MS, RN, LMT
Clinical Nurse Specialist/Nursing Advisor
Otterbein College
Cleveland, Ohio

Denice Economou, RN, MN, AOCN®
Senior Research Specialist–Project Director
Survivorship Education
City of Hope
Duarte, California

Anne Fedoroff, RN, BSN
Clinical Research Nurse
Department of Neuro-Oncology
University of California at San Francisco
San Francisco, California

Cathy Fortenbaugh, RN, MSN, AOCN®, APN, C
Oncology Clinical Nurse Specialist
Capital Health System
Trenton, New Jersey

Ruth Canty Gholz, RN, MS, AOCN®
Oncology Clinical Nurse Specialist
Cincinnati Veterans Affairs Medical Center
Cincinnati, Ohio

Barbara Holmes Gobel, RN, MS, AOCN®
Oncology Clinical Nurse Specialist
Northwestern Memorial Hospital
Adjunct Faculty
Rush University College of Nursing
Chicago, Illinois

Carolyn Grande, MSN, CRNP, AOCNP®
Nurse Practitioner
Abramson Cancer Center
Hospital of the University of Pennsylvania
Philadelphia, Pennsylvania

Debra E. Heidrich, MSN, RN, ACHPN®, AOCN®
Clinical Nurse Specialist, Palliative Care
Bethesda North Hospital
Tri Health, Inc.
Cincinnati, Ohio

Margaret Hickey, RN, MSN, MS, OCN®, CORLN
Associate Director
Novartis Oncology
Florham Park, New Jersey

Kyle-Ann Hoyer, RN, BSN, MSN, AOCNS
Oncology Clinical Coordinator
Genentech BioOncology
South San Francisco, California

Melanie N. Hurst, APRN, BC, FNP
Hematology-Oncology Nurse Practitioner
Associates in Hematology-Oncology, PC
Crozier Regional Cancer Center
Upland, Pennsylvania

Brenda Keith, RN, MN, AOCNS®
Oncology Clinical Coordinator
Genentech BioOncology
Phoenix, Arizona

Paula R. Klemm, PhD, RN, OCN®
Professor
School of Nursing
University of Delaware
Newark, Delaware

Linda U. Krebs, RN, PhD, AOCN®, FAAN
Associate Professor
University of Colorado Denver
Anschutz Medical Campus
School of Nursing
Aurora, Colorado

Nancy J. Leahy, RN, MSN, CRNP, AOCN®
Nurse Practitioner
Albert Einstein Cancer Center
Philadelphia, Pennsylvania

Suzanne M. Mahon, RN, DNSC, AOCN®, APNG
Clinical Professor
Division of Hematology/Oncology
Department of Internal Medicine
Clinical Professor
School of Nursing
Doisy College of Health Professions
Saint Louis University
Saint Louis, Missouri

Joyce Marrs, RN, MS, CNP, FNP-BC, AOCNP®
Oncology Nurse Practitioner
Dayton Physicians, Hematology and Oncology
Dayton, Ohio

Deborah Mast, RN, BSN, OCN®
Clinical Coordinator
Northwestern Memorial Hospital
Chicago, Illinois

Sandra A. Mitchell, CRNP, MScN, AOCN®
Predoctoral Fellow,
National Institutes of Health, Clinical Center
Oncology Nurse Practitioner
National Cancer Institute
Bethesda, Maryland
Doctoral Candidate
Distance Education PhD in Cancer Research
University of Utah College of Nursing
Salt Lake City, Utah

Barbara J. Murphy, RN, MN, AOCN®
Consultant
Oncology Nurse Educator
Ashburn, Virginia

Mary Murphy, MS, RN, AOCN®, ACHPN
Director of Clinical Systems–CNS Oncology
Hospice of Dayton
Dayton, Ohio

Michele L. Musella, RN, MSN, DOCTOR OF INTEGRATIVE MEDICINE
Division Director
Women's and Children's Services
Potomac Hospital
Woodbridge, Virginia

Susan Newton, RN, MS, AOCN®, AOCNS®
Oncology Advanced Practice Nurse
Project Leader, Innovex
Dayton, Ohio

Kristi Orbaugh, RN, MSN, RNP, AOCN®
Indiana Community Cancer Care
Indianapolis, Indiana

Margaretta S. Page, MS, RN
Clinical Nurse Specialist
Department of Neuro-oncology
University of California San Francisco
San Francisco, California

Yvette Payne, RN, MSN, MBA
Director Medical Science Liaisons
Cephalon Oncology, Inc.
Frazer, Pennsylvania

Sandra E. Remer, RN, BS, OCN®, CCRP®
Neuro–Oncology Coordinator
Hermelin Brain Tumor Center
Henry Ford Hospital System
Detroit, Michigan

Jeanene (Gigi) Robison, MSN, RN, AOCN®
Oncology Clinical Nurse Specialist
The Christ Hospital
Cincinnati, Ohio

Mary Garlick Roll, RN, BSN, MS
Oncology Clinical Coordinator
Genentech BioOncology
Williamsville, New York

Jean Rosiak, RN, MSN, ANP-BC, AOCNP®
Nurse Practitioner
Aurora Health Care/ Aurora Medical Group
Milwaukee, Wisconsin

Jason M. Rothaermel, RN, BSN, OCN®
Cleveland Clinic Taussig Cancer Center
Genitourinary Oncology Program Coordinator
Cleveland, Ohio

Jennifer K. Simpson, PhD, MSN, CRNP
Co–Promotion Alliance Director/Product Director
Oncology Sales & Marketing
Ortho Biotech, LLC
Bridgewater, New Jersey

Marta M. Smith-Zamiska, RN, BSN, OCN®
Genentech BioOncology
South San Francisco, California

Roberta Anne Strohl, RN, MN, AOCN®
Senior Training Manager
Schering-Plough
Kenilworth, New Jersey

Dawn Tiedemann, APRN, MSN, AOCN®
Advanced Practice Nurse
Medical Oncology and Hematology, PC
Meriden, Connecticut

Wendy H. Vogel, MSN, FNP, AOCNP®
Oncology Nurse Practitioner
Blue Ridge Medical Specialists, PC
Bristol, Tennessee

Jimmie G. Wells, MSN, RN, OCN®
Nurse Manager/Educator
University of Mississippi Medical Center
Jackson, Mississippi

Laura S. Wood, RN, MSN, OCN®
Renal Cancer Research Coordinator
Cleveland Clinic Taussig Cancer Center
Cleveland, Ohio

Reviewers

Carol S. Blecher, MS, APN, C, AOCN®, CSB
Advanced Practice Nurse/Clinical Educator
Trinitas Comprehensive Cancer Center
Elizabeth, New Jersey

Denise Scott Korn, RN, MSN, OCN®
Staff Educator, Oncology: Organizational Development
High Point Regional Health System
High Point, North Carolina

Maureen E. O'Rourke, RN, PhD
Associate Clinical Professor of Nursing
School of Nursing
University of North Carolina, Greensboro
Greensboro, North Carolina
Adjunct Assistant Professor of Medicine-Hematology/Oncology
Wake Forest University
Winston-Salem, North Carolina

PHARMACOLOGY REVIEWER

Michael J. Berger, PharmD, BCOP
Arthur G. James Cancer Hospital and Richard J. Solove
   Research Institute
Ohio State University Medical Center
Columbus, Ohio

Foreword

Nearly ten years ago we published the first edition of *Oncology Nursing: Assessment and Clinical Care*. The focus of this book was to guide oncology nurses through the expanding scope of nursing practice and care venues of a new century of oncology research and practice. Our goal was to present a comprehensive discussion of oncologic disease with current and emerging treatments, and excellence in symptom management. This approach addressed management of the patient with cancer from time of diagnosis to end of life and in care settings of ambulatory and inpatient care. Our goal was successful and resulted in a tome of almost 1800 pages.

Since that time our world has changed. We have entered a fast moving pace of learning that includes hand held computers, web based learning, and distance learning. Electronic medical records and charting are rapidly replacing hand written physician orders, patient prescriptions, and multidisciplinary notes. Cultural diversity is rapidly expanding and oncology nurses are caring for patients with diverse beliefs about their health, their values, and their customs. Additionally, we are experiencing the greatest shortage of nurses in the history of our country. Time is precious for learning the complex emerging treatments such as gene therapy, cancer vaccines, stem cell therapy, and new applications of older chemotherapy agents to use in dose intensive therapy.

These shifts led us to believe that oncology nurses now require a learning vehicle that is portable, concise, and incorporates oncology information in a succinct manner. Thus we have asked our colleagues to move forth with a book that retains the original intent of our textbook to one that meets the needs of the oncology nurse today. The editors, Susan Newton, RN, MS, AOCN©, AOCNS®, Margie Hickey, RN, MSN, MS, OCN®, CORLN, and Joyce Marrs, RN, MS, CNP, FNP-BC, AOCNP® have compiled a book that presents comprehensive and rapidly-accessed information on oncologic disease, its treatment, and evidence-based symptom management. We believe this book to be an important tool for all oncology nurses.

Christine Miaskowski, RN, PhD, FAAN
Professor of Physiological Nursing
Associate Dean
University of California at San Francisco
San Francisco, California

Patricia C. Buchsel, RN, MSN, FAAN
Instructor
Seattle University College of Nursing
Seattle, Washington

Preface

Welcome to the first edition of a new textbook designed for the busy nurse who needs easy-to-access clinical information on a full range of oncology topics. This book evolved secondary to the foundation laid by our esteemed oncology colleagues, Christine Miaskowski and Patricia Buchsel. They were the editors of *Oncology Nursing: Assessment and Clinical Care* (1999). A second edition was needed, and Christine and Patricia in their generosity passed the torch to us. We wish to thank Christine and Patricia for their confidence in us, and particularly Patricia for her guidance and support along the way. Pat, you provided the inspiration that made this book a reality.

Thanks to the creative ideas from the staff of Elsevier and a desire to meet the needs of the busy practicing nurse in today's fast-paced oncology environment, this book is quite different from the *Oncology Nursing: Assessment and Clinical Care* textbook. With sections such as major cancers, chemotherapy drugs, and symptom management, nurses can access nearly any oncology topic and find streamlined, evidence-based information in a concise format. This innovative format should provide the basic information necessary to guide practice. References are listed for further in-depth study.

Nursing, in particular oncology nursing, is our passion. Working on this text has provided a venue to allow us to contribute to the oncology nursing body of knowledge. It also allowed us to work with some of the brightest and best of oncology nurses across the nation. We would like to thank the contributing authors whose expertise and willingness to share their knowledge made this book possible. The contributing authors are truly content experts in their topic areas, and they showed great patience and persistence through the entire writing and editing process. While we, Susie, Margie, and Joyce, are oncology advanced practice nurses with varied clinical backgrounds, it is the expertise and diverse experiences of the many contributing authors who made this text a solid resource for nurses.

Susie Newton, RN, MS, AOCN®, AOCNS®

Margie Hickey, RN, MSN, MS, OCN®, CORLN

Joyce Marrs, RN, MS, CNP, FNP-BC, AOCNP®

Contents

SECTION SEVEN: PATIENT TEACHING

Appendix

Newly Released Oncology Drugs 515
Joyce Marrs

Mosby's

ONCOLOGY NURSING ADVISOR

A Comprehensive Guide to Clinical Practice

Introduction

Cancer Epidemiology
Implications for Prevention, Early Detection, and Treatment

Suzanne M. Mahon

OVERVIEW

Cancer continues to be a significant public health problem in the United States and throughout the world. Each year the American Cancer Society (ACS) estimates the number of new cancer cases and deaths expected in the United States in the current year. This report is an epidemiologic report of cancer in the United States that provides insight into trends in cancer and its care. For example, in 2007 the ACS reported that the number of cancer deaths decreased for the second consecutive year in the United States (Jemal et al., 2007).

Epidemiology is defined as the study of how disease is distributed in a population, factors that influence its distribution in a population, and trends over time. Although it often receives little attention in formal educational programs, an understanding of epidemiology is critical to understanding the biology of a disease and its possible risk factors and ultimately to developing prevention and treatment strategies. The study of epidemiology encompasses not only the basis of disease but also the impact of treatment, screening, and preventive measures on the natural history of the disease.

Epidemiologists believe that illness, disease, or poor health are not necessarily random events. Some persons have risk factors that place them at risk for development of disease. Thus risk assessment is a significant component of epidemiology. General goals of epidemiology and commonly used epidemiologic terms are shown in the boxes below and on page 4.

TYPES OF EPIDEMIOLOGY

Two basic types of epidemiology are often applied in cancer. These include descriptive epidemiology and analytic epidemiology.

Focus of Epidemiologic Studies

- Determine the extent of disease in a community, region, or defined area.
- Identify potential etiologic sources of a disease and risk factors for the disease.
- Study the natural history of the disease.
- Study the prognosis of the disease with and without treatment or intervention.
- Evaluate both existing and new prevention and treatment measures and methods of health care delivery.
- Examine the cost-effectiveness of various prevention and treatment strategies.
- Provide the basis for public health policy and regulatory decisions regarding health care spending and environmental issues.

Common reasons for using epidemiology in health care. Based on information from Gordis L. (2000). *Epidemiology* (2nd ed.). Philadelphia: W.B. Saunders.

Descriptive Epidemiology

Descriptive epidemiology provides information about the occurrence of disease in a population or its subgroups and trends in the frequency of disease over time. In particular, this entails incidence and mortality rates and survival data. Sources of data include death certificates, cancer registries, surveys, and population censuses (Jennings-Dozier & Foltz, 2002). Descriptive measures are useful for identifying populations and subgroups at high and low risk of disease and for monitoring time trends for specific diseases. They provide the leads for analytic studies designed to investigate factors responsible for such disease profiles. Several common descriptive epidemiologic terms are described.

Incidence. Incidence refers to the number of new cases of disease that occur during a specified period of time in a defined population at risk for development of the disease (ACS, 2007). Incidence rates also provide information about the risk for development of a disease or condition just by virtue of being a member of a specified population. The ACS publishes projected incidence rates annually for common cancers in its annual *Cancer Facts & Figures* publication (ACS, 2007).

The table on page 5 illustrates that the most commonly diagnosed cancers in the United States for women are cancers of the breast, lung, colon, lymphoma, and melanoma. For men the most commonly diagnosed cancers are cancers of the prostate and lung, lymphoma, and melanoma. The ACS estimates that overall there will be about 1.44 million new cases of cancer in the United States in 2007 (Jemal et al., 2007).

Mortality Rates. The table on page 5 also shows the projected number of deaths from cancer in the United States. The mortality rate is the number of persons who are estimated to die from a particular cancer during a particular time. The ACS (2007) estimates that approximately 559,650 Americans will die from cancer during 2007. This translates to about 1,500 deaths per day (Jemal et al., 2007). For men, those cancers associated with the highest mortality rates are cancers of the lung, prostate, and colon, and for women the cancers with the highest mortality rates are associated with cancers of the lung, breast, and colon. These four cancers account for half the total cancer deaths among men and women (ACS, 2007).

Many epidemiologists consider the incidence and mortality rates together when making public health decisions. For example, breast cancer affects one in eight women (178,480 new cases) and results in 40,460 deaths annually. It accounts for 26% of new cases of cancer in women and 15% of deaths annually. Compare this with the figures

Definitions of Terms Used in Cancer Epidemiology

Absolute risk: the occurrence of the cancer in the general population (either incidence or mortality rate)

Asymptomatic: the person being screened and the examiner are unaware of any signs or symptoms of cancer in the individual before the screening test was initiated

Attributable risk: the number of cases of cancer that could be prevented with the manipulation of known risk factors

Cancer screening test: a method or strategy used to detect a specific target cancer. It may be a single modality, but often is a combination of tests. Laboratory tests of blood or body fluids, imaging tests, physical examination, and invasive procedures are all sometimes used for screening tests.

Cost-effectiveness: a financial indicator that is achieved if the costs of the screening program are less than the costs in the unscreened group

Diagnostic tests: tests used in those with symptoms of cancer or abnormal screening tests. The purpose of diagnostic testing is to determine the cause of symptoms or abnormal screening test results.

Effectiveness: a measure determined by comparing the outcomes to determine whether the benefits outweigh the risks and harms and the actual costs of the benefits

False negative: a test result indicating that the tested person does not have a particular characteristic but the individual actually does (a negative mammogram in a woman with early breast cancer)

False positive: a test result indicating that the tested person does have a particular characteristic but the person actually does not (a very suspicious mammogram in a woman who does not have breast cancer)

Incidence: the number of cancers that develop in a population during a defined period of time, such as a year

Mortality rate: the number of persons who die of a particular cancer during a defined period of time, such as 1 year

Outcomes: health and economic results that occur related to screening. Outcomes may include the benefits, harms, and costs of screening or genetic testing and its incurred diagnostic evaluations. These may be short or long term in nature.

Prevalence: the number of cancers that exist in a defined population at a given point in time

Primary cancer prevention: measures to avoid carcinogen exposure, improve health practices, and, in some cases, the use of chemoprevention agents. Primary prevention may also include the use of prophylactic surgery to prevent or significantly reduce the development of a malignancy.

Relative risk: a statistical estimate that is a comparison of the likelihood of development of a cancer with a specific risk factor with a person who does not have the specific risk factor

Secondary cancer prevention: identification of persons at risk for development of malignancy and implementing appropriate screening recommendations. Terms often used interchangeably with secondary cancer prevention are early detection and cancer screening.

Sensitivity: ability of a screening test to detect individuals with the characteristic being screened for. It is calculated by dividing the total number of true positives by the total number of the population.

Target population: number of persons in a defined group who are capable of developing the disease and would be appropriate candidates for screening. Population may refer to the general population, or a specific group of people defined by geographic, physical, or social characteristics. For example, nurses who provide cancer genetics counseling need to assess whether a person is of Ashkenazi Jewish background. This special population of Jewish people is at higher risk for three specific mutations for hereditary breast cancer (Struewing et al., 1997).

Tertiary cancer prevention: efforts aimed at persons with a history of malignancy and includes monitoring for and preventing recurrence and screening for second primary cancers. In many cases, those who have had a diagnosis of cancer and who carry a mutation in a cancer susceptibility gene are at significantly higher risk for development of a second malignancy.

True negative: test result indicating that the tested person does not have the trait tested for and the person indeed does not (a woman has a negative mammogram and cancer does not develop in the next 12 to 24 months)

True positive: test result indicating that the tested person has the characteristic tested for and indeed the person does have it (a woman has a suspicious mammogram and a biopsy demonstrates the area is indeed a malignancy)

Validity: measure of how well a test measures what it is supposed to measure

---

for ovarian cancer. Ovarian cancer affects approximately one in 66 women (22,430 new cases) and results in 15,280 deaths annually. Thus it accounts for 3% of new cases of cancer in women but 6% of deaths annually. Examination of these figures suggests that ovarian cancer is either diagnosed at a later stage on average than breast cancer, or treatment is less effective, or both.

Age-Specific Rates. Age-specific rates provide valuable information and insight about how disease risks vary among groups and populations. Often this information is extremely helpful when conveying information about risk

to an individual. The table on page 6 provides an example of age-specific rates from the ACS for commonly diagnosed cancers.

Prevalence. The prevalence of a disease or condition is the proportion of individuals in a specific population who have the disease or condition at a specific point or during a defined period of time. Prevalence includes both newly diagnosed and existing (previously diagnosed or current) cases of a given disease. Cancer prevalence data provide information on the current impact that cancer has on a population and often have implications for the scope

Estimated New Cancer Cases and Deaths by Sex for All Sites, United States, 2007*

	Estimated New Cases			Estimated Deaths		
	Both Sexes	*Male*	*Female*	*Both Sexes*	*Male*	*Female*
All sites	1,444,920	766,860	678,060	559,650	289,550	270,100
Oral cavity & pharynx	34,360	24,180	10,180	7,550	5,180	2,370
Tongue	9,800	6,930	2,870	1,830	1,180	650
Mouth	10,660	6,480	4,180	1,860	1,110	750
Pharynx	11,800	9,310	2,490	2,180	1,620	560
Other oral cavity	2,100	1,460	640	1,680	1,270	410
Digestive system	271,250	147,390	123,860	134,710	74,500	60,210
Esophagus	15,560	12,130	3,430	13,940	10,900	3,040
Stomach	21,260	13,000	8,260	11,210	6,610	4,600
Small intestine	5,640	2,940	2,700	1,090	570	520
Colon†	112,340	55,290	57,050	52,180	26,000	26,180
Rectum	41,420	23,840	17,580			
Anus, anal canal, & anorectum	4,650	1,900	2,750	690	260	430
Liver & intrahepatic bile duct	19,160	13,650	5,510	16,780	11,280	5,500
Gallbladder & other biliary organs	9,250	4,380	4,870	3,250	1,260	1,990
Pancreas	37,170	18,830	18,340	33,370	16,840	16,530
Other digestive organs	4,800	1,430	3,370	2,200	780	1,420
Respiratory system	229,400	127,090	102,310	164,840	92,910	71,930
Larynx	11,300	8,960	2,340	3,660	2,900	760
Lung & bronchus	213,380	114,760	98,620	160,390	89,510	70,880
Other respiratory organs	4,720	3,370	1,350	790	500	290
Bones & joints	2,370	1,330	1,040	1,330	740	590
Soft tissue (including heart)	9,220	5,050	4,170	3,560	1,840	1,720
Skin (excluding basal & squamous)	65,050	37,070	27,980	10,850	7,140	3,710
Melanoma-skin	59,940	33,910	26,030	8,110	5,220	2,890
Other non-epithelial skin	5,110	3,160	1,950	2,740	1,920	820
Breast	180,510	2,030	178,480	40,910	450	40,460
Genital system	306,380	228,090	78,290	55,740	27,720	28,020
Uterine cervix	11,150		11,150	3,670		3,670
Uterine corpus	39,080		39,080	7,400		7,400
Ovary	22,430		22,430	15,280		15,280
Vulva	3,490		3,490	880		880
Vagina & other genital, female	2,140		2,140	790		790
Prostate	218,890	218,890		27,050	27,050	
Testis	7,920	7,920		380	380	
Penis & other genital, male	1,280	1,280		290	290	
Urinary system	120,400	82,960	37,440	27,340	18,100	9,240
Urinary bladder	67,160	50,040	17,120	13,750	9,630	4,120
Kidney & renal pelvis	51,190	31,590	19,600	12,890	8,080	4,810
Ureter & other urinary organs	2,050	1,330	720	700	390	310
Eye & orbit	2,340	1,310	1,030	220	110	110
Brain & other nervous system	20,500	11,170	9,330	12,740	7,150	5,590
Endocrine system	35,520	9,040	26,480	2,320	1,030	1,290
Thyroid	33,550	8,070	25,480	1,530	650	880
Other endocrine	1,970	970	1,000	790	380	410
Lymphoma	71,380	38,670	32,710	19,730	10,370	9,360
Hodgkin lymphoma	8,190	4,470	3,720	1,070	770	300
Non-Hodgkin lymphoma	63,190	34,200	28,990	18,660	9,600	9,060
Multiple myeloma	19,900	10,960	8,940	10,790	5,550	5,240
Leukemia	44,240	24,800	19,440	21,790	12,320	9,470
Acute lymphocytic leukemia	5,200	3,060	2,140	1,420	820	600
Chronic lymphocytic leukemia	15,340	8,960	6,380	4,500	2,560	1,940
Acute myeloid leukemia	13,410	7,060	6,350	8,990	5,020	3,970
Chronic myeloid leukemia	4,570	2,570	2,000	490	240	250
Other leukemia‡	5,720	3,150	2,570	6,390	3,680	2,710
Other & unspecified primary sites‡	32,100	15,720	16,380	45,230	24,440	20,790

*Rounded to the nearest 10; estimated new cases exclude basal and squamous cell skin cancers and in situ carcinomas except urinary bladder. About 62,030 female carcinoma in situ of the breast and 48,290 melanoma in situ will be newly diagnosed in 2007. †Estimated deaths for colon and rectum cancers are combined. ‡More deaths than cases suggests lack of specificity in recording underlying causes of death on death certificates.
Source: Estimated new cases are based on 1995-2003 incidence rates from 41 states as reported by the North American Association of Central Cancer Registries (NAACCR), representing about 86% of the US population. Estimated deaths are based on data from US Mortality Public Use Data Tapes, 1969 to 2004, National Center for Health Statistics, Centers for Disease Control and Prevention, 2006.
From American Cancer Society. (2007). *Cancer facts & figures 2007.* Atlanta, GA: American Cancer Society.

of cancer health services needed in a specific community or population.

Case-Fatality Rates. Cancer case-fatality rates are often an important indicator of the effectiveness of a particular cancer detection or treatment method and the impact of the cancer in a defined population. Cancer case-fatality rates provide information about the likelihood of dying from cancer among those diagnosed with the disease (Jennings-Dozier & Foltz, 2002). Case-fatality rates are different than mortality rates in that the mortality rate represents an entire population at risk from dying from a cancer and includes those who do and do not have the cancer. Cancer case-fatality rates include only those who have the disease.

Risk Factor. A risk factor is a trait or characteristic that is associated with a statistically significant and an increased likelihood of development of a disease (Mahon, 2002). It is important to note, however, that having a risk factor does not mean a person will develop a disease or malignancy, nor does the absence of a risk factor mean one will not develop a disease or malignancy.

Absolute Risk. Absolute risk is a measure of the occurrence of cancer, either incidence (new cases) or mortality (deaths), in the general population. Absolute risk is helpful when a patient needs to understand what the chances are for all persons in a population having a particular disease. Absolute risk can be expressed either as the number of cases for a specified denominator (e.g., 131 cases of breast cancer per 100,000 women annually) or as a cumulative risk up to a specified age (e.g., one in eight women will develop breast cancer if they live to age 85 years) (ACS, 2007).

Another way to express absolute risk is to discuss the average risk of having breast cancer at a certain age. For example, a woman's risk for development of breast cancer may be 2% at age 50 years but at age 85 years it might be 13%. Risk estimates will be much different for a 50-year-old woman than for an 85-year-old woman because approximately 50% of the cases of breast cancer occur after the age of 65 years. This is illustrated in the table below.

Individuals need to understand that certain assumptions are made to reach an absolute risk figure for a particular cancer. For example, the one-in-eight figure describes the "average" risk of breast cancer in white American women and is calculated to take into consideration other causes of death over the life span. This figure overestimates breast cancer risk for some women with no risk factors and underestimates the risk for women with several risk factors. What this statistic actually means is that the average woman's breast cancer risk is just 0.048% to age 40 years, 3.98% from 40 to 60 years, 3.65% from age 60 to 69 years, and 4.56% from age 70 years on. The 12.67% or one-in-eight risk is obtained by adding the risk in each age category (0.048 + 3.98 + 3.65 + 4.56 = 12.67%). When a woman who has an average risk reaches age 40 years without a diagnosis of breast cancer, she has passed through 0.048% of her risk, so her lifetime risk is 12.67% minus 0.48%, which equals 12.19%. When she reaches age 70 years without a diagnosis of breast cancer her risk is 12.67% − 0.048% − 3.98 − 3.65% = 4.52%. Time must always be considered for the absolute risk figure to be meaningful.

Relative Risk. The term relative risk refers to a comparison of the incidence or deaths among those with a particular risk factor compared with those without the risk

Probability of Development of Invasive Cancer Over Selected Age Intervals by Sex, United States, 2001-2003*

		Birth to 39 (%)	40 to 59 (%)	60 to 69 (%)	70 and Older (%)	Birth to Death (%)
All sites [†]	Male	1.42 (1 in 70)	8.69 (1 in 12)	16.58 (1 in 6)	39.44 (1 in 3)	45.31 (1 in 2)
	Female	2.03 (1 in 49)	9.09 (1 in 11)	10.57 (1 in 9)	26.60 (1 in 4)	37.86 (1 in 3)
Urinary bladder[‡]	Male	.02 (1 in 4381)	.41 (1 in 241)	.96 (1 in 105)	3.41 (1 in 29)	3.61 (1 in 28)
	Female	.01 (1 in 9527)	.13 (1 in 782)	.26 (1 in 379)	.96 (1 in 105)	1.14 (1 in 87)
Breast	Female	.48 (1 in 210)	3.98 (1 in 25)	3.65 (1 in 27)	6.84 (1 in 15)	12.67 (1 in 8)
Colon & rectum	Male	.07 (1 in 1342)	.93 (1 in 107)	1.67 (1 in 60)	4.92 (1 in 20)	5.79 (1 in 17)
	Female	.07 (1 in 1469)	.73 (1 in 138)	1.16 (1 in 86)	4.45 (1 in 22)	5.37 (1 in 19)
Leukemia	Male	.16 (1 in 640)	.22 (1 in 452)	.35 (1 in 286)	1.17 (1 in 86)	1.49 (1 in 67)
	Female	.12 (1 in 820)	.14 (1 in 694)	.20 (1 in 491)	.75 (1 in 132)	1.05 (1 in 95)
Lung & bronchus	Male	.03 (1 in 3146)	1.09 (1 in 92)	2.61 (1 in 38)	6.76 (1 in 15)	8.02 (1 in 12)
	Female	.04 (1 in 2779)	.85 (1 in 117)	1.84 (1 in 54)	4.52 (1 in 22)	6.15 (1 in 16)
Melanoma of the skin	Male	.13 (1 in 775)	.53 (1 in 187)	.56 (1 in 178)	1.32 (1 in 76)	2.04 (1 in 49)
	Female	.21 (1 in 467)	.42 (1 in 237)	.29 (1 in 347)	.62 (1 in 163)	1.38 (1 in 73)
Non-Hodgkin lymphoma	Male	.14 (1 in 735)	.45 (1 in 222)	.57 (1 in 176)	1.56 (1 in 64)	2.14 (1 in 47)
	Female	.08 (1 in 1200)	.32 (1 in 313)	.44 (1 in 229)	1.30 (1 in 77)	1.83 (1 in 55)
Prostate	Male	.01 (1 in 10373)	2.59 (1 in 39)	7.03 (1 in 14)	13.83 (1 in 7)	17.12 (1 in 6)
Uterine cervix	Female	.16 (1 in 631)	.29 (1 in 346)	.14 (1 in 695)	.20 (1 in 512)	.73 (1 in 138)
Uterine corpus	Female	.06 (1 in 1652)	.70 (1 in 142)	.81 (1 in 124)	1.28 (1 in 78)	2.49 (1 in 40)

*For people free of cancer at beginning of age interval. [†]All sites exclude basal and squamous cell skin cancers and in situ cancers except urinary bladder. [‡]Includes invasive and in situ cancer cases.
Source: DevCan: Probability of Developing or Dying of Cancer Software, Version 6.1.0. Statistical Research and Applications Branch, National Cancer Institute, 2006. www.srab.cancer.gov/devcan
From American Cancer Society. (2007.) *Cancer facts & figures 2007.* Atlanta, GA: American Cancer Society.

factor. By using relative risk factors, individuals can determine their risk factors and thus better understand their personal chances of development of a specific cancer compared with an individual without such risk factors. If the risk for a person with no known risk factors is 1.0%, the risk for those with known risk factors can be evaluated in relation to this figure.

This can be illustrated by considering several of the relative risk factors for breast cancer. A woman who has her first menstrual period before age 12 years has a 1.3% relative risk for development of breast cancer compared with a woman who has her first menstrual period after age 15 years (Singletary, 2003). For the woman with two first-degree relatives with premenopausal breast cancer, the relative risk is estimated to be 7.1% compared with the woman with no relatives with premenopausal breast cancer. This means she is 7.1 times more likely to develop breast cancer than is the woman without risk factors.

Attributable Risk. Attributable risk is the amount of disease within the population that could be prevented by alteration of a risk factor. Attributable risk has important implications for public health policy. A risk factor could be associated with a very large relative risk but be restricted to a few individuals; so changing it would only benefit a small group. Conversely, some risk factors that can be altered could potentially decrease the morbidity and mortality rates associated with malignancy in a large number of people. Smoking is a perfect example. The ACS estimates that one in five premature deaths (438,000 deaths) in the United States can be attributed to smoking (ACS,

2007). An additional 8.6 million persons are affected by chronic disease related to smoking. Smoking accounts for 30% of all cancer deaths and 87% of lung cancer deaths. Clearly altering this risk factor could significantly alter the morbidity and mortality associated with cancer in the future. The figure below illustrates the attributable risk associated with tobacco use in the United States.

Odds Ratio. The odds ratio is a measure of association that provides information similar to that found in relative risk calculations. Odds ratios are an estimate or measure of the chance of having exposure (usually to an environmental agent) among those with the disease compared with the odds of having the exposure among those who do not have the disease. It is most commonly used in cohort studies to address the question of whether an association exists between the exposure and the disease (Jennings-Dozier & Foltz, 2002).

Analytic Epidemiology

Descriptive epidemiology helps to identify variations and trends in the distribution of cancer in a population. When analyzed, descriptive epidemiology provides information to formulate hypotheses about the health of a population. Analytic epidemiology provides strategies to test these hypotheses in an attempt to find the reasons or determinants that are associated with variations noted in descriptive epidemiology (Jennings-Dozier & Foltz, 2002). In general, analytic epidemiology strives to determine whether an association exists between a particular exposure or carcinogen and disease status.

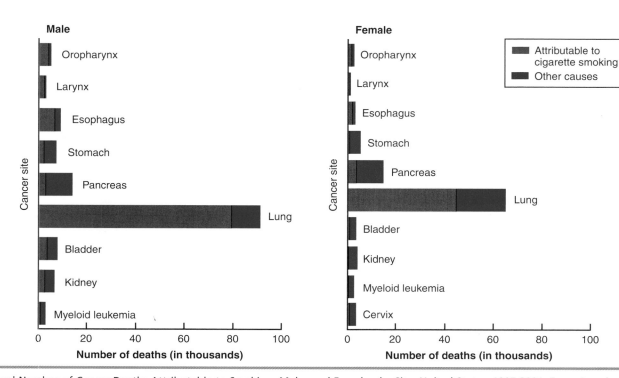

Annual Number of Cancer Deaths Attributable to Smoking, Males and Females, by Site, United States, 1997-2001. From American Cancer Society. (2007). *Cancer facts and figures 2007.* Atlanta, GA: American Cancer Society.

Analytic epidemiologic studies can be either observational or interventional in nature. Observational studies include cohort, case control, and cross-sectional studies. Cohort studies follow a group of people during a period of time. They can be retrospective or prospective in design. A case control study is a retrospective study in which exposures and risk factors in persons with a disease are compared with persons who do not have a disease. In interventional studies, participants receive or do not receive a specific exposure (drug, treatment, lifestyle change) and then compare changes in disease status. Interventional studies are often referred to as clinical trials and may be randomized or blinded.

RISK ASSESSMENT

Basic elements of a cancer risk assessment may include a review of medical history, a history of exposures to carcinogens in daily living, and a detailed family history. Once all information is gathered, it must be interpreted to the patient in understandable terms. Often this is accomplished by using various risk calculations such as absolute risk, relative risk, attributable risk, or specific risk models for various cancers.

Family History

A family history should focus on first- and second-degree relatives and include at least three generations. This includes an assessment of both paternal and maternal sides because many autosomal dominant syndromes can be passed through either the father or mother (Greco & Mahon, 2004). This is typically displayed in a pedigree (figure below). First-degree relatives include parents, siblings, and children. Because first-degree relatives share 50% of their

genes, these will be the relatives most likely to inherit similar genetic information. Information about second-degree relatives can also be helpful. Second-degree relatives include grandparents, aunts, and uncles. Second-degree relatives have 25% of their genes in common. In particular, older second-degree relatives can provide important information about genetic risk because they would have been expected to manifest an early-onset cancer if a hereditary trait is present in the family. The pedigree should also include nieces and nephews because these younger family members can provide information about childhood cancers, which also has implications for the genetic risk assessment. Third-degree relatives (cousins, great-aunts, great-uncles, and great grandparents) can also be included, although the accuracy of reports on these relatives is not always high. These relatives share 12.5% of the same genes. Once all this information is documented, it should be stored in a standard pedigree format (see figure). This pedigree can be helpful in families with multiple cases of malignancy to teach concepts of genetics, clarify relationships, and provide a quick reference. The recent availability of software to draw these pedigrees has made updating the information quite simple.

The family history provides an organized way to document the risk factors related to family history, such as whether a relative is alive or dead, age at death if applicable, significant medical diagnoses, or a diagnosis of cancer. Space can be provided to describe in detail the specific type of cancer, age at diagnosis, and other characteristics such as if a breast cancer was premenopausal or bilateral. Specific knowledge may influence recommendations for screening. Taking a detailed family history is not only useful for cancer risk assessment, but it is also the first step in identifying families with a possible hereditary predisposition to malignancy and other illnesses. Health care providers should ask patients about specific relatives and their health individually rather than asking a more general question such as "Have any of your relatives been diagnosed with cancer?" After gathering the family history, it is important to recheck whether any of the patient's relatives have been diagnosed with these cancers. It is amazing how often patients forget to provide this information, and reiterating this question provides valuable information. Those with multiple members diagnosed with cancer, especially at a younger age, should be referred to a health care provider with expertise in genetics.

Medical History and Lifestyle Factors

Assessment of medical history and personal history factors that may increase the risk for development of cancer should be documented. This can include information such as menstrual history, hormonal exposures, or exposure to other carcinogens such as ultraviolet light or tobacco. Many of these risk factors are not within an individual's control and are not amenable to primary prevention efforts (such as age at menarche). Some lifestyle factors are often within the control of the individual and provide

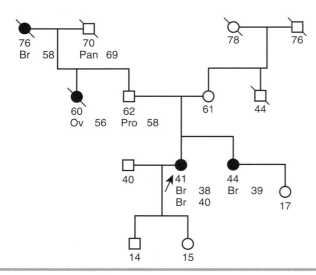

Example of a Pedigree. Example of a typical pedigree constructed to evaluate hereditary risk. Squares represent males and circles represent females. The arrow represents the proband or spokesperson for the family. Slashes represent deceased persons. Filled in circles and squares represent persons affected with cancer. The age and site of diagnosis is recorded.

a framework for providing education about primary prevention efforts.

After all the risk data are collected, the clinician must assimilate the risk factors mentally and provide information about them for each of the major cancers to the patient (Mahon, 2003). For example, the risk factors of early menarche, nulliparity, and late menopause are risk factors for both breast and endometrial cancer. The communication of risk should include a discussion of the risk for development of both these cancers. Risk can be communicated to patients in several different formats. Often it is best to use several means. This can include absolute, relative, and attributable risk.

LEVELS OF CANCER PREVENTION

There are three levels of cancer prevention. Primary prevention refers to the prevention of disease such as immunization against childhood diseases, avoiding tobacco products, or reducing exposure to ultraviolet rays. Primary prevention measures for malignancy reduce the risk for development of cancer but do not provide a guarantee that the person will not go on to develop malignancy.

Secondary prevention refers to the early detection and treatment of subclinical, asymptomatic, or early disease in persons without signs or symptoms of cancer. Forms of secondary cancer prevention include the use of a Papanicolaou (Pap) smear to detect cervical cancer or a mammogram to detect a nonpalpable breast cancer. Cancer screening is aimed at asymptomatic persons with the goal of finding disease when it is most easily treated.

Screening tests seek to decrease the morbidity and mortality rates associated with cancer. After a positive screening test result, further diagnostic testing is required to determine whether a malignancy exists. This is the traditional definition of cancer screening. Some also consider screening for genetic or molecular markers that put the individual at high risk for development of cancer as a specialized form of cancer screening.

Tertiary prevention refers to the management of an illness such as cancer to prevent progression, recurrence, or other complications. In cancer care, examples of tertiary prevention include monitoring for early signs of recurrence by use of tumor markers or detecting second primary malignancies early in long-term survivors.

SCREENING TEST ACCURACY MEASUREMENT

In addition to communicating about cancer risk, nurses must communicate to patients about the accuracy of screening tests. It is not enough to simply recommend a screening test. Patients need to understand what the possibilities are regarding a truly positive or a truly negative test result.

Individuals often inquire about recommendations for a specific cancer screening test such as mammography or Pap smear. Specific recommendations for a screening test often vary among organizations such as the ACS, the United States Preventive Services Task Force (USPSTF), or

the National Cancer Institute (NCI). These recommendations are readily available for comparison at *www.guidelines.gov*. The specific criteria each of these organizations uses to make recommendations may vary, which is why the recommendations are not universal and very confusing to the general public.

There are, however, generally agreed on requirements and characteristics of acceptable screening tests. When screening recommendations are presented to individuals, it is important to include the rationale and strengths and limitations of the test and to present this information in light of the individual's risk for development of cancer. These are shown in the box below.

The accuracy of screening tests is described by a number of terms. A true-positive (TP) test result is a normal test result for cancer in an individual who actually has cancer. A true-negative (TN) test result is a normal or negative screening result for cancer in an individual who is subsequently found not to have cancer within a defined period after the last test. A false-negative (FN) test result is a normal test result for cancer in an individual who actually has cancer. A false-positive (FP) test result is an abnormal test result for cancer screening in an individual who actually does not have cancer.

Considerations for Cancer Screening Tests

- ***The disease should be an important health problem.*** There is little doubt that cancer is a significant health problem. Cancer is not just one disease. Some types of cancer are more significant health problems than other types. For example, the incidence of breast cancer is an estimated 180,570 new cases annually and lung cancer is an estimated 213,380 new cases, which make both of these cancers very significant. The mortality rate associated with these cancers is also high, with an estimated 40,910 deaths annually from breast cancer and an estimated 160,390 deaths annually from lung cancer. Clearly, both these cancers are significant health problems.
- ***The disease should have a preclinical stage before symptoms are obvious.*** In breast cancer, mammography is able to detect breast cancers before the cancer is palpable. Although lung cancer has a high incidence, at present there is no obvious preclinical stage.
- ***The disease should be treatable, and there should be a recognized treatment for lesions identified after screening.*** Breast cancer is clearly a disease that responds to surgery, chemotherapy, and radiation therapy, especially when the disease is detected early (ACS, 2007). Even more important, when breast cancer is detected early, it can often be treated with less-radical surgery such as lumpectomy. The same is not true of lung cancer.
- ***The test must be clinically relevant.*** The test must be able to detect a condition for which intervention at a preclinical stage can improve outcome. The test must be accurate. The sensitivity and specificity must be acceptable. The test must be acceptable to individuals being screened. Highly invasive, painful, or risky procedures are generally unacceptable. The test must be widely available and easily accessible. The test must be cost-effective. Most women are willing to tolerate the discomfort and risks associated with mammography. Undergoing bronchoscopy with the hope of a random biopsy detecting lung cancer is significantly risk laden.

Sensitivity

An understanding of true and false test results is necessary to calculate information about sensitivity and specificity. The sensitivity of a screening test is its ability to detect those individuals with cancer. It is calculated by taking the number of TPs and dividing it by the total number of cancer cases (TP + FN). For example, a screening test given to 1,000 persons with 85 TPs and 15 FNs would have a sensitivity of 0.85. This would be calculated as 85/(85 + 15) = 0.85. Most people are unwilling to accept a test with a high FN rate because many cancers will be missed.

Specificity

The specificity of a test is its ability to identify those individuals who actually do not have cancer. It is calculated by dividing the TN by the sum of the TN and FP cases. For example if a test is given to 1,000 persons and there are 775 TNs and 225 FPs, the specificity would be 0.78. This would be calculated as 775/(775 + 225) = 0.78. A high FP test rate can result in unnecessary follow-up testing and anxiety in persons who have a positive screening result.

Positive Predictive Value

The positive predictive value is the measure of the validity of a positive test. It is the proportion of positive tests that are TP cases. The predictive value of a test depends on the disease prevalence. As the prevalence of a cancer increases in the population, the positive predictive value of the screening tests increases, although its sensitivity and specificity remain unchanged. The negative predictive value is the measure of the validity of a negative test. This refers to the proportion of negative tests that are TNs.

Bias

Bias is another factor that affects screening tests. Selection bias occurs during clinical trials that evaluate the effectiveness of screening tests. Ideally, those screened should be similar to those not screened to determine the effectiveness of the tests. This problem is minimized with randomization. Lead time bias refers to the bias that arises by adding the time gained as a result of early diagnosis to survival time. Length bias occurs because of the preferential diagnosis of more indolent cases of cancer through screening. This may be especially true with in situ cancers that never really become a health threat. Persons with length time bias have indolent cancers diagnosed early, but these cancers may take years to progress, and thus it appears they have longer survival times. Overdiagnosis bias occurs with excess screening. FP rates and overzealous screeners may inflate the actual detection and diagnosis of early-stage cancers.

Outcomes

Outcomes of cancer screening are also considered in epidemiologic studies. When there are no differences in outcome, particularly in respect to morbidity and mortality rates, often it is inappropriate to offer a screening maneuver. Similarly, some agencies consider cost-benefit analyses to determine purely on a financial basis whether years of life saved and costs of treatment are reduced with early detection of cancer through a screening test. Quality of life can be another significant outcome.

Selection of a Screening Test

Understanding these principles is necessary to help patients understand the strengths and limitations of the test they are using to screen for a particular cancer. Individuals need to realize that the perfect screening test does not exist. Even mammography will fail to detect 6% to 10% of all breast cancers (Colditz, 2005). Other considerations drive the screening recommendations. The cancer being screened for should have a high prevalence and incidence and significant mortality and morbidity rates and cost, with a hope for effective treatment if detected early.

Many individuals, however, will still choose to undergo a screening examination, even if a test has a lower sensitivity and specificity in hopes that it will be effective for them. Screening for ovarian cancer is an excellent example. Highly specific and sensitive screening tests are currently unavailable for the early detection of ovarian cancer. Many women, however, will still want an annual pelvic examination to assess for ovarian masses. The test is relatively inexpensive to perform and is usually tolerated fairly well by women. Some clinicians are better at detecting ovarian masses than others and many ovarian cancers cannot be detected by this examination, even when it is performed by skilled clinicians. As long as a woman realizes the test may fail to detect ovarian cancer and is willing to accept this limitation, the pelvic examination may be considered to be effective by some.

There are some steps that can be taken by health care providers to improve the accuracy of screening tests. The establishment of certification and federal guidelines in the area of radiology and laboratory services is one such example. Guidelines are now in place for mammography centers and laboratories providing cancer screening services to ensure that a minimum acceptable standard is met to help ensure the screen is as accurate as possible.

The person conducting the examination or interpreting the laboratory or radiologic test results also affects the effectiveness of a cancer screening test. For example, it is well known that some health care professionals are better at performing clinical examinations than others and are more likely to detect a subtle physical change. Monitoring the quality of clinical examinations is important. Monitoring and improving the quality of physical examinations in the clinical setting is far more challenging but important to improve the sensitivity and specificity of the examination.

Screening quality may also be improved by developing standardized instructions for patient preparation. This may not only improve patient compliance but also help obtain the best possible screen. An example might be scheduling a breast screening a week after the menses begin, avoiding the use of deodorant before mammography, or instructing a patient to avoid douching for 24 hours before a Pap smear.

CANCER SCREENING RECOMMENDATIONS

A screening protocol or recommendation defines how cancer screening tests should be used. The table below illustrates the current ACS recommendations for the early detection of cancer in asymptomatic individuals. This is an example of a screening protocol. Such recommendations can vary among organizations and practitioners. A recommendation generally describes the target population being served, the screening recommendation to be applied, and the interval at which the test should be applied.

Screening guidelines change over time. The ACS has been publishing guidelines for the early detection of cancer for more than 20 years (Jemal et al., 2007). Although specific guidelines have changed over the years, the focus of the guidelines has changed very little. The focus is still that health care providers will use the guidelines to select the best screening tests for an individual of average risk and that the guidelines should be modified in some cases, if an individual has a particularly high risk for a specific malignancy. For example, a woman with a known hereditary predisposition gene for hereditary nonpolyposis colorectal cancer (HNPCC) should begin having an annual colonoscopy at age 25 years instead of the population

Screening Guidelines for the Early Detection of Cancer in Asymptomatic People

Site	Recommendation
Breast	• Yearly mammograms are recommended starting at age 40. The age at which screening should be stopped should be individualized by considering the potential risks and benefits of screening in the context of overall health status and longevity. • Clinical breast exam should be part of a periodic health exam about every 3 years for women in their 20s and 30s, and every year for women 40 and older. • Women should know how their breasts normally feel and report any breast change promptly to their health care providers. Breast self-exam is an option for women starting in their 20s. • Women at increased risk (e.g., family history, genetic tendency, past breast cancer) should talk with their doctors about the benefits and limitations of starting mammography screening earlier, having additional tests (i.e., breast ultrasound and MRI), or having more frequent exams.
Colon & Rectum	Beginning at age 50, men and women should begin screening with 1 of the examination schedules below: • A fecal occult blood test (FOBT) or fecal immunochemical test (FIT) every year • A flexible sigmoidoscopy (FSIG) every 5 years • Annual FOBT or FIT and flexible sigmoidoscopy every 5 years* • A double-contrast barium enema every 5 years • A colonoscopy every 10 years *Combined testing is preferred over either annual FOBT or FIT, or FSIG every 5 years, alone. People who are at moderate or high risk for colorectal cancer should talk with a doctor about a different testing schedule.*
Prostate	The PSA test and the digital rectal examination should be offered annually, beginning at age 50, to men who have a life expectancy of at least 10 years. Men at high risk (African American men and men with a strong family history of one or more first-degree relatives diagnosed with prostate cancer at an early age) should begin testing at age 45. For both men at average risk and high risk, information should be provided about what is known and what is uncertain about the benefits and limitations of early detection and treatment of prostate cancer so that they can make an informed decision about testing.
Uterus	**Cervix:** Screening should begin approximately 3 years after a woman begins having vaginal intercourse, but no later than 21 years of age. Screening should be done every year with regular Pap tests or every 2 years using liquid-based tests. At or after age 30, women who have had 3 normal test results in a row may get screened every 2 to 3 years. Alternatively, cervical cancer screening with HPV DNA testing and conventional or liquid-based cytology could be performed every 3 years. However, doctors may suggest a woman get screened more often if she has certain risk factors, such as HIV infection or a weak immune system. Women aged 70 years and older who have had 3 or more consecutive normal Pap tests in the last 10 years may choose to stop cervical cancer screening. Screening after total hysterectomy (with removal of the cervix) is not necessary unless the surgery was done as a treatment for cervical cancer. **Endometrium:** The ACS recommends that at the time of menopause all women should be informed about the risks and symptoms of endometrial cancer, and strongly encouraged to report any unexpected bleeding or spotting to their physicians. Annual screening for endometrial cancer with endometrial biopsy beginning at age 35 should be offered to women with or at risk for hereditary nonpolyposis colon cancer (HNPCC).
Cancer-Related Checkup	For individuals undergoing periodic health examinations, a cancer-related checkup should include health counseling and, depending on a person's age and gender, might include examinations for cancers of the thyroid, oral cavity, skin, lymph nodes, testes, and ovaries, as well as for some nonmalignant diseases.

American Cancer Society guidelines for early cancer detection are assessed annually in order to identify whether there is new scientific evidence sufficient to warrant a reevaluation of current recommendations. If evidence is sufficiently compelling to consider a change or clarification in a current guideline or the development of a new guideline, a formal procedure is initiated. Guidelines are formally evaluated every 5 years regardless of whether new evidence suggests a change in the existing recommendations. There are 9 steps in this procedure, and these "guidelines for guideline development" were formally established to provide a specific methodology for science and expert judgment to form the underpinnings of specific statements and recommendations from the Society. These procedures constitute a deliberate process to ensure that all Society recommendations have the same methodological and evidence-based process at their core. This process also employs a system for rating strength and consistency of evidence that is similar to that employed by the Agency for Health Care Research and Quality (AHCRQ) and the US Preventive Services Task Force (USPSTF).
From American Cancer Society. (2007). *Cancer facts & figures 2007.* Atlanta, GA: American Cancer Society.

recommendation for every 5 to 10 years beginning at age 50 years. Her risk for development of colorectal cancer approaches 85% over a lifetime, and individuals with this mutation can have colon cancer develop in as little as 12 to 18 months after the development of a polyp. These polyps lead to an increased risk of colorectal cancer in HNPCC; at least 25% by age 50 years and up to 82% by age 70 years, so aggressive screening is imperative to decrease the morbidity and mortality rates associated with the disease (Giardiello, Brensinger, & Petersen, 2001).

Clinicians must remember that screening protocols are guidelines. Screening recommendations are not practice standards to be used with every individual. The goal of the ACS standards is the detection of malignancy. The USPSTF uses very strict criteria for evidence of effectiveness. Cost-effectiveness of the screening recommendations is an important consideration for this group. When providing information on cancer screening recommendations, nurses need to inform the individual why a certain recommendation is being selected.

MEANS TO EXPRESS CANCER PROGNOSIS AND OUTCOMES

Patient survival is one of the primary means of assessing the effectiveness of not only screening tests but also the effectiveness of treatment. Because patients will usually have had cancer for varying lengths of time, survival rates are often expressed separately by stage. See the table below for an example of relative survival rates by stage at diagnosis.

The difference of living 6 months or 10 years after diagnosis is important to both patients and health care providers. Length of survival is often a function of disease stage at diagnosis, clinical characteristics of the disease, comorbidities, and treatment used to manage the disease.

The observed survival rate, which is also known as the overall survival rate, is a measure of the proportion of patients who survive all causes of death after a cancer diagnosis for a defined period of study. The cause- or disease-specific survival rate is a measure of the proportion of persons who do not die from specific disease, such as cancer, under study during a defined period of time.

The relative survival rate is a ratio of the observed survival rate to the expected survival rate for a patient cohort. It is the observed survival rate of individuals with a specific cancer relative to the survival rate that is expected for people of similar age, race, and sex in the general population during the same period of observation. (See the table).

The 5-year survival rate represents the proportion of patients who did not experience a defined event (usually death) during the first 5 years after diagnosis. The selection of the 5-year mark is actually arbitrary (Jemal et al., 2007). Because a significant number of persons historically have died during the first 5 years after diagnosis, health care providers have traditionally used this time period as an indicator of successful treatment and management of the disease.

ETHNIC DIFFERENCES

Knowledge of the overall trends in cancer incidence and mortality rates, particularly among individuals in certain age groups or racial/ethnic groups, can help oncology nurses identify populations at risk. These populations may require specialized prevention or early detection programs. If these individuals live within certain communities, efforts can be made to provide more targeted prevention

Five-Year Relative Survival Rates* by Stage at Diagnosis, 1996-2002

Site	All Stages %	Local %	Regional %	Distant %	Site	All Stages %	Local %	Regional %	Distant %
Breast (female)	88.5	98.1	83.1	26.0	Ovary‡	44.7	93.1	69.0	29.6
Colon & rectum	64.1	90.4	68.1	9.8	Pancreas	5.0	19.6	8.2	1.9
Esophagus	15.6	33.6	16.8	2.6	Prostate§	99.9	100.0	--	33.3
Kidney	65.6	90.4	61.7	9.5	Stomach	23.9	61.9	22.2	3.4
Larynx	64.1	83.5	50.4	13.7	Testis	95.7	99.5	96.3	70.1
Liver†	10.5	21.9	7.2	3.3	Thyroid	96.7	99.7	96.9	56.4
Lung & bronchus	15.0	49.3	15.5	2.1	Urinary bladder	80.8	93.7	46.0	6.2
Melanoma of the skin	91.5	99.0	64.9	15.3	Uterine cervix	71.6	92.0	55.5	14.6
Oral cavity & pharynx	58.8	81.3	51.7	26.4	Uterine corpus	83.2	95.7	66.9	23.1

*Rates are adjusted for normal life expectancy and are based on cases diagnosed in the SEER 17 areas from 1996-2002, followed through 2003. †Includes intrahepatic bile duct. ‡Recent changes in classification of ovarian cancer, specifically excluding borderline tumors, have affected survival rates. §The rate for local stage represents local and regional stages combined.
Local: an invasive malignant cancer confined entirely to the organ of origin. **Regional:** a malignant cancer that 1) has extended beyond the limits of the organ of origin directly into surrounding organs or tissues; 2) involves regional lymph nodes by way of the lymphatic system; or 3) has both regional extension and involvement of regional lymph nodes. **Distant:** a malignant cancer that has spread to parts of the body remote from the primary tumor either by direct extension or by discontinuous metastasis to distant organs, tissues, or via the lymphatic system to distant lymph nodes.
Source: Surveillance, Epidemiology, and End Results Program, 1975-2003, Division of Cancer Control and Population Sciences, National Cancer Institute, Bethesda, MD, 2006.
From American Cancer Society. (2007). *Cancer facts & figures 2007.* Atlanta, GA: American Cancer Society.

and early detection intervention strategies that are culturally acceptable.

Data on differences in stage of diagnosis, prognosis, incidence, and mortality rate is readily available both from the Surveillance, Epidemiology, and End Results Program (SEER) data and from the ACS. The table below illustrates differences in mortality rates and incidence in several ethnic groups. This information can be particularly helpful when screening programs targeted at populations at risk are developed.

EPIDEMIOLOGY RESOURCES

Each year the ACS publishes *Cancer Facts and Figures*. This is a helpful and quick reference nurses can use to quickly gather incidence data about estimated cancer cases. The information is presented in several different formats,

Incidence and Mortality Rates* by Site, Race, and Ethnicity, United States, 1999-2003

Incidence	White	African American	Asian American and Pacific Islander	American Indian and Alaska Native	Hispanic Latino[†]
All sites	555.0	639.8	385.5	359.9	444.1
Males	421.1	383.8	303.3	305.0	327.2
Females					
Breast (female)	130.8	111.5	91.2	74.4	92.6
Colon & rectum					
Males	63.7	70.2	52.6	52.7	52.4
Females	45.9	53.5	38.0	41.9	37.3
Kidney & renal pelvis					
Males	18.0	18.5	9.8	20.9	16.9
Females	9.3	9.5	4.9	10.0	9.4
Liver & bile duct					
Males	7.2	11.1	22.1	14.5	14.8
Females	2.7	3.6	8.3	6.5	5.8
Lung & bronchus					
Males	88.8	110.6	56.6	55.5	52.7
Females	56.2	50.3	28.7	33.8	26.7
Prostate	156.0	243.0	104.2	70.7	141.1
Stomach					
Males	9.7	17.4	20.0	21.6	16.1
Females	4.4	9.0	11.4	12.3	9.1
Uterine cervix	8.6	13.0	9.3	7.2	14.7

Mortality	White	African American	Asian American and Pacific Islander	American Indian and Alaska Native	Hispanic/Latino[†‡]
All sites					
Males	239.2	331.0	144.9	153.4	166.4
Females	163.4	192.4	98.8	111.6	108.8
Breast (female)	25.4	34.4	12.6	13.8	16.3
Colon & rectum					
Males	23.7	33.6	15.3	15.9	17.5
Females	16.4	23.7	10.5	11.1	11.4
Kidney & renal pelvis					
Males	6.2	6.1	2.6	6.8	5.3
Females	2.8	2.8	1.2	3.3	2.4
Liver & bile duct					
Males	6.3	9.6	15.5	7.8	10.7
Females	2.8	3.8	6.7	4.0	5.0
Lung & bronchus					
Males	73.8	98.4	38.8	42.9	37.2
Females	42.0	39.8	18.8	27.0	14.7
Prostate	26.7	65.1	11.8	18.0	22.1
Stomach					
Males	5.4	12.4	11.0	7.1	9.2
Females	2.7	6.0	6.7	3.7	5.2
Uterine cervix	2.4	5.1	2.5	2.6	3.4

*Per 100,000, age-adjusted to the 2000 US standard population. †Persons of Hispanic/Latino origin may be of any race. ‡Excludes deaths from Minnesota, New Hampshire, and North Dakota due to unreliable data.
Source: Incidence (except American Indian and Alaska Native): Howe HL, Wu X, Ries LAG, et al. Annual report to the nation on the status of cancer 1975-2003, featuring cancer among US Hispanic/Latino populations. *Cancer.* 2006;107:1643-1658. Incidence (American Indian and Alaska Native 1999-2002): Ries LAG, Harkins D, Krapcho M, et al.(eds). SEER Cancer Statistics Review, 1975-2003, National Cancer Institute, Bethesda, MD, www.seer.cancer.gov/csr/1975_2003/, 2006. Mortality:SEER Program (www.seer.cancer.gov) SEER*Stat Database: Mortality – All COD, Public-Use With State, Total US (1990-2003), National Cancer Institute, DCCPS, Surveillance Research Program, Cancer Statistics Branch, released April 2006. Underlying mortality data provided by NCHS.
From American Cancer Society. (2007). *Cancer facts & figures 2007.* Atlanta, GA: American Cancer Society.

including the estimated projected number of new cases of specific cancer (incidence) and estimated mortality rates. The incidence rates are also given by state. Oncology nurses can obtain this publication free of charge from the local unit of the ACS and may find it helpful to review to better understand the incidence of specific cancers in the geographic areas of the country in which they practice. The publication also offers detailed information about primary and secondary cancer prevention of the major tumors and projected survival data by stage. Once familiarized with the format of the publication, oncology nurses will find this to be an invaluable resource.

Another source of commonly cited data is the SEER data. Currently, SEER data include incidence, mortality rates, and survival data from 1973 through 2003 (Ries et al., 2006). Data from the SEER geographic areas are used to represent an estimated 9.5% of the U.S. population. Currently, the database contains information on 3.3 million cases diagnosed since 1973. Approximately 125,000 new cases are added yearly. This information can be obtained easily at the NCI Web site (www.seer.ims. nci.nih.gov/).

CONCLUSION

A knowledge of and integration of epidemiologic concepts is essential in oncology nursing practice. These concepts have implications for risk assessment, prevention recommendations, screening strategies, and monitoring the effectiveness of various therapies.

Epidemiologic data are presented in numerous formats. Nurses can use this information when educating patients, devising screening or prevention programs, conducting clinical research, and monitoring the effectiveness of therapy.

REFERENCES

American Cancer Society. (2007). *Cancer facts & figures 2007*. Atlanta, GA: American Cancer Society.

Colditz, G. A. (2005). Epidemiology and prevention of breast cancer. *Cancer Epidemiology, Biomarkers & Prevention, 14*, 768-772.

Giardiello, F. M., Brensinger, J. D., & Petersen, G. M. (2001). AGA technical review on hereditary colorectal cancer and genetic testing. *Gastroenterology, 121*,198-213.

Greco, K. E., & Mahon, S. (2004). Common hereditary cancer syndromes. *Seminars in Oncology Nursing, 20*, 164-177.

Gordis L. (2000). *Epidemiology* (2nd ed.). Philadelphia: W.B. Saunders.

Jemal, A., Siegel, R., Ward, E., et al. (2007). Cancer statistics, 2007. *CA: A Cancer Journal for Clinicians, 57*, 43-66.

Jennings-Dozier, K. & Foltz, A. (2002). An epidemiological approach to cancer prevention and control. In K. Jennings-Dozier & S. M. Mahon (Eds), *Cancer prevention, detection, and control: A nursing perspective* (pp. 33-78). Pittsburgh, PA: Oncology Nursing Society.

Mahon, S. M. (2002). Overview. In K. Jennings-Dozier & S. M. Mahon (Eds.), *Cancer prevention, detection, and control: A nursing perspective* (pp. 385-387). Pittsburgh, PA: Oncology Nursing Society.

Mahon, S. M. (2003). Cancer-risk assessment: considerations for cancer genetics. In A. S. Tranin, A. Masny, & J. Jenkins (Eds.), *Genetics in oncology practice: Cancer risk assessment* (pp. 77-138). Pittsburgh, PA: Oncology Nursing Society.

Ries, L. A. G., Harkins, D., Krapcho, M., et al. (eds). (2006). *SEER Cancer statistics review, 1975-2003*, National Cancer Institute, Bethesda, MD. Retrieved September 13, 2007 from http://seer.cancer.gov/csr/1975_2003/, based on November 2005 SEER data submission, posted to the SEER Web site, 2006.

Singletary S. E. (2003). Rating the risk factors for breast cancer. *Annals of Surgery. 237*, 474-482.

Struewing, J. P., Hartge, P., Wacholder, S., et al. (1997). The risk of cancer associated with specific mutations of BRCA1 and BRCA2 among Ashkenazi Jews. *The New England Journal of Medicine, 336*, 1401-1408.

Cancer Pathophysiology

Paula R. Klemm and Melanie N. Hurst

Cancer is a genetic disease in which the regulation, characteristics, and functions of normal cells are altered. Genes provide the instructions for making proteins and regulate when and where a protein will be produced. Proteins perform many functions essential for normal cellular functioning. During protein synthesis, deoxyribonucleic acid (DNA) serves as codes for the production of amino acids and proteins. Genetic mutations may occur during DNA and protein synthesis, which allow malignant cells to gain a selection advantage over normal cells, enabling them to grow uncontrollably. Malignant transformation is influenced by multiple factors, including oncogenes, overexpression of growth factors (GFs), defective intracellular signal transducers, and cell membrane changes.

The development of cancer (carcinogenesis) is a multistep process, governed by a series of genetic or epigenetic changes that take place over a period of many years. This phenomenon is called the multihit concept of tumor development. Although some cancers are inherited, most occur by a series of somatic mutations. Environmental and personal factors can play a role in the development of cancer as well. Exposure to chemicals, radiation, and viral agents can cause genetic mutations leading to the development of a malignancy. In addition, dietary influences, personal factors, immune function, and genetic predisposition often play a role in carcinogenesis.

NORMAL CELLULAR BIOLOGY

Cancer pathophysiology depends on genetic and external factors that cause changes in normal cell biology. To provide insight into this process, the regulatory, anatomic, and functional characteristics of normal cells, embryonic cells, nonmalignant neoplastic cells (benign cells), and malignant cells are compared.

Normal Cells

Growth Characteristics. Cell division is a tightly regulated and orderly process. Normal cells capable of mitosis divide only for one of two reasons: to develop normal tissue and to replace lost or damaged normal tissues. Even when cell loss has occurred and tissue replacement is needed, normal cells capable of mitosis will divide only if conditions for optimum growth are present. These conditions include the presence of specific cell GFs, adequate nutrition, sufficient blood supply, existence of inducing tissues, and appropriate space. If one of these requirements is missing or less than optimum, cell division is diminished or absent. Once the cause for cell division is addressed (e.g., skin lost in a partial-thickness burn injury has been replaced), cell division ceases so that redundant tissue does not form. This characteristic is demonstrated in vitro as density-dependent contact inhibition of cell growth in tissue culture. Once a cell is in direct contact on all sides with like cells, mitosis ceases and normal cell division contact is halted (i.e., contact inhibition).

Cell Cycle. The cell cycle, an essential sequence of events, promotes cellular division and tissue growth. The cell cycle consists of four phases, each of which is unique and vital for cellular survival. This four-phase process includes the synthesis (S), mitosis (M), GAP 1 (G_1), and GAP 2 (G_2) phases (see figure below). During the mitosis (cellular division) phase, which lasts about 1 hour, the chromatids (i.e., daughter strands of a duplicated chromosome) split to form two identical cells. Mitosis consists of a five-phase progression that leads to the final separation of all intracellular components and the formation of two new daughter cells. Each daughter cell consists of a complete identical set of chromosomes and the essential components of the original cell. On completion of mitosis, the cell either begins a new cycle by entering the GAP 1 phase or proceeds to the G_0 phase, also called resting the stage or quiescence.

In GAP 1, which lasts 4 to 6 hours, the nucleus enlarges and the cell performs the processes of transcription and translation essential for the replication of DNA. The next phase is the S or synthesis phase, during which cells perform DNA replication and produce a set of chromatids. On completion of DNA replication, the cells enter the GAP 2 phase, lasting from 2 to 8 hours. GAP 2 is characterized by intense synthesis of protein and cellular organelles. It is during this phase that cells become committed to entering mitotic division.

Cell Cycle Checkpoints. During the cell cycle, there are specific monitors (checkpoints) in the cell cycle that must be passed before the cell can progress to the next phase. These checkpoints are controlled by a family of proteins called cyclins, which are active at three points in the cell cycle. The cyclins provide checkpoints between GAP 1 and S, S and GAP 2, and GAP 2 and M. Normal cells must accurately complete the synthesis phase before entering or exiting mitosis. The checkpoints serve as a preventive approach to potential errors in the replication of DNA. During the GAP 2 and M phases, another checkpoint identifies DNA replication errors or centrosomes (i.e., primary microtubule organizing center of animal cells) that are defective.

Phenotypic Characteristics. Mature normal cells are functionally and morphologically differentiated, have a specific morphology, and at least one specific function. For example, neurons receive, process, and transmit information; erythrocytes deliver oxygen to the body through the blood; myocytes contract in response to nerve stimulation; and melanocytes produce pigment that determines eye, skin, and hair color.

Except for erythrocytes, leukocytes, and thrombocytes, which are supposed to be mobile, normal cells within a tissue tightly adhere to one another, preventing migration. This is accomplished by adhesion proteins located on the surface of cells that bind normal cells of one type firmly together. Thus, each cell type remains within its organ of origin and does not migrate from one organ to another.

Genotypic Characteristics. Gene storage and activity occurs in the nucleus of cells. Each normal cell contains all the genetic material (i.e., genes or DNA) that is appropriate for the species. During the M phase of the cell cycle, genes can be visualized as condensed matter, called chromosomes. Euploid is the term that signifies the normal number of chromosomes for a species. In humans, the euploid number of chromosomes is 46. The exception to this is the unfertilized egg and sperm, which contain 23 chromosomes. Therefore, normal human cells contain 46 chromosomes (22 pairs of [nonsex] autosomes, and one pair of sex chromosomes). The sex cells are considered haploid because they contain only half of each pair of chromosomes. Mature erythrocytes have extruded

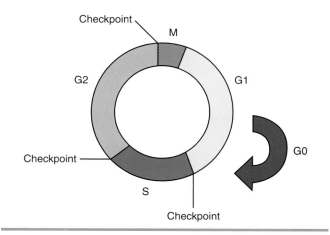

Cell Cycle.

their nuclei during the maturation process and contain no chromosomes.

Although all normal cells contain a full complement of human genes, not all genes in every cell are active. For example, only the beta cells of the pancreas synthesize insulin, although all cells have the gene for insulin. The insulin gene is suppressed or maintained in an inactive state in all cells except the pancreatic beta cells, where the insulin gene is permitted to be expressed.

The size of the nucleus of normal cells is relatively small because each cell contains one copy of each pair of genes. By contrast, the cytoplasmic areas of normal differentiated cells are large because this is the location of a great deal of intracellular activity. Thus, normal differentiated cells have a small nuclear/cytoplasmic ratio.

Embryonic Cells

The concept of each normal, mature cell having a specific morphology and function (or set of functions) is astounding when one considers that all humans started life as a single cell. Although human embryonic cells, those present from conception until postconception day 8 are clearly normal, for a short period of time their behavior and characteristics are very different from the behavior and characteristics of mature differentiated cells.

Growth Characteristics. The main activity for an early embryonic cell is to undergo mitosis and expand the size and cell numbers of the embryo. Cell division for early embryonic cells is controlled but very rapid.

Cell Cycle. Early embryonic cells move through each phase of the cell cycle in a specific sequence. Conditions surrounding the embryo are so favorable that as quickly as a cell completes mitosis, it is ready to re-enter the cell cycle. Although these cells are under restriction point control (checkpoints), they do not spend a significant amount of time in G_0. It appears that early embryonic cells continue to enter the cell cycle even when contacted on all surfaces by other cells. Thus, they do not exhibit density-dependent contact inhibition.

Phenotypic Characteristics. Early embryonic cells are functionally and morphologically undifferentiated. Anatomic features that distinguish the future neuron from the future myocyte are absent. Early embryonic cells appear small and round (anaplastic morphology) and are unable to perform differentiated functions. In addition, they do not synthesize any of the intracellular or cell-surface proteins found on normal differentiated cells. As a result, they loosely adhere to each other and continually reposition themselves within the growing embryonic ball. At this developmental stage, embryonic cells have the potential to mature into any kind of differentiated cell. This flexible state is referred to as pluripotent, multipotent, or totipotent. The characteristic of pluripotency coupled with rapid mitosis allows early embryonic cells to survive

and progress even when conditions are unfavorable. If exposed to lethal conditions at this stage, resulting in the destruction of 90% of the embryo, the remaining 10% continue mitosis and simply replace the lost cells. Such a situation would delay but not disrupt cellular development.

Genotypic Characteristics. All normal human early embryonic cells are euploid, containing only the normal diploid chromosome number. These cells are in an almost constant state of mitosis in which the DNA content must be duplicated; therefore, the nuclei of embryonic cells appear larger than those of normal differentiated cells. Embryonic cells have no differentiated function; thus the cytoplasmic space of the cells is smaller than that of differentiated cells (i.e., large nuclear/cytoplasmic ratio). In the early embryonic cell, all genes are duplicated during cell division. Although these early embryonic cells contain the same genes that mature differentiated human cells contain, only a relatively few genes in the early embryo are expressed. The expressed genes are believed to regulate the growth and characteristics of the embryo at this stage while all other genes are suppressed.

Commitment. At a predetermined point in early embryonic development, the cells initiate the steps to become differentiated. This is thought to occur on or about postconception day 8 (National Institutes of Health [NIH], 2001). In response to an unknown signal(s), each cell commits itself to a specific maturational outcome and positions itself within a group of cells that will eventually take on a specific morphology and functional behavior. Differentiation does not involve the loss of any genes because all committed cells retain the same number of genes present in the fertilized egg. Differentiation is a function of the selective suppression and expression of individual genes. Commitment also involves suppression (turning off) of the specific genes that regulated and directed the rapid growth of early embryonic cells and expression (turning on) of other specific genes to initiate cellular differentiation (e.g., nerve cells, bone cells, muscle cells). The genes that are selectively expressed determine the specific type of tissue that each embryonic cell will become.

GENETICS AND CANCER
Molecular Genetics

Genes, the smallest functional units of inherited information in living organisms, are the controlling factors for cellular development and function. Genes provide the instructions for making proteins, using different combinations of amino acids, and regulate when and where a protein will be produced (regulatory sequence). The process of making proteins is called protein synthesis. Proteins perform a host of biological functions. Some proteins, called enzymes, act to catalyze (speed up) chemical reactions within or between cells. Other proteins support the cytoskeleton of the cell, play a role in immune responses, or participate in the storage or transport of ligands.

Some cells transport proteins that are used by other cells or used to direct the activity of other cells. In short, proteins play essential roles in cellular maintenance, growth, and function (see table below).

DNA Synthesis

DNA is a nucleic acid located in the nucleus of each cell as a condensed, compact structure that contains codes for the construction of every protein made in the body. The helix-shaped form of DNA is actually a pair of molecules consisting of polymers (long chains) of interlocking nucleotides called chromatin. The nucleotide molecules are chemical building blocks consisting of a phosphate, a five-carbon sugar, and a base (adenine [A], guanine [G], thymine [T], or cytosine [C]). The arrangement of the bases can be likened to a genetic alphabet that is used to create the language of intercellular and intracellular communication. (See figure on page 18).

The two strands of DNA are aligned as two complementary threads, held in close proximity by hydrogen bonds. These bonds are disrupted when the cell undergoes DNA or protein synthesis. The bases in the two adjoining strands can only pair up with one single predetermined base. Two nucleotides, paired together are termed a base pair. A pairs with thymine; T and G pair with C. The only possible combinations of the bases are A and T, T and A, C and G, and G and C. A on one strand of DNA can only pair up or mate with the T on the complementary strand. Therefore, if the sequence of nucleotides on one DNA strand is known, the order of the complementary DNA strand can be predicted accurately. One additional nucleotide, uracil (U) is rarely seen in DNA except in some viruses, where it can replace T (see figure on page 19). There are approximately three billion base pairs in the human genome. Base pairing ensures the structural integrity of DNA and is essential for the storage, retrieval, and transference of genetic information.

During mitosis, the DNA content of the dividing cell must first replicate through the process of DNA synthesis, which takes place within the nucleus of the cell. The original strands of DNA are the templates for the construction of new DNA. An enzyme, topoisomerase, is initially responsible for unwinding the double helix by cleaving a single strand of DNA. Then, other enzymes called helicases disassociate the hydrogen bonds that connect the two strands. The unwinding of the two strands of DNA, with each one acting as a template for a new strand, is known as semiconservative replication. The DNA relaxes, unwinds, slightly straightens, and separates the two strands.

The intertwined double strands of DNA are antiparallel (run in opposite directions) with the asymmetric ends (referred to as "five prime" [5'] and "three prime" [3'])

Common Terms Used in Molecular Genetics

Component	Function
Amino acid	Basic building units from which all proteins formed. There are 20 standard and two nonstandard amino acids in the genetic code.
Base pairs	The DNA nucleotide is composed of a molecule each of phosphoric acid, sugar, and a base. The bases are coded with the letters A, T, G, and C. These letters represent, respectively, the chemicals adenine, thymine, guanine, and cytosine.
Cadherin	Protein expressed on the surface of the cell. Plays an important role in cell adhesion
Codon	A group of three bases in an RNA strand located on mRNA. Each codon represents a particular amino acid. Each codon on mRNA has a complementary **anticodon** on tRNA so that tRNA recognizes the correct binding site.
DNA	Deoxyribonucleic acid. Codes for amino acids, which form proteins that carry out cell functions. Composed of a phosphate, base (cytosine, guanine, adenine, guanine), and a sugar (deoxyribose).
Enzyme	A protein that catalyzes (speeds up) chemical reactions in cells
Exon	Region of a gene that contains part of the code for producing protein. Each exon codes for a specific portion of the complete protein.
Gene	Repository of heredity. Located in DNA and RNA and encoded with genetic information.
Growth factor	Protein that binds to receptors of the surface of a cell that stimulates cellular proliferation and differentiation
Hilacases	Enzymes that split the hydrogen bonds that connect the two strands of DNA together
Integrin	Protein that plays a role in the attachment of a cell to the ECM and in signal transduction from the ECM to the cell
Intron	Section of RNA that is deleted because it is not needed during protein synthesis
Ligand	A molecule that interacts with a protein by binding to the protein
Nucleic acid	A complex molecule made up of nucleotide chains that transmit genetic information (e.g., DNA, ribonucleic acid)
Nucleotide	Basic unit of a polynucleic chain made up of a phosphate, a base (cytosine, guanine, adenine, guanine), and a sugar. Cytosine pairs with guanine; adenine pairs with thymine. Uracil takes the place of thymine in RNA.
Peptide	Small molecules formed by the linking (in a specific sequence) of amino acids
Polymer	Molecules composed of repeating structural units connected by covalent chemical bonds (e.g., proteins are polymers of amino acids)
Protein	Organic compound consisting of amino acids joined by peptide bonds. Proteins are polypeptide molecules or consist of polypeptide subunits.
RNA	Ribonucleic acid. Composed of a phosphate, a base (uracil, cytosine, adenine, guanine), and a sugar (ribose)
mRNA	Messenger ribonucleic acid. Carries a copy of the genetic information stored in DNA to the ribosomes, to be made into protein
rRNA	Ribosomal RNA. A structural component of the ribosome that has complementary sequences that bind to regions of mRNA.
tRNA	Transfer ribonucleic acid. Carries the amino acid components of a protein to the appropriate place as coded for on mRNA

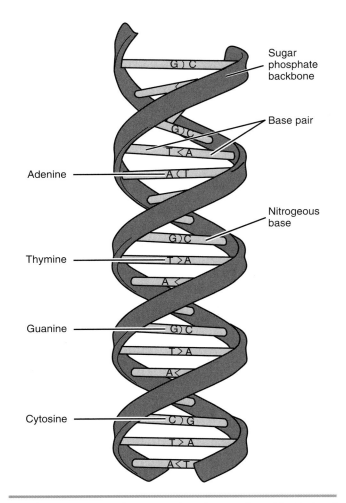

DNA molecule. From the National Institutes of Health: National Human Genome Research Institute: www.genome.gov.

[Labels on figure:]
Sugar phosphate backbone
Base pair
Adenine
Nitrogeous base
Thymine
Guanine
Cytosine

winding around a helix axis in a right-handed spiral. In a vertical double helix, 3′ is designated as "ascending" and 5′ is designated as "descending." A polymerizing enzyme attaches itself to one strand and descends from the 5′ to the 3′ direction. As the enzyme moves along the strand, it "reads" the base sequence and forms a new string of DNA complementary to the template strand. After the strands of DNA are replicated, they condense into supercoiled chromosome sets that split to become part of two new daughter cells.

Protein Synthesis

Protein synthesis is the process by which DNA genes serve as codes for the production of amino acids and proteins. This activity occurs in the ribosomes, which are ribonucleoprotein complexes found in the cytoplasm of the cell. Proteins are formed by peptide bonds joined to individual amino acids together in a linear strand. To accomplish protein synthesis, a particular DNA gene sequence for a specific protein is transcribed into a piece of ribonucleic acid (RNA). RNA consists of a sugar-phosphate

backbone with a nucleotide attached. Although RNA is similar to DNA, it uses the nucleotide base U instead of T and has a hydroxyl group attached to its ribose sugar.

Protein synthesis consists of two phases: transcription and translation. Initially, the cells receive a message to produce a specific protein. During transcription, the portion of the DNA that contains the genetic code for producing the protein uncoils ("unzips") as occurs during cell division. Nucleotides then move along the strand of exposed gene and transcribe the subunits of DNA. The new strand is an RNA molecule referred to as messenger RNA (mRNA). The exposed DNA "zips" closed and remains in the nucleus of the cell. Before the transcribed mRNA moves into the cytoplasm, nuclear enzymes remove introns (noncoding sections, also called "junk DNA") and splice together exons (the working sequences that code for proteins) (see figure on page 20).

Next, the genetic copies (i.e., mRNA) enter the cytoplasm through channels (pores) in the nucleus, bind to ribosomal RNA (rRNA) found in the cytoplasm, and are decoded. The mRNA is encoded with information on the particular arrangement of amino acids that will make up each protein. During translation, a molecule of transfer RNA (tRNA) matches up to the strand of mRNA and carries the correct amino acids to the ribosome (see figure on page 20). Three nucleotide bases (codons) are read at a time, each representing a specific amino acid (see figure on page 20). As each codon is decoded, the corresponding amino acid is activated. The amino acids are brought into the proper sequence once the entire message is read, and the newly formed polypeptide chain folds into its final three-dimensional shape. The total number of amino acids in a specific protein and the exact code that links them together determines the nature and activity of the protein. Different sequences of amino acids change the shape of the proteins and therefore their functions (see figure on page 21).

Neoplasia

Neoplasia is a term designated to signify a new growth of cells in the body. Although all neoplasms are considered to be abnormal, they are designated as either benign (non-cancerous) or malignant (cancerous). All tumors, whether benign or malignant, share two things in common: a parenchyma (functional part) that contains proliferating neoplastic cells and a stroma (supportive structure) consisting of connective tissue and blood vessels (Kumar, Abbas, & Fausto, 2005).

Benign Neoplasia. Benign neoplastic cells enter and progress through the phases of the cell cycle in the same fashion as normal cells. Benign neoplastic cells arise from normal cells and tend to retain most of the properties of the cells from which they arose. At the microscopic level, benign cells are euploid, containing the normal chromosome complement. However, because their behavior is not completely normal, it is likely that some alteration in gene regulation is present. Benign neoplastic cells are

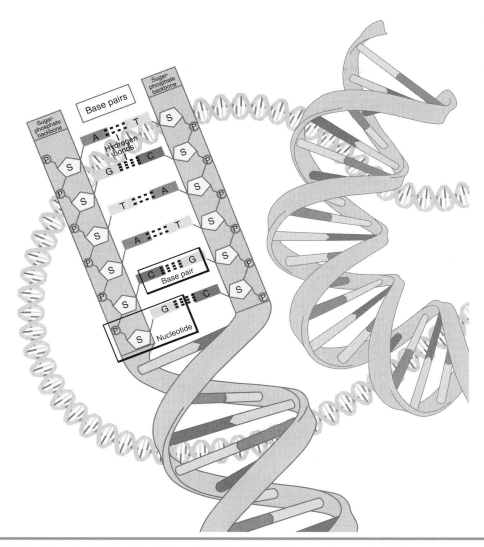

DNA replication. From the National Institutes of Health: National Human Genome Institute: www.genome.gov.

characterized by increased proliferation or decreased apoptosis (programmed cell death). A major difference in growth characteristics between benign neoplastic cells and normal cells is that density-dependent contact inhibition has been lost. Therefore, benign neoplastic cells continue to grow by expansion into the surrounding tissue.

Although benign neoplastic cells have lost some degree of growth control, they have not developed the ability to metastasize (spread to other organs), which is the hallmark of a malignant neoplasm. The suffix "-oma" is generally assigned to designate a benign neoplasm on the basis of the cell of origin (e.g., fibroma [fibroblastic cell], osteoma [bone cell]). Additionally, the type of pattern that it displays may be used to name a benign neoplasm. For example, an adenoma generally displays a glandular pattern, but it may arise from several different types of cells (e.g., epithelium, glandular).

Benign neoplastic tissues are typically well differentiated. In essence, they are morphologically and functionally similar to the normal tissues from which they arose. They retain a small nuclear/cytoplasmic ratio and continue to synthesize fibronectin, as do normal cells. Like normal cells, benign neoplastic cells adhere tightly and do not metastasize. Even so, benign neoplastic growth can cause physiological dysfunction and death. For example, a benign tumor can exert pressure on nerves and blood vessels or obstruct lumens (e.g., trachea, colon) (Kumar, Abbas, & Fausto, 2005).

Malignant Neoplasia. Proteins play an important role in the development of malignant disease. The normal cell cycle is regulated by proteins called cyclins, cyclin-dependent kinases, and cyclin-dependent kinase inhibitors. The role of these proteins is to provide cell-cycle checkpoints to control the signals that coordinate cell reproduction. Checkpoints occur in late G1 before DNA synthesis, during the S phase when DNA content is duplicated, and in G2 before cells become completely

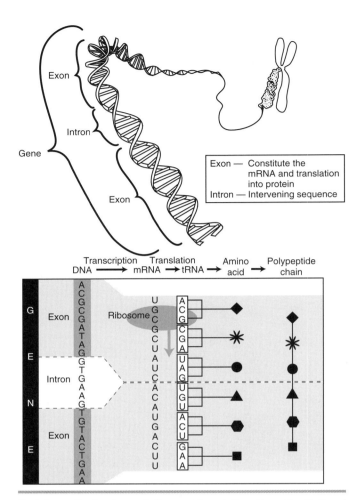

Transcription → Translation → Amino → Polypeptide
DNA → mRNA → tRNA → acid → chain

Protein synthesis—transcription and translation. From the National Institutes of Health: National Human Genome Research Institute: www.genome.org.

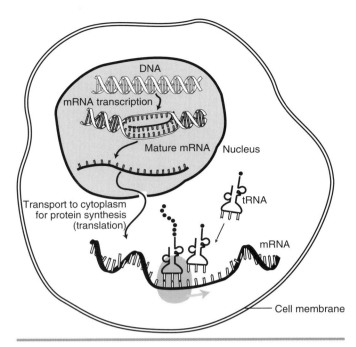

Protein synthesis within the cell. From the National Institutes of Health: National Genome Institute: www.genome.gov.

committed to mitosis. These checkpoints occur at times during the cell cycle when cells are most vulnerable to the harmful effects of DNA (genetic) damage. The checkpoints allow cells to make DNA repairs and remove damaged molecules before they threaten the survival of the organism (Reed, 2005; Rettig & Sawicki, 2001; Skaar & DeCaprio, 2006).

Normal cells have multiple copies of specific DNA sequences and proteins at the ends of their chromosomes, called telomeres. Each time a cell divides, it loses a telomere, thus shortening the chromosome. When the chromosome is shortened to a predetermined length, the cell is signaled to enter the resting stage, also known as senescence. The cell remains viable but stops reproducing (Kashima et al., 2006). Normal cells in a culture plate have a limited life span and a specific number of doubling times before they enter senescence. In addition, they display contact inhibition. Once the cells reach the boundary of the culture dish, they stop proliferating.

Normal cells are anchorage dependent. With the exception of hematopoietic cells, they must be attached to a surface (substratum) to proliferate. Malignant (cancer) cells,

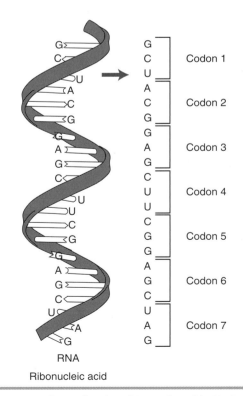

Codones. From the National Institutes of Health: National Human Genome Institute: www.genome.gov.

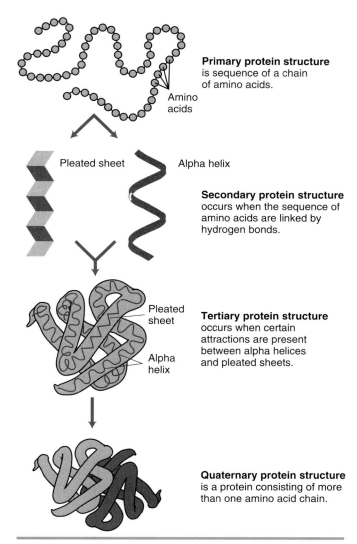

Primary protein structure is sequence of a chain of amino acids.

Amino acids

Pleated sheet

Alpha helix

Secondary protein structure occurs when the sequence of amino acids are linked by hydrogen bonds.

Pleated sheet

Tertiary protein structure occurs when certain attractions are present between alpha helices and pleated sheets.

Alpha helix

Quaternary protein structure is a protein consisting of more than one amino acid chain.

Protein structures. From the National Institutes of Health: National Human Genome Institute: www.genome.gov.

by contrast, are immortal. In a culture medium, growth is not confined to the surface of the culture dish. When malignant cells reach the edges of the culture dish, they continue to grow on top of each other. Malignant neoplastic cells are also capable of growing without a supporting substratum. They grow easily in suspension in an agarose or other medium, whereas normal cells must adhere to the surface of the culture plate to grow. Thus, malignant cells have a loss of anchorage dependence.

Cancer cells range from well differentiated to anaplastic (undifferentiated). Anaplasia, or lack of differentiation, is a classic sign of malignant transformation. As cancer progresses, the cells become increasingly anaplastic until they no longer resemble the parent tissue and most differentiated functions are lost. Cancer cells continually undergo mitosis and perform fewer and fewer differentiated functions. As a result, cancer cells have a large nuclear/cytoplasmic ratio, whereas the reverse is true for normal cells.

The nomenclature for malignant neoplasms is the same as that used for benign tumors. Cancerous tumors of epithelial cell origin are called carcinomas (e.g., bronchogenic carcinoma [respiratory], renal cell carcinoma [kidney], hepatocellular carcinoma [liver]). Adenocarcinoma is a term reserved for tumors that display a glandular pattern. Cancers arising from smooth muscle are called leiomyosarcomas, whereas the term leukemia refers to a hematopoietic malignancy.

MALIGNANT TRANSFORMATION: CARCINOGENESIS

The process by which normal cells become cancer cells is called malignant transformation or carcinogenesis. Carcinogenesis is a multistep process that may take years to complete, and it is governed by a series of genetic or epigenetic changes. Genetic mutations may occur by deletion, duplication, inversion, insertion, or translocation (Baltzell, Eder, & Wrensch, 2005; Calvo, Petricoin, & Liotta, 2005; Rettig & Sawicki, 2001; Smith, Marks, & Lieberman, 2005) (see figure on page 22).

Genetic mutations are not uncommon and are usually repaired by cellular mechanisms. Cancer arises when defects in the genes that regulate cellular proliferation and differentiation, suppress tumor growth, target irreparably damaged cells for apoptosis, or repair damaged DNA are not corrected. As a result of these defects, cancer cells are not governed by the signals that regulate cell growth and may consequently exhibit uncontrolled proliferation (Calvo, Petricoin, & Liotta, 2005; Hoeijmakers, 2001; Taniwaki et al., 2006). Although cancer is sometimes caused by passing a defective gene to offspring, it is most often caused by mutations that occur over the course of a lifetime. These somatic (acquired, sporadic) mutations may result from a variety of factors that include physical, environmental, or chemical agents; ultraviolet (UV) radiation; viruses; or errors in replication that can cause base changes or breaks in the DNA strands. Acquired mutations are not passed on to offspring because these mutations are only found in the malignant neoplastic cell (Smith, Marks, & Lieberman, 2005; Stetler-Stevenson, 2005).

Oncogenes

Two types of genes are responsible for the development of cancer: oncogenes and tumor suppressor genes. Oncogenes are mutations of normal genes called proto-oncogenes that govern growth factors (GFs), GF receptors (GFRs), signal transducers, transcription factors, apoptosis regulators, and cell cycle regulators (see table on page 22). Defects in any of these can provide a "gain of function" and cause a cell to grow out of control. For example, GFs serve as ligands that bind to receptors on the surface of cells. If a GF, or GFR, is overproduced by an oncogene, the target cells may experience uncontrolled proliferation (Carpenter & Cantley, 2005; Connolly et al., 2006; Smith, Marks, & Lieberman, 2005). Other oncogenes can affect signal transduction in cells and activate a series of protein

Types of mutation

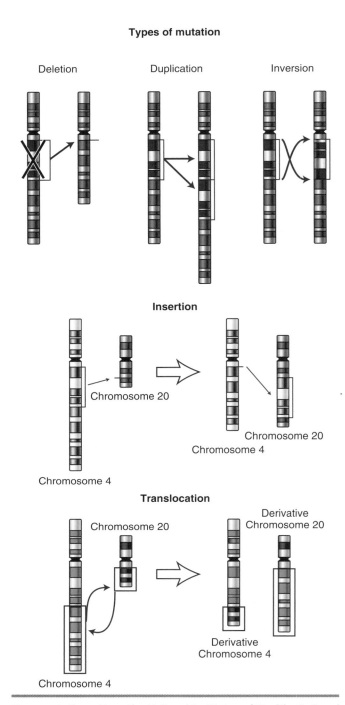

Gene mutations. From the National Institutes of Health: National Human Genome Institute: www.genome.gov.

kinases, leading to uncontrolled cell proliferation. However, the mutation only occurs in one copy of a proto-oncogene.

Subsequent mutations are required for cancer to develop. This phenomenon is referred to as the multihit concept of tumor development. Examples of oncogenes that are altered in many types of cancers include *myc* (leukemia, lymphoma, lung cancer), *ras* (bladder, lung, breast, ovarian cancer), *sis* (glioma), and HER-2/*neu* (breast cancer, cervical cancer). GFs and GFRs function as ligands and regulate cell proliferation by binding to receptors on the plasma membrane.

Selected Oncogenes

Oncogene	Function	Malignancy
abl	Tyrosine kinase activity	Chronic myelogenous leukemia
akt-2	Cell cycle progression	Ovarian and pancreatic cancer
c-myc	DNA synthesis	Breast, cervical, colorectal, and lung cancer; leukemia, neuroblastoma, glioblastoma
egfr	Tyrosine kinase	Squamous cell carcinoma
*erb*B	Tyrosine kinase	Brain tumors; squamous cell carcinoma
*erb*B-2 (formerly *neu*)	Tyrosine kinase	Breast and ovarian cancer, cancer of the salivary gland
ets-1	Transcription factor	Lymphoma
fos	Transcription factor	Osteosarcoma
HER-2/*neu*	Fusion gene	Breast and cervical cancer
hst	Growth factor	Breast cancer; squamous cell carcinoma
int-2	Growth factor	Breast cancer; squamous cell carcinoma
jun	Transcription factor	Sarcoma
kit	Tyrosine kinase	Sarcoma
L-*myc*	DNA synthesis	Lung cancer
mdm-2	p53 inhibitor	Sarcoma

If excessive GF is produced because of genetic mutation, cells may proliferate inappropriately. In essence, the signal for cellular reproduction is constantly "on."

Growth Factor Receptors

Mutations in GFRs cause multiple copies of a gene to be made (amplification) leading to overexpression of cellular proteins. For example, HER-2/*neu* is a GFR that, when amplified, causes overexpression of the HER-2/*neu* protein in some breast and other cancers. A greater degree of amplification is correlated with a poorer prognosis (Hill, 2001; Rettig & Sawicki, 2001).

Intracellular Signal Transducers (Kinases)

Kinases encode proteins that are active in GF signal transduction. Mutations in signal transducers can lead to uncontrolled proliferation. Nuclear transcription factors regulate the expression of genes that are involved in cellular growth, proliferation, metabolism, differentiation, and apoptosis. Overexpression of the transcription factor *myc* is one of the most common mutations among people with cancer, causing uncontrolled growth and a loss of apoptosis.

Tumor Suppressor Genes

Tumor suppressor (TS) genes (normal growth suppressor genes) are designed to limit cell division, promote apoptosis, or repair defective DNA. Defects in limiting cell proliferation, cell death, or DNA repair contribute to uncontrolled proliferation of neoplastic cells (Calvo, Petricoin, & Liotta, 2005; Lembo et al., 2006). Defects in TS genes are referred to as "loss of function" mutations. Both a gain of function

Selected Tumor Suppressors

Tumor Suppressor	Function	Malignancy
APC	Controls specific transcription factors	Familial adenomatous polyposis colorectal stomach, pancreatic cancers
BRCA1, BRCA2	DNA repair	Inherited breast cancers; ovarian cancers

in an oncogene and a corresponding loss of function in TS genes, repair enzymes, or activators of apoptosis are necessary to promote malignant neoplasia (Smith, Marks, & Lieberman, 2005). When both proto-oncogenes and TS genes are mutated, there is little to prevent cancer cells from proliferating. Cancer cells speed up the rate of tissue growth because they spend very little time in G_0, before proceeding through the cell cycle (Hill, 2001; Reed, 2005; Smith, Marks, & Lieberman, 2005) (see table above).

The first TS gene to be identified was the retinoblastoma gene Rb1, which predisposes those affected to the development of osteosarcoma and retinoblastoma. The best-known mutated gene in humans is the tumor-suppressor gene that codes for p53, found on chromosome 17. p53 plays a role in blocking proliferation in G_1, apoptosis, and DNA repair. If an individual inherits only one working copy of the gene, he or she is predisposed to cancer. A lack of p53 allows cells with genetic mutations to propagate and is found in many people with malignancies, including cancer of the lung, breast, esophagus, liver, bladder, ovary, and brain and sarcoma, lymphoma, and leukemia. Up to 70% of cancers contain a mutation in p53 or mdm2 (the gene that regulates p53) (Loescher & Whitesell, 2003; Papakosta et al., 2006; Rettig & Sawicki, 2001; Rudin & Thompson, 2002).

DNA Repair Enzymes. Normal cell mitosis and activity are dependent on the accurate transcription of DNA. Redundant molecular genetic "backup" mechanisms exist that examine newly transcribed DNA, check for damaged or mismatched base pairs, and ensure that accurate transcription has occurred. Damage to DNA can occur, as a result of chemical toxins, exposure to sunlight, and errors in replication. One type of tumor suppressor gene, the DNA repair enzymes, makes repairs to DNA before cell replication takes place.

Repair to DNA can take place by several mechanisms. Some common types of damage to DNA base pairs can be repaired by the cellular subsystem itself. When only one strand of DNA is damaged, the second strand can be used as a template to make the necessary repairs. These types of repairs may include base excision repair, nucleotide excision repair, and mismatch repair mechanisms. If both strands of DNA are damaged, nonhomologous end-joining and template-assisted repair (homologous recombination repair)

mechanisms are used (Reed, 2005; Rettig & Sawicki, 2001). Examples of mutated tumor suppressor genes that cause cancer are the BRCA-1 and BRCA-2 genes that predispose some women to the development breast cancer, p53 (bladder, breast, liver, lung, prostate, ovarian cancer), APC (familial adenomatous and noninherited colorectal cancer), and Rb1 (retinoblastoma, sarcoma, bladder cancer, breast cancer, lung cancer). BRCA-1 and BRCA-2 account for up to 90% of familial breast cancers (Bangsi et al., 2006; Dominguez et al., 2005; Haffty et al., 2006; Hill, 2001).

Surface and Membrane Changes

Some of the acquired characteristics of cancer cells involve surface and membrane changes. The cells that make up a multicellular organism interact with each other and with the extracellular matrix (ECM). The structure of the ECM (a three-dimensional, noncellular medium) differs by tissue type, but it is essential for the growth and survival of normal cells. For example, the components that make up ECM interact and combine with GFs, thereby controlling their availability to the cells. Without interactions with the ECM, normal cells undergo apoptosis. However, malignant neoplastic cells can survive and reproduce without the usual interactions with the ECM. Cancer cells produce plasminogen activator, which helps break down plasminogen to plasmin. Plasmin, in turn, can cause the release of GFs in cancer cells, thereby leading to greater proliferation of these mutant cells (i.e., gain of function) (Egeblad & Werb, 2002; Hojilla, Mohammed, & Khokha, 2003; Stamenkovic, 2003; Stetler-Stevenson, 2005).

Matrix Metalloproteinases

Matrix metalloproteinases (MMPs) are a family of proteases (enzymes that degrade proteins) that help regulate the microenvironment of cells by controlling GFs and GFRs and are active in cell adhesion and apoptosis. They can degrade the protein components of the ECM and basement membranes, as well. Some MMPs may generate specific signals that promote tumor development and the growth of new blood vessels to support tumor growth. Increased expression of MMPs is correlated with poor prognosis and more invasive malignant disease (Bissell & Radisky, 2001; Connolly et al., 2006; Hojilla, Mohammed, & Khokha, 2003; Stamenkovic, 2003).

Cell Adhesion Molecules

Normal cells express a variety of cell adhesion molecules (CAMs) on their surface. Integrins span the plasma membrane of the cell, bind to specific ECM proteins, and play a vital role in cell-ECM interactions (Hill, 2001). Cadherins are CAMs that regulate signal transduction within the cell and in interactions between similar cells. Some members of the immunoglobulin family also play a role in cellular adhesion. Changes in the expression of integrins and cadherins increase the ability of cancer cells to metastasize and foster more aggressive disease (Hill, 2001; Kute et al., 1998; Watson-Hurst & Becker, 2006).

Surface Antigens

Cancer cells express different membrane surface components, particularly receptors and proteins (antigens), than do the normal cells from which they arose (Polyak & Meyerson, 2006; Rettig & Sawicki, 2001). Some cancer cells express cell surface antigens that are unlike surface antigens of normal differentiated cells. Cancer antigens may be ordinary protein products that are synthesized by normal cells at an earlier developmental period but are not expressed by mature cells or are expressed only in small quantities (Abbas & Lichtman, 2003). Examples of normal cellular antigens include prostate specific antigen, alpha-fetoprotein, carcinoembryonic antigen, human chorionic gonadotropin, lactate dehydrogenase, and alkaline phosphatase. Elevated levels of these can indicate the presence of a malignancy.

Cancer cells may express surface antigens that are found only on malignant cells. Such proteins are termed tumor-specific antigens (TSAs) and can be used as markers to identify and quantify the amount of tumor present (Abbas & Lichtman, 2003). Examples include the HER-2 protein (breast cancer) and the CD20 antigen (non-Hodgkin's lymphoma). Antibodies directed against TSAs are being used for cancer therapy and prevention. For example, trastuzumab (Herceptin) targets the HER-2 protein that is overexpressed in a small percentage of women with breast cancer (Plosker & Keam, 2006; Tokunaga et al., 2006). Rituximab (Rituxan), ibritumomab tiuxetan (Zevalin), and tositumomab (Bexxar) are used to treat individuals with non-Hodgkin's lymphoma who overexpress the CD20 antigen (Cvetkovic & Perry, 2006; Nowakowski & Witzig, 2006).

Metastasis

A hallmark of malignant cells is their ability to initiate the growth of tumors in other parts of the body (metastasis). The process of metastatic spread is pathophysiologically complex and involves a multistage progression of events. Cancer may spread by local invasion, lymphatic spread, or through the blood. To disseminate by the hematogenous route, malignant cells must be able to break away from the original tumor by a process called intravasation. Then they must enter blood vessels, survive travel through the circulatory system, exit the circulation (extravasation), migrate into interstitial spaces, and initiate new tumor growth (Hill, 2001; Kumar, Abbas, & Fausto, 2005; McDonnell & Wellstein, 2006; Rettig & Sawicki, 2001; Skaar & DeCaprio, 2006).

Metastasis requires that cancer cells penetrate the stroma surrounding the malignant growth. Cancer cells may express higher levels of proteolytic enzymes, which break down the cell membrane and ECM components. This breakdown in the cytoskeleton enables cancer cells to migrate to distant sites and proliferate. Once the basement membrane of the tumor is breached, tumor cells can travel into the blood vessels or lymphatics. However, to do this, malignant cells must be able to translocate. This is made possible by a number of cellular proteins (i.e., GFs, ECM molecules) found in cancer cells that stimulate the growth of pseudopodia, allowing cancer cells to move through the circulatory system (Jia et al., 2005). Once cancer cells have reached the target organ, they must exit the circulation and initiate new growth. MMPs help degrade the ECM that cancer cells must penetrate in the target organ to initiate metastatic development. Metastatic spread also depends on cell-to-cell and cell-to-matrix interactions between the circulating metastatic cells and the target organ (Egeblad & Werb, 2002; Hill, 2001; Hojilla, Mohammed, & Khokha, 2003; Kute et al., 1998; McDonnell & Wellstein, 2006; Skaar & DeCaprio, 2006; Stamenkovic, 2003; Thompson et al., 2005).

The metastatic process can only be accomplished by a small number of cells within the primary tumor. One model of metastasis formation suggests that mutations in oncogenes or inactivation of TS genes may result in a selective growth advantage for tumor cells. As additional mutations occur, advantageous phenotypes develop and become dominant, thus conferring a growth advantage and metastatic competence to all cells within the tumor. Another explanation of metastatic development purports that aggressive tumor cells, capable of metastasis, comprise only a small percentage of the primary tumor's cells. Although tumors slough off many malignant cells that then travel through the circulatory system, only a few are capable of stimulating a metastatic growth. The low metastatic potential of the shed tumor cells may be attributed to the fact that most of these are undergoing apoptosis as they disengage from the primary tumor (Swartz et al., 1999). Some studies have indicated that cancer cells vary in their metastatic proclivity and are influenced by genetic mutations in GFs, GFRs, TS genes, and other proteins (Flatmark et al., 2004; Hessel et al., 2004; Lev, Kiriakova, & Price, 2003; Stetler-Stevenson, 2005). Metastatic activity is also influenced by tumor-host interactions and the microenvironment of the target organ (Fidler, 2003; Fidler et al., 2005; Killion & Fidler, 2005; McDonnell & Wellstein, 2006).

Cancer Stem Cells. Recent evidence suggests that the growth of undifferentiated cells arises from stem cells present in all specialized tissues (Clarke & Weissman, 2004; Kumar, Abbas, & Fausto, 2005; Lawson et al., 2005; Wang et al., 2001). Stem cells are undifferentiated cells that have the ability to divide and renew themselves over long periods and give rise to specialized cells to take the place of those that have been lost. The renewal of stem cells is a highly regulated process in which chemical signals play an important role in renewing or repairing damaged tissue (Armanios & Greider, 2005; NIH, 2006). Defects in signaling pathways allow cancer stem cells within malignant neoplasms to regrow tumor cells (Beachy, Karhadkar, & Berman, 2004; Kalirai & Clarke, 2006; Liu, Dontu, & Wicha, 2005; Reya & Clevers, 2005; Taipale & Beachy, 2001). Only a small percentage of cells within a tumor are thought to consist of stem cells, but their presence would help explain the fact that some tumors recur even after aggressive treatment (Calvo, Petricoin, & Liotta, 2005; Clarke & Weissman, 2004).

Angiogenesis. Primary and metastatic tumors need an adequate blood supply to grow and survive. The process by which vascular networks are created to sustain malignant tumors is called angiogenesis. An independent vascular network provides malignant tumors with easy access to the circulatory system. In addition to supplying the tumor with nutrients, a convenient blood supply facilitates metastasis to distant sites. Angiogenesis may be an important step in tumor initiation; research has provided evidence of angiogenesis in transformed tissue before the appearance of malignant tumor masses (Ecsedy & Hunter, 2002; Genis et al., 2006).

Angiogenesis differs from vasculogenesis, the formation of new blood vessels in developing embryos. Angiogenesis involves the formation of blood vessels from preexisting ones. The budding of vascular networks that arise from existing tumors provides malignant cells with easy access to the circulatory system and facilitates tumor spread. The process of developing new blood vessels depends on a variety of proangiogengenic (e.g., interferons, tissue inhibitors of metalloproteinases) and antiangiogenic influences (e.g., vascular endothelial growth factor [VEGF], epidermal growth factor). For example, early in the metastatic process quiescent endothelial cells are activated and begin to migrate or proliferate. The production of VEGF provides the stimulus for epithelial cells to proliferate and enhances vascular permeability. Tumor necrosis factor stimulates the migration of tumor cells. In addition, basement membranes are degraded through the actions of MMPs. This is crucial to local invasion and metastasis of tumor cells (Ecsedy & Hunter, 2002; Pallares et al., 2006).

CAUSES OF CARCINOGENESIS

Carcinogenesis refers to the process by which cancer develops and generally includes multiple steps. This process generally requires time and an interaction among several influences that may include both environmental and personal factors. Environmental causes of cancer include exposure to chemicals, radiation, viruses, personal lifestyle characteristics, and dietary influences.

Environmental Factors

Cancer development in the United States is usually the result of exposure to environmental or extrinsic factors (Jemal et al., 2007). Environmental carcinogens include chemicals, radiation, viruses, personal lifestyle characteristics, and dietary influences. Exposure to these agents can occur in the home, workplace, or other geographic settings (Shields, 2006).

Chemical Carcinogenesis. Most instances of chemical carcinogenesis were identified through clinical observations.

In 1775, English physician Percival Pott noted an unusually high incidence of scrotal cancer in men who were employed as chimney sweeps in childhood. He correctly surmised that the cancer was directly attributable to soot exposure and suggested that chimney sweeps bathe daily as a means of prevention. More than a century later, Japanese pathologists induced skin tumors in rabbits by the repeated application of coal tar to the ears. Such early experiments gave rise to the notion that environmental factors can be responsible for the development of cancer, especially with repeated exposures over time.

Other evidence in support of chemically induced carcinogenesis has been demonstrated by comparing cancer incidences in different parts of the world. Some cancers are more prevalent in certain geographical locations. For example, there are significantly higher rates of cervical cancer in developing nations (e.g., Latin America, Africa) but higher incidence of prostate cancer in developed countries (Parkin et al., 2002). Gastric cancer is relatively rare in the United States but common in Japan. Studies over two generations of Japanese immigrants to the United States found that patterns of cancer development became similar to those prevalent in Western society. This change implicates environmental factors in the pattern of cancer development.

Epidemiologic evidence supports the idea of chemically induced carcinogenesis. Chemical carcinogens can react with the cell's DNA to induce certain genetic mutations by altering the function of regulatory genes. Some chemical agents stimulate cell proliferation through increased cell division. Many chemical carcinogens can induce genetic mutations and increase cell proliferation by acting either directly or indirectly. Direct-acting chemicals do not require a chemical transformation to induce carcinogenesis. Indirect-acting chemicals, or procarcinogens, require metabolic conversion in the host to be capable of malignant transformation. Both direct-acting and metabolically converted chemicals have electron-deficient atoms that react with electron-rich sites within the cell, including DNA and RNA. Tobacco and ethanol are examples of chemicals capable of inducing carcinogenesis.

Smoking. Although research evidence links cigarette use to the development of lung cancer, smoking remains the number one cause of malignancy in humans. Cigarettes contain more than 60 chemicals known to cause cancer (National Cancer Institute, 2004a). Smoking can be linked to nearly one third of all cancer deaths. In addition, smoking has been linked to a variety of cancers, including lung, oral cavity, larynx, esophagus, kidney, pancreas, cervix, stomach, and bladder. Tobacco is a potent carcinogen, containing benzo(a)pyrene, dimethylnitrosamine, and nickel compounds, which can lead to malignant transformation of cells.

The prevalence of tobacco use, in the form of cigarettes, pipes, cigars, and chewing tobacco persists, despite warnings from the U.S. Surgeon General (Department of Health & Human Services, 2006). Recently, lung cancer incidence has declined in men and leveled off in women (Jemal et al., 2007). However, cancer of the lung and bronchus accounts for approximately 31% of cancer-related deaths (Jemal et al., 2007). There is a relatively long latency period between the onset of smoking and the development of lung cancer that can span 20 or more years. The risk for development of lung cancer depends largely on the quantity and duration of tobacco use. Recent research indicates that passive smoking is associated with an increased risk of lung cancer and may increase the risk for development of breast cancer (Department of Health & Human Services, 2006; Hill et al., 2007; Johnson, 2005).

Alcohol. The mechanism by which excessive alcohol intake may influence the subsequent development of cancer is uncertain. However, it may act to potentiate the action of other carcinogens. Ingestion of excessive ethanol has been linked to the development of cancers of the breast, liver, esophagus, mouth, and larynx. There is evidence to suggest that cancers of the colon and rectum are associated with excessive alcohol intake (Bongaerts et al., 2006). Alcohol, as a cocarcinogen, acts in conjunction with tobacco to greatly increase the risk for cancer development. The combination of tobacco and alcohol use can be attributed as a cause of 75% of all cancers of the oral cavity (American Cancer Society, 2006a).

Radiation Carcinogenesis. Radiant energy is able to induce malignant transformation in experimental animals and humans. The two most common forms of radiant energy are ionizing radiation and UV radiation.

Ionizing Radiation. Radiation is energy emitted and transferred through matter or space. Ionizing radiation creates enough energy to change a stable atom to an unstable one by ejecting orbital electrons. Examples of ionizing radiation include x-rays, gamma rays, and particulate radiation. Sources of exposure to ionizing radiation include nuclear accidents, occupational exposure, and medial treatments. Ionizing radiation interacts with tissue and can cause somatic (tissues), biological (cells), and hereditary (offspring) damage.

The effects of nuclear explosions were documented in the survivors of the atomic bomb blasts, who had acute and chronic myelocytic leukemias. In the early part of the 20th century, radiologists who had frequent exposure to x-rays incurred a threefold to fourfold risk for development of leukemia. Both healthy tissue and tumors are affected by radiation. Some cells remain undamaged, some recover over time, and other cells die. Radiation therapy for malignancies, although one of the most common treatments for cancer, has been shown to lead to the development of secondary cancers (American Cancer Society, 2006b; Friedman & Constine, 2006; Ganz, 2001; Paulino, 2004).

Ionizing radiation appears to exert its effects directly on the double helix, causing damage to DNA by breaking the nucleotide and phosphate backbone of the molecule. Before 1985, radiation dose was measured in *rads* (radiation-absorbed doses). Currently, the dose unit of radiation therapy is termed a gray (*Gy*). One *Gy* is equivalent to 100 *rads* and one centigray (*cGy*) is equal to one *rad* (National Cancer Institute, 2004b). In living systems, radiation is absorbed randomly by atoms and molecules in cells. Extended exposure to ionizing radiation can play a role in the development of many types of human cancers. The risk for development of a radiation-associated cancer depends on the type, dose, and the amount of exposure to which individuals are subjected (Norval, 2006). Ionizing radiation has a temporal relationship of exposure, meaning the effects of this type of radiation are cumulative (Kuster et al., 2006; Takashima et al., 2006).

Ultraviolet Radiation. Solar radiation is the primary source of UV radiation and is the major cause of skin cancer worldwide (Cadet, Sage, & Douki, 2005; Hussein, 2005). UV rays affect the skin with several effects on the cells of the skin. UVA and UVB sunlight can lead to carcinogenesis individually and synergistically by adversely affecting TS genes, cell-cycle control signaling pathways, cellular enzymes, and pyrimidine dimers in DNA. Epidemiologic evidence suggests that the risk for cancer of the skin depends on the intensity and type of exposure and the distribution of melanin (American Cancer Society, 2006e; Tadokoro et al., 2005). The effects of UV exposure tend to be cumulative. Risk factors for skin cancer include fair skin, unprotected and repeated exposure to UV radiation, repeated severe sunburns as a child, certain types of moles, family history, immune suppression, sex, and age (American Cancer Society, 2006c).

According to the American Cancer Society, one million cases of nonmelanoma (basal and squamous cell) skin cancers are diagnosed each year in the United States (American Cancer Society, 2006d; Jemal et al., 2007). In 2006, more than 62,000 people were diagnosed with melanoma, the most serious form of skin cancer. Although basal cell carcinoma is fairly infrequent, it is an aggressive disease and accounts for most skin cancer deaths.

Chronic Irritation. The role of chronic irritation in the development of cancer was proposed as early as the mid-19th century, although the exact mechanism by which this occurs is elusive (Mueller, 2006). Mutations in some of the contributors to tissue repair (e.g., GFs, ECM proteins, angiogenesis factors) have been shown to play a role in carcinogenesis (Hill, 2001; Hojilla, Mohammed, & Khokha, 2003). A number of inflammatory disorders are associated with malignancies, including lupus erythematosus, osteomyelitis, perineal inflammatory disease, leg ulceration, and burn scars (Gupta, Barman, & Saify, 2005; Gur et al., 1997; Kowal-Vern & Criswell, 2005).

Viral Agents. Viruses play a role in the development of certain cancers. For example: the human papilloma virus (HPV) is linked to the development of cervical and vulvar cancer; the Epstein-Barr virus is associated with nasopharyngeal and anal cancer; and the hepatitis B virus (HBV) and hepatitis C virus (HCV) increase the risk of liver cancer. Recently, HPV has been linked to colorectal cancer (Bodaghi et al., 2005). When viruses infect body cells, they break the DNA chain and inset their own genetic material into it. Breaking the DNA, coupled with the viral gene insertion, mutates the normal cell's DNA and can either activate an oncogene or repress a suppressor gene. Viruses capable of causing cancer are known as oncoviruses. Although any type of virus has the potential to enter a cell and mutate the DNA, leading to oncogene activation, infection with retroviruses is more likely to be oncogenic.

Three vaccines are currently approved by the Food and Drug Administration to prevent the formation of cancer. The HBV prevents infection with the hepatitis B virus, which can cause liver cancer (Lavanchy, 2005). Gardasil and Cervarix prevent several types of HPV that can cause cervical cancer (Schmiedeskamp & Kockler, 2006). The vaccines are produced from the purified proteins that are expressed in papillomaviruses. The body's immune response to the genetically engineered proteins protect against infection from the actual viruses.

Dietary Influences. Dietary practices or combinations of dietary practices and environmental exposures are thought to be associated with carcinogenesis. However, the relationship between diet and carcinogenesis is poorly understood and the process by which carcinogenesis occurs is controversial (Davis, 2007; Hecht et al., 2004; Rock, 2007). Dietary considerations are usually not independent of other possible carcinogenic agents and personal influences. In addition, preservatives, contaminants, preparation methods, and additives (dyes, flavorings) have the potential for carcinogenic effects.

Personal Factors

Immune Function. The immune system provides protection against the development of cancer. Malignant cells are considered foreign (nonself) because they are no longer completely normal. These cells often express cell surface antigens that are different from normal cells, allowing recognition by macrophages, helper T lymphocytes, and natural killer cells. Once malignant cells have been recognized as foreign, defensive and offensive actions are initiated by the immune system to eliminate or destroy them. This continuing protection, or immunosurveillance, is crucial in suppressing cancer development.

The vital role of the immune system in preventing cancer development is supported by cancer incidence statistics in immunosuppressed people. Children younger than 2 years and adults older that 60 years have immune systems that function at less than optimal levels, and both groups have a higher incidence of cancer compared with

that of the general population. People receiving immunosuppressive therapy (e.g., organ transplant recipients) to reduce the risk of organ rejection or those with significant autoimmune disease in which chronic immunosuppression is the only means of controlling disease progression also have higher incidences of cancer. Among people with human immunodeficiency virus/acquired immunodeficiency syndrome who are immunocompromised, the actual incidence of cancer development may be as high as 70%.

Therefore, individuals whose immune system functions at less than optimum level have an increased cancer risk. In addition, immune function can be compromised as a result of aging, cytotoxic therapy, injury to marrow-forming bone areas, surgical removal of primary or secondary lymphoid tissues (thymectomy, splenectomy), or exposure to chronic low-dose radiation. Recent research has shown that survivors of childhood cancer who were treated with chemotherapy have a higher risk for development of cancer later in life (Friedman & Constine, 2006; Kenney et al., 2004). Cancer patients treated with high-dose chemotherapy (which can cause immunosuppression) are at higher risk for a second malignancy (Friedman & Constine, 2006; Ganz, 2001; Kenney et al., 2004; Livi et al., 2006; Robison et al., 2005).

Advancing age is probably the most common risk factor related to the development of cancer. More than 50% of all malignancies in the United States occur in people more than 65 years old (Jemal et al., 2007). The higher incidence of cancer in this age group reflects both the life-long accumulation of DNA mutations resulting in transformation and the diminishing immune response. Additionally, the efficiency of DNA repair mechanisms can be compromised as individuals age and the body may not be able to repair even minor mutations.

Surveillance Failure

An intact immune system provides the body with constant surveillance and detects the presence of foreign invaders and altered self-cells (including malignant cells). Macrophages, T lymphocytes, and natural killer cells are the most active cell types involved in this protective function. However, even when these are performing at an optimal level, the protection afforded to the body is not always perfect. The immune surveillance system is most effective at identifying and attacking those cancer cells that have been induced by viral and chemical carcinogenic events. The system appears to have little protective value against those tumors that are a result of inheritance or spontaneous DNA replication error. A likely explanation for the selectivity in the immune surveillance system is the difference in cell surface properties of malignant cells caused by different types of carcinogenic or mutational events. Malignancies arising from viral or chemical carcinogenesis have new cell surface proteins unique to the cancer cells and are more easily recognized by immunoreactive cells as foreign. Several mechanisms have been proposed for cancer surveillance failure among immunocompetent individuals. These proposed mechanisms include those discussed in the next sections.

Malignant Cell "Mimic." Some cancer cells may initially have a less malignant phenotype and more normal cell surface characteristics. Such properties may not be sufficient to trigger an immune response. Thus, cancer cells might go undetected by the immune system until significant proliferation has occurred.

Decoy Jamming. Some cancer cells that synthesize specific surface proteins capable of triggering an immune response shed these tumor-specific antigens. Thus, an immune response is directed toward the loose antigens rather than toward the malignant cell.

Bone Marrow Invasion. Bone marrow invasion by cancer cells makes it less able to carry on normal immune and inflammatory functions. Therefore, the number of cells available to mount an immune response is decreased, generally resulting in both lymphopenia and neutropenia.

Enhanced Lymphocyte Suppression Activity. Some tumors release factors that selectively enhance the activity and number of T-suppressor cells so that the T suppressors constitute a larger percentage of circulating leukocytes. T suppressors can compromise the immune response and favor tumor growth by suppressing the proliferative response of other T lymphocytes, macrophages, and natural killer cells or by suppressing immunoglobulin production.

Immune Blockade. Some cancer cells are capable of releasing factors that specifically suppress natural killer cells, which play a major role in the rejection of tumors and cells infected with viruses. If these are suppressed, the ability of cancer cells to reproduce is enhanced.

Subclinical Dose. The initial malignant colony contains so few cells that initially they are not capable of signaling or triggering the immune system. This delay allows the original cells to become well established and grow unnoticed until they reach a size that is detected by the immune system. At this point the malignancy may be so large that the immune system cannot effectively destroy or inactivate these cells.

Increased Prostaglandin Production. Certain cancers are able to increase the production and release prostaglandins (either directly in the cancer cells or by stimulating some normal tissue to increase the production and release of prostaglandin) (Marks, Furstenberger, & Muller-Decker, 2007). Prostaglandins inhibit the ability of most lymphocytes to respond to lectins and other mitogenic agents so that there is a decrease in the production of lymphocytes and an overall immunosuppressive effect.

Down-Regulation of Tumor-Specific Antigens. As cancer cells progress toward an increasingly malignant state, some of them undergo antigenic modulation as part of this process. This modulation may involve loss of tumor-specific antigens, thereby decreasing the likelihood of an immune response. Another type of modulation is to continually change the nature of the tumor-specific antigens, requiring a corresponding change in immune surveillance before recognition and elimination can occur.

Immunoprivileged Sites. Malignant transformation occurs in areas of the body that have less active immune functions compared with the rest of the body. These immunoprivileged sites (e.g., testis, brain) may differ with the developmental stage of the host. Initiation or metastasis in such a place would allow establishment of cancer cells and a relatively large tumor burden before recognition by the immune system.

Genetic Predisposition

Although damage to a tumor-suppressor gene or a change from a proto-oncogene to an oncogene can be caused by exposure to carcinogens, genetic predisposition influences the carcinogenic process as well. In humans, the efficiency of DNA repair mechanisms is inherited and can be decreased over time as a result of disease, toxins, aging, and other genotoxic events. A proto-oncogene needs to be damaged or altered to allow for expression of the oncogene. In some people, the location of specific proto-oncogenes within the genome is different and may provide an increased susceptibility to mutation or activation. In others, the position of the oncogene may be normal, but the tumor-suppressor gene that controls the oncogene's activity may be abnormal or translocated (Smith, Marks, & Lieberman, 2005; Stetler-Stevenson, 2005).

Although most mutations in cancer cells are somatic, about 1% of all cancers are inherited (germ line cancer). In these cases, the mutation is carried in the genetic code of each cell in the body. Families with inherited cancer syndromes generally display cancer in an autosomal dominant pattern in two or more generations. More than 20 types of inherited cancer syndromes have been identified (see box on page 29) (Hill, 2001; Rettig & Sawicki, 2001). Most of these tumors are caused by tumor-suppressor genes, although some are caused by oncogenes. Other tumors arise from mutations in DNA repair genes (e.g., hereditary breast cancer, hereditary nonpolyposis colorectal cancer). Inheriting one mutated gene is usually not enough to cause cancer, although it is sufficient to transmit a trait or characteristic (phenotype).

However, individuals with one mutated gene are at increased risk for the development of cancer because one allele has already been compromised. A mutation in the second allele triggers the growth of a malignant neoplasm (Ecsedy & Hunter, 2002; Rettig & Sawicki, 2001).

Gene activity is dependent on how well one or both genes of a pair functions. For example, the BCRA1 gene is a suppressor gene. Faulty functioning of this gene is associated with the development of an inherited form of breast cancer. If both BRCA1 genes of this pair are normal in structure and location, the woman is at normal risk for the development of breast cancer. However, if a woman inherits one mutated gene and one normal gene, her risk for development of breast cancer increases by as much as 50%. If she inherits two faulty BRCA1 genes, her risk for development of breast cancer may increase to almost 100% (Ecsedy & Hunter, 2002; Rettig & Sawicki, 2001). For other types of cancer, a familial tendency may be noted, but no specific pattern of inheritance is evident.

Familial cancers may be limited to a particular type (e.g., colorectal cancer, breast cancer), or there may be a prevalence of different types of cancers. These are called cancer family syndromes. The ontogeny of this kind of genetic predisposition can be difficult to elucidate and is often multifactorial in nature. Multiple small gene mutations may be responsible, or even normal exposure to carcinogenic events enhances a basal level of genetic predisposition to cancer.

Race is a genetically determined characteristic that plays a role in cancer incidence. For example, African American men in the United States have a higher incidence of prostate cancer than do Caucasian Americans. The incidence of breast cancer in the United States is highest among Caucasian women, followed by African American, Asian American/Pacific Islander, Hispanic, and American Indian/Alaskan native women (Smigal et al., 2006). Ashkenazi women are at increased risk for breast cancer because of a higher incidence of BRCA1 or BRCA2 gene mutations (Dominguez et al., 2005). Gastroesophageal cancer rates are higher among Asian Americans than among any other Americans (El-Serag & Sonnenberg, 1999). Although race/ethnicity plays a role in the development of cancer, these should not be considered in isolation. Behaviors related to culture or ethnic group, geographical location, diet, and socioeconomic factors must be considered as well (Angwafo, 1998; El-Serag & Sonnenberg, 1999). The American Cancer Society has reported that cancer incidence and survival are often related to socioeconomic

factors, such as the availability of health care services or the belief that seeking early health care has a positive effect on the outcome of a cancer diagnosis.

MALIGNANCY QUANTIFICATION
Grading of Malignancy

A system of grading tumor cells was established to accurately qualify the malignant characteristics of individual tumors diagnosed in humans. This system compares cancer cells with their normal counterparts on appearance and cellular activity. Some cancer cells retain more of their normal appearance and functions and are thus considered low grade. Others are more aggressive and treatment resistant and are classified as high-grade tumors.

Staging of Malignancy

Staging is a step-by-step process to determine the location of a cancer and the degree to which it has spread. In general, the smaller the tumor at the time of diagnosis and the less it has spread, the greater the potential for cure or control. Therefore, to determine the best treatment options for a specific malignancy, the stage of that malignancy must be determined. Three methods are used to stage a malignancy: clinical staging, pathological staging, and restaging.

Clinical Staging. Clinical staging provides an estimate of the size and extent of tumor. This is determined by physical examination and other diagnostic measures and may include laboratory tests (blood work), imaging tests (e.g., computed tomographic scan, magnetic resonance imaging), biopsy, endoscopy, or laparoscopy. Some cancers may require surgery to determine the extent of the cancer. The choice of diagnostic tests is based on the type of cancer that is being evaluated.

Pathological Staging. Tumor size, number of sites, and degree of metastasis are determined by pathological examination of tissue obtained at surgery. Pathological examination provides the clinician with information about the cellular characteristics of the tumor.

Restaging. Although not common, surgery may be done for recurrent disease to help determine the extent of recurrence and the best treatment options. It is important to note that cancer staging does not change, even if the cancer recurs or spreads to other areas of the body.

The TNM System for Staging Malignancy. Survival rates are usually higher for individuals whose tumors are localized. This observation gave rise to the notion that malignant tumors progress over time, perhaps influenced by the type of cancer and other host factors. Although several systems for grading tumor cells are available, the TNM system is commonly used to stage malignancies and characterize their pattern of growth and spread. The T signifies the extent or size of the tumor, the N indicates the presence or absence of lymph node involvement, and the

---

Selected Hereditary Cancer Syndromes

Beckwith-Wiedmann syndrome (Wilms' tumor, liver cancer)
Bloom syndrome (solid tumors)
Cowden syndrome (breast, thyroid, head and neck cancer)
Familial adenomatous polyposis
Familial melanoma
Familial breast cancer
Hereditary nonpolyposis colorectal cancer
Hereditary prostate cancer
Li-Fraumeni syndrome (brain tumor, sarcoma, breast cancer)
Peutz-Jeghers syndrome (colorectal, breast, ovarian cancer)
Von Hippel-Lindau syndrome (renal cancer)
Wilms' tumor (pediatric kidney cancer)
Xeroderma pigmentosum (skin cancer)

Grading System for Malignancy

Grade	Characteristics
GX	Grade cannot be determined
G1	Cells are well differentiated, closely resembling the tissue from which they arose. Considered a "low-grade" tumor.
G2	Cells are moderately differentiated, still resemble normal cells somewhat, but exhibit more malignant characteristics.
G3	Cells are poorly differentiated, few normal cellular characteristics are retained, but the tissue of origin may still be established.
G4	Cells are undifferentiated, no normal cellular characteristics can be found, and determining the tissue of origin is very difficult

From Workman, M. L., & Visovsky, C. G. (1999). Cancer pathophysiology. In C. Miaskowksi, & P. Buchsel (Eds.), *Oncology nursing: assessment and clinical care.* St. Louis: Mosby.

M denotes the presence or absence of metastases. Additionally, the subscript numbers assigned to any of these components is indicative of an increase in tumor size, nodal involvement, or metastases. This classification system serves several purposes: to examine the extent of the particular cancer as related to the natural course of the disease, to provide standardization on which to base treatment options, and to indicate prognosis. The table above provides an example of the TNM staging system. Other staging systems are used for some childhood cancers, lymphomas, leukemias, colorectal cancer, and cancers of the cervix, ovary, uterus, vagina, and vulva.

CONCLUSION

The process of carcinogenesis is multifactorial, with significant interactions between personal and environmental factors. Not all people are at equal risk for the development of cancer. The roles played by immune function, genetic predisposition, and environmental exposure to mutagenic events vary widely among individuals. Immune and genetic factors cannot, as of yet, be altered to prevent cancer development. However, manipulation of environmental exposure to carcinogenic events could reduce the incidence of cancer by as much as 50% (Jemal et al., 2007).

REFERENCES

Abbas, A., & Lichtman, A. (2003). Immunity to tumors. In *Cellular and molecular immunology* (5th ed., pp. 391-410). Philadelphia: W. B. Saunders.

American Cancer Society. (2006a). *Alcohol and cancer.* Retrieved September 12, 2007, from http://www.cancer.org/downloads/PRO/alcohol.pdf.

American Cancer Society. (2006b). *Childhood cancer: late effects of cancer treatment.* Retrieved September 12, 2007, from http://www.cancer.org/docroot/CRI/content/CRI_2_6x_Late_Effects_of_Childhood_Cancer.asp

American Cancer Society. (2006c). *Overview skin cancer—melanoma.* Retrieved September 12, 2007, from http://www.cancer.org/docroot/CRI/content/CRI_2_2_2X_What_causes_melanoma_skin_cancer_50.asp?sitearea=.

American Cancer Society. (2006d.) *Skin cancer facts.* Retrieved September 12, 2007, from http://www.cancer.org/docroot/PED/content/ped_7_1_What_You_Need_To_Know_About_Skin_Cancer.asp?sitearea=&level=.

American Cancer Society. (2006e). *UV radiation and cancer.* Retrieved September 12, 2007, from http://www.cancer.org/downloads/PRO/UV.pdf.

Angwafo, F. (1998). Migration and prostate cancer: An international perspective. *Journal of the National Medical Association, 90*(Suppl), S7230723.

Armanios, M., & Greider, C. (2005). Telomerase and cancer stem cells. *Cold Spring Harbor Symposia on Quantitative Biology, 70,* 205-208.

Baltzell, K., Eder, S., & Wrensch, M. (2005). Breast carcinogenesis—Can the examination of ductal fluid enhance our understanding? *Oncology Nursing Forum, 32,* 33-39.

Bangsi, D., Zhou, J., Sun, Y., et al. (2006). Impact of a genetic variant in CYP3A4 on risk and clinical presentation of prostate cancer among white and African-American men. *Urologic Oncology, 24,* 21-27.

Beachy, P., Karhadkar, S., & Berman, D. (2004). Tissue repair and stem cell renewal in carcinogenesis. *Nature, 432,* 324-331.

Bissell, M., & Radisky, D. (2001). Putting tumours in context. *Nature Reviews Cancer, 1,* 45-54.

Bodaghi, S., Yamanegi, K., Xiao, S., et al. (2005). Colorectal papillomavirus infection in patients with colorectal cancer. *Clinical Cancer Research, 11,* 2862-2867.

Bongaerts, B., deGoeij, A., van den Brandt, P., et al. (2006). Alcohol and the risk of colon and rectal cancer with mutations in the K-ras gene. *Alcohol, 38,* 147-154.

Cadet, J., Sage, E., & Douki, T. (2005). Ultraviolet radiation-mediated damage to cellular DNA. *Mutation Research, 571,* 3-17.

Calvo, K., Petricoin III, E., & Liotta, L. (2005). Genomics and proteomics. In V. DeVita, S. Hellman, & S. Rosenberg (Eds.), *Cancer: principles and practice of oncology* (7th ed., Vol. 1, pp. 51-73). Philadelphia: Lippincott Williams & Wilkins.

Carpenter, C., & Cantley, L. (2005). Molecular targets in oncology: signal transduction systems. In V. DeVita, S. Hellman, & S. Rosenberg (Eds.), *Cancer: principles and practice of oncology* (7th ed., Vol. 1, pp. 51-83). Philadelphia: Lippincott Williams & Wilkins.

Clarke, M., & Weissman, I. (2004). Stem cells, cell differentiation, & cancer. In M. Abeloff, J. Armitage, J. Niederhuber, et al. (Eds.), *Clinical oncology* (3rd ed., pp. 139-149). Philadelphia: Elsevier.

Connolly, J., Goldsmith, J., Wang, J., et al. (2006). Principles of cancer pathology. In D. Kufe, J. R. Bast, W. Hait, et al. (Eds.), *Holland-Frei: cancer medicine 7* (7th ed., pp. 437-454). Hamilton, ON: BC Decker.

Cvetkovic, R., & Perry, C. (2006). Spotlight on rituximab in non-hodgkin lymphoma and chronic lymphocytic leukemia. *BioDrugs Clinical Immunotherapeutics, Biopharmaceuticals, and Gene Therapy, 20,* 253-257.

Davis, C. (2007). Nutritional interactions: credentialing of molecular targets for cancer prevention. *Experimental Biology and Medicine, 232,* 176-183.

Department of Health & Human Services. (2006). *Health consequences of involuntary exposure to tobacco smoke: a report of the Surgeon General.* Washington, D.C.: U.S. Department of Health and Human Services.

Dominguez, F., Jones, J., Zabicki, K., et al. (2005). Prevalence of hereditary breast/ovarian carcinoma risk in patients with a personal history of breast or ovarian carcinoma in a mammography population. *Cancer, 104,* 1849-1853.

Ecsedy, J., & Hunter, D. (2002). The origin of cancer. In H. Adami, D. Hunter, & D. Trichopoulos (Eds.), *Textbook of cancer epidemiology* (pp. 29-53). New York: Oxford University Press.

Egeblad, M., & Werb, Z. (2002). New functions for the matrix metalloproteinases in cancer progression. *Nature Reviews Cancer, 2,* 161-174.

El-Serag, H., & Sonnenberg, A. (1999). Ethnic variations in the occurrence of gastroesophageal cancers. *Journal of Clinical Gastroenterology, 28,* 135-139.

Fidler, I. (2003). The pathogenesis of cancer metastasis: the "seed and soil" hypothesis revisited. *Nature Reviews Cancer, 3,* 453-458.

Fidler, I., Langley, R., Kerbel, R., et al. (2005). Angiogenesis. In V. DeVita, S. Hellman, & S. Rosenberg (Eds.), *Cancer: principles and practice of oncology* (7th ed., Vol. 1, pp. 129-138). Philadelphia: Lippincott Williams & Wilkins.

Flatmark, K., Maelandsmo, G., Martinsen, M., et al. (2004). Twelve colorectal cancer cell lines exhibit highly variable growth and metastatic capacities in an orthotopic model in nude mice. *European Journal of Cancer, 40,* 1593-1598.

Friedman, D. L., & Constine, L. S. (2006). Late effects of treatment for Hodgkin lymphoma. *Journal of the National Comprehensive Cancer Network, 4,* 249-257.

Ganz, P. A. (2001). Late effects of cancer and its treatment. *Seminars in Oncology Nursing, 17,* 241-248.

Genis, L., Galvez, B., Gonzalo, P., et al. (2006). MT1-MMP: universal or particular player in angiogenesis? *Cancer Metastasis Reviews, 25,* 77-86.

Gupta, U., Barman, K., & Saify, K. (2005). Squamous cell carcinoma complicating an untreated chronic discoid lupus erythematosus (CDLE) lesion in a black female. *Journal of Dermatology, 32,* 1010-1013.

Gur, E., Neligan, P., Shafir, R., et al. (1997). Squamous cell carcinoma in perineal inflammatory disease. *Annals of Plastic Surgery, 38,* 653-657.

Haffty, B. G., Silber, A., Matloff, E., et al. (2006). Racial differences in the incidence of BRCA1 and BRCA2 mutations in a cohort of early onset breast cancer patients: African American compared to white women. *Journal of Medical Genetics, 43,* 133-137.

Hecht, S., Carmella, S., Kenney, P., et al. (2004). Effects of cruciferous vegetable consumption on urinary metabolites of the tobacco-specific lung carcinogen 4-(methylnitrosamino)-1-(3-pyridyl)-1-butanone in Singapore Chinese. *Pharmacological Research, 13,* 997-1004.

Hessel, F., Krause, M., Helm, A., et al. (2004). Differentiation status of human squamous cell carcinoma xenografts does not appear to correlate with the repopulation capacity of clonogenic tumour cells during fractionated irradiation. *International Journal of Radiation Oncology, Biology, and Physics, 80,* 719-727.

Hill, R. (2001). The biology of cancer. In P. Robin (Ed.), *Clinical oncology: a multidisciplinary approach for physicians and students* (8th ed., pp. 32-45). Philadelphia: W. B. Saunders.

Hill, S., Blakely, T., Kawachi, I., et al. (2007). Mortality among lifelong nonsmokers exposed to secondhand smoke at home: cohort data and sensitivity analysis. *American Journal of Epidemiology, 165,* 530-540.

Hoeijmakers, J. (2001). Genome maintenance mechanisms for preventing cancer. *Nature, 411,* 366-374.

Hojilla, C., Mohammed, F., & Khokha, R. (2003). Matrix metalloproteinases and their tissue inhibitors direct cell fate during cancer development. *British Journal of Cancer, 89,* 1817-1821.

Hussein, J. (2005). Ultraviolet radiation and skin cancer: molecular mechanisms. *Journal of Cutaneous Pathology, 32,* 191-205.

Jemal, A., Siegel, R., Ward, E., et al. (2007). Cancer statistics, 2007. *CA: A Cancer Journal for Clinicians, 57,* 43-66.

Jemal, A., Ward, E., Cokkinides, V., et al. (2006). Trends in breast cancer by race and ethnicity: update 2006. *CA: A Cancer Journal for Clinicians, 56,* 168-183.

Jia, Z., Barbier, L., Stuart, H., et al. (2005). Tumor cell pseudopodial protrusions: Localized signaling domains coordinating cytoskeleton remodeling, cell adhesion, glycolysis, RNA translocation, and protein translation. *Journal of Biological Chemistry, 280,* 30564-30573.

Johnson, K. (2005). Accumulating evidence on passive and active smoking and breast cancer risk. *International Journal of Cancer, 117,* 619-628.

Kalirai, H., & Clarke, R. (2006). Human breast epithelial stem cells and their regulation. *The Journal of Pathology, 208,* 7-16.

Kashima, K., Nanashima, A., Yasutake, T., et al. (2006). Decrease telomeres and increase of interstitial telomeric sites in chromosomes of short-term cultured gastric carcinoma cells detected by fluorescence in situ hybridization. *Anticancer Research, 26,* 2849-2855.

Kenney, L. B., Yutaka, Y., Inskip, P. D., et al. (2004). Breast cancer after childhood cancer: a report from the Childhood Cancer Survivor Study. *Annals of Internal Medicine, 141,* 590-597.

Killion, J., & Fidler, I. (2005). Cancer growth, progression, and metastasis. In A. Shaw, B. Riedel, A. Burton, et al. (Eds.), *Acute care of the cancer patient* (pp. 1-10). Boca Raton: Taylor & Francis Group.

Kowal-Vern, A., & Criswell, B. (2005). Burn scar neoplasms: a literature review and statistical analysis. *Burns, 31,* 403-413.

Kumar, V., Abbas, A., & Fausto, N. (2005). Neoplasia. In *Robbins and Cotran pathologic basis of disease.* (7th ed., pp. 269-342). Philadelphia: Elsevier.

Kuster, N., Berdiñas Torres, V., Nikoloski, N., et al. (2006). Methodology of detailed dosimetry and treatment of uncertainty and variations for in vivo studies. *Bioelectromagnetics, 27,* 378-391.

Kute, T., Grondahl-Hansen, J., Shao, S., et al. (1998). Low cathepsin D and low plasminogen activator type 1 inhibitor in tumor cytosols defines a group of node negative breast cancer patients with low risk of recurrence. *Breast Cancer Research and Treatment, 47,* 9-16.

Lavanchy, D. (2005). Worldwide epidemiology of HBV infection, disease burden, and vaccine prevention. *Journal of Clinical Virology, 34*(1 Suppl), S1-3.

Lawson, D., Xin, L., Lukacs, R., et al. (2005). Prostate stem cells and prostate cancer. *Cold Spring Harbor Symposia on Quantitative Biology, 70,* 187-196.

Lembo, D., Donalisio, M., Cornaglia, M., et al. (2006). *Effect of high-risk human papillomavirus oncoproteins on p53R2 gene expression after DNA damage.* Retrieved September, 2007, from http://www.ncbi.nlm.nih.gov/sites/entrez?Db=pubmed&Cmd=ShowDetailView&TermToSearch=16872707&ordinalpos=1&itool=EntrezSystem2.PEntrez.Pubmed.Pubmed_ResultsPanel.Pubmed_RVDocSum

Lev, D., Kiriakova, G., & Price, J. (2003). Selection of more aggressive variants of the gI101A human breast cancer cell line: a model for analyzing the metastatic phenotype of breast cancer. *Clinical and Experimental Metastasis, 20,* 515-523.

Liu, S., Dontu, G., & Wicha, M. (2005). Mammary stem cells, self-renewal pathways, and carcinogenesis. *Breast Cancer Research, 7,* 86-95.

Livi, L., Santoni, R., Paiar, F., et al. (2006). Late treatment-related complications in 214 patients with extremity soft-tissue sarcoma treated by surgery and postoperative radiation therapy. *American Journal of Surgery, 191,* 230-234.

Loescher, L., & Whitesell, L. (2003). The biology of cancer. In A. Tranin, A. Masny, & J. Jenkins (Eds.), *Genetics in oncology practice* (pp. 23-55). Pittsburgh: Oncology Nursing Society.

Marks, F., Furstenberger, G., & Muller-Decker, K. (2007). Tumor promotion as a target of cancer prevention. *Recent Results in Cancer Research, 174,* 37-47.

McDonnell, K., & Wellstein, A. (2006). Cancer metastasis. In A. Chang, P. Ganz, Hayes, D. F., et al. (Eds.), *Oncology: an evidence-based approach* (pp. 244-250). New York: Springer.

Mueller, M. (2006). Inflammation in epithelial skin tumours: old stories and new ideas. *European Journal of Cancer, 42*, 735-744.

National Cancer Institute. (2004a). *Cigarette smoking and cancer: questions and answers.* Retrieved September 12, 2007, from: http://www.cancer.gov/cancertopics/factsheet/Tobacco/cancer.

National Cancer Institute. (2004b). *Radiation therapy for cancer: questions and answers.* Retrieved September 12, 2007, from http://www.cancer.gov/PDF/FactSheet/fs7_1.pdf.

National Institutes of Health. (2001). *Stem cell information: early development.* Retrieved September 12, 2007, from: http://stemcells.nih.gov/info/scireport/appendixa.asp#figure1.

National Institutes of Health. (2005). *Stem cell basis.* Retrieved September 12, 2007, from: http://stemcells.nih.gov/info/basics/basics2.asp.

Norval, M. (2006). The mechanisms and consequences of ultraviolet-induced immunosuppression. *Progress in Biophysics and Molecular Biology, 92*, 108-118.

Nowakowski, G., & Witzig, T. (2006). Radioimmunotherapy for B-cell non-Hodgkin lymphoma. *Clinical Advances in Hematology and Oncology, 4*, 225-231.

Pallares, J., Rojo, F., Iriarte, J., et al. (2006). Study of microvessel density and the expression of the angiogenic factors VEGF, bFGF and the receptors Flt-1 and FLK-1 in benign, premalignant and malignant prostate tissues. *Histology and Histopathology, 21*, 857-865.

Papakosta, V., Vairaktaris, E., Vylliotis, A., et al. (2006). The co-expression of c-*myc* and p53 increases and reaches a plateau early in oral oncogenesis. *Anticancer Research, 26*, 2957-2962.

Parkin, D., Bray, F., Ferlay, J., et al. (2002). Global cancer statistics, 2002. *CA: A Cancer Journal for Clinicians, 55*, 74-108.

Paulino, A. C. (2004). Late effects of radiotherapy for pediatric extremity sarcomas. *International Journal of Radiation Oncology, Biology, & Physics, 60*, 265-274.

Plosker, G., & Keam, S. (2006). Spotlight on trastuzumab in the management of HER2-positive metastatic and early-stage breast cancer. *BioDrugs: Clinical Immunotherapeutics, Biopharmaceuticals, and Gene Therapy, 20*, 259-262.

Polyak, K., & Meyerson, M. (2006). Molecular biology, genomics, proteomics, and mouse models of human cancer. In D. Kufe, J. R. Bast, W. Hait, et al. (Eds.), *Cancer medicine 7* (pp. 9-26). Hamilton: BC Decker.

Reed, S. (2005). Cell cycle. In V. DeVita, S. Hellman, & S. Rosenberg (Eds.), *Cancer: principles and practice of oncology* (Vol. 1, pp. 83-94). Philadelphia: Lippincott Williams & Wilkins.

Rettig, M., & Sawicki, M. (2001). Biology of cancer. In C. Haskell (Ed.), *Cancer treatment* (5th ed., pp. 9-28). Philadelphia: W. B. Saunders.

Reya, T., & Clevers, H. (2005). Wnt signaling in stem cells and cancer. *Nature, 434*, 843-850.

Robison, L. L., Green, D. M., Hudson, M., et al. (2005). Long-term outcomes of adult survivors of childhood cancer: results from the Childhood Cancer Survivor Study. *Cancer, 104*(11 Suppl), 2557-2564.

Rock, C. (2007). Primary dietary prevention: is the fiber story over? *Recent Results in Cancer Research, 174*, 171-177.

Rudin, C., & Thompson, C. (2002). Apoptosis and cancer. In B. Vogelstein & K. Kinzler (Eds.), *The genetic basis of human cancer* (2nd ed., pp. 163-175). New York: McGraw-Hill.

Schmiedeskamp, M., & Kockler, D. (2006). Human papillomavirus vaccines. *The Annals of Pharmacotherapy, 40*, 1344-1352.

Shields, P. (2006). Understanding population and individual risk assessment: the case of polycholinated biphenyls. *Cancer Epidemiology Biomarkers and Prevention, 15*, 830-839.

Skaar, J., & DeCaprio, J. (2006). Fundamental aspects of the cell cycle and signal transduction. In A. Chang, P. Ganz, D. Hayes, et al. (Eds.), *Oncology: an evidence-based approach* (pp. 207-213). New York: Springer.

Smith, C., Marks, A., & Lieberman, M. (2005). The molecular biology of cancer. In C. Smith, A. Marks, & M. Lieberman (Eds.), *Marks' basic medical biochemistry: a clinical approach* (2nd ed., pp. 317-336). Philadelphia: Lippincott Williams & Wilkins.

Stamenkovic, I. (2003). Extracellular matrix remodelling: the role of matrix metalloproteinases. *Journal of Pathology, 200*, 448-464.

Stetler-Stevenson, W. (2005). Invasion and metastases. In V. DeVita, S. Hellman, & S. Rosenberg (Eds.), *Cancer: principles and practice of oncology* (7th ed., Vol. 1, pp. 113-128). Philadelphia: Lippincott Williams & Wilkins.

Swartz, M., Kristensen, C., Melder, R., et al. (1999). Cells shed from tumours show reduced clonogenicity, resistance to apoptosis, and in vivo tumorigenicity. *British Journal of Cancer, 81*, 756-759.

Tadokoro, T., Yamaguchi, Y., Batzer, J., et al. (2005). Mechanisms of skin tanning in different racial/ethnic groups in response to ultraviolet radiation. *The Journal of Investigative Dermatology, 124*, 1326-1332.

Taipale, J., & Beachy, P. (2001). The Hedgehog and Wnt signaling pathways in cancer. *Nature, 411*, 349-354.

Takashima, Y., Hirose, H., Koyama, S., et al. (2006). Effects of continuous and intermittent exposure to RF fields with a wide range of SARs on cell growth, survival, and cell cycle distribution. *Bioelectromagnetics, 27*, 392-400.

Taniwaki, M., Daigo, Y., Ishikawa, N., et al. (2006). Gene expression profiles of small-cell lung cancers: molecular signatures of lung cancer. *International Journal of Oncology, 29*, 567-575.

Thompson, C., Bauer, D., Lum, J., et al. (2005). How do cancer cells acquire the fuel needed to support cell growth? *Cold Spring Harbor Symposia on Quantitative Biology, 70*, 357-362.

Tokunaga, E., Oki, E., Nishida, K., et al. (2006). Trastuzubab and breast cancer: developments and current status. *International Journal of Clinical Oncology, 11*, 199-208.

Wang, Y., Hayward, S., Cao, M., et al. (2001). Cell differentiation lineage in the prostate. *Differentiation, 68*, 270-279.

Watson-Hurst, K., & Becker, D. (2006). The role of N-cadherin, MCAM and beta3 integrin in melanoma progression, proliferation, migration and invasion. *Cancer Biology and Therapy, 5*, 1375-1382.

Major Cancers

Breast Cancer

Yvette Payne

Invasive Breast Cancer

DEFINITION

Invasive breast cancer, also referred to as infiltrating breast cancer, has spread beyond the basement membrane of the duct or lobule of the breast and into the surrounding tissue. The diagnosis of invasive breast cancer is considered to be systemic, not localized, because of its ability to spread through the vascular system. The breast includes the following specific anatomical areas:

- Nipple
- Areola
- Ducts
- Lobules
- Adipose tissue
- Pectoralis major and minor muscles
- Associated lymph nodes

INCIDENCE

Breast cancer is the most common form of cancer among women in industrialized countries. The incidence of breast cancer increases with age, beginning slowly between the ages of 45 and 50 years and then rising steadily each year thereafter. More than 70% of breast cancers occur in women 50 years of age and older. In 2007, 178,480 new cases of breast cancer are expected to be diagnosed in women living in the United States. Breast cancer is the leading cause of cancer deaths for women between 20 and 59 years of age with a projected death rate of 40,910 in 2007. Male breast cancer accounts for less than 1% of all breast cancers, with an estimated 2,030 new cancers diagnosed and 450 breast cancer deaths in 2007.

ETIOLOGY AND RISK FACTORS

There is no single cause of breast cancer. It is a heterogeneous disease likely developing as a result of multiple factors. Broad generalizations about the risk of breast cancer are often published; however, the future for an individual woman who has breast cancer is unpredictable. The following factors are those most commonly suspected to increase the probability of a woman having breast cancer:

- Sex—>99% of cases occur in women
- Age—risk increases with age
- Personal history of breast cancer—threefold to fourfold increased risk of second primary cancer
- Family history of breast cancer—the risk is particularly great if:
  ○ The affected relative is on the maternal side of the family
  ○ Two first-degree relatives are affected
  ○ The relative has bilateral breast cancer
  ○ The relative's breast cancer was diagnosed before the age of 50 years
- Genetic influences:
  ○ BRCA1 (17q21)
  ○ BRCA2 (13q14)
  ○ CHEK2 thought to activate BRCA1
  ○ TP53 germ line mutations
  ○ EMSY thought to interact with BRCA2
- History of receiving ionizing radiation
- Hormonal factors:
  ○ Postmenopausal obesity
  ○ Early menarche (before age 12 years) and late menopause (after age 50 years)
  ○ Nulliparity
  ○ First term pregnancy after 30 or 35 years of age
  ○ Use of oral contraceptives before age 20 years with use lasting 6 or more years
  ○ Hormone replacement therapy with estrogen plus progestin

- Proliferative breast disease, atypical hyperplasia
- Ingestion of 15 g (two drinks) or more alcohol each day

SIGNS AND SYMPTOMS

Breast cancer in its early stages is usually asymptomatic. Later signs and symptoms include the following:

- Pain is uncommon in early disease
- Changes in the size or shape of the breast
- Pink or bloody spontaneous unilateral nipple discharge may occur
- Arm edema (lymphedema)
- Skin changes—dimpling, edema, erythema, ulceration
- Nipple changes—inversion, scaling, ulceration
- Symptoms of metastases (i.e., shortness of breath), cough. Loss of appetite, abnormal liver function tests, headaches, and many others

DIAGNOSTIC WORKUP

Diagnostic mammogram for early detection of breast lesions:

- Workup may include ultrasonography, positron emission tomographic scan, or magnetic resonance imaging of the breast.
- Clinical breast examination to include bilateral breasts, axilla, and supraclavicular and infraclavicular areas
- Biopsy for a pathological diagnosis (see table on page 36)
- Imaging studies may include bone scan, computed tomographic scan of the chest and abdomen or others depending on the presenting signs and symptoms to rule out metastases
- Laboratory tests to include hematological chemistry evaluations and tests for tumor markers CA15-3 and CA27.29

Breast Biopsy Techniques

Type of Biopsy	Method of Analysis	Palpable Lesion	Nonpalpable Lesion
Needle	Cytology	Fine-needle aspiration	Stereotactic fine-needle aspiration
	Histology	Core biopsy	Stereotactic core biopsy
Open	Histology	Incisional/excisional biopsy	Needle localization breast biopsy

From Bernice, M. (2005). Nursing care of the client with breast cancer. In J. K. Itano & K. N. Taoka (Eds.), *Core curriculum for oncology nursing* (4th ed., p. 497). St. Louis: Elsevier Saunders.

HISTOLOGY

Breast cancer is a heterogeneous disease with 24 distinct histological subtypes. Some of the more common subtypes of breast cancer are the following:

- Invasive ductal carcinoma—70% to 80% of all breast cancers
- Invasive lobular carcinoma—10% to 15% of all breast cancers
- Medullary carcinomas—5% to 7% of malignant breast tumors
- Other less common subtypes include tubular, mucinous, sarcomas, and papillary carcinomas

Inflammatory breast cancer is not a subtype but a special manifestation typically presenting with dramatic and diffuse skin edema, erythema, hyperemia, and induration of the underlying tissue.

The identification of prognostic factors is critical in determining the appropriate treatment of an individual woman's breast cancer:

- Axillary lymph node status—prognosis worsens with increased involvement
- Tumor size—increased risk of recurrence with increasing size
- Hormone receptor status—estrogen receptor (ER)- and progesterone receptor (PR)-negative tumors are associated with a worse prognosis
- Deoxyribonucleic acid (DNA) ploidy—aneuploid tumors, those with an abnormal amount of DNA have a poorer prognosis
- High S-phase fraction predicts poorer outcome
- Histopathological considerations take into account the nuclear pattern, morphologic features, and mitotic activity. The higher the grade the worse the prognosis
- Molecular and biological factors that may be associated with a poor prognosis include the following:
  - Loss of functioning of tumor suppression genes, p53, nm23
  - Overexpression of oncogenes, HER-2/neu and epidermal growth factor receptor (EGFR)
  - Proteases such as cathepsin D and urokinase plasminogen activator

CLINICAL STAGING

Clinical staging is based on the characteristics of the primary tumor, the physical examination of the axilla, and distant metastases. These three factors determine the stage, I to IV (see table on pages 36-38). Pathological staging is more accurate and recommended by the American Joint Committee on Cancer Staging (AJCC).

TREATMENT

There are many treatment choices available to men and women with breast cancer on the basis of multiple individual factors. Most breast cancer treatment involves local and systemic measures. The goal of local treatments is to remove or eradicate cancer cells in the breast or axilla.

Local surgical primary treatments include lumpectomies, segmental resections, mastectomies, and axillary lymph node dissections (see table on page 38). Surgery may be used as a palliative treatment and in the

Clinical Staging: Invasive Breast Cancer

Definition of TNM

Primary Tumor (T)

TX	Primary tumor cannot be assessed
T0	No evidence of primary tumor
Tis	Carcinoma in situ
Tis (DCIS)	Ductal carcinoma in situ
Tis (LCIS)	Lobular carcinoma in situ
Tis (Paget's)	Paget's disease of the nipple with no tumor

Note: Paget's disease associated with a tumor is classified according to the size of the tumor

T1	Tumor 2 cm or less in greatest dimension
T1mic	Microinvasion 0.1 cm or less in greatest dimension
T1a	Tumor more than 0.1 cm but not more than 0.5 cm in greatest dimension
T1b	Tumor more than 0.5 cm but not more than 1 cm in greatest dimension
T1c	Tumor more than 1 cm but not more than 2 cm in greatest dimension
T2	Tumor more than 2 cm but not more than 5 cm in greatest dimension
T3	Tumor more than 5 cm in greatest dimension
T4	Tumor of any size with direct extension to (a) chest wall or (b) skin, only as described below
T4a	Extension to chest wall, not including pectoralis muscle
T4b	Edema (including peau d'orange) or ulceration of the skin of the breast, or satellite skin nodules confined to the same breast
T4c	Both T4a and T4b
T4d	Inflammatory carcinoma

Regional Lymph Nodes (N)

Clinical

NX	Regional lymph nodes cannot be assessed (e.g., previously removed)
N0	No regional lymph node metastasis
N1	Metastasis to movable ipsilateral axillary lymph node(s)

Clinical Staging: Invasive Breast Cancer—cont'd

Regional Lymph Nodes (N)—cont'd

N2	Metastases in ipsilateral axillary lymph nodes fixed or matted or in clinically apparent* ipsilateral internal mammary nodes in the *absence* of clinically evident axillary lymph node metastasis
N2a	Metastasis in ipsilateral axillary lymph nodes fixed to one another (matted) or to other structures
N2b	Metastasis only in clinically apparent* ipsilateral internal mammary nodes and in the *absence* of clinically evident axillary lymph node metastasis
N3	Metastasis in ipsilateral infraclavicular lymph node(s) with or without axillary lymph node involvement, or in clinically apparent* ipsilateral internal mammary lymph node(s) and in the *presence* of clinically evident axillary lymph node metastasis; or metastasis in ipsilateral supraclavicular lymph node(s) with or without axillary or internal mammary lymph node involvement
N3a	Metastasis in ipsilateral infraclavicular lymph node(s)
N3b	Metastasis in ipsilateral internal mammary lymph node(s) and axillary lymph node(s)
N3c	Metastasis in ipsilateral supraclavicular lymph node(s)

Clinically apparent is defined as detected by imaging studies (excluding lymphoscintigraphy) or by clinical examination or grossly visible pathologically.

Pathologic (pN)[a]

pNX	Regional lymph nodes cannot be assessed (e.g., previously removed or not removed for pathologic study)
pN0	No regional lymph node metastasis histologically, no additional examination for isolated tumor cells (ITC)

Note: ITC are defined as single tumor cells or small cell clusters not greater than 0.2 mm, usually detected only by immunohistochemical (IHC) or molecular methods but which may be verified on H&E stains. ITCs do not usually show evidence of malignant activity e.g., proliferation or stromal reaction.

pN0 (i -)	No regional lymph node metastasis histologically, negative IHC
pN0 (i +)	No regional lymph node metastasis histologically, positive IHC, no IHC cluster greater than 0.2 mm
pN0 (mol -)	No regional lymph node metastasis histologically, negative molecular findings (RT-PCR)[b]
pN0 (mol +)	No regional lymph node metastasis histologically, positive molecular findings (RT-PCR)[b]

[a]Classification is based on axillary lymph node dissection with or without sentinel lymph node dissection. Classification based solely on sentinel lymph node dissection without subsequent axillary lymph node dissection is designated (sn) for "sentinel node, "e.g., pN0(i +) (sn).
[b]RT-PCR: reverse transcriptase/polymerase chain reaction.

pN1	Metastasis in 1 to 3 axillary lymph nodes or in internal mammary nodes with microscopic disease detected by sentinel lymph node dissection but not clinically apparent**
pN1mi	Micrometastasis (greater than 0.2 mm, none greater than 2.0 mm)
pN1a	Metastasis in 1 to 3 axillary lymph nodes
pN1b	Metastasis in internal mammary nodes with microscopic disease detected by sentinel lymph node dissection but not clinically apparent**
pN1c	Metastasis in 1 to 3 axillary lymph nodes and in internal mammary lymph nodes with microscopic disease detected by sentinel lymph node dissection but not clinically apparent.** (If associated with greater than 3 positive axillary lymph nodes, the internal mammary nodes are classified as pN3b to reflect increased tumor burden.)
pN2	Metastasis in four to nine axillary lymph nodes, or in clinically apparent* internal mammary lymph nodes in the *absence* of axillary lymph node metastasis.
pN2a	Metastasis in four to nine axillary lymph nodes (at least one tumor deposit greater than 2.0 mm)
pN2b	Metastasis in clinically apparent * internal mammary lymph nodes in the *absence* of axillary lymph node metastasis
pN3	Metastasis in 10 or more axillary lymph nodes, or in infraclavicular lymph nodes, or in clinically apparent* ipsilateral internal mammary lymph nodes in the *presence* of one or more positive axillary lymph nodes; or in more than three axillary lymph nodes with clinically negative microscopic metastasis in internal mammary lymph nodes; or in ipsilateral supraclavicular lymph nodes

Continued

prevention, diagnosis, staging, and rehabilitation of the patient with breast cancer.

After breast-conserving surgeries, radiation therapy (RT) may be given to achieve local control and to reduce the risk of local recurrence. New operative approaches, such as Mammosite, have been developed to provide targeted RT to the tumor bed to reduce radiation exposure to healthy tissue. RT also has a palliative role in metastatic breast cancer and is used to reduce the pain from bone metastases and to control symptoms from central nervous system disease.

The goal of systemic treatment is to destroy or control cancer cells throughout the body. Systemic treatments, chemotherapies, hormonal therapies, and biological therapies may be given in the neoadjuvant, adjuvant, and metastatic settings. Treatments are chosen on the basis of multiple individual factors such age, health, size of tumor, nodal involvement, hormone receptor status, HER-2/neu status and varied other factors. Hormonal therapies provide a response rate of between 50% to 70% in women with ER- and PgR-positive tumors. Common therapies include anastrozole, letrozole, tamoxifen plus numerous others.

Chemotherapy may be given to reduce the size of a tumor before surgery, to eliminate occult tumor cells after primary surgery, or for palliation in the metastatic setting. Agents commonly used and combined in the adjuvant and neoadjuvant setting are doxorubicin, epirubicin, paclitaxel, docetaxel, cyclophosphamide, fluorouracil, and methotrexate. In the metastatic setting the same agents may be used as single agents. Other agents frequently used are capecitabine, gemcitabine, and vinorelbine.

Biological therapies selectively target various steps in a pathway necessary for tumor growth. An example is trastuzumab, an anti-HER-2/neu monoclonal antibody that is widely used in the metastatic setting. This and other biological agents are being investigated in earlier stage breast cancer.

Clinical Staging: Invasive Breast Cancer—cont'd

Pathologic (pN)ᵃ—cont'd

pN3a	Metastasis in 10 or more axillary lymph nodes (at least one tumor deposit greater than 2.0 mm), or metastasis to the infraclavicular lymph nodes
pN3b	Metastasis in clinically apparent* ipsilateral internal mammary lymph nodes in the *presence* of one or more positive axillary lymph nodes; or in more than three axillary lymph nodes and in internal mammary lymph nodes with microscopic disease detected by sentinel lymph node dissection but not clinically apparent.**
pN3c	Metastasis in ipsilateral supraclavicular lymph nodes

*Clinically apparent is defined as detected by imaging studies (excluding lymphoscintigraphy) or by clinical examination.
**Not clinically apparent is defined as not detected by imaging studies (excluding lymphoscintigraphy) or by clinical examination.

Distant Metastasis (M)

MX	Distant metastasis cannot be assessed
M0	No distant metastasis
M1	Distant metastasis

Stage Grouping

Stage 0	Tis	N0	M0
Stage I	T1*	N0	M0
Stage IIA	T0	N1	M0
	T1*	N1	M0
	T2	N0	M0
Stage IIB	T2	N1	M0
	T3	N0	M0
Stage IIIA	T0	N2	M0
	T1*	N2	M0
	T2	N2	M0
	T3	N1	M0
	T3	N2	M0
Stage IIIB	T4	N0	M0
	T4	N1	M0
	T4	N2	M0
Stage IIIC	Any T	N3	M0
Stage IV	Any T	Any N	M1

*T1 includes T1mic
Note: Stage designation may be changed if post-surgical imaging studies reveal the presence of distant metastases, provided that the studies are carried out within 4 months of diagnosis in the absence of disease progression and provided that the patient has not received neoadjuvant therapy.
Used with the permission of the American Joint Committee on Cancer (AJCC), Chicago, Illinois. The original source for this material is the *AJCC Cancer staging manual*, Sixth Edition (2002) published by Springer Science and Business Media LLC, www.springerlink.com.

Breast Cancer Surgical Procedures

Breast-Conserving Surgeries*	Surgical Procedure(s)
Lumpectomy	Excision of tumor with small margin of normal tissue around it
Segmental resection (tylectomy, quadrantectomy, partial mastectomy)	Excision of tumor with a wider margin of surrounding tissue
Mastectomies	
Subcutaneous mastectomy	Removes all breast tissue except overlying skin and nipple-areolar complex
Skin sparing	Removes above plus limited overlying skin at risk biopsy scar, nipple-areolar complex
Total (simple) mastectomy	Removes all breast tissue including skin, gland, nipple-areolar complex
Modified radical mastectomy	Removes above plus axillary node dissection
Radical mastectomy	Removes above plus underlying pectoral muscles

From J. K. Itano & K. N. Taoka (Eds.). (2005). *Core curriculum for oncology nursing* (4th ed., p. 499). St. Louis: Elsevier Saunders.
*Usually done in conjunction with axillary node biopsy or dissection through a second incision.

PROGNOSIS

The prognosis of breast cancer depends on many factors, both known and unknown. Some more common factors that affect prognosis are stage of disease, the histologic diagnosis and grade of the cancer, hormone receptor status, HER-2/neu status, menopausal status, and the overall health of the individual. Among the many known factors, stage of disease is one of the best indicators of prognosis. Five-year survival rates for individuals with breast cancer who receive appropriate treatment are as follow:

- Stage I—88%
- Stage II—66%
- Stage III—36%
- Stage IV—7%

PREVENTION

Breast cancer screening includes both clinical and self-evaluation and mammograms:

- Screening mammograms between the ages of 35 and 40 years, every 1 to 2 years between the ages of 40 and 49 years, and yearly for women 50 years of age and older
- The American Cancer Society (ACS) recommends instruction and information about breast self-examination (BSE) for women beginning in their 20s. BSE effectiveness may be improved with Mammosite or the BSE pad.
- The ACS recommends clinical breast examination by a health care professional at least every 3 years from ages 20 to 39 years and then annually.
- A number of trials have been conducted within the breast cancer arena to determine prevention methods.
- The Breast Cancer Prevention Trial (BCPT or NSABP-1) showed a 49% risk reduction of breast cancer for women with a known high risk for breast cancer taking 20 mg of tamoxifen daily versus those taking a placebo.

- The STAR trial (NSABP-P2) is a randomized study of tamoxifen and raloxifene in women with a high risk of breast cancer, examining the risk reduction and side effects of each agent.
- The MORE (Multiple Outcomes of Raloxifene Evaluation) trial examined the effects of raloxifene versus placebo on osteoporosis. The data showed a 76% reduction in relative risk for invasive breast cancer in the patients treated with raloxifene.
- Prophylactic mastectomy or oophorectomy may be appropriate for some women with a high genetic risk for development of breast cancer.

BIBLIOGRAPHY

Baum, M., & Schipper, H. (2005). *Fast facts—breast cancer* (3rd ed.). Oxford: Health Press.

Bernice, M. (2005). Nursing care of the client with breast cancer. In J. K. Itano & K. N. Taoka, (Eds.) *Core curriculum for oncology nursing* (4th ed., pp. 492-511). St. Louis: Elsevier Saunders.

Breast cancer. (2002). In C. H. Yarbro, M. H. Frogge, & M. Goodman (Eds.), *Clinical guide to cancer nursing* (5th ed., pp. 226-239). Sudbury, MA: Jones & Bartlett.

Breast cancer (PDQ): treatment. Retrieved November 29, 2006, from http://www.cancer.gov/cancertopics/pdq/treatment/breast/patient.

Levin, M. *Breast cancer.* VeriMed Health Network. Retrieved November 29, 2006, from http://www.nlm.nih.gov/medlineplus/ency/article/000913.htm Updated October 21, 2005.

Chapman, D. D., & Moore, S. (2005). In C. H. Yarbro, M. H. Frogge, & M. Goodman, M. (Eds.), *Cancer nursing principles and practice* (6th ed., pp. 1022-1088). Sudbury, MA: Jones & Bartlett.

Jemal, A., Siegel, R., Ward, E., et al. (2007). Cancer statistics, 2007. *Cancer Journal for Clinicians. 57,* 43-66.

Noninvasive Breast Cancer

DEFINITION

Noninvasive breast cancers, also referred to as in situ cancers, are precancerous lesions confined to the duct or lobule within the breast. The two types of in situ carcinomas are ductal carcinoma in situ (DCIS) and lobular carcinoma in situ (LCIS). DCIS is a precancerous condition in which abnormal cells are found in the lining of a breast duct. DCIS may become invasive cancer and spread to other tissues. In LCIS, the abnormal cells are found only in the lobules of the breast. LCIS is a warning sign of increased risk for development of an invasive breast cancer in the same or the opposite breast.

INCIDENCE

The incidence of noninvasive breast cancers is thought to be the same as invasive breast cancer (see Invasive Breast Cancer). DCIS accounts for about 20% of all new breast cancer cases and occurs in about 5% of male breast cancers. The incidence of LCIS is difficult to estimate because it is generally an incidental finding and is therefore likely to be underdiagnosed.

ETIOLOGY AND RISK FACTORS

The etiology of noninvasive breast cancers is thought to be the same as for invasive breast cancer (see Invasive Breast Cancer).

SIGNS AND SYMPTOMS

Most women with noninvasive breast cancer do not have palpable lesions or symptoms. Rarely a woman with DCIS will be seen for a lump, nipple discharge, or Paget's disease of the breast. LCIS, although uncommon, occurs predominantly in premenopausal patients at an average age around 45 years. LCIS is asymptomatic and usually found by chance from tissue obtained during a breast biopsy or other surgical procedure.

DIAGNOSTIC WORKUP

DCIS is typically diagnosed from routine mammograms. The mammogram will show an unusual cluster of microcalcifications. A needle localization or needle core biopsy may be required. Although not standard of care, some centers will conduct sentinel node biopsies in high-grade DCIS because there are reports of positive nodes in some cases. LCIS is usually diagnosed coincidently from tissue taken after a biopsy or breast surgery.

HISTOLOGY

DCIS is a precancerous condition in which abnormal cells are found in the lining of a breast duct. DCIS may become invasive cancer and spread to other tissues, although it is not known at this time how to predict which lesions will become invasive. DCIS is further divided into noncomedo and comedo carcinoma and into low-, intermediate-, or high-grade lesions.

LCIS is a precancerous condition in which abnormal cells are found in the lobules of the breast. This condition seldom becomes invasive cancer; however, having LCIS in situ in one breast increases the risk for development of breast cancer in either breast.

Women with DCIS or LCIS carry an 8-fold to 10-fold risk for development of an invasive breast cancer. DCIS classified as noncomedo and low-grade carcinoma carries a better prognosis than a high-grade comedo carcinoma. LCIS is associated with a small but increased risk for development of invasive breast cancer.

CLINICAL STAGING

On the basis of the AJCC staging classification system for breast cancer, a noninvasive cancer is a Stage 0.

TREATMENT

Treatment for DCIS depends on several factors, such as the extent and grade of disease, the classification, the patient's health, and medical history. Surgery, lumpectomy or simple mastectomy, is the standard treatment for DCIS and is intended to completely remove all cancer cells. Adjuvant treatments, such as radiation therapy and hormonal therapy, may be given to reduce the risk of DCIS recurring.

Women with LCIS may be given the option of a lumpectomy or mastectomy. Many clinicians advocate for a local excision with close follow-up that includes mammography twice yearly and a clinical examination

Major Cancers

every 3 to 4 months. Women with LCIS may be given hormone therapy to reduce the risk of recurrence in both the affected breast and the bilateral breast.

PROGNOSIS

The prognosis for women with non-invasive beast cancer is near a 100% 5-year survival rate.

PREVENTION

The prevention of noninvasive breast cancers is not specifically reported but is thought to be the same as for invasive breast cancer (see Invasive Breast Cancer).

BIBLIOGRAPHY

Breast cancer. (2002). In C. H. Yarbro, M. H. Frogge, & M. Goodman (Eds.), *Clinical guide to cancer nursing* (5th ed., pp. 226-239). Sudbury, MA: Jones & Bartlett.

Breast cancer (PDQ): treatment. Retrieved November 29, 2006, from http://www.cancer.gov/cancertopics/pdq/treatment/breast/patient.

Levin, M. *Breast cancer.* VeriMed Health Network. Retrieved November 29, 2006, from http://www.nlm.nih.gov/medlineplus/ency/article/000913.htm. Updated October 21, 2005.

Chapman, D. D., & Moore, S. (2005). In C. H. Yarbro, M. H. Frogge, & M. Goodman, M. (Eds.), *Cancer nursing principles and practice.* (6th ed., pp. 1022-1088). Sudbury, MA: Jones & Bartlett.

Ductal carcinoma in-situ (DCIS). (2006). Retrieved November 29, 2006, from http://cancer.stanford.edu/breastcancer/dcis.html.

Lobular carcinoma in-situ (LCIS). (2006). Retrieved November 29, 2006, from http://cancer.stanford.edu/breastcancer/lcis.html.

Central Nervous System

Margaretta S. Page and Anne Fedoroff

Central Nervous System Malignancies: Overview

DEFINITION

Central nervous system (CNS) malignancies refer to a heterogeneous group of cancers of the brain and spinal cord. These cancers originate from neural tissue (considered primary brain tumors) or other non-neural tissue or they can be metastatic tumors. This section provides a general overview and the following sections will address specific adult CNS malignancies in more detail.

INCIDENCE

The Central Brain Tumor Registry of the United States estimated 43,800 new cases of primary nonmalignant and malignant CNS tumors to be diagnosed in 2005. An additional 170,000 cases of metastatic brain tumors will be diagnosed. The American Cancer Society predicts that 20,500 new cases of malignant brain and central nervous system tumors will be diagnosed in the United States in 2007. The age of onset and male/female predisposition vary significantly on the basis of tumor type. For example, the average age of onset is 62 years for glioblastoma and meningioma and 16 years for medulloblastoma. The figure below shows the incidence of primary brain tumors by major histological types.

ETIOLOGY AND RISK FACTORS

There is no known cause for brain tumors; however, the following are considered risk factors:
- Exposure to therapeutic ionizing radiation
- Genetic disorders, including neurofibromatosis type I and II, tuberous sclerosis, Von-Hippel Lindau syndrome, and Li-Fraumeni syndrome

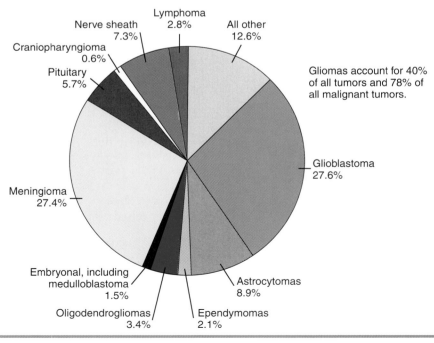

Gliomas account for 40% of all tumors and 78% of all malignant tumors.

Distribution of Central Nervous System Tumors by Histological Type. From Central Brain Tumor Registry of the United States. (2005). *Statistical report: primary brain tumors in the United States, 1998-2002* (p. 18). CBTRUS.

SIGNS AND SYMPTOMS

General signs and symptoms that are related to increased mass in the cranial vault and increased intracranial pressure include headache, nausea, vomiting, altered level of consciousness, and seizures. The individual sections will outline signs and symptoms specific to the tumor type. Focal signs and symptoms related to tumor location include seizures, weakness, sensory changes, personality changes, and endocrine abnormalities (see table below).

DIAGNOSTIC WORKUP

- Neurological examination
- Imaging of brain or spine
  - Magnetic resonance imaging (MRI)
  - Magnetic resonance spectroscopy (MRS)
  - Positron emission tomography (PET)
- Biopsy/craniotomy for tissue diagnosis

HISTOLOGY

Brain tumors are classified according to the World Health Organization Classification of Central Nervous System Tumors, which incorporates morphologic features, cytogenetics, molecular genetics, and immunologic markers. Malignancy is established on the basis of histological features. (See box at right.)

CLINICAL STAGING

Because of the very low incidence of metastases, not all CNS tumors require staging. In CNS malignancies staging involves imaging of the spine and obtaining cerebrospinal fluid to identify evidence of metastasis.

TREATMENT

Treatment varies on the basis of tumor type but includes surgery, radiation, and chemotherapy. The following sections will outline specific treatment dependent on tumor type. Concomitant medications used in brain tumors often include steroids, specifically dexamethasone for control of cerebral edema or symptom management, and anticonvulsants for patients who are in the acute postoperative period or who have seizures.

World Health Organization Grading of Tumors

- **WHO grade I:** Lesions with low proliferative potential and cure is possible with surgical resection.
- **WHO grade II:** Infiltrating lesions with low mitotic activity that have a tendency to recur. Some tumors may progress to higher grades.
- **WHO grade III:** Lesions with evidence of malignancy usually seen in mitotic activity, infiltrative ability, and anaplasia.
- **WHO grade IV:** Lesions that high mitotic activity, are prone to necrosis and usually are associated with a rapid disease seen both preoperatively and postoperatively

Adapted from National Cancer Institute. *Adult brain tumors, PDQ treatment: classification.* Retrieved March 11, 2007, from http://www.cancer.gov/cancertopics/pdq/treatment/adultbrain/HealthProfessional/page2.

PROGNOSIS

Prognosis is variable and depends on the tumor type.

BIBLIOGRAPHY

Central Brain Tumor Registry of the United States. (2005-2006). *Primary brain tumors in the United States, statistical report.* Retrieved on March 11, 2007, from http://www.cbtrus.org/reports//2005-2006/2006report.pdf.

Fox, S. W., & Mitchell, S. A. (2006). Cognitive impairment in patients with brain tumors: assessment in the clinical setting. *Clinical Journal of Oncology Nursing, 10,* 169-182.

Hickey, J. (2002). *Clinical practice of neurological and neurosurgical nursing.* Philadelphia: Lippincott Williams & Wilkins.

National Cancer Institute. (2007). *Adult brain tumors PDQ for health professionals.* Retrieved March 11, 2007 from www.cancer.gov/cancertopics/pdq/treatment/adultbrain/Healthprofessional.

Prados, M. (2006). Primary neoplasms of the central nervous system. In D. W. Kufe, R. C. Bast, W. N. Hait, et al. (Eds.), *Adults in cancer medicine* (pp. 1037-1065). Hamilton, ON: BC Decker.

Wrensch, M. R., Minn, Y., & Bondy, M. (2000). Epidemiology. In M. Berstein & M. Berger, (Eds.), *Neuro-oncology: the essentials* (pp. 2-17). New York: Thieme Medical.

Brain Lobe Function and Associated Symptoms on the Basis of Lesion Location

Location	Function	Symptom
Frontal	Motor movement, thought, reasoning, behavior, executive functioning, memory, motor aspect of speech, and bowel and bladder control. Dominant hemisphere controls language and writing	Personality changes, short-term memory loss, judgment, confusion, other mental changes, contralateral weakness, seizures, impaired speech or smell, visual field cuts, urinary frequency and urgency
Temporal	Behavior, long-term memory, hearing and vision pathways, understanding of speech, emotion, sensation, abstract concepts	Receptive aphasia, seizures, vision impairment, poor memory
Parietal	Sensory perceptions, spatial relations, reasoning, memory	Sensory deficits, seizures, inability to read, spatial disorders, difficulty with math, difficulty with complex reasoning, impaired memory
Occipital	Vision, reading	Visual hallucinations, visual disturbances, blindness, inability to read
Cerebellum	Balance, coordination	Ataxia, slurred speech
Brain stem Midbrain Pons Medulla	Basic life functions, heart rate, blood pressure, breathing, consciousness, attachment for cranial nerves	Vomiting and headaches in the morning, ataxia, cranial nerve palsy, weakness, double vision

Astrocytoma, World Health Organization Grade I

DEFINITION

Astrocytomas are the most common type of gliomas; they arise from astrocytes (the star-shaped supporting cells for the neurons). Astrocytomas make up about half of all primary brain tumors. Astrocytomas are classified by grade according to level of malignancy according to World Health Organization (WHO) criteria.

INCIDENCE

WHO grade I astrocytomas are most common in children and young adults. They include pilocytic astrocytoma and subependymal giant cell astrocytoma.

ETIOLOGY AND RISK FACTORS

There is no known cause for brain tumors; however the following are considered risk factors:

- Exposure to therapeutic ionizing radiation
- Genetic disorders, including neurofibromatosis type I and II, tuberous sclerosis, Von-Hippel Lindau syndrome, and Li-Fraumeni syndrome

SIGNS AND SYMPTOMS

Signs and symptoms are location dependent (see the table on page 41 in the Central Nervous System Malignancies Overview section). Because of the slow-growing nature of these tumors, symptoms may be subtle.

DIAGNOSTIC WORKUP

- Neurological examination
- Imaging of brain or spine
  - Magnetic resonance imaging
  - Magnetic resonance spectroscopy
  - Positron emission tomography
- Biopsy/craniotomy for tissue diagnosis

HISTOLOGY AND CLINICAL STAGING

WHO grade I lesions are those with low proliferative potential that are frequently discrete in nature, and cure is possible with surgical resection alone. Because of the very low incidence of metastasis, staging is not usually done with this tumor type.

TREATMENT

- Surgery may involve a craniotomy or biopsy depending on tumor location; it is often curative alone.
- Radiation may be administered if resection is suboptimal or if the tumor recurs.

PROGNOSIS

With complete resection, prognosis is excellent.

BIBLIOGRAPHY

Central Brain Tumor Registry of the United States. (2005-2006). *Primary brain tumors in the United States: statistical report*. Retrieved March 11, 2007, from http://www.cbtrus.org/reports//2005-2006/2006report.pdf.
National Cancer Institute. (2007). *Adult brain tumors PDQ for health professionals*. Retrieved March 11, 2007, from www.cancer.gov/cancertopics/pdq/treatment/adultbrain/Healthprofessional.
Prados, M. (2006). Primary neoplasms of the central nervous system. In D. W. Kufe, R. C. Bast, W. N. Hait, et al. (Eds.), *Adults in cancer medicine* (pp. 1037-1065). Hamilton, ON: BC Decker.
Wrensch, M. R., Minn, Y., & Bondy, M. (2000). Epidemiology. In M. Berstein, & M. Berger (Eds.), *Neuro-oncology: the essentials* (pp. 2-17). New York: Thieme Medical.

Astrocytoma, World Health Organization Grade II

DEFINITION

Astrocytomas are the most common type of gliomas; they arise from astrocytes (the star-shaped supporting cells for the neurons). Astrocytomas make up about half of all primary brain tumors. Astrocytomas are classified by grade according to level of malignancy by use of World Health Organization (WHO) criteria. WHO grade II astrocytomas are also referred to as low-grade astrocytomas or astrocytomas.

INCIDENCE

WHO grade II astrocytomas, also known simply as astrocytomas or low-grade astrocytomas, make up 26% of all primary glial tumors. They most commonly occur between 20 and 50 years of age. The median age at diagnosis is 37 years.

ETIOLOGY AND RISK FACTORS

There is no known cause for brain tumors; however, the following are considered risk factors:

- Exposure to therapeutic ionizing radiation
- Genetic disorders, including neurofibromatosis type I and II, tuberous sclerosis, Von-Hippel Lindau syndrome, and Li-Fraumeni syndrome

SIGNS AND SYMPTOMS

Seizures are the most common presenting symptom, but there may also be headaches or focal neurological deficits (see the table on page 41 in the Central Nervous System Malignancies Overview section).

DIAGNOSTIC WORKUP

- Neurological examination
- Imaging of brain or spine
  - Magnetic resonance imaging
  - Magnetic resonance spectroscopy

○ Positron emission tomography
- Biopsy/craniotomy for tissue diagnosis

HISTOLOGY

WHO grade II astrocytomas are generally infiltrating and low in mitotic activity but tend to recur. They consist of uniform cells, showing increased cellularity and minimal pleomorphism. They are composed of well-differentiated fibrillary or gemistocytic neoplastic astrocytes. Three histologic variants include: fibrillary astrocytoma, gemistocytic astrocytoma, and protoplasmic astrocytoma. Some of these tumor types tend to progress to higher grades of malignancy.

CLINICAL STAGING

Because of the very low incidence of metastasis, staging is not usually done with this tumor type.

TREATMENT

- Surgery may involve a craniotomy or biopsy, depending on tumor location.
- Radiation: Because of the slow-growing nature of tumor and the potential for toxicity, radiation at diagnosis is controversial. If gross total resection has been obtained, radiation may be deferred. Patients can be monitored with serial scans. Radiation is recommended, regardless, for patients >35 years of age. Recommended dose is 54 Gy in single fractions to the tumor volume and small surrounding margins.
- Chemotherapy may be administered at diagnosis in an effort to defer radiation. Currently this strategy remains investigational. Temozolomide or nitrosoureas are the recommended agents at diagnosis or recurrence.

PROGNOSIS

Median survival is 4.7 years. Eighty percent of patients survive 2 years, 46% survive 5 years, and 17% survive 10 years. Median survival at recur-

rence is 16 months. Prognosis is better for patients under 40 years of age at diagnosis, with a positive seizure history and absence of enhancement. It is now thought that mutation or deletion of the p53 gene is a negative prognostic indicator and, conversely, that vascular endothelial growth factor expression correlates positively with survival.

BIBLIOGRAPHY

Central Brain Tumor Registry of the United States. (2005-2006) *Primary brain tumors in the United States statistical report*. Retrieved March 11, 2007, from http://www.cbtrus.org/reports//2005-2006/2006report.pdf.

National Cancer Institute. (2007). *Adult brain tumors PDQ for health professionals*. Retrieved March 11, 2007, from www.cancer.gov/cancertopics/pdq/treatment/adultbrain/Healthprofessional.

Prados, M. (2006). Primary neoplasms of the central nervous system. In D. W. Kufe, R. C. Bast, W. N. Hait, et al. (Eds.), *Adults in cancer medicine* (pp. 1037-1065). Hamilton, ON: BC Decker.

Wrensch, M. R., Minn, Y., & Bondy, M. (2000). Epidemiology. In M. Berstein & M. Berger (Eds.), *Neuro-oncology: the essentials* (pp. 2-17). New York: Thieme Medical.

Astrocytoma, World Health Organization Grade III

DEFINITION

Astrocytomas are the most common type of gliomas; they arise from astrocytes (the star-shaped supporting cells for the neurons). Astrocytomas make up about half of all primary brain tumors. Astrocytomas are classified by grade according to level of malignancy by use of World Health Organization (WHO) criteria. WHO grade III astrocytomas are also referred to as anaplastic astrocytomas.

INCIDENCE

This astrocytic tumor type is faster growing than a grade II astrocytoma

and is considered "malignant." Grade III astrocytomas or anaplastic astrocytomas commonly occur in patients between 30 and 50 years of age. The mean age at diagnosis is 45 years. They are slightly more common in men than women and make up 4% of all brain tumors.

ETIOLOGY AND RISK FACTORS

There is no known cause for brain tumors; however, the following are considered risk factors:
- Exposure to therapeutic ionizing radiation
- Genetic disorders, including neurofibromatosis type I and II, tuberous sclerosis, Von-Hippel Lindau syndrome, and Li-Fraumeni syndrome

SIGNS AND SYMPTOMS

Signs and symptoms vary and are related to tumor location (see table in the Central Nervous System Malignancies Overview section on page 41).

DIAGNOSTIC WORKUP

- Neurological examination
- Imaging of brain or spine
  - Magnetic resonance imaging
  - Magnetic resonance spectroscopy
  - Positron emission tomography
- Biopsy/craniotomy for tissue diagnosis

HISTOLOGY

Anaplastic astrocytomas are highly cellular with increased nuclear and cellular pleomorphism and mitoses.

CLINICAL STAGING

Because of the very low incidence of metastasis, staging is not usually done with this tumor type.

TREATMENT

- Surgery is done to establish diagnosis and debulk as much tumor as possible
- Radiation is the single most effective therapy at this time. Recommended dose is 60 Gy in

single fractions to the tumor volume and small surrounding margins

- Chemotherapy includes temozolomide and nitrosoureas.

PROGNOSIS

Median time to tumor progression is 2 years; and median survival is 2.5 to 4 years.

BIBLIOGRAPHY

Central Brain Tumor Registry of the United States. (2005-2006). *Primary brain tumors in the United States statistical report*. Retrieved on March 11, 2007, from http://www.cbtrus.org/reports//2005-2006/2006report.pdf.

National Cancer Institute. (2007). *Adult brain tumors PDQ for health professionals*. Retrieved March 11, 2007, from www.cancer.gov/cancertopics/pdq/treatment/adultbrain/Healthprofessional.

Prados, M. (2006). Primary neoplasms of the central nervous system. In D. W. Kufe, R. C. Bast, W. N. Hait, et al. (Eds.), *Adults in cancer medicine* (pp. 1037-1065). Hamilton, ON: BC Decker.

Wrensch, M. R., Minn, Y., & Bondy, M. (2000). Epidemiology. In M. Berstein & M. Berger (Eds.), *Neuro-oncology: the essentials* (pp. 2-17). New York: Thieme Medical.

Astrocytoma, World Health Organization Grade IV

DEFINITION

Astrocytomas are the most common type of gliomas and arise from astrocytes (the star-shaped supporting cells for the neurons). Astrocytomas make up about half of all primary brain tumors. Astrocytomas are classified by grade according to level of malignancy using World Health Organization (WHO) criteria.

WHO grade IV astrocytoma is also known as glioblastoma multiforme (GBM). This is a highly malignant astrocytic tumor that can evolve from a lower-grade tumor through malignant degeneration, called a secondary glioblastoma, or can be a GBM at the outset, known as primary, or de novo, glioblastoma.

INCIDENCE

The peak incidence occurs between 65 and 74 years of age. The mean age at diagnosis is 54 years. They are slightly more common in men than women. GBMs make up 23% of all brain tumors and 50% of astrocytomas.

ETIOLOGY AND RISK FACTORS

There is no known cause for brain tumors; however, the following are considered risk factors:

- Exposure to therapeutic ionizing radiation
- Genetic disorders, including neurofibromatosis type I and II, tuberous sclerosis, Von-Hippel Lindau syndrome, and Li-Fraumeni syndrome

SIGNS AND SYMPTOMS

Signs and symptoms are location dependent (see table in the Central Nervous System Malignancies Overview section on page 41).

DIAGNOSTIC WORKUP

- Neurological examination
- Imaging of brain or spine
  - ○ Magnetic resonance imaging
  - ○ Magnetic resonance spectroscopy
  - ○ Positron emission tomography
- Biopsy/craniotomy for tissue diagnosis

HISTOLOGY

WHO grade IV GBM includes lesions that have poorly differentiated, often pleomorphic astrocytic cells, marked with brisk mitotic activity, endothelial or microvascular proliferation, and necrosis. The presence of necrosis is the hallmark for this tumor. Two histological variants include giant cell glioblastoma and gliosarcoma.

CLINICAL STAGING

Because of the very low incidence of metastasis, staging is not usually done with this tumor type.

TREATMENT

- Surgery to establish diagnosis and debulk as much of the tumor as possible
- Radiation is the single most effective therapy for this tumor type. Total dose given in single fractions to 60 Gy.
- Adjuvant chemotherapy includes temozolomide or nitrosoureas. Adjuvant chemotherapy is recommended in patients <40 years of age, with minimal disease and minimal dysfunction.
- Investigational treatments such as vaccine therapy or small molecule therapies may be considered at diagnosis or recurrence. Investigational therapies may target growth factor receptors, platelet-derived growth factor receptors, epidermal growth factor receptor, vascular endothelial growth factor receptor, or various cell-signaling pathways.

PROGNOSIS

Patients with grade IV astrocytomas or GBM have a very poor prognosis. Median survival is 15 months with radiation therapy and temozolomide, although it may be longer for patients <40 years of age who have undergone gross total resection and who have good performance status.

BIBLIOGRAPHY

Central Brain Tumor Registry of the United States. (2005-2006). *Primary brain tumors in the United States, statistical report*. Retrieved March 11, 2007, from http://www.cbtrus.org/reports//2005-2006/2006report.pdf.

National Cancer Institute. (2007). *Adult brain tumors PDQ for health professionals*. Retrieved March 11, 2007, from www.cancer.gov/cancertopics/pdq/treatment/adultbrain/Healthprofessional.

Prados, M. (2006). Primary neoplasms of the central nervous system. In D. W. Kufe, R. C. Bast, W. N. Hait, et al. (Eds.), *Adults in cancer medicine* (pp. 1037-1065). Hamilton, ON: BC Decker.

Wrensch, M. R., Minn, Y., & Bondy, M. (2000). Epidemiology. In M. Berstein & M. Berger (Eds.), *Neuro-oncology: the essentials* (pp. 2-17). New York: Thieme Medical.

Benign Brain Tumors

DEFINITION

Benign brain tumors are slow-growing brain tumors that can be removed or destroyed if in a surgically accessible location. The border or edge of a benign brain tumor can be clearly seen. Cells from benign tumors do not invade tissues around them or spread to other parts of the body. However, benign tumors can press on sensitive areas of the brain and cause serious health problems. Many of the tumors in this category grow inside the skull but outside the brain. Many histological types of brain tumors are considered to be benign. They include meningiomas, craniopharyngiomas, acoustic neuromas, and pituitary adenomas.

INCIDENCE

Meningiomas, pituitary adenomas, craniopharyngiomas, and nerve sheath tumors make up 45% of all primary brain tumors.

ETIOLOGY AND RISK FACTORS

The causes for these tumors remain unknown:

- Prior radiation predisposes patients to meningioma.
- Neurofibromatosis type 2 predisposes patients to bilateral acoustic neuromas and meningiomas.

SIGNS AND SYMPTOMS

- Signs and symptoms are related to tumor location (see table on page 41 in the Central Nervous System Malignancies Overview section).
- Craniopharyngiomas and pituitary adenomas occur near the pituitary gland or axis, so patients may present with hormonal abnormalities or visual disturbances.
- Acoustic neuromas occur along the acoustic nerve and can cause vertigo, dizziness, or loss of hearing.

HISTOLOGY

Histological diagnosis varies on the basis of tumor type. Typically these tumors are well circumscribed and slow growing.

CLINICAL STAGING

Staging is not necessary because these lesions do not tend to disseminate.

TREATMENT

- Surgery: resection of tumor is often curative.
- Radiation: if incomplete resection is obtained or tumor is in a surgically inaccessible area, radiosurgery may be administered. Radiation therapy may be recommended in the rare cases of recurrence.
- Long-term follow-up with endocrinologist is required if pituitary gland/area is involved.

PROGNOSIS

The prognosis is usually very good. However, because of the nature of the location where these tumors occur, patients can have significant neurological or endocrine sequelae from the tumor or from treatments.

BIBLIOGRAPHY

Central Brain Tumor Registry of the United States. (2005-2006). *Primary brain tumors in the United States, statistical report*. Retrieved March 11, 2007, from http://www.cbtrus.org/reports//2005-2006/2006report.pdf.

National Cancer Institute. (2007). *Adult brain tumors PDQ for health professionals*. Retrieved March 11, 2007, from www.cancer.gov/cancertopics/ pdq/treatment/adultbrain/Healthprofessional.

Prados, M. (2006). Primary neoplasms of the central nervous system. In D. W. Kufe, R. C. Bast, W. N. Hait, et al. (Eds.), *Adults in cancer medicine* (pp. 1037-1065). Hamilton, ON: BC Decker.

Wrensch, M. R., Minn, Y., & Bondy, M. (2000). Epidemiology. In M. Berstein & M. Berger (Eds.), *Neuro-oncology: the essentials* (pp. 2-17). New York: Thieme Medical.

Ependymoma

DEFINITION

An ependymoma is a glial tumor that develops from the neuroepithelial lining of the cerebral ventricles and the central canal of the spinal cord. This lining is known as the ependyma. Ependymomas can be classified as a World Health Organization grade I-III tumor. Included are myxopapillary ependymoma, subependymoma, and anaplastic ependymoma.

INCIDENCE

Ependymomas are more common in the pediatric population, making up 10% of childhood central nervous system tumors. In adults, ependymomas account for 5% of intracranial gliomas and 50% to 60% of spinal cord tumors. Sixty percent of these tumors occur infratentorially, most commonly in the posterior fossa. Peak incidence is at 5 years of age and again at 34 years of age.

ETIOLOGY AND RISK FACTORS

Spinal ependymomas can be associated with neurofibromatosis.

SIGNS AND SYMPTOMS

Because of the high incidence of infratentorial location, signs and symptoms often include those associated with hydrocephalus: morning headaches, vomiting, ataxia, cranial nerve deficits, and decreased level of consciousness. Because of their propensity to occur in the spinal cord, ependymomas can be associated with paresthesias, hemiplegias, and pain. Focal findings are related to tumor location (see table on page 41 in the Central Nervous System Malignancies Overview section).

DIAGNOSTIC WORKUP

- Neurological examination
- Cytological examination of cerebrospinal fluid (CSF)
- Imaging of brain or spine
  ○ Magnetic resonance imaging

○ Magnetic resonance spectroscopy
○ Positron emission tomography
• Biopsy/craniotomy for tissue diagnosis

HISTOLOGY

Most are cellular tumors consisting of uniform polygonal cells in a collagenous background with well-defined cytoplasmic borders. They may also contain areas of cysts, calcifications, and occasional hemorrhage. Anaplastic ependymomas have features that resemble glioblastoma multiforme, with high mitotic activity, endothelial proliferation, and necrosis. Ependymomas can be divided into supratentorial and infratentorial tumors.

CLINICAL STAGING

Because of location in or near the CSF pathways, the staging process is critical for this tumor type to determine whether the tumor has metastasized. Staging includes a spinal magnetic resonance imaging and obtaining a CSF sample for cytological examination.

TREATMENT

• Surgery may be performed for maximal resection and relief of hydrocephalus if present. A ventriculoperitoneal shunt may be placed, if needed. For patients older than 3 years of age with low-grade tumors in the brain and spine, gross total resection is considered complete therapy.
• Radiation: focal radiation may be given for residual disease, unless the disease has disseminated along CSF pathways; then craniospinal radiation is required.
• Chemotherapy: adjuvant chemotherapy does not improve survival but may be used at recurrence.

PROGNOSIS

Prognosis depends on a number of factors including age, tumor location, and extent of surgical resection. The overall 5-year survival rate is 57%.

Patients <3 years of age who have undergone a subtotal resection and have grade III tumors have a significantly worse, if not poor, prognosis.

BIBLIOGRAPHY

Central Brain Tumor Registry of the United States. (2005-2006). *Primary brain tumors in the United States, statistical report*. Retrieved March 11, 2007, from http://www.cbtrus.org/reports//2005-2006/2006report.pdf.

National Cancer Institute. (2007). *Adult brain tumors PDQ for health professionals*. Retrieved March 11, 2007, from www.cancer.gov/cancertopics/pdq/treatment/adultbrain/Healthprofessional.

Prados, M. (2006). Primary neoplasms of the central nervous system. In D. W. Kufe, R. C. Bast, W. N. Hait, et al. (Eds.), *Adults in cancer medicine* (pp. 1037-1065). Hamilton, ON: BC Decker.

Wrensch, M. R., Minn, Y., & Bondy, M. (2000). Epidemiology. In M. Berstein & M. Berger (Eds.), *Neuro-oncology: the essentials* (pp. 2-17). New York: Thieme Medical.

Metastatic Brain Tumors

DEFINITION

Metastatic brain tumors are tumors from other parts of the body, called primary tumors, that have metastasized to the brain.

INCIDENCE

Metastatic brain tumors make up greatest number of central nervous system tumors. Most metastatic tumors arise from lung, breast, colon, skin (melanoma), and kidney and are often multifocal.

ETIOLOGY AND RISK FACTORS

Metastatic brain tumors occur as a result of the development of a primary cancer, particularly lung, breast, colon, skin (melanoma), and kidney cancer.

DIAGNOSTIC WORKUP

• Neurological examination
• Imaging of brain or spine
○ Magnetic resonance imaging

○ Magnetic resonance spectroscopy
○ Positron emission tomography
• Biopsy/craniotomy for tissue diagnosis

SIGNS AND SYMPTOMS

Signs and symptoms vary depending on tumor size and location (see the table on page 41 in the Central Nervous System Malignancies Overview section).

HISTOLOGY

It can never be assumed that a brain lesion in the context of a history of prior cancer is a metastatic lesion nor that a primary lesion is known when a metastatic lesion is discovered. For this reason, biopsy or craniotomy to obtain tissue diagnosis of a brain tumor is essential.

CLINICAL STAGING

All cancers are to be considered stage IV when distant metastasis is present.

TREATMENT

The status of a patient's primary disease is critical in determining treatment options for a metastatic brain lesion. A patient with a newly diagnosed brain lesion must undergo a thorough workup to assess status of the primary disease before treatment decisions are made regarding the brain lesion. If the primary disease is controlled, surgery and radiation therapy are the recommended treatments. Depending on the primary disease, chemotherapy may or may not be added.

PROGNOSIS

Prognosis is disease dependent. Most patients die from uncontrolled primary disease, not the brain lesions.

BIBLIOGRAPHY

Lallana, E. C., & DeAngelis, L. (2005). Lymphomas and hemopoietic neoplasms. In M. Berger & M. Prados (Eds.). *Textbook of neuro-oncology* (pp. 301-309). St. Louis: Elsevier.

National Cancer Institute. (2007). *Adult brain tumors PDQ for health professionals*. Retrieved March 11, 2007, from www.cancer.gov/cancertopics/pdq/treatment/adultbrain/Healthprofessional.

Prados, M. (2006). Primary neoplasms of the central nervous system. In D. W. Kufe, R. C. Bast, W. N. Hait, et al. (Eds.), *Adults in cancer medicine* (pp. 1037-1065). Hamilton, ON: BC Decker.

Wrensch, M. R., Minn, Y., & Bondy, M. (2000). Epidemiology. In M. Berstein & M. Berger (Eds.), *Neuro-oncology: the essentials* (pp. 2-17). New York: Thieme Medical.

Mixed Glioma

DEFINITION

A glioma that contains two or more glioma cell types: astrocytes, oligodendrocytes, or ependymal cells.

INCIDENCE

Mixed tumors are most commonly found in patients 20 to 50 years old and make up 1% of all brain tumors.

ETIOLOGY AND RISK FACTORS

There is no known cause for brain tumors; however, the following are considered risk factors:

- Exposure to therapeutic ionizing radiation
- Genetic disorders, including neurofibromatosis type I and II, tuberous sclerosis, Von-Hippel Lindau syndrome, and Li-Fraumeni syndrome

SIGNS AND SYMPTOMS

Signs and symptoms are location dependent (see table on page 41 in the Central Nervous System Malignancies Overview section).

DIAGNOSTIC WORKUP

- Neurological examination
- Imaging of brain or spine
  - Magnetic resonance imaging
  - Magnetic resonance spectroscopy
  - Positron emission tomography
- Biopsy/craniotomy for tissue diagnosis

HISTOLOGY

The histological features of mixed gliomas differ on the basis of the grade and types of cells present. They can include astrocytes, oligodendrocytes, and ependymal cells with varying degrees of malignant or nonmalignant features. The most aggressive type of cell found in the tumor specimen determines the tumor grade.

CLINICAL STAGING

Because of the very low incidence of metastasis, staging is not usually done with this tumor type.

TREATMENT

Mixed gliomas are treated by using the recommended treatment for the most aggressive/anaplastic cell type found in the tumor.

PROGNOSIS

The prognosis for mixed gliomas depends on the most aggressive/anaplastic part of the mixed tumor.

BIBLIOGRAPHY

Central Brain Tumor Registry of the United States. (2005-2006). *Primary brain tumors in the United States, statistical report*. Retrieved March 11, 2007, from http://www.cbtrus.org/reports//2005-2006/2006report.pdf.

National Cancer Institute. (2007). *Adult brain tumors PDQ for health professionals*. Retrieved March 11, 2007, from www.cancer.gov/cancertopics/pdq/treatment/adultbrain/Healthprofessional.

Prados, M. (2006). Primary neoplasms of the central nervous system. In D. W. Kufe, R. C. Bast, W. N. Hait, et al. (Eds.), *Adults in cancer medicine* (pp. 1037-1065). Hamilton, ON: BC Decker.

Wrensch, M. R., Minn, Y., & Bondy, M. (2000). Epidemiology. In M. Berstein & M. Berger (Eds.), *Neuro-oncology: the essentials* (pp. 2-17). New York: Thieme Medical.

Oligodendroglioma

DEFINITION

An oligodendroglioma is a tumor that develops from the oligodendrocytes, which are supporting glial cells in the brain. Oligodendrogliomas represent about 5% of all gliomas.

INCIDENCE

Oligodendrogliomas are most common in patients between 20 and 40 years old and are more common in men than women. They make up <3% of all brain tumors and 5-10% of gliomas.

ETIOLOGY AND RISK FACTORS

There is no known cause for brain tumors, however the following are considered risk factors.

- Exposure to therapeutic ionizing radiation
- Genetic disorders, including neurofibromatosis type I and II, tuberous sclerosis, Von-Hippel Lindau syndrome, and Li-Fraumeni syndrome

SIGNS AND SYMPTOMS

Signs and symptoms are location-dependent (see table on page 41 in the Central Nervous System Malignancies Overview section).

HISTOLOGY

The histology of oligodendrogliomas differs based on grade or type. They are classified as grade II or III using the World Health Organization (WHO) classification for tumors of the central nervous system (See box on page 41 in the Central Nervous System Malignancies section). Oligodendrogliomas are considered WHO grade II and anaplastic oligodendrogliomas are WHO grade III. Due to the very low incidence of metastasis staging is not usually done with this tumor type.

DIAGNOSTIC WORKUP

- Neurological exam
- Imaging of brain and/or spine
  - Magnetic resonance imaging (MRI)

○ Magnetic resonance spectroscopy (MRS)
○ Positron emission tomography (PET)
• Biopsy/craniotomy for tissue diagnosis

TREATMENT

Appropriate treatment depends on the grade of the tumor and may include:

• Surgery is recommended for all oligodendrogliomas to establish diagnosis and minimize tumor burden. It may be the only therapy necessary for lower grade tumors if resection is complete.
• Radiation is used to treat more aggressive grade III and grade IV tumors and/or at recurrence of lower grade tumors.
• Chemotherapy: oligodendrogliomas are thought to be more sensitive to chemotherapy than malignant astrocytomas. Anaplastic oligodendrogliomas show exceptional chemosensitivity. This is thought to be related to the loss of 1p and 19 q chromosomes. Agents used are temozolomide and nitrosureas.

PROGNOSIS

Prognosis is dependent on the grade of the tumor, but is generally better than for astrocytomas of similar grade. Median survival for low-grade oligodendroglioma is 9.8 years; 93% of patients survive 2 years, 73% survive 5 years, and 49% survive 10 years. Positive predictors of outcome appear to be associated with 1p or 19q chromosomal losses.

BIBLIOGRAPHY

Central Brain Tumor Registry of the United States. (2005-2006). *Primary brain tumors in the United States, statistical report*. Retrieved March 11, 2007, from http://www.cbtrus.org/reports//2005-2006/2006report.pdf.
National Cancer Institute. (2007). *Adult brain tumors PDQ for health professionals*. Retrieved March 11, 2007, from www.cancer.gov/cancertopics/pdq/treatment/adultbrain/Healthprofessional.
Prados, M. (2006). Primary neoplasms of the central nervous system. In D. W. Kufe, R. C. Bast, W. N. Hait, et al. (Eds.), *Adults in cancer medicine* (pp. 1037-1065). Hamilton, ON: BC Decker.
Wrensch, M. R., Minn, Y., & Bondy, M. (2000). Epidemiology. In M. Berstein & M. Berger (Eds.), *Neuro-oncology: the essentials* (pp. 2-17). New York: Thieme Medical.

Primitive Neuroectodermal Tumor

DEFINITION

Primitive neuroectodermal tumor (PNET) is a grade IV embryonal tumor that arises from the neural crest. Some PNETs occur in the brain, whereas others (the peripheral PNETs) occur in sites outside the brain such as in the extremities, pelvis, and the chest wall. Only tumors of the central nervous system are discussed here; peripheral PNETs are part of the Ewing family of tumors (see Ewing's sarcoma on page 123).

PNET of the central nervous system can be divided grossly into infratentorial tumors (medulloblastoma or iPNET) and supratentorial tumors (sPNET). The latter occur rarely (25:1); however, they are more common in young adults. This section discusses sPNET only.

INCIDENCE

PNETs are more common in children than adults. These tumors account for less than 0.5% of primary supratentorial brain tumors in adults. Most sPNETs diagnosed in adults occur in young adults aged between 21 and 30 years.

ETIOLOGY AND RISK FACTORS

• Exposure to therapeutic ionizing radiation
• Genetic disorders including Turcot syndrome and Li-Fraumeni syndrome

SIGNS AND SYMPTOMS

• Usually related to increased intracranial pressure and tumor location (see table on page 41)
• Cranial nerve palsies and spinal cord symptoms if disseminated in the brain or spinal cord.

DIAGNOSTIC WORKUP

• Neurological examination
• Imaging of brain or spine
  ○ Magnetic resonance imaging
  ○ Magnetic resonance spectroscopy
  ○ Positron emission tomography
• Biopsy/craniotomy for tissue diagnosis

HISTOLOGY

PNETs, medulloblastomas, and pineoblastomas are histologically the same tumor in different locations. They comprise a predominant population of round to oval undifferentiated blue cells.

CLINICAL STAGING

These tumors are fast growing with a propensity to disseminate along cerebral spinal fluid (CSF) pathways. Staging is critical for this tumor type to detect whether the lesion has metastasized. Staging includes CSF cytologic examination either before surgery or 2 to 3 weeks after surgery to examine for evidence of dissemination.

TREATMENT

• Surgery: craniotomy or biopsy depending on tumor location
• Radiation of the entire neuroaxis is required because of the high propensity of the tumor to disseminate through the CSF.
• Chemotherapy includes nitrosoureas and platinum-based regimens.

PROGNOSIS

The mean survival is 86 months with a 3-year survival rate of 75%.

BIBLIOGRAPHY

Central Brain Tumor Registry of the United States. (2005-2006). *Primary brain tumors in the United States, statistical report*. Retrieved March 11,

2007, from http://www.cbtrus.org/reports//2005-2006/2006report.pdf.

Ghosh, S., & Jichici, D. (2006). Primitive *neuroectodermal tumors of the central nervous system*. Retrieved March 11, 2007, from http://www.emedicine.com/neuro/topic326.htm.

National Cancer Institute. (2007). *Adult brain tumors PDQ for health professionals*. Retrieved March 11, 2007, from www.cancer.gov/cancertopics/pdq/treatment/adultbrain/Healthprofessional.

Prados, M. (2006). Primary neoplasms of the central nervous system. In D. W. Kufe, R. C. Bast, W. N. Hait, et al. (Eds.), *Adults in cancer medicine* (pp. 1037-1065). Hamilton, ON: BC Decker.

Wrensch, M. R., Minn, Y., & Bondy, M. (2000). Epidemiology. In M. Berstein & M. Berger (Eds.), *Neuro-oncology: the essentials* (pp. 2-17). New York: Thieme Medical.

Recurrent Glial Tumor

DEFINITION

A recurrent glioma is one that has recurred despite surgery, radiation, or chemotherapy. Growth is demonstrated by changes in volume or enhancement on serial magnetic resonance images or neurological decline. It may require additional scanning (positron emission tomography, magnetic resonance spectroscopy) to differentiate among tumor, necrosis, and treatment effect.

INCIDENCE

The incidence of glial tumors (gliomas) recurring is very high.

ETIOLOGY AND RISK FACTORS

There is no known cause for the development of a primary brain tumor. Recurrent glial tumors discussed in this section are subsequent to a prior diagnosis of glial tumors.

SIGNS AND SYMPTOMS

Signs and symptoms will vary depending on tumor size and location (see table on page 41 in the Central Nervous System Malignancies Overview section).

DIAGNOSTIC WORKUP

- Neurological examination
- Imaging of brain or spine
  - Magnetic resonance imaging
  - Magnetic resonance spectroscopy
  - Positron emission tomography
- Biopsy/craniotomy for tissue diagnosis

HISTOLOGY

Recurrent gliomas usually show necrotic areas, mixed with nuclear atypia, mitotic activity, and anaplasia. It is not uncommon for a tumor to recur as a more aggressive or malignant type of glioma (i.e., glioblastoma).

CLINICAL STAGING

Staging is not usually done in this tumor type.

TREATMENT

- Surgery is done to debulk the tumor, therefore decreasing tumor burden and alleviating symptoms.
- Radiation therapy depends on the location of recurrence, prior radiation treatment, and type of radiation to be delivered. Stereotactic radiosurgery is often used in this context.
- Chemotherapy or other cytostatic agents such as temozolomide or nitrosoureas may be administered if they had not been used in the adjuvant setting. Other standard chemotherapy agents include etoposide or carboplatin.
- Other options include investigational therapies.

PROGNOSIS

Median survival at recurrence is grim. It varies from 2 to 3 months for older, incapacitated patients to 1 year in younger, neurologically intact patients. Important factors when considering further therapy include age, performance status, and tumor histologic diagnosis.

BIBLIOGRAPHY

Central Brain Tumor Registry of the United States. (2005-2006). *Primary brain tumors in the United States, statistical report*. Retrieved March 11, 2007, from http://www.cbtrus.org/reports//2005-2006/2006report.pdf.

National Cancer Institute. (2007). *Adult brain tumors PDQ for health professionals*. Retrieved March 11, 2007, from www.cancer.gov/cancertopics/pdq/treatment/adultbrain/Healthprofessional.

Prados, M. (2006). Primary neoplasms of the central nervous system. In D. W. Kufe, R. C. Bast, W. N. Hait, et al. (Eds.), *Adults in cancer medicine* (pp. 1037-1065). Hamilton, ON: BC Decker.

Wrensch, M. R., Minn, Y., & Bondy, M. (2000). Epidemiology. In M. Berstein & M. Berger (Eds.), *Neuro-oncology: the essentials* (pp. 2-17). New York: Thieme Medical.

Major Cancers

Gastrointestinal System

Anal Cancer

Carolyn Grande

DEFINITION

Anal cancers are uncommon tumors located in the anus. The anus is the proximal end of the large intestine that connects to the outside of the body. It measures approximately an inch and a half and opens to allow passage of stool from the body.

INCIDENCE

The incidence of anal cancer has increased since the 1980s. This is theorized to be due, in part, to the rise in sexual transmission of the human papilloma virus (HPV). This theory suggests that squamous cell cancer of the anus could be preventable.

In 2007, there will be an estimated 4,650 cases of anal cancer diagnosed in the United States and approximately 690 people will die from this disease. Women are diagnosed with anal cancer slightly more frequently than men. Diagnosis of anal cancer generally occurs in adults over the age of 35 years.

ETIOLOGY AND RISK FACTORS

- HPV, particularly HPV type 16, may be implicated in the development of squamous cell carcinoma of the anus
- Multiple sex partners is a risk factor for women
- Engaging in anal intercourse is a risk factor for both men and women
- Smokers are at a four-times-higher risk for development of anal cancer than are those who never smoked
- Immunocompromised people who have undergone transplants or have human immunodeficiency virus (HIV) are at greater risk
- Long-term medical problems in the anal area such as anal fistulas or other benign conditions increase risk

SIGNS AND SYMPTOMS

- Bleeding or itching around the anus
- Pain in the anal area
- Change in caliber of stool; stool may be narrower
- Abnormal discharge from the anus
- Enlarged/swollen lymph nodes in the groin or anal area

DIAGNOSTIC WORKUP

- Rectal examination to feel for lumps or growths
- Swabbing the anal lining and review of cells under a microscope
- Anal biopsy
- Computerized tomography scan of the abdomen and pelvis

HISTOLOGY

The anus is lined with squamous cells; thus squamous cell carcinoma is the most common form of anal cancer diagnosed in 47% of patients. Cloacogenic or transitional carcinoma, diagnosed in 27% of patients, is a type of squamous cell carcinoma that develops in the cloaca portion of the anus. Fifteen percent of anal cancers are adenocarcinomas that develop in the glands of the anal area. Other histologic diagnoses include basal cell carcinoma identical with that seen in other areas of the skin, Paget's disease, Bowen's disease, and melanoma.

CLINICAL STAGING

Clinical staging is essential for determining extent of disease and associated treatment strategies. Staging is done using the American Joint Committee on Cancer (AJCC) tumor, node, and metastasis (TNM) system (see table on page 51).

TREATMENT

Treatment decisions are based on several factors, including tumor location and type and stage of disease. The three main modes of treatment are surgery, radiation therapy, and chemotherapy. Historically surgery was the only therapeutic option; however, progress has been made. Combined modality therapy or chemoradiation is the most commonly used approach.

If surgery is an option, several surgical approaches are available depending on the type and location of the tumor:

- **Local resection** involves removal of only the tumor with a slim margin of noncancerous tissue around the tumor
- **Abdominoperineal resection** is an extensive procedure used in treatment of cancer of the anal canal. After this procedure, patients will have a permanent colostomy. This procedure can often be avoided by using chemoradiation

Radiation therapy can be used as neoadjuvant therapy in combination with chemotherapy or as primary treatment. External beam radiation is the most common method of delivery of high-energy waves. Other forms of radiation include the following:

- Internal radiation
- Brachytherapy
- Interstitial radiation

The chemotherapy agents used to treat anal cancer are as follows:

- Mitomycin and fluorouracil
- Cisplatin and fluorouracil

PROGNOSIS

The most important prognostic factor for anal cancer is the clinical stage. Seventy percent of anal cancers are stage I or II at presentation; most patients at this stage will be cured. Twenty percent of anal cancers have positive lymph nodes on presentation and 30% to 63% have positive nodes at surgery. The local failure rates of T3 and T4 tumors are approximately 50% after combined modality therapy.

Clinical Staging: Anal Cancer

Definition of TNM

Primary Tumor (T)

TX	Primary tumor cannot be assessed
T0	No evidence of primary tumor
Tis	Carcinoma in situ
T1	Tumor 2 cm or less in greatest dimension
T2	Tumor more than 2 cm but not more than 5 cm in greatest dimension
T3	Tumor of more than 5 cm in greatest dimension
T4	Tumor of any size invades adjacent organ(s) (e.g., vagina, urethra, bladder)*

Regional Lymph Nodes (N)

NX	Regional lymph nodes cannot be assessed
N0	No regional lymph node metastasis
N1	Metastasis in perirectal lymph node(s)
N2	Metastasis in unilateral internal iliac and/or inguinal lymph node(s)
M3	Metastasis in perirectal and inguinal lymph nodes and/or bilateral internal iliac and/or inguinal lymph node(s)

Distant Metastasis (M)

MX	Distant metastasis cannot be assessed
M0	No distant metastasis
M1	Distant metastasis

Stage Grouping

Stage 0	Tis	N0	M0
Stage I	T1	N0	M0
Stage II	T2	N0	M0
	T3	N0	M0
Stage IIIA	T1	N1	M0
	T2	N1	M0
	T3	N1	M0
	T4	N0	M0
Stage IIIB	T4	N1	M0
	Any T	N2	M0
	Any T	N3	M0
Stage IV	Any T	Any N	M1

*Note: Direct invasion of the rectal wall, perirectal skin, subcutaneous tissue, or the sphincter muscle(s) is not classified as T4.

Used with the permission of the American Joint Committee on Cancer (AJCC), Chicago, Illinois. The original source for this material is the *AJCC Cancer staging manual,* Sixth Edition (2002) published by Springer Science and Business Media LLC, www.springerlink.com.

PREVENTION

The causes of many anal cancers remain unknown. Because HPV and HIV infections are known risk factors for the development of anal cancer, reduction in sexual practices that carry a high risk for contracting these infections should be used. Practices to avoid include the following:

- Multiple sex partners
- Unprotected sex
- Anal intercourse

A vaccine to protect against HPV types 16 and 18 has recently been approved by the Food and Drug Administration. It is indicated for use in women before they become sexually active to protect against HPV, which is a risk factor for cervical cancer. Studies are continuing to ascertain use in males.

Smoking is also a known risk factor for anal cancer; therefore, smoking cessation can reduce the likelihood of development of anal cancer and other types of cancer.

BIBLIOGRAPHY

American Cancer Society. (2006). *Learn about cancer, anal cancer.* Retrieved December 1, 2006, from www.cancer.gov.

American Cancer Society. (2007). *Cancer facts and figures 2007.* Retrieved January 22, 2007, from www.cancer.org.

Greene, F., Page, D., Fleming, I., et al. (Eds.). (2002). Anal cancer. In *AJCC cancer staging handbook* (6th ed., pp. 126-127). New York: Springer-Verlag.

Minsky, B. D., Hoffman, J. P., Kelson, D. P. (2001). Cancer of the anal region. In DeVita, V.T., Hellman, S., & Rosenberg, S.A. (Eds.), *Cancer: principles and practice of oncology* (pp. 1319-1342). Philadelphia: Lippincott Williams & Wilkins.

National Comprehensive Cancer Network. (2007). *NCCN clinical practice guidelines in oncology-rectal cancer,* version 1.2007. Retrieved January 23, 2007, from http://www. NCCN.org.

Biliary (Extrahepatic Bile Duct) and Gallbladder Cancers

Kyle-Anne Hoyer

DEFINITION

Cancer of the biliary tract includes the gallbladder and the extrahepatic biliary ducts from the canals of Hering to the ampulla of Vater. Metastasis most frequently occurs through spreading into local lymph nodes and perineural invasion.

INCIDENCE

It is expected that approximately 9,250 Americans will be diagnosed and 3,250 will die from cancers of the gallbladder and other biliary sites in 2007. The populations at greatest risk are women and Native Americans.

ETIOLOGY AND RISK FACTORS

The exact etiology is unknown for extrahepatic biliary duct cancer, although ulcerative colitis and primary sclerosing cholangitis are predisposing conditions. The etiology of gallbladder cancer is also unknown, although 75% of patients with a diagnosis of gallbladder cancer have a medical history that is positive for gallstones. It is important to note that cancer of the gallbladder will develop in only 1% of patients with gallstones, and therefore gallstones are not considered a risk factor. Risk factors for gallbladder cancer include calcification of the gallbladder (porcelain gallbladder), and there is a sixfold increase in risk among typhoid carriers.

Major Cancers

SIGNS AND SYMPTOMS
Extrahepatic Bile Ducts

Presenting symptoms may include the following:

- Pain, jaundice, fever, pruritus
- Light-colored stools (most common)
- Bilirubinemia (early sign)
- Deep discomfort in the right upper quadrant
- Progressive weight loss resulting from anorexia
- Icterus and hepatomegaly on physical examination

Gallbladder

Presenting symptoms may include the following:

- Pain, obstructive jaundice, fever
- Right upper quadrant pain similar to biliary colic but more persistent
- Acute cholecystitis

DIAGNOSTIC WORKUP

- Endoscopic retrograde cholangiopancreatography
- Imaging studies: abdominal ultrasonography, computed tomography scan, magnetic resonance cholangiopancreatography, and percutaneous transhepatic cholangiography
- Blood work: complete blood cell count, chemistry panel, liver function tests, carcinoembryonic antigen, CA19-9
- Physical examination
- Biopsy (incisional or fine needle)

HISTOLOGY

Most cancers of the extrahepatic biliary ducts and gallbladder are adenocarcinomas. Other histologic types include carcinoma in situ, papillary carcinoma, mucinous, signet ring, clear cell, oat cell, and squamous cell variants. A differential diagnosis between a primary biliary cancer versus a metastatic adenocarcinoma is determined by the following criteria:

- The presence of in situ carcinoma in the ducts near the tumor
- Modulation from bile duct to parenchyma liver cells

(cells resemble biliary epithelium without bile production versus hepatocytes from the liver)
- Ducal plate configuration within the tumor
- Histologic grade as illustrated in the box below.

Histologic Grade

GX: Grade cannot be assessed
G1: Well differentiated
G2: Moderately differentiated
G3: Poorly differentiated
G4: Undifferentiated

From American Joint Committee on Cancer. (2002). *AJCC staging manual* (6th ed.). Chicago: American Joint Committee on Cancer.

CLINICAL STAGING

Staging is clinically based and is the best possible estimate of the extent of disease before treatment. Staging should be done by the TNM classification published by the American Joint Committee on Cancer. See the tables on pages 52 and 53.

TREATMENT
Extrahepatic Bile Duct

- Classified as being resectable or unresectable
- Surgical procedure varies according to location of tumor and is usually extensive (i.e., Whipple procedure) with a 5% to 10% mortality rate and a cure rate of ≈5%.
- Palliative surgical interventions are similar to those for cancer of the gallbladder.
- External beam radiation may be used in conjunction with surgical intervention.
- Clinical trials

Clinical Staging: Extrahepatic Bile Duct Cancer

Definition of TNM

Primary Tumor (T)

TX	Primary tumor cannot be assessed
T0	No evidence of primary tumor
Tis	Carcinoma in situ
T1	Tumor confined to the bile duct histologically
T2	Tumor invades beyond the wall of the bile duct
T3	Tumor invades the liver, gallbladder, pancreas, or unilateral branches of the portal vein (right or left) or hepatic artery (right or left)
T4	Tumor invades any of the following: main portal vein or its branches bilaterally, common hepatic artery, or other adjacent structures, such as the colon, stomach, duodenum, or abdominal wall

Regional Lymph Nodes (N)

NX	Regional lymph nodes cannot be assessed
N0	No regional lymph node metastasis
N1	Regional lymph node metastasis

Distant Metastasis (M)

MX	Distant metastasis cannot be assessed
M0	No distant metastasis
M1	Distant metastasis

Stage Grouping

Stage 0	Tis	N0	M0
Stage I	T1	N0	M0
Stage IB	T2	N0	M0
Stage IIA	T3	N0	M0
Stage IIB	T1	N1	M0
	T2	N1	M0
	T3	N1	M0
Stage III	T4	Any N	M0
Stage IV	Any T	Any N	M1

Used with the permission of the American Joint Committee on Cancer (AJCC), Chicago, Illinois. The original source for this material is the *AJCC Cancer staging manual,* Sixth Edition (2002) published by Springer Science and Business Media LLC, www.springerlink.com.

Clinical Staging: Gallbladder Cancer

Definition of TNM

Primary Tumor (T)

TX	Primary tumor cannot be assessed
T0	No evidence of primary tumor
Tis	Carcinoma in situ
T1	Tumor invades lamina propria or muscle layer
T1a	Tumor invades lamina propria
T1b	Tumor invades muscle layer
T2	Tumor invades perimuscular connective tissue; no extension beyond serosa or into liver
T3	Tumor perforates the serosa (visceral peritoneum) or directly invades the liver or one other adjacent organ or structure, such as the stomach, duodenum, colon, or pancreas, omentum, or extrahepatic bile ducts
T4	Tumor invades main portal vein or hepatic artery or invades multiple hepatic organs or structures

Regional Lymph Nodes (N)

NX	Regional lymph nodes cannot be assessed
N0	No regional lymph node metastasis
N1	Regional lymph node metastasis

Distant Metastasis (M)

MX	Distant metastasis cannot be assessed
M0	No distant metastasis
M1	Distant metastasis

Stage Grouping

Stage 0	Tis	N0	M0
Stage IA	T1	N0	M0
Stage IB	T2	N0	M0
Stage IIA	T3	N0	M0
Stage IIB	T1	N1	M0
	T2	N1	M0
	T3	N1	M0
Stage III	T4	Any N	M0
Stage IV	Any T	Any N	M1

Used with the permission of the American Joint Committee on Cancer (AJCC), Chicago, Illinois. The original source for this material is the *AJCC Cancer staging manual*, Sixth Edition (2002) published by Springer Science and Business Media LLC, www.springerlink.com.

Gallbladder

- Stage II-IV gallbladder cancer is considered unresectable.
- Surgical cure not possible for T2 and greater tumors.
- Palliative surgical intervention
  - Extended surgical resection with partial hepatectomy and portal lymph node dissection
  - Biliary bypass
  - Percutaneous transhepatic biliary drainage
- Stent placed to relieve jaundice
- Radiation may be internal or external depending on stage of disease.
- Clinical trials

PROGNOSIS
Extrahepatic Bile Ducts

Prognosis is poor with <10% being curable. Prognosis depends on anatomical location of the tumor, which affects resectability. The more proximal the tumor is to the gallbladder, the poorer the prognosis. Perineural invasion at the time of diagnosis has a negative impact on survival.

Gallbladder

The cure rate for asymptomatic pathological tumors diagnosed at surgery performed for reasons other than for treatment of suspected cancer is 80% but decreases to 5% if patient is symptomatic at the time of surgery. Lymph node–negative T2-T4 tumors have an anticipated 5-year survival rate of approximately 42%. Lymph node–positive T2-T4 tumors have an anticipated 5-year survival rate of 31%.

PREVENTION

There is no early detection or screening methods for biliary and gallbladder cancers. Adherence to treatment regimens for managing ulcerative colitis and prevention of gallstones may reduce risk, but no effective prevention strategies have been identified.

BIBLIOGRAPHY

American Cancer Society. (2007). *Cancer facts and figures 2007*. Retrieved January 28, 2007, from http://www.cancer.org/docroot/STT/stt_0.asp.

Coleman, J. (2005). Gallbladder and bile duct cancer. In C. H. Yarbro, M. H. Frogge, & M. Goodman (Eds.), *Cancer nursing principles and practice* (6th ed., pp. 1276-1291). Sudbury, MA: Jones & Bartlett.

Greene, F., Page, D., Fleming, I. et al. (Eds.). (2002). *AJCC cancer staging handbook* (6th ed.). New York: Springer-Verlag.

National Cancer Institute. (2006). *Gallbladder cancer*. Retrieved on January 28, 2007, from http://cancer-net.nci.nih.gov/cancertopics/pdq/prevention/oral/healthprofessional.

National Cancer Institute. (2006). *What you need to know about extrahepatic bile duct cancer*. Retrieved on June 2, 2006, from www.cancer.gov/cancer-topics/wyntk/oral.

Colon and Rectal Cancer

Carolyn Grande

DEFINITION

Colon cancer includes cancer of the ascending colon, transverse colon, descending colon, and sigmoid colon. Rectal cancer can develop anywhere between the rectosigmoid junction and the anal canal. Metastasis occurs when tumor invades through the bowel wall and travels to lymph nodes or distant organs, particularly the liver, lungs, and peritoneum.

INCIDENCE

Colorectal (CRC) cancer is the third most common cancer in both men and women. In 2007, an estimated 112,340 cases of colon and 41,420 cases of rectal cancer are expected to occur in the United States. It is expected that 52,180 Americans will die from colon or rectal cancer in 2007.

Major Cancers

ETIOLOGY AND RISK FACTORS

- The risk for development of CRC increases with age. Ninety percent of cases are diagnosed in individuals more than 50 years old.
- Risk is increased in individuals with a personal or family history of colon cancer or polyps or a personal history of inflammatory bowel disease. Inherited genetic syndromes including familial adenomatous polyposis and hereditary nonpolyposis colon cancer are associated with significantly increased risk for development of CRC.
- Additionally, modifiable risk factors in personal lifestyle and environmental exposures contribute to the risk for development of sporadic CRC. These include obesity; a diet high in fat, red meat, or processed foods and low in fruits and vegetables; heavy alcohol consumption; smoking; and physical inactivity.

SIGNS AND SYMPTOMS

Presenting symptoms may vary depending on the location of the tumor:

- Right side of the colon (cecum and ascending colon)
  - Dull, vague abdominal pain
  - Palpable mass in right lower quadrant
  - Melena
  - Anemia
  - Anorexia/weight loss
  - Indigestion
- Transverse colon
  - Changes in bowel habits
  - Blood in stool
- Left side of the colon (descending colon)
  - Change in bowel habits
  - Cramps/flatulence
  - Decreased stool caliber
  - Bright red blood in stool
  - Incomplete evacuation
- Rectum
  - Gross bleeding
  - Pain
  - Tenesmus
  - Constipation
  - Incomplete evacuation
  - Decreased stool caliber

DIAGNOSTIC WORKUP

- If CRC is suspected a comprehensive general history should be obtained. Individual and family risks, prior surgery, medical history, and social factors are critical components. Family history of cancer including type of cancer (especially colorectal, uterine, ovarian, ureter, or bladder) and age at diagnosis are important factors in identifying potential hereditary or familial syndromes. Thorough review of systems can provide insight to early or late signs of malignancy.
- A complete physical examination with emphasis on lymph nodes, abdomen, breast, and rectum should be performed.
- Laboratory tests should include a complete blood cell count, liver function tests, coagulation profile, and carcinoembryonic antigen (CEA). CEA is a glycoprotein that is present in gastrointestinal mucosa cells. Overexpression is suspicious for malignancy. It is not a tumor marker but rather a tumor-associated marker.
- Endoscopic examination is performed after the completion of the history and physical examination when a better sense of tumor location may be identified. Methods include a sigmoidoscopy, either flexible, which allows visualization to just above the rectosigmoid junction (20 cm), or a rigid sigmoidoscopy, which visualizes to the proximal end of the sigmoid colon (60 cm). A colonoscopy visualizes the entire colon. Biopsy of the tumor can be obtained at this time.
- Transrectal ultrasonography is a good tool for staging rectal carcinomas.
- A noninvasive examination of the colon can be performed with a double contrast barium enema.
- Diagnostic imaging studies are completed to ascertain the presence of metastatic disease.

Chest x-ray examination is appropriate at time of diagnosis if computerized tomography (CT) of the chest has not been obtained. CT of the abdomen and pelvis can determine the presence of extracolonic disease. Magnetic resonance imaging is a good follow-up to questionable findings in the liver on CT.

HISTOLOGY

The majority of CRCs are adenocarcinomas. Moderate to well-differentiated tumors are most common. Poorly differentiated or undifferentiated tumors, vascular invasion, or lymphatic spread of tumors are poor prognostic signs.

CLINICAL STAGING

Accurate staging is essential for adjuvant treatment decision making and development of prognosis. Staging is done according to the American Joint Committee on Cancer guidelines by the TNM classification system (see table on page 55). In CRC, staging relates to the depth of tumor invasion through the bowel wall, involvement of regional lymph nodes, and the presence of distant metastasis.

TREATMENT
Colon Cancer

- Surgical removal of the primary tumor and lymph node resection is the initial therapy. If there is presence of synchronous metastasis that is deemed unresectable at any point along the cancer trajectory, a limited colon resection to relieve blockage may be performed.
- Adjuvant chemotherapy depends on the stage of disease and the prognostic risk factors.
  - Chemotherapy in stage II disease is a topic of controversy and requires informed decision making on the part of the patient.
  - Adjuvant chemotherapy in stage III is given for a 6-month period.

Clinical Staging: Colon and Rectal Cancers

Definition of TNM

Primary Tumor (T)

TX	Primary tumor cannot be assessed
T0	No evidence of primary tumor
Tis	Carcinoma in situ: intraepithelial or invasion of lamina propria*
T1	Tumor invades submucosa
T2	Tumor invades muscularis propria
T3	Tumor invades through the muscularis propria into the subserosa, or into nonperitonealized pericolic or perirectal tissues
T4	Tumor directly invades other organs or structures or perforates visceral peritoneum**, ***

*Note: Tis includes cancer cells confined within the glandular basement membrane (intraepithelial) or the lamina propria (intramucosal) with no extension through the muscularis mucosae into the submucosa.

**Note: Direct invasion in T4 includes invasion of other segments of the colorectum by way of the serosa; for example, invasion of the sigmoid colon by a carcinoma of the cecum.

***Tumor that is adherent to other organs or structures macroscopically is classified T4. However, if no tumor is present in the adhesion microscopically the classification should be pT3. The V and L substaging should be used to identify the presence or absence of vascular or lymphatic invasion.

Regional Lymph Nodes (N)

NX	Regional lymph nodes cannot be assessed
N0	No regional lymph node metastasis
N1	Metastasis in one to three regional lymph nodes
N2	Metastasis in four or more regional lymph nodes

Note: A tumor module in the pericolorectal adipose tissue of a primary carcinoma without histologic evidence of residual lymph node in the nodule is classified in the pN category as a regional lymph node metastasis if the nodule has the form and smooth contour of a lymph node. If the nodule has an irregular contour, it should be classified in the T category and also coded as V1 (microscopic venous invasion) or as V2 (if it was grossly evident) because there is a strong likelihood that it represents venous invasion.

Distant Metastasis (M)

MX	Distant metastasis cannot be assessed
M0	No distant metastasis
M1	Distant metastasis

Stage Grouping

Stage	T	N	M	Dukes*	MAC*
0	Tis	N0	M0	—	—
I	T1	N0	M0	A	A
	T2	N0	M0	A	B1
IIA	T3	N0	M0	B	B2
IIB	T4	N0	M0	B	B3
IIIA	T1-T2	N1	M0	C	C1
IIIB	T3-T4	N1	M0	C	C2/C3
IIIC	Any T	N2	M0	C	C1/C2/C3
IV	Any T	Any N	M1	—	D

*Dukes B is a composite of better (T3, N0, M0) and worse (T4, N0, M0) prognostic groups, as is Dukes C (Any TN1, M0 and Any T, N2, M0). MAC is the modified Astler-Coller classification.

Note: The y prefix is to be used for those cancers that are classified after pretreatment, whereas the r prefix is to be used for those cancers that have recurred.

Used with the permission of the American Joint Committee on Cancer (AJCC), Chicago, Illinois. The original source for this material is the *AJCC Cancer staging manual*, Sixth Edition (2002) published by Springer Science and Business Media LLC, www.springerlink.com.

- In stage IV, with evidence of measurable disease, chemotherapy in combination with biological therapy is given indefinitely with the potential for treatment breaks.

- Approved chemotherapy regimens for stage II and stage III disease include the following:
  - 5-fluorouracil (5-FU)/leucovorin/oxiliplatin (FOLFOX)
  - 5-FU/ leucovorin
  - Capecitabine
- Approved treatment for stage IV or recurrent disease includes the following:
  - 5-FU/leucovorin/oxaliplatin (FOLFOX) + bevacizumab
  - 5-FU/leucovorin/irinotecan (FOLFIRI) + bevacizumab
  - Capecitabine/oxiliplatin (CAPEOX) + bevacizumab
  - Single-agent irinotecan
  - Cetuximab with or without irinotecan
  - Panitumumab
- Radiation therapy (RT) has a limited role in colon cancer. It may be recommended for patients who have had a bowel perforation in attempt to improve local control. Additionally, it may be used for palliation of painful metastasis.

Rectal Cancer

- Surgical resection by either a transanal or a transabdominal approach is primary treatment for T1-2 lesions in the low rectum.
- Neoadjuvant chemoradiation may be used to reduce the tumor size before surgery for T3, T4, or T1-4 lesions with nodal involvement.
- Adjuvant chemotherapy should be given for at least 6 months after surgery for all patients who received preoperative therapy regardless of pathological staging.
- Combined modality neoadjuvant therapy for rectal cancer is as follows:
  - Infusional 5-FU +RT
  - 5-FU/leucovorin + RT
  - Capecitabine + RT
- Adjuvant therapy and therapy for metastatic or recurrent rectal cancer includes regimens outlined in the treatment of colorectal cancer.

PROGNOSIS

Five-year overall survival is 93.2%, in stage I, 72% to 85% in stage II, 44% to 83% in stage III, and 8.1% in metastatic or stage IV. The range in overall survival results from the subdivisions of stage II and III disease; there is a decrease in survival as the stage of disease worsens.

Major Cancers

PREVENTION

Modifiable lifestyle prevention strategies include the following:

- Eating more fruits and vegetables
- Reducing high-fat foods, particularly animal fat
- Minimizing alcohol intake, avoiding beer and beverages with a high percentage of alcohol that contain nitrosamines, which can be carcinogenic to the colon
- Maintaining weight within healthy range
- Engaging in 30 minutes of exercise a day

Those who have a family history of colon cancer or a genetic predisposition for colorectal cancer should use routine screening practices as directed by their physicians.

BIBLIOGRAPHY

American Cancer Society. (2007). *Cancer facts and figures 2007*. Retrieved January 22, 2007, from www.cancer.org.

Greene, F., Page, D., Fleming, I., et al. (Eds.). (2002). *AJCC cancer staging handbook* (6th ed.). New York: Springer-Verlag.

National Comprehensive Cancer Network. (2007). *NCCN clinical practice guidelines in oncology-rectal cancer*, version 1.2007. Retrieved January 23, 2007, from http://www.NCCN.org.

O'Connell, J. B., Maggard, M. A., & Ko, C. Y. (2004). Colon cancer survival rates with the new American Joint Committee on Cancer sixth edition staging. *Journal of National Cancer Institute, 96*, 1420-1425.

Skibber, J. M., Minsky, B. D., & Hoff, P. M. (2001). Cancer of the colon. In V. T. DeVita, S. Hellman, & S. A. Rosenberg (Eds.), *Cancer principles and practice of oncology*. (pp. 1216-1271). Philadelphia: Lippincott.

Skibber, J. M., Minsky, B. D., & Hoff, P. M. (2001). Cancer of the rectum. In V. T. DeVita, S. Hellman, & S. A. Rosenberg, S.A. (Eds.), *Cancer principles and practice of oncology*. (pp. 1271-1319). Philadelphia: Lippincott.

Sweede, M. R., & Meropol, N. J. (2001). Assessment, diagnosis and staging. In D. T. Berg, (Ed.), *Contemporary issues in colorectal cancer: A nursing perspective*. (pp. 65-80). Sudbury, MA: Jones & Bartlett.

Esophageal Cancer

Brenda Keith

DEFINITION

Cancer that begins in the esophagus is divided into two major types:

- **Squamous cell carcinoma** arises in the squamous cells that line the esophagus. These cancers usually occur in the upper and middle part of the esophagus
- **Adenocarcinoma** usually develops in the glandular tissue in the lower part of the esophagus

At diagnosis, approximately 50% of patients with esophageal cancer will have metastatic disease. Metastasis most frequently occurs through spread into local lymph nodes. The liver, lungs, and pleura are the most common sites of distant metastases.

INCIDENCE

It is estimated that 15,560 Americans will be diagnosed and 13,940 will die of esophageal cancer in 2007. Three times as many cases occur in men than in women. Esophageal cancer is a disease of middle to older age, with most cases occurring over the age of 60 years. Although it is the ninth most common malignancy in the world with most cases arising in developing countries, the incidence of esophageal cancer is infrequent in the United States, constituting 1% of all malignancies. However, the incidence continues to rise each year in the United States.

- Squamous cell carcinomas
  - Worldwide, squamous cell carcinomas are the most common
  - African American males are six times more likely than white males to develop squamous cell carcinoma.
- Adenocarcinomas
  - In North America and Europe, adenocarcinomas are more common than squamous cell carcinomas.
  - Adenocarcinoma of the esophagus has the fastest

growing incidence rate of all cancers in the United States.
  - Patients diagnosed with adenocarcinoma are predominantly white men.

ETIOLOGY AND RISK FACTORS

The exact cause of esophageal cancer is unknown.

- Risk factors for squamous cell carcinoma:
  - *Tobacco*: smoking cigarettes or using smokeless tobacco is one of the major risk factors for esophageal cancer
  - *Alcohol*: long-term or heavy use of alcohol. There is a synergistic effect when combined with tobacco.
  - *Diet*: a diet that is low in fruits, vegetables, and vitamins A, B_{12}, and C increases the risk for esophageal cancer. Other potential contributing factors include frequent ingestion of hot liquids or foods or smoked, nitrate-cured, and salt-cured foods.
  - *Esophageal strictures*: achalasia (spasms of esophageal sphincter); caustic injury to the esophagus (e.g., ingestion of lye).
  - *Previous cancers of lung or head and neck*: other cancers associated with risk factors of tobacco and alcohol result in increased risk of a secondary primary esophageal cancer.
- Risk factors for adenocarcinoma:
  - *Gastroesophageal reflux disease (GERD)*: the presence of GERD is associated with an increased risk for development of adenocarcinoma of the esophagus. Long-standing GERD predisposes to Barrett's esophagus, in which epithelial changes occur in the lower esophagus as a result of esophageal damage from GERD.
  - *Obesity*: there is a strong relationship between body mass index and adenocarcinoma of the esophagus, with the risk of esophageal cancer up to

threefold in overweight individuals

SIGNS AND SYMPTOMS

Early esophageal cancer usually does not cause symptoms. However, as the cancer grows, symptoms may include the following:

- Dysphagia is the most common symptom—initially experienced with solids and then progresses to include liquids.
- Weight loss is the second most common symptom.
- Heartburn
- Regurgitation of food
- Epigastric or retrosternal pain
- Hoarseness or chronic cough
- Vomiting
- Hemoptysis

DIAGNOSTIC WORKUP

Imaging studies such as a chest x-ray film, barium swallow, and esophagoscopy (or esophagogastroduodenoscopy [EGD]). Endoscopy and biopsy must follow to determine the invasiveness of the tumor, the integrity of the esophageal wall, and the tumor tissue type. Once the diagnosis is confirmed, computed tomography or magnetic resonance imaging to evaluate the extent of disease of the chest, abdomen, and pelvis; bone scan; and bronchoscopy are performed. Additional techniques may include endoscopic ultrasonography, laparoscopy, or thoracoscopy. A positron emission tomographic scan is sometimes used to detect distant metastases.

HISTOLOGY

The most common histologic types of esophageal cancer are squamous cell carcinoma and adenocarcinoma. Most adenocarcinomas are located in the distal esophagus. Most squamous cell carcinomas are located in the proximal or mid esophagus. Tumor grade is as recommended by the American Joint Commission on Cancer (see box at right).

CLINICAL STAGING

Only the depth of penetration into the esophagus wall and nodal status

Tumor Grade

GX: Grade cannot be assessed
G1: Well differentiated
G2: Moderately differentiated
G3: Poorly differentiated
G4: Undifferentiated

From American Joint Committee on Cancer. (2002). *AJCC cancer staging manual* (6th Ed.). Chicago: American Joint Committee on Cancer.

are considered in staging, regardless of the length of extension over mucosal surfaces. Staging of carcinoma of the esophagus is based on the TNM classification developed by the American Joint Committee on Cancer (see table at right).

TREATMENT

Treatment goals (cure versus palliation) are based on the clinical stage of the disease and the feasibility of surgical resection of the tumor. Surgery, radiation therapy, and chemotherapy are all useful treatment modalities, with surgery being the primary approach whenever possible.

Surgery

- The gold standard for the treatment of localized esophageal cancer. The goal of surgery is to provide a definitive cure and to provide palliation of symptoms.
- Most tumors require a partial esophagogastrectomy. The remaining esophagus is then reconstructed with the use of the stomach or a segment of intestinal tissue.

Radiation Therapy

- May be combined with surgery preoperatively or postoperatively
- May be combined with chemotherapy and surgery
- May be used to alleviate obstruction, control pain, or restore swallowing

Chemotherapy

- Agents such as 5-fluorouracil (5-FU) or cisplatin may be combined with simultaneous radiation therapy.

Clinical Staging: Esophageal Tumor

Definition of TNM

Primary Tumor (T)

TX	Primary tumor cannot be assessed
T0	No evidence of primary tumor
Tis	Carcinoma in situ
T1	Tumor invades lamina propria or submucosa
T2	Tumor invades muscularis propria
T3	Tumor invades adventitia
T4	Tumor invades adjacent structures

Regional Lymph Nodes (N)

NX	Regional lymph nodes cannot be assessed
N0	No regional lymph node metastasis
N1	Regional lymph node metastasis

Distant Metastasis (M)

MX	Distant metastasis cannot be assessed
M0	No distant metastasis
M1	Distant metastasis

Tumors of the lower thoracic esophagus

M1a	Metastasis in celiac lymph nodes
M1b	Other distant metastasis

Tumors of the midthoracic esophagus

M1a	Not applicable
M1b	Nonregional lymph nodes or other distant metastasis

Tumors of the upper thoracic esophagus

M1a	Metastasis in cervical nodes
M1b	Other distant metastasis

Stage Grouping

Stage	T	N	M
Stage 0	Tis	N0	M0
Stage I	T1	N0	M0
Stage IIA	T2	N0	M0
	T3	N0	M0
Stage IIB	T1	N1	M0
	T2	N1	M0
Stage III	T3	N1	M0
	T4	Any N	M1
Stage IV	Any T	Any N	M1a
Stage IVA	Any T	Any N	M1b
Stage IVB	Any T	Any N	

Used with the permission of the American Joint Committee on Cancer (AJCC), Chicago, Illinois. The original source for this material is the *AJCC Cancer staging manual*, Sixth Edition (2002) published by Springer Science and Business Media LLC, www.springerlink.com.

- Adjuvant therapy protocols consist of paclitaxel and cisplatin in those who had total removal of the disease with negative margins.

Major Cancers

- Preoperative chemotherapy is under clinical evaluation.
- Metastatic disease regimens include the use of: 5-FU and cisplatin; irinotecan and cisplatin; paclitaxel and cisplatin; or single-agent paclitaxel.

Photodynamic Therapy

- Used in superficial and mucosal lesions and to palliate dysphagia
- Principles from laser treatment are used. A light-sensitizing agent is administered intravenously. The injected chemical is taken up by the esophageal tumor, a laser light is administered at the tumor site, and tumor necrosis occurs.

Symptom Management

- Esophageal dilatation may be done to maintain esophageal patency and improve dysphagia.
- A stent is inserted to maintain esophageal patency and improve symptoms of dysphagia.
- Nutritional support is indicated in any patient undergoing treatment for esophageal cancer.

PROGNOSIS

Surgical treatment of resectable esophageal cancers results in 5-year survival rates of 5% to 20%, with higher survival rates in patients with early-stage cancers. The 5-year relative survival rate for all stages combined is 15%. Histologic type is not a prognostic factor (see table below).

PREVENTION

There are no current recommendations for screening and early detection programs for esophageal cancer. High-risk candidates are those who use tobacco and alcohol, have poor dietary habits, or have a history of GERD. Measures to prevent esophageal cancer include avoidance or limited intake of alcohol, cessation of smoking and smokeless tobacco products, and management of GERD with antireflux medications and measures.

Squamous Cell Carcinomas

On the basis of solid evidence, avoidance of tobacco and alcohol would help decrease the risk of squamous cell cancer. Diets high in cruciferous (cabbage, broccoli, cauliflower) and green and yellow vegetables and fruits *may* be associated with a decreased risk of squamous cell esophageal cancer. Epidemiological studies have found that aspirin or nonsteroidal anti-inflammatory drug (NSAID) use *may* be associated with a decreased risk of developing or dying from squamous cell esophageal cancer.

Adenocarcinomas

Surveillance EGD and biopsy in people with Barrett's esophagus may lead to early detection and improved survival. People diagnosed with Barrett's esophagus should see a gastroenterologist (gastrointestinal specialist) at least every year. Epidemiological studies have found that aspirin or NSAID use *may* be associated with decreased risk of developing or dying from esophageal cancer.

BIBLIOGRAPHY

American Cancer Society. (2007). *Cancer facts and figures*. Atlanta: American Cancer Society.

Blot, W., & McLaughlin, J. (1999). The changing epidemiology of esophageal cancer. *Seminars in Oncology, 26*(5 Suppl 15), 2-8.

Corley, D., Kerlikowske, K., Verma, R., et al. (2003). Protective association of aspirin/NSAIDs and esophageal cancer: a systematic review and meta-analysis. *Gastroenterology 124,* 47-56.

Devesa, S., Blot, W., & Fraumeni, Jr., J. (1998). Changing patterns in the incidence of esophageal and gastric carcinoma in the United States. *Cancer, 83,* 2049-53.

Digestive system: esophagus. (2002). In F. Greene, D. Page, I., Fleming, et al. (Eds.), *AJCC cancer staging handbook* (6th ed.). New York: Springer-Verlag.

Grund, S. (2004). *Medical encyclopedia, esophageal cancer*. Retrieved June 2, 2006, from http://www.nlm.nih. gov/medlineplus/ency/article/ 000283.htm.

Heath, E. Heitmiller, R., & Forastiere, A. (2000). Esophageal cancer. In R. Lenhard Jr., R. Osteen, & T. Gansler, (Eds.), *The American Cancer Society's clinical oncology* (pp. 331-343). Atlanta: American Cancer Society.

Lagergren, J., Bergström, R., Lindgren, A., et al. (1999). Symptomatic gastroesophageal reflux as a risk factor for esophageal adenocarcinoma. *New England Journal of Medicine, 340,* 825-831.

Lagergren, J., Bergstrom, R., & Nyren, O. (1999). Association between body mass and adenocarcinoma of the esophagus and gastric cardia. *Annals of Internal Medicine, 130,* 883-890.

National Cancer Institute. (2006). *Esophageal cancer*. Retrieved on January 28, 2007, from http:// www. cancernet.nci.nih.gov/cancer-topics/pdq/prevention/esophageal/ healthprofessional

National Cancer Institute. *What you need to know about cancer of the esophagus*. (2006). Retrieved on May 30, 2006, from http://www.cancer. gov/cancertopics/wyntk/esophagus.

Patti, M., & Tedesco, P. *Esophageal cancer*. (2005). Retrieved on June 2, 2006, from http://www.emedicine.com/med/topi c741.htm.

Strohl, R. (2005). Nursing care of the client with cancers of the gastrointestinal tract. In J. Itano & K. Taoka (Eds.), *Core curriculum for oncology nursing* (4th ed., pp. 524-531). St. Louis: Elsevier.

Surveillance, epidemiology and end results cancer statistics review, 1975-2001. Retrieved on June 5, 2006, from http://seer.cancer.gov/csr/1975_2001/.

Volker, D. (2004). Other cancers. In C. Varricchio (Ed.). *A cancer source book for nurses* (8th ed., pp. 309-312). Boston: Jones & Bartlett.

5-year Relative Survival Rate for Esophageal Cancer

Stage	Percent diagnosed survival rate	5-year relative
Localized (I and II)	26	29.3
Regional (III)	30	13.3
Distant (IV)	27	3.1

Data from Surveillance, Epidemiology, and End Results (SEER) Program (www.seer.cancer.gov). SEER stat database: incidence—SEER 17 regs limited use, Nov 2006 sub (1973-2004 varying), National Cancer Institute, DCCPS Surveillance Research Program, Cancer Statistics Branch, released April 2007, based on the November 2006 submission.

Gastric Cancer

Carolyn Grande

DEFINITION

Gastric cancer is also referred to as stomach cancer. The stomach is divided into five sections and cancers originating in different sections may have different symptoms and outcomes. The five sections of the stomach are as follows:

- Cardia or proximal stomach, the upper portion closest to the esophagus
- Fundus
- Distal stomach, the lower portion closest to the intestines
- Antrum, where food is mixed with gastric juice
- Pylorus, which acts as a valve controlling emptying of the stomach contents

Stomach cancers can spread in several ways

- Growth through the wall of the stomach into nearby organs
- Spread to the lymph system, including lymph nodes and vessels

INCIDENCE

An estimated 21,260 Americans will be diagnosed with stomach cancer in 2007; it is expected that 11,210 people will die of this disease in 2007. A person's lifetime risk for development of stomach cancer is 1 in 100. Two thirds of the people diagnosed are generally older than 65 years. The male/ female ratio is 2:1.

Gastric cancer is much more common worldwide, particularly in underdeveloped countries. It is believed that the rates are lower in the United States because of frequent use of antibiotics in children that also kill the bacteria *Helicobacter pylori (H pylori)*, which is believed to be a major cause of stomach cancer.

ETIOLOGY AND RISK FACTORS

The role of diet in association with stomach cancer has been investigated. Dietary factors associated with increased risk of gastric cancer include the following:

- High salt consumption
- High nitrate consumption
- Low dietary vitamins A and C
- Poor food preparation (smoked or salt cured)
- Lack of refrigeration
- Poor drinking water (well water)

Occupational risks include the following:

- Coal and rubber workers

Other risk factors include the following:

- Cigarette smoking
- Radiation exposure
- *H pylori*
- Epstein-Barr virus
- Prior gastric surgery for ulcer disease

Genetic risk factors include the following:

- Type A blood
- Pernicious anemia
- Family history
- Hereditary nonpolyposis colon cancer
- Li-Fraumeni syndrome

SIGNS AND SYMPTOMS

Only about 10% to 20% of gastric cancers are diagnosed in the early stage. The vague, nonspecific symptoms of gastric cancer result in most patients in the United States being diagnosed with advanced stage disease.

The signs and symptoms of gastric cancers include the following:

- Unintended weight loss
- Anorexia
- Early satiety
- Nausea
- Vomiting with or without blood
- Heartburn
- Indigestion
- Sense of fullness in the upper abdomen
- Dysphagia

It is important to note that certain symptoms may guide the clinician to the location of the tumor in the stomach.

DIAGNOSTIC WORKUP

- Complete history and physical examination
- Upper endoscopy with biopsy
- Upper gastrointestinal x-ray series with barium
- Endoscopic ultrasonography can determine tumor size and invasion
- Computerized tomography scan with contrast
- Positron emission tomography
  - useful in identifying cancer that has spread beyond the stomach and cannot be removed with surgery
- Magnetic resonance imaging
- Chest x-ray film
- Complete blood cell count, fecal occult blood, liver function tests
- Laparoscopy in preparation for surgery to ascertain whether all the tumor is resectable

HISTOLOGY

Approximately 95% of malignant gastric neoplasms are adenocarcinomas. Other malignant tumors are rare and can include squamous cell carcinoma, adenoacanthoma, carcinoid tumors, leiomyosarcoma, and lymphoma. Lauren's classification is a widely used classification in gastric cancer (see box below), dividing gastric cancer into intestinal or diffuse forms.

Lauren's Classification of Gastric Cancer

INTESTINAL FORM
A differentiated cancer with a tendency to form glands

DIFFUSE FORM
Exhibits very little cell cohesion and has affinity for submucosal spread and early metastasis

CLINICAL STAGING

Clinical staging is essential for determining the extent of disease and associated treatment strategies. Staging is done according to the American Joint Committee on Cancer tumor, node, and metastasis (TNM) system (see table on page 60).

TREATMENT

Laparoscopic findings will determine whether patients have locoregional or metastatic carcinoma. Surgery is recommended for medically fit patients with

Clinical Staging: Gastric Cancer

Definition of TNM

Primary Tumor (T)

TX	Primary tumor cannot be assessed
T0	No evidence of primary tumor
Tis	Carcinoma in situ; intraepithelial tumor without invasion of the lamina propria
T1	Tumor invades lamina propria or submucosa
T2	Tumor invades muscularis propria or subserosa*
T2a	Tumor invades muscularis propria
T2b	Tumor invades subserosa
T3	Tumor penetrates serosa (visceral peritoneum) without invasion of adjacent structures**, ***
T4	Tumor invades adjacent structures**, ***

*A tumor may penetrate the muscularis propria with extension into the gastrocolic or gastrohepatic ligaments, or into the greater or lesser omentum, without perforation of the visceral peritoneum covering these structures. In this case, the tumor is classified as T2. If there is perforation of the visceral peritoneum covering the gastric ligaments or the omentum, the tumor should be classified as T3.

**Note: The adjacent structures of the stomach include the spleen, transverse colon, liver, diaphragm, pancreas, abdominal wall, adrenal gland, kidney, small intestine, and retroperitoneum.

***Note: Intramural extension to the duodenum or esophagus is classified by the depth of the greatest invasion in any of these sites, including the stomach.

Regional Lymph Nodes (N)

NX	Regional lymph node(s) cannot be assessed
N0	No regional lymph node metastasis*
N1	Metastasis in one to six regional lymph nodes
N2	Metastasis in seven to 15 regional lymph nodes
N3	Metastasis in more than 15 regional lymph nodes

*Note: A designation of pN0 should be used if all examined lymph nodes are negative, regardless of the total number removed and examined.

Distant Metastasis (M)

MX	Distant metastasis cannot be assessed
M0	No distant metastasis
M1	Distant metastasis

Stage Grouping

Stage 0	Tis	N0	M0
Stage IA	T1	N0	M0
Stage IB	T1	N1	M0
	T2a/b	N0	M0
Stage II	T1	N2	M0
	T2a/b	N1	M0
	T3	N0	M0
Stage IIIA	T2a/b	N2	M0
	T3	N1	M0
	T4	N0	M0
Stage IIIB	T3	N2	M0
Stage IV	T4	N1-3	M0
	T1-3	N3	M0
	Any T	Any N	M1

Used with the permission of the American Joint Committee on Cancer (AJCC), Chicago, Illinois. The original source for this material is the *AJCC Cancer staging manual,* Sixth Edition (2002) published by Springer Science and Business Media LLC, www.springerlink.com.

resectable (stages I to III). Goals of surgery are to achieve curative resection. For carcinomas in the distal stomach a subtotal gastrectomy is preferred. For proximal carcinomas total gastrectomy is recommended. Recent studies suggest that preoperative induction chemotherapy followed by chemoradiotherapy obtains a substantial pathologic response resulting in durable survival time.

Adjuvant therapy in patients with surgical pathological T1, N0, M0, and R0 (negative margins) may be observed without adjuvant therapy. Patients with an R0 resection who have T2, N0 with high-risk features should receive adjuvant chemoradiotherapy (5-fluorouracil [5-FU]–based/ radiation therapy [RT]).

Gastric cancer is considered unresectable if there is evidence of peritoneal involvement, distant metastasis, or invasion/encasement of blood vessels.

For unresectable locoregional cancer, combined modality therapy is used with radiation and 5-FU for radiosensitization. If the patient is considered medically unfit, he or she may also be offered combined modality therapy or salvage chemotherapy.

Salvage chemotherapy agents include the following:

- 5-FU/leucovorin
- Epirubicin/cisplatin/5-FU
- 5-FU based, capecitabine
- Cisplatin based
- Oxaliplatin based
- Irinotecan based
- Taxane based

PROGNOSIS

The 5-year overall survival rate for patients with gastric cancer in the United States is about 24%. This is due to the diagnosis being made in the relatively later stages of the disease. Cancers in the lower part of the stomach may have better outcomes than those in the higher part of the stomach.

PREVENTION

Although the exact cause of stomach cancer is not known, there are certain lifestyle behaviors that can lower risk, including the following:

- A diet high in fresh fruits and vegetables (five servings/day)
- Moderate consumption of red meat
- Limited use of alcoholic beverages, if at all
- Smoking cessation

Other approaches to lowering risk include the following:

- Daily aspirin may decrease the risk of gastric and colon cancer.
- Early diagnosis and intervention for *H pylori* infection

BIBLIOGRAPHY

American Cancer Society. (2006). *Learn about cancer, stomach cancer.*

Retrieved December 1, 2006, from www.cancer.gov.

Stomach cancer. (2002). In F. Greene, D. Page, I. Fleming, et al. (Eds.), *AJCC cancer staging handbook* (6th ed., p. 101). New York: Springer-Verlag.

Karpeh, M. S., Kelsen, D. P., & Tepper, J. (2001).Cancer of the stomach. In V. T. DeVita, S. Hellman, & S. A. Rosenberg (Eds.), *Cancer principles and practice of oncology* (pp. 1092-1126). Philadelphia: Lippincott.

National Comprehensive Cancer Network. (2006). *NCCN clinical practice guidelines in oncology-rectal cancer*, version 2.2006. Retrieved July 1, 2006, from http://www. NCCN.org.

Gastrointestinal Stromal Tumor

Carolyn Grande

DEFINITION

Gastrointestinal stromal tumors (GISTs) develop from precursors of connective tissue in the gastrointestinal (GI) tract. These tumors can arise anywhere in the GI tract:

- Stomach, 60%-70% of cases
- Small intestine, 20%-25% of cases
- Colon, 5% of cases
- Esophagus, <5% of cases

INCIDENCE

GISTs are relatively uncommon; therefore, the exact number of cases per year is not known. A study of malignant GISTs done in the United States found the incidence to be 7 cases per million people or approximately 1,500 cases per year. The majority of cases are diagnosed in persons more than 50 years old. GISTs are slightly more common in men with a higher incidence in African Americans than in whites.

ETIOLOGY AND RISK FACTORS

There are no known risk factors for GIST. The exact cause of GIST is unknown although there is an abnormality in a gene called *c-kit* in most patients with GIST. There are rare cases where several family members have GIST. Under these circumstances

they may have inherited a gene mutation; however, the majority of GIST diagnoses are sporadic.

SIGNS AND SYMPTOMS

Presenting symptoms are related to the tumor site and may include the following:

- Bleeding into the intestinal tract
- Hematemesis
- Melena
- Abdominal discomfort
- Palpable abdominal mass
- Dysphagia
- Nausea/vomiting

DIAGNOSTIC WORKUP

Diagnostic workup will include testing directed toward the presumed origin of the tumor:

- Thorough history and physical examination
- Upper GI series (barium swallow)
- Lower GI series (barium enema)
- Upper endoscopy
- Lower endoscopy (colonoscopy)
- Endoscopic ultrasonography
- Computerized tomography
- Magnetic resonance imaging
- Positron emission tomography
- Biopsy by endoscopy or laparoscopy
- Complete blood cell count and liver function tests

HISTOLOGY

Histologic grading can help predict whether the GIST is a benign or a malignant tumor.

A GIST diagnosis is made through immunohistochemistry. The tissue sample is treated with laboratory antibodies that can adhere to the KIT protein (CD117). Color changes to the surface of the cells confirm the presence of KIT proteins, thus distinguishing GIST from other GI tumors.

CLINICAL STAGING

There is no clinical staging system for GIST. Prognostic features are used to evaluate treatment decisions and outcomes for patients include the following:

- Size of tumor (tumors >2 inches have worse outcomes)
- Tumor location
- Histologic grading (can determine low-, intermediate- or high-risk tumors)

TREATMENT

Surgery is frontline treatment for GIST. If the tumor is completely resected, no further therapy is needed. For unresectable or widespread metastatic disease, neoadjuvant treatment with imatinib mesylate can be initiated, assessing therapeutic response within 3 months of therapy. If response is noted, consider surgical resection or continue imatinib. In the presence of progressive disease, radiofrequency ablation or chemoembolization may be an option. Additionally, therapy with sunitinib can be considered.

PROGNOSIS

The 5-year overall survival rate for malignant GIST is 45%. The percentage of relative 5-year survival rate considering other prognostic factors is as follows:

- Tumor confined to the organ of origin, 64%
- Tumor has grown into nearby tissue, 30%
- Tumor has spread to distant sites, 13%

PREVENTION

No risk factors have been identified to prevent GIST; therefore, it is not possible to identify prevention strategies.

BIBLIOGRAPHY

American Cancer Society. (2006). *Learn about cancer, gastrointestinal stromal tumors*. Retrieved December 1, 2006, from www.cancer.gov.

Brennan, M. F., Alektiar, K. M., & Maki, R. G. (2001). Sarcomas of the soft tissue and bone. In V. T. DeVita, S. Hellman, & S. A. Rosenberg (Eds.), *Cancer principles and practice of oncology* (pp. 1848 & 1854). Philadelphia: Lippincott.

National Comprehensive Cancer Network. (2006). *NCCN clinical practice guidelines in oncology-rectal cancer*, version.2.2006. Retrieved July 1, 2006, from http://www. NCCN.org.

VonMehren, M. (2006). *New approaches to the management of gastrointestinal stromal tumors* [brochure]. New York: McMahon.

Hepatocellular Carcinoma

Brooke M. Aghajani

DEFINITION

Hepatocellular cancer (HCC) is a primary tumor of the liver. Tumors in the liver generally comprise two major cell types: hepatocellular carcinoma (liver cell carcinoma) and cholangiocarcinoma (intrahepatic bile duct carcinoma).

INCIDENCE

More than 1 million new cases of hepatocellular cancer are diagnosed each year worldwide, making it the seventh most commonly diagnosed cancer and the most commonly diagnosed cancer in men. However, in the United States it is much less common, with an estimated 19,160 new cases and 16,780 deaths projected from liver and intrahepatic bile duct cancer for 2007. These rates have been rising steadily over the last two decades, possibly because of an increase in the number of individuals in the United States with chronic hepatitis C infection (HCV). HCC generally occurs in individuals with chronic liver disease, especially those with viral hepatitis. In the United States, HCC is more common in individuals over the age of 50 years and it affects at least twice as many men as women.

ETIOLOGY AND RISK FACTORS

- Cirrhosis of the liver is associated in up to 80% of all patients with HCC and increases an individual's risk for development of HCC up to 2% per year.
- Hepatitis B (HBV) and C (HCV) account for 30% to 40% of HCC. The time period between contracting the virus and development of HCC has a wide variation of 30 to 50 years. This latency period between viral exposure and cancer development may be shortened if an individual consumes alcohol regularly. The risk for development of HCC is greater in patients who have both HBV and HCV.
- The mycotoxin, aflatoxin, is most commonly found on foods such as peanuts, soybeans, and corn and has been associated with mutations in the tumor suppressor gene p53.
- Hereditary hemochromatosis, an inherited disorder, can ultimately lead to cirrhosis of the liver and can confer up to a 20-fold increase in HCC.
- Alcohol has been associated with exacerbation of certain risk factors such as HBV and HCV but is not itself an independent risk factor.

SIGNS AND SYMPTOMS

HCC is difficult to diagnose because most individuals with HCC have underlying liver disease. In the case where a patient has a history of compensated cirrhosis (cirrhosis without complication of liver disease) the following may indicate a progression to HCC:

- Upper abdominal pain
- Palpable mass
- Enlarged, tender liver
- Ascites
- Unexplained weight loss or fevers
- Jaundice
- Esophageal varices
- Hepatic bruit (caused by turbulent blood flow into the hepatic artery)
- Watery diarrhea

HCC most commonly metastasizes to the lung and less frequently to the bone and brain. Associated symptoms such as dyspnea, bone pain, or central nervous system disturbances may occur with advanced disease.

DIAGNOSTIC WORKUP

Because the majority of patients with HCC have cirrhosis, abnormal liver function tests are not necessarily diagnostic. A rise in the tumor marker alpha-fetoprotein (AFP), however, is present in many patients (60% to 90%) and warrants imaging studies such as ultrasonography (US), computerized tomography (CT) scan, or magnetic resonance imaging (MRI). If a mass is found, fine-needle aspiration or biopsy may be done to confirm the histologic diagnosis, although there are bleeding risks associated with percutaneous biopsies of the liver. If no tumor is found in a patient with a rising AFP level, reimaging and a repeat AFP test are recommended every 3 months. In the minority of patients who have a mass and no history of cirrhosis or other liver disease, imaging studies (US, CT, or MRI) are indicated as well as comprehensive blood tests including a hepatitis panel and an AFP level.

HISTOLOGY

Tumors in the liver are primarily adenocarcinomas. They consist of the following:

- HCC (primary liver cancer including fibrolamellar variant)
- Cholangiocarcinoma (intrahepatic bile duct carcinoma)
- Mixed hepatocellular cholangiocarcinoma
- Undifferentiated

Tumor grading for primary liver cancer is recommended on the basis of the Edmondson and Steiner classification (see box below). There is no standard grading classification for intrahepatic bile duct carcinoma (cholangiocarcinoma).

Histologic Tumor Grading (Edmondson and Steiner's System)

G1: Well differentiated
G2: Moderately differentiated
G3: Poorly differentiated
G4: Undifferentiated.

From Edmondson H. A. & Steiner, P. E. (1954). Primary carcinoma of the liver: a study of 100 cases among 48,900 necropsies. *Cancer, 7,* 462-503.

CLINICAL STAGING

Staging for hepatocellular carcinoma classifies extent of disease before any treatment by looking at tumor size, extent of nodal involvement, and presence or absence of metastatic disease (TNM scale) according to the American Joint Committee on Cancer (see table below).

TREATMENT

Surgery, including resection and transplantation, remains the only curative modality in HCC. Resection, with or without adjuvant therapy, is generally appropriate in those patients who have limited disease

Child-Pugh Score

Scores (Points) for Increasing Abnormality	1	2	3
Encephalopathy	None	1-2	3-4
Ascites	None	Slight	Moderate
Albumin (g/dL)	>3.5	2.8-3.5	<2.8
Prothrombin time prolonged (seconds)	1-4	4-6	>6
Bilirubin (mg/dL)	1-2	2-3	>3
For primary biliary cirrhosis	1-4	4-10	>10

Child-Pugh score (sometimes the Child-Turcotte-Pugh score) is used to assess the prognosis of chronic liver disease, mainly cirrhosis.
Class A = 5-6 points; Class B = 7-9 points; Class C= 10-15 points
Class A: Good operative risk
Class B: Moderate operative risk
Class C: Poor operative risk
From Pugh, R. N. H., Murray-Lyon, I. M., Dawson, J. L., Pietroni, M. C., & Williams R. (1973). Transection of the esophagus in bleeding oesophageal varices. *British Journal of Surgery, 60*, 648-52.

Clinical Staging: Hepatocellular Carcinoma

Definition of TNM

Primary Tumor (T)

TX	Primary tumor cannot be assessed
T0	No evidence of primary tumor
T1	Solitary tumor without vascular invasion
T2	Solitary tumor with vascular invasion or multiple tumors none more than 5 cm
T3	Multiple tumors more than 5 cm or tumor involving a major branch of the portal or hepatic vein(s)
T4	Tumor(s) with direct invasion of adjacent organs other than the gallbladder or with perforation of visceral peritoneum

Regional Lymph Nodes (N)

NX	Regional lymph nodes cannot be assessed
N0	No regional lymph node metastasis
N2	Regional lymph node metastasis

Distant Metastasis (M)

MX	Distant metastasis cannot be assessed
M0	No distant metastasis
M1	Distant metastasis

Stage Grouping

Stage I	T1	N0	M0
Stage II	T2	N0	M0
Stage IIIA	T3	N0	M0
Stage IIIB	T4	N0	M0
Stage IIIC	Any T	N1	M0
Stage IV	Any T	Any N	M1

Used with the permission of the American Joint Committee on Cancer (AJCC), Chicago, Illinois. The original source for this material is the *AJCC Cancer staging manual*, Sixth Edition (2002) published by Springer Science and Business Media LLC, www.springerlink.com.

(stage I or II) and adequate liver reserve and who are reasonable surgical candidates. Patients who have cirrhosis are at high risk for surgical complications and must be assessed accordingly. The Child-Pugh score (refer to table above) and fibrosis score (see box below) are included in assessments of these surgical candidates. Portal vein embolization may also make surgery more possible for patients with cirrhosis. Patients who are cirrhotic or who would have limited reserve after resection may be candidates for transplantation provided that they do not have vascular invasion or nodal involvement with their disease.

Treatment options for patients who are not surgical candidates or who refuse surgery include interferon treatment, ablation with radiofrequency, alcohol, cryotherapy or microwave chemoembolization, radiotherapy, radiotherapy with chemotherapy, or systemic chemotherapy alone in a clinical trial setting.

Fibrosis Score (F)

The fibrosis score is recommended because of its prognostic value in overall survival. This scoring system uses a 0-6 scale.
F0: Fibrosis score of 0-4 (none to moderate fibrosis)
F1: Fibrosis score 5-6 (severe fibrosis or cirrhosis)

From Ishak, K., Baptista, A., Bianchi, L., Callea, F., De Groote, J., Gudat, F., et al. (1995). Histological grading and staging of chronic hepatitis. *Journal of Hepatology, 22*, 696-699.

PROGNOSIS

The 5-year survival rates for patients with resected disease range from 30% to 50%. Patients who have undergone transplantation have 5-year survival rates as high as 75%. Although it is clear that survival rates are vastly increased if patients are diagnosed with localized disease, the efficacy of screening for those at high risk for HCC (hepatitis B Sag positive, HCV positive, or patients with cirrhosis) is still under review.

PREVENTION

Because viral hepatitis is the largest single contributor to cirrhosis, and thus HCC, infectious disease control is instrumental in decreasing the worldwide incidence of HCC.

BIBLIOGRAPHY

Edmondson, H. A., Steiner, P. E. (1954). Primary carcinoma of the liver: a study of 100 cases among 48,900 necropsies. *Cancer, 7*, 462-503.

Greene, F., Page, D., Fleming, I., et al. (Eds.), (2002). *AJCC cancer staging handbook* (6th ed.). New York: Springer-Verlag.

Ishak, K., Baptista, A., Bianchi, L., et al. (1995). Histological grading and staging of chronic hepatitis. *Journal of Hepatology, 22*, 696-699.

National Cancer Institute (2006). *Adult primary liver cancer treatment*. Retrieved on January 28, 2007, from http://www.cancer.gov/cancertopics/pdq/treatment/adult-primary-liver/HealthProfessional/.

National Comprehensive Cancer Network. (2006). *Hepatobiliary cancers*. Retrieved May 30, 2006, from

Major Cancers

http://www.nccn.org/professionals/physician_gls/PDF/hepatobiliary.pdf.

Pugh, R. N. H., Murray-Lyon, I. M., Dawson, J. L., et al. (1973). Transection of the esophagus in bleeding oesophageal varices. *British Journal of Surgery, 60*, 648-52.

UpToDate. (2006). *Assessing surgical risk in patients with liver disease.* Retrieved June 9, 2006, from http://www.utdol.com/utd/content/topic.do?topicKey=cirrhosi/10733.

Pancreatic Cancer

Marta M. Smith-Zamiska and Mary Garlick Roll

DEFINITION

Pancreatic cancer is a primary tumor of the pancreas, an organ that is 5 to 6 inches in length, lying horizontally in the upper abdomen. The pancreas is divided into the head, neck, body, and tail. The head lies in the C-shaped curve of the duodenum. The body crosses the midline of the abdomen. The tail extends toward the spleen.

INCIDENCE

In the United States, pancreatic cancer ranks tenth in cancer incidence for both men and women. Although the overall incidence has slowly decreased over the past two decades, survival has not significantly improved, as evidenced by the fact that in 2007 there will be approximately 37,170 new cases of pancreatic cancer with 33,370 deaths.

ETIOLOGY AND RISK FACTORS

The exact cause of pancreatic cancer is unknown.

- Age is the most significant risk factor for pancreatic cancer, with an 80% peak incidence occurring between the ages of 60 and 80 years.
- Smoking is the most common manageable risk factor. Smokers have a 1.5 greater risk for development of pancreatic cancer. Smokers constitute 20% to 30% of all pancreatic cancers.
- Race: seen more frequently in African American men, who also have higher mortality rates.

- Diabetes: a sudden onset of type 2 diabetes in adults over the age of 50 years increases risk.
- Family history: although hereditary genetic factors are complex, it is thought they may contribute between 10% to 20% of all pancreatic cancers. These syndromes may include hereditary pancreatitis, familial breast cancers linked to BRCA-2, familial atypical multiple mole melanoma, and hereditary nonpolyposis.
- High-fat diet
- Obesity/sedentary lifestyle
- Chronic pancreatitis
- Sporadic (noninherited) gene mutations: several mutations have been identified; the most widely recognized are p53, the tumor suppressor gene, and *ras*, an oncogene.
- Growth factors: overexpression of certain growth factors has been associated with pancreatic cancer. These growth factors include: epidermal growth factor, vascular endothelial growth factor, and insulin-like growth factor I.

SIGNS AND SYMPTOMS

Early pancreatic cancer does not have obvious signs and symptoms. Symptoms occur as the disease develops with subsequent invasion or obstruction of nearby structures.

- Classic triad consists of jaundice, weight loss, and abdominal pain.
- Tumors in the head of the pancreas: jaundice, weight loss, cachexia, abdominal pain, anorexia, nausea, diarrhea, acute pancreatitis
- Tumors in the body or tail: upper left abdominal pain, weight loss, cachexia, palpable mass, indigestion, vomiting, acute pancreatitis
- Thrombosis may develop as a result of venous involvement.

The most common sites of metastatic disease are liver and peritoneum, followed by lung, duodenum, diaphragm, adrenal gland, spleen, kidney, and small intestines. There is often perineural

infiltration and vascular and lymphatic involvement.

DIAGNOSTIC WORKUP

Tissue biopsy or peritoneal washings are necessary to correctly diagnose pancreatic cancer. The workup should include a detailed personal and family history and a physical examination.

- Laboratory values are often within normal ranges unless there has been obstruction of an organ. Laboratory tests should include the following:
  - Complete blood cell count to evaluate normochromatic anemia
  - Liver profile to evaluate elevated bilirubin and other elevated liver enzymes
  - Tumor markers: there are no 100% reliable markers for pancreatic cancer. CA19-9 is the only one that is Food and Drug Administration approved for monitoring. Levels >90 units/mL are 80% predictive of advanced pancreatic cancer.
  - CEA is nonspecific but is used as a digestive tumor marker.
- Noninvasive imaging studies may include computed tomographic scan, ultrasonography, magnetic resonance imaging, or positron emission tomography.
- Invasive imaging studies may be preformed as well, including endoscopic ultrasonography, endoscopic retrograde cholangiopancreatography, angiography, laparoscopy, or percutaneous transhepatic cholangiography.

HISTOLOGY

The pancreas has two distinct functions and cell types restricted to separate compartments in the gland.

- The exocrine pancreas synthesizes and secretes precursor forms of digestive enzymes into the duodenum through a duct.
- The endocrine pancreas, composed of cluster of cells called islets of Langerhans, synthesizes and secretes

hormones (such as insulin) into the blood. These hormones regulate glucose, lipid, and protein metabolism.

Pancreatic cancer can arise in either the exocrine or endocrine portions of the pancreas.

- 90% are in the exocrine pancreas as an infiltrating ductal adenocarcinoma
- 60%-70% of tumors arise in the head, obstructing the bile duct
- 15% arise in the tail
- The remainder is diffused throughout the pancreas.

CLINICAL STAGING

Staging is important because it guides the treatment options. Pancreatic staging is based on the TNM classification developed by the American Joint Committee on Cancer (see table below).

TREATMENT

Pancreatic cancer remains one of the most difficult cancers to treat. Options depend on the stage, symptoms, and performance status and include surgery, radiation, chemotherapy, and targeted therapy.

Resectable or Locally Advanced Resectable Tumors with No Metastases

- Surgical resection of the tumor and surrounding pancreatic tissue is the only curative therapy for pancreatic cancer. The National Comprehensive Cancer Network has developed guidelines for surgical resectability criteria, with resectable tumors defined as T1, T2, and T3 (stage IA, IB, IIA, IIB) with a clear fat plane around the celiac axis and the superior mesenteric artery. In addition, the superior mesenteric vein and the portal vein cannot be circled by tumor. Temporary stents can be placed if jaundice is present, followed by curative intent surgery. For right-sided tumors in the head of the pancreas, the Whipple (pancreaticoduodenectomy) procedure may be preformed. For tumors on the left side in the tail, an option is a distal pancreatectomy.
- Neoadjuvant chemoradiation is a newer option, but currently survival data are similar to those for chemoradiation after surgery.
- Adjuvant chemotherapy options: clinical trials, 5-fluorouracil–based chemoradiation with or with out gemcitabine-based chemotherapy or gemcitabine-based chemotherapy alone.

Locally Advanced or Unresectable Tumors

- More than 80% of patients with pancreatic cancer have unresectable disease.
- Good performance status: permanent stent if jaundice present, clinical trial, chemoradiation with or with out gemcitabine-based chemotherapy, or gemcitabine-based chemotherapy alone.
- Poor performance status: permanent stent if jaundice present, gemcitabine, best supportive care

Metastatic disease

- Treatment: clinical trial, gemcitabine plus erlotinib, or best supportive care
- Salvage therapy: clinical trial, fluorinated pyrimidine–based therapy, or best supportive care

PROGNOSIS

Pancreatic cancer has one of the lowest survival rates of any cancer. The median survival time for all patients is 4 to 6 months, with a range of 2 to 10 months. Prognosis depends on stage at diagnosis, with the average 5-year survival for all stages at 4.4% (see table on page 66).

Clinical Staging: Pancreatic Cancer

Definition of TNM

Primary Tumor (T)

TX	Primary tumor cannot be assessed
T0	No evidence of primary tumor
Tis	Carcinoma in situ*
T1	Tumor limited to the pancreas, 2 cm or less in greatest dimension
T2	Tumor limited to the pancreas, more than 2 cm in greatest dimension
T3	Tumor extends beyond the pancreas but without involvement of the celiac axis or the superior mesenteric artery
T4	Tumor involves the celiac axis or the superior mesenteric artery (unresectable primary tumor)

Regional Lymph Nodes (N)

NX	Regional lymph nodes cannot be assessed
N0	No regional lymph node metastasis
N1	Regional lymph node metastasis

Distant Metastasis (M)

MX	Distant metastasis cannot be assessed
M0	No distant metastasis
M1	Distant metastasis

*This also includes the "PanInIII" classification.

Stage Grouping

Stage 0	Tis	N0	M0
Stage IA	T1	N0	M0
Stage IB	T2	N0	M0
Stage IIA	T3	N0	M0
Stage IIB	T1	N1	M0
	T2	N1	M0
	T3	N1	M0
Stage III	T4	Any N	M0
Stage IV	Any T	Any N	M1

Prognosis at Stage of Diagnosis: Pancreatic Cancer

Stage	Resectability	Patients at Diagnosis (%)	5-Year Survival (%)
Stage IA Stage IB	Resectable	7%	15.2%
Stage IIA Stage IIB	Potentially resectable	39%	6.8%
Stage III Stage IV	Unresectable/locally advanced Unresectable/metastatic disease	54%	1.8%

From Freelove, R., Walling, A.D. (2006). Pancreatic cancer: Diagnosis and management. *American Family Physician 73(3)*, 485-92.

PREVENTION

There are no current recommendations for screening or early detection, although patients who have jaundice of unknown origin or acute pancreatitis should be evaluated for pancreatic cancer.

The following are some general lifestyle recommendations for prevention:

- Smoking cessation
- Maintain a healthy weight
- Regular exercise program
- Healthy diets lower in fat and higher in fruits and vegetables.

BIBLIOGRAPHY

Evans, J. (2001). Cancer of the pancreas. In V. DeVita, S. Hellman, & S. Rosenberg (Eds.), *Cancer: principles and practice of oncology* (pp.1126-1161). Philadelphia: Lippincott.

Frogge, M. (2005). Gastrointestinal cancers. In C. Yarbro, M. Frogge, & M. Goodman (Eds.), *Cancer nursing: principles and practice* (6th ed., pp. 933-966). Boston: Jones & Bartlett.

Greene, F., Page, D., Fleming, I., et al. (Eds.). (2002). *AJCC cancer staging handbook* (6th ed.). New York: Springer-Verlag.

Hawkins, B. (1999). Pancreatic cancer. In C. Miaskowski & P. Buchsel (Eds.), *Oncology nursing assessment and clinical care* (pp. 955-975). St. Louis: Mosby.

Jemal, A., Siegel, R., Ward, E., et al. (2007). Cancer statistics, 2007. *CA:A Cancer Journal for Clinicians*, 57, 43-66.

Mayo Clinic. (2006). *Pancreatic cancer*. Retrieved December 6, 2006, from http://www.mayoclinic.com/health/pancreatic-cancer/DS00357.

National Cancer Institute. (2006). *Pancreatic cancer PDQ treatment*. Retrieved December 6, 2006, from http://www.cancer.gov/cancertopics/pdq/treatment/pancreatic/HealthProfessional.

National Comprehensive Cancer Network. *NCCN clinical practice guidelines in oncology, pancreatic adenocarcinoma*, version 2.2006. Retrieved December 6, 2006, from http://www.nccn.org/professionals/physician_gls/PDF/pancreatic.pdf.

Genitourinary Cancers

Bladder Cancer

Mary Collins

DEFINITION

Bladder cancer is the fourth most common cancer in men and the ninth most common cancer in women. Alterations in deoxyribonucleic acid from viruses, chemical carcinogens, or exposure to other chemical agents will influence who has bladder cancer. Bladder cancer is often described as a field-change disease, which involves the urothelium from the renal pelvis to the urethra. Metastasis occurs through the lymphatic system to the regional lymph nodes. Bladder cancer may also metastasize to the bones, liver, and lungs.

INCIDENCE

Bladder cancer is the second most common urologic malignancy. It is estimated more than 67,160 Americans will be diagnosed with bladder cancer in 2007 and more than 13,750 will die from this disease. Bladder cancer occurs twice as frequently in men than in women. The average age at diagnosis is between 65 and 70 years.

ETIOLOGY AND RISK FACTORS

Risk factors include the following:

- Increasing age (>65 years)
- White race and male sex
- Cigarette smoking
  - At least 50% of bladder cancer in men is attributed to cigarette smoking. Men and women who smoke have two to three times the risk for development of bladder cancer compared with nonsmokers.
- Exposure to industrial chemicals
  - Most bladder carcinogens are aromatic amines. Individuals working in the rubber, paint, leather, petroleum, and printing industry are at an increased risk for development of bladder cancer.
  - Other occupations that involve organic chemicals such as rope making and dry cleaning and barbers and beauticians may also be at increased risk.
- Patients with indwelling catheters, chronic urinary infections, and renal calculi may be prone to development of the disease.
- Cyclophosphamide administered over an extended period of time, in particular to patients with upper tract bladder outlet obstruction, has been reported to increase the incidence of bladder cancer.

SIGNS AND SYMPTOMS

- Frequency
- Dysuria

- Urgency
- Altered stream

Advanced disease

- Palpable mass
- Bone pain
- Flank/rectal/pelvic pain

DIAGNOSTIC WORKUP

Diagnostic workup includes a urine specimen for cytologic study, which may include saline solution irrigation of the bladder (bladder washings) for more accurate results and an excretory urogram (intravenous pyelogram). Definitive diagnosis is made with cystoscopy and biopsy. To rule out advanced disease, chest x-ray films, computed tomography scans, bone scans, and magnetic resonance imaging may be ordered.

HISTOLOGY

Approximately 90% of all bladder cancers are transitional cell or urothelial carcinomas. Squamous cell carcinoma accounts for 3% to 7% and adenocarcinoma represents 2% of malignant bladder tumors. Bladder cancer is typically divided into two groups: superficial or muscle invasive. Superficial bladder cancer, T1, Tis or Ta, is usually low grade and noninvasive, whereas muscle invasive disease, T2 to T4 tends to be more aggressive and invades the muscularis propria. The degree of cellular differentiation determines histological tumor grade. A grade 1 tumor is well differentiated, grade 2 is moderately differentiated, and grade 3 to 4 is poorly differentiated or undifferentiated.

CLINICAL STAGING

Information obtained before definitive treatment may be included for clinical staging. Two staging systems are used for bladder cancer: the Jewett Marshall system and the TNM (tumor, node, metastasis) system based on the American Joint Committee for Cancer Staging. The TNM system is the most accurate and is also the preferred system (see table at right). Histologic grade (G) is the grading system for bladder cancer (see box at right).

Clinical Staging: Bladder Cancer

Definition of TNM

Primary Tumor (T)

TX	Primary tumor cannot be assessed
T0	No evidence of primary tumor
Ta	Noninvasive papillary carcinoma
Tis	Carcinoma in situ: "flat tumor"
T1	Tumor invades subepithelial connective tissue
T2	Tumor invades muscle
pT2a	Tumor invades superficial muscle (inner half)
pT2b	Tumor invades deep muscle (outer half)
T3	Tumor invades perivesical tissue
pT3a	Microscopically
pT3b	Macroscopically (extravesical mass)
T4	Tumor invades any of the following: prostate, uterus, vagina, pelvic wall, abdominal wall
T4a	Tumor invades prostate, uterus, vagina
T4b	Tumor invades pelvic wall, abdominal wall

Regional Lymph Nodes (N)

Regional lymph nodes are those within the true pelvis; all others are distant lymph nodes

NX	Regional lymph nodes cannot be assessed
N0	No regional lymph node metastasis
N1	Metastasis in a single lymph node, 2 cm or less in greatest dimension
N2	Metastasis in a single lymph node, more than 2 cm but not more than 5 cm in greatest dimension; or multiple lymph nodes, none more than 5 cm in greatest dimension
N3	Metastasis in lymph node, more than 5 cm in greatest dimension

Distant Metastasis (M)

MX	Distant metastasis cannot be assessed
M0	No distant metastasis
M1	Distant metastasis

Stage Grouping

Stage 0a	Ta	N0	M0
Stage 0is	Tis	N0	M0
Stage I	T1	N0	M0
Stage II	T2a	N0	M0
	T2b	N0	M0
Stage III	T3a	N0	M0
	T3b	N0	M0
	T4a	N0	M0
Stage IV	T4b	N0	M0
	Any T	N1	M0
	Any T	N2	M0
	Any T	N3	M0
	Any T	Any N	M1

Used with the permission of the American Joint Committee on Cancer (AJCC), Chicago, Illinois. The original source for this material is the *AJCC Cancer staging manual,* Sixth Edition (2002) published by Springer Science and Business Media LLC, www.springerlink.com.

Histologic Grading System

GX: Grade cannot be assessed
G1: Well differentiated
G2: Moderately differentiated
G3-4: Poorly differentiated or undifferentiated

From American Joint Committee on Cancer. (2002). *AJCC cancer staging manual* (6th Ed.). Chicago: American Joint Committee on Cancer.

TREATMENT
Medical Treatment

Often for high-grade lesions or lesions suspected of recurring, intravesical therapy may be warranted. Immunotherapy such as Bacille Calmette-Guérin (BCG) or chemotherapy is used to decrease recurrence, prevent progression, and eradicate the residual disease after transurethral resection. Intravesical BCG is the standard treatment for superficial bladder cancer. Treatment with BCG is weekly for 6 weeks, and maintenance therapy is usually monthly or every 3 months. Subcutaneous interferon may be used in patients who have failed BCG. Interferon response rates have been reported at 20% to 43%. Interferon may also be effective in preventing recurrence of superficial disease. Intravesical chemotherapy is generally given for low-grade disease. Mitomycin, doxorubicin, or thiotepa is recommended to be administered at surgery or at least within 6 hours of resection. The role of gene therapy for superficial bladder cancer is currently being investigated.

Radiation Therapy

The role of radiation therapy is limited in bladder cancer. Clinical trials indicate a high recurrence rate of 90% within 5 years when used for Ta disease. Higher grade lesions (grades 3 and 4) have been reported to have better response rates. Patients who are not candidates for surgery may be offered radiation therapy.

Surgery

Transurethral resection of the bladder followed by observation is generally all that is required for superficial low-grade tumors. Cystectomy for superficial disease is recommended in patients who have failed intravesical therapy or who have persistent recurrent disease. Radical cystectomy remains the gold standard for muscle-invasive bladder cancer without metastatic disease. This procedure includes removal of bilateral pelvic lymph nodes, bladder, the prostate gland, and seminal vesicles in men and the uterus, fallopian tubes, ovaries, bladder, urethra, and a segment of the interior vaginal wall in women. After surgical removal of the bladder, patients will require either an ileal conduit or a continent urinary diversion such as a Kock pouch or an Indiana pouch.

Chemotherapy

Systemic chemotherapy may be given neoadjuvantly to downstage a tumor before surgery or as adjuvant therapy after cystectomy for muscle-invasive lesions or metastatic disease. In advanced disease, methotrexate, vincristine, doxorubicin, and cisplatin (MVAC) have achieved reported response rates from 40-65% with median survival rates of approximately 1 year. Newer agents such as paclitaxel, docetaxel, and gemcitabine have also produced similar response rates with less toxicity.

PROGNOSIS

The incidence and mortality rates of bladder cancer have continued to decline over the last several years. Radical cystectomy results in the lowest recurrence rate for invasive disease, although high-grade lesions (grade 3) progress in at least 50% of patients. Patients who fail the initial treatment for muscle-invasive disease are predicted to die of their disease within 3 years of diagnosis. The prognosis is poor for metastatic disease.

PREVENTION

Avoiding tobacco and limiting exposure to environmental carcinogens may decrease the risk for development of bladder cancer.

BIBLIOGRAPHY

Green, F. L., Page, D. L., Fleming, I. D., et al. (2002). *AJCC cancer staging manual* (6th ed.). New York: Springer-Verlag.

Grossfield, G., & Carroll, P. (2004). Urothelial carcinoma: cancers of the bladder, ureter and renal pelvis. In E. Tanagho & J. McAninch (Eds.), *Smith's general urology* (6th ed., pp. 324-345). New York: McGraw-Hill.

Jemal, A., Siegel, R., Ward, E., et al. (2007). Cancer statistics, 2007. *CA: A Cancer Journal for Clinicians, 57;* 43-66.

Lamm, D. L., McGee, W., & Hale, K. (2005). Bladder cancer: current optimal intravesical treatment. *Urologic Nursing, 25,* 323-333.

Malkowicz, S. (2002). Management of superficial bladder cancer. In P. C. Walsh, A. B. Retik, E. D. Vaughan, et al. (Eds.). *Campbell's urology* (8th ed., pp. 2785-2802). Philadelphia: W. B. Saunders.

Nieder, A. M., Brausi, M., Lamm, D., et al. (2005). Management of stage 1 tumors of the bladder: international consensus panel. In M. Soloway (Ed.) *Urology, 66*(6A Suppl), 108-125.

Raghavan, D., Skinner, E. (2004). Genitourinary cancer in the elderly. *Seminars in Oncology, 31,* 249-263.

Schoenberg, M. (2002). Management of invasive and metastatic bladder cancer. In P. C. Walsh, A. B. Retik, E. D. Vaughan, et al. (Eds.), *Campbell's urology* (8th ed., pp. 2803-2817). Philadelphia: W. B. Saunders.

Shipley, W., Kaufman, D., McDougal, W., et al. (2005). Cancer of the bladder, urether, and renal pelvis. In V. DeVita, S. Hellman, S. Rosenberg (Eds.), *Cancer principles and practice* (7th ed., pp. 1168-1192). Philadelphia: Lippincott Williams & Wilkins.

Skinner, D., Stein, J., Ross, R., et al. (2002). Cancer of the bladder. In J.Y. Gillenwater, J. T. Grayhack, S. S. Howards, et al. (Eds.), *Adult and pediatric urology* (4th ed., pp. 1298-1362). Philadelphia: Lippincott Williams & Wilkins.

Wood, L., & Clabrese, D. (2005). Bladder and renal cancers. In C. Yarbro, M. Frogge, M. Goodman (Eds.). *Cancer nursing* (6th ed., pp. 1005-1021). Boston: Jones & Bartlett.

Penile Cancer

*Patty Woods Bunch
and Mary Collins*

DEFINITION

Carcinoma of the penis is an uncommon malignancy in the United States. Ninety-five percent of cancers of the penis are squamous cell carcinoma that may evolve from the prepuce, glans, or shaft of the penis. Metastasis occurs primarily in regional lymph nodes (femoral, inguinal, pelvic, iliac) and rarely spreads to distant sites such as lung, liver, bone, or brain.

INCIDENCE

Carcinoma of the penis comprises less that 1% of all malignancies in men. Approximately one to two cases per 100,000 occur annually. The peak incidence is in the sixth and seventh decades of life. It is estimated there will be 1,280 men diagnosed in the United States with penile cancer in 2007 and 290 will die of the disease. Although the incidence is low in North America and Europe, penile malignancies are higher in Africa, South America, and Asian countries.

ETIOLOGY AND RISK FACTORS

The etiology of penile carcinoma is controversial. Risk factors include the following:

- Increasing age—most diagnoses are made after 60 years of age.

- The presence of a foreskin. It is rare to find cancer of the penis in a man who was circumcised at birth
- Phimosis (tightness of the foreskin that prevents retraction)
  - 25% to 75% of men with penile cancer have had phimosis
- Exposure to human papillomavirus (HPV)
- Multiple sex partners
- Prior history of sexually transmitted diseases, including human immunodeficiency virus
- Poor personal hygiene practices
- Tobacco use
- Psoriasis patients treated with ultraviolet radiation in combination with oral 8-methoxypsoralen
- Premalignant lesions associated with squamous cell carcinoma of the penis include the following:
  - Balanitis xerotica obliterans
  - Cutaneous horn
  - Giant condyloma
  - Bowenoid papulosis

SIGNS AND SYMPTOMS

The presenting penile lesions may be quite variable, ranging from a small papule or pustule that does not heal to a large exophytic, fungating lesion. These lesions occur most commonly on the glans (48%) and prepuce (21%) and less commonly on the coronal sulcus and penile shaft. These lesions are usually painless. A reddish rash or persistent, foul-smelling discharge under the foreskin may also be present.

DIAGNOSTIC WORKUP

The following diagnostic tools are crucial in the diagnosis and staging of penile cancer:

- Complete physical examination
- Biopsy from the penile lesion
- Imaging such as ultrasonography, computed tomographic scan, and magnetic resonance imaging

HISTOLOGY

Ninety-five percent of penile cancers are squamous cell carcinoma. Squamous cell carcinoma is graded according to Broders' classification: well, moderately, and poorly differentiated. The distinction as to degree of differentiation

is an important predictor for risk of metastatic disease to the groin and even more powerful when combined with the depth of tumor invasion. The remaining 5% of malignancies include the sarcomas, melanoma, basal cell carcinoma, and lymphoma.

CLINICAL STAGING

No universal staging system has been established for penile cancer, but the AJCC TNM system is preferred. Combining the TNM system with differentiation gives the predictive ability for regional nodal involvement (see table below).

TREATMENT

Because the incidence is so rare, treatment management decisions may

be difficult. Depending on the stage of the disease at diagnosis, the following treatments may be used:

- Small superficial tumors: Mohs' micrographic surgery, laser beam therapy, radiation therapy, and in some cases, topical fluorouracil
- Tumors involving only the prepuce: circumcision
- Invasive tumors: partial or total penectomy
- Advanced stages: single-agent or combination chemotherapy
- Approximately half of the patients with penile cancer present with lymphadenopathy.
  - Frequently this is the result of inflammation and a course of antibiotics is recommended.

Clinical Staging: Penile Cancer

Definition of TNM

Primary Tumor (T)

TX	Primary tumor cannot be assessed
T0	No evidence of primary tumor
Tis	Carcinoma in situ
Ta	Noninvasive verrucous carcinoma
T1	Tumor invades subepithelial connective tissue
T2	Tumor invades corpus spongiosum or cavernosum
T3	Tumor invades urethra or prostate
T4	Tumor invades other adjacent structures

Regional Lymph Nodes (N)

NX	Regional lymph nodes cannot be assessed
N0	No regional lymph node metastasis
N1	Metastasis in a single superficial, inguinal lymph node
N2	Metastasis in multiple or bilateral superficial inguinal lymph nodes
N3	Metastasis in deep inguinal or pelvic lymph node(s) unilateral or bilateral

Distant Metastasis (M)

MX	Distant metastasis cannot be assessed
M0	No distant metastasis
M1	Distant metastasis

Additional descriptor: The **m suffix** indicates the presence of multiple primary tumors and is recorded in parentheses–e.g., pTA(m)N0M0

Stage Grouping

Stage 0	Tis	N0	M0
	Ta	N0	M0
Stage I	T1	N0	M0
Stage II	T1	N1	M0
	T2	N0	M0
	T2	N1	M0
Stage III	T1	N2	M0
	T2	N2	M0
	T3	N0	M0
	T3	N1	M0
	T2	N2	M0
Stage IV	T4	Any N	M0
	Any T	N3	M0
	Any T	Any N	M1

Used with the permission of the American Joint Committee on Cancer (AJCC), Chicago, Illinois. The original source for this material is the *AJCC Cancer staging manual,* Sixth Edition (2002) published by Springer Science and Business Media LLC, www.springerlink.com.

○ If the lymphadenopathy does not resolve after the antibiotics, patients should have a biopsy and treatment.

Other than 5-fluorouracil, which has been used to treat superficial penile cancer, chemotherapy has had a limited role. Cisplatin, bleomycin, and methotrexate have been the only drugs used with modest activity.

• Combination therapy of surgery, chemotherapy, and radiation has been used with some encouraging results in patients with advanced disease.

PROGNOSIS

Prognosis is primarily related to the presence or absence of inguinal node metastasis. The prognosis is worse if lymph node involvement is present. Untreated patients with inguinal metastases rarely survive 2 years. In patients with clinically palpable adenopathy and histologically proven metastases, 20% to 50% are alive 5 years after inguinal lymphadenectomy. An 82% to 88% 5-year survival rate has been reported when only one to three lymph nodes are involved.

PREVENTION

• Good genital hygiene in men who have not been circumcised
• Avoiding sexual practices likely to result in HPV or HIV infection
• Avoid tobacco use

BIBLIOGRAPHY

Brosman, S. A. (2006). *Penile cancer.* Retrieved on June 13, 2006 from http://www.emedicine.com/med/topic3046.htm.

Green, F. L., Page, D. L., Fleming, I. D., et al. (2002). *AJCC cancer staging manual* 6th Ed.). New York: Springer-Verlag.

Jemal, A., Siegel, R., Ward, E., et al. (2007). Cancer statistics, 2007. *CA: A Cancer Journal for Clinicians, 57,* 43-66.

Misra, S., Chaturvedi, A., & Misra, N. (2004). Penile carcinoma: a challenge for the developing world. *The Lancet, 5,* 240-247.

Presti, J. Genital tumors. (2004). In E. Tanagho & J. McAninch (Eds.) *Smith's general urology* (6th Ed., pp. 386-399), New York: McGraw-Hill.

Razdan, S., & Gomella, L. (2005). *Cancer of the urethra and pelvis.* In V. DeVita,

S. Hellman, & S. Rosenberg (Eds). *Cancer principles and practice* (7th ed., pp. 1260-1267). Philadelphia: Lippincott Williams & Wilkins.

Sanchez-Ortiz, R., & Pettaway, C. (2003). National history, management, and surveillance of recurrent squamous cell penile carcinoma: a risk-based approach. *Urological Clinics of North America, 30,* 853-867.

Stotts, R. C. (2004). Cancers of the prostate, penis, and testicles: epidemiology, prevention, and treatment. *Nursing Clinics of North America, 39,* 327-340.

Vogelzang, N. J., Scardina, P. T., Shipley, W. U., et al. (2006). Comprehensive textbook of genitourinary oncology. In N. J. Vogelzang, P. T. Scardino, W. U. Shipley, et al. (Eds.), *Penile cancer: clinical signs and symptoms* (pp. 805-830). Philadelphia: Lippincott Williams & Wilkins.

Prostate Cancer

Mary Collins

DEFINITION

Prostate cancer is the most frequently diagnosed noncutaneous cancer in men. Typically, there is a long interval between time of diagnosis and death. Prostate cancer spreads initially by extending through the capsule into the seminal vesicles. Metastasis occurs to the bones of the pelvis, axial skeleton, lymph nodes, lungs, liver, bladder, and adrenal glands.

INCIDENCE

Despite a reduction in the mortality rate over the years, prostate cancer remains the third leading cause of cancer death in men. It is estimated that there will be 218,890 new cases of prostate cancer diagnosed in 2007 and 27,050 will die of the disease. The median age at diagnosis is 72 years and there is a higher incidence in African American men. African Americans have twice the risk of death from prostate cancer than white males do.

ETIOLOGY AND RISK FACTORS

• Age: risk increased after 50 years
• Race: African Americans are at higher risk than white Americans; Hispanic Americans are at similar

risk to whites; and Asian Americans are at lower risk than whites
• More common in North America and Northwestern Europe than Asia, Africa, Central America, and South America.
• Family history of prostate cancer
  ○ Father or brother with prostate cancer doubles the risk (higher if brother)
  ○ Higher risk with several family members affected, particularly if young at diagnosis
  ○ Risk higher in the presence of BRCA1 and BRCA2 gene mutations (infrequent occurrence)
• Diet high in red meat and high-fat dairy products
• Controversy regarding increased risk from vasectomy, particularly if vasectomy was performed before the age of 35 years
• History of high-grade prostatic intraepithelial neoplasia

SIGNS AND SYMPTOMS

• Urinary frequency, hesitancy, decreased stream, urgency and nocturia
• Abnormal digital rectal examination
• Elevated prostate-specific antigen (PSA)
• Bone pain, particularly in the ribs, back, and hips, may be presenting symptom in patients with metastatic disease.

DIAGNOSTIC WORKUP

• Screening for prostate cancer includes a prostate specific antigen (PSA) test and a digital rectal examination.
  ○ PSA is also used to monitor patients because an elevation of PSA after normalization following treatment can be evidence of disease recurrence.
• Ultrasonography of the prostate with biopsy is used to confirm the diagnosis.
• The Partin Table combines PSA, clinical stage, and Gleason score to predict the probability of the final pathological stage.

- Prostatic acid phosphatase is elevated in greater than 60% of patients with extracapsular disease.
- Bone scans, computed tomography, and magnetic resonance imaging evaluate the presence of metastatic disease.
- Pelvic lymphadenectomy provides the most accurate staging information related to lymph node status.

HISTOLOGY

Adenocarcinoma of the prostate comprises approximately 95% of all prostate cancers. Carcinosarcomas, nonepithelial neoplasms, and germ cell tumors make up the remaining 5% of prostate tumors.

CLINICAL STAGING

Clinical staging for prostate cancer uses the Tumor Node Metastasis system, also known as the Staging System of the American Joint Committee on Cancer along with the tumor grade or Gleason score. The TNM system describes the extent of the primary tumor (T), whether the cancer has spread to nearby lymph nodes (N), and the absence or presence of distant metastasis (M) (see table, right). The Gleason score ranges from 2 to 10. A pathologist scores the two most prominent patterns (primary and secondary) in a biopsy specimen. The primary and secondary patterns are graded from 1 (well differentiated) to 5 (undifferentiated). The Gleason score is the sum of these two.

TREATMENT
Surgical Procedures

Radical prostatectomy using a perineal or retropubic approach, is the gold standard for organ-confined prostate cancer. Cryosurgery may also be used. This is a process that freezes prostatic tissue, thereby destroying cancer cells. Long-term outcomes are not known for this procedure.

Radiation Therapy

Radiation has typically been reserved for older men or patients who are not surgical candidates. Younger men are also choosing radiation because it is

Clinical Staging: Prostate Cancer

Definition of TNM

Primary Tumor (T)

Clinical

TX	Primary tumor cannot be assessed
T0	No evidence of primary tumor
T1	Clinically inapparently tumor neither palpable nor visible by imaging
T1a	Tumor incidental histologic finding in 5% or less of tissue resected
T1b	Tumor incidental histologic finding in more than 5% of tissue resected
T1c	Tumor identified by needle biopsy (e.g., because of elevated prostate-specific antigen level))
T2	Tumor confined within prostate*
T2a	Tumor involves one half of one lobe or less
T2b	Tumor involves more than one half of one lobe but not both lobes
T2c	Tumor involves both lobes
T3	Tumor extends through the prostate capsule**
T3a	Extracapsular extension (unilateral or bilateral)
T3b	Tumor invades seminal vesicle(s)
T4	Tumor is fixed or invades adjacent structures other than seminal vesicles: bladder neck, external sphincter, rectum, levator muscles, or pelvic wall

*Tumor found in one or both lobes by needle biopsy, but not palpable or reliably visible by imaging, is classified as T1c.
**Invasion into the prostatic apex or into (but not beyond) the prostatic capsule is classified not as T3 but as T2.

Pathologic (pT)

pT2*	Organ confined
pT2a	Unilateral, involving one half of one lobe or less
pT2b	Unilateral involving more than one half of one lobe but not both lobes
pT2c	Bilateral disease
pT3	Extraprostatic extension
pT3a	Extraprostatic extension**
pT3b	Seminal vesicle invasion
pT4	Invasion of bladder, rectum

*There is no pathologic T1 classification.
**Positive surgical margin should be indicated by an R1 descriptor (residual microscopic disease).

Regional Lymph Nodes (N)

Clinical

NX	Regional lymph nodes were not assessed
N0	No regional lymph node involvement
N1	Metastases in regional lymph node(s)

Pathologic

pNX	Regional lymph nodes not sampled
pN0	No positive regional nodes
pN1	Metastases in regional node(s)

Distant Metastasis (M)*

MX	Distant metastasis cannot be assessed (not evaluated by any modality)
M0	No distant metastasis
M1	Distant metastasis
M1a	Nonregional lymph node(s)
M1b	Bone(s)
M1c	Other site(s) with or without bone disease

*When more than one site of metastasis is present, the most advanced category is used. pM1c is most advanced.

Histologic Grade (G)

Gleason Score = _____ + _____	
Gx	Grade cannot be assessed
G1	Well differentiated (slight anaplasia) (Gleason 2-4)
G2	Moderately differentiated (moderate anaplasia) (Gleason 5-6)
G3-4	Poorly differentiated/undifferentiated (marked anaplasia) (Gleason 7-10)

Continued

Clinical Staging: Prostate Cancer—cont'd

Stage Grouping

Stage I	T1a	N0	M0	G1
Stage II	T1a	N0	M0	G2, 3-4
	T1b	N0	M0	Any G
	T1c	N0	M0	Any G
	T1	N0	M0	Any G
	T2	N0	M0	Any G
Stage III	T3	N0	M0	Any G
Stage IV	T4	N0	M0	Any G
	Any T	N1	M0	Any G
	Any T	Any N	M1	Any G

Used with the permission of the American Joint Committee on Cancer (AJCC), Chicago, Illinois. The original source for this material is the *AJCC Cancer staging manual*, Sixth Edition (2002) published by Springer Science and Business Media LLC, www.springerlink.com.

less invasive than surgery with less chance of resulting incontinence or immediate impotence. External beam radiation is used to treat disease confined to the prostate or surrounding tissue. Brachytherapy prostate seed implant is the process of using radioactive seeds implanted into the prostate. This therapy is designated for early-stage, low-volume, well-differentiated to moderately differentiated cancers.

Hormonal Therapy

Hormones suppress testosterone, which feeds the cancer cells. It is never given as a curative form of therapy. It is first-line therapy for metastatic disease. Hormonal therapy consists of luteinizing-hormone releasing hormone agonist alone or in combination with an antiandrogen. Orchiectomy, surgical removal of the testes, is a permanent form of hormonal therapy.

Chemotherapy

Chemotherapy is given for metastatic disease that is hormone refractory or that no longer responds to hormonal therapy. Currently, front-line chemotherapy includes docetaxel or mitoxantrone in combination with prednisone. New agents, including other cytotoxics, antiangiogenic therapies, immune-based therapies, and gene therapy, are currently being investigated.

PROGNOSIS

Mortality rates have improved in recent years for patients with prostate cancer; however, prostate cancer remains the third most common cause of cancer death in men. There is a 40-month median survival expectancy in patients with hormone-refractory prostate cancer with bone metastasis and a 68-month median survival for those without skeletal disease.

PREVENTION

- There is no definite evidence to prevent prostate cancer.
- Controversy exists regarding screening for prostate cancer and if there is clear evidence that it improves survival. The American Cancer Society recommends annual PSA and digital rectal examination starting at age of 50 years old. The National Cancer Institute and the U.S. Preventive Services Task Force do not endorse screening for prostate cancer
- Prevention studies have evaluated dietary factors, vitamins, trace elements, and hormonal agents.
  ○ The SELECT trial is a national prostate cancer prevention trial comparing vitamin E and selenium. Results will not be known for several years.

BIBLIOGRAPHY

Burgess, E. F., & Roth, B. (2006). Changing perspectives of the role of chemotherapy in advanced prostate cancer. *Urologic Clinics of North America, 33*, 227-236.

Cash, J. (2006). Cellular characteristics, pathophysiology and disease manifestations. In J. Held-Warmkessel (Ed.), *Contemporary issues in prostate cancer: a nursing perspective* (2nd ed., pp. 60-78) Boston: Jones & Bartlett.

Collins, M. (2006). Staging of prostate cancer. In J. Held-Warmkessel (Ed.), *Contemporary issues in prostate cancer: a nursing perspective* (2nd ed., pp. 107-124) Boston: Jones & Bartlett.

Desai, P., Jimenez, J., Kao, C., et al. (2006). Future innovations in treating advanced prostate cancer. *Urologic Clinics of North America, 33*, 247-272.

Eastham, J., & Scardino, P. (2002). Radical prostatectomy. In P. C. Walsh, A. B. Ratik, E. D. Vaughan, et al. (Eds.), *Campbell's urology* (8th ed., pp. 3080-3106). Philadelphia: W. B. Saunders.

Ferrini, R.,& Woolf, S. (2005). *Screening for prostate cancer in American men*. American College of Preventive Medicine Practice Policy Statement. Retrieved February, 2005, from http://www.acpm.org/prostate.htm.

Green, F. L., Page, D. L., Fleming I.D., et al. (2002). *AJCC cancer staging manual* (6th ed.). New York: Springer-Verlag.

Jemal, A., Siegel, R., Ward, E., et al. (2007). Cancer statistics, 2007. *CA: A Cancer Journal for Clinicians, 57*, 43-66.

National Cancer Institute. (2007). *Prostate cancer, PDQ*. Retrieved February 24, 2007 from http://www.cancer.gov/cancertopics/pdq/treatment/prostate/healthprofessional.

Presti, J. (2004). Neoplasms of the prostate. In E. Tanagho & J. McAninch (Eds.). *Smith's general urology* (16th ed., pp. 367-385). New York: McGraw-Hill.

Scher, H., Leibel, S., Fuks, Z., et al. (2005). Cancer of the prostate. In V. DeVita, S. Hellman, & S. Rosenberg (Eds.). *Cancer principles and practice* (7th ed., pp. 1192-1259). Philadelphia: Lippincott Williams & Wilkins.

Stotts, R. C. (2004). Cancers of the prostate, penis, and testicles: epidemiology, prevention, and treatment. *Nursing Clinics of North America, 39*, 327-340.

Renal Cancer

Mary Collins

DEFINITION

Renal cancer comprises various types of cancer with different histologic features and disease courses. Renal cell carcinoma (RCC) is the most common type of kidney cancer. It accounts for more than 90% of malignant kidney tumors. Transitional cell carcinoma accounts for 5% to 10% of kidney cancers. Five to six percent of kidney cancer is Wilms' tumors; these are almost always found in children and very rare in adults. Less than 1% of kidney cancers are renal sarcomas (see Soft Tissue Sarcoma, page 127). Renal cell cancer occurs equally in the right and left kidneys. Approximately 2% of renal cancer results from inherited syndromes. The most common metastatic sites are bone, liver, lung, brain, and distant lymph nodes. About 20% to 30% of patients are diagnosed with metastatic disease present.

INCIDENCE

Renal cancer accounts for approximately 3% of all adult malignancies. It is estimated that there will be 51,190 new cases diagnosed in 2007, 31,590 men and 19,600 women; 12,890 deaths are expected from the disease in 2007. Renal cancer is most commonly diagnosed in patients between 55 and 84 years of age. The incidence of renal cancer has slowly been increasing, particularly in men.

ETIOLOGY AND RISK FACTORS

- Hereditary renal cell cancer involves bilateral kidneys and usually occurs at younger ages than does nonhereditary or sporadic renal cell cancer. Renal cell cancer will develop in approximately 40% of patients with von Hippel-Lindau disease.
- Acquired cystic kidney disease is associated with end-stage renal disease.
- Tobacco use
- Chronic misuse of certain pain medicines, including over-the-counter pain medicines
- Obesity and hypertension have also been linked with RCC.

SIGNS AND SYMPTOMS

Presenting symptoms include flank pain, hematuria, and a palpable abdominal mass; however, approximately 50% of renal cancers are discovered as an incidental finding on an x-ray film. Other symptoms may include weight loss, fatigue and anemia.

DIAGNOSTIC WORKUP

- Laboratory studies: complete blood cell count, comprehensive metabolic panel, acetate dehydrogenase, prothrombin time, partial thromboplastin time, and urinalysis
- Chest x-ray film
- Chest, abdominal, and pelvic computed tomographic scans to differentiate between benign and malignant masses and evaluate lymph node status
- Magnetic resonance imaging may be done if the inferior vena cava is involved, to help determine the need for vascular surgery.
- Biopsy

HISTOLOGY

There are five histologic RCC subgroups:

- Clear cell (75%-80%)
- Papillary (10%-15%), which arises in the proximal tubules
- Chromophobe (5%)
- Collecting duct (very rare)
- Unclassified (5%)

Transitional cell carcinoma, also known as urothelial carcinoma, begins in the renal pelvis and looks and acts very much like bladder cancer.

CLINICAL STAGING

RCC is staged according to the American Joint Committee on Cancer, or the TNM (Tumor, Node, Metastasis) system. See the table on page 74.

TREATMENT

Radical nephrectomy that includes removal of the kidney, ipsilateral adrenal gland, and regional lymph nodes is the standard of care for RCC. Newer procedures include partial nephrectomy or nephron-sparing surgery, laparoscopic nephrectomy, and radiofrequency heat ablation or cryoablation. Radiation is indicated for symptomatic treatment of disease such as bone metastasis.

Chemotherapy has limited activity in RCC. Newer targeted therapies and biological response modifiers are the only therapies currently approved by the Food and Drug Administration. Sunitinib is a tyrosine kinase inhibitor approved for advanced RCC, and interleukin-2 is approved for metastatic disease. Multiple agents and combinations are currently under investigation.

PROGNOSIS

The prognosis for RCC is based on grade and stage of the disease. Renal cell carcinoma can often be cured if it is diagnosed and treated when localized to the kidney and to the immediate surrounding tissue. Because RCC is often diagnosed early in the disease, there is an overall 40% survival at 5 years. The 5-year survival rate for disease confined to the kidney is 90%, for locally advanced disease 60%, and 5% for metastatic disease.

Poor prognostic factors for advanced or metastatic disease include poor performance status, anemia, elevated lactate dehydrogenase (>1.5 times the upper limit of normal), and metastasis noted in less than 1 year from initial diagnosis.

PREVENTION

Nurses are in a unique position to educate patients regarding smoking cessation, obesity, and hypertension, which may reduce the risk for RCC. Education materials are available from the American Cancer Society and the National Cancer Institute. A family history of RCC, particularly in individuals less than 50 years old, may indicate a hereditary predisposition to the disease. Patients with a family history or hereditary RCC (i.e., von Hippel-Lindau disease) should be closely monitored.

BIBLIOGRAPHY

Atkins, M., & Garnick, M. (2000). Renal neoplasia. In Brenner B. (Ed.). *The kidney* (pp. 1844-1868). Philadelphia: W. B. Saunders.

Cohen, H., & McGovern, F. (2005). Renal-cell carcinoma. *New England Journal of Medicine, 353,* 2477-90.

Creel, T. (2005). *Medical management of patients with renal cell carcinoma.* Presented at the meeting of the Oncology Nursing Society's Institute of Learning, Orlando, FL.

Curti, B. (2004). Renal cell carcinoma. *Journal of the American Medical Association, 292,* 97-100.

Green, F. L., Page, D. L., Fleming, I. D., et al. (2002). *AJCC cancer staging, annual* (6th ed.). New York: Springer-Verlag.

Hamsiworth, J., Sosman, J., Spigel, D., et al. (2005). Treatment of metastatic renal

Clinical Staging: Renal Cancer

Definition of TNM

Primary Tumor (T)

TX	Primary tumor cannot be assessed
T0	No evidence of primary tumor
T1	Tumor 7 cm or less in greatest dimension, limited to the kidney
T1a	Tumor 4 cm or less in greatest dimension, limited to the kidney
T1b	Tumor more than 4 cm but not more than 7 cm in greatest dimension, limited to the kidney
T2	Tumor more than 7 cm in greatest dimension, limited to the kidney
T3	Tumor extends into major veins or invades adrenal gland or perinephric tissues but not beyond Gerota's fascia
T3a	Tumor directly invades adrenal gland or perirenal or renal sinus fat but not beyond Gerota's fascia
T3b	Tumor grossly extends into the renal vein or its segmental (muscle-containing) branches, or vena cava below the diaphragm
T3c	Tumor grossly extends into vena cava above diaphragm or invades the wall of the vena cava
T4	Tumor invades beyond Gerota's fascia

Regional Lymph Nodes (N)*

NX	Regional lymph nodes cannot be assessed
N0	No regional lymph node metastases
N1	Metastases in a single regional lymph node
N2	Metastasis in more than one regional lymph node

*Laterality does not affect the N classification.
Note: If a lymph node dissection is performed, then pathological evaluation would ordinarily include at least eight nodes.

Distant Metastasis (M)

MX	Distant metastasis cannot be assessed
M0	No distant metastasis
M1	Distant metastasis

Stage Grouping

Stage	T	N	M
Stage I	T1	N0	M0
Stage II	T2	N0	M0
Stage III	T1	N1	M0
	T2	N1	M0
	T3	N0	M0
	T3	N1	M0
	T3a	N0	M0
	T3a	N1	M0
	T3b	N0	M0
	T3b	N1	M0
	T3c	N0	M0
	T3c	N1	M0
Stage IV	T4	N0	M0
	T4	N1	M0
	Any T	N2	M0
	Any T	Any N	M1

Used with the permission of the American Joint Committee on Cancer (AJCC), Chicago, Illinois. The original source for this material is the *AJCC Cancer staging manual*, Sixth Edition (2002) published by Springer Science and Business Media LLC, www.springerlink.com.

cell carcinoma with a combination of bevacizumab and erlotinib. *Journal of Clinical Oncology, 23,* 7889-7896.

Jemal, A., Siegel, R., Ward, E., et al. (2007). Cancer statistics, 2007. *CA: A Cancer Journal for Clinicians, 57,* 43-66.

Lam, J., Shvarts, O., Leppert, J., et al. (2005). Renal cell carcinoma 2005: new frontiers in staging, progno-stication and targeted molecular therapy. *Journal of Urology, 173,* 1853-1862.

Lee, F., & Patel, H. (2002). Kidney cancer: current management guidelines. *Hospital Medicine, 63,* 214-217.

Linehan, W. M., Bates, S., & Yang, J. (2005). Cancer of the kidney. In V. DeVita, S. Hellman, & S. Rosenberg (Eds.). *Cancer principles & practice* (7th ed., 1139-1168). Philadelphia: Lippincott Williams & Wilkins.

National Cancer Institute. (2007). *Renal cell cancer, PDQ.* Retrieved February 25, 2007 from http://www.cancer.gov/cancertopics/pdq/treatment/renalcell/HealthProfessional.

National Cancer Institute. (2007). *Transitional cell cancer of the renal pelvis and ureter, PDQ.* Retrieved February 25, 2007 from http://www.cancer.gov/cancertopics/pdq/treatment/transitionalcell/Health Professional.

Novick, A., & Campbell, S. (2002). Renal tumors. In P. C. Walsh, A. B. Retik, E. D. Vaughan, et al. (Eds.). *Campbell's urology* (8th ed., pp. 2672-2731) Philadelphia: W. B. Saunders.

Wood, L. (2005). *Renal cell carcinoma: overview advances in the treatment of renal cell carcinoma.* Presented at the meeting of the Oncology Nursing Society's Institute of Learning, Orlando, FL.

Testicular Cancer

Patty Woods Bunch and Mary Collins

DEFINITION

Testicular cancer, although relatively rare, is the most common malignancy among men aged 15 to 35 years. Germ cell tumors (GCTs) account for 98% of all testicular malignancies, of which 40% are seminomas and 60% are non-seminomas. The other 2% are made up of stromal cell tumors and secondary testicular tumors. Testicular cancer metastasizes through the lymphatic system to the retroperitoneal lymph nodes. Distant metastasis sites include the lungs, liver, skeleton, and brain.

INCIDENCE

It is estimated that 7,920 men will be diagnosed with testicular cancer in 2007 in the United States and 380 will die from the disease. The worldwide incidence of testicular cancer has increased in the last 30 years, primarily in industrialized regions. Scandinavia, Switzerland, Germany, and New Zealand report the highest incidence of testicular cancer. The rates in the United States and the United Kingdom are intermediate and Africa and Asia have the lowest rates.

- Testicular cancer accounts for 1% of all malignancies in men.
- The incidence in whites is greater than that in African Americans (4:1).
  - However, the lifetime probability of having testicular cancer is only 0.2% for a white male in the United States.
- Incidence peaks at three stages of life: infancy, 25-40 years old, and 60 years or older.

○ Peak frequency is early adulthood
○ Testicular cancer is uncommon after the age of 40 years.

ETIOLOGY AND RISK FACTORS

The exact cause of testicular cancer is unknown, but several risk factors have been suggested for the development of this malignancy:

- Cryptorchidism (undescended testicles)
  ○ More common in the right testes
  ○ 5%-10% of patients with unilateral cryptorchidis have tumor in the descended testicle
- Testicular cancer in the contralateral testis
- Klinefelter's syndrome
  ○ Genetic disorder manifested by testicular atrophy, gynecomastia, and absence of spermatogenesis
  ○ Increased risk of mediastinal GCTs
- Positive for human immunodeficiency virus
- Family history/genetics
- Environmental and dietary factors
- Hormones

SIGNS AND SYMPTOMS

Early signs of testicular cancer are asymptomatic nodule or swelling, testicular mass, feeling of heaviness, pain, or hardness. Patients with advanced disease may have back or abdominal pain, weight loss, gynecomastia (from elevated beta-human chorionic gonadotropin levels), supraclavicular lymphadenopathy, superior vena cava syndrome, urinary obstruction, dyspnea and hemoptysis, bone pain, and headaches or seizures.

DIAGNOSTIC WORKUP

Ultrasonography with high-frequency transducer has become the imaging modality of choice for examining the scrotum. Other evaluations include the following:

- Chest radiograph to rule out pulmonary metastases
- Computed tomographic scans of chest, abdomen, and pelvis to establish the extent of disease

- Magnetic resonance imaging when results of physical examination and ultrasonography are equivocal and if there are central nervous system symptoms suggestive of brain metastases.
- Biochemical markers: serum alpha-fetoprotein, serum beta-human chorionic gonadotropin, serum lactate dehydrogenase
  ○ Used also to monitor for recurrent disease
  ○ Elevated levels of alpha-fetoprotein (50%-70%) and human chorionic gonadotropin (40%-60%) are seen in patients with nonseminomatous testis tumors
  ○ Lactate dehydrogenase is elevated in approximately 60% of patients with nonseminoma with metastatic disease and 8% advanced disease
- High inguinal orchiectomy with complete removal of the testis and spermatic cord through the inguinal ring is the procedure of choice for pathological evaluation. Biopsy is not recommended because of concerns about local and nodal dissemination of tumor.

HISTOLOGY

GCTs comprise about 95% of testicular tumors and non-germ-cell tumors account for 5%. GCTs are classified into two histologic categories: seminomas and nonseminomas. Seminoma peaks in men in the fourth decade, whereas nonseminoma occurs between 25 and 35 years of age. Nonseminomas are further classified into embryonal carcinoma, teratoma, choriocarcinoma, and yolk sac tumor. GCTs are believed to be more responsive to chemotherapy (and in the case of seminoma, to radiation therapy) because of their high tumor cell–doubling time. The spread of these cancers is generally predictable, with the initial spread occurring to the retroperitoneal lymph nodes.

CLINICAL STAGING

Several systems classify and stage testicular cancer; they are institution dependent. The International Germ Cell Collaborative Group developed a

prognostic system in 1997 that remains a standard (see box below). Staging is also assessed according to the Tumor, Node, and Metastasis System (TNM) in conjunction with serum tumor markers, lactate dehydrogenase, human chorionic gonadotropin, and alpha-fetoprotein. The American Joint committee on Cancer provides this staging system. (See the table on pages 76-77). Radiographic evaluation of the chest, abdomen, and pelvis determine the N and M status. Examination of the orchiectomy specimens is used for the T classification.

International Germ Cell Consensus Prognostic Classification System for Testicular Cancer

GOOD PROGNOSIS
Nonseminoma
Testis or retroperitoneal primary
No nonpulmonary visceral metastases
Alpha-fetoprotein <1000 ng/mL, human chorionic gonadotropin <5000 IU/L, and lactate dehydrogenase <1.5 times upper limit of normal.

Seminoma
Any primary site
No nonpulmonary visceral metastases
Normal alpha-fetoprtein; any human chorionic gonadotropin or lactate dehydrogenase

INTERMEDIATE PROGNOSIS
Nonseminoma
Testis or retroperitoneal primary
No nonpulmonary visceral metastases
Any of: alpha-fetoprotein 1000-10,000 ng/mL, human chorionic gonadotropin 5000-50,000 IU/L, or lactate dehydrogenase 1.5-10 times upper limit of normal

Seminoma
Testis or retroperitoneal primary site
Normal alpha-fetoprotein; any human chorionic gonadotropin or lactate dehydrogenase
Nonpulmonary visceral metastases

POOR PROGNOSIS
Nonseminoma Only
Any of the following criteria:
    Mediastinal primary
    Nonpulmonary visceral metastases
    Alpha-fetoprotein >10,000 ng/mL, human chorionic gonadotropin >50,000 IU/L, or lactate dehydrogenase >10 times upper limit of normal

Adapted from Richie, J., & Steele, G. (2002). Neoplasms of the testis. In *Campbell's urology* (8th Ed., p. 2902). Philadelphia: W. B. Saunders.

TREATMENT

Radical orchiectomy is performed to stage and treat testicular cancer. Further therapy depends on whether it is seminoma or nonseminoma. Surgery alone is used for early-stage nonseminoma disease. Retroperitoneal lymph node dissection after orchiectomy is considered primary therapy for nonseminomatous tumors. Patients who do have relapses, 5% to 10% for low-volume disease, have a high cure rate with chemotherapy. Cisplatin-based chemotherapy is recommended for patients with stage II and III disease.

Early-stage seminoma is very sensitive to radiotherapy. Both stages I and II are treated with external beam irradiation after orchiectomy. Bulky stage IIC and disseminated disease are treated primarily with chemotherapy. Approximately 20% to 30% of patients with advanced disease may have a relapse after conventional chemotherapy. Cure rates for this population are anywhere from 0% to 78%. Ifosfamide, cisplatin, etoposide, or vinblastine may be used in these situations, and 25% to 35% may have a complete response. High-dose chemotherapy and autologous stem cell support have been used in poor-risk patients with fairly good response rates of 50% disease free at 5 years.

PROGNOSIS

The percentage of embryonal carcinoma and vascular invasion appear to be the most significant prognosticators for GCTs. Virtually all patients with stage I or II seminomas and nonseminomas should survive their disease. Prognosis is closely correlated with stage of disease and tumor burden. The International Germ Cell Cancer Collaborative Group risk classification found in the box on page 75 also predicts 5-year progression-free and overall survival.

Although the majority of men are cured of their disease, patients with a poor prognosis can have rapidly progressive disease. Approximately 15% of patients will not be cured of their disease. Metastatic nonseminoma may have an annual relapse rate of 1% to 2% continuing even beyond 10 years.

Clinical Staging: Testicular Cancer

Definition of TNM

Primary Tumor (T)

The extent of primary tumor is usually classified after radical orchiectomy, and for this reason, a *pathological* stage is assigned.

pTX*	Primary tumor cannot be assessed
pT0	No evidence of primary tumor (e.g., histologic scar in testis)
pTis	Intratubular germ cell neoplasia (carcinoma in *situ*)
pT1	Tumor limited to the testis and epididymis without vascular/lymphatic invasion; tumor may invade into the tunica albuginea but not the tunica vaginalis
pT2	Tumor limited to the testis and epididymis with vascular/lymphatic invasion, or tumor extending through the tunica albuginea with involvement of the tunica vaginalis
pT3	Tumor invades the spermatic cord with or without vascular/lymphatic invasion
pT4	Tumor invades the scrotum with or without vascular/lymphatic invasion

*Except for pTis and pT4, extent of primary tumor is classified by radical orchiectomy. TX may be used for other categories in the absence of radical orchiectomy.

Regional Lymph Nodes (N)

Clinical

NX	Regional lymph nodes cannot be assessed
N0	No regional lymph node metastasis
N1	Metastasis with a lymph node mass 2 cm or less in greatest dimension; or multiple lymph nodes, none more than 2 cm in greatest dimension
N2	Metastasis with a lymph node mass more than 2 m but not more than 5 cm in greatest dimension; or multiple lymph nodes, any one mass greater than 2 cm but not more than 5 cm in greatest dimension
N3	Metastasis with a lymph node mass more than 5 cm in greatest dimension

Pathologic (pN)

pNX	Regional lymph nodes cannot be assessed
pN0	No regional lymph node involvement
pN1	Metastasis with a lymph node mass 2 cm or less in greatest dimension and less than or equal to five nodes positive, none more than 2 cm in greatest dimension
pN2	Metastasis with a lymph node mass more than 2 cm but not more than 5 cm in greatest dimension; or more than five nodes positive, none more than 5 cm; or evidence of extranodal extension of tumor
pN3	Metastasis with a lymph node mass more than 5 cm in greatest dimension

Distant Metastasis (M)

MX	Distant metastasis cannot be assessed
M0	No distant metastasis
M1	Distant metastasis
M1a	Nonregional nodal or pulmonary metastasis
M1b	Distant metastasis other than to nonregional lymph nodes and lungs

Serum Tumor Markers (S)

SX	Marker studies not available or not performed
S0	Marker study levels within normal limits
S1	Lactate dehydrogenase <1.5× N* **AND** Human chorionic gonadotropin (mIU/mL) <5000 **AND** Alpha-fetoprotein (ng/mL) <1000
S2	Lactate dehydrogenase 1.5-10× N **OR** Human chorionic gonadotropin (mIU/mL) 5000-50,000 **OR** Alpha-fetoprotein (ng/mL) 1000-10,000
S3	Lactate dehydrogenase >10× N **OR** Human chorionic gonadotropin (mIU/mL) >50,000 **OR** Alpha-fetoprotein (ng/mL) >10,000

*N indicates the upper limit of normal for the LDH assay.

Clinical Staging: Testicular Cancer—cont'd

Stage Grouping

Stage 0	pTis	N0	M0	S0
Stage I	pT1-4	N0	M0	SX
Stage IA	pT1	N0	M0	S0
Stage IB	pT2	N0	M0	S0
	pT3	N0	M0	S0
	pT4	N0	M0	S0
Stage IS	Any pT/Tx	N0	M0	S1-3
Stage II	Any pT/Tx	N1-3	M0	SX
Stage IIA	Any pT/Tx	N1	M0	S0
	Any PT/Tx	N2	M0	S1
Stage IIB	Any pT/Tx	N2	M0	S0
	Any pT/Tx	N2	M0	S1
Stage IIC	Any pT/Tx	N3	M0	S0
	Any pT/Tx	N3	M0	S1
Stage III	Any pT/Tx	Any N	M1	SX
Stage IIIA	Any pT/Tx	Any N	M1a	S1
	Any pT/Tx	Any N	M1a	S1
Stage IIIB	Any pT/Tx	N1-3	M0	S2
	Any pT/Tx	Any N	M1a	S2
Stage IIIC	Any pT/Tx	N1-3	M0	S3
	Any pT/Tx	Any N	M1a	S3
	Any pT/Tx	Any N	M1b	Any S

Used with the permission of the American Joint Committee on Cancer (AJCC), Chicago, Illinois. The original source for this material is the *AJCC Cancer staging manual,* Sixth Edition (2002) published by Springer Science and Business Media LLC, www.springerlink.com.

PREVENTION

Education on the risk factors and the importance of testicular self-examination beginning during the teen years is the most important prevention method. The American Cancer Society recommends a testicular examination every 3 years for men over 20 years and annually for those over 40 years. Educational pamphlets can guide men to do a self-testicular examination. The U.S. Preventive Task Force recommends that young men seek medical care promptly if they notice any abnormality in the scrotal area.

Long-term follow-up is essential because relapses may occur several years after therapy, including the development of a second testicular cancer. Patients should also be discouraged from smoking and should limit their exposure to the sun. Continued follow-up is also needed to address fertility issues that may develop after chemotherapy.

BIBLIOGRAPHY

Abraham, J., Gulley, J., & Allegra, C. (2005). Testicular carcinoma. In *Bethesda handbook of clinical oncology* (pp. 211-222). Philadelphia: Lippincott Williams & Wilkins.

Bosl, G., Bajorin, D., Sheinfeld, J., et al. (2005). Cancer of the testis. In V. DeVita, S. Hellman, & S. Rosenberg (Eds.). *Cancer principles and practice* (7th ed., pp. 1269-1293). Philadelphia: Lippincott Williams & Wilkins.

Green, F. L., Page, D. L., Fleming, I. D., et al. (2002). *AJCC cancer staging manual* (6th ed.) New York: Springer-Verlag.

Huyghe, E., Matsuda, T., & Thonneav, P. (2003). Increasing incidence of testicular cancer worldwide: a review. *Journal of Urology, 170,* 5-11.

Jemal, A., Siegel, R., Ward, E., et al. (2007). Cancer statistics, 2007. *CA: A Cancer Journal for Clinicians, 57,* 43-66

Lee, F., Hamid, R., Arya, M., et al. (2002). Testicular cancer: current update and controversies. *Hospital Medicine, 63,* 615-620.

Presti, J. (2004). Genital tumors. In E. Tanagho & J. McAninch J. (Eds.), *Smith's general urology* (6th ed., 386-399). New York: Lange.

Richie, J., & Steele, G. (2002). Neoplasms of the testis. In P. C. Walsh, A. B. Retik, E. D. Vaughan, et al (Eds.), *Campbell's urology* (8th ed., pp. 2876-2919). Philadelphia: W. B. Saunders.

Stotts, R. C. (2004). Cancers of the prostate, penis, and testicles: epidemiology, prevention, and treatment. *Nursing Clinics of North America, 39,* 327-340.

Vaughn, D., Gignac, G., & Meadows A. (2002). Long-term medical care of testicular cancer survivors. *Annals of Internal Medicine, 136,*463-468.

Warde, P., Specht, L., Horwich, A., et al. (2002). Prognostic factors for relapse in stage 1 seminoma managed by surveillance: a pooled analysis. *Journal of Clinical Oncology, 20,* 4448-4452.

Yarbro, C. H., Frogge, M. H., & Goodman, M. (2005). Testicular germ cell cancer. In *Cancer nursing principles and practice* (pp. 1630-1643). Sudbury, MA: Jones & Bartlett.

Gynecological Cancer

Patty Woods Bunch

Cervical Cancer

DEFINITION

Cervical cancer consists of several cell types, but the most common, approximately 85% to 90%, are squamous cell carcinoma. Most of the remaining 10% to 15% are adenocarcinomas. Human papillomavirus (HPV) is strongly associated with cervical cancer, therefore leading to the conclusion that cervical cancer is a sexually transmitted disease associated with chronic infection by oncogenic types of HPV.

The main routes of spread of carcinoma of the cervix are as follows:

- Into the vaginal mucosa, then
- Into the myometrium, then
- Into the paracervical lymphatics, then
- Into common lymph nodes

INCIDENCE

There are approximately 12,800 new cases per year and around 4,600 deaths per year in the United States. There are approximately 50,000 new cases of carcinoma in situ per year.

The incidence appears to be less frequent in rural areas than in metropolitan areas; underdeveloped countries have a greater incidence of cervical cancer than that of developed countries. Approximately 93% are squamous cell cancers and contain HPV deoxyribonucleic acid; 90% of these are subtypes 16/18, which are the most virulent.

ETIOLOGY AND RISK FACTORS

Many of the risks factors for cervical cancer are the same as those for sexually transmitted disease:

- Early age at onset of sexual activity
- Multiple pregnancies
- Multiple sexual partners
- Long-term use of oral contraceptives
- Tobacco smoking

Cervical carcinoma is the sixth most common malignant tumor in women in the United States; black and Hispanic women are disproportionately affected. The incidence and mortality rates of this disease in North America have declined during the last half century because of both increased availability of Papanicolaou (Pap) smear screening and a decrease in fertility rate. These declines in incidence have slowed in recent years, and there is a trend toward increasing incidence in some populations of white women in the United States.

SIGNS AND SYMPTOMS

Presenting symptoms may include the following:

- Increased amount and duration of regular thin, watery, blood-tinged vaginal discharge
- Painless spotting only postcoitally or after douching
- As the malignancy enlarges, bleeding episodes become heavier and more frequent. Menstrual flow eventually becomes continuous.

Late symptoms include the following:

- Pain referred to the flank or leg
- Dysuria
- Hematuria
- Rectal bleeding
- Persistent edema in lower extremities
- Massive hemorrhage and development of uremia (occasionally this is the initial presenting symptom)

DIAGNOSTIC WORKUP

Recommendations of the American Cancer Society are that asymptomatic and low-risk women aged 20 years and older and sexually active women under the age of 20 years have annual Pap smears for 2 consecutive years and every 3 years until age 65 years. Biopsy should be performed on any suspicious lesion of the cervix to an adequate depth, preferably at the margin, to confirm the diagnosis of invasive carcinoma. Specimens should be obtained from any suspicious area in all four quadrants of the cervix and from suspicious areas in the vagina.

If biopsy is necessary, patients should also have the following studies performed:

- Complete peripheral blood evaluation
- Complete chemistry profile
- Urinalysis
- Imaging studies such as computed tomography scan, magnetic resonance imaging, or positron emission tomography

HISTOLOGY

Cervical cancer consists of several cell types, but the most common (85%-90%) are squamous cell. Most of the remaining is adenocarcinoma.

CLINICAL STAGING

The staging of cervical cancer is a clinical appraisal. Because of the advantage of having several examiners and the benefit of muscular relaxation, pelvic examination under anesthesia is recommended. The International Federation of Gynecology and Obstetrics staging system is widely used for cervical cancer. A parallel TNM staging system has been proposed by the American Joint Committee Commission on Cancer (see table on page 79).

TREATMENT

Specific therapeutic measures in the treatment of cervical cancer are usually governed by the age and general health of the patient, by the extent of the cancer, and by the presence and nature of any complicating abnormalities.

- Stage 0, carcinoma in situ (CIS), is often treated with a total hysterectomy. In cases where women wish to have more children, CIS may be treated conservatively with a therapeutic conization, laser ablation, or cryotherapy.
- Stage I and stage IIa cervical cancer may be treated with surgery or radiotherapy. Surgery for stage I and IIa may be reserved for young patients in whom preservation of ovarian function is desired and improved vaginal preservation is expected.
- Stages IIB and III tumors are best treated with concurrent chemoradiation or, in some cases, with irradiation alone. Radiation may be either external beam or brachytherapy. The chemotherapy of choice in this setting is cisplatinum. There are two rationales for using concurrent chemoradiation: (1) to increase the sensitivity of the tumor to the effects of the irradiation and (2) to eradicate systemic disease.
- Stage IVA disease (bladder or rectal invasion) can be treated either with irradiation or with pelvic exenteration.
- Combination chemotherapy involving bleomycin, cyclophosphamide, doxorubicin, cisplatinum, and methotrexate is used in patients where surgery and radiotherapy failed.

PROGNOSIS

The prognosis for patients with cervical cancers varies greatly with factors including age, race, socioeconomic status, and general health at the time of diagnosis. Race and socioeconomic

International Federation of Gynecology and Obstetrics and Parallel TNM Staging System Proposed by American Joint Committee on Cancer: Cervical Cancer

TNM Categories	FIGO Stages	
Primary Tumor (T)		
TX		Primary tumor cannot be assessed
T0		No evidence of primary tumor
Tis	0	Carcinoma in situ
T1	I	Cervical carcinoma confined to uterus (extension to corpus should be disregarded)
T1a*	IA	Invasive carcinoma diagnosed only be microscopy. Stromal invasion with a maximum depth of 5.0 mm measured from the base of the epithelium and a horizontal spread of 7.0 mm or less. Vascular space involvement, venous or lymphatic, does not affect classification
T1a1	IA1	Measured stromal invasion 3.0 mm or less in depth and 7.0 mm or less in horizontal spread
T1a2	IA2	Measured stromal invasion more than 3.0 mm and not more than 5.0 mm with a horizontal spread 7.0 mm or less
T1b	IB	Clinically visible lesion confined to the cervix or microscopic lesion greater than T1a/IA2
T1b1	IB1	Clinically visible lesion 4.0 cm or less in greatest dimension
T1b2	IB2	Clinically visible lesion more than 4.0 cm in greatest dimension
T2	II	Cervical carcinoma invades beyond uterus but not to pelvic wall or to lower third of vagina
T2a	IIA	Tumor without parametrial invasion
T2b	IIB	Tumor with parametrial invasion
T3	III	Tumor extends to pelvic wall or involves lower third of vagina or causes hydronephrosis or nonfunctioning kidney
T3a	IIIA	Tumor involves lower third of vagina, no extension to pelvic wall
T3b	IIIB	Tumor extends to pelvic wall or causes hydronephrosis or nonfunctioning kidney
T4	IVA	Tumor invades mucosa of bladder or rectum or extends beyond true pelvis (bullous edema is not sufficient to classify a tumor as T4)

*All macroscopically visible lesions—even with superficial invasion—are T1b/IB.

Regional Lymph Nodes (N)	
NX	Regional lymph nodes cannot be assessed
N0	No regional lymph node metastasis
N1	Regional lymph node metastasis

Distant Metastasis (M)		
MX		Distant metastasis cannot be assessed
M0		No distant metastasis
M1	IVB	Distant metastasis

Stage Grouping

Stage	T	N	M
Stage 0	Tis	N0	M0
Stage I	T1	N0	M0
Stage IA	T1a	N0	M0
Stage IA1	T1a1	N0	M0
Stage IA2	T1a2	N0	M0
Stage IB	T1b	N0	M0
Stage IB1	T1b1	N0	M0
Stage IB2	T1b2	N0	M0
Stage II	T2	N0	M0
Stage IIA	T2a	N0	M0
Stage IIB	T2b	N0	M0
Stage III	T23	N0	M0
Stage IIIA	T3a	N0	M0
Stage IIIB	T1	N1	M0
	T2	N1	M0
	T3a	N1	M0
	T3b	Any N	M0
Stage IVA	T4	Any N	M0
Stage IVB	Any T	Any N	M1

Used with the permission of the American Joint Committee on Cancer (AJCC), Chicago, Illinois. The original source for this material is the *AJCC Cancer staging manual*, Sixth Edition (2002) published by Springer Science and Business Media LLC, www.springerlink.com; Benedet, J. L., Bender, H., Jones III, H., Ngan, H. Y., & Pecorelli, S. (2000). FIGO staging classifications and clinical practice guidelines in the management of gynecologic cancers: FIGO Committee on Gynecologic Oncology. *International Journal of Gynaecology and Obstetrics, 70*, 209-262.

characteristics are believed to be factors because of greater exposure to other risk factors, more advanced disease at diagnosis, and the fact that these patients are less likely to undergo curative therapy.

Five-year survival by stage is as follows:

- Stage IA: 95%
- Stage IB or IIA: 70%-85%
- Stage IIB, III, and IVA: 65%, 40%, and 20%, respectively
- Stage IVB: 10%

PREVENTION

A wealth of epidemiological and molecular evidence has led to the conclusion that virtually all cases of cervical cancer and its precursor intraepithelial lesions are a result of infection with one or other of a subset of genital HPVs, suggesting that prevention of infection by prophylactic vaccination would be an effective anticancer strategy. Decreasing exposure to risk factors may also possibly prevent cervical carcinoma.

BIBLIOGRAPHY

American Society for Colposcopy and Cervical Pathology. (2005). *Practice recommendations: practice management*. Retrieved on May 20, 2006, from http://www.asccp.org/edu/practice/cervix/cancer.shtml.

Denny, L., Hacker, N. F., Gori, J., et al. (Eds.) (2000). Staging classifications and clinical practice guidelines for gynaecologic cancers. (3rd ed.). *International Journal of Gynecology and Obstetrics 70*, 207-312. Elsevier.

Greene, F., Page, D., Fleming, I., et al. (Eds.). (2002). *AJCC cancer staging handbook* (6th ed.). New York: Springer-Verlag.

Stehman, F. B., Perez, C. A., Karman, R. J., et al. Uterine cervix. (2005). In W. J. Hoskins, C. A. Perez, R. C. Young, et al. (Eds.), *Principles and practice of gynecologic oncology* (pp.743-767). Philadelphia: Lippincott Williams & Wilkins.

National Cancer Institute. (2006). *Human papillomavirus vaccines*. Retrieved May 20, 2006, from http://www.ncbi.nlm.nih.gov/entrez/query.fcgi?cmd.

Zorab, R., et al. (2002). Invasive cervical cancer. In P. J. DiSaia & W. T. Creasman (Eds.), *Clinical gynecologic oncology* (pp. 53-61). St. Louis: Mosby.

Endometrial Cancer

DEFINITION

Endometrial cancer arises from the lining of the uterus. It is primarily a disease of the postmenopausal woman; only 25% of the cases occur in premenopausal patients, and in most cases the tumor is confined to the uterine corpus (body of the uterus) at the time of diagnosis. A small percentage are sarcomas arising from either endometrial glands and stroma or from the uterine muscle (leiomyosarcoma). The usual carcinoma of the endometrium is easily diagnosed, but the well-differentiated cancers may be difficult to separate from advanced atypical hyperplasia. In the past 10 years, helpful criteria have been adopted to permit differentiation of the two conditions into a benign lesion (atypical hyperplasia) and a neoplasm that is progressive (well-differentiated carcinoma).

INCIDENCE

Currently, endometrial carcinoma is the fourth most common cancer in women. The American Cancer Society estimates 39,080 new cases of endometrial cancer will be diagnosed in the United States in 2007 and 7,400 deaths from this disease. Endometrial adenocarcinomas are the most common, with endometrial sarcomas accounting for only about 6% of all of the endometrial cancer cases in the United States. Endometrial cancer occurs most commonly in postmenopausal women, although 25% of cases occur before menopause and 5% in patients younger than 40 years.

ETIOLOGY AND RISK FACTORS

The occurrence of endometrial cancer is higher in Western countries than Eastern ones. In the United States, white women have a twofold higher risk for development of this disease than African American women, and it is more common among urban than rural residents. The genetic syndrome of hereditary nonpolyposis colon cancer (HNPCC) has been associated with ovarian and endometrial cancer.

Factors for increased risk of endometrial carcinoma include the following:

- Unopposed estrogens
- Obesity
- Nulliparity
- Menopause after age 52 years
- Hypertension
- Diabetes mellitus
- Diet (possible relationship to high fat intake)
- Complex endometrial hyperplasia
- Use of tamoxifen

SIGNS AND SYMPTOMS

Symptoms of early endometrial carcinoma are few. However, 90% of patients have abnormal vaginal discharge; 80% of these show abnormal bleeding, usually postmenopausal, and 10% show leukorrhea. Signs and symptoms of more advanced disease include pelvic pressure and other symptoms indicative of uterine enlargement or extrauterine tumor spread.

DIAGNOSTIC WORKUP

The standard method of assessing abnormal uterine bleeding and diagnosing uterine carcinoma remains fractional curettage. This procedure involves curetting the endocervix, followed by sounding, in which a thin rod is used to determine the length of the uterus. The cervix is then dilated, and systematic curetting of the entire endometrial cavity is performed. Outpatient endometrial biopsy or aspiration curettage that avoids general anesthesia may be performed before formal curettage, but because this sampling type is random and does not include the entire endometrium, these tests would only be definitive if they were positive for cancer.

HISTOLOGY

Adenocarcinoma is the most common histologic subtype that may originate in the endometrium.

Classification of endometrial carcinoma is as follows:

- Endometroid adenocarcinoma
  - Papillary villoglandular
  - Secretory
  - Ciliated cell
  - Adenocarcinoma with squamous differentiation
- Mucinous carcinoma
- Serous carcinoma
- Clear-cell carcinoma
- Squamous carcinoma
- Undifferentiated carcinoma
- Mixed types
- Miscellaneous carcinomas
- Metastatic carcinoma
- Sarcoma

CLINICAL STAGING

The prognostic value of surgicopathologic staging has been confirmed in multiple studies of large numbers of patients. Stage of the disease is often the single strongest predictor of outcome for women with endometrial adenocarcinoma. See the box on page 81 for the International Federation of Gynecology and Obstetrics staging system for endometrial carcinoma.

TREATMENT

Endometrial cancer seems to have more advocates for different treatment plans than any other female pelvic malignancy does. The standard treatment is a total abdominal hysterectomy. However, through the years, preoperative and postoperative irradiation and, occasionally, chemotherapy and hormonal therapy have also been used. With improved preoperative and postoperative care, surgical techniques, and knowledge of tumor spread, the current treatment trend is to avoid preoperative irradiation or chemotherapy and to stage all patients surgically. Postoperative treatment, whether with chemotherapy or radiation therapy or both, is reserved for those who are found to have poor prognostic factors after the surgicopathologic material is reviewed.

PROGNOSIS

Many patients with endometrial adenocarcinoma have a mixture of good

International Federation of Gynecology and Obstetrics Classification of Endometrial Carcinoma

IA G1,2,3	Tumor limited to endometrium
IB G1,2,3	Invasion to less than half of the myometrium
IC G1,2,3	Invasion to more than half of the myometrium
IIA G1,2,3	Endocervical glandular involvement only
IIB G1,2,3	Cervical stromal invasion
IIIA G1,2,3	Tumor invades serosa or adnexa or positive peritoneal cytologic findings
IIIB G1,2,3	Vaginal metastasis
IIIC G1,2,3	Metastasis to pelvic or para-aortic lymph nodes
IVA G1,2,3	Tumor invades bladder or bowel mucosa
IVB	Distant metastasis including intra-abdominal or inguinal lymph nodes

HISTOPATHOLOGY: DEGREE OF DIFFERENTIATION

Cases of carcinoma of the corpus should be grouped according to the degree of differentiation of the adenocarcinoma as follows:

G1	5% or less of a nonsquamous or nonmorular solid growth pattern
G2	6% to 50% of a nonsquamous or nonmorular solid growth pattern
G3	More than 50% of a nonsquamous or nonmorular solid growth pattern

Data from Benedet, J.L., Bender, H., Jones, H., 3rd, Ngan, H.Y., & Pecorelli, S. (2000), FIGO staging classifications and clinical practice guidelines in the management of gynecologic cancers. FIGO Committee on Gynecologic Oncology. *International Journal of Gynaecology and Obstetrics, 70*(2), 206-62.

and bad prognostic factors and do not fall into categories for which either the prognosis or need for adjuvant therapy is clear. It should be noted that the survival for most women with early surgical stage disease is excellent. The 1-year relative survival rate is 94%; the 5-year survival rate for patients with stage I-IIA disease is 96%, for stage IIB-IIIB it is 66%, and for stage IIIC-IV disease it is 25%. Essentially all reports agree that differentiation (grade) of tumor and depth of invasion are important prognostic considerations.

PREVENTION

- All women at menopause should be informed about the risks and symptoms of endometrial cancer. They should be encouraged to report any unexpected bleeding or spotting to their physicians.
- Annual screening with endometrial biopsy beginning at age 35 years should be offered to women with or at risk for HNPCC.
- Increasing data suggest that the use of combination oral contraceptives decreases the risk for development of endometrial cancer. This protection was most notable for nulliparous women.
- Although obesity is a controllable risk factor, the type of obesity in patients with endometrial cancer has been evaluated. Researchers have concluded that upper-body fat localization is a significant risk factor for these patients.
- Significant protection was noted with an elevated intake of most vegetables, fresh fruits, whole-grain bread, and pasta.
- The addition of progestin in the use of estrogen appears to be protective against endometrial cancer.

BIBLIOGRAPHY

Denny, L., Hacker, N. F., Gori, J., et al. (2000). Staging classifications and clinical practice guidelines for gynaecologic cancers. *International Journal of Gynecology and Obstetrics, 70,* 207-312.

Jemal, A., Siegel, R., Ward, E., et al. (2007). Cancer Statistics, 2007. *CA:A Cancer Journal for Clinicians.* 57(1);p.21.

Hoskins, W.J., et al. (2005). Corpus epithelial tumors. In W. J. Hoskins, C. A. Perez, R. C. Young, et al. (Eds.), *Principles and practice of gynecologic oncology* (pp. 823-842). Philadelphia: Lippincott Williams & Wilkins.

Endometrial cancer. (2002). In R. R. Barakat, M. W. Bevers, D. M. Gershenson, et al. (Eds.), *Memorial Sloan-Kettering Cancer Center & MD Anderson Cancer Center handbook of gynecologic oncology* (pp. 283-290). London: Martin Dunitz.

Zorab, R., et al. (2002). Adenocarcinoma of the uterus. In P. J. DiSaia, & W. T. Creasman, *Clinical gynecologic oncology* (pp.137-163). St. Louis: Mosby.

Gestational Trophoblastic Neoplasia

DEFINITION

Gestational trophoblastic disease (GTD) applies to tumors that arise in the fetal chorion. Although these tumors most commonly follow a molar pregnancy, they may develop after any gestation. GTDs include benign partial and complete hydatidiform moles, persistent invasive or metastatic moles, placental-site trophoblastic tumors, and gestational choriocarcinomas. Whether hydatidiform moles are classified as complete (malignant) or partial (rarely malignant) is based on gross morphological features, histopathological examination, and karyotype. This section focuses on gestational trophoblastic neoplasia (GTN), which is recognized as the most curable gynecological malignancy.

INCIDENCE

The reported incidence of GTDs varies around the world. The incidence of molar gestation in the United States is about 1 per 1,500 live births. The frequency of molar pregnancy in Asian countries is seven to ten times greater than that reported in North America or Europe. These variations in incidence rates are thought to result partly from the use of different reporting methods.

ETIOLOGY AND RISK FACTORS

Risk factors may include the following:
- Age (an increase in incidence has been seen in women <15 years old and >40 years old)
- Increased risk in women with a prior molar pregnancy
- Prior use of oral contraceptives
- History of prior spontaneous abortion and infertility

SIGNS AND SYMPTOMS

Almost all patients with a complete hydatidiform mole have delayed

Major Cancers

menses, and most patients are considered to be pregnant. Vaginal bleeding usually occurs during the first trimester. The most significant symptom of a complete mole is acute respiratory distress that may be the result of the embolization of molar tissue to the pulmonary vasculature. Other factors such as cardiovascular complications of thyroid storm, preeclampsia, or massive fluid replacement may also contribute to this condition. Other signs of a complete mole are as follows:

- Excessive uterine size for gestational age
- Hyperemesis
- Preeclampsia
- Hyperthyroidism

DIAGNOSTIC WORKUP

Ultrasonography has become the test of choice in the diagnosis of a molar pregnancy. It notes multiple echoes that are formed by the interface between the molar villi and the surrounding tissue without the normal gestational sac or fetus present. In rare cases, a fetus may coexist with a mole. Human chorionic gonadotropin (hCG) levels may be markedly elevated with a complete mole and therefore may also be used along with ultrasonography for diagnosis.

HISTOLOGY

Complete hydatidiform moles are diploid conceptions of paternal origin that are characterized by generalized diffuse hyperplasia of both cytotrophoblast and syncytiotrophoblast elements.

CLINICAL STAGING

The International Federation of Gynecology and Obstetrics reports data on gestational trophoblastic tumors according to an anatomical staging system (see box on right). International staging enables comparable reporting of data.

TREATMENT

If preservation of fertility is not desired, hysterectomy may be performed. Hysterectomy eliminates the risks of local invasion, but it does not prevent metastasis. If the patient

---

International Federation of Gynecology and Obstetrics Anatomic Staging for Gestational Trophoblastic Neoplasia

Stage I:	Disease confined to the uterus
Stage II:	Disease extends outside of the uterus but is limited to the genital structures (adnexa, vagina, broad ligament)
Stage III:	Disease extends to the lungs, with or without known genital tract involvement
Stage IV:	All other metastatic sites

Data from Benedet, J.L., Bender, H., Jones, H., 3rd, Ngan, H.Y., & Pecorelli, S. (2000), FIGO staging classifications and clinical practice guidelines in the management of gynecologic cancers. FIGO Committee on Gynecologic Oncology. *International Journal of Gynaecology and Obstetrics*, 70(2), 206-62.

---

desires to preserve fertility, suction curettage is the preferred method of evacuation regardless of uterine size. All patients must be followed up with hCG measurements to ensure remission. Chemotherapy is started immediately if hCG titer rises or plateaus during follow-up or if metastases are detected at any time. Single-agent methotrexate or actinomycin D is the treatment of choice for nonmetastatic GTN.

PROGNOSIS

Treatment of nonmetastatic GTN has been 100% successful. Patients with GTN who are found to have metastatic disease are categorized as good prognosis when **none** of the following is present:

- Brain or liver metastasis
- Urinary hCG titer >100,000 IU/24 hr or serum beta-hCG titer greater than 40,000 mIU/mL
- Previous chemotherapy
- Symptoms (antecedent pregnancy) longer than 4 months

When patients are found to have any of the above, the prognosis is considered poor and treatment is a major challenge. Multiple-agent chemotherapy is recommended with a combination therapy of methotrexate, dactinomycin, and chlorambucil. Patients with brain or liver metastasis

---

are treated with the above chemotherapy concurrently with whole brain or liver radiation.

PREVENTION

Avoid pregnancy before the age of 15 years or after the age of 40 years and avoid use of oral contraceptives because these are the only controllable risk factors documented for this disease.

BIBLIOGRAPHY

Denny, L., Hacker, N. F., Gori, J., et al. (2000). Staging classifications and clinical practice guidelines for gynaecologic cancers. *International Journal of Gynecology and Obstetrics*, 70, 207-312.

Hoskins, W. J., et al. Gestational trophoblastic diseases. (2005). In W. J. Hoskins, C. A. Perez, R. C. Young, et al. (Eds.). *Principles and practice of gynecologic oncology* (pp.1055-1063). Philadelphia: Lippincott Williams & Wilkins.

Gestational trophoblastic disease. (2002). In R. R. Barakat, M. W. Bevers, D. M. Gershenson, et al. (Eds.). *Memorial Sloan-Kettering Cancer Center & MD Anderson Cancer Center handbook of gynecologic oncology* (pp.341-351). Philadelphia: Lippincott Williams & Wilkins.

Zorab, R., et al. (2002). Gestational trophoblastic neoplasia. In P. J. DiSaia, & W. T. Creasman (Eds.). *Clinical gynecologic oncology* (pp.185-200). St. Louis: Mosby.

Ovarian Cancer

DEFINITION

Ovarian cancer is the leading cause of death from gynecological cancer in the United States. The majority (85%-90%) of malignant ovarian tumors seen in the United States are epithelial neoplasms. The remaining percentages consist of ovarian germ cell tumors and sex cord–stromal tumors.

INCIDENCE

Approximately 23% of gynecologic cancers are of ovarian origin, but 47% of all deaths from cancer of the female genital tract occur in women who have ovarian cancer. The American

Cancer Society estimates that in 2007, 22,430 women will be diagnosed with ovarian cancer with 15,280 deaths from the disease in the United States alone. It has been estimated that, in the United States, one woman in 70 will have ovarian cancer. In African American women the average incidence is 10 per 100,000 compared with 13 to 15 in white women. The rate of ovarian cancer may be on the decline because there was a 0.7% decreased rate per year noted from 1985 through 2002.

ETIOLOGY AND RISK FACTORS

The molecular events leading to the development of epithelial ovarian cancer are unknown. Epidemiological studies have identified endocrine, environmental, and genetic factors as being important in the development of ovarian cancer.

Epidemiologically established risk factors include the following:
- Nulliparity
- Family history (probably 10% of all epithelial ovarian carcinomas result from a hereditary predisposition)
- Genetic mutations or syndromes including BRCAI, BRCAII and hereditary nonpolyposis colon cancer
- Early menarche and late menopause
- White race
- Increasing age
- Residence in Western industrialized countries

SIGNS AND SYMPTOMS

Early-stage disease may remain asymptomatic until ovarian masses are quite large. As the neoplasm enlarges, it begins to rise out of the pelvis and may account for abdominal enlargement. Early symptoms often include the following:
- Vague abdominal discomfort
- Dyspepsia
- Mild digestive disturbances

These early symptoms may be present for several months before the diagnosis. These complaints are usually recognized as nothing more than indigestion. These vague symptoms unfortunately result in more than half of the women who have ovarian cancer presenting with late stage (stage III-IV) disease at diagnosis.

DIAGNOSTIC WORKUP

Although routine pelvic examinations detect only one case of ovarian cancer in 10,000 asymptomatic women, it still remains the most practical means of detecting early disease. There is no evidence available yet that transvaginal ultrasonography or screening for serum CA125 can be used to reduce deaths from ovarian cancer. Serum CA125 levels, although not exclusive to ovarian cancer, may reflect volume of disease and can be a powerful tool in monitoring for tumor response and relapse.

HISTOLOGY

Epithelial ovarian malignancies are adenocarcinomas that can have a variety of histologic appearances, including the following:
- Serous   42%
- Mucinous   12%
- Endometroid   15%
- Undifferentiated 17%
- Clear cell   6%

There is limited prognostic significance to the histologic type of malignant epithelial ovarian cancer independent of clinical stage, extent of residual disease, and histologic grade.

STAGING

The staging of ovarian cancer is surgical and based on the operative findings at the start of the procedure. See the table on page 84 for International Federation of Gynecology and Obstetrics staging.

TREATMENT

The recommended treatment includes primary surgery for diagnosis, staging, and cytoreduction, followed by chemotherapy. The goal of primary surgery is to reduce the burden of ovarian cancer to no or minimal residual disease. Surgical treatment usually includes a total abdominal hysterectomy and bilateral salpingo-oophorectomy.

- In younger women with very early disease (stage IA) who may wish to have children, surgery may only include removal of one ovary.
- There are several treatment choices for stage IIa, IIb, and IIc disease. The most commonly used treatment plan is surgery, total abdominal hysterectomy, and bilateral salpingo-oophorectomy, followed by a platinum-taxane chemotherapy. Another option would be to follow surgery with instillation of phosphorus 32, postoperative abdominal and pelvic irradiation, or the combination of pelvic irradiation and systemic chemotherapy.
- For patients with stage III disease, in addition to the removal of the uterus and both adnexa, every effort should be made to remove the bulk of the tumor, including the large omental cakes. Unlike many other solid tumors, effective cytoreduction or debulking results in a survival benefit. Surgery is followed by platinum-taxane chemotherapy given intravenously. For patients who have had their tumors optimally debulked and who have <1 cm residual tumor, intravenous plus intraperitoneal platinum-taxane therapy may be used.
- For stage IV disease, the tumor should be optimally debulked and again a platinum-taxane combination therapy should be administered postoperatively.
- In all stages, the value of omentectomy remains inconclusive, but omentectomy does serve as a valuable diagnostic tool.

PROGNOSIS

The 5-year survival rate of patients with epithelial ovarian cancer is directly correlated with the tumor stage. Overall 1-year and 5-year survival rates for women diagnosed with ovarian cancer are 76% and 45%, respectively. The rates of 5-year survival diminish greatly with the advancing stages of the disease. Patients with early or local disease

TNM and International Federation of Gynecology and Obstetrics Clinical Staging: Ovarian Cancer

The definitions of the T categories correspond to the stages accepted by the International Federation of Gynecology and Obstetrics (FIGO). Both systems are included for comparison.

TNM Categories	FIGO Stages	Definitions
Primary Tumor (T)		
TX		Primary tumor cannot be assessed
T0		No evidence of primary tumor
T1	I	Tumor limited to ovaries (one or both)
T1a	IA	Tumor limited to one ovary; capsule intact, no tumor on ovarian surface. No malignant cells in ascites or peritoneal washings*
T1b	IB	Tumor limited to both ovaries; capsules intact, no tumor on ovarian surface. No malignant cells in ascites or peritoneal washings*
T1c	IC	Tumor limited to one or both ovaries with any of the following: capsule ruptured, tumor on ovarian surface, malignant cells in ascites or peritoneal washings*
T2	II	Tumor involves one or both ovaries with pelvic extension or implants
T2a	IIA	Extension or implants on uterus and/or tube(s). No malignant cells in ascites or peritoneal washings
T2b	IIB	Extension to or implants on other pelvic tissues. No malignant cells in ascites or peritoneal washings
T2c	IIC	Pelvic extension or implants (T2a or T2b) with malignant cells in ascites or peritoneal washings
T3	III	Tumor involves one or both ovaries with microscopically confirmed peritoneal metastasis outside the pelvis
T3a	IIIA	Microscopic peritoneal metastasis beyond pelvis (no macroscopic tumor)
T3b	IIIB	Macroscopic peritoneal metastasis beyond pelvis 2 cm or less in greatest dimension
T3c	IIIC	Peritoneal metastasis beyond pelvis more than 2 cm in greatest dimension or regional lymph node metastasis

*NOTE: The presence of nonmalignant ascites is not classified. The presence of ascites does not affect staging unless malignant cells are present.
NOTE: Liver capsule metastasis T3/Stage III; liver parenchymal metastasis M1/Stage IV. Pleural effusion must have positive cytological findings for M1/Stage IV.

Regional Lymph Nodes (N)		
NX		Regional lymph nodes cannot be assessed
N0		No regional lymph node metastasis
N1	IIIC	Regional lymph node metastasis

Distant Metastasis (M)		
MX		Distant metastasis cannot be assessed
M0		No distant metastasis
M1	IV	Distant metastasis (excludes peritoneal metastasis)

pTNM Pathological Classification

The pT, pN, and PM categories correspond to the T, N, and M categories.

Stage Grouping

Stage I	T1	N0	M0
Stage IA	T1a	N0	M0
Stage IB	T2b	N0	M0
Stage IC	T1c	N0	M0
Stage II	T2	N0	M0
Stage IIA	T2a	N0	M0
Stage IIB	T2b	N0	M0
Stage IIC	T2c	N0	M0
Stage III	T3	N0	M0
Stage IIIA	T3s	N0	M0
Stage IIIB	T3b	N0	M0
Stage IIIC	T3c	N0	M0
	Any T	N1	M0
Stage IV	Any T	Any N	M1

have a 5-year survival rate of 94%; however, only about 19% of all ovarian cancers are diagnosed this early in the disease. For regional and distant disease, the 5-year survival rates fall to 68% and 29%. Relative survival also varies by age; younger women <65 years old are twice as likely to survive 5 years than older women, 57% and 28%, respectively. The volume of residual disease after cytoreductive surgery also correlates with survival. Patients whose tumors have been optimally cytoreduced have a 22-month improvement in median survival compared with those patients undergoing less than optimum resection.

PREVENTION

When different cultures, such as Japanese and Americans, are examined, there is a strong suggestion that causative factors for ovarian cancer are probably in the immediate environment, such as food and personal customs. But to date there are no clues as to which dietary items or other environmental contacts might be specifically carcinogenic for the ovary. Controllable factors that are being studied closely at this point are as follows:

- Parity (increased number of term pregnancies shows decreased number of ovarian cancer cases)
- Oral contraceptive use (increased duration of use shows decreased number of ovarian cancer cases)

The theory of incessant ovulation suggests that the epithelial lining of the ovary may be sensitive to the constant trauma of ovulation.

BIBLIOGRAPHY

Armstrong, D. K, Bundy, B., Wenzel, L., et al. (2006). Intraperitoneal cisplatin and paclitaxel in ovarian cancer. *New England Journal of Medicine, 354,* 34-43.

Denny, L., Hacker, N. F., Gori, J., et al. (2000). Staging classifications and clinical practice guidelines for gynaecologic cancers. *International Journal of Gynecology and Obstetrics 70,* 207-312.

Hoskins, W. J., et al. (2005). Epithelial ovarian cancer. In W. J. Hoskins, C. A. Perez, R. C. Young, et al.

(Eds.). *Principles and practice of gynecologic oncology* (pp. 895-920). Philadelphia: Lippincott Williams & Wilkins.

Jemal, A., Siegel, R., Ward, E., et al. (2007). Cancer Statistics, 2007. *CA: A Cancer Journal for Clinicians.* 57(1);p. 15-16.

Zorab, R. et al. (2002). Epithelial ovarian. In P. J. DiSaia, & W. T. Creasman, (Eds.). *Clinical gynecologic oncology* (pp. 289-312). St. Louis: Mosby.

Vaginal Cancer

DEFINITION

The vaginal tissues are relatively immune to malignant change. When primary vaginal cancer does occur, it is usually in the upper third of the vagina. Any malignancy involving both the cervix and vagina that is histologically compatible with origin in either organ is classified as cervical cancer.

INCIDENCE

Vaginal cancer is rare, representing only 1% to 2% of all female genital tract malignancies. The majority of vaginal neoplasms are metastases from other primary sites such the cervix, vulva, and endometrium. More rigid diagnostic criteria to determine the site of the primary lesion has decreased the number of vaginal cancers recently reported.

ETIOLOGY AND RISK FACTORS

The cause of vaginal carcinoma is basically unknown. Some of the possible risk factors include the following:

- Socioeconomic status
- History of human papillomavirus infection
- Chronic vaginal irritation
- Prior Papanicolaou smear with cervical intraepithelial neoplasia
- Prior treatment for cervical cancer
- In utero exposure to diethylstilbestrol during the first 12 weeks of pregnancy is associated with an increased incidence of clear-cell adenocarcinoma of the vagina

Carcinoma of the vagina has been associated with advanced age, and there has been an increase incidence in younger women. This is possibly due to increased incidences of human papillomavirus infection.

SIGNS AND SYMPTOMS

Vaginal discharge, frequently bloody, is the most common reported symptom. Postcoital spotting, irregular or postmenopausal bleeding, and dysuria are also seen. Pelvic pain is a relative late symptom and is generally related to tumor extended beyond the vagina.

DIAGNOSTIC WORKUP

Patients with suspected vaginal malignancy should undergo the following:

- Thorough physical examination
- Detailed speculum inspection
- Digital palpation
- Colposcopy and cytological evaluation
- Biopsy

HISTOLOGY

Eighty to ninety percent of primary vaginal carcinomas are squamous cell neoplasms. The remaining are made up of adenocarcinomas, melanomas, and mesenchymal tumors.

CLINICAL STAGING

At present, all primary malignancies of the vagina are staged clinically. Chest radiograph, bimanual and rectovaginal examination, cystoscopy, proctoscopy, and intravenous pyelogram are allowed by International Federation of Gynecology and Obstetrics to determine the extent of disease. See the table on page 86 for staging.

TREATMENT

Specific treatment plans are based on the stage and extent of disease. Very early stage (stage 0 and stage I) cases may be treated with surgery alone. The majority of cases of primary vaginal carcinoma are treated with radiation therapy. Both external beam and brachytherapy are used. The type of radiation used is tailored to both the stage and extent of disease. Concomitant chemoradiotherapy agents such as 5-fluorouracil, mitomycin, and cisplatinum have some promise in advanced disease, but more studies are needed for these combination regimens. Chemotherapy alone is used only is salvage therapy.

PROGNOSIS

The prognosis depends on the stage of the disease, but the number of patients who survive vaginal cancer has increased significantly. Reports have indicated survival rates are similar to those seen in patients with cervical cancer.

PREVENTION

Many women have no known risk factors, making prevention very difficult, if not impossible.

BIBLIOGRAPHY

Denny, L., Hacker, N. F., Gori, J., et al. (2000). Staging classifications and clinical practice guidelines for gynaecologic cancers. *International Journal of Gynecology and Obstetrics, 70*, 207-312.

Hoskins, W. J., et al. Vagina. (2005). In W. J. Hoskins, C. A. Perez, R. C. Young, et al. (Eds.). *Principles and practice of gynecologic oncology* (pp. 707-714). Philadelphia: Lippincott Williams & Wilkins.

Gestational trophoblastic disease (2002). In R. R. Barakat, M. W. Bevers, D. M. Gershenson, et al. (Eds.), *Memorial Sloan-Kettering Cancer Center & MD Anderson Cancer Center handbook of gynecologic oncology* (pp. 223-229). London: Martin Dunitz.

Zorab, R., et al. Invasive cancer of the vagina and urethra. (2002). In P. J. DiSaia & W. T. Creasman, (Eds.), *Clinical gynecologic oncology* (pp. 241-248). St. Louis: Mosby.

Vulvar Cancer

DEFINITION

Primary malignant tumors of the vulva are uncommon neoplasms that account for only 3% to 4% of all gynecologic cancers. The vulva consists of the external genital organs including the mons pubis, labia minora and

American Joint Committee on Cancer and International Federation of Gynecology and Obstetrics Clinical Staging: Vaginal Cancer

The definitions of the T categories correspond to the stages accepted by the International Federation of Gynecology and Obstetrics (FIGO). Both systems are included for comparison.

TNM Categories	FIGO Stages	Definition
Primary Tumor (T)		
TX		Primary tumor cannot be assessed
T0		No evidence of primary tumor
Tis	0	Carcinoma in situ
T1	I	Tumor confined to vagina
T2	II	Tumor invades paravaginal tissues but not to pelvic wall
T3	III	Tumor extends to pelvic wall*
T4	IVA	Tumor invades mucosa of the bladder or rectum or extends beyond the true pelvis (bullous edema is not sufficient evidence to classify a tumor as T4/IVA)

*Pelvic wall is defined as muscle, fascia, neurovascular structures, or skeletal portions of the bony pelvis.

Regional Lymph Nodes (N)		
NX		Regional lymph nodes cannot be assessed
N0		No regional lymph node metastasis
N1	IVB	Pelvic or inguinal lymph node metastasis

Distant Metastasis (M)		
MX		Distant metastasis cannot be assessed
M0		No distant metastasis
M1	IVB	Distant metastasis

Stage Grouping			
Stage 0	Tis	N0	M0
Stage I	T1	N0	M0
Stage II	T2	N0	M0
Stage III	T1-T3	N1	M0
	T3	N0	M0
Stage IVA	T4	Any N	M0
Stage IVB	Any T	Any N	M1

Used with the permission of the American Joint Committee on Cancer (AJCC), Chicago, Illinois. The original source for this material is the *AJCC Cancer staging manual*, Sixth Edition (2002) published by Springer Science and Business Media LLC, www.springerlink.com.

majora, clitoris, vaginal vestibule, perineal body, and their supporting subcutaneous tissues.

INCIDENCE

Malignant tumors of the vulva are rare and account for less than 5% of all cancers of the female genital tract. Most vulvar cancers occur in post-menopausal women, but recent reports show a trend toward younger age at diagnosis.

ETIOLOGY AND RISK FACTORS

The cause of vulvar cancer is unknown and the rarity of this disease site makes a detailed investigation of the epidemiological risk factors difficult. A number of potential associations have been suggested:

- History of preinvasive genital neoplasia
- Human papillomavirus infection
- Herpes simplex virus infection
- Syphilis
- Lichen sclerosus
- Hypertrophic dystrophy
- Diabetes mellitus
- Hypertension
- Obesity
- Immunosuppression
- Cigarette smoking
- Prior genital tract neoplasia

SIGNS AND SYMPTOMS

Most women with vulvar cancer present with pruritus and a recognizable lesion. Many women ignore or deny obvious symptoms and lesions for long periods of time and present with advanced disease. The presentation in these cases is generally local pain, bleeding, and surface drainage from the tumor.

DIAGNOSTIC WORKUP

Initial evaluation includes the following:

- Detailed physical examination with measurements of the primary tumor
- Assessment for extension to adjacent mucosal or bony structures
- Assessment for possible involvement of the inguinal lymph nodes

Presentation with small cancers and clinically negative groin nodes requires few diagnostic studies other than those for preoperative clearance. Additional radiographic and endoscopic studies should be considered for those with large primary tumors or suspected metastases. Neoplasia of the female genital tract is often multifocal, so evaluation of the vagina and cervix, including cervical cytological screening, should always be performed in women with vulvar neoplasms.

HISTOLOGY

The vulva is covered by keratinized squamous epithelium; therefore the majority (85%) of malignant vulvar tumors are squamous cell carcinomas. Melanoma is the second most common, accounting for 5% to 10% of cases. The remaining tumors are a diverse set of rare lesions that include basal cell carcinoma, adenocarcinomas, Paget's disease, and sarcomas arising from connective tissue.

STAGING

The International Federation of Gynecology and Obstetrics uses a modified TNM and surgical staging scheme for vulvar carcinoma. This staging system incorporates the major identified prognostic factors of increasing primary tumor volume, lymph node metastasis, and distant spread (see table on page 87).

American Joint Committee on Cancer and International Federation of Gynecology and Obstetrics Staging: Vulvar Carcinoma

The definitions of the T categories correspond to the stages accepted by the International Federation of Gynecology and Obstetrics (FIGO). Both systems are included for comparison.

TNM Categories	FIGO Stages	Definitions
Primary Tumor		
TX		Primary tumor cannot be assessed
T0		No evidence of primary tumor
Tis	0	Carcinoma in situ
T1	I	Tumor confined to the vulva or vulva and perineum, 2 cm or less in greatest dimension
T1a	IA	Tumor confined to the vulva or vulva and perineum, 2 cm or less in greatest dimension, and with stromal invasion to greater than 1 mm*
T1b	IB	Tumor confined to the vulva or vulva and perineum, 2 cm or less in greatest dimension, and with stromal invasion greater than 1 mm*
T2	II	Tumor confined to the vulva or vulva and perineum, more than 2 cm in greatest dimension
T3	III	Tumor of any size with contiguous spread to the lower urethra or vagina or anus
T4	IVA	Tumor invades any of the following: upper urethra, bladder mucosa, rectal mucosa, or is fixed to the pubic bone

*NOTE: The depth of invasion is defined as the measurement of the tumor from the epithelial-stromal junction of the adjacent most superficial dermal papilla to the deepest point of invasion

Regional Lymph Nodes (N)		
NX		Regional lymph nodes cannot be assessed
N0		No regional lymph node metastasis
N1	III	Unilateral regional lymph node metastasis
N2	IVA	Bilateral regional lymph node metastasis

Every effort should be made to determine the site and laterality of lymph node metastasis. However, if "regional lymph node metastases, NOS" is the final diagnosis, then the disease should be staged as N1.

Distant Metastasis (M)		
MX		Distant metastasis cannot be assessed
M0		No distant metastasis
M1	IVB	Distant metastasis (including pelvic lymph node metastasis)

Stage Grouping

Stage 0	Tis	N0	M0
Stage I	T1	N0	M0
Stage IA	T1a	N0	M0
Stage IB	T1b	N0	M0
Stage II	T2	N0	M0
Stage III	T1	N1	M0
	T2	N1	M0
	T3	N0	M0
	T3	N1	M0
Stage IVA	T1	N2	M0
	T2	N2	M0
	T3	N2	M0
	T4	Any N	M0
Stage IVB	Any T	Any N	M1

Used with the permission of the American Joint Committee on Cancer (AJCC), Chicago, Illinois. The original source for this material is the *AJCC Cancer staging manual,* Sixth Edition (2002) published by Springer Science and Business Media LLC, www.springerlink.com.

or low-risk disease. Most surgeons now limit the initial procedure to radical vulvectomy and bilateral inguinal lymphadenectomy and do not proceed with pelvic node therapy unless metastasis is demonstrated in the inguinal node area. If the presence of tumor is documented in the inguinal nodes, a pelvic lymphadenectomy is an option for therapy, on the involved side only. Some gynecologists now recommend pelvic lymph node irradiation for patients with positive inguinal nodes, but controversy still surrounds this approach.

Combined radiation therapy and surgery, as well as radiation alone and local surgery alone, have been applied to this disease. No adequate prospective studies comparing various therapies or combinations of such are available for analysis. Chemotherapy has been used primarily as a salvage therapy.

PROGNOSIS

Survival in cancer of the vulva is directly related to the extent of disease at the time diagnosis is made and treatment is started. It has been reported that in patients with negative nodes, irrespective of size of primary lesion, the 5-year survival rate is 90%. Only one fifth of patients with deep pelvic node metastasis survive 5 years.

PREVENTION

Combining the facts that vulvar cancer is a rare disease and the cause is truly unknown, it is difficult to determine what factors may prevent this disease.

BIBLIOGRAPHY

Denny, L., Hacker, N. F., Gori, J., et al. (2000). Staging classifications and clinical practice guidelines for gynaecologic cancers. *International Journal of Gynecology and Obstetrics, 70,* 207-312.

Hoskins, W. J., et al. (2005). Vulva. In W. J. Hoskins, C. A. Perez, R. C. Young, et al. (Eds.). *Principles and practice of gynecologic oncology* (pp. 665-672). Philadelphia: Lippincott Williams & Wilkins.

TREATMENT

Surgical emphasis has evolved to an individualized approach for tumors. Smaller vulvar tumors can be managed by less-radical surgical approaches than used in the past. More limited resections are proposed for certain subsets considered to represent early

Major Cancers

Zorab, R., et al. Invasive cancer of the vulva. (2002). In P. J. DiSaia & W. T. Creasman (Eds.). *Clinical gynecologic oncology* (pp. 211-229). St. Louis: Mosby.

Vulvar cancer. (2002). In R. R. Barakat, M. W. Bevers, D. M. Gershenson, et al. (Eds.). *Memorial Sloan-Kettering Cancer Center & MD Anderson Cancer Center handbook of gynecologic oncology.* (pp. 213-220). London: Martin Dunitz

Head and Neck Cancers

Roberta Anne Strohl

Laryngeal Cancer

DEFINITION

The larynx is divided into three anatomical regions:

- **Supraglottic larynx** includes the epiglottis, false vocal cords, ventricles, aryepiglottic folds, and arytenoids; approximately 34% of laryngeal cancers occur in this region.
- **Glottis** includes the true vocal cords and the anterior and posterior commissures; approximately 65% of laryngeal cancers occur in this region.
- **Subglottic region** begins about 1 cm below the true vocal cords and extends to the lower border of the cricoid cartilage or the first tracheal ring; approximately 1% of laryngeal cancers occur in this region.

INCIDENCE

The global incidence of cancers of the oral cavity, pharynx, and larynx is about 500,000 cases per year with 270,000 deaths. In the United States, the estimated incidence of new cases of cancer of the larynx for 2007 is 11,300 with 3,660 deaths estimated to occur. Men are nearly four times more likely to be diagnosed and die from the disease than women. The incidence also increases with age.

ETIOLOGY AND RISK FACTORS

It has been estimated that more than three fourths of head and neck cancers in the United States are related to tobacco and alcohol use. Risk factors include the following:

- Cigarette smoking is the single most important risk factor in head and neck cancer. The smoking attributable risk for laryngeal cancer is 79% in men and 87% in women.
- The combined use of alcohol and tobacco increases the risk of laryngeal cancer by about 50%. Alcohol and tobacco are believed to act synergistically. Alcohol itself is not a known carcinogen, and it may be that it damages the mucosa to allow increased cellular permeability to known carcinogens.
- Occupational exposure to wood dust
- Exposure to organic chemicals, coal products, cement, paint, varnish, and lacquer also increase risk.
- The human papillomavirus has been identified in some head and neck cancers.
- Personal history of laryngeal cancer—second primary tumors have been reported in up to 25% of patients whose initial lesion was controlled

SIGNS AND SYMPTOMS
Supraglottic

- Sore throat
- Painful swallowing
- Referred ear pain
- Change in voice quality
- Enlarged neck nodes
- Weight loss
- Aspiration

Glottic

- Hoarseness
- Difficulty swallowing
- Dyspnea
- Stridor
- Irritation of throat

Subglottic

- Dyspnea
- Hemoptysis
- Stridor

DIAGNOSTIC WORKUP

- Physical examination of oral cavity and neck
- Thorough palpation of neck for evidence of metastatic disease
- Mirror examination and endoscopy, if indicated
- Computed tomography and magnetic resonance imaging with contrast
- Biopsy of suspicious lesions

HISTOLOGY

Most head and neck cancers are squamous cell carcinomas.

CLINICAL STAGING

Staging is based on the best possible estimate of the extent of the disease before treatment according to the American Joint Committee on Cancer TNM classification (see table on pages 89-90).

TREATMENT

- Treatment often involves a multimodal approach. The choice of treatment is determined by the anticipated functional and cosmetic results and by the availability of the medical expertise required.
- Consideration is given to the efficacy of treatment and quality-of-life issues, such as preservation of voice in laryngeal tumors.
- Treatment for patients with recurrent lesions depends on the location and size of the recurrent lesion and on prior treatment.

Chemotherapy

- Historically, surgery and radiation therapy have formed the basis of therapy in head and neck tumors, with chemotherapy playing a minor role.
  - This has changed; platinum-based chemotherapy concurrent with radiation has become a new standard of care for locally advanced nonresectable lesions and laryngeal lesions.
  - Postoperative chemotherapy is often used in patients with a high-risk of recurrence: T3-4 lesions, positive nodes, or inadequate resection.
- Molecularly targeted therapies are available for head and neck cancers as well.
  - Epidermal growth factor is expressed in the majority of head and neck tumors.
  - Cetuximab, a monoclonal antibody, binds to the epidermal growth factor receptor and appears to be a promising agent in combination with paclitaxel and carboplatin.
- Neoadjuvant therapy for locally advanced head and neck cancer is undergoing investigation. In this case, chemotherapy is given before surgery to facilitate organ preservation.
  - Cisplatin/5-fluorouracil combination therapy is most commonly used.

Radiation

- Although most early lesions can be cured by either radiation or surgery, radiation may be reasonable to preserve the voice, leaving surgery for salvage if needed.
- Radiation therapy is most commonly external beam, treating the primary site and regional lymph nodes.
- Intensity-modulated radiation therapy has become more widely available as a technique to limit normal tissue reactions, which can be considerable in the head and neck region.
- Patients who smoke while on radiation therapy appear to have

Clinical Staging: Laryngeal Cancer

Definition of TNM

Primary Tumor (T)

TX	Primary tumor cannot be assessed
T0	No evidence of primary tumor
Tis	Carcinoma in situ

Supraglottis

T1	Tumor limited to one subsite of supraglottis with normal vocal cord ability
T2	Tumor invades mucosa of more than one adjacent subsite of supraglottis or glottis or region outside the supraglottis (e.g., mucosa of base of tongue, vallecula, medial wall or pyriform sinus) without fixation of the larynx
T3	Tumor limited to larynx with vocal cord fixation or invades any of the following: postcricoid area, pre-epiglottic tissues, paraglottic space, or minor thyroid cartilage erosion (e.g., inner cortex)
T4a	Tumor invades through the thyroid cartilage or invades tissues beyond the larynx (e.g. tracha, soft tissues of neck including deep extrinsic muscle of the tongue, strap muscles, thyroid, or esophagus)
T4b	Tumor invades prevertebral space, encases carotid artery, or invades mediastinal structures

Glottis

T1	Tumor limited to the vocal cord(s) (may involve anterior or posterior commissure) with normal mobility
T1a	Tumor limited to one vocal cord
T1b	Tumor involves both vocal cords
T2	Tumor extends to supraglottis or subglottis, or with impaired vocal cord mobility
T3	Tumor limited to the larynx with vocal cord fixation or invades paraglottic space, or minor thyroid cartilage erosion (e.g., inner cortex)
T4a	Tumor invades through the thyroid cartilage or invades tissues beyond the larynx (te.g, trachea, soft tissues of neck including deep extrinsic muscle of the tongue, strap muscles, thyroid, or esophagus)
T4b	Tumor invades prevertebral space, encases carotid artery, or invades mediastinal structures

Subglottis

T1	Tumor limited to the subglottis
T2	Tumor extends to the vocal cord(s) with normal or impaired mobility
T3	Tumor limited to larynx with vocal cord fixation
T4a	Tumor invades cricoid or thyroid cartilage or invades tissues beyond the larynx (e.g., trachea, soft tissues of neck including deep extrinsic muscles of the tongue, strap muscles, thyroid, or esophagus)
T4b	Tumor invades prevertebral space, encases carotid artery, or invades mediastinal structures

Regional Lymph Nodes (N)

NX	Regional lymph nodes cannot be assessed
N0	No regional lymph node metastasis
N1	Metastasis in single ipsilateral lymph node, 3 cm or less in greatest dimension
N2	Metastasis in a single ipsilateral lymph node, more than 3 cm but not more than 6 cm in greatest dimension, or in multiple ipsilateral lymph nodes, none more than 6 cm in greatest dimension, or in bilateral or contralateral lymph nodes, none more than 6 cm in greatest dimension
N2a	Metastasis in single ipsilateral lymph node, more than 3 cm but not more than 6 cm in greatest dimension
N2b	Metastasis in multiple ipsilateral lymph nodes, none more than 6 cm in greatest dimension
N2c	Metastasis in bilateral or contralateral lymph nodes, none more than 6 cm in greatest dimension
N3	Metastasis in a lymph node, more than 6 cm in greatest dimension

Distant Metastasis (M)

MX	Distant metastasis cannot be assessed
M0	No distant metastasis
M1	Distant metastasis

Major Cancers

Continued

Clinical Staging: Laryngeal Cancer—cont'd

Stage Grouping

Stage 0	Tis	N0	M0
Stage 1	T1	N0	M0
Stage II	T2	N0	M0
Stage III	T3	N0	M0
	T1	N1	M0
	T2	N1	M0
	T3	N1	M0
Stage IVA	T4a	N0	M0
	T4a	N1	M0
	T1	N2	M0
	T2	N2	M0
	T3	N2	M0
	T4a	N2	M0
Stage IVB	T4b	Any N	M0
	Any T	N3	M0
Stage IVC	Any T	Any N	M1

Used with the permission of the American Joint Committee on Cancer (AJCC), Chicago, Illinois. The original source for this material is the *AJCC Cancer staging manual,* Sixth Edition (2002) published by Springer Science and Business Media LLC, www.springerlink.com.

lower response rates and shorter survival durations than those who do not; therefore, patients should be counseled to stop smoking before beginning radiation therapy.

- Research suggests that there is a significant loss of local control when radiation therapy was not delivered according to planned schedule; therefore, lengthening of the radiation schedule should be avoided whenever possible

Surgery

- Surgical excision must encompass gross tumor and microscopic disease.
- If positive regional nodes are present, node dissection is usually done.
- Postoperatively, rehabilitation, including voice aids for laryngectomized patients, is important to ensure the best quality of life.

PROGNOSIS

The most important adverse prognostic factors for laryngeal cancers include tumor size, invasiveness and the presence or absence of positive lymph nodes. Other prognostic factors may include sex, age, performance status, and a variety of pathological features of the tumor, including grade and depth of invasion. Metastasis to bone and lymph nodes does occur; however, the consequences of local-regional disease, malnutrition, and cachexia remain the most difficult to manage.

The prognosis for small laryngeal cancers that have not spread to lymph nodes is very good, with cure rates of 75% to 95%. Locally advanced lesions are poorly controlled with surgery, radiation therapy, or combined modality treatment. Distant metastases are common, even if the primary tumor is controlled. Intermediate lesions have intermediate prognoses, depending on site, T status, N status, and performance status. Patients treated for laryngeal cancers are at the highest risk of recurrence in the first 2 to 3 years. Recurrences after 5 years are rare and usually represent new primary malignancies.

PREVENTION

Primary prevention of head and neck cancer requires cessation of alcohol and tobacco use. Individuals who have had one cancer in this region are at an increased risk for development of other cancers related to these risk factors, including other head and neck cancers, lung and esophageal tumors. Patients should be referred for counseling and support to address issues related to tobacco and alcohol use. Individuals with a history of head and neck cancer who cease tobacco and alcohol use retain a risk of a second primary at a rate of 3% to 7% per year. This has led to exploration of other preventive strategies such as vitamin A and the retinoids as chemoprevention. Clinical trials are in progress.

BIBLIOGRAPHY

Clarke, L. K. & Dropkin, M. J. (Eds.). (2006). *Site specific cancer series: head and neck cancer.* Pittsburgh, PA: Oncology Nursing Society.

Jemal, A., Siegel, R., Ward, E., et al. (2007). Cancer statistics, 2007. *CA: A Cancer Journal for Clinicians, 57,* 43-66.

National Cancer Institute. *Laryngeal cancer PDQ.* (2006). Retrieved Jan. 11, 2007, from http://www.cancer.gov/cancertopics/pdq/treatment/laryngeal/HealthProfessional.

Shah, J. (2001). *American Cancer Society atlas of clinical oncology: cancer of the head and neck.* London: BC Decker.

Oral Cavity Cancer

DEFINITION

Cancer of the oral cavity encompasses the following structures:

- Lip
- Anterior two thirds of tongue
- Buccal mucosa
- Floor of mouth
- Lower gingival
- Retromolar trigone
- Upper gingival
- Hard palate

INCIDENCE

Global incidence of cancers of the oral cavity, pharynx and larynx is about 500,000 cases per year with 270,000 deaths. In the United States, it is estimated that there will be 22,560 new cases of oral cavity in 2007, which includes 9,800 cases of cancer of the tongue; 10,660 new cases of mouth cancer; and 2,100 new cases of other oral cancers. Deaths from oral cavity cancer are estimated to be 5,370. Men are more likely to be diagnosed with oral cancer than women and the incidence also increases with age.

ETIOLOGY AND RISK FACTORS

It has been estimated that over three quarters of head and neck cancers in the United States are related to tobacco and alcohol use. Alcohol and tobacco are believed to act synergistically. Alcohol itself is not a known carcinogen and it may be that it damages the mucosa to allow increased cellular permeability to known carcinogens. Risk factors include:

- Cigarette smoking is the single most important risk factor in head and neck cancer.
  - In men, 90% of cancer risk for oral cancer is attributed to tobacco use. The risk for women is lower at 59%.
- Smokeless tobacco results in a 4- to 6-fold increase in cancers of the alveolar ridge and buccal mucosa.
- Occupational exposure to wood dust
- Exposure to organic chemicals, coal products, cement, paint, varnish, and lacquer
- Personal history of head and neck cancers have an increased chance of developing a second primary tumor
- The human papilloma virus (HPV 16)
- HIV
- Herpes simplex
- Diet low in fruits and vegetables
- Sun exposure increases risk of cancer of the lip

SIGNS AND SYMPTOMS

Presenting signs and symptoms may include:
- Leukoplakia
- Ulcer
- Lump or thickening
- Feeling of fullness in throat
- Dysphagia
- Jaw swelling
- Unilateral otalgia without hearing loss
- Pain
- Bleeding

DIAGNOSTIC WORK-UP

- Physical exam of oral cavity and neck.
  - Thorough palpation of neck for evidence of metastatic disease.
- Mirror exam and endoscopy if indicated.
- CT and MRI with contrast.
- Biopsy of suspicious lesions.

HISTOLOGY

More than 90% of oral cavity tumors are squamous cell carcinoma. Verrucous carcinoma is a type of squamous cell carcinoma accounting for less than 5% of oral cavity tumors. It rarely metastasizes but can spread deeply into surrounding tissue.

CLINICAL STAGING

Staging is done with the American Joint Committee on Cancer (AJCC) TNM classification (see table on page 92).

TREATMENT

- Treatment often involves a multimodal approach. Depending on the site and extent of the primary tumor and the status of the lymph nodes, the treatment of lip and oral cavity cancer may be by surgery alone, radiation therapy alone, or a combination of these.
- Early cancers (stage I and stage II) are highly curable by surgery or radiation therapy.
- The choice of treatment is determined by the anticipated functional and cosmetic results and by the availability of the medical expertise required.
- Most patients with stage III or stage IV tumors require multimodality approach of surgery and radiation therapy. Because of the risk of local recurrence and/or distant metastases in these patients, they should be considered for clinical trials.
- Treatment for patients with recurrent lesions will be dependent upon the location and size of the recurrent lesion as well as prior treatment.

Surgery

- For lesions of the oral cavity, surgical excision must encompass gross tumor as well as the microscopic disease.
- If positive regional nodes are present, cervical node dissection is usually done.
- Post-operatively, prosthodontic rehabilitation is important to assure the best quality of life.

Radiation

- Radiation therapy may be external-beam or brachytherapy using interstitial implants.
  - Local implants can be successful in treating small superficial cancers.
  - Larger lesions can be managed external-beam radiation therapy of the primary site and regional lymph nodes.
- Patients who smoke while on radiation therapy appear to have lower response rates and shorter survival durations than those who do not; therefore, patients should be counseled to stop smoking before beginning radiation therapy.

PROGNOSIS

Prognostic factors relate to the size, thickness, invasiveness, and vascular invasion, margins of resection, mitotic index, and morphology of the tumor as well as to the presence or absence of positive lymph nodes. If nodes are positive, prognostic factors include the number of positive nodes, the size of the largest node, laterality of nodes and the presence or absence of extracapsular extension.

Survival for head and neck cancers is stage dependent. Although metastatic disease to bone and lymph nodes does occur, the consequences of local-regional disease, malnutrition, and cachexia remain the most difficult to manage. Five-year survival rates for T1-2 lesions of the oral cavity ranges 70-90% and stage IV disease is less than 20%.

PREVENTION

Primary prevention of head and neck cancer requires cessation of alcohol and tobacco use. Individuals who have had one cancer in this region are at an increased risk to develop other cancers related to these risk factors including other head and neck cancers as well as lung and esophageal tumors. Patients should be referred for counseling and support to address issues related to tobacco and alcohol use. Individuals with a history of head and neck

Major Cancers

Clinical Staging: Cancers of the Oral Cavity

Definition of TNM

Primary Tumor (T)

TX	Primary tumor cannot be assessed
T0	No evidence of primary tumor
Tis	Carcinoma in situ
T1	Tumor 2 cm or less in greatest dimension
T2	Tumor more than 2 cam but not more than 4 cm in greatest dimension
T3	Tumor more than 4 cm in greatest dimension
T4*	(lip) Tumor invades through critical bone, inferior alveolar nerve, floor of mouth, or skin of face (i.e., chin or nose)
T4a	(oral cavity) Tumor invades adjacent structures (e.g., through cortical bone, into deep [extrinsic] muscle or tongue [genioglossus, hyoglossus, palatoglossus, and styloglossus], maxillary sinus, skin of face)
T4b	Tumor invades masticator space, pterygoid plates, or skull base and/or encases internal carotid artery

*NOTE: Superficial erosion alone of bone/tooth socket by gingival primary is not sufficient to classify a tumor as T4.

Regional Lymph Nodes (N)

NX	Regional lymph nodes cannot be assessed
N0	No regional lymph node metastasis
N1	Metastasis in single ipsilateral lymph node, 3 cm or less in greatest dimension
N2	Metastasis in a single ipsilateral lymph node, more than 3 cm but not more than 6 cm in greatest dimension; or in multiple ipsilateral lymph nodes, none more than 6 cm in greatest dimension; or in bilateral or contralateral lymph nodes, none more than 6 cm in greatest dimension
N2a	Metastasis in single ipsilateral lymph node more than 3 cm but not more than 6 cm in greatest dimension
N2b	Metastasis in multiple ipsilateral lymph nodes, none more than 6 cm in greatest dimension
N2c	Metastasis in bilateral or contralateral lymph nodes, none more than 6 cm in greatest dimension
N3	Metastasis in a lymph node more than 6 cm in greatest dimension

Distant Metastasis (M)

MX	Distant metastasis cannot be assessed
M0	No distant metastasis
M1	Distant metastasis

Stage Grouping

Stage 0	Tis	N0	M0
Stage I	T1	N0	M0
Stage II	T2	N0	M0
Stage III	T3	N0	M0
	T1	N1	M0
	T2	N1	M0
	T3	N1	M0
Stage IVA	T4a	N0	M0
	T4a	N1	M0
	T1	N2	M0
	T2	N2	M0
	T3	N2	M0
	T4a	N2	M0
Stage IVB	Any T	N3	M0
	T4b	Any N	M0
Stage IVC	Any T	Any N	M1

Used with the permission of the American Joint Committee on Cancer (AJCC), Chicago, Illinois. The original source for this material is the *AJCC Cancer staging manual,* Sixth Edition (2002) published by Springer Science and Business Media LLC, www.springerlink.com.

cancer that cease tobacco and alcohol use retain a risk of a second primary at a rate of 3-7% per year. This has led to exploration of other preventive strategies such as Vitamin A and the retinoids as chemoprevention. Clinical trials are ongoing.

BIBLIOGRAPHY

Clarke, L. K., & Dropkin, M. J. (Eds.) (2006). Site Specific Cancer Series: *Head and Neck Cancer.* Pittsburgh, PA: Oncology Nursing Society.

Jemal, A., Siegel, R., Ward, E., et al. (2007). Cancer Statistics, 2007. *CA: A Cancer Journal for Clinicians,* 57(1), 43-66.

National Cancer Institute. *Lip and Oral Cavity Cancer PDQ(r).* (2006). Retrieved Jan. 11, 2007, from http://www. cancer.gov/cancertopics/ pdq/treatment/lip-and-oral-cavity/ Health Professional

Shah, J. (2001). *American Cancer Society Atlas of Clinical Oncology Cancer of the Head and Neck.* London: BC Decker.

Pharyngeal Cancer

DEFINITION

Pharyngeal cancer encompasses the following structures:

- The **nasopharynx** is behind the nose and is the upper part of the throat. The nares lead into the nasopharynx. Two openings on the side of the nasopharynx lead into the ear. Cancer of the nasopharynx most commonly starts in the cells that line the oropharynx.
- The **oropharynx** is the middle part of the throat. The oropharynx includes the soft palate, the base of the tongue, and the tonsils.
- The **hypopharynx** is the bottom part of the throat.

INCIDENCE

The global incidence of cancers of the oral cavity, pharynx, and larynx is about 500,000 cases per year with 270,000 deaths. In the United States, it is estimated that there will be 11,800 new cases of pharyngeal cancer in 2007 with 2,180 deaths from the disease. Men are nearly four times more likely to be diagnosed with pharyngeal cancer than women and nearly three times more likely to die from the disease. The incidence of oropharyngeal cancer is higher in African Americans than in whites. The incidence also increases with age.

ETIOLOGY AND RISK FACTORS

It has been estimated that more than three fourths of head and neck cancers in the United States are related to tobacco and alcohol use. Alcohol and tobacco are believed to act synergistically. Alcohol itself is not a known carcinogen and it may be that it damages the mucosa to allow increased cellular permeability to known carcinogens.

Risk factors include the following:

- Cigarette smoking is the single most important risk factor in head and neck cancer.
- After adjustment for tobacco use, the relative risk of pharyngeal cancer rises with increased alcohol consumption.
- Occupational exposure to wood dust
- Exposure to organic chemicals, coal products, cement, paint, varnish, and lacquer
- Those with a personal history of head and neck cancers have an increased chance for development of a second primary tumor.
- The rising incidence of oropharyngeal cancer in younger individuals without an alcohol and tobacco history is associated with human papillomavirus types 16, 18, 31, 33, and 35.
- Epstein-Barr viruses have been linked to nasopharyngeal cancer.
- Diet low in fruits and vegetables

SIGNS AND SYMPTOMS
Nasopharynx

- Neck mass
- Nasal obstruction
- Change in voice quality
- Serous otitis media

Oropharynx

- May be asymptomatic
- Sore throat
- Difficulty swallowing
- Foreign-body sensation in throat
- Altered voice
- Ear pain
- Neck lump is presenting sign in more than 50% of patients

Hypopharynx and Cervical Esophagus

- Dysphagia
- Hoarseness
- Neck mass
- Weight loss

DIAGNOSTIC WORKUP

- Physical examination of oral cavity and neck
  - Thorough palpation of neck for evidence of metastatic disease
- Mirror examination and endoscopy if indicated
- Computed tomography and magnetic resonance imaging with contrast
- Biopsy of suspicious lesions

HISTOLOGY

Most pharyngeal cancers are squamous cell carcinomas. Other oropharyngeal cancers include minor salivary gland tumors, lymphomas, and lymphoepitheliomas. Also, a wide variety of malignant tumors may arise in the nasopharynx; however, only squamous cell carcinoma is considered in this discussion because management of the others varies widely with histologic features.

CLINICAL STAGING

Staging is done with the American Joint Committee on Cancer TNM classification (see the table on pages 94-95). Staging is the same for hypopharyngeal and oropharyngeal cancer. Nasopharyngeal cancer is staged somewhat differently. Staging is not used to report the results of radiation therapy for nasopharyngeal carcinoma. Locoregional control and survival are usually reported by T status and N status separately or by specific T and N subgroupings.

TREATMENT

- Treatment often involves a multimodal approach.
- The choice of treatment is determined by the anticipated functional and cosmetic results and by the availability of the medical expertise required.
- Consideration is given to the efficacy of treatment and quality-of-life issues.
- Treatment for patients with recurrent lesions will depend on the location and size of the recurrent lesion and on prior treatment.

Chemotherapy

- Historically, surgery and radiation therapy have formed the basis of

therapy in head and neck tumors, with chemotherapy playing a minor role. Early cancers (stage I and stage II) are highly curable by surgery or radiation therapy.
- Platinum-based chemotherapy concurrent with radiation has become a new standard of care for locally advanced nonresectable lesions, nasopharyngeal lesions, and oropharyngeal lesions.
- Postoperative chemotherapy is often used in patients with a high risk of recurrence: T3-4 lesions, positive nodes, or inadequate resection. Molecularly targeted therapies are available for head and neck cancers as well.
  - Epidermal growth factor is expressed in the majority of head and neck tumors.
  - Cetuximab, a monoclonal antibody, binds to the epidermal growth factor receptor and appears to be a promising agent in combination with paclitaxel and carboplatin.
- Neoadjuvant therapy for locally advanced head and neck cancer is undergoing investigation.
  - In this case, chemotherapy is given before surgery; to facilitate organ preservation.
  - Cisplatin/5-fluorouracil combination therapy is most commonly used.

Surgery

- Surgical excision must encompass gross tumor and the microscopic disease.
- If positive regional nodes are present, node dissection is usually done.
- Postoperatively, rehabilitation is important to ensure the best quality of life.

Radiation

- Radiation therapy may be external beam or brachytherapy with interstitial implants. Local implants can be successful in treating small superficial cancers. Larger lesions can be managed with external beam radiation therapy of the primary site and regional lymph nodes.

- Intensity-modulated radiation therapy has become more widely available as a technique to limit normal tissue reactions, which can be considerable in the head and neck region.
- Patients who smoke while on radiation therapy appear to have lower response rates and shorter survival durations than those who do not; therefore, patients should be counseled to stop smoking before beginning radiation therapy.
- Research suggests that there is a significant loss of local control when radiation therapy was not delivered according to planned schedule; therefore, lengthening of the radiation schedule should be avoided whenever possible.

PROGNOSIS

Prognostic factors relate to the size, thickness, invasiveness and vascular invasion, margins of resection, mitotic index, and morphologic features of the tumor as well as to the presence or absence of positive lymph nodes. If nodes are positive, the number of positive nodes, the size of the largest node, laterality of nodes, and the presence or absence of extracapsular extension further affect prognosis.

Survival for head and neck cancers is stage dependent. Although metastatic disease to bone and lymph nodes does occur, the consequences of local-regional disease, malnutrition, and cachexia, remain the most difficult to manage. Outcomes are shown in the table on page 95.

PREVENTION

Primary prevention of head and neck cancer requires cessation of alcohol and tobacco use. Individuals who have had one cancer in this region are at an increased risk for development of other cancers related to these risk factors, including other head and neck cancers and lung and esophageal tumors. Patients should be referred for counseling and support to address issues related to tobacco and alcohol use.

Individuals with a history of head and neck cancer who cease tobacco

Clinical Staging: Pharyngeal Cancer

Definition of TNM

Primary Tumor (T)

TX	Primary tumor cannot be assessed
T0	No evidence of primary tumor
Tis	Carcinoma in situ

Nasopharynx

T1	Tumor confined to the nasopharynx
T2	Tumor extends to soft tissues
T2a	Tumor extends to the oropharynx or nasal cavity without parapharyngeal extension
T2b	Any tumor with parapharyngeal extension*
T3	Tumor involves bony structures or paranasal sinuses
T4	Tumor with intracranial extension and/or involvement of cranial nerves, infratemporal fossa, hypopharynx, orbit, or masticular space

*NOTE: Parapharyngeal extension denotes posterolateral infiltration of tumor beyond the pharyngobasilar fascia.

Oropharynx

T1	Tumor cm or less in greatest dimension
T2	Tumor more than 2 cm but not more than 4 cm in greatest dimension
T3	Tumor more than 4 cm in greatest dimension
T4a	Tumor invades the larynx, deep/extrinsic muscle of tongue, medial pterygoid, hard palate, or mandible
T4b	Tumor invades lateral pterygoid muscle, pterygoid plates, lateral nasopharynx, or skull base or encases carotid artery

Hypopharynx

T1	Tumor limited to one subsite of hypopharynx and 2 cm or less in greatest dimension
T2	Tumor invades more than one subsite of hypopharynx or an adjacent site, or measures more than 2 cm but not more than 4 cm in greatest diameter without fixation of hemilarynx
T3	Tumor more than 4 cm in greatest dimension or with fixation of hemilarynx
T4a	Tumor invades thyroid/cricoid cartilage, hyoid bone, thyroid gland, esophagus, or central compartment soft tissue*
T4b	Tumor invades prevertebral fascia, encases carotid artery, or involves mediastinal structures

*NOTE: Central compartment soft tissue includes prelaryngeal strap muscles and subcutaneous fat.

Regional Lymph Nodes (N)

Nasopharynx

The distribution and the prognostic impact of regional lymph node spread from nasopharynx cancer, particularly of the undifferentiated type, are different from those of other head and neck cancers and justify the use of a different N classification scheme.

NX	Regional lymph nodes cannot be assessed
N0	No regional lymph node metastasis
N1	Unilateral metastasis in lymph node(s), 6 cm or less in greatest dimension, above the supraclavicular fossa*
N2	Bilateral metastasis in lymph node(s), 6 cm or less in greatest dimension, above the supraclavicular fossa*
N3	Metastasis in a lymph node(s)(n >6 cm and/or to supraclavicular fossa
N3a	Greater than 6 cm in dimension
N3b	Extension to the supraclavicular fossa**

*NOTE: Midline nodes are considered ipsilateral nodes.

**Supraclavicular zone or fossa is relevant to the staging of nasopharyngeal carcinoma and is the triangular region defined by three points: (1) the superior margin of the sternal end of the clavicle, (2) the superior margin of the lateral end of the clavicle, (3) the point where the neck meets the shoulder. Note that this would include caudal portions of Levels IV and V. All cases with lymph nodes (whole or part) in the fossa are considered N3b.

Oropharynx and Hypopharynx

NX	Regional lymph nodes cannot be assessed
N0	No regional lymph node metastasis
N1	Metastasis in a single ipsilateral lymph node, 3 cm or less in greatest dimension

Clinical Staging: Pharyngeal Cancer—cont'd

N2	Metastasis in a single ipsilateral lymph node, more than 3 cm not more than 6 cm in greatest dimension, or in multiple ipsilateral lymph nodes, none more than 6 cm in greatest dimension, or in bilateral or contralateral lymph nodes, none more than 6 cm in greatest dimension
N2a	Metastasis in a single ipsilateral lymph node more than 3 cm but not more than 6 cm in greatest dimension
N2b	Metastasis in multiple ipsilateral lymph nodes, none more than 6 cm in greatest dimension
N2c	Metastasis in bilateral or contralateral lymph nodes, none more than 6 cm in greatest dimension
N3	Metastasis in a lymph node more than 6 cm in greatest dimension

Distant Metastasis (M)

MX	Distant metastasis cannot be assessed
M0	No distant metastasis
M1	Distant metastasis

Stage Grouping: Nasopharynx

Stage	T	N	M
Stage 0	Tis	N0	M0
Stage I	T1	N0	M0
Stage IIA	T2a	N0	M0
Stage IIB	T1	N1	M0
	T2	N1	M0
	T2a	N1	M0
	T2b	N0	M0
	T2v	N1	M0
Stage III	T1	N2	M0
	T2a	N2	M0
	T2b	N2	M0
	T3	N0	M0
	T3	N1	M0
	T3	N2	M0
Stage IVA	T4	N0	M0
	T4	N1	M0
	T4	N2	M0
Stage IVB	Any t	N3	M0
Stage IVC	Any T	Any N	M1

Stage Grouping: Oropharynx, Hypopharynx

Stage	T	N	M
Stage 0	Tis	N0	M0
Stage I	T1	N0	M0
Stage II	T2	N0	M0
Stage III	T3	N0	M0
	T1	N1	M0
	T2	N1	M0
	T3	N1	M0
Stage IVA	T4a	N0	M0
	T4a	N1	M0
	T1	N2	M0
	T2	N2	M0
	T3	N2	M0
	T4a	N2	M0
Stage IVB	T4b	Any N	M0
	Any T	N3	M0
Stage IVC	Any T	Any N	M1

Used with the permission of the American Joint Committee on Cancer (AJCC), Chicago, Illinois. The original source for this material is the *AJCC Cancer staging manual*, Sixth Edition (2002) published by Springer Science and Business Media LLC, www.springerlink.com.

Survival for Pharyngeal Cancer

Base of tongue (oropharynx)	2-yr survival: T1: 96% T2: 57%-92%	2-yr survival: T3: 45%-72% T4: 23%-40%
Tonsil (oropharynx)	5-yr survival: Stage I: 93%-100% Stage II: 57%-77%	5-yr survival: Stage III: 27%-52% Stage IV: 17%-29%
Nasopharynx	5-yr survival: T1: 76% T2: 68%	5-yr survival: T3: 58% T4: 0%-42%

and alcohol use retain a risk of a second primary at a rate of 3% to 7% per year. This has lead to exploration of other preventive strategies such as vitamin A and the retinoids as chemoprevention. Clinical trials are in progress.

BIBLIOGRAPHY

Clarke, L. K., & Dropkin, M. J. (Eds.). (2006). *Site specific cancer series: head and neck cancer*. Pittsburgh, PA: Oncology Nursing Society.

Jemal, A., Siegel, R., Ward, E., et al. (2007). Cancer statistics, 2007. *CA: A Cancer Journal for Clinicians, 57*, 43-66.

National Cancer Institute. (2006). *Hypopharyngeal cancer PDQ*. Retrieved Janurary 11, 2007, from http://www.cancer.gov/cancertopics/pdq/treatment/hypopharyngeal/ healthprofessional.

National Cancer Institute. (2006). *Nasopharyngeal cancer PDQ*. Retrieved January 11, 2007, from http://www.cancer.gov/cancertopics/pdq/treatment/nasopharyngeal/healthprofessional.

National Cancer Institute. (2006). *Oropharyngeal cancer PDQ*. Retrieved January 11, 2007, from http://www.cancer.gov/cancertopics/pdq/treatment/oropharyngeal/healthprofessional.

Shah, J. (2001). *American Cancer Society atlas of clinical oncology: cancer of the head and neck*. London: BC Decker.

Salivary Gland Cancer

DEFINITION

Tumors of the salivary glands can involve either the major glands or the minor glands. The three major glands include the following:

- **Parotid:** largest salivary glands, found in front of and just below the ear. Approximately 70% to 80% of major salivary gland tumors begin in this gland.
- **Submandibular:** glands found below the jawbone
- **Sublingual:** glands found under the tongue in the floor of the mouth

There are hundreds of minor salivary glands found in the oral mucosa, palate, uvula, floor of mouth, posterior tongue, retromolar area and peritonsillar area, pharynx, larynx, or paranasal sinuses. Most of the minor salivary gland tumors begin in the palate.

More than half of salivary gland tumors are benign. The frequency of malignant lesions vary by site of origin with approximately 20% to 25% of parotid tumors, 35% to 40% of submandibular tumors, 50% of palate tumors, and more than 90% of sublingual gland tumors.

INCIDENCE

Neoplasms of the salivary glands are rare, with an overall incidence in the Western world of approximately 2.5 to 3.0 cases per 100,000 per year. Malignant salivary gland neoplasms account for <0.5% of all malignancies and approximately 3% to 5% of all head and neck cancers. Most patients are diagnosed in the sixth or seventh decade of life

ETIOLOGY AND RISK FACTORS

Little is available about the etiology of malignant salivary gland tumors. Factors associated with increased risk include the following:

- Increased age
- Prior radiation therapy to the head and neck area
- Tobacco use may be a risk factor for squamous cell cancer but does not likely increase the risk for other salivary gland tumor types.
- A diet high in animal fat and deplete of vegetables has been suggest to increase the risk.
- Occupations associated with an increased risk for salivary gland cancers include rubber products manufacturing, asbestos mining, plumbing, and some types of woodworking.

SIGNS AND SYMPTOMS

- Painless swelling of the parotid, submandibular, or sublingual glands
- Numbness or weakness in the face
- Persistent facial pain

DIAGNOSTIC WORKUP

- Physical examination and history
- Imaging studies: magnetic resonance imaging, computed tomography scan, positron emission tomography scan, or ultrasonography
- Endoscopy
- Biopsy of suspicious lesions.

HISTOLOGY

Salivary gland neoplasms are histologically diverse with almost 40 histologic types of epithelial tumors. Salivary gland carcinomas include the following:

- Mucoepidermoid carcinoma— the most common malignant major and minor salivary gland tumor
- Adenoid cystic carcinoma
- Adenocarcinomas
- Malignant mixed tumors
- Rare carcinomas

Histologic grading of salivary gland carcinomas aids in determining treatment. Grading is used primarily for mucoepidermoid carcinomas, adenocarcinomas (not otherwise specified), adenoid cystic carcinomas, and squamous cell carcinomas. In most instances, the histologic type defines the grade (i.e., salivary duct carcinoma is high grade and basal cell adenocarcinoma is low grade.)

CLINICAL STAGING

Various other salivary gland carcinomas can also be categorized according to histologic grade as follows. Staging is done according to the American Joint Committee on Cancer TNM classification (see table on page 97).

TREATMENT

Salivary gland tumors may be cured with surgery alone. Large bulky tumors or high-grade tumors carry a poorer prognosis, and treatment should include surgical resection with postoperative adjuvant radiation therapy. Postoperative radiation is also used if tumor cells are found in or close to the surgical margins or lymph node involvement is present. Neutron beam radiation is more effective than conventional x-ray radiotherapy.

Primary radiation therapy may be given for tumors that are inoperable, unresectable, or recurrent. Fast neutron beam radiation or accelerated hyperfractionated photon beam are reported to be more effective than conventional x-ray radiation therapy.

Patients with stage IV salivary gland cancer should be considered for clinical trials. Their cancers may be responsive to aggressive combinations of chemotherapy and radiation. Single-agent or combination chemotherapy with doxorubicin, cisplatin, cyclophosphamide, and 5-fluorouracil has modest response rates.

PROGNOSIS

Prognosis depends on the following:
- Salivary gland of origin
- Histologic features
- Grade
- Stage
- Involvement of facial nerve, fixation to the skin or deep structures, or spread to the lymph nodes or distant sites

As with other head and neck cancers, clinical stage, particularly tumor size, may be the crucial factor to determine treatment outcome. Early-stage low-grade malignant salivary gland tumors are usually curable with adequate surgical resection. The prognosis is more favorable when the tumor is in a major salivary gland. The parotid gland has the most favorable prognosis, followed by the submandibular gland, and the least favorable sites are the sublingual and minor salivary glands.

PREVENTION

Because the etiology of this malignancy is not understood, no specific recommendations for prevention are available, although avoiding risk factors may have some effect.

BIBLIOGRAPHY

American Cancer Society. (2007). *Detailed guide: salivary gland cancer*. Retrieved June 11, 2007 from http://documents. cancer.org/187.00/187.00.pdf.

Clarke, L. K., & Dropkin, M. J. (Eds.). (2006). *Site specific cancer series: head and neck cancer*. Pittsburgh, PA: Oncology Nursing Society.

Mendenhall, W. M., Riggs, C. E., & Cassisi, N. J. (2005). Treatment of head and neck. In V. T. Devik, S. Hellman, & S. A. Rosenberg (Eds.). *Cancer: principles and practice*

Clinical Staging: Primary Salivary Gland Tumors

Definition of TNM

Primary Tumor (T)

TX	Primary tumor cannot be assessed
T0	No evidence of primary tumor
T1	Tumor 2 cm or less in greatest dimension without extraparenchymal extension*
T2	Tumor more than 2 cm but not more than 4 cm in greatest dimension without extraparenchymal extension*
T3	Tumor more than 4 cm or tumor having extraparenchymal extension*
T4a	Tumor invades skin, mandible, ear canal, or facial nerve
T4b	Tumor invades skull base or pterygoid plates or encases carotid artery

*NOTE: Extraparenchymal extension is clinical or macroscopic evidence of invasion of soft tissues. Microscopic evidence alone does not constitute extraparenchymal extension for classification purposes.

Regional Lymph Nodes (N)

NX	Regional lymph nodes cannot be assessed
N0	No regional lymph node metastasis
N1	Metastasis in a single ipsilateral lymph node, 2 cm or less in greatest dimension
N2	Metastasis in a single ipsilateral lymph node, more than 3 cm but not more than 6 cm in greatest dimension, or in bilateral or contralateral lymph nodes, none more than 6 cm in greatest dimension
N2a	Metastasis in a single ipsilateral lymph node, more than 3 cm but not more than 6 cm in greatest dimension
N2b	Metastasis in multiple ipsilateral lymph nodes, none more than 6 cm in greatest dimension
N2c	Metastasis in bilateral or contralateral lymph nodes, none more than 6 cm in greatest dimension
N3	Metastasis in a lymph node, more than 6 cm in greatest dimension

Distant Metastasis (M)

MX	Distant metastasis cannot be assessed
M0	No distant metastasis
M1	Distant metastasis

Stage Grouping

Stage	T	N	M
Stage I	T1	N0	M0
Stage II	T2	N0	M0
Stage III	T3	N0	M0
	T1	N1	M0
	T2	N1	M0
	T3	N1	M0
Stage IVA	T4a	N0	M0
	T4a	N1	M0
	T1	N2	M0
	T2	N2	M0
	T3	N2	M0
	T4a	N2	M0
Stage IVB	T4b	Any N	M0
	Any T	N3	M0
Stage IVC	Any T	Any N	M1

Used with the permission of the American Joint Committee on Cancer (AJCC), Chicago, Illinois. The original source for this material is the *AJCC Cancer staging manual*, Sixth Edition (2002) published by Springer Science and Business Media LLC, www.springerlink.com.

(pp. 662-732). Philadelphia: Lippincott Williams & Wilkins.

National Cancer Institute. (2005). *Salivary gland cancer PDQ*. Retrieved June 11, 2007 from http://www. cancer.gov/cancertopics/pdq/treatment/ salivarygland/HealthProfessional.

Shah, J.(2001). American Cancer Society atlas of clinical oncology: cancer of the head and neck. London: BC Decker.

Speight, P. M., & Barrett, A. W. (2002). Salivary gland tumours. *Oral Disease, 8*, 229-240.

Thyroid and Parathyroid Tumors

DEFINITION

- The **thyroid gland** is located in the base of the neck on both sides of the lower part of the larynx and upper part of the trachea.

- The **parathyroid glands** are most often located on the posterior surface of the thyroid gland. Each of the four parathyroid glands weighs about 35 mg.

The thyroid gland consists of two lateral lobes connected by an isthmus. It is composed of a large number of follicles containing colloid, which contains an iodine-containing protein known as thyroglobulin. Thyroglobulin contains several active factors, including thyroxin.

The parathyroid glands secrete a substance known as parathormone, which regulates calcium and phosphorus metabolism.

INCIDENCE

In 2007, the estimated number of new cases in the United States was 33,550 with 1,530 estimated deaths. Thyroid cancer is more common in women; 25,480 new cases are estimated in women and 8,070 in men.

ETIOLOGY AND RISK FACTORS

- A history of radiation to the neck increases the risk for thyroid cancer.
  - Historically, radiation was used for the treatment of benign conditions such as tonsillitis, acne, and enlarged thymus to a dose of 800 to 1,200 cGy. These lower doses appear to cause more mutagenesis than the higher doses given for tumors.
- Benign thyroid disease is more common in middle age.
- Thyroid cancer is more common in the young and the elderly.
- Family history of medullary carcinoma of the thyroid increases risk in patients with type I or II multiple endocrine neoplasia (MEN).
  - In familial medullary thyroid cancer a mutation in the RET proto-oncogene has been identified. In families with MEN, screening for this mutation can be done as early as age 5 or 6 years and those testing positive are considered candidates for prophylactic total thyroidectomy.
  - MEN I and II are autosomal dominant inherited genetic deficits that produce hyperplasia

Major Cancers

or malignant tumors in several endocrine glands. In MEN I, tumors occur in the parathyroid, pancreatic islet cells, adrenal cortex, and thyroid. In MEN II, tumors are medullary thyroid, pheochromocytoma, and parathyroid hyperplasia.

SIGNS AND SYMPTOMS
Thyroid

- Solitary thyroid mass
- Diffuse enlargement of thyroid
- Vocal cord paralysis—the recurrent laryngeal nerve surrounds the thyroid gland
- Neck node

Parathyroid

- Hypercalcemia
- Fatigue
- Weight loss
- Forgetfulness
- Renal stones
- Low phosphorus levels
- High parathormone serum levels

DIAGNOSTIC WORKUP

- Fine-needle aspiration is the standard for solitary thyroid nodules.
- Chest x-ray film
- Thyroid scan
- Ultrasonography, magnetic resonance imaging, or positron emission tomography
- Thyroid function studies
  - Thyroid function studies most often have normal results in cancer of the thyroid.
- Indirect laryngoscopy
- Laboratory tests for parathyroid tumors include calcium, phosphorus, parathormone, chloride-p ratio, and ionized calcium.
- Bone analysis of metacarpal bone thickness, and photon beam bone densitometry may also be indicated.

HISTOLOGY

Parathyroid tumors are usually single-gland, well-differentiated adenomas (85% of tumors).

There are four main cell types of thyroid cancer: papillary, follicular, medullary, and anaplastic:

- Papillary tumors are the most common. They are often multicentric and metastasize to

Clinical Staging: Thyroid and Parathyroid Tumors

Definition of TNM

Primary Tumor (T)

All categories may be subdivided: (a) solitary tumor, (b) multifocal tumor (the largest determines the classification).

TX	Primary tumor cannot be assessed
T0	No evidence of primary tumor
T1	Tumor 2 cm or less in greatest dimension limited to the thyroid
T2	Tumor more than 2 cm but not more than 4 cm in greatest dimension limited to the thyroid
T3	Tumor more than 4 cm in greatest dimension limited to the thyroid or any tumor with minimal extrathyroid extension (e.g., extension to sternothyroid muscle or perithyroid soft tissues)
T4a	Tumor of any size extending beyond the thyroid capsule to invade subcutaneous soft tissues, larynx, trachea, esophagus, or recurrent laryngeal nerve
T4b	Tumor involves pervertebral fascia or encases carotid artery or mediastinal vessels

All anaplastic carcinomas are considered T4 tumors

T4a	Intrathyroidal anaplastic carcinoma—surgically respectable
T4b	Extrathyroidal anaplastic carcinoma—surgically unresectable

Regional Lymph Nodes (N)

Regional lymph nodes are the central compartment, lateral cervical, and upper mediastinal lymph nodes.

NX	Regional lymph nodes cannot be assessed
N0	No regional lymph metastasis
N1	Regional lymph node metastasis
N1a	Metastasis to level VI (pretracheal, paratracheal, and prelaryngeal/delphian lymph nodes)
N1b	Metastasis to unilateral, bilateral, or contralateral cervical or superior mediastinal lymph nodes

Distant Metastasis (M)

MX	Distant metastasis cannot be assessed
M0	No distant metastasis
M1	Distant metastasis

Stage Grouping

Separate stage groupings are recommended for papillary or follicular, medullary, and anaplastic (undifferentiated) carcinoma.

Papillary or Follicular: Under 45 Years

Stage I	Any T	Any N	M0
Stage II	Any T	Any N	M1

Papillary or Follicular: 45 Years and Older

Stage I	T1	N0	M0
Stage II	T2	N0	M0
Stage III	T3	N0	M0
	T1	N1a	M0
	T2	N1a	M0
	T3	N1a	M0
Stage IVA	T4a	N0	M0
	T4a	N1a	M0
	T1	N1b	M0
	T2	N1b	M0
	T3	N1b	M0
	T4a	N1b	M0
Stage IVB	T4b	Any N	M0
Stage IVC	Any T	Any N	M1

Medullary Carcinoma

Stage I	T1	N0	M0
Stage II	T2	N0	M0
Stage III	T3	N0	M0
	T1	N1a	M0
	T2	N1a	M0
	T3	N1a	M0
Stage IVA	T4a	N0	M0
	T4a	N1a	M0
	T1	N1b	M0
	T2	N1b	M0
	T3	N1b	M0

Clinical Staging: Thyroid and Parathyroid Tumors—cont'd

Stage IVB	T4a	N1b	M0
Stage IVB	T4b	Any N	M0
Stage IVC	Any T	Any N	M1

Anaplastic Carcinoma

All anaplastic carcinomas are considered stage IV.

Stage IVA	T4a	Any N	M0
Stage IVB	T4b	Any N	M0
Stage IVC	Any T	Any N	M1

Used with the permission of the American Joint Committee on Cancer (AJCC), Chicago, Illinois. The original source for this material is the *AJCC Cancer staging manual,* Sixth Edition (2002) published by Springer Science and Business Media LLC, www.springerlink.com.

lymph nodes (70% of thyroid cancers).

- Follicular thyroid cancer has a high likelihood of hematogenous spread and prevalence of distant metastatic disease ($\approx$15% of thyroid cancers).
  - Hürthle cell tumors are an independent group consisting of an oncocytic cell. Although considered a variant of follicular tumors, they carry a worse prognosis.
- Medullary thyroid cancer presents in a sporadic or familiar form. It arises from parafollicular C cells, which produce calcitonin (5%-8% of thyroid cancers).
- Anaplastic thyroid cancer is a rare yet aggressive tumor, often with lymph node and metastatic sites (0.5%-1.5% of thyroid cancers).

For clinical management, thyroid cancer is generally divided into two categories: well differentiated or poorly differentiated. The most common malignant tumors of the thyroid are well differentiated and include papillary, follicular, mixed, and Hürthle cell tumors.

CLINICAL STAGING

The American Joint Commission on Cancer has established the TNM classification for clinical staging based on primary tumor size, nodal involvement and presence or absence of metastatic disease. Thyroid cancer is unique among solid tumors in that disease staging is recommended by tumor type. In patients with papillary and follicular tumors staging is age driven. Patients less than 45 years of age at diagnosis with papillary or follicular thyroid cancer are considered to be stage I or stage II regardless of tumor

size, nodal involvement or metastatic disease. TNM categories determine the clinical stage in patients 45 years of age and older with papillary and follicular tumors and all patients with medullary cancer. All anaplastic thyroid tumors are considered to be stage IV. See the table on pages 98-99 for further details.

TREATMENT

- The primary treatment for thyroid and parathyroid cancer is surgery.
  - Surgical exploration of the neck with parathyroidectomy is the primary treatment for parathyroid tumors. The glands are not easily located, although the use of scan-guided surgery and quick parathormone assays has aided surgical techniques.
- The most common adjuvant therapy for thyroid cancer is radioactive iodine.
- External beam radiotherapy may be used if there is extensive nodal or mediastinal disease or gross residual tumor after surgery or for the management of bone or brain metastases.
- Chemotherapy has not played a role in well-differentiated tumors

and is usually reserved for anaplastic tumors with metastatic disease.

PROGNOSIS

Parathyroid cancer is a rare disease, so data are limited. About one third of patients will have recurrent disease, 17% regional nodal disease, and 25% metastatic disease to lung, bones, or liver. In a review of 286 patients, the National Cancer Database reported that the 5- year survival rate was 86% and the 10-year survival rate49%. (See table below.)

PREVENTION

There are no specific prevention measures as most patients who are diagnosed do not have any known risk factors. Genetic testing and counseling for individuals with family history of medullary cancer should be done. A prophylactic thyroidectomy may be indicated or the disease can be identified and treated earlier.

BIBLIOGRAPHY

Clarke, L. K., & Dropkin, M. J. (Eds.). (2006). *Site specific cancer series: head and neck cancer*. Pittsburgh, PA: Oncology Nursing Society.

Jemal, A., Siegel, R., Ward, E., et al. (2007). Cancer statistics, 2007. *CA: A Cancer Journal for Clinicians, 57,* 43-66.

National Cancer Institute. (2006). *Parathyroid cancer PDQ.* Retrieved January 11, 2007, from http://www.cancer.gov/cancertopics/pdq/treatment/parathyroid/HealthProfessional.

National Cancer Institute. (2006). *Thyroid cancer PDQ. (2006).* Retrieved January 11, 2007, from http://www.cancer.gov/cancertopics/pdq/treatment/thyroid/HealthProfessional.

Shah, J. (2001). *American Cancer Society atlas of clinical oncology: cancer of the head and neck.* London: BC Decker.

Prognosis for Thyroid Cancer Patients

Risk	Low Risk	Intermediate Risk		High Risk
Age (yr)	<45	<45	>45	>45
Distant metastases	None	Present	None	Present
Tumor size	T1-T2: <4 cm	T3-T4: >4 cm	T1-T2: <4 cm	T3-T4: >4 cm
Histologic diagnosis and grade	Papillary	Follicular or high grade	Papillary	Follicular or high grade
5-yr survival	100%	96%	96%	72%
20-yr survival	99%	85%	85%	57%

Data from National Cancer Institute. (2008). *Thyroid cancer treatement (PDQ®).* Accessed on January 15, 2008 from http://www.cancer.gov/cancertopics/pdq/treatment/thyroid/HealthProfessional/page4. Bethesda, Md.:NCI.

The Leukemias

Jennifer K. Simpson

Acute Lymphocytic Leukemia

DEFINITION

Leukemias are malignant neoplasms characterized by abnormal proliferation and development of leukocytes and their precursors, which infiltrate the bone marrow, peripheral blood, and other organs resulting in altered normal cell differentiation. Leukemias are classified according to cell type (lymphoid or myeloid) and can be acute or chronic. Acute leukemias are characterized by a block in differentiation resulting in massive accumulation of immature cells or blasts; onset is acute. Acute lymphocytic leukemia (ALL) is a cancer of lymphoblasts. ALL can be divided into two subtypes. The majority of ALL patients, 85%, have B-cell subtype and 15% of patients are diagnosed with T-cell subtype.

INCIDENCE

- In the United States, a total of 5,200 new cases of ALL are estimated for 2007 with 1,420 deaths.
- Most common form of leukemia in children <19 years of age
- >30% of new cases of ALL are in children
- Incidence in 1- to 4-year-old children is more than nine times the rate for young adults aged 20 to 24 years.
- Male > female
- Whites >African Americans

ETIOLOGY AND RISK FACTORS

- Radiation exposure linked with development of ALL, although only found in Japanese atomic bomb survivors
- Congenital diseases are linked with ALL: Down syndrome
- Cytogenetic abnormalities—possible involvement of oncogenes
- Prior treatment with intensive immunosuppressive therapies

SIGNS AND SYMPTOMS

- Generally abrupt presentation
  - Malaise
  - Fatigue
  - Bony pain—especially sternal
  - Sweats
  - Bleeding; easy bruising
- Physical findings
  - Pallor
  - Petechiae
  - Ecchymoses
  - Lymphadenopathy
  - Splenomegaly
  - Hepatomegaly
  - Mediastinal mass generally with T-cell subtype
  - Abdominal adenopathy with Burkitt's type

DIAGNOSTIC WORKUP

- Medical history and physical examination
- Laboratory tests
  - Complete blood cell count with differential
    - Pancytopenia as a result of marrow replacement by tumor
    - Two thirds of patients have white blood cell count >100,000
    - 10% will have normal white blood cell count
- Serum chemistry panel:
  - Elevated lactate dehydrogenase, uric acid correlates with large tumor burden
- Cytogenetic analysis:
  - Permits identification of chromosomes or gene abnormalities in the cells
  - t(9;22) Philadelphia (Ph) chromosome most common abnormality in adult ALL (17%-25% of cases)
- Immunophenotyping:
  - Enables the physician to determine the type of disease that is present in the patient
- Bone marrow aspirate/biopsy
- Lumbar puncture—to identify malignant cells in the cerebrospinal fluid
- Chest x-ray film

CLINICAL STAGING

No clinical staging is performed for ALL.

TREATMENT

Average length of treatment varies between 1.5 and 3 years. There are three phases to the treatment of ALL:

- **Remission induction** – typically requires hospitalization for approximately 4 weeks:
  - Common agents include:
    - Prednisone
    - Vincristine
    - Anthracycline
    - Asparaginase
    - Cyclophosphamide
    - Etoposide
    - Methotrexate
    - Cytarabine
    - Imatinib (if Ph +)
  - Complete response rates range from 60% to 90% with these induction regimens.
- **Consolidation or intensification**
  - Patients must be in remission to begin this phase.
  - Typically lasts 1-3 months
  - Treatment is still fairly intense and many of the same agents administered during induction are utilized.
  - High risk patients may be considered for transplant at this time. This includes:
    - Allogeneic stem cell transplant
    - Autologous stem cell transplant
- **Maintenance**
  - Lasts approximately 2 years
  - Typical agents include:
    - Methotrexate
    - 6-mercaptopurine (6-MP)
    - Vincristine
    - Prednisone

- **Central nervous system prophylaxis**
  - Typically completed during the induction phase but may extend throughout therapy
  - Common agents include:
    - Methotrexate
    - Hydrocortisone
    - Cytarabine
    - Cranial/spinal irradiation
    - High dose IV methotrexate
- Patients who have relapsed after induction chemotherapy or maintenance therapy are unlikely to be cured by further chemotherapy alone.
  - Reinduction chemotherapy followed by allogeneic bone marrow transplantation should be considered.
  - Patients who do not have an HLA-matched donor may be considered for an unrelated stem cell/bone marrow transplant
  - Clinical trials should also be considered

PROGNOSIS

- Overall 5-year survival:
  - Adults 64%
  - Children 85%
- Long-term follow-up of 30 patients with ALL in remission for at least 10 years has demonstrated 10 cases of secondary malignancies.
- Of 31 long-term female survivors of ALL or acute myeloid leukemia under 40 years of age, 26 resumed normal menstruation after completion of therapy. Among 36 live offspring of survivors, two congenital problems occurred.

PREVENTION

There are no known preventive measures for ALL.

BIBLIOGRAPHY

American Cancer Society. (2007). *Leukemia—acute lymphocytic.* Retrieved June. 11, 2007, from http://www.cancer.org/docroot/lrn/lrn_0.asp.

Jemal, A., Murray, T., Ward, E., et al. (2005). Cancer statistics, 2005. *CA: A Cancer Journal for Clinicians, 55,* 10-30.

Leukemia and Lymphoma Society (2007). *Acute lymphocytic leukemia.* Retrieved June. 11, 2007, from http://www.leukemia-lymphoma.org/all_page?item_id=7049.

National Cancer Institute. (2007). *Adult acute lymphoblastic leukemia (PDQ).* Retrieved June. 11, 2007, from http://www.cancer.gov/cancertopics/pdq/treatment/adultALL/HealthProfessional/page1#Reference1.19.

Micallef, I. N., Rohatiner, A. Z., Carter, M., et al. (2001). Long-term outcome of patients surviving for more than ten years following treatment for acute leukaemia. *British Journal of Haematology, 113,* 443-445.

Acute Myelogenous Leukemia

DEFINITION

Acute myelogenous leukemia (AML) is a cancer of the blood and bone marrow specifically involving the myeloid progenitor cells. Most AML is distinguished from other related blood disorders such as myelodysplastic syndrome by the presence of more than 20% blasts in the blood and bone marrow. AML results from the failure of the myeloid progenitor cells to mature. The mechanism causing the arrest of cell maturation is not fully understood; however, it may often involve the activation of abnormal genes through chromosomal translocations and other genetic abnormalities. This developmental arrest results in a marked decrease in the production of normal blood cells, resulting in varying degrees of anemia, thrombocytopenia, and neutropenia. Second, the immature cells (blasts) begin to accumulate in the blood, bone marrow, and frequently the liver and spleen as a result of their rapid proliferation and reduction in apoptosis (programmed cell death).

INCIDENCE

- In the United States, a total of 13,410 new cases of AML are expected in 2007, with more than 90% of the cases diagnosed in adults.
- 8,990 deaths from the disease are estimated for 2007 in the U.S.
- Affects all age groups with median age at diagnosis of 65 years. There is an increased prevalence with age.
- More common in whites
- More common in men than women, particularly in older patients

ETIOLOGY AND RISK FACTORS

The specific etiology or cause of AML is unknown. Of all leukemias, AML has the strongest link to an increased risk seen in patients who have had prior radiation and toxin exposure.

- The most common risk factor is the presence of an antecedent hematologic disorder, usually high-risk myelodysplastic syndrome.
- Radiation exposure: increased risk seen in patients exposed to atomic bomb explosion in Japan; early radiologists (before appropriate shielding); and patients irradiated for ankylosing spondylitis
- Prior chemotherapy, particularly alkylating agents and topoisomerase II inhibitors
- Period between drug or radiation exposure and evidence of acute leukemia approximately 3 to 5 years for alkylating agents or radiation exposure but only 9 to 12 months for topoisomerase II inhibitors
- Tobacco use: It is estimated that one fifth of cases of AML are related to smoking.
- Congenital disorders resulting in development of AML during childhood, although some may develop as adults
  - Bloom syndrome, Down syndrome, congenital neutropenia, Fanconi anemia, and neurofibromatosis
- Increased risk with age: risk increases tenfold between 30 and 70 years of age

SIGNS AND SYMPTOMS

Presenting symptoms are related to bone marrow failure with resulting anemia, neutropenia, and thrombocytopenia or organ infiltration with leukemic cells. Common sites include the spleen, liver, and gums. Organ infiltration occurs most commonly in patients with monocytic subtypes.

Patient Complaints

- Fatigue
- Weakness
- Shortness of breath
- Weight loss
- Fever
- Bleeding and easy bruising
- Early satiety and fullness in right upper quadrant (from splenomegaly)
- Bone pain resulting from high leukemic cell burden and increased pressure in the marrow
- Respiratory distress and altered mental status from leukostasis, which is a medical emergency and requires immediate treatment

Physical Findings

- Pallor
- Petechiae or ecchymoses
- Hepatosplenomegaly
- Signs of infection, including pneumonia
- Gingivitis
- Rash resulting from skin infiltration

DIAGNOSTIC WORKUP

- Medical history and physical examination
- Laboratory tests:
  - Complete blood cell count with differential
  - Serum chemistry panel
  - Elevated lactate dehydrogenase, uric acid: correlates with large tumor burden
  - Cytogenetics
    - Permits identification of chromosomes or gene abnormalities in the cells
- Additional studies:
  - Bone marrow aspirate/biopsy
  - Immunophenotyping
    - Helps determine the type of disease that is present in the patient through identification of antigens (proteins) on the cell surface and the antibodies produced

by the body that match the antigen
- Imaging studies
  - Chest x-ray film

CLINICAL STAGING

Clinical staging is not done in AML.

HISTOLOGY

Determination of the subtype of AML helps to predict prognosis and suggest treatment implications. However, for all practical purposes the treatment is similar for all subtypes. Classification of AML has been revised under the auspices of the World Health Organization (WHO) and replaces the older French American British (FAB) classification. The WHO classification for AML incorporates and interrelates morphology, cytogenetics, molecular genetics, and immunological markers in an attempt to construct a classification that is universally applicable and prognostically valid. Elements of the

FAB classification that were specific to disease morphology have been retained. The WHO classification is outlined in the box below.

TREATMENT

Treatment is delivered in two phases: induction to attain remission and postremission therapy to maintain the remission. Intensive consolidation therapy is effective when given either immediately after remission or when delayed.

Induction Therapy

Various induction regimens may be used. The most common one is often called "3 and 7." Three days of an anthracycline is combined with cytarabine (araC) as a 24-hour infusion for 7 days. Approximately 50% of patients achieve a remission with one course of therapy and another 10% to 15% enter remission after the second course. High-dose araC combined with an anthracycline may also be

---

World Health Organization Classification—Acute Myelogenous Leukemia

- AML with characteristic genetic abnormalities
  - AML with t(8;21)(q22;q22) (AML/ETO)
  - AML with inv(16)(p13q22) or t(16;16)(p13;q22) (CBFβ/MYH11)
  - Acute promyelocytic leukemia—AML with t(15;17)(q22;q12) (PML/RARa) and variants
  - AML with 11q23 (MLL) abnormalities
- AML with FLT3 mutation
- AML with multilineage dysplasia
  - AML with multilineage dysplasia after myelodysplastic syndrome (>20% blasts in the blood or bone marrow) (defined in FAB MDS criterion as refractory anemia with excess blasts in transformation [RAEB-t])
- AML and MDS, therapy related
  - Alkylating agent–related AML and MDS
  - Topoisomerase II inhibitor–related AML
- AML not otherwise categorized (morphology based and reflects the older French, American, and British morphology-based classification with a few changes)
  - Acute myeloblastic leukemia, minimally differentiated (FAB classification M0)
  - Acute myeloblastic leukemia, without maturation (FAB classification M1)
  - Acute myeloblastic leukemia with maturation (FAB classification M2)
  - Acute myelomonocytic leukemia (FAB classification M4)
  - Acute monoblastic leukemia and acute monocytic leukemia (FAB classifications M5a and M5b)
  - Acute erythroid leukemias (FAB classifications M6a and M6b)
  - Acute megakaryoblastic leukemia (FAB classification M7)
- AML/transient myeloproliferative disorder in Down syndrome
  - Acute basophilic leukemia
  - Acute panmyelosis with myelofibrosis
  - Myeloid sarcoma
- Acute leukemias of ambiguous lineage

AML, Acute myelogenous leukemia; *MDS*, myelodysplastic syndrome; *FAB*, French, American, and British classification.
Adapted from National Cancer Institute. (2007). *Adult acute myeloid leukemias (PDQ): treatment health professional version.* Retrieved June 14, 2007, from http://www.cancer.gov/cancertopics/pdq/treatment/adultAML/HealthProfessional/page2.

used as induction therapy in younger patients. A remission is defined as a normal peripheral blood cell count and normocellular marrow with less than 5% blasts in the marrow and no signs or symptoms of the disease. The majority of patients with AML meeting this remission criteria often still have residual leukemia, which led to modifications of the definition of complete remission to include cytogenetic remission, in which a previously abnormal karyotype reverts to normal, and molecular remission, in which interphase fluorescence in situ hybridization (FISH) or multiparameter flow cytometry are used to detect minimal residual disease. Immunophenotyping and interphase FISH have greater prognostic significance than the conventional criteria for remission.

Postremission Therapy

Postremission therapy is indicated when curative intent is the goal. Current postremission therapy or consolidation therapy includes short-term, relatively intensive chemotherapy with cytarabine-based regimens, high-dose chemotherapy or chemoradiation therapy with autologous bone marrow rescue, and high-dose marrow-ablative therapy with allogeneic bone marrow rescue.

PROGNOSIS

- Overall 5-year survival rate is 33% for adults under 65 years of age but only 4% for adults >65 years of age.
- Nontransplant consolidation therapy with cytarabine-containing regimens has treatment-related death rates that are usually less than 10% to 20% and have yielded reported disease-free survival rates from 20% to 50%.
- Allogeneic bone marrow transplantation results in the lowest incidence of leukemic relapse. Disease-free survival rates with allogeneic transplantation in first complete remission have ranged from 45% to 60%. Use of allogeneic bone marrow

transplantation as primary postremission therapy is limited by the need for a human leukocyte antigen (HLA)-matched sibling donor and the increased mortality from allogeneic bone marrow transplantation of patients who are older than 50 years. The mortality from allogeneic bone marrow transplantation that uses an HLA-matched sibling donor ranges from 20% to 40%.
- Autologous bone marrow transplantation results in disease-free survival rates between 35% and 50% in patients with AML in first remission. This approach is more limited due to concern of persistent leukemia cells in the collected marrow.

PREVENTION

The etiology of AML is not fully understood; therefore, specific measures to prevent AML cannot be identified. Limiting controllable risk factors such as exposure to toxins and radiation and tobacco use should be used. Individuals with exposure to known toxins and radiation should be monitored. It is important to note that most people who have known risk factors do not get leukemia.

BIBLIOGRAPHY

Bennett, J., Catovsky, D., Daniel, M., et al. (1976). Proposals for the classification of the acute leukemias: French-American-British (FAB) co-operative group. *British Journal of Haematology, 33*, 451-458.

Bostrom, B., Brunning, R. D., McGlave, P., et al. (1985). Bone marrow transplantation for acute nonlymphocytic leukemia in first remission: analysis of prognostic factors. *Blood, 65*, 1191-1196.

Brunning, R. D., Matutes, E., Harris, N. L., et al. (2001). Acute myeloid leukaemia: introduction. In E. S. Jaffe, N. L. Harris, H. Stein, et al. (Eds.). *Pathology and genetics of tumours of haematopoietic and lymphoid tissues* (pp. 77-80). Lyon, France: IARC Press.

Cassileth, P. A., Andersen, J., Lazarus, H. M., et al. (1993). Autologous bone marrow transplant in acute myeloid leukemia in first remission. *Journal of Clinical Oncology, 11*, 314-319.

Chao, N. J., Stein, A. S., Long, G. D., et al. (1993). Busulfan/etoposide—initial experience with a new preparatory regimen for autologous bone marrow transplantation in patients with acute nonlymphoblastic leukemia. *Blood, 81*, 319-323.

Clift, R. A., Buckner, C. D., Thomas, E. D., et al. (1987). The treatment of acute non-lymphoblastic leukemia by allogeneic marrow transplantation. *Bone Marrow Transplantation, 2*, 243-258.

Gorin, N. C., Aegerter, P., Auvert, B., et al. (1990). Autologous bone marrow transplantation for acute myelocytic leukemia in first remission: a European survey of the role of marrow purging. *Blood, 75*, 1606-1614.

Jemal, A., Siegel, R., Ward, E., et al. (2007). Cancer statistics, 2007. *CA: A Cancer Journal for Clinicians, 57*, 43-66.

Jones, R. J., & Santos, G. W. (1990). Autologous bone marrow transplantation with 4-hydroperoxycyclophosphamide purging. In R. P. Gale RP (Ed.). *Acute myelogenous leukemia: progress and controversies* (pp. 411-419). Proceedings of a Wyeth-Ayerst-UCLA Symposia Western Workshop Held at Lake Lanier, Georgia, November 28–December 1, 1989. New York: Wiley-Liss.

Linker, C. A., Ries, C. A., Damon, L. E., et al. (1993). Autologous bone marrow transplantation for acute myeloid leukemia using busulfan plus etoposide as a preparative regimen. *Blood, 81*, 311-318.

Mayer, R. J., Davis, R. B., Schiffer, C. A., et al. (1994). Intensive postremission chemotherapy in adults with acute myeloid leukemia: cancer and leukemia group B. *New England Journal of Medicine, 331*, 896-903.

National Cancer Institute. (2007). *Adult acute myeloid leukemia (PDQ): treatment, health professional version*. Retrieved June 14, 2007, from http://www.cancer.gov/cancertopics/pdq/treatment/adultAML/HealthProfessional/page2.

Reiffers, J., Gaspard, M. H., Maraninchi, D., et al. (1989). Comparison of allogeneic or autologous bone marrow transplantation and chemotherapy in patients with acute myeloid leukaemia in first remission: a prospective controlled trial. *British Journal of Haematology, 72*, 57-63.

Robertson, M. J., Soiffer, R. J., Freedman, A. S., et al. (1992). Human bone marrow depleted of CD33-positive cells mediates delayed but durable reconstitution of hematopoiesis: clinical trial of MY9 monoclonal antibody-purged autografts for the treatment of acute myeloid leukemia. *Blood, 79*, 2229-2236.

Sanz, M. A., de la Rubia, J., Sanz, G. F., et al. (1993). Busulfan plus cyclophosphamide followed by autologous blood stem-cell transplantation for patients with acute myeloblastic leukemia in first complete remission: a report from a single institution. *Journal of Clinical Oncology, 11*, 1661-1667.

Vardiman, J., Harris, N., & Brunning, R. (2002). The World Health Organization (WHO) classification of the myeloid neoplasms. *Blood, 100*, 2292-2302.

Chronic Lymphocytic Leukemia

DEFINITION

Chronic lymphocytic leukemia (CLL), an indolent cancer of the B cells, is the most common type of leukemia, characterized by lymphocytosis, lymphadenopathy, and splenomegaly. It results from an acquired injury to the deoxyribonucleic acid (DNA) of a lymphocyte in the bone marrow causing uncontrolled growth of CLL cells in the marrow, leading to an increased concentration in the blood. Lymphocyte counts are usually >5,000/mm^3 with a characteristic immunophenotype (CD5- and CD23-positive B cells). CLL cells in the marrow do not impede normal blood cell production to the extent that is the case with acute lymphocytic leukemia. This important distinction from acute leukemia accounts for the less severe early course of the disease.

INCIDENCE

- In 2007, 15,340 new cases are expected (8960 men and 6380 women) to be diagnosed in the U.S. with 4,500 expected deaths
- Affects middle aged or elderly adults:
  ○ Median age is 72 years
  ○ Most are >55 years old; CLL almost never affects children
- Affects whites more often than African Americans

ETIOLOGY AND RISK FACTORS

- It is not understand what induces the change to the lymphocyte DNA.
- Risk factors include the following:
  ○ Smoking
  ○ Long-term exposure to herbicides or pesticides (e.g., Agent Orange during the Vietnam War)
  ○ Increasing age
  ○ Family history of CLL or cancer of the lymph system
  ○ Russian or Eastern European Jewish descent

SIGNS AND SYMPTOMS

- Symptoms are generally present with advanced disease.
- Diagnosis is typically made during routine blood work.
- Presenting symptoms include the following
  ○ Fatigue
  ○ Shortness of breath with exertion
  ○ Weight loss
  ○ Night sweats
  ○ Frequent infections of the skin, lungs, kidneys, or other sites
- Physical findings may include the following
  ○ Ecchymosis
  ○ Lymphadenopathy
  ○ Splenomegaly

DIAGNOSTIC WORKUP

- Medical history and physical examination
- Laboratory tests
  ○ Complete blood cell count with differential
    ▪ 35% will present with anemia
    ▪ 25% will present with thrombocytopenia
  ○ Serum chemistry panel
    ▪ Elevated lactate dehydrogenase, uric acid correlate with large tumor burden
  ○ Evaluation of immunoglobulins (gamma globulins). Patients with CLL may not have enough of these proteins, which may lead to repeated infections.
- Cytogenetics for identification of chromosomes or gene abnormalities in the cells
  ○ Fluorescence in situ hybridization to evaluate chromosome changes. This can be used to monitor response to treatment.
  ○ Immunophenotyping (also known as flow cytometry) helps to identify whether the CLL began with a B lymphocyte or a T lymphocyte. B lymphocyte (or B-cell CLL) is most common.
- Additional studies
  ○ Bone marrow aspirate/biopsy
- Imaging studies
  ○ Chest x-ray film
  ○ Computed tomography scan
  ○ Magnetic resonance imaging

CLINICAL STAGING

Staging is useful to predict prognosis and to stratify patients. Anemia and thrombocytopenia are the major adverse prognostic variables. There is no standard staging system. The table on page 105 outlines the Rai staging system and the Binet classification.

TREATMENT

CLL usually occurs in elderly patients, progresses slowly, and is generally not curable; therefore, treatment is usually conservative. Treatment should be individualized and based on the clinical behavior of the disease. Treatment decisions are dependent on the patient's symptoms, prognostic factors, stage of disease, disease recurrence, and response to prior therapies. In asymptomatic patients, treatment may be deferred until the patient becomes symptomatic. The rate of disease progression is patient specific and there may be long periods of stable disease and sometimes spontaneous regressions; frequent and careful observation is required to monitor the clinical course. Treatment may range from watchful waiting with treatment for complications as needed to a variety of therapeutic options including steroids;

Staging of Chronic Lymphocytic Leukemia (CLL)

RAI STAGING SYSTEM

Stage 0	Absolute lymphocytosis (>15,000/mm3) without adenopathy, hepatosplenomegaly, anemia or thrombocytopenia
Stage I	Absolute lymphocytosis with lymphadenopathy without hepatosplenomegaly, anemia or thrombocytopenia
Stage II	Absolute lymphocytosis with either hepatomegaly or splenomegaly, with or without lymphadenopathy
Stage III	Absolute lymphocytosis and anemia (hg <11 g/dL) with or without lymphadenopathy, hepatomegaly or splenomegaly
Stage IV	Absolute lymphocytosis and thrombocytopenia (<100,000/mm3) with or without lymphadenopathy, hepatomegaly, splenomegaly or anemia

BINET CLASSIFICATION

Clinical stage A	No anemia or thrombocytopenia and <3 areas of lymphoid involvement
Clinical stage B	No anemia or thrombocytopenia with > 3 areas of lymphoid involvement
Clinical stage C	Anemia and/or thrombocytopenia regardless of the number of areas of lymphoid enlargement

Adapted from National Cancer Institute (2/7/2007). Chronic Lymphocytic Leukemia (PDQ®): Treatment, Health Professional Version. Retrieved on June 14, 2007 from http://www.cancer.gov/cancertopics/pdq/treatment/CLL/HealthProfessional/page2.

chemotherapy, alkylating agents, purine analogs, or combinations; monoclonal antibodies; radiation; or transplantation.

PROGNOSIS

The overall 5-year survival rate for patients with CLL is 73%. Data from older trials of the 1970s and 1980s report median survival for all patients ranging from 8 to 12 years. There is a large variation in survival among individual patients, ranging from several months to a normal life expectancy.

PREVENTION

There are no guidelines for preventing CLL.

BIBLIOGRAPHY

Jemal, A., Siegel, R., Ward, E., et al. (2007). Cancer sStatistics, 2007. *CA: A Cancer Journal for Clinicians, 57,* 43-66.

National Cancer Institute. (2007). *Chronic lymphocytic leukemia (PDQ): treatment, health professional version.* Retrieved June 14, 2007, from http://www.cancer.gov/cancertopics/pdq/treatment/CLL/HealthProfessional.

Rai, K. R., Sawitsky, A., Cronkite, E. P., et al. (1975). Clinical staging of chronic lymphocytic leukemia. *Blood, 46,* 219-234.

Sokal, J. E., Cox, E. B., Baccarani, M., et al. (1984). Prognostic discrimination in "good-risk" chronic granulocytic leukemia. *Blood, 63,* 789-799.

Chronic Myelogenous Leukemia

DEFINITION

Chronic myelogenous leukemia (CML) is a cancer of the granulocytes or monocytes. It is considered a myeloproliferative disorder and causes a rapid growth of the myeloid precursors in the bone marrow, peripheral blood, and body tissues. The Philadelphia chromosome (Ph1) can be seen in more than 95% of patients diagnosed with CML. The Ph1 results from a reciprocal translocation between the long arms of chromosomes 9 and 22. This translocation transfers the Abelson (ABL) on chromosome 9 oncogene to an area of chromosome 22 termed the breakpoint cluster region (BCR), creating a fused BCR/ABL gene leading to the production of an abnormal tyrosine kinase protein that causes CML.

INCIDENCE

- Affects one to two people per 100,000 and accounts for 7% to 20% of cases of leukemia
- 4,570 new cases and 490 deaths estimated in 2007 in the United States
- About 21,501 people in the United States are living with CML
- Median age at diagnosis is 66 years; 80% of patients diagnosed are over the age of 45 years.
- Only 2.6% of leukemias in children aged 0 to 19 years are CML

ETIOLOGY AND RISK FACTORS

On the basis of the Surveillance Epidemiology and End Result (SEER) rates from 2002 to 2004, 0.15% of men and women born today will be diagnosed with CML at some time during their lifetimes. High-dose radiation exposure may contribute to the development of the Ph1 chromosome. Most with CML have not been exposed to radiation and many exposed to high dose radiation do not have CML.

SIGNS AND SYMPTOMS

Symptoms usually develop gradually and are generally present with advanced disease. Diagnosis is often made during routine blood examination for other reasons.

Patient complaints

- Fatigue
- Malaise
- Fever
- Weight loss
- Night sweats

Physical findings

- Ecchymosis
- Lymphadenopathy
- Splenomegaly in approximately 50% of patients

DIAGNOSTIC WORKUP

- Medical history and physical examination
- Laboratory tests
  - Complete blood cell count with differential
- Serum chemistry panel
  - Elevated lactate dehydrogenase, uric acid correlates with large tumor burden

Major Cancers

- Cytogenetics to identify chromosomes or gene abnormalities in the cells
- Polymerase chain reaction—Highly sensitive test of blood cells to detect as little as one BCR/ABL-positive cell in a background of about 500,000 normal cells.
- Additional studies
  ○ Bone marrow aspirate/biopsy
- Imaging studies
  ○ Chest x-ray film
  ○ Computed tomographic scan
  ○ Magnetic resonance imaging

CLINICAL STAGING

CML can have three phases: chronic, accelerated, and blast. Transition from the chronic phase to the accelerated phase and later the blastic phase may occur gradually over a period of 1 year or more, or it may appear abruptly (blast crisis).

Chronic-Phase Chronic Myelogenous Leukemia

Most patients are in chronic-phase CML at diagnosis characterized by bone marrow and cytogenetic findings with less than 10% blasts and promyelocytes in the peripheral blood and bone marrow.

Accelerated-Phase Chronic Myelogenous Leukemia

This phase is characterized by 10% to 19% blasts in either the peripheral blood or bone marrow.

Blastic-Phase Chronic Myelogenous Leukemia

A total of 20% or more blasts may be found in the peripheral blood or bone marrow. When the patient has fever, malaise, and splenomegaly with >20% blasts, this is considered blast crisis. The annual rate of progression from chronic phase to blast crisis is 5% to 10% in the first 2 years and 20% in subsequent years.

TREATMENT

- The goal for treatment in the chronic phase is to return hematologic values to normal and eliminate BCR/ABL. Treatment goals for a patient in the accelerated phase or blast crisis phase is to eliminate cells with the BCR/ABL gene and return patient's disease to the chronic phase.
- Leukapheresis or hydroxyurea to reduce white blood cell counts may be used.
- Treatment of choice is a tyrosine kinase inhibitors. Imatinib mesylate is usually the first choice with alternative tyrosine kinase inhibitors such as dasatinib or nilotinib used if the disease progresses or the patient cannot tolerate imatinib.

Transplant

- Allogeneic bone marrow or stem cell transplant is the only potentially curative treatment to date, but it is not without significant morbidity and mortality rates. Transplantation is most successful in younger patients. Patients up to about 60 years of age who have a matched donor may be candidates.
- Nonmyeloablative stem cell transplant or minitransplant is being investigated as well as autologous stem cell transplants, which may be beneficial to patients not eligible for a traditional allogeneic transplant.
- Cord blood stem cell transplants are under investigation.

Donor Lymphocyte Infusion

- In patients who have a relapse after allogeneic stem cell transplant, treatment alternatives may be a second transplant, a tyrosine kinase inhibitor, or donor lymphocyte infusion from the original stem cell donor.

PROGNOSIS

The overall 5-year relative survival rate for 1996 to 2003 from 17 SEER geographical areas was 47.5%. The median survival is 4 to 6 years, with a range of less than 1 year to more than 10 years. Survival after development of an accelerated phase is usually less than 1 year and after blastic transformation only a few months.

PREVENTION

There are no prevention guidelines for CML.

BIBLIOGRAPHY

Jemal, A., Siegel, R., Ward, E., et al. (2007). Cancer statistics, 2007. *CA: A Cancer Journal for Clinicians, 57,* 43-66.

National Cancer Institute. (2007). *Chronic myelogenous leukemia (PDQ): treatment, health professional version.* Retrieved June 14, 2007, from http://www.cancer.gov/cancertopics/pdq/treatment/CML/HealthProfessional.

National Cancer Institute. (2007). *Treatment statement for health professionals: chronic myelogenous leukemia.* Retrieved June 27, 2007, from http://www.meb.uni-bonn.de/cancer.gov/CDR0000062876.html.

Ries, L. A. G., Melbert, D., Krapcho, M., et al. (Eds.). (2006). *SEER cancer statistics review, 1975-2004, National Cancer Institute.* Bethesda, MD.. Retrieved June 17, 2007, from http://seer.cancer.gov/csr/1975_2004/.

Sawyers, C. L. (1999). Chronic myeloid leukemia. *New England Journal of Medicine, 340,* 1330-40.

Sokal, J. E., Baccarani, M., Russo, D., et al. (1988). Staging and prognosis in chronic myelogenous leukemia. *Seminars in Hematology, 25,* 49-61.

Myelodysplastic Syndromes

DEFINITION

Myelodysplastic syndromes (MDS) are a group of acquired bone marrow stem cell malignancies that result in ineffective hematopoiesis in one or more myeloid lineages. Although technically not cancer, over time MDS may transform into leukemia and are therefore often referred to as preleukemia. In patients with this disorder, the marrow produces too few red blood cells, white blood cells, and often platelets

INCIDENCE

- Prevalence is estimated to be 55,000 patients in the United States.

- 15,000 to 25,000 new cases diagnosed per year
- Median age between 60 and 70 years; 70% of patients are >50 years old
- Occurs in men more often than in women

ETIOLOGY AND RISK FACTORS

MDS can present either de novo (primary) or secondary to treatment with chemotherapy or radiation therapy for other diseases.

Risk factors include the following:

- Age >60 years
- Male sex
- Alcohol use
- Cigarette smoking
- Exposure to ionizing radiation
- Immunosuppressive therapy
- Viral infection

- Benzene and other environmental/occupational exposures

SIGNS AND SYMPTOMS

Symptoms usually develop gradually and are generally present with advanced disease. Disease usually presents as a result of marrow failure in one or more cell lines. Diagnosis is often made during routine blood examination.

Symptoms include the following:

- Fatigue
- Malaise
- Fever
- Shortness of breath with exertion
- Weight loss

Physical findings include the following:

- Pallor
- Ecchymosis or bleeding

- Infection

DIAGNOSTIC WORKUP

- Medical history and physical examination
- Laboratory tests
  - Complete blood cell count with differential
  - Cytogenetics—permits identification of chromosomes or gene abnormalities in the cells
- Additional studies
  - Bone marrow aspirate/biopsy is critical to the diagnosis.
- Imaging studies
  - Chest x-ray film
  - Computed tomographic scan
  - Magnetic resonance imaging

Major Cancers

Classification Systems of Myelodysplastic Syndromes

French, American, and British	International Prognostic Scoring System		World Health Organization
(1) Refractory anemia: cytopenia of one peripheral blood lineage; normocellular or hypocellular marrow with dysplasias; <1% blasts in peripheral blood and <5% bone marrow blasts	(1) Marrow blast (%) <5 5-10 11-20 21-30	Score 0 0.5 1.5 2.0	Myelodysplastic syndromes (1) Refractory anemia (2) Refractory cytopenia with multilineage dysplasia
(2) Refractory anemia with ringed sideroblasts: cytopenia, dysplasia, and the same % blast involvement as refractory anemia; >15% ringed sideroblasts in bone marrow	(2) Cytogenic karyotype Good prognosis: (–Y, 5q–, 2-q–, normal) Intermediate prognosis: (trisomy 8) Poor prognosis (abn 7, complex)	Score 0 0.5 1.0	(3) Refractory cytopenia with ringed sideroblasts (4) Refractory cytopenia with multilineage dysplasia, ringed sideroblasts
(3) Refractory anemia with excess blasts: cytopenia of two or more peripheral blood lineages; dysplasia involving all three lineages; <5% peripheral blood blasts and 5%-20% bone marrow blasts	(3) Cytopenia: None or one lineage Two or three lineages	Score 0 0.5	(5) Refractory anemia with excess blasts 1: 5%-10% blasts (6) Refractory anemia with excess blasts 2: 10%-20% blasts (7) Myelodysplastic syndrome with isolated 5q-: (5q- syndrome) (8) Myelodysplastic syndrome unclassified
(4) Refractory anemia with excess blasts in transformation: hematologic features identical to refractory anemia with excess blasts; >5% blasts in peripheral blood or 21%-30% blasts in bone marrow or the presence of Auer rods in blasts	(4) Overall score Low 0 Intermediate 1 Intermediate 2 High 2.5 or more	Median survival 5.7 yr 3.5 yr 1.2 yr 0.4 yr	Acute myelogenous leukemia: (1) With recurrent genetic abnormalities (2) With multilineage dysplasia (3) In transformation and myelodysplastic syndrome in transformation (4) Not otherwise categorized Myelodysplastic/myeloproliferative diseases: (1) Chronic myelomonocytic leukemia (2) Atypical chronic myelogenous leukemia (3) Juvenile myelomonocytic leukemia
(5) Chronic myelomonocytic leukemia: monocytosis in peripheral blood; <5% blasts in peripheral blood and up to 20% bone marrow blasts			

Adapted from National Cancer Institute. (2007). *Chronic lymphocytic leukemia (PDQ): treatment, health professional version*. Retrieved June 14, 2007, from http://www.cancer.gov/cancertopics/pdq/treatment/CLL/HealthProfessional/page2.

HISTOLOGY

In general the marrow is normocellular or hypercellular.

CLINICAL STAGING

No clinical staging is applied. Classification of the disease to predict prognosis and to guide therapy has been difficult. In 1982, a French, American, and British (FAB) classification was agreed on based on morphological criteria of the marrow. The International Prognostic Scoring System (IPSS) described in 1996 defined survival and risk of progression to acute myelogenous leukemia (AML) better than FAB. Limitations continued to be present and in 1997 the World Health Organization classification was defined. All three of these classifications systems can be seen in the table on page 107.

TREATMENT

The principle of MDS treatment is to individualize therapy for the patient. Therapy for MDS has historically been supportive care for the majority of patients. The only curative treatment is allogeneic stem cell transplant; however, intensive chemotherapy and transplants are used only in those patients with available donors, higher

risk disease, younger age, and adequate performance status—a minority of the patients with MDS.

- Supportive care:
  - ○ Transfusions to correct anemia and thrombocytopenia
  - ○ Antibiotics
  - ○ Hematopoietic growth factors, recombinant erythropoietin, granulocyte colony-stimulating factor, or granulocyte-macrophage colony-stimulating factor
- Immunomodulatory agents: lenalidomide
- Hypomethylating agents: 5-azacitidine and decitabine

PROGNOSIS

Secondary myelodysplasia usually has a poorer prognosis than does de novo myelodysplasia. Prognosis is directly related to the number of bone marrow blast cells and to the amount of peripheral blood cytopenias. MDS transforms to AML in about 30% of patients. IPSS, which was developed from a multivariate analysis, predicts median time to AML transformation and overall survival per risk group determined by the IPSS classification, which stratifies patients into four risk groups: low risk, intermediate-1,

intermediate-2, and high risk. The time to AML transformation in the risk groups was 9.4 years, 3.3 years, 1.1 years, and 0.2 years, respectively. Median survival for the groups was 5.7 years, 3.5 years, 1.2 years, and 0.4 years, respectively.

PREVENTION

There are no recommended measures for prevention of MDS.

BIBLIOGRAPHY

Bennett, J. M., Catovsky, D., Daniel, M. T., et al. (1982). Proposals for the classification of the myelodysplastic syndromes. *British Journal of Haematology, 51*, 189.

Catenacci, D. V. T., & Schiller, G. J. (2005). Myelodysplasic syndromes: a comprehensive review. *Blood Reviews, 19*, 301-319.

List, A. F., Vardiman, J., Issa, J. P., et al. (2004). Myelodysplastic syndromes. *Hematology*, 297-319.

National Cancer Institute. (2006). *Myelodysplastic syndromes (PDQ): treatment, health professional version*. Retrieved July 12, 2007, from http:// www.cancer.gov/cancertopics/ pdq/treatment/myelodysplastic/Health Professional/page1.

Vardiman, J., Harris, N., & Brunning, R. (2002). The World Health Organization (WHO) classification of the myeloid neoplasms. *Blood, 100*, 2292-302.

The Lymphomas

Jennifer K. Simpson

Hodgkin Lymphoma

DEFINITION

Lymphomas are cancers of the B or T lymphocytes or natural killer cells that originate in the lymphatic system. The lymphomas are divided into two major categories: Hodgkin lymphoma (HL) and all other lymphomas, called non-Hodgkin lymphomas. HL is an uncommon neoplasm arising from B lymphocytes and marked by a diagnostic tumor cell called the Reed-Sternberg cell. HL

is also commonly referred to as Hodgkin disease.

INCIDENCE

- HL will represent about 11.4% of all lymphomas diagnosed in 2007.
- 8,190 (4,470 males and 3,720 females) new cases in the United States are expected to be diagnosed in 2007, with 1,070 deaths from the disease
- Bimodal distribution with the first peak at 15 to 34 years of age and the second at >50 years of age

ETIOLOGY AND RISK FACTORS

- The etiology of HL is uncertain.
- History of infectious mononucleosis caused by the Epstein-Barr virus is associated with nearly half of cases. Risk can be up to 20 years after infection and is more frequently associated with childhood and older adult cases.
- Infection with human immunodeficiency virus (HIV) also has an increased probability of development of HL.
- Measles virus exposure in childhood increases risk in young adults.

- Personal history of autoimmune conditions may be linked to increased risk.
- Familial HL represents approximately 5% of new cases
  - First-degree relative with HL results in a threefold increased risk. Risk is stronger at younger age, in males, and in siblings.

SIGNS AND SYMPTOMS

- Approximately one third of patients are symptomatic.
- B symptoms (absence or presence is key in staging):
  - Unexplained loss of more than 10% of body weight in the 6 months before diagnosis
  - Unexplained fever with temperatures >101.5° F (38° C) for more than 3 days
  - Drenching night sweats
- Pruritus
- Less common: pain in involved areas after ingestion of alcohol
- Physical findings:
  - Painless adenopathy, commonly in the supraclavicular or cervical areas
  - Splenomegaly

DIAGNOSTIC WORKUP

- History and physical examination
- Laboratory tests:
  - Complete blood cell count with differential
  - Erythrocyte sedimentation rate
  - Serum chemistries
  - HIV
- Bone marrow aspirate and biopsy
  - Biopsy indicated in the presence of constitutional B symptoms or anemia, leukopenia, or thrombocytopenia (bone marrow involvement occurs in 5% of patients)
- Imaging studies:
  - Chest x-ray film
  - Skeletal survey
  - Neck, thoracic, and abdominal/pelvic computerized tomographic scans
  - Positron emission tomography scans, sometimes combined with computed tomographic

scans, have replaced gallium scans and lymphangiography for clinical staging.
  - Magnetic resonance imaging may provide information on bone marrow involvement.

HISTOLOGY

The World Health Organization modification of the Revised European-American Lymphoma classification is currently used. Two clinicopathological entities are described: nodular lymphocyte predominance HL (NLPHL) and classical HL (CHL). NLPHL is distinct from CHL: the profile for NLPHL is CD15$^-$, CD20$^+$, CD30$^-$, CD45$^+$, whereas the profile for CHL is CD15$^+$, CD20$^-$, CD30$^+$, CD45$^-$.

- NLPHL
  - Approximately 5% of HL cases
  - Typically diagnosed in asymptomatic young men with cervical or inguinal lymph nodes without mediastinal involvement
  - Typical immunophenotype is CD15$^-$, CD20$^+$, CD30$^-$, CD45$^+$ B cell lymphocytes.
  - Patients usually diagnosed with earlier-stage disease, longer survival, and fewer treatment failures
- CHL
  - Accounts for 95% of cases
  - Typical immunophenotype is CD15$^+$, CD20$^-$, CD30$^+$, CD45$^-$ B cell lymphocytes.
  - Four subtypes:
    - Nodular sclerosis (grade I and II)
      - 75% of HL cases in United States
      - Equal distribution between sexes
      - More prominent in patients <50 years of age
      - Common anterior mediastinal involvement
      - Grade I, 75% of nodules contain scattered H-RS cells
      - Grade 2, 25% contain numerous H-RS cells surrounded with necrosis
    - Mixed cellularity
      - More prominent in males

      - Frequently associated with HIV and Epstein-Barr virus infection
      - Classic H-RS cells with inflammatory rich background of lymphocytes, plasma cells, and eosinophils
    - Lymphocyte rich
      - More common in males
      - Most with stage I or II disease with rare B symptoms
      - Infrequent H-RS cells background of small lymphocytes
    - Lymphocyte depleted
      - Least common subtype with <5% of cases
      - More common in men
      - Typically advanced stage disease and B symptoms at presentation
      - H-RS cells predominant in background of depleted lymphocytes.

STAGING

The staging classification that is currently used was adopted in 1971 at the Ann Arbor Conference with some modifications at the Cotswolds meeting 18 years later. This staging system is based on the number and location of involved lymph nodes and extranodal involvement. The current practice is to assign a clinical stage on the basis of the findings of the clinical evaluation and a pathological stage on the basis of the findings of invasive procedures. Pathological confirmation of noncontiguous extralymphatic involvement is strongly suggested.

Stages I, II, III, and IV can be subclassified into A and B categories: A for those without B symptoms and B for those with defined B symptoms. The E designation is also used in stages I-III. The E designation notes the presence of extralymphatic disease resulting from direct extension of an involved lymph node region. It is not appropriate to use this designation in the presence of widespread disease or diffuse extralymphatic disease.

- **Stage I.** Involvement of a single lymph node region (I) or localized involvement of a single extralymphatic organ or site (IE).
- **Stage II.** Involvement of more than two lymph node regions on the same side of the diaphragm (II) or localized involvement of a single associated extralymphatic organ or site and its regional lymph node(s) with or without involvement of other lymph node regions on the same side of the diaphragm (IIE).
- **Stage III.** Involvement of lymph node regions on both sides of the diaphragm (III), which may also be accompanied by localized involvement of an associated extralymphatic organ or site (IIIE).
- **Stage IV.** Disseminated (multifocal) involvement of one or more extralymphatic organs, with or without associated lymph node involvement, or isolated extralymphatic organ involvement with distant (nonregional) nodal involvement.

A prognostic staging system can also be used that is particularly useful in clinical trials. This risk system uses three major groups on the basis of prognostic features. The European Organization for Research and Treatment of Cancer defines favorable and unfavorable features for stage I and II disease and the International Prognostic Factors Project has developed an International Prognostic Index with seven adverse factors for advanced stages (stage III and IV). These are described in the box on right.

TREATMENT

- Treatment is based on stage and prognostic factors.
- Standard treatment is intensive combination chemotherapy and involved-field radiation therapy, which yields a >90% cure rate.
- Front-line chemotherapy agents are usually given in combination and may include the following:
  - Cyclophosphamide
  - Procarbazine

Risk-Based Staging System

EARLY FAVORABLE (EUROPEAN ORGANIZATION FOR RESEARCH AND TREATMENT OF CANCER PROGNOSTIC DEFINITIONS)
- <50 years of age
- Clinical stage I and II
- No B symptoms or elevated erythrocyte sedimentation rate
- B symptoms + erythrocyte sedimentation rate <30 mm/h
- Involvement of <3 lymph node areas
- Mediastinal involvement <33% of the thoracic width on the chest x-ray, <10 cm on computed tomographic scan

EARLY UNFAVORABLE (EUROPEAN ORGANIZATION FOR RESEARCH AND TREATMENT OF CANCER PROGNOSTIC DEFINITIONS)
- Age >50 years
- Clinical stage II
- Elevated erythrocyte sedimentation rate >50 mm/hr or >30 mm/hr in the presence of B symptoms
- Involvement in >3 lymph node areas.
- Mediastinal involvement >33% of the thoracic width on the chest x-ray, >10 cm on computed tomographic scan

ADVANCED (IPI FOR PATIENTS WITH CLINICAL STAGE III OR IV)
- Albumin level <4.0 g/dL
- Hemoglobin <10.5 g/dL
- Male sex
- Age >45 years
- Stage IV disease
- White blood cell count at least 15,000/mm^3
- Absolute lymphocytic count <600/mm^3 or a lymphocyte count < 8% of the total white blood cell count

Adapted from Mullen, E., & Zhong, Y. (2007). Hodgkin lymphoma: an update, *The Journal for Nurse Practitioners*, 398.

  - Vincristine or vinblastine
  - Prednisone or dexamethasone
  - Doxorubicin
  - Bleomycin
  - Dacarbazine
  - Etoposide
  - Methotrexate
  - Cytosine arabinoside
  - Mechlorethamine
- Rituximab is being investigated, particularly for patients with NLPHL (CD20$^+$).
- Salvage treatments:
  - In late recurrences the same regimen used for front-line therapy may be effective.

Early recurrence should be treated with different agents.
  - A number of chemotherapy drugs not generally used in the initial treatment have demonstrated efficacy in recurrent disease, including:
    - Moderate- or high-dose cytarabine
    - Carboplatin/cisplatin
    - Ifosfamide
    - Etoposide
    - Vinorelbine
    - Gemcitabine
    - Vinblastine.
  - Radiation to sites not previously irradiated

PROGNOSIS

- HL is considered a curable disease with the overall 5-year survival rate of 86%.
- The mortality rate in the United States has fallen more rapidly for adult HL than for any other malignancy.
- HL is the primary cause of death over the first 15 years after treatment. By 15 to 20 years after therapy, the cumulative mortality from a second malignancy will exceed the cumulative mortality from HL.
- Patients with advanced favorable disease, zero to three adverse risk factors, have a 60% to 80% freedom-from-progression at 5 years with first-line chemotherapy.
- Patients with the very highest risk, advanced unfavorable disease and four to seven adverse factors, showed a 42% to 51% freedom-from-progression at 5 years with first-line therapy.

PREVENTION

Because the etiology of HL is unknown, there are no known preventive measures. There are no specific screening tests, and regular physical examination is currently the best method for early diagnosis.

BIBLIOGRAPHY

Jemal, A., Siegel, R., Ward, E., et al. (2007). Cancer statistics, 2007. *CA: A Cancer Journal for Clinicians*, *57*, 43-66.

Leukemia Lymphoma Society. (2007). *Hodgkin lymphoma*. Retrieved June 25, 2007, from http://www.leukemia-lymphoma.org/all_page?item_id=7085.

Mullen, E., & Zhong, Y. (2007). Hodgkin lymphoma: an update. *The Journal for Nurse Practitioners, 3*, 393-403.

National Cancer Institute. (2007). *Adult Hodgkin's lymphoma (PDQ): treatment, health professional version*. Retrieved July 3, 2007, from http://www.cancer.gov/cancertopics/pdq/treatment/adulthodgkins/HealthProfessional.

National Cancer Institute. (2007). *Childhood Hodgkin's lymphoma (PDQ): treatment, health professional version*. Retrieved July 3, 2007, from http://www.cancer.gov/cancertopics/pdq/treatment/childhodgkins/Health Professional.

Skarin, A.T., & Dorfman, D. M. (1997). Non-Hodgkin's lymphomas: current classification and management. *CA; A Cancer Journal for Clinicians, 47*, 351-372.

Non-Hodgkin Lymphoma

DEFINITION

Lymphomas are cancers of the B or T lymphocytes or natural killer cells that originate in the lymphatic system. The lymphomas are divided into two major categories: Hodgkin lymphoma and all other lymphomas, called non-Hodgkin lymphomas (NHL). NHL is a diverse group of cancers of the immune system. NHL can be divided into aggressive and indolent types and can be classified as either B-cell or T-cell NHL. B-cell NHLs include Burkitt's lymphoma, diffuse large B-cell lymphoma, follicular lymphoma, immunoblastic large cell lymphoma, precursor B-lymphoblastic lymphoma, and mantle cell lymphoma. T-cell NHLs include mycosis fungoides, anaplastic large cell lymphoma, and precursor T-lymphoblastic lymphoma.

INCIDENCE

- Fifth most common cancer in men and women in the United States.
- 63,190 (34,200 men and 28,990 women) new cases in the United States are expected to be diagnosed in 2007 with 18,660 deaths from the disease
- Incidence increases with age; median age at diagnosis is 67 years of age.
- Occurs more often in whites than in blacks and is more common among men than women

ETIOLOGY AND RISK FACTORS

- The etiology of NHL is unknown. A number of risk factors are related to the either a chronic decrease or increase in immune response.
- Risk factors related to viral exposure include the following:
  - MALT (mucosa-associated lymphoid tissue) lymphoma is associated with *Helicobacter pylori* infection.
  - Epstein-Barr virus is associated with 30% of Burkitt's lymphoma.
  - Human T-cell leukemia/lymphoma virus 1
  - Human herpes virus 8
  - Hepatitis C virus
- Increased risks factors resulting from chronic suppression of the immune system include the following:
  - Human immunodeficiency virus (HIV) infection
  - Organ or bone marrow transplant (requiring immune suppression medications)
  - Rheumatoid arthritis
  - Inherited immune deficiencies
- Positive association between exposure to pesticides and herbicides and NHL
- Increasing age; rates are much higher among persons over the age of 65 years (68 for every 100,000 people).

SIGNS AND SYMPTOMS

- Most common early symptom is painless lymphadenopathy (generally in the neck, armpit, groin, or abdomen)
- B symptoms (absence or presence is key in staging)
  - Unexplained loss of more than 10% of body weight in the 6 months before diagnosis.
  - Unexplained fever with temperatures >101.5° F (38° C) for more than 3 days
  - Drenching night sweats
- Fatigue
- Pruritus
- Given the heterogeneity of NHL, signs and symptoms can vary greatly depending on the areas of the body that are affected.
  - MALT lymphoma affects the stomach lining and can cause nausea, vomiting, and abdominal pain.
  - Cutaneous T-cell lymphoma affects the skin and can cause redness, itching, or raised patches on the skin.

DIAGNOSTIC WORKUP

- Complete medical history and physical examination
- Laboratory tests
  - Complete blood cell count with differential
  - Erythrocyte sedimentation rate
  - Serum chemistries
  - Lactate dehydrogenase (LDH) and uric acid: elevated levels correlate with large tumor burden
  - Beta2-microglobulin
  - HIV
  - Cytogenetics
    - Permits identification of chromosome or gene abnormalities in the cells
  - Immunophenotyping
  - Cerebrospinal fluid assessment for malignant cells
  - Bone marrow aspirate and biopsy
- Imaging studies
  - Chest x-ray film
  - Thoracic and abdominal/pelvic computerized tomographic (CT) scans or magnetic resonance imaging
  - Positron emission tomography scans, sometimes combined with CT scans, have replaced gallium scans and lymphangiography for clinical staging

- Biopsy of involved lymph node
  - Only definitive method to diagnose NHL
  - Necessary to determine presence of disease and type of lymphoma

HISTOLOGY

The World Health Organization (WHO) modification of the Revised European American Lymphoma classification system recognizes three major categories of lymphoid malignancies on the basis of morphology and cell lineage: B-cell neoplasms, T-cell/natural killer–cell neoplasms, and Hodgkin lymphoma. Both lymphomas and lymphoid leukemias are included in this classification because both solid and circulating phases are present in many lymphoid neoplasms and distinction between them is artificial. Within the B-cell and T-cell categories, two subdivisions are recognized: precursor neoplasms, which correspond to the earliest stages of differentiation, and more mature differentiated neoplasms. These classifications can be found in the box on right.

The more than 20 clinicopathological entities described by the WHO classification can be divided into the more clinically useful indolent or aggressive lymphomas. These are listed in the box on page 113. Indolent or low-grade classifications account for approximately 35% of NHL diagnoses, whereas the remaining 65% are aggressive (called intermediate or high-grade NHL). In the United States, B-cell lymphomas account for about 90% of all NHL cases.

CLINICAL STAGING

Current practice is to assign a clinical stage on the basis of the findings of the clinical evaluation and a pathological stage on the basis of the findings of invasive procedures beyond that of the initial biopsy. The Ann Arbor staging system is commonly used and stages I-IV can be subclassified into A and B categories: A for those without B symptoms and B for those with defined B symptoms (refer to Signs and Symptoms). The E designation is

World Health Organization Modification of the REAL Classification of Lymphoid Tumors

B-CELL NEOPLASMS
I. **Precursor B-cell neoplasm:** precursor B-acute lymphoblastic leukemia/lymphoblastic lymphoma
II. **Peripheral B-cell neoplasms.**
 A. B-cell chronic lymphocytic leukemia/small lymphocytic lymphoma
 B. B-cell prolymphocytic leukemia
 C. Lymphoplasmacytic lymphoma/immunocytoma
 D. Mantle cell lymphoma
 E. Follicular lymphoma
 F. Extranodal marginal zone B-cell lymphoma of mucosa-associated lymphatic tissue (MALT) type
 G. Nodal marginal zone B-cell lymphoma (± monocytoid B-cells)
 H. Splenic marginal zone lymphoma (± villous lymphocytes)
 I. Hairy cell leukemia
 J. Plasmacytoma/plasma cell myeloma
 K. Diffuse large B-cell lymphoma
 L. Burkitt's lymphoma

T-CELL NEOPLASMS
III. **Precursor T-cell neoplasm:** precursor T-acute lymphoblastic leukemia/LBL
IV. **Peripheral T-cell and natural killer cell neoplasms**
 A. T-cell chronic lymphocytic leukemia/prolymphocytic leukemia
 B. T-cell granular lymphocytic leukemia
 C. Mycosis fungoides/Sézary syndrome
 D. Peripheral T-cell lymphoma, not otherwise characterized
 E. Hepatosplenic gamma/delta T-cell lymphoma
 F. Subcutaneous panniculitis-like T-cell lymphoma
 G. Angioimmunoblastic T-cell lymphoma
 H. Extranodal T-/natural killer cell lymphoma, nasal type
 I. Enteropathy-type intestinal T-cell lymphoma
 J. Adult T-cell lymphoma/leukemia (human T-lymphotrophic virus [HTLV -1+)
 K. Anaplastic large cell lymphoma, primary systemic type
 L. Anaplastic large cell lymphoma, primary cutaneous type
 M. Aggressive natural killer cell leukemia

Adapted from Pileri, S. A., Milani, M., Fraternali-Orcioni, G., et al. (1998). From the R.E.A.L. Classification to the upcoming WHO scheme: a step toward universal categorization of lymphoma entities? *Annals of Oncology, 9,* 608.

also used in stages I-III. The E designation notes the presence of extralymphatic disease resulting from direct extension of an involved lymph node region. It is not appropriate to use this designation in the presence of widespread disease or diffuse extralymphatic disease.

- **Stage I.** Involvement of a single lymph node region (I) or localized involvement of a single extralymphatic organ or site (IE)
- **Stage II.** Involvement of more than two lymph node regions on the same side of the diaphragm (II) or localized involvement of a single associated extralymphatic organ or site and its regional lymph node(s) with or without involvement of other lymph node regions on the same side of the diaphragm (IIE)
- **Stage III.** Involvement of lymph node regions on both sides of the diaphragm (III), which may also be accompanied by localized involvement of an associated extralymphatic organ or site (IIIE)
- **Stage IV.** Disseminated (multifocal) involvement of one or more extralymphatic organs, with or without associated lymph node involvement, or isolated extralymphatic organ involvement with distant (nonregional) nodal involvement

Note: A different staging system is used for cutaneous T-cell lymphoma, mycosis fungoides.

TREATMENT

Treatment depends on the stage, histologic type, and indolent or aggressive nature of the disease. Chemotherapy is the most commonly used treatment. Other therapies include immunotherapy and radioimmunotherapy. Radiation therapy use is limited to treat localized disease or symptomatic areas. Surgery is generally used to establish the diagnosis; exceptions to this are early-stage gastrointestinal lymphomas and testicular lymphomas.

Listing of Indolent and Aggressive Non-Hodgkin Lymphomas

I. **Indolent lymphoma/leukemia**
   A. Follicular lymphoma (follicular small-cleaved cell [grade 1], follicular mixed small-cleaved and large cell [grade 2], diffuse small-cleaved cell)
   B. Small lymphocytic lymphoma
   C. Lymphoplasmacytic lymphoma (Waldenström's macroglobulinemia)
   D. Extranodal marginal zone B-cell lymphoma (mucosa-associated lymphoid tissue [MALT] lymphoma)
   E. Nodal marginal zone B-cell lymphoma (monocytoid B-cell lymphoma)
   F. Splenic marginal zone lymphoma (splenic lymphoma with villous lymphocytes)
   G. Mycosis fungoides/Sézary syndrome
   H. Primary cutaneous anaplastic large cell lymphoma/lymphomatoid papulosis (CD30+)
II. **Aggressive lymphoma/leukemia**
   A. Diffuse large cell lymphoma (includes diffuse mixed-cell, diffuse large cell, immunoblastic, T-cell rich large B-cell lymphoma)
      1. Mediastinal large B-cell lymphoma
      2. Follicular large cell lymphoma (grade 3)
      3. Anaplastic large cell lymphoma (CD30+)
      4. Extranodal natural killer cell/T-cell lymphoma, nasal type/aggressive natural killer cell leukemia/blastic natural killer cell lymphoma
      5. Lymphomatoid granulomatosis (angiocentric pulmonary B-cell lymphoma)
      6. Angioimmunoblastic T-cell lymphoma
      7. Peripheral T-cell lymphoma, unspecified
      8. Subcutaneous panniculitis-like T-cell lymphoma
      9. Hepatosplenic T-cell lymphoma
      10. Enteropathy-type T-cell lymphoma
      11. Intravascular large B-cell lymphoma
   B. Burkitt's lymphoma/ Burkitt's-like lymphoma
   C. Precursor B-cell or T-cell lymphoblastic lymphoma
   D. Primary central nervous system lymphoma
   E. Adult T-cell lymphoma (HTLV 1+)
   F. Mantle cell lymphoma
   G. Polymorphic posttransplantation lymphoproliferative disorder
   H. Acquired immunodeficiency syndrome–related lymphoma
   I. True histiocytic lymphoma
   J. Primary effusion lymphoma

Adapted from National Cancer Institute. (2007). *Cellular classification: adult non-Hodgkin's lymphoma (PDQ): treatment, health professional version.* Retrieved July 4, 2007, from http://www.cancer.gov/cancertopics/pdq/treatment/adult-non-hodgkins/HealthProfessional/page2# Reference2.11.

Indolent, Stage I and Contiguous Stage II

Localized disease is uncommon in patients with NHL and any of the following treatments may be used:

- Watchful waiting in asymptomatic patients until disease progression or patient becomes symptomatic
- Involved-field radiation therapy (IF-XRT)
- Extended (regional) radiation therapy to cover adjacent nodes
- Chemotherapy with radiation therapy
- Rituximab, an anti-CD20 monoclonal antibody, either alone or in combination with chemotherapy
- Other therapies as designated for patients with advanced-stage disease

Aggressive, Stage I and Contiguous Stage II

- Chemotherapy with or without IF-XRT:
  ○ Rituximab plus cyclophosphamide, doxorubicin, vincristine, and prednisone (R-CHOP) (four to eight cycles)
  ○ Rituximab + doxorubicin + cyclophosphamide + vindesine + bleomycin + prednisone is being evaluated

Indolent, Noncontiguous Stage II/III/IV

- Optimal treatment of advanced stages of low-grade lymphoma is controversial because of the low cure rates with current therapies.
- Watchful waiting in asymptomatic patients until disease progression or until patient becomes symptomatic

- Rituximab as single agent or in combination
- Chemotherapy usually in combination purine nucleoside analog (fludarabine or 2-chlorodeoxyadenosine)
- Radioimmunotherapy with yttrium 90–labeled ibritumomab tiuxetan and iodine 131–labeled tositumomab for patients with minimal (<25%) or no marrow involvement
- Intensive therapy with chemotherapy with or without total body irradiation or high-dose chemotherapy followed by autologous or allogeneic bone marrow transplantation or peripheral stem cell transplantation is under clinical evaluation
- Extended-field radiation therapy (stage III patients only)

Aggressive, Noncontiguous Stage II/III/IV

- Combination chemotherapy, either alone or with local-field radiation therapy
  ○ Doxorubicin-based combination chemotherapy produces long-term disease-free survival in 35% to 45% of patients.
  ○ Rituximab may be used for B-cell NHL with CD20+ cells.
- Bone marrow or stem cell transplantations for patients at high risk of relapse is under clinical evaluation.
- Central nervous system (CNS) prophylaxis (usually with four to six injections of methotrexate intrathecally) is recommended for patients with paranasal sinus or testicular involvement.

Adult Lymphoblastic Lymphoma

Lymphoblastic lymphoma is a very aggressive form of NHL that most often occurs in younger patients. It is commonly associated with large mediastinal masses and often disseminates to the bone marrow and the CNS, much like acute lymphocytic leukemia (ALL).

- Treatment is usually patterned after ALL (see pages 100-101).
- Intensive combination chemotherapy with CNS prophylaxis is the standard therapy.

- Radiation is sometimes used to treat bulky tumor areas.

Diffuse Small Noncleaved-Cell/Burkitt's Lymphoma

Patients with diffuse small non-cleaved-cell/Burkitt's lymphoma have a 20% to 30% lifetime risk of CNS involvement. CNS prophylaxis is recommended for all patients.

PROGNOSIS

Overall survival rates are 53%, 43%, and 37% at 5, 10, and 15 years, respectively. Patients with indolent NHL have a relatively good prognosis with a median survival up to 10 years, but the disease is usually not curable in advanced clinical stages. Aggressive NHL has a shorter natural history, but 30% to 60% of patients can be cured. The majority of relapses occur in the first 2 years after therapy.

Five significant risk factors of overall survival for patients with NHL have been identified. Patients with two or more risk factors have a less than 50% chance of relapse-free and overall survival at 5 years:

- Age (<60 years versus >60 years)
- Performance status (0 or 1 versus 2-4)
- Serum LDH (normal versus elevated)
- Stage (stage I or stage II versus stage III or stage IV)
- Extranodal site involvement (0 or 1 versus 2-4).

An increased risk for relapse has also been linked to specific sites of involvement, including bone marrow, central nervous system, liver, lung, and spleen.

PREVENTION

Because no one knows the specific cause for NHL, there are no known measures to prevent it.. The factors that increase risk are generally not things that can be avoided, making it difficult to decrease risk.

BIBLIOGRAPHY

Jemal, A., Siegel, R., Ward, E., et al. (2007). Cancer statistics, 2007. *CA: A Cancer Journal for Clinicians, 57*, 43-66.

Leukemia and Lymphoma Society. (2007). *Non-Hodgkin lymphoma facts and statistics*. Retrieved July 3, 2007, from http://www.leukemia.org/all_page?item_id=8965.

National Cancer Institute. (2007). *Adult non-Hodgkin's lymphoma (PDQ): treatment, health professional version*. Retrieved July 3, 2007, from http://www.cancer.gov/cancertopics/pdq/treatment/adult-non-hodgkins/Health Professional/page1.

National Cancer Institute. (2006). *AIDS-related lymphoma (PDQ): treatment, health professional version*. Retrieved July 3, 2007, from http://www.cancer.gov/cancertopics/pdq/treatment/AIDS-related-lymphoma/Health Professional.

Pileri, S. A., Milani, M., Fraternali-Orcioni, G., et al. (1998). From the R.E.A.L. Classification to the upcoming WHO scheme: a step toward universal categorization of lymphoma entities? *Annals of Oncology, 9*, 607-612.

Skarin, A. T., & Dorfman, D. M. (1997). Non-Hodgkin's lymphomas: current classification and management. *CA: A Cancer Journal for Clinicians, 47*, 351-372.

Vachani, C. (2006). *Non-Hodgkin's lymphoma: the basics*. OncoLink. Retrieved July 3, 2007, from http://www.oncolink.com/types/article.cfm?c?10&s=36&ss=820&id=9539.

Multiple Myeloma

Jennifer K. Simpson

DEFINITION

Multiple myeloma is a cancer that belongs to a group of B-cell disorders, specifically a cancer of the plasma cell. It is characterized by an excess of abnormal plasma cells in the bone marrow and an increased production of monoclonal immunoglobulin (IgG, IgA, IgD, IgG) or Bence-Jones protein (free monoclonal κ or λ light chains).

INCIDENCE

- Accounts for 1% of all cancers and 14% of hematological malignancies (second most prevalent hematological cancer after non-Hodgkin lymphoma)
- In 2007, it is expected that 19,900 new cases of multiple myeloma will be diagnosed in 10,960 men and in 8,940 women.
- Death is expected from multiple myeloma in 10,790 (5,550 men and 5,240 women) in 2007.

- The 5-year relative survival rate for multiple myeloma is approximately 32%.

ETIOLOGY AND RISK FACTORS

- Age
  - >65 years
  - Median age at diagnosis is 65 years
  - 2% are <40 years old
- Race
  - Highest incidence: African Americans and native Pacific Islanders
  - Lowest incidence: Asians
  - African Americans more than twice as likely than white Americans to be diagnosed with multiple myeloma
- Family history
  - Fourfold risk if sibling or parent has disease
- Obesity
- Other plasma cell diseases

  - Monoclonal gammopathy of undetermined significance
  - Olitary plasmacytoma
- Etiology is unknown
  - Herbicides, insecticides, petroleum products, heavy metals, plastics, and asbestos may increase the risk of multiple myeloma.
- Radiation exposure victims (e.g., survivors of atomic bomb explosions in Japan) have an increased risk, although this number is small.

SIGNS AND SYMPTOMS

- Typically no symptoms in early stages
- Pain is a common early symptom as a result of osteoporosis and fractures, usually in the lower back and ribs. Other sites of osteoporosis include the pelvis and skull.

- Fatigue from anemia
- Recurrent infection, particularly pneumonia.
- Hypercalcemia
- Renal damage and potential renal failure

DIAGNOSTIC WORKUP

- Diagnosis requires presence of one major and one minor criteria or three minor criteria with multiple myeloma symptoms.
  - Major criteria
    - Biopsy-proven plasmocytoma
    - Elevated monoclonal immunoglobulin levels in the serum or urine
    - 30% or greater plasma cells on a bone marrow examination
  - Minor criteria
    - 10%-30% plasma cells on a bone marrow examination
    - Minor monoclonal immunoglobulin levels in the serum or urine
    - Lytic bone lesions or generalized osteoporosis
    - Abnormally low serum antibody levels (excluding antibodies produced by myeloma cells)
- The foundation of the diagnostic workup includes a thorough history and physical examination in conjunction with laboratory tests as outlined below.

Laboratory Tests

- Complete blood cell count with differential
- Serum chemistries (calcium, albumin, lactate dehydrogenase, uric acid)
- Renal function (serum blood urea nitrogen, creatinine)
- 24-hour urine and urine protein electrophoresis to determine protein and creatinine clearance
- Serum beta2-microglobulin (reflects tumor mass)
- Serum protein electrophoresis to identify M spike
- Quantitative immunoglobulins to determine concentration of the various immunoglobulin subtypes
- Bone marrow aspirate and biopsy

Imaging Studies

- Avoid contrast studies because they may worsen renal failure.
- Chest x-ray film
- Skeletal survey
- Magnetic resonance imaging may provide information on bone marrow involvement.

Additional Studies

- C-reactive protein; surrogate marker for interleukin-6, considered a growth factor for myeloma cells
- Plasma cell labeling index
- Cytogenetic testing, including fluorescence in situ hybridization; specific attention to translocations or deletions of 13q because the presence of this abnormality is predictive of a poorer prognosis.

CLASSIFICATION

Patients may be classified into one of three myeloma categories:

- Monoclonal gammopathy of undetermined significance
- Asymptomatic multiple myeloma
- Symptomatic multiple myeloma.

The International Myeloma Working Group has identified the following criteria that must be met to establish the diagnosis:

- Symptomatic multiple myeloma
  - Presence of serum or urinary monoclonal protein
  - Presence of clonal plasma cells in the bone marrow or a plasmacytoma
  - Presence of end-organ damage felt related to the plasma cell dyscrasia
  - Hypercalcemia
  - Lytic bone lesions
  - Anemia
  - Renal failure
- Asymptomatic or smoldering multiple myeloma
  - Serum monoclonal protein >3 g/dL or bone marrow plasma cells >10%
  - No end-organ damage related to plasma cell dyscrasia (see list above)
- Monoclonal gammopathy of undetermined significance
  - Serum monoclonal protein <3 g/dL
  - Bone marrow plasma cells <10%
  - No end-organ damage related to plasma cell dyscrasia or B-cell lymphoproliferative disorder (see list above)

CLINICAL STAGING

The Durie-Salmon Staging System outlines three stages of the disease:

- Stage I (low disease burden)
  - Hemoglobin greater than 10.0 g/dL.
  - Serum calcium = 12 mg/dL
  - Normal bone x-rays or the presence of a solitary bone lesion
  - Low monoclonal (or myeloma) protein (M protein) production as shown by
    - IgG less than 5.0 g/dL
    - IgA less than 3.0 g/dL
    - Urine M-protein less than 4 g/24 hours
- Stage II
  - Stage II fits neither stage I nor stage III.
- Stage III
  - One or more of the following
    - Hemoglobin less than 8.5 g/dL
    - Serum calcium greater than 12.0 mg/dL
    - Advanced bone lytic lesions
    - IgG greater than 7.0 g/dL
    - IgA greater than 5.0 g/dL
    - Urine M-protein greater than 12.0 g/24 hours
- Patients are further subclassified as:
  - A: serum creatinine less than 2.0 mg/dL and
  - B: serum creatinine = 2.0 mg/dL

The majority of symptomatic patients with myeloma fall into stage III by the Durie/Salmon criteria; this staging system has not proved to be very useful. In 2005, the International Myeloma Working Group studied more than 11,000 treated with either high-dose therapy (2,901) or standard-dose therapy (8,270) and established a new International Staging System (ISS) as follows:

- Stage I
  - Serum beta2-microglobulin less than 3.5 mg/L
  - Serum albumin greater than or equal to 3.5 g/dL
- Stage II
  - Serum beta2-microglobulin greater 3.5 mg/L but serum albumin less than 3.5 g/dL
  - Serum beta2-microglobulin 3.5 to less than 5.5 mg/L irrespective of the serum albumin level
- Stage III
  - Beta2-microglobulin greater than or equal to 5.5 mg/dL

TREATMENT

- Therapy is not initiated unless the patient is symptomatic. Nonsymptomatic patients are closely monitored, typically every 3 months, until evidence of disease progression.
- Bisphosphonates
- Supportive care including appropriate pain medication and possible radiation therapy or surgical interventions for problematic bone lytic lesions
- Therapy for newly diagnosed symptomatic patients includes systemic chemotherapy.
- Chemotherapy is selected depending on the performance status and renal compromise as

well as disease stage and potential for the patient to receive a stem cell transplant.
- Chemotherapy choices may include the following:
  - Dexamethasone alone or in combination
  - Doxorubicin/vincristine/ dexamethasone or pegylated liposomal doxorubicin/ vincristine/dexamethasone
  - Thalidomide/dexamethasone
  - Melphalan/prednisone (usually not given if a patient is a potential stem cell transplant candidate)
- Stem cell transplantation may follow induction chemotherapy— single or double autologous transplant.
- Additional chemotherapy regimens for relapsed/refractory multiple myeloma include the following:
  - Lenolidomide/ dexamethasone
  - Velcade alone or in combination with dexamethasone
  - Velcade/pegylated liposomal doxorubicin

PROGNOSIS

- Multiple myeloma is seldom curable; the overall 5-year survival rate is 32%.
- Stage I (ISS): median survival of 62 months

- Stage II (ISS): median survival of 44 months
- Stage III (ISS): median survival of 29 months

PREVENTION

Because the etiology is not understood, no specific recommendations for prevention are available, although avoiding risk factors may have some effect.

BIBLIOGRAPHY

American Cancer Society. (2006). *Multiple myeloma*. Retrieved September 29, 2006, from http://www.cancer.org/.

Ghobrial, I. M., Lockridge, L., & Richardson, P. G. (2006). The emerging role of novel therapeutic agents in the management of patients with multiple myeloma. *Community Oncology, 3*, 575-582.

Greipp, P. R., San Miguel, J., & Durie, B. G. M. (2005). International staging system for multiple myeloma. *Journal of Clinical Oncology, 23*, 3412-3420.

Jemal, A., Murray, T., Ward, E., et al. (2005). Cancer statistics, 2005. *CA: A Cancer Journal for Clinicians, 55*, 10-30.

National Cancer Institute. (2007). *Multiple myeloma and other plasma cell neoplasms (PDQ)*. Retrieved June 11, 2007, from http://www.cancer.gov/cancertopics/pdq/treatment/myeloma/HealthProfessional/page1.

Sagar, L. (2005). *About myeloma*. Retrieved September 29, 2006, from http://www.multiplemyeloma.org/about_myeloma/index.html.

Smith, A., Wisloff, F., & Samson, D. (2006). Guidelines on the diagnosis and management of multiple myeloma. *British Journal of Haematology, 132*, 410-451.

Lung Cancer

Dawn Tiedemann

Non–Small Cell Lung Cancer

DEFINITION

Lung cancer is the development of cancer in any area of the lungs or bronchus, generally in the bronchial endothelium. Lung cancer is generally divided into two major types: small cell lung cancer (SCLC) and non–small cell lung cancer (NSCLC).

INCIDENCE

Lung cancer will be the second most commonly diagnosed cancer in men and women in 2007. According to the American Cancer Society, estimated new cases for 2007 are almost 213,380 with 160,390 expected deaths from the disease. Incidence is finally declining significantly in men, and since 1998, after a long period of increases,

the rate has been stable in women. It is the leading cause of cancer-related deaths in the United States and worldwide. NSCLC is the most common lung cancer type, representing about 87% of lung cancer diagnoses.

ETIOLOGY AND RISK FACTORS

- Tobacco is the primary risk factor. Long-term exposure to cigarette or cigar smoking is the major risk factor in development of lung cancer. Risk increases with number of years of smoking, number of cigarettes smoked, young age when smoking started, increased degree of inhalation, high tar and nicotine content, and use of unfiltered cigarettes. Risk does decrease after cessation. Second-hand smoke exposure contributes to a lesser extent.

- Environmental and occupational exposures to arsenic, benzene, radon, asbestos (especially in smokers), copper, silica, lead, diesel exhaust, chromium, and air pollution
- Radiation exposure from occupational, medical, and environmental sources
- Current and former smokers who take pharmacological doses of beta-carotene
- Scars from tuberculosis or inflammatory processes
- Although evidence is increasing that genetic factors can contribute to risk, no genetic abnormality has been found that causes lung cancer.

SIGNS AND SYMPTOMS

Unfortunately there are few to no symptoms of early stage lung cancer. Symptoms that occur as the cancer progresses include the following:

- Persistent cough
- Shortness of breath
- Sputum streaked with blood
- Chest pain
- Hoarseness
- Recurrent pneumonia or bronchitis

Later-stage symptoms include pain from bone metastasis, fatigue, anorexia, central nervous system changes from brain metastasis, and weight loss. Paraneoplastic syndromes, which are more common in lung cancer than in any other kind of cancer, may cause humoral hypercalcemia of malignancy (especially in squamous cell), hypercoagulable states, and skin conditions such as acanthosis nigricans (in adenocarcinoma).

DIAGNOSTIC WORKUP

The purpose of the diagnostic workup is to determine where the primary cancer is, where a biopsy can be done, and whether there are sites of metastatic disease.

- History and physical examination to determine signs and symptoms of lung cancer and metastatic disease. Smoking and carcinogenic exposure history is important.
- Chest x-ray is probably the most helpful initial examination, but peripheral nodules must be 1 cm or larger to be visualized on radiographs. Other changes include lymphadenopathy, atelectasis, and pleural effusions.
- Computed tomographic (CT) scan of chest, abdomen, and pelvis to identify location of primary tumor and sites of metastatic disease (lymph nodes, liver, adrenal glands, bones)
- Biopsy under CT scan guidance, or bronchoscopy
- Mediastinoscopy to determine whether tumor has spread to mediastinal nodes if surgical resection is to be considered.
- Brain magnetic resonance imaging and bone scan looking for metastatic disease.
- Positron emission tomographic scans have become increasingly popular to find metastatic disease.
- Laboratory testing: alkaline phosphatase (bone/liver disease), calcium (hypercalcemia), complete blood cell count, kidney function, and liver function tests
- Pulmonary function tests to determine whether patient can tolerate removal of part of the lung

HISTOLOGY

There are three common histologies:

- Adenocarcinoma is the most common type (about 40%), and the incidence is increasing. Adenocarcinoma is associated with irritation and scarred areas. About one half of cases are not resectable at diagnosis. Includes subtypes of acinar, papillary, and bronchoalveolar
- Squamous carcinoma compromise about 30% of all lung cancers and are generally associated with smoking. These tend to be slow growing and therefore stay localized for a longer period. It usually presents as masses in large bronchi with local extension that may result in atelectasis and pneumonitis. When detected early, squamous carcinoma may be resectable and can be associated with longer survival.
- Large cell carcinoma represents about 10% to 15% of lung cancers. It is more undifferentiated and difficult to treat. It usually arises as peripheral nodules and metastasizes early, often to the gastrointestinal tract. It can be further classified into clear cell and giant cell, but they are treated the same.

CLINICAL STAGING

Lung cancers have predictable patterns of growth, and can spread locally, by lymphatic invasion, and through the bloodstream. NSCLC spreads locally initially and can occlude the bronchial lumens; grow into the pleura and chest wall; spread to hilar, mediastinal, and supraclavicular lymph nodes; and finally to bone, liver, adrenal glands, and the brain.

The purpose of staging is to determine how far the cancer has spread, so that appropriate treatment can be offered and a prognosis can be estimated. Patients can be divided into cases that are resectable and those that are not because only in the early stages can surgery be considered. NSCLC uses the TNM (tumor size, lymph nodes, and metastasis) system adopted by the American Joint Commission on Cancer. Histology or type of cancer is not a factor in staging. The stage of cancer determines the most appropriate treatment. See the table on page 118 for staging of lung cancer.

TREATMENT

When the cancer is localized and small (stages I, II, and some IIIA), surgery is usually the treatment of

Clinical Staging: Non–Small Cell Lung Cancer

Definition of TNM

Primary Tumor (T)

TX	Primary tumor cannot be assessed, or tumor proven by the presence of malignant cells in sputum or bronchial washings but not visualized by imaging or bronchoscopy
T0	No evidence of primary tumor
Tis	Carcinoma *in situ*
T1	Tumor 3 cm or less in greatest dimension, surrounded by lung or visceral pleura, without bronchoscopic evidence of invasion more proximal than the lobar bronchus* (i.e., not in the main bronchus)
T2	Tumor with any of the following features of size or extent: More than 3 cm in greatest dimension Involves main bronchus, 2 cm or more distal to the carina Invades the visceral pleura Associated with atelectasis or obstructive pneumonitis that extends to the hilar region but does not involve the entire lung
T3	Tumor of any size that directly invades any of the following: chest wall (including superior sulcus tumors), diaphragm, mediastinal pleura, parietal pericardium; or tumor in the main bronchus less than 2 cm distal to the carina, but without involvement of the carina; or associated atelectasis or obstructive pneumonitis of the entire lung
T4	Tumor of any size that invades any of the following: mediastinum, heart, great vessels, trachea, esophagus, vertebral body, carina; or separate tumor nodules in the same lobe; or tumor with malignant pleural effusion**

*Note: The uncommon superficial tumor of any size with its invasive component limited to the bronchial wall, which may extend proximal to the main bronchus, is also classified T1.

**Note: Most pleural effusions associated with lung cancer are due to tumor. However, there are a few patients in whom multiple cytopathological examinations of pleural fluid are negative for tumor. In these cases, fluid is nonbloody and is not an exudate. Such patients may be further evaluated by videothoroscopy and direct pleural biopsies. When these elements are clinical judgment dictate that the effusion is not related to the tumor, the effusion should be excluded as a staging element, and the disease should be staged as T1, T2, or T3.

Regional Lymph Nodes (N)

NX	Regional lymph nodes cannot be assessed
N0	No regional lymph node metastasis
N1	Metastasis to ipsilateral peribronchial or ipsilateral hilar lymph nodes including involvement by direct extension of the primary tumor
N2	Metastasis to ipsilateral mediastinal or subcarinal lymph node(s)
N3	Metastasis to contralateral mediastinal, contralateral hilar, ipsilateral or contralateral scalene, or supraclavicular lymph node(s)

Distant Metastasis (M)

MX	Distant metastasis cannot be assessed
M0	No distant metastasis
M1	Distant metastasis present
M1	includes a separate tumor nodule(s) in a different lobe (ipsilateral or contralateral).

Stage Grouping

Occult carcinoma	TX	N0	M0
Stage 0	Tis	N0	M0
Stage IA	T1	N0	M0
Stage IB	T2	N0	M0
Stage IIA	T2	N1	M0
Stage IIB	T2	N1	M0
	T3	N0	M0
Stage IIIA	T1	N2	M0
	T2	N2	M0
	T3	N1	M0
	T3	N2	M0
Stage IIIB	Any T	N3	M0
	T4	Any N	M0
Stage IV	Any T	Any N	M1

Used with the permission of the American Joint Committee on Cancer (AJCC), Chicago, Illinois. The original source for this material is the *AJCC Cancer staging manual*, Sixth Edition (2002) published by Springer Science and Business Media LLC, www.springerlink.com.

choice if the patient is a good surgical risk and can have a good quality of life after removal of that part of the lung (adequate pulmonary function tests). Surgical procedures include a wedge resection that removes small peripheral nodules (most conservative), segmentectomy that removes part of a lobe of the lung, lobectomy that removes a lobe of the lung (most common), or pneumonectomy that removes either the right or left lung. Only about 25% of patients with NSCLC are operable at diagnosis. Recent studies have shown that adjuvant chemotherapy after surgery in localized NSCLC can improve survival.

Unfortunately, some patients who are surgical candidates are found during surgery to have tumors that cannot be totally removed. These patients will require further treatment with radiation or chemotherapy. Patients who are not surgical candidates or who refuse surgery can receive radiation therapy, which can be curative in some patients with stage I or II disease. Adjuvant radiation therapy may be used after surgery for stage IIIA disease and as primary therapy for unresectable stage IIIA disease. Patients with stage IIIB disease generally receive a combination of chemotherapy and radiation therapy.

Neoadjuvant therapy (chemotherapy with or without radiation before surgery) has been an area of intense study in recent years as a way of treating undetectable metastatic disease and shrinking the tumor to improve successful resection and improve survival. Although survival rates have improved in stages IB through IIIA with neoadjuvant therapy, it does carry a greater risk of complications.

Stage IIIB and IV NSLC is considered to be inoperable. At times, solitary metastatic lesions in the lung and brain can be resected.

Most patients with NSLC will receive chemotherapy because many are initially seen with unresectable disease and 80% of those with resectable disease will have relapses. Treatment with chemotherapy alone for metastatic disease produces only moderate response rates (up to 30% with the newer drugs) and a median survival time of 25 to 30 weeks.

First-line regimens of choice are usually combination therapies including carboplatin/paclitaxel, paclitaxel/cisplatin, vinorelbine/cisplatin, docetaxel/cisplatin, docetaxel/carboplatin, docetaxel/ gemcitabine, gemcitabine/cisplatin, or gemcitabine/vinorelbine. Bevacizumab recently received Food and Drug Administration approval for use in non–squamous cell non–small cell cancers with carboplatin and paclitaxel as first-line treatment. Contraindications are brain metastasis or hemoptysis. Patients with poor performance status are generally treated with either single agents or with supportive care.

Once the disease progresses, single agents such as docetaxel, gemcitabine, topotecan, vinorelbine, and pemetrexed are used, depending on which drugs have already been given. Targeted therapies, those that target specific aspects of tumor development at the molecular level, are the latest group of drugs to become available. Because they target specifically the tumor, it is hoped these will be more effective and less toxic to the rest of the body. These include the epidermal growth factor receptors that are expressed in the majority of NSCLC tumors, of which gefitinib (Iressa) and erlotinib (Tarceva) are examples. Finally, participation in a clinical trial should be considered.

Palliative radiation is done for symptomatic treatment of bone pain, spinal cord compression, brain metastasis, and postobstructive pneumonia.

PROGNOSIS

Lung cancer remains the leading cause of cancer-related deaths in the United States and worldwide because so many patients are found to have advanced stages at diagnosis. Despite many advances in treatment, effective treatment for lung cancer remains elusive, especially in the later stages. Five-year survival rates remain low and almost unchanged over the last 30 years at 15%.

Stage of disease is the most important prognostic factor, with earlier stages having better response to treatment and longer survival. Poor prognostic factors include weight loss, poor performance status, male sex, elevated lacate dehydrogenase levels, and bone or liver metastasis. Survival rates depend on stage:

- Stage I: 5-year survival rate 60%-80%
- Stage II: 5-year survival rate 25%-50%
- Stage IIIA: 5-year survival rate 10%-40%
- Stage IIIB: 5-year survival rate less than 5%
- Stage IV: 5-year survival rate less than 5%

PREVENTION

If smoking products were removed from the marketplace, 85% of lung cancers would not develop. Smoking cessation for current smokers can reduce their likelihood for development of lung cancer, depending on how much and how long they have smoked. Education, behavioral therapy, and smoking cessation products offer some effective methods, but success rates vary. Avoidance of exposures to the other occupational and environmental agents is important, especially in smokers. Unfortunately, efforts to find a method of early detection have not demonstrated any reduction in mortality rates.

BIBLIOGRAPHY

Chu, E., et al. (2006). Common chemotherapy regimens in clinical practice. In E. Chu E. & V. DeVita (Eds.). *Cancer chemotherapy drug manual 2006* (pp. 437-440). Sudbury, MA: Jones & Bartlett.

Flannery, M. (2005). Nursing care of the client with lung cancer. In J. Itano & K. Taoka (Eds.). *Core curriculum for oncology nursing* (4th ed., pp. 512-523). St. Louis: Elsevier Saunders.

Govindan, R. (2004). *Locally advanced non-small cell lung cancer.* Manhasset, NY: CMP Healthcare Media.

Ingle, R. (2000). Lung cancers. In C. Yarbro, M. Frogge, M. Goodman, et al. (Eds.). *Cancer nursing principles and practice* (5th ed., pp. 1298-1328). Sudbury, MA: Jones & Bartlett.

Jemal, A., Siegel, R., Ward, E., et al. (2007). Cancer statistics, 2007. *CA: A Cancer Journal for Clinicians, 57,* 43-66.

National Cancer Institute. (2006). *Non-small cell lung cancer, PDQ.* Retrieved January 11, 2007, from http://www.cancer.gov/cancertopics/pdq/treatment/non-small-cell-lung/Health Professional.

Schramp, D., Altorki, N., Henschke, C., et al. (2005). Non-small cell lung cancer. In V. DeVita, S. Hellman, & S. Rosenberg (Eds.). *Cancer principles and practice of oncology* (7th ed., pp. 753-809). Philadelphia: Lippincott Williams & Wilkins.

Small Cell Lung Cancer

DEFINITION

Lung cancer is the development of cancer in any area of the lungs or bronchus, generally in the bronchial endothelium. Lung cancer is generally divided into two major types: small cell lung cancer (SCLC) and non–small cell lung cancer (NSCLC). SCLC is discussed in this section.

INCIDENCE

Lung cancer will be the second most commonly diagnosed cancer in men and women in 2007. According to the American Cancer Society, estimated new cases for 2007 are almost 213,380 with 160,390 expected deaths from the disease. Incidence is finally declining significantly in men, and since 1998, after a long period of increases, the rate has been stable in women. It is the leading cause of cancer-related deaths in the United States and worldwide. SCLC represents about 13% of lung cancer cases.

ETIOLOGY AND RISK FACTORS

- Tobacco is the primary risk factor. Long-term exposure to cigarette or cigar smoking is the major risk factor in development of lung cancer. Risk increases with number of years of smoking, number of cigarettes smoked, young age when smoking started,

increased degree of inhalation, high tar and nicotine content, and use of unfiltered cigarettes. Risk does decrease after cessation. Second-hand smoke exposure contributes to a lesser extent.
- Environmental and occupational exposures to arsenic, benzene, radon, asbestos (especially in smokers), copper, silica, lead, diesel exhaust, chromium, and air pollution
- Radiation exposure from occupational, medical, and environmental sources
- Although evidence is increasing that genetic factors can contribute to risk, no genetic abnormality has been found that causes lung cancer.

SIGNS AND SYMPTOMS

Unfortunately there are few to no symptoms of early-stage lung cancer. Symptoms that occur as the cancer progresses include the following:
- Persistent cough
- Shortness of breath
- Sputum streaked with blood
- Chest pain
- Hoarseness
- Recurrent pneumonia or bronchitis

Later-stage symptoms include pain from bone metastasis, fatigue, anorexia, central nervous system changes from brain metastasis, and weight loss. Paraneoplastic syndromes, which are more common in lung cancer than in any other kind of cancer, may cause syndrome of inappropriate antidiuretic hormone, peripheral neuropathy, Eaton-Lambert syndrome (proximal muscle weakness), and skin conditions such as acanthosis nigricans, which is associated with adenocarcinomas. A complication of SCLC present in about 10% of patients at diagnosis is superior vena cava syndrome, which occurs when the tumor compromises blood flow through the superior vena cava.

DIAGNOSTIC WORKUP

The purpose of the diagnostic workup is to determine the primary cancer site, locate a potential biopsy site, and identify any metastatic disease.
- History and physical examination to determine symptoms of lung cancer and metastatic disease. Smoking and carcinogenic exposure history is important.
- Chest radiography is probably the most helpful initial examination, but peripheral nodules must be 1 cm or larger to be visualized. Other changes include lymphadenopathy, atelectasis, and pleural effusions.
- Computed tomographic (CT) scan of chest, abdomen, and pelvis to identify location of primary tumor and sites of metastatic disease (lymph nodes, liver, adrenal glands, bones)
- Biopsy under CT scan guidance or bronchoscopy
- Brain magnetic resonance imaging and bone scan looking for metastatic disease. Bone marrow biopsy may be done in SCLC looking for metastatic disease.
- Positron emission tomographic scans have become increasingly popular to find metastatic disease.
- Laboratory testing: alkaline phosphatase (bone/liver disease), serum lactate dehydrogenase (LDH), complete blood count, kidney function, and liver function tests

HISTOLOGY

The current classifications of SCLC subtypes are pure small cell carcinoma and two less common subtypes: mixed small cell/large cell carcinoma and combined small cell carcinoma (i.e., SCLC combined with neoplastic squamous or glandular components). SCLC is considered a more aggressive type of lung cancer because it metastasizes early; however, it is generally more responsive to chemotherapy. It used to be commonly known as oat cell carcinoma.

CLINICAL STAGING

Lung cancers have predictable patterns of growth and can spread locally, by lymphatic invasion, and through the bloodstream. SCLC is usually centrally located, around a main bronchus, with metastasis to distant sites occurring in more than 60% of patients at diagnosis, and it can be found in bone, bone marrow, liver, brain, lymph nodes, pleura, and adrenal glands. The purpose of staging is to determine how far the cancer has spread so that appropriate treatment can be offered and a prognosis can be estimated.

Although the American Joint Committee on Cancer has recommended a TNM staging system for SCLC, most clinicians use a simple limited-stage and extensive-stage determination. Limited-stage tumor is confined to one hemithorax and regional lymph nodes with or without pleural effusion that can be treated with a single radiation therapy port. About 30% to 40% of patients at diagnosis have limited-stage disease. The remaining 60% to 70% have extensive disease, which means tumor that has spread beyond these areas. As with NSCLC, staging is useful in determining treatment and prognosis.

TREATMENT

For many years, patients with limited-stage SCLC with a small solitary peripheral nodule were considered surgical candidates. However, many of these recurred or were later found to have metastatic disease. If a patient does have surgery for SCLC, which is very rare, postoperative chemotherapy or radiation therapy may increase the chance of cure.

SCLC is very sensitive to chemotherapy and radiation. In patients with limited-stage disease, radiation to the primary tumor and chemotherapy are generally done. Despite high sensitivity to chemotherapy with response rates of up to 90% in limited-stage disease, long-term survival at 5 years is less than 10%; and it is 0% for extensive-stage disease. Patients generally receive four to six cycles of chemotherapy. Combination therapies such as etoposide/cisplatin, etoposide/carboplatin, irinotecan/cisplatin, or cyclophosphamide/doxorubicin/vincristine are used. When a patient progresses, single agents such as topotecan, oral etoposide, gemcitabine, or irinotecan are used. Eventually the tumor becomes resistant to chemotherapy.

Prophylactic brain radiation has been controversial and may be done in patients with a complete response to help decrease the chance of brain metastasis, despite the risk of potentially serious side effects such as dementia and gait problems. Palliative radiation is done for symptomatic treatment of bone pain, superior vena cava syndrome, spinal cord compression, brain metastasis, and post obstructive pneumonia.

PROGNOSIS

The prognosis for SCLC is more favorable for those with limited-stage disease, but the overall 5-year survival rate is about 5%. Other factors associated with better prognosis include performance status, female sex, and normal LDH levels at diagnosis.

Few patients are cured. The median survival for limited stage disease with maximum treatment with combined chemotherapy and radiation is 15 to 26 months. For extensive-stage disease, it is 7 to 11 months. If untreated, survival is 6 to 12 weeks.

PREVENTION

If smoking products were removed from the marketplace, 85% of lung cancers would not develop. Smoking cessation for current smokers can reduce the likelihood of development of lung cancer, depending on how much and how long they have smoked. Education, behavioral therapy, and smoking cessation products offer some effective methods, but success rates vary. Avoidance of exposures to the other occupational and environmental agents is important, especially in smokers. Unfortunately, efforts to find a method of early detection have not demonstrated any reduction in mortality.

BIBLIOGRAPHY

Chu, E., Noronha, V., Roy, S., et al. (2006). Common chemotherapy regimens in clinical practice. In E. Chu & V. DeVita (Eds.). *Cancer chemotherapy drug manual 2006* (pp. 441-442). Sudbury, MA: Jones & Bartlett.

Flannery, M. (2005). Nursing care of the client with lung cancer. In J. Itano & K. Taoka (Eds.). *Core curriculum for oncology nursing* (4th ed., pp. 512-523). St. Louis: Elsevier Saunders.

Ingle, R. (2000). Lung cancers. In C. Yarbro, M. Frogge, M. Goodman, et al. (Eds.). *Cancer nursing principles and practice.* (5th ed., pp. 1298-1328). Sudbury, MA: Jones & Bartlett.

Jemal, A., Siegel, R., Ward, E., et al. (2007). Cancer statistics, 2007. *CA: A Cancer Journal for Clinicians, 57*, 43-66.

Murren, J., Turrisi, A., & Pass, H. (2005). Small cell cancer of the lung. In V. DeVita, S. Hellman, & S. Rosenberg (Eds.). *Cancer principles and practice of oncology* (7th ed., pp. 810-844). Philadelphia: Lippincott Williams & Wilkins.

National Cancer Institute. (2006). *Small cell lung cancer, PDQ.* Retrieved January 11, 2007, from http://www.cancer.gov/cancertopics/pdq/treatment/small-cell-lung/Health Professional.

Major Cancers

Sarcomas

Chondrosarcoma

Nancy J. Leahy

DEFINITION

Chondrosarcoma is one type of primary bone cancer that derives its name on the basis of its histologic origin, the cartilage. Primary bone cancers demonstrate wide clinical heterogeneity and are often curable with proper treatment.

INCIDENCE

- Primary bone cancers are extremely rare, accounting for less than 0.2% of all cancers.
- Chondrosarcoma is the second most common form of bone cancer, accounting for 30% of bone cancers in the United States.
- An estimated 4,720 new cases will be diagnosed in 2007 in the United States and 790 people will die from the disease.
- Chondrosarcoma is usually found in middle-aged and older adults.

ETIOLOGY AND RISK FACTORS

Chondrosarcomas characteristically produce cartilage matrix from neoplastic tissue devoid of osteoid. Conventional chondrosarcomas are divided into two groupings: primary or central lesions arising from previously normal-appearing bone preformed from cartilage; secondary or peripheral tumors that arise or develop from preexisting benign cartilage lesions, such as enchondromas, or from the cartilaginous portion of osteochondroma. Malignant transformation has been reported in lesions in patients with Ollier's disease (enchondromatosis).

SIGNS AND SYMPTOMS

Symptoms of chondrosarcoma are usually mild and depend on tumor size and location. Patients with pelvic or axial lesions are typically diagnosed later in the disease course because the associated pain has a more insidious onset and often occurs when the tumor has reached a significant size.

DIAGNOSTIC WORKUP

Imaging of the primary lesions includes the following:

- X-ray films

- ○ Show cortical destruction and loss of medullary bone trabeculations
- ○ Evidence of calcification and destruction.
- Magnetic resonance imaging
  - ○ Shows intramedullary involvement and extraosseous extension of the tumor.
- Serial radiographs
  - ○ Demonstrate a slow increase in size of the osteochondroma or enchondroma.
- A cartilage "cap" measuring greater than 2 cm on a preexisting lesion or documented growth after skeletal maturity should raise the suspicion of sarcomatous transformation.

HISTOLOGY

The histologic grade of chondrosarcoma and location are important in treatment decisions. Dedifferentiated chondrosarcomas are high-grade lesions and should be treated as osteosarcoma. Mesenchymal chondrosarcomas are treated as Ewing's sarcoma as a function of their grade.

GX: Grade cannot be assessed
G1: Well differentiated—low grade
G2: Moderately differentiated—low grade
G3: Poorly differentiated—high grade
G4: Undifferentiated—high grade

CLINICAL STAGING

The American Joint Committee on Cancer TNM Staging System for Bone Sarcomas is used for all bone sarcomas. See the table below for the clinical staging of chondrosarcoma by the AJCC system.

TREATMENT

- Surgery
  - ○ Patients with resectable low-grade lesions are treated with intralesional excision or wide excision with negative margins.
  - ○ High-grade lesions (grade II, III or clear cell) surgically treated and obtaining a wide margin.
- Chemotherapy
  - ○ Some low-grade lesions treated with intralesional excision will receive adjuvant chemotherapy.
- Radiation
- High-dose photons are used to treat unresectable high and low-grade lesions.
- Proton beam radiation therapy
  - ○ Also used in unresectable high and low-grade lesions.
- Surveillance
  - ○ Low-grade lesions
    - Physical examination
    - Imaging of the lesion and chest radiograph every 6 to 12 months for 2 years and then yearly as appropriate
  - ○ High-grade lesions
    - Physical examination
    - Primary site or cross-sectional imaging as indicated
    - Chest imaging every 3 to 6 months for the first 5 years and yearly thereafter for a minimum of 10 years
- Relapse
- Local recurrence or relapse should be treated with wide excision with or without radiation therapy depending on margin status.
- Radiation therapy should be considered after excision with positive surgical margins. Negative surgical margins should be observed.
- Unresectable recurrences are treated with either conventional or proton beam radiation therapy.
- Surgical excision is an option for systemic relapse of a high-grade lesion.
- Patients should also be considered for participation in a clinical trial.

PROGNOSIS

Late metastases and recurrences after 5 years are more common with

Clinical Staging: Chondrosarcoma

Definition of TNM

Primary Tumor (T)

TX	Primary tumor cannot be assessed
T0	No evidence of primary tumor
T1	Tumor 8 cm or less in greatest dimension
T2	Tumor more than 8 cm in greatest dimension
T3	Discontinuous tumors in the primary bone site

Regional Lymph Nodes (N)

NX	Regional lymph nodes cannot be assessed
N0	No regional lymph node metastasis
N1	Regional lymph node metastasis

Note: Because of the rarity of lymph node involvement in sarcomas, the designation NX may not be appropriate and should be considered N0 if no clinical involvement is evident.

Distant Metastasis (M)

MX	Distant metastasis cannot be assessed
M0	No distant metastasis
M1	Distant metastasis
M1a	Lung
M1b	Other distant sites

Stage Grouping

Stage IA	T1	N0	M0	G1, 2 Low grade
Stage IB	T2	N0	M0	G1, 2 Low grade
Stage IIA	T1	N0	M0	G3, 4 High grade
Stage IIB	T2	N0	M0	G3, 4 High grade
Stage III	T3	N0	M0	Any G
Stage IVA	Any T	N0	M1a	Any G
Stage IVB	Any T	N1	Any M	Any G
	Any T	Any N	M1b	Any G

chondrosarcoma than with other sarcomas.

The higher the grade of chondrosarcoma the worse the prognosis with increased risk for early metastases. Grade I and II tumors five year survival rate is 80-90% with a low potential for metastases. Grade III tumors five year survival rate is reported to be 29% with greater than a 50% potential for metastasis. The Grade IV or undifferentiated tumors have the greatest metastatic potential with a survival rate of less than 10% at one year.

BIBLIOGRAPHY

Bovee, J. V., Cleton-Jansen, A. M., Taminiau, A. H., et al. (2005). Emerging pathways in the development of chondrosarcoma of bone and implications for targeted treatment. *Lancet Oncology, 6*, 599-607.

Bruns, J., Elbracht, M., & Niggemeyer, O. (2001). Chondrosarcoma of bone: an oncological and functional follow-up study. *Annals of Oncology, 84*, 93-99.

Fiorenza, F., Abudu, A., Grimer, R. J., et al. (2002). Risk factors for survival and local control in chondrosarcoma of bone. *Journal of Bone and Joint Surgery British, 84*, 93-99.

Hug, E. B., & Slater, J. D. (2000). Proton radiation therapy for chordomas and chondrosarcomas of the skull base. *Neurosurgery Clinics of North America, 11*, 627-638.

Lee, F. Y., Mank, H. J., Fondren, G., et al. (1999). Chondrosarcomas of bone: an assessment of outcome. *Journal of Bone and Joint Surgery American 81*, 326-338.

Mankin, H. J., Cantley, K. D., Lipielo, L., et al. (1980). The biology of human chondrosarcoma, I: description of cases, grading, and biochemical analyses. *Journal of Bone and Joint Surgery American, 62*, 160-176.

Mankin, H. J., Cantley, K. D., Schiller, A. L., et al. (1980). The biology of human chondrosarcoma, II: variation in chemical composite among types and subtypes of benign and malignant cartilage tumors. *Journal of Bone and Joint Surgery American 62*, 176-188.

Terek, R. M. Recent advances in basic science of chondrosarcoma. (2006). *Orthopedic Clinics of North America, 37*, 9-14.

Ewing's Sarcoma

Nancy J. Leahy

DEFINITION

Ewing's sarcoma is one type of primary bone cancer that has an unknown histologic origin. Primary bone cancers demonstrate wide clinical heterogeneity and are often curable with proper treatment. Ewing's sarcoma family of tumors (ESFT) includes Ewing's sarcoma, primitive neuroectodermal tumor (PNET), Askin's tumor, PNET of bone, and extraosseous Ewing's sarcoma.

INCIDENCE

Ewing's sarcoma is the third most common form of bone cancer and accounts for 16% of all bone cancer cases. Ewing's sarcoma develops mainly in adolescents and young adults.

ETIOLOGY AND RISK FACTORS

Ewing's sarcoma and PNET are small round cell neoplasms developing in bone and soft tissue. They exhibit chromosomal translocation, t(11;22)(q24;q12), and closely related variants. Ewing's sarcoma is poorly differentiated and is also characterized by strong expression of cell-surface glycoprotein CD99. The most common sites of primary Ewing's sarcoma are the femur, pelvic bones, and the bones of chest wall, although any bone may be affected. Presentation in a long bone most frequently involves the diaphysis. The bone has been described as mottled on imaging. Periosteal reaction is classic and is referred to as "onion skin" by radiologists.

SIGNS AND SYMPTOMS

- Localized pain or swelling.
- Constitutional symptoms such as fever, weight loss, and fatigue are occasionally noted on presentation.
- Nearly 25% of patients have metastatic disease on diagnosis.

DIAGNOSTIC WORKUP

If ESFT is suspected as a diagnosis, the patient should undergo a complete staging before biopsy.

- Imaging of the primary lesions
  - Plain radiographs of primary site
  - Computed tomography (CT) or magnetic resonance imaging (MRI) of the entire involved bone or area
  - CT of the chest
  - Bone scan
  - Positron emission tomographic scan can also be considered; it is still considered experimental by most insurance companies.
  - MRI of spine and pelvis should be considered.
- Laboratory values most often elevated in Ewing's sarcoma:
  - Lactate dehydrogenase (a prognostic value as a tumor marker)
  - Leukocytosis
- Cytogenetic analysis of the biopsy specimen to evaluate the t(11;22) translocation
- Bone marrow biopsy should be considered to complete the workup.

HISTOLOGY

GX: Grade cannot be assessed
G1: Well differentiated— low grade
G2: Moderately differentiated—low grade
G3: Poorly differentiated—high grade
G4: Undifferentiated—high grade
  Note: Ewing's sarcoma is classified as G4.

CLINICAL STAGING

The American Joint Committee on Cancer (AJCC) TNM Staging System for Bone Sarcomas is used for all bone sarcomas. See the table on page 122 for stages of Ewing's sarcoma according to the AJCC system.

TREATMENT

- Surgery
  - For local control; includes wide excision
  - Amputation may be required in some cases.

- Chemotherapy
  - A combination of at least three of the following agents:
    - Ifosfamide and/or cyclophosphamide
    - Etoposide
    - Doxorubicin
    - Vincristine
  - If patient responds, he or she is treated with further adjuvant chemotherapy after surgery or radiation.
  - Chemotherapy should be given for a total of 36 weeks, including chemotherapy received before local therapy.
- Radiation therapy with or without surgery followed by chemotherapy or best supportive care is recommended for unresponsive or progressive disease.
- Investigational approaches should be considered in patients with recurrent and metastatic disease.
- Surveillance
  - Every 2 to 3 months
  - Physician examination
  - Chest x-ray film
  - Local imaging
  - Increase interval after 2 years
  - Long-term surveillance should be completed annually after 5 years.

PROGNOSIS

In the past, Ewing's sarcoma was associated with a poor prognosis. The development of multiagent chemotherapy regimens for both neoadjuvant and adjuvant treatment has improved the prognosis greatly for patients with Ewing's sarcoma: 60% to 75% progression-free survival has been observed in patients with localized Ewing's sarcoma. Even patients diagnosed with metastatic disease at presentation are able to achieve a cure.

BIBLIOGRAPHY

Avigad, S., Cohen, I. J., Zilberstein, J., et al. (2004). The predictive potential of molecular detection in the nonmetastatic Ewing family of tumors. *Cancer, 100*, 1053-1058.

Bernstein, M., Cover, H., Paulsen, M., et al. (2006). Ewing's sarcoma family of tumors: current management. *Oncologist, 11*, 503-519.

Cotterill, S. O., Ahrens, S., Paulussen, M., et al. (2000). Prognostic factors in Ewing's tumor of bone: analysis of 975 patients form the European Intergroup Cooperative Ewing's sarcoma study group. *Journal of Clinical Oncology, 18*, 3108-3114.

De Alva, E., & Gerald, W. L. (2000). Molecular biology of the Ewing's sarcoma/PNET. *Journal of Clinical Oncology, 18*, 204-213.

DeAlva, E., Kawai, A., Healy, J. H., et al. (1998). EWS-FLI1 fusion transcript structure is an independent determinant of prognosis in Ewing's sarcoma. *Journal of Clinical Oncology, 16*, 1248-1255.

Denny, C. T. (1996). Gene rearrangements in Ewing's sarcoma. *Cancer Investigation, 14*, 83-88.

Hawking, D. S., Schuetze, S. M., Butrynski, J. E., et al. (2005). 18F-fluorodeoxyglucose positron emission tomography predicts outcome for Ewing sarcoma family of tumors. *Journal of Clinical Oncology, 23*, 8828-8834.

Zoubeck, A., Codkhonr-Dworniczak, B., Delattre, O., et al. Does expression of different EWS chimeric transcripts define clinically distinct risk groups of Ewing's tumor patients? *Journal of Clinical Oncology 12*, 1245-1251.

Kaposi's Sarcoma

Nancy J. Leahy

DEFINITION

Kaposi's sarcoma (KS) is a tumor caused by Kaposi's sarcoma–associated herpes virus (KSHV), also known as human herpes virus 8. Despite its name, it is generally not considered a true sarcoma, which is a tumor arising from connective tissue. KS actually arises as a cancer of lymphatic endothelium and forms vascular channels that fill with blood cells, giving the tumor its characteristic bruise-like appearance.

INCIDENCE

KS was historically very rare and found mainly in older men of Mediterranean, Jewish, or African origin (classic KS) or in patients with severely weakened immune systems, such as after an organ transplant (immunosuppressive treatment– related KS). In the early 1980s KS began to be seen in patients with acquired immunodeficiency syndrome (AIDS). This led to the belief that AIDS weakened the immune system. KSHV is responsible for all forms of KS. The percentage of people in the United States infected with this virus is unknown. Studies suggest an infection rate of 3.5% to 25% varied by geography.

ETIOLOGY AND RISK FACTORS

- Sex
  - Men are much more likely than women to have this disease.
  - White men are the most likely group to be affected.
- Sexual activity
  - Men who have sex with men
  - Women who have sex with these men
- Immune deficiency
  - A defect in the immune system increases the risk of KS in those with human immunodeficiency virus (HIV) infection.
  - There have been reports of some drugs used to block immunity leading to KS.
- Patient whose immune system is suppressed due to AIDS or after organ transplant.

SIGNS AND SYMPTOMS

- Red to brown to purple growth on the skin—found mostly on the legs and face
- Mouth and throat lesions, mainly on the roof of the mouth
- The throat may be tender and sore and may bleed. Eating, breathing, or swallowing may be uncomfortable.
- Lesions can contribute to dental problems, including tooth loss.
- Possible abdominal discomfort
  - Intestinal tract common site for disease at diagnosis
  - Lesions in the gastrointestinal tract do not usually cause symptoms.
  - Bleeding and pain are sometimes seen.
  - Gastrointestinal lesions may interfere with digestion and absorption of nutrients from

food, which may lead to diarrhea.
- Lymphedema is seen in some people; it may appear with or without skin lesions.
- May develop in the lung and produce cough, shortness of breath, and fever

DIAGNOSTIC WORKUP
- Complete medical history
  - Sexual history
  - Exposure to KSHV
  - Exposure to HIV
- Physical examination
  - Thorough skin assessment
  - Rectal examination
- Biopsy of lesion(s)
  - Punch biopsy
  - Excisional biopsy
- Chest x-ray film
- Endoscopy with biopsy of lesions
- Bronchoscopy, especially if bloody sputum is present

HISTOLOGY
KS lesions contain tumor cells with a characteristic abnormal elongated shape, called spindle cells. The tumor is highly vascular, containing abnormally dense and irregular blood vessels, which leak red blood cells into the surrounding tissue and give the tumor its dark color. Inflammation around the tumor may produce swelling and pain.

Although KS may be suspected from the appearance of lesions and the patient's risk factors, a definite diagnosis can only be made by biopsy and microscopic examination, which will show the presence of spindle cells. Detection of the viral protein LANA in tumor cells confirms the diagnosis.

CLINICAL STAGING
The AIDS Clinical Trials Group (ACTG) proposed a staging classification for AIDS-related KS in 1988. The ACTG system considers three criteria:

Tumor Status (T)
T0: localized tumor (good risk)
T1: disseminated/widespread tumor (poor risk)

Immune System Status (I)
I0: CD4 cell count > 200 cells per cubic mm (good risk)
I1: CD4 count < 200 cells per cubic mm (poor risk)

Systemic Illness Status (S)
S0: no systemic illness present—no history of opportunistic infections or thrush; no B symptoms (fever, night sweats, >10% weight loss or diarrhea >2 weeks); Karnofsky performance status score (KPS) >70 (good risk)
S1: systemic illness present—history of opportunistic infections or thrush; B symptoms (1 or more); KPS <70; other HIV-related illness (poor risk)

TREATMENT
- Surgical procedures
  - Local excision
    - The lesion and some of the surrounding tissue is cut out.
  - Electrodesiccation and curettage
    - The lesion is burned and removed with a sharp instrument.
  - Cryotherapy
    - Freezes and kills the tumor
- Chemotherapy
  - Oral
  - Intravenous
  - Intramuscular
  - Intralesional
  - Radiation therapy
  - External beam
- Biological therapy
  - Biological response modifier therapy
  - Immunotherapy

PROGNOSIS
Patients who are at good risk in any of the categories live longer. The 5-year survival rate for patients with combined T and I good risk is 90%. For patients with combined T and I poor risk the 5-year survival rate is 50%. If the lung is involved, the 5-year survival rate is 30%.

BIBLIOGRAPHY
Antman, K., & Chang, Y. (2000). Kaposi's sarcoma. *New England Journal of Medicine, 342*, 1027-1038.
Boshoff, C., & Weiss, R. (2002). AIDS-related malignancies. *Nature Review of Cancer, 2*, 373-382.
Di Lorenzo, G., Konstantinopoulos, P., Pantanowitz, L., et al. (2007). Management of AIDS-related Kaposi's sarcoma. *The Lancet Oncology, 8*, 167-176.
Edelman, D. C. (2005). Human herpesvirus 8—a novel human pathogen. *Virology Journal, 2*, 78.
Yarchoan, R., Tosato, G., & Little, R. F. (2005). Therapy insight: AIDS-related malignancies—the influence of antiviral therapy on pathogenesis and management. *Nature Clinical Practice of Oncology, 2*, 406-415.

Osteosarcoma

Nancy J. Leahy

DEFINITION
Osteosarcoma is one type of primary bone cancer that derives its name on the basis of its histologic origin, the bone. Primary bone cancers demonstrate wide clinical heterogeneity and are often curable with proper treatment.

INCIDENCE
Primary bone cancers are extremely rare, accounting for less than 0.2% of all cancers. An estimated 4,720 new cases will be diagnosed in 2007 in the United States and 790 people will die from the disease. Osteosarcoma is the most common form of bone cancer, accounting for 35% of bone cancers in the United States. Osteosarcoma is the most common primary malignant bone tumor in young adults. The median age for all osteosarcoma patients is 20 years.

ETIOLOGY AND RISK FACTORS
There are 11 known variants of osteosarcoma with variable natural histories. Classic osteosarcoma comprises 80% of osteosarcoma; the most frequent sites are the metaphyseal areas of the distal femur or proximal tibia, which are the sites of maximal growth. Medullary parosteal lesions are juxtacortical and occur mostly in the posterior distal femur. The juxtacortical variant that is a periosteal osteosarcoma involves the tibia.

- Trauma has been implicated in the development of sarcoma, but a cause-and-effect relationship has not been identified.
- Li-Fraumeni syndrome is a family cancer syndrome in which there is a germline mutation of the p53 gene that results in familial sarcomas, including osteosarcoma.
- Specific genetic alterations also play a role in osteosarcoma pathogenesis.
- Variants of osteosarcoma may be the result of:
  - Paget's disease
  - Prior irradiation
- Patients with retinoblastoma are at an increased risk for development of a very aggressive variant of osteosarcoma.

SIGNS AND SYMPTOMS

Pain and swelling are the most frequent early symptoms of osteosarcoma. Pain in the beginning is often described as intermittent and is often considered to be growing pains. Osteosarcomas spread hematogenously, with the lung being the most common metastatic site.

DIAGNOSTIC WORKUP

Osteosarcoma usually presents as a local lesion; however, there is concern for distant metastasis.

- Imaging of the primary lesions includes:
  - X-ray films: show cortical destruction and irregular reactive bone formation
  - Magnetic resonance imaging (MRI):
    - The best study to define the extent of the lesion in the bone and in the soft tissues
  - Computed tomography (CT) and bone scan:
    - Usually uniformly abnormal at the lesion, but may be useful in identifying any additional synchronous lesions
  - Positron emission tomographic (PET) scan can also be considered; still considered experimental by most insurance companies

- Laboratory values most often elevated in osteosarcoma include alkaline phosphatase (Alk Phos) and lactate dehydrogenase (LDH)

HISTOLOGY

Classic osteosarcoma is a high-grade spindle cell tumor that produces osteoid or immature bone. Medullary parosteal lesions metastasize later than the classic form and are considered low grade. The juxtacortical variant, which is a periosteal osteosarcoma involving the tibia, is intermediate grade in its severity.

CLINICAL STAGING

The American Joint Committee on Cancer (AJCC) TNM staging system for bone sarcomas is used for all bone sarcomas. See the table below for AJCC clinical staging of osteosarcoma.

The Surgical Staging System (SSS) is also used for staging musculoskeletal sarcomas. SSS outlines three stages and, similar to the AJCC system, SSS determines stage on the basis of tumor, tumor grade, and the presence of metastasis:

- Stage I: low grade, intracompartmental or extracompartmental lesions
- Stage II: high grade, intracompartmental or extracompartmental lesions
- Stage III: any grade, intracompartmental or extracompartmental lesions with regional or distant metastasis

Clinical Staging: Osteosarcoma

Definition of TNM

Primary Tumor (T)

TX	Primary tumor cannot be assessed
T0	No evidence of primary tumor
T1	Tumor 8 cm or less in greatest dimension
T2	Tumor more than 8 cm in greatest dimension
T3	Discontinuous tumors in the primary bone site

Regional Lymph Nodes (N)

NX	Regional lymph nodes cannot be assessed
N0	No regional lymph node metastasis
N1	Regional lymph node metastasis

Note: Because of the rarity of lymph node involvement in sarcomas, the designation of NX may not be appropriate and could be considered N0 if no clinical involvement is evident.

Distant Metastasis (M)

MX	Distant metastasis cannot be assessed
M0	No distant metastasis
M1	Distant metastasis
M1a	Lung
M1b	Other distant sites

Staging Grouping

Stage IA	T1	N0	M0	G1,2 Low grade
Stage IB	T2	N0	M0	G1,2 Low grade
Stage IIA	T1	N0	M0	G3,4 High grade
Stage IIB	T2	N0	M0	G3,4 High grade
Stage III	T3	N0	M0	Any G
Stage IVA	Any T	N0	M1a	Any G
Stage IVB	Any T	N1	Any M	Any G
	Any T	Any N	M1b	Any G

Histologic Grade

GX	Grade cannot be assessed
G1	Well differentiated—Low Grade
G2	Moderately differentiated—Low Grade
G3	Poorly differentiated—High Grade
G4	Undifferentiated—High Grade

Note: Ewing's sarcoma is classified as G4

TREATMENT

- Surgery: Patients with periosteal and low-grade (intramedullary and surface) osteosarcomas, such as parosteal lesions, are treated with wide excision.
- Chemotherapy: Neoadjuvant and adjuvant chemotherapy are effective for localized disease at diagnosis. Chemotherapy can be given either intravenously or intra-arterially and should include at least two of the following drugs: doxorubicin, cisplatinum, ifosfamide, and high-dose methotrexate. Drug doses should be sufficiently high to mandate the use of myeloid growth factors.
  - Preoperative chemotherapy is preferred for high-grade osteosarcoma and many of the variants as well, including periosteal lesions, although selected elderly patients may benefit from immediate surgery.
  - Patients with pathological findings of high-grade disease after wide excision for suspected low-grade or periosteal sarcomas should be given postoperative chemotherapy.
  - For high-grade osteosarcoma, after wide excision patients with a good histologic response should continue to receive several more cycles of the same chemotherapy, whereas patients with a poor response should be considered for further chemotherapy with a second-line regimen.
- Radiation therapy followed by adjuvant chemotherapy is recommended for unresectable high-grade osteosarcoma.
- Novel therapies should be considered for patients with unresectable pulmonary or any bone metastasis because prognosis is poor for this group of patients.
- Surveillance: Every 3 months for the first 2 years, then every 4 months for the third year, and then every 6 months for the fourth and fifth years and then continue annually. The surveillance should include a complete physical examination, chest imaging, and plain films of the extremity.

PROGNOSIS

In the past, osteosarcoma was associated with a poor prognosis. A generation ago, 80% of patients with osteosarcoma would have metastatic disease and succumb to the disease. All patients with extremity osteosarcomas were treated with amputation. The development of multiagent chemotherapy regimens for both neoadjuvant and adjuvant treatment has improved the prognosis greatly for patients with osteosarcoma. Approximately 75% of osteosarcoma patients are cured. Almost 90% of adult patients with osteosarcoma can be treated successfully with limb-sparing surgery rather than amputation. Even patients diagnosed with metastatic disease at time of presentation are able to achieve a cure. Patients with one or a few resectable pulmonary metastases have a survival rate that approaches that of patients with no metastatic disease.

BIBLIOGRAPHY

Bacci, G., Ferrari, S., Longhi, A., et al. (2001). Neoadjuvant chemotherapy for high-grade osteosarcoma of the extremities: long-term results for patients treated according to Rizzoli IOR/OS-3b protocol. *Journal of Chemotherapy, 13*, 93-99.

Bacci, G., Briccoli, A., Rocca, M., et al. (2003). Neoadjuvant chemotherapy for osteosarcoma of the extremities with metastases at presentation: recent experiences at the Rizzoli Institute in 57 patients treated with cisplatin, doxorubicin, and a high dose of methotrexate and ifosfamide. *Annals of Oncology: Official Journal of the European Society for Medical Oncology/ ESMO, 14*, 1126-1134.

Bielack, S. S., Kempf-Bielack, B., Delling, G., et al. (2002). Prognostic factors in high-grade osteosarcoma of the extremities or trunk: an analysis of 1,702 patients treated on neoadjuvant cooperative osteosarcoma study group protocols. *Journal of Clinical Oncology: Official Journal of the American Society of Clinical Oncology, 20*, 776-790.

Enneking, W. F., Spanier, S. S., & Goodman. M.A. (1980). A system for the surgical staging of musculoskeletal sarcoma. *Clinical Orthopaedics and Related Research, 153*, 106-120.

Gorlick, R. G., Meyers, P. A., & Marina, N. (2006). Osteosarcoma: a review of current management and future clinical trial directions. In American Society of Clinical Oncology (ASCO), *2006 Educational Book* (pp. 558-561). Alexandria, VA: ASCO.

Meyers, P. A., Schwartz, C. L., Krailo, M., et al. (2005). Osteosarcoma: a randomized, prospective trial of the addition of ifosfamide and/or muramyl tripeptide to cisplatin, doxorubicin, and high-dose methotrexate. *Journal of Clinical Oncology: Official Journal of the American Society of Clinical Oncology, 23*, 2004-2011.

Saeter, G., Hoie, J., Stenwig, A. E., et al. (1995). Systemic relapse of patients with osteogenic sarcoma: prognostic factors for long-term survival. *Cancer 75*, 1084-1093.

Yasko, A. W. & Warren Chow, W. (2005). Bone sarcomas. In R. Pazdur, W. J. Hoskins, L. R. Coia, et al. (Eds.). *Cancer management: a multidisciplinary approach*, (9th ed.) (pp. 573- 584). Melville, NY: CMP United Business Media.

Soft Tissue Sarcoma

Cathy Fortenbaugh

DEFINITION

Adult soft tissue sarcoma occurs in the supporting structures and soft tissues of the body, including the following:

- Muscles
- Fat
- Blood vessels
- Lymph vessels
- Nerves, ligaments
- Tissues around joints
- Fibrous tissues.

Soft tissue sarcomas can occur anywhere in the body:

- Arms and legs: 50%-60%
- Trunk: 15%-20%
- Head and neck: 8%-10%
- Internal organs or retroperitoneum: 15%

There are approximately 50 subtypes of soft tissue sarcomas. Adult soft tissue sarcomas are classified by the type of tissue cells they arise from.

INCIDENCE

Soft tissue sarcoma is a relatively rare cancer.

- 9,220 new cases of soft tissue sarcoma are expected to be diagnosed in adults and children in the United States in 2007; a total of 3,560 are expected to die of the disease.
- 5,050 will be in men and 4,710 in women
- From 2000-2003, the median age at diagnosis was 56 years.

ETIOLOGY AND RISK FACTORS

- Exposure to ionizing radiation
  - Accounts for less than 5% of all soft tissue sarcomas
  - Number is expected to decline because radiation therapy techniques have steadily improved
  - Most common form is radiation used to treat other primary cancers such as lymphoma, breast cancer, and cervical cancer
  - The time between the exposure to radiation and the diagnosis of soft tissue sarcoma is approximately 10 years.
- Family history
  - Neurofibromatosis
    - One or more will develop into a peripheral nerve sheath tumor in 5% of patients with neurofibromatosis.
  - Gardner's syndrome
    - An inherited genetic disorder that leads to benign polyps, colon cancer, desmoid tumors in the abdomen, and benign bone tumors
  - Li-Fraumeni syndrome
    - Increases the risk for development of breast cancer, brain tumors, leukemias, adrenal cancer, and bone and soft tissue sarcoma
    - Patients with Li-Fraumeni syndrome who have received radiation for cancer are at very high risk for development soft tissue sarcoma in the area of the body where they received the radiation
  - Retinoblastoma
    - Children with the inherited form of retinoblastoma at increased risk for development of both bone and soft tissue sarcomas
- Impaired lymph drainage
  - Lymphangiosarcoma can occur rarely in parts of the body where lymph nodes have been removed or damaged by radiation.
- Having one or more of any of the above risk factors increases an individual's risk for development of soft tissue sarcoma.
- People with a family history of these inherited conditions or a strong family history of sarcomas may wish to discuss genetic testing with their physicians.
- There is no evidence to date that exposure to chemicals or injury causes soft tissue sarcoma.

SIGNS AND SYMPTOMS

- Symptoms vary depending on what part of the body is affected.
  - Sarcomas that develop in the extremities usually begin as a painless lump that grows over a period of weeks to months.
  - Sarcomas that present elsewhere in the body such as the chest or abdomen may also begin as painless lumps.
  - Retroperitoneal or sarcomas that develop within the abdomen or chest begin with more vague symptoms such as abdominal pain, bowel obstruction, or bleeding.
- About 50% of patients will have lung metastasis on diagnosis. Respiratory symptoms vary depending on the extent of lung involvement.

DIAGNOSTIC WORKUP

- Any soft tissue mass that is two inches or more in diameter that has not gone away in a month should be evaluated.
- Complete medical history and physical examination.
  - Computed tomographic (CT) scans and magnetic resonance imaging
    - Determine the size of the tumor
    - Determine nodal involvement
    - Detect the presence of metastasis
    - Usually repeated 3 months after treatment started to determine response
  - Chest x-ray film
    - May determine the presence of lung metastases
  - Positron emission tomography scans
    - Are not yet used in the routine evaluation of sarcoma
    - They are useful when metastasis is suspected but not definitively found.
- Biopsy
  - Diagnosis of soft tissue sarcoma cannot take place without biopsy.
  - Best performed by an orthopedic surgeon with extensive experience in sarcoma surgery
  - Specimen is sent to the pathology department for evaluation.
  - Several types of biopsies—depends on size and location of mass.
    - Fine-needle aspiration (FNA)
      - When mass can be felt and is near body surface
      - Can be done as an office procedure
      - CT-guided FNA if mass is too deep to feel
      - Disadvantage of FNA: there may not be enough cells to determine the exact type and grade of sarcoma if present
      - FNA useful in ruling out other conditions such as other types of cancer, benign tumors, or infection
      - If FNA leads to a sarcoma diagnosis, usually another

biopsy is needed to yield further information.

- ○ Core needle biopsy
  - ■ Takes more of a tissue sample than a FNA
  - ■ Usually contains enough tissue to adequately make a soft tissue sarcoma diagnosis
  - ■ CT scans can be used to guide core needle biopsies when the mass cannot be palpated
- ○ Excisional biopsy
  - ■ When tumor is small and not located next to any critical structures
  - ■ Entire tumor and a margin of surrounding normal tissue are removed, combining diagnostic biopsy and surgical treatment in one procedure
  - ■ For large mass that cannot be completely removed
- If the mass is soft tissue sarcoma, the biopsy must be carefully planned
  - ○ Later wide excision removes soft tissue sarcoma and wide enough margins without extensive damage to normal structures or resulting in limb removal.
- The biopsy specimen is sent to the pathology department.

HISTOLOGY

- Muscle sarcoma is the most common soft tissue sarcoma.
  - ○ Smooth muscle sarcomas
    - ■ Rhabdomyosarcomas
      - □ Occur in the skeletal muscles
      - □ Children are affected more than adults
      - □ Occur most frequently in the arms and legs
      - □ May be found in the head and neck area, reproductive, or urinary organs (e.g., vagina or bladder).
  - ○ Skeletal muscle sarcomas
    - ■ Leiomyosarcomas
    - ■ Involve involuntary smooth muscle tissue

- ■ Occur primarily in older adults
- ■ Occur anywhere in the body
- ■ Most commonly found in the retroperitoneum, internal organs, and blood vessels
- ■ Leiomyosarcoma of the uterus is common
- ■ May develop in the deep soft tissues of the arms and legs
- Synovial tissue (tissues that surround the joints) sarcoma
  - ○ Synovial sarcoma
    - ■ Knees and ankles are most common locations
    - ■ May occur in shoulders and hips
- Fibrous tissue (tendons and ligaments that cover bones and other organs) sarcoma
  - ○ Fibrosarcoma
    - ■ Affects adults most commonly between the ages of 20 and 60 years
    - ■ Some physicians classify desmoid tumors as a type of low-grade fibrosarcoma
    - ■ Musculoaponeurotic fibromatosis are closely attached to skeletal tissue
    - ■ Tumors do not metastasize but they are invasive and are sometimes fatal.
  - ○ Malignant fibrohistiocytoma
    - ■ Tends to grow locally but can metastasize
    - ■ Most commonly found in the arms and legs
    - ■ Less commonly found in the retroperitoneum
    - ■ Occurs most frequently in older adults
- Fat tissue sarcoma
  - ○ Liposarcomas
    - ■ Develop almost anywhere in the body
    - ■ Commonly found in the thigh, behind the knee, or in the retroperitoneum
    - ■ Most prevalent in middle-aged adults from 50-65 years of age
    - ■ Range from slow growing to very aggressive

- Blood vessel sarcoma
  - ○ Hemangiopericytoma is a tumor of the perivascular tissue.
    - ■ Can be benign or malignant
    - ■ Develops in the legs, pelvis, and retropentoneum
    - ■ Does not usually metastasize but recurs locally
  - ○ Hemangiosarcoma
    - ■ Angiosarcoma that develops from blood vessels
    - ■ Can develop in previously irradiated part of the body
- Lymph vessel sarcoma
  - ○ Lymphangiosarcomas
    - ■ Can develop in a part of the body that has been previously irradiated
    - ■ Common example: angiosarcoma of the breast or arm on the same side of a breast that has received radiation therapy
- Nerve sarcoma
  - ○ Malignant schwannomas
  - ○ Neurofibrosarcomas
  - ○ Neurogenic sarcomas
    - ■ Include the cells that surround the peripheral nervous system
- Malignant mesenchymoma.
  - ○ Contains some features of fibrosarcoma and at least two other types of cancer
- Alveolar soft-part sarcoma affects young adults and occurs primarily in the legs.
- Clear cell sarcoma develops in the tendons of the arms or legs.
  - ○ Has some features of malignant melanoma.
- Desmoplastic small cell tumor
  - ○ Characterized by small round cells surrounded by scar-like tissue
  - ○ Found in the retroperitoneum
  - ○ Most often seen in adolescents and young adults
- Soft tissue sarcomas of uncertain tissue type are tumors that cannot be linked to any specific type of normal soft tissue. They are all rare types of sarcoma.

CLINICAL STAGING

Staging has an important role in determining the most effective treatment

Major Cancers

of soft tissue sarcomas and estimating prognosis. American Joint Committee on Cancer criteria of tumor size, nodal status, grade, and metastasis (TNGM) is used in the staging process. (See table below.) Nodal involvement is rare and occurs in less than 3% of soft tissue sarcomas.

Intracompartmental or extracompartmental extension of extremity sarcomas is also important for surgical decision making. For complete staging, a thorough physical examination, x-rays, laboratory studies, and careful review of all biopsy specimens (including those from the primary tumor, lymph nodes, or other suspicious lesions) are essential.

G stands for histologic grade on the basis of how the cells look under the microscope. This helps determine how likely the tumor will metastasize and is divided into the following categories:

GX: Grade cannot be assessed
G1: Well differentiated
G2: Moderately differentiated
G3: Poorly differentiated
G4: Poorly differentiated or undifferentiated (four-tiered systems only)

TREATMENT

- Treatment varies depending on the site and stage of the disease.
- Low-grade soft tissue sarcoma with low metastatic potential can be treated with surgery and radiation therapy.
- It is essential that surgical oncologists, medical oncologists, and radiation oncologists have experience and expertise in sarcoma treatment and collaborate in the treatment plan.
- Studies have shown that patients who are treated at centers that have experience in sarcoma treatment have better outcomes than those who are not.

- Almost all patients, regardless of stage of disease, are treated with surgery. In the past, half of sarcomas located in the extremities were treated with surgery.
- Now limb-sparing surgery combined with radiation and chemotherapy is the treatment of choice, depending on the stage of the disease.
- Amputations are only done when the treatment would leave a limb that cannot function or that will result in chronic pain.
- Neoadjuvant chemotherapy and radiation may be done before surgery to shrink the tumor to allow complete resection.
- A combination of adjuvant radiation with surgery is also used when the tumor is high grade and there is a risk that the patient will have metastasis.
- If the tumor has metastasized to the lung, the site of the metastasis can be surgically removed.
- About one third of patients who undergo surgical resection or lung metastasis will survive 5 years.
- Palliative radiation is used for metastatic disease.
- Brachytherapy may be used to treat recurrent sarcoma if external beam radiation has already been used.
- The most commonly used chemotheraputic agents:
  ○ Ifosfamide
  ○ Doxorubicin
- Other chemotherapeutic agents:
  ○ Cyclophosphamide
  ○ Dacarbazine
  ○ Methotrexate
  ○ Irinotecan
  ○ Vincristine
  ○ Cisplatin
  ○ Paclitaxel
  ○ Docetaxel
  ○ Gemcitabine
- Clinical trials are being done to evaluate the use of targeted therapies.

PROGNOSIS

The prognosis is primarily determined by the grade, size, and depth of the tumor and the presence or absence of tumor at the surgical margins.

Clinical Staging: Soft Tissue Sarcoma

Definition of TNM

Primary Tumor (T)

TX	Primary tumor cannot be assessed
T0	No evidence of primary tumor
T1	Tumor 5 cm or less in greatest dimension
	T1a Superficial tumor
	T1b Deep tumor
T2	Tumor more than 5 cm in greatest dimension
	T2a Superficial tumor
	T2b Deep tumor

Note: Superficial tumor is located exclusively above the superficial fascia without invasion of the fascia; deep tumor located either exclusively beneath the superficial fascia, superficial to the fascia with invasion of or through the fascia, or both superficial yet beneath the fascia. Retroperitoneal, mediastinal, and pelvic sarcomas are classified as deep tumors.

Regional Lymph Nodes (N)

NX	Regional lymph nodes cannot be assessed
N0	No regional lymph node metastasis
N1*	Regional lymph node metastasis

*Note: Presence of positive nodes (N1) is considered stage IV.

Distant Metastasis (M)

MX	Distant metastasis cannot be assessed
M0	No distant metastasis
M1	Distant metastasis

Stage Grouping

Stage I	T1a, 1b, 2a, 2b	N0	M0	G1-2	G1	Low
Stage II	T1a, 1b, 2a	N0	M0	G3-4	G2-3	High
Stage III	T2b	N0	M0	G3-4	G2-3	High
Stage IV	Any T	N1	M0	Any G	Any G	High or low
	Any T	N0	M1	Any G	Any G	High or low

Large high-grade tumors have a higher incidence of local and distant recurrence. Metastasis free five year survival rates for patients with lesions less than 5 cm is 81%; 5-9 cm is 64%; and > 10 cm is 48%.

PREVENTION

The only way to prevent soft tissue sarcoma is to avoid exposure to risk factors. Most soft tissue sarcomas develop in individuals with no known risk factors. For people receiving radiation therapy, the benefits of the treatment outweigh the risks of subsequent development of sarcoma.

BIBLIOGRAPHY

American Cancer Society. (2006). *Can soft tissue sarcomas be found early?* Retrieved March 17, 2007, from http://www.cancer.org/docroot/CRI/content/CRI_2_4_3X_Can_Sarcoma_Be_Found_Early_38.asp?sitearea=.

American Cancer Society. (2006). *Can soft tissue sarcoma be prevented?* Retrieved March 17, 2007, from http://www.cancer.org/docroot/CRI/content/CRI_2_4_2X_Can_sarcoma_be_prevented_38.asp?sitearea=.

American Cancer Society. (2006). *Do we know what causes soft tissue sarcoma?* Retrieved March 17, 2007, from http://www.cancer.org/docroot/CRI/content/CRI_2_4_2X_Do_we_know_what_causes_sarcoma_38.asp?sitearea=.

American Cancer Society. (2006). *How are soft tissue sarcomas diagnosed?* Retrieved March 17, 2007 from http://www.cancer.org/docroot/CRI/content/CRI_2_4_3X_How_is_sarcoma_diagnosed_38.asp?sitearea=.

American Cancer Society. (2006). *How are soft tissue sarcomas staged?* Retrieved March 17, 2007, from http://www.cancer.org/docroot/CRI/content/CRI_2_4_3X_How_is_sarcoma_staged_38.asp?sitearea=.

American Cancer Society. (2006). *What are the key statistics about soft tissue sarcoma?* Retrieved March 17, 2007, from http://www.cancer.org/docroot/CRI/content/CRI_2_4_1X_What_are_the_key_statistics_for_sarcoma_38.asp?sitearea=.

American Cancer Society. (2006). *What are the risk factors for soft tissue sarcoma?* Retrieved March 17, 2007, from http://www.cancer.org/docroot/CRI/content/CRI_2_4_2X_What_are_the_risk_factors_for_sarcoma_38.asp?sitearea=.

American Cancer Society. (2006). *What is a soft tissue sarcoma?* Retrieved March 17, 2007, from http://www.cancer.org/docroot/CRI/content/CRI_2_4_1X_What_is_sarcoma_38.asp?sitearea.

American Joint Committee on Cancer. (1997). Soft tissue sarcoma. In *AJCC cancer staging manual* (5th ed., pp. 149-156). Philadelphia: Lippincott-Raven.

Brennan, M., Alektiar, K., & Maki, R. (2005). Soft tissue sarcoma. In V. Devita, S. Hellman, & S. Rosenberg (Eds.). *Cancer principles and practice of oncology* (6th Ed., pp. 1841-?). Philadelphia: Lippincott Williams Wilkins.

Clark, A., Fisher, C., Judson, I., et al. (2005). Soft-tissue sarcomas in adults. *New England Journal of Medicine, 353,* 701-711.

Kilpatrick, S., Cappellari, J., Bos, G., et al. (2001). Is fine-needle aspiration a practical alternative to open biopsy for the primary diagnosis of sarcoma? Experience with 140 patients. *American Journal of Clinical Pathology, 11,* 59-68.

Knapp, E. L., Kransdorf, M. J., & Letson, G. D. (2005). Diagnostic imaging update: soft tissue sarcomas. *Cancer Control, 12,* 27-35. Retrieved March 25, 2007, from http://www.medscape.com/viewarticle/498750.

Memorial Sloan-Kettering Cancer Center. (2004). *Soft tissue sarcoma: treatment.* Retrieved March 31, 2007, from http://www.mskcc.org/mskcc/html/443.cfm.

Memorial Sloan-Kettering Cancer Center. (2006). *Our clinical trials for soft-tissue sarcoma.* Retrieved March 31, 2007, from http://www.mskcc.org/mskcc/html/14449.cfm.

National Cancer Institute. (1999). *Adult soft tissue sarcoma.* Retrieved March 25, 2007, from http://www.meds.com/pdq/sarcoma_pro.html.

National Cancer Institute. (2006). *General information about adult soft tissue sarcoma.* Retrieved March 13, 2007, from http://www.cancer.gov/cancertopics/pdq/treatment/adult-soft-tissue-sarcoma/patient/.

Sarcoma Foundation of America. *Sarcoma—cancer of the connective tissues.* Retrieved March 16, 2007, from http://www.curesarcoma.org/subtypes.htm.

Siteman Cancer Center. (2006). *Adult soft tissue sarcoma.* Retrieved Mach 25, 2007, from http://www.siteman.wustl.edu/PDQ.aspx?id=672&xml=CDR62681.xml.

Surveillance Epidemiology and End Results. *Cancer of the soft tissue including heart.* Retrieved March 25, 2007, from http://seer.cancer.gov/statfacts/html/soft.html.

Skin Cancer

Dawn Tiedemann

Melanoma

DEFINITION

The three main types of cells in the outer layer of the skin (epidermis) are squamous cells, basal cells, and melanocytes. Skin cancers are malignant lesions that occur in these cells, including the less aggressive basal cell and squamous cell carcinomas and the more aggressive malignant melanoma. Melanoma is a malignant tumor of melanocytes. Melanocytes are the cells that make the pigment melanin and they are derived from the neural crest. Although most melanomas arise in the skin, they may develop on mucosal surfaces or at other sites to which neural crest cells migrate.

INCIDENCE

The American Cancer Society estimates 59,940 cases of melanoma will be diagnosed in 2007. During the 1970s, the incidence of melanoma increased by about 6% per year. Since 1980, the rate of increase has slowed to slightly less than 3% per year, perhaps because of increased awareness and promotion of preventive measures. Melanoma is primarily a disease of whites; the incidence is 10 times greater than in blacks.

ETIOLOGY AND RISK FACTORS

Skin cancers are generally associated with exposure to ultraviolet light found in sunlight but can be found anywhere on the skin.

- Prior melanoma
- Family history of melanoma
- Nevi (moles), particularly if numerous, large, or unusual
- Fair complexion
- History of unprotected or excessive sun exposure
- Severe sunburns as a child
- Use of tanning beds
- More common in the southern latitudes of the Northern Hemisphere
- Exposure to coal tar, pitch, creosote, arsenic compounds, or radium
- History of radiation or ultraviolet treatments
- Individuals with immune suppression from disease or medical treatment

SIGNS AND SYMPTOMS

Generally a change in the size, shape, color, or diameter of an existing skin lesion or the appearance of a new lesion causes the suspicion of a skin cancer to be raised. They usually occur on sun-exposed areas but can occur anywhere.

Melanoma: signs are usually promoted as "ABCD":

A: Asymmetry (one half of the mole does not match the other)
B: Border (irregular)
C: Color, such as blue, black, or variation in the same mole
D: Diameter greater than 6 mm

DIAGNOSTIC WORKUP

Skin cancer screening is by self-examination and clinical visual examination of the skin to identify any suspicious lesions. It is often difficult to distinguish a benign pigmented lesion from an early melanoma. A biopsy, preferably by local excision of the entire lesion, should be performed to make a definitive diagnosis. A suspicious pigmented lesion should never be shaved off or cauterized. Additionally, computed tomographic scans are done to identify any potential sites of metastasis: brain, lung, liver, regional lymph nodes, and skin.

HISTOLOGY

Following is a list of clinicopathologic cellular subtypes of malignant melanoma. These subtypes should be considered descriptive terms only. They do not have any prognostic or therapeutic significance:

- Superficial spreading, which commonly arises in preexisting nevi and usually presents with irregular borders; scaly, crusty surface; and in a variety of colors
- Nodular, which is raised, usually blue-black in color, and has a rapid vertical growth phase
- Lentigo maligna is a large freckle-like lesion, tan to black in color, or a raised nodule with notched borders.
- Acral lentiginous (palmar/plantar and nailbed) is usually flat and irregular in shape, varies in color, may be smooth or ulcerated, raised or flat.
- Miscellaneous unusual types:
  ○ Mucosal lentiginous (oral and genital)
  ○ Desmoplastic
  ○ Verrucous

STAGING

Various methods have been used to stage melanoma. Currently vertical thickness, presence or absence of ulceration, lymph node involvement, and distant metastasis are factors used in staging. Several systems are used:

- Clark's level: scores the primary melanoma lesion according to levels I-V that describe penetration into the various layers of the skin
- Breslow thickness: measures the actual vertical thickness of the lesion in millimeters
- TNM (tumor, nodes, metastasis): uses the Clark level and Breslow thickness measurements and involvement of lymph nodes, presence of ulceration, and distant metastasis, to assign stages. (See table on pages 133-134).

TREATMENT

- Surgical excision with a wide margin if possible (depending on tumor thickness) is the primary treatment for melanoma. Skin grafting may be needed to close the wound.

- Regional lymph node dissection is done in the case of palpable lymph nodes, to identify regional spread, and to assist in controlling the disease through lymphatic spread. In the case of nonpalpable lymph nodes where the primary melanoma is 1 to 4 mm thick, the "sentinel" lymph node is identified and this node is examined to determine the presence of disease before additional nodes are removed. This technique helps to avoid extensive lymph node dissections. The "sentinel" node is identified through lymphoscintigraphy and identifies the first lymph node that drains the tumor bed.
- Surgery may also be done for palliation of painful or draining lesions.
- Radiation is generally not used because melanoma can be resistant to radiation but may be done if the tumor is small or in cases of brain metastasis.
- Chemotherapy with interferon alfa-2b may be used as adjuvant therapy. For metastatic disease, dacarbazine, temozolomide, cisplatin, thalidomide, interferon alfa-2b, interleukin-2, or carmustine have been used.

PROGNOSIS

The American Cancer Society estimates that in 2007 there will be approximately 8,110 deaths from melanoma. The 5-year survival rates for localized melanoma are 98% but drop to 64% and 16% for regional and distant metastatic stages. A number of factors affect the prognosis, including clinical and histologic features and the location of the lesion. These factors include the thickness or level of invasion of the melanoma, mitotic index, presence of tumor infiltrating lymphocytes, number of regional lymph nodes involved, and ulceration or bleeding at the primary site. Patients who are younger, female, and who have melanomas on the extremities generally have a better prognosis.

PREVENTION

- High-risk individuals should have a yearly skin examination by a dermatologist (individuals with multiple nevi, personal or family history of melanoma).
- Skin screening should be done to identify lesions early, including monthly self-examination and examination of suspicious areas by a physician.
- The following guidelines help to prevent overexposure to ultraviolet rays:
  - Limit exposure to sun during midday (10 AM–4 PM).
  - Use protection with a hat shading the face, neck, and ears; long sleeves and pants; sunglasses; sunscreen with sun protection factor of 15 or higher
  - Avoid tanning beds and sun lamps

BIBLIOGRAPHY

Balch, C., Atkins, M., & Sober, A. (2005). Cutaneous melanoma. In V. DeVita, S. Hellman, & S. Rosenberg (Eds.). *Cancer principles and practice of oncology* (7th ed. pp. 1754-1808) Philadelphia: Lippincott Williams & Wilkins.

Chu, E., Noronha, V., Roy, S., et al. (2006). Common chemotherapy regimens in clinical practice. In E. Chu & V. DeVita (Eds.), *Cancer chemotherapy drug manual 2006* (pp. 453-455). Sudbury, MA: Jones & Bartlett.

Greene, F., Page, D., Fleming, I., et al. (Eds.). (2002). *AJCC cancer staging handbook* (6th ed.). New York: Springer-Verlag.

Jemal, A., Siegel, R., Ward, E., et al. (2007). Cancer statistics, 2007. *CA: A Cancer Journal for Clinicians, 57*, 43-66.

Longman, A. (2005). Nursing care of the client with skin cancer. In J. Itano & K. Taoka (Eds.). *Core curriculum for oncology nursing* (4th ed., pp. 615-623). St. Louis: Elsevier Saunders.

National Cancer Institute. (2006). *Melanoma, PDQ*. Retrieved January 14, 2007, from http://www.cancer.gov/cancertopics/pdq/treatment/Melanoma/HealthProfessional.

Clinical Staging: Melanoma of the Skin

Definition of TNM

Primary Tumor (T)

TX	Primary tumor cannot be assessed (e.g., shave biopsy or regressed melanoma)
T0	No evidence of primary tumor
Tis	Carcinoma in situ
T1	Melanoma ≤1.0 mm in thickness with or without ulceration
T1a	Melanoma ≤1.0 mm in thickness and level II or III, no ulceration
T1b	Melanoma ≤1.0 mm in thickness and level IV or V or with ulceration
T2	Melanoma 1.01-2.0 mm in thickness with our without ulceration
T2a	Melanoma 1.01-2.0 mm in thickness, no ulceration
T2b	Melanoma 1.01-2.0 mm in thickness, with ulceration
T3	Melanoma 2.01-4 mm in thickness with or without ulceration
T3a	Melanoma 2.01-4 mm in thickness, no ulceration
T3b	Melanoma 2.01-4 mm in thickness, with ulceration
T4	Melanoma greater than 4.0 mm in thickness with or without ulceration
T4a	Melanoma >4.0 mm in thickness, no ulceration
T4b	Melanoma >4.0 mm in thickness, with ulceration

Regional Lymph Nodes (N)

NX	Regional lymph nodes cannot be assessed
N0	No regional lymph node metastasis
N1	Metastasis in one lymph node
N1a	Clinically occult (microscopic) metastasis
N1b	Clinically apparent (macroscopic) metastasis
N2	Metastasis in two to three regional nodes or intralymphatic regional metastasis without nodal metastases
N2a	Clinically occult (microscopic) metastasis
N2b	Clinically apparent (macroscopic) metastasis
N2c	Satellite or in-transit metastasis *without* nodal metastasis
N3	Metastasis in for or more regional nodes, or matted metastatic nodes, or in-transit metastasis or satellite(s) *with* metastasis in regional node(s)

Distant Metastasis (M)

MX	Distant metastasis cannot be assessed
M0	No distant metastasis
M1	Distant metastasis
M1a	Metastasis to skin, subcutaneous tissues or distant lymph nodes
M1b	Metastasis to lung
M1c	Metastasis to all other visceral sites or distant metastasis at any site associated with an elevated serum lactate dehydrogenase

Clinical Stage Grouping

Stage 0	Tis	N0	M0
Stage IA	T1a	N0	M0
Stage IB	T1b	N0	M0
	T2a	N0	M0
Stage IIA	T2b	N0	M0
	T3a	N0	M0
Stage IIB	T3b	N0	M0
	T4a	N0	M0
Stage IIC	T4b	N0	M0
Stage III	Any T	N1	M0
	Any T	N2	M0
	Any T	N3	M0
Stage IV	Any T	Any N	M1

Note: Clinical staging includes microstaging of the primary melanoma and clinical/radiological evaluation for metastases. By convention, it should be used after complete excision of the primary melanoma with clinical assessment for regional metastases.

Continued

Clinical Staging: Melanoma of the Skin—cont'd

Pathological Stage Grouping

Stage 0	Tis	N0	M0
Stage IA	T1a	N0	M0
Stage IB	T1b	N0	M0
	T2a	N0	M0
Stage IIA	T2b	N0	M0
	T3a	N0	M0
Stage IIB	T3b	N0	M0
	T4a	N0	M0
Stage IIC	T4b	N0	M0
Stage IIIA	T1-4a	N1a	M0
	T1-4a	N2a	M0
Stage IIIB	T1-4b	N1a	M0
	T1-4b	N2a	M0
	T1-4a	N1b	M0
	T1-4a	N2b	M0
	T1-4a/b	N2c	M0
Stage IIIC	T1-4b	N1b	M0
	T1-4b	N2b	M0
	Any T	N3	M0
Stage IV	Any T	Any N	M1

Note: Pathologic staging includes microstaging of the primary melanoma and pathologic information about the regional lymph nodes after partial or complete lymphadenectomy. Pathologic stage 0 or stage IA patients are the exception; they do not require pathologic evaluation of their lymph nodes.

Used with the permission of the American Joint Committee on Cancer (AJCC), Chicago, Illinois. The original source for this material is the AJCC Cancer staging manual, Sixth Edition (2002) published by Springer Science and Business Media LLC, www.springerlink.com.

Non–Melanoma Skin Cancer: Basal Cell Carcinoma and Squamous Cell Carcinoma

DEFINITION

The three main types of cells in the outer layer of the skin (epidermis) are squamous cells, basal cells, and melanocytes. Skin cancers are malignant lesions that occur in these cells, including the less aggressive basal cell and squamous cell carcinomas and the more aggressive malignant melanoma.

INCIDENCE

More than one million basal cell or squamous cell carcinomas of the skin will be diagnosed in 2007 according to the American Cancer Society with 2,800 deaths contributed to the disease. Although these are the most common malignancies, they account for fewer than 0.1% of patient deaths caused by cancer.

ETIOLOGY AND RISK FACTORS

Basal cell and squamous cell carcinoma are generally associated with exposure to ultraviolet light and most commonly found on sun-exposed areas such as the face, ear, neck, lips, and the backs of the hands. However, they can be found anywhere on the body. Other risk factors include the following:

- Fair complexion
- History of unprotected or excessive sun exposure
- Severe sunburns as a child
- Use of tanning beds
- Residence in the southern latitudes of the Northern Hemisphere
- Exposure to coal tar, pitch, creosote, arsenic compounds, or radium
- History of radiation or ultraviolet treatments
- Individuals with immune suppression from disease or medical treatment (such as organ transplantation)
- Family history
- Prior history of skin cancer
  - 36% of patients with basal cell carcinoma will have a second primary within the next 5 years

SIGNS AND SYMPTOMS

Generally a change in the size, shape, color, or diameter of an existing skin lesion or the appearance of a new lesion causes the suspicion of a skin cancer to be raised. They usually occur on sun-exposed areas but can occur anywhere. Squamous cell carcinomas that arise in areas of non–sun-exposed skin or that originate de novo on areas of sun-exposed skin have a worse prognosis because these have a greater tendency to metastasize.

- Basal cell carcinoma may be nodular–flat, firm, and pale or a small raised pink or red lesion. They may also present as nodular ulcerative lesions, a translucent shiny area that bleeds easily or a sore that does not heal. The nose is the most frequent site.
- Squamous cell carcinomas usually present as growing lumps with a rough surface or a flat reddish patch that grows slowly. They can present as a sore that does not heal.

DIAGNOSTIC WORKUP

Skin cancer screening is done by self-examination and clinical visual examination of the skin. A definitive diagnosis of skin cancer requires a biopsy of the suspicious lesion. The biopsy can be an excisional biopsy in which the entire lesion is removed; a punch biopsy in which a small portion of the lesion is lifted; or a shave biopsy in which a thin slice of the lesion is removed. Basal cell carcinoma rarely metastasizes, and thus a metastatic workup is usually not necessary. Regional lymph nodes evaluation should be done in some cases of squamous cell carcinoma, such as those that occur in the high-risk areas such as lips, ears, genitals, or hands or in previously radiated skin. Additionally, computed tomographic scans may be done for large, neglected, or aggressive lesions to identify any sites of metastasis: brain, lung, liver, and regional lymph nodes.

HISTOLOGY

- Basal cell carcinoma and squamous cell carcinoma are both of epithelial origin.
- Basal cell carcinoma represents about 75% of all non-melanoma skin cancers. They have a low metastatic potential but can be quite destructive with local invasion.
- Squamous cell carcinoma represents about 25% of non-melanoma skin cancers. The deeper the lesion, the more likely it will recur. Larger lesions are associated with higher rates of metastasis.

STAGING

Squamous cell carcinoma is graded 1 to 4 on the basis of the proportion of differentiating cells present, the degree of atypical tumor cells, and the depth of tumor penetration. Basal cell and squamous cell skin cancers are further defined by stage. Stage I is any tumor 2 cm or less in size. Stage II is any tumor greater than 2 cm. Stage III is any size tumor that invades cartilage, muscle, bone, or regional lymph nodes. Stage IV is any size tumor with distant metastasis. See the American Joint Committee on Cancer TNM staging table on right.

TREATMENT

Localized basal cell and squamous cell carcinomas of the skin are highly curable. The traditional methods of treatment involve the use of cryosurgery, radiation therapy, electrodesiccation and curettage, and simple excision. Mohs' micrographic surgery has the highest 5-year cure rate for both primary and recurrent tumors. Treatment decision depends on multiple factors including those specific to the lesion such as: location, lesion size, possible extension into nearby structures, and factors specific to the patient such as age, general condition, any prior cancer treatments, and desired cosmetic results.

Clinical Staging: Non-Melanoma Skin Cancer

Definition of TNM

Primary Tumor (T)

TX	Primary tumor cannot be assessed
T0	No evidence of primary tumor
Tis	Carcinoma in situ
T1	Tumor 2 cm or less in greatest dimension
T2	Tumor more than 2 cm, but not more than 5 cm, in greatest dimension
T3	Tumor more than 5 cm in greatest dimension
T4	Tumor invades deep extradermal structures (i.e., cartilage, skeletal muscle, or bone)

Note: In case of multiple simultaneous tumors, the tumor with the highest T category will be classified and the number of separate tumors will be indicated in parentheses, e.g., T2 (5).

Regional Lymph Nodes (N)

NX	Regional lymph nodes cannot be assessed
N0	No regional lymph node metastasis
N1	Regional lymph node metastasis

Distant Metastasis (M)

MX	Distant metastasis cannot be assessed
M0	No distant metastasis
M1	Distant metastasis

Stage Grouping

Stage 0	Tis	N0	M0
Stage I	T1	N0	M0
Stage II	T2	N0	M0
	T3	N0	M0
Stage III	T4	N0	M0
	Any T	N1	M0
Stage IV	Any T	Any N	M1

Used with the permission of the American Joint Committee on Cancer (AJCC), Chicago, Illinois. The original source for this material is the *AJCC Cancer staging manual,* Sixth Edition (2002) published by Springer Science and Business Media LLC, www.springerlink.com.

- Simple excision with frozen or permanent sectioning for margin evaluation relies on surgical margins ranging from 3 to 10 mm, depending on the diameter of the original tumor. Only a fraction of the total tumor is examined pathologically and subsequently the tumor may recur.
- Electrodesiccation and curettage should be limited to very small tumors. It is a quick method for destroying the tumor, but it is limited because the surgeon cannot visualize the depth of the tumor invasion.
- Cryosurgery may be used for clinically well-defined or in situ tumors. This procedure may also be useful for debilitated patients whose medical conditions preclude other procedures.
- Mohs' micrographic surgery uses repeated progressive removal of tissue in thin layers under micrographic control examining each layer for tumor cells. This procedure provides the greatest tumor control while maximizing cosmetic results.
- External beam radiation can be used on lesions greater than 1 mm but less than 10 mm, in areas where surgical resection is difficult, or in cases of recurrence.
- Topical chemotherapy with 5-fluorouracil can be used for premalignant lesions (actinic keratoses), lesion recurrences, or lesions that cannot be managed by radiation or surgery.

- Systemic chemotherapy of cisplatin or doxorubicin may be used for metastatic disease.

PROGNOSIS

The overall cure rate for basal cell carcinoma and squamous cell carcinoma is directly related to the stage of the disease and the type of treatment used. Because neither basal cell carcinoma nor squamous cell carcinomas are reportable diseases, precise 5-year cure rates are not known.

Basal cell carcinoma 5-year cure rates range from 85% to 96%; however, 36% of patients will have a second primary within 5 years. Cure rates for squamous cell carcinoma of the skin depend on the size of the lesion and the aggressiveness. The cure rate for small lesions is about 90%. There is an increase in metastasis in squamous cell lesions that occur on the lip, ears, and palms of the hands or soles of the feet.

PREVENTION

Skin screening should be done to identify lesions early, including monthly self-examination, and suspicious areas should be examined by a physician. High-risk individuals should have a yearly skin examination by a dermatologist. The following guidelines help to prevent overexposure to ultraviolet rays:

- Limit exposure to sun during midday (10 AM–4 PM).
- Use protection with a hat shading the face, neck, and ears; long sleeves and pants; sunglasses; sunscreen with a sun protection factor of 15 or higher.
- Avoid tanning beds and sun lamps.
- Extra attention should be given to minimize risk of sunburns and sun exposure for children.

BIBLIOGRAPHY

Aasi, S., & Leffell, D. (2005). Cancer of the skin. In V. DeVita, S. Hellman, & S. Rosenberg (Eds.). *Cancer principles and practice of oncology* (7th ed. pp. 1717-1744). Philadelphia: Lippincott Williams & Wilkins.

Greene, F., Page, D., Fleming, I., et al. (Eds.). (2002). *AJCC cancer staging handbook* (6th ed.). New York: Springer-Verlag.

Jemal, A., Siegel, R., Ward, E., et al. (2007). Cancer statistics, 2007. *CA: A Cancer Journal for Clinicians, 57*, 43-66.

Longman, A. (2005). Nursing care of the client with skin cancer. In J. Itano, & K. Taoka (Eds). *Core curriculum for oncology nursing* (4th ed., pp. 615-623). St. Louis: Elsevier Saunders.

National Cancer Institute. (2006). *Skin cancer, PDQ.* Retrieved January 14, 2007, from http://www.cancer.gov/cancertopics/pdq/treatment/skin/HealthProfessional.

Principles of Cancer Management

Continued

Surgical Therapy

Yvette Payne

Surgery was the earliest form of cancer therapy and today 60% of cancer patients will be treated with surgery alone or surgery in combination with other treatment modalities. Surgeons must be knowledgeable about current therapeutic approaches to the treatment of particular cancers and about specific tumor, patient, and environmental factors when making surgical decisions. Surgery is part of a multidisciplinary approach to therapy, and surgical oncologists must carefully consider the impact surgery will have on future treatment decisions in the overall care of a patient. Surgery is used in the prevention, diagnosis, staging, and treatment of cancer and in restoration or rehabilitation.

PREVENTION

As our knowledge of tumorigenesis has increased, so has the use of surgery to prevent cancer. Surgery is used to remove nonvital benign or precancerous tissue that may predispose an individual to cancer. The National Comprehensive Cancer Network (NCCN) has written consensus guidelines that include the prevention and risk reduction of cancer. Examples of surgical interventions used for cancer prevention include removal of precancerous polyps. This is a common procedure to prevent colon cancer. Less commonly seen, but recommended by the NCCN for a small subset of women at high risk for development of ovarian cancer is a bilateral salpingo-oophorectomy.

DIAGNOSIS

Surgery is the primary therapy used to obtain the tissue or cells necessary for the definitive diagnosis of cancer. Surgical oncologists use multiple techniques to obtain tissue for diagnosis. Incisional and excisional biopsies and the use of endoscopy to obtain tissue or cells are common procedures in the diagnosis of cancer. In an effort to obtain tissue in a less invasive way, some newer technologies being used to diagnose cancer include image guided or stereotactic biopsies and nipple fluid aspirate to collect cells in individuals suspected of having breast cancer.

STAGING OF DISEASE

An adequate staging workup is required to determine which therapies will benefit the patient. Exploratory surgeries can help define the extent of tumor involvement that cannot be gained from our current radiographic technology. An example is an exploratory laparotomy in the staging of ovarian cancer. Sentinel lymph node biopsy, which carries less morbidity than complete lymph node dissection, has replaced complete lymph node dissection in some cancers.

TREATMENT OF DISEASE AS A CURE

Surgery usually represents the best option of treatment when cancer is diagnosed at an early stage. The surgical approach, especially when the goal is cure, is to remove all of the tumor while maintaining function and appearance. Early-stage solid tumors and in situ tumors lend themselves to traditional en bloc resections where the entire tumor and surrounding tumor-free margin are removed. If the primary tumor is larger or invades a functional area, it may be surgically resected and followed by radiation or chemotherapy to meet the goal of cure.

TREATMENT OF ADVANCED DISEASE

Surgery is used in advanced cancer to remove solitary or limited disease to extend survival and increase the quality of survival in the palliative setting. The most commonly removed solitary lesions include lung, liver, and brain nodules. These may be removed for both symptom control and in some cases to attempt a cure. If used with the hope for a cure, the surgery will usually be followed by radiation or chemotherapy. Surgery is often used to palliate symptoms in the advanced setting, particularly in cases where a long survival is possible with a goal of quality of life. As an example, a gastrojejunostomy bypass may be indicated to relieve gastric outlet obstruction or an ommaya reservoir may be placed to relieve pressure related to central nervous system metastasis.

RECONSTRUCTION

The goals of reconstructive surgery are to improve function and restore cosmetic appearance. Considerable advances have been made in the field of restorative and rehabilitative surgery. Specialized expertise may be required, depending on the extent, location, and type of surgery being performed. Surgical reconstruction is commonly used for cosmesis after mastectomies for breast cancer. Gynecologic, gastrointestinal, and urinary cancers may require surgery for restoration of function and cosmesis. Reconstruction for some cancers, such as head and neck cancers, while a challenge for both the surgeon and patient, may greatly enhance the individual's functionality, cosmetic appearance, and body image.

SURGICAL DECISION-MAKING

Surgical decision-making involves the analysis of considerable data, including tumor characteristics, patient characteristics, and environmental factors. The surgeon must be knowledgeable of the cancer diagnosis, biological features, and natural history of the tumor and the current

Cancer Management

presurgery and postsurgery therapies that are available to the patient. The growth rate, invasiveness, and metastatic potential may drive the treatment decision or the sequence of therapies. Additionally, the individual's age, health status, performance status, prior therapies, health history, and emotional state must be considered to ensure that the patient is a suitable surgical candidate. Environmental factors may contribute to the decision for surgery. Environmental factors include the patient's living arrangements, emotional and physical support systems in place, and availability to required expert care, equipment, and drugs after surgery. The decision for surgical therapy involves multiple factors and all must be considered to reach the optimal overall goal of the surgery.

CONSIDERATIONS FOR NURSING CARE

Approximately 75% of surgical procedures performed today are in the ambulatory setting. This presents unique challenges for nurses caring for oncology patients. One of the greatest challenges is the short amount of time available for patient teaching. Teaching should involve a family member or significant other beginning in the preoperative setting and continuing through follow-up. Written instructions should be both reviewed and given to the patient. Some patients wish to donate blood before surgery and the nurse can assist in evaluating the patient for and teaching the patients about blood donation. In addition to the immediate preoperative and postoperative periods, surgical

education of the patient should include teaching about the following:

- Pain: expectations of pain control and both pharmacologic and nonpharmacologic interventions
- Anxiety: fear of the unknown should be addressed
- Nutritional support: individualized on the basis of the patient's nutritional status and the surgical procedure to be performed

CONCLUSION

Surgical oncologists perform a variety of procedures for multiple purposes including prevention, diagnosis, staging, and treatment of cancer. Nursing care is essential to reaching the short- and long-term surgical outcomes.

BIBLIOGRAPHY

Gillespie, T. W. (2005). Surgical Therapy. In C. H. Yarbro, M. H. Frogge, & M. Goodman (Eds.). *Cancer nursing principles and practice* (6th ed., pp. 212-228). Sudbury, MA: Jones & Bartlett.

National Comprehensive Cancer Network. (2007). *NCCN Clinical Practice Guidelines in Oncology: NCCN breast cancer physician guidelines, v.1.* Retrieved October 11, 2007 from http://www.nccn.org/professional/physician_gls/PDF/breast_risk.pdf.

Surgical oncology. Retrieved October 11, 2007, http://www.surgeryencyclopedia.com/St-Wr/Surgical-Oncology.html. (2007).

Surgical therapy. (2002). In C. H. Yarbro, M. H. Frogge, & M. Goodman (Eds.). *Clinical guide to cancer nursing* (5th ed., pp. 39-44). Sudbury, MA: Jones & Bartlett.

Radiation Therapy

Roberta Anne Strohl

DEFINITION

Radiation therapy is a local treatment for cancer. It is the use of high-energy particles or x-rays, which possess sufficient energy to create ionizing radiation by ejecting electrons from their orbit. The effects of radiation occur because of physical, chemical, and biochemical factors. Physical factors consist of the energy of the radiation that is able to eject electrons, creating instability. Chemical reactions occur because ionization creates powerful oxidizing and reducing agents, known as free radicals, in cellular fluid. The target of radiation effect is cellular deoxyribonucleic acid (DNA). Radiation results in biochemical damage of the chemical bonds, which loosely hold DNA together. Double-strand breaks in DNA are the most important effect of radiation on cells.

RADIOBIOLOGY

Apoptotic, or programmed, cell death is enhanced by radiation. Radiation damage most often occurs at the time the cell attempts to divide. Cells are most sensitive to radiation damage during the G2 and M phases of the cell cycle and

least sensitive during S phase. Cells that have a higher mitotic index are more sensitive to radiation damage.

Normal cells have a better ability to recover and repair from radiation damage than do cancer cells. Despite this ability, there is a maximally tolerated radiation dose for normal cells, and treatment above that dose may result in irreparable damage. The delivery of radiation must balance the dose of radiation needed to treat the given tumor cell line and the dose that is tolerated by the surrounding normal tissues. When there is a wide margin between the dose that must be given and the tolerance of the surrounding tissue, the treatment course may be short and will be better tolerated than when that margin is narrow. For example, cancers in the head and neck area require a high radiation dose, which is difficult for the mitotically active oral mucosa to tolerate.

RADIATION DELIVERY
External Beam Therapy

This is the most common delivery system for radiation. The linear accelerator is a treatment machine, which generates ionizing radiation by accelerating electrons along a tube. In this form of radiation, the patient is positioned on a treatment couch and through a sophisticated system of planning; the radiation beam is directed to the tumor site. The total dose of radiation required is achieved through equal daily fractions of radiation, usually given one a day, 5 days per week, until the total dose is reached. Patients receiving this form of radiation are not radioactive.

Brachytherapy

Radioactive material is placed into the tumor or near the tumor site. This is implant treatment. The implant may be temporary or permanent. Temporary implants are more common and are used in clinical situations where a local radiation dose required is higher than can be achieved with external beam therapy because it would exceed the normal tissue tolerance. Implants deposit most of the radiation dose in a small-volume area. The radioactive sources are sealed in metal carriers. Patients having implants are radioactive for the period of time that the source is in them. Because the radiation source is sealed, there is no contamination of the body fluids. Nurses caring for these individuals are instructed to observe the precautions of time, distance, and shielding to protect themselves from radiation exposure. This means spending a defined amount of time at a defined distance from the source and to use shielding as available.

Permanent implants are the insertion of radioactive materials that are not removed. The sources used are weak emitters of gamma radiation yielding low surface doses. Iodine 125 used in prostate cancer is the most common permanent implant in cancer care.

Radioisotope Therapy

This therapy uses unsealed sources of radiation. Patients are hospitalized for a period determined by the activity of the isotope because body fluids are radioactive. Radioactive iodine for thyroid cancer is the most common use of isotope therapy.

Stereotactic Radiosurgery

Despite the name, stereotactic radiosurgery is a nonsurgical procedure. It is a technique is used to deliver highly precise radiation beams to a small volume of tissue. Gamma knife radiation, used in the management of brain tumors, is an example of this treatment. The gamma knife has 201 cobalt sources from which are selected a configuration to deliver a high dose in a single treatment.

MEASURING RADIATION DOSE

Absorbed dose or radiation absorbed dose, RAD, has been used to measure the dose of radiation delivered. The preferred measure is the gray (GY). One GY is equal to 100 centigrays (cGY). One cGY equals 1 RAD.

THE ROLE OF RADIATION IN CANCER CARE

It has been estimated that 60% of patients with cancer receive radiation therapy at some point during the treatment of the disease. Radiation may be used as a single treatment but is often combined with surgery or chemotherapy. Terms used to describe the role of radiation therapy in patient treatment include the following:

- Definitive therapy is used with curative intent as in early head and neck, cervical, and prostate cancers.
- Neoadjuvant is given before primary therapy as in esophageal cancer where radiation is given preoperatively with the goal of rendering the tumor operable.
- Adjuvant therapy is treatment given after primary surgical therapy as in breast or lung cancer.
- Prophylactic therapy is used when there is no evidence of disease but the risk of disease presenting is high, as in cranial radiation in small cell lung cancer.
- Palliative therapy is used to alleviate symptoms as in treatment for brain metastases and bone pain.

SIDE EFFECTS

Because radiation is a local therapy, many side effects are related to the specific area being treated. The one general side effect is fatigue. Skin reactions with erythema progressing to desquamation may occur, depending on the dose and the amount of radiation received by the skin. Selected site-specific side effects are listed in the table below. The reference provided in the bibliography will provide a more thorough review of the side effects and specific management measures. Because radiation is often given with other treatment modalities, the nurse involved in patient care must coordinate symptom management strategies.

Site-Specific Side Effects

Site	Radiation Effect	Management
Brain	Alopecia, late cognitive changes	Avoid irritants to scalp, assess neurocognitive function
Head and neck	Xerostomia, mucositis, dental caries, dysphagia	Soft bland food, saliva substitutes, analgesics, prophylactic dental care
Chest	Cough, pneumonitis, late fibrosis	Expectorants, corticosteroids
Abdomen	Nausea and vomiting	Antiemetics, bland diet, maintaining fluids
Pelvis	Diarrhea, cystitis, infertility	Maintain fluids, antidiarrheals, fertility counseling
Skin	Erythema, dry and moist desquamation	Avoid trauma, protect skin, creams and lotions as prescribed

BIBLIOGRAPHY

Watkins-Bruner, D., Haas, M., & Gosselin-Acomb, T. (Eds). (2005). *Radiation oncology nursing practice and education.* Pittsburgh, PA: Oncology Nursing Society.

Cancer Management

Hematopoietic Stem Cell Transplantation

Sandra A. Mitchell

INTRODUCTION AND OVERVIEW

Over the past 20 years, hematopoietic stem cell transplantation (HSCT) has evolved from an experimental treatment for patients with advanced acute leukemia to a therapeutically effective modality that is now standard therapy for selected diseases. HSCT, which is known to be curative in several malignant and nonmalignant disorders, is a transplant of hematopoietic stem cells at various stages of differentiation and maturation.

Astute nursing care of transplant recipients is essential to prevent treatment-related complications and death. Even when a patient is cured of the original disease, he or she may have delayed and long-term complications that can shorten or negatively affect the quality of his or her remaining life. These complications include infections, thyroid dysfunction, pulmonary complications, cataracts, and the development of second malignancies. Allogeneic HSCT recipients may also have chronic graft-versus-host disease (GVHD). In general, autologous transplantation has fewer long-term complications, largely because no GVHD is associated with autologous transplantation.

Advances in histocompatibility matching, safer preparative regimens, improvements in stem cell collection and cryopreservation techniques, and the development of pharmacological agents to accelerate the recovery of hematopoiesis, manage bacterial, viral, and fungal infections, and prevent and treat acute and chronic GVHD after transplant have contributed to the success of HSCT. This chapter reviews the principles of caring for patients undergoing autologous or allogeneic HSCT.

Rationale for High-Dose Therapy With Stem Cell Transplantation

HSCT involves replacing diseased, destroyed, or nonfunctioning hematopoietic cells with healthy hematopoietic progenitor cells, also called stem cells. Stem cells are primitive hematopoietic cells capable of self-renewal, and they are pluripotent, meaning that they are capable of maturing into a red blood cell (RBC), a white blood cell (WBC), or a platelet. These stem cells may be collected directly from the bone marrow spaces by a bone marrow harvest procedure or from the peripheral blood by apheresis. Stem cells can also be harvested from the placenta immediately after delivery.

In both autologous and allogeneic HSCT, peripheral blood stem cells have become the preferred source of hematopoietic stem cells for grafting. Collection of cells through apheresis is easier and less costly and may also result in a more rapid recovery of neutrophil and platelet counts. In unrelated allogeneic transplantation, the source of stem cells may be either a bone marrow harvest procedure or a peripheral blood stem cell collection.

Types of Hematopoietic Stem Cell Transplantation

The various types of HSCTs can be differentiated in terms of the hematopoietic stem cell donor, the method used to collect the cells, and the intensity of the conditioning regimen. Each type of HSCT has relative advantages and disadvantages, as summarized in the table below. In an autologous stem cell transplant, the patient serves as his or her own donor of stem cells, whereas for an allogeneic transplant the donor is either related (typically a sibling) or unrelated. If an identical twin donor is available, the transplant is termed a syngeneic transplant. The source of the stem cells may be the peripheral blood stream (peripheral blood stem cell transplant), or the cells may be collected directly from the bone marrow spaces (bone marrow transplant) or from a placenta (cord blood transplant). Transplants can also be differentiated on the basis of the intensity of the conditioning regimen. A myeloablative transplant provides high doses of radiation or chemotherapy to treat the underlying malignancy and ablate the bone marrow, thereby causing myelosuppression that would be irreversible without stem cell support. A reduced-intensity transplant delivers lower doses of radiation or chemotherapy, typically causing less severe myelosuppression and less nonhematologic toxicity.

Comparison of Techniques for Harvesting Hematopoietic Stem Cells

Technique	Advantages/Disadvantages
Bone marrow harvest	Harvest-related pain General anesthesia required May be more cost-effective and more convenient for donors
Peripheral blood stem cells	Easier collection for autologous patients and potentially for allogeneic donors Shorter duration of myelosuppression in stem cell transplant recipients Incidence of graft-versus-host disease may be higher
Cord blood	Plentiful and relatively easy to harvest by obstetricians trained in the procedure Inexpensive Excellent source to increase pool of unrelated donors May be associated with less graft-versus-host disease Currently limited to individuals weighing less than 50-70 kg. With ex vivo expansion techniques may become more widespread

Indications for and Outcomes of Hematopoietic Stem Cell Transplantation

HSCT represents an important advance in restoring hematopoietic function in patients whose bone marrow has been destroyed by radiation or high-dose chemotherapy to treat an underlying malignancy. Many factors influence the indications for and patient eligibility for transplantation. HSCT is used when bone marrow is defective or destroyed by a disease process or as a result of treating an underlying disease. The box below lists the diseases for which adults are currently treated with autologous or allogeneic HSCT.

Factors that may affect the outcomes of HSCT include the type and stage of disease at the time of transplantation, the type of transplant (allogeneic versus autologous), the degree of human leukocyte antigen (HLA) matching in allogeneic transplants, the intensity of the conditioning regimen, the ages of both the donor and the recipient, and the experience of the transplantation center. In general, the transplant-related mortality risk in allogeneic HSCT is about 20% to 30% higher than in autologous HSCT. At most transplant centers, the transplant-related mortality rate in autologous HSCT is less than 5%.

Disease-free survival at 5 years after HSCT varies substantially, depending on the age of the recipient, the underlying disease, disease status at the time of transplantation, the type of HSCT procedure, and the extent of prior treatment. Depending on these factors, disease-free survival can range from 10% to 75% (Baron & Storb, 2007; Brunstein, Baker, & Wagner, 2007; Chantry et al., 2006; Koreth et al., 2007; Nademanee & Forman, 2006; Tabbara et al., 2002; Yakoub-Agha et al., 2006).

Diseases Treated With Hematopoietic Stem Cell Transplantation

AUTOLOGOUS HEMATOPOIETIC STEM CELL TRANSPLANTATION
- Acute myelogenous leukemia
- Acute lymphoblastic leukemia
- Chronic myelogenous leukemia
- Non-Hodgkin lymphoma
- Chronic lymphocytic leukemia
- Hodgkin lymphoma
- Multiple myeloma
- Selected solid tumors, within clinical trials: germ cell tumors, sarcoma, neuroblastoma, melanoma, breast cancer

ALLOGENEIC HEMATOPOIETIC STEM CELL TRANSPLANTATION
- Acute myelogenous leukemia
- Acute lymphocytic leukemia
- Chronic myelogenous leukemia
- Non-Hodgkin lymphoma
- Chronic lymphocytic leukemia
- Hodgkin lymphoma
- Multiple myeloma
- Severe aplastic anemia
- Selected solid tumors, within clinical trials: renal cell

OVERVIEW OF THE PROCESS AND IMPLICATIONS FOR NURSING CARE

Pretransplant Evaluation of the Recipient and Donor

The pretransplant evaluation of the recipient includes physical and psychosocial evaluation, an evaluation of the adequacy of insurance coverage, and family support and education about the transplant process to permit informed consent for the procedure. Evaluation before final selection of a donor includes confirmatory high-resolution tissue typing, an assessment of viral serology, and an evaluation of overall health. The components of the evaluation of recipient and donor are summarized in the box on page 144.

In selecting an individual to serve as an allogeneic HSCT donor, histocompatibility testing (tissue typing) is performed to evaluate the human leukocyte antigen (HLA) match between antigens of the donor and that of the recipient. A person's tissue type is coded by genes of the major histocompatibility complex. These genes contain information for cell surface antigens that differentiate self from nonself. The major histocompatibility complex involved in the immune response include class I antigens (A, B) and class II, the DR antigens. Each person has two A-, B-, and DR-locus antigens that are inherited as a haplotype (i.e., a single unit) from each parent. Many possible antigens may occur at each locus, resulting in a large number of HLA combinations. The higher the number of antigens that match, the higher the likelihood of compatibility, and the lower the risk of acute and chronic GVHD and graft rejection.

Selection of a donor for HSCT is based on the type and stage of the underlying disease, donor and recipient age, and comorbidities, together with HLA- and mixed leukocyte culture (MLC)-matched donor. MLC is performed to observe for interaction between the potential donor's cells and recipient cells. Low reactivity indicates greater compatibility. A related donor is usually a sibling (siblings have the greatest chance of matching on both HLA and on other minor and as yet unrecognized antigens). If more than one donor is HLA identical to the patient, donor selection is based on sex, ABO compatibility, negative viral titers, younger donor age, and donor nulliparity because all these factors are associated with an improved outcome of HSCT (Confer & Miller, 2007). Into the future, there is a potential role for non-HLA genetics in donor selection, based on the insights into the immunobiology of HSCT complications provided by genotyping for non-HLA genes (Dickinson, 2007).

If the patient does not have a suitable family donor, a search for an unrelated donor may be undertaken. The National Marrow Donor Program, a donor registry developed in 1986, allows patients without a related donor to find an HLA-matched unrelated donor. Umbilical cord blood is another potential stem cell source, particularly in pediatric allogeneic transplantation.

Mismatch in ABO blood group between patient and donor does not preclude successful HSCT. Depending on

Pretransplant Evaluation of Recipient and Donor

EVALUATION OF THE HEMATOPOIETIC STEM CELL TRANSPLANT RECIPIENT
Pretreatment testing and evaluation of the patient undergoing hematopoietic stem cell transplantation includes the following:

- History of current illness, including presenting signs and symptoms; previous therapies; initial diagnosis; pathology and staging; complications; relapses or progressions; current disease status; transfusion history
- Medical history, including major illnesses, chronic illnesses, recurring illnesses, surgical history, childhood illnesses, and infectious disease exposure. For women, the medical history should also include menarche, onset of menopause or date of last menstrual period, pregnancies, and outcomes.
- Current medications
- Allergies
- Social and family history
- Performance status
- Current laboratory studies, including liver function tests, renal function, and complete blood cell count (CBC)
- Infectious disease serologies, including human immunodeficiency virus (HIV), hepatitis B and C, cytomegalovirus (CMV), herpes simplex virus (HSV), human T-cell leukemia/lymphoma virus (HTLV)-1, Epstein-Barr virus (EBV), toxoplasma titer, and ABO and Rh typing
- Human leukocyte antigen typing and deoxyribonucleic acid procurement for future engraftment studies (allogeneic transplant recipients)
- Chest x-ray film
- Electrocardiogram
- Multiple gated acquisition (MUGA) scan
- Pulmonary function tests, including single-breath diffusing capacity
- 24-Hour urine for creatinine clearance
- Computed tomography (CT) of chest and sinuses periodically for surveillance and if there are symptoms or a history of repeated infections
- Disease restaging, including radiographic studies (computed tomography (CT), nuclear medicine studies), bone marrow aspirate and biopsy, cytogenetics, molecular diagnostics, and measures of minimal residual disease
- Dental evaluation, including full-mouth x-rays and cleaning
- Sperm/fertilized embryo banking
- Autologous stem cell backup if undergoing unrelated or mismatched transplantation
- Informed consent for treatment, transfusion support, clinical trials
- Nutritional evaluation, if appropriate
- Consultations with radiation therapy, infectious disease, pulmonary, cardiology, or renal services, if clinically indicated
- Financial screening
- Psychosocial evaluation

EVALUATION OF THE HEMATOPOIETIC STEM CELL DONOR
Pretreatment testing and evaluation of the hematopoietic stem cell donor usually includes the following:

- History and physical examination, noting history of serious or chronic illnesses, history of hematological problems including bleeding tendencies, cancer history and transfusion history, current medications, allergies, and pregnancy history for females.
- The presence of any risk factors for HIV or viral hepatitis infection are noted
- Physical examination for any abnormalities and an assessment of the adequacy of peripheral veins
- CBC with differential, chemistries, liver and renal function tests, coagulation studies, ABO and Rh typing; pregnancy test
- Confirmatory HLA typing, deoxyribonucleic acid procurement for future engraftment studies (allogeneic donors only)
- Infectious disease serologies, including VDRL, HIV, hepatitis B and C, CMV, HSV, HTLV-1, EBV, toxoplasma titer

the direction of the incompatibility (major versus minor incompatibility), the hematopoietic stem cell product may have to be depleted of RBCs to prevent a hemolytic reaction caused by ABO antibodies still circulating in the patient's bloodstream. After engraftment and approximately 100 days after transplantation, the recipient of an ABO-mismatched transplant will seroconvert to the ABO type of the donor.

Stem Cell Harvesting, Mobilization, and Collection

Stem cells are most numerous in the bone marrow spaces, and some circulate in the peripheral blood. The process of harvesting and collecting hematopoietic stem cells differs depending on the type of transplant. Progenitor cells may be obtained through a bone marrow harvest or collected through the peripheral blood. Immediately after delivery, hematopoietic stem cells may also be collected from the placental cord and cryopreserved for subsequent use.

When stem cells are obtained from the donor's bone marrow, the harvesting procedure is performed in the operating room under spinal or general anesthesia. Multiple aspirations are obtained from each posterior iliac crest with large-bore needles until a total of 2 to 3×10^8 nucleated cells per kilogram of recipient's body weight is obtained. The total volume of aspirate is 1 to 2 L. The marrow is placed in a heparinized tissue culture medium and filtered for the removal of fat and bone particles, and the cells are taken directly to the recipient's room for infusion or cryopreserved for subsequent infusion. The bone marrow harvest procedure usually takes 1 to 2 hours, and the donor is often hospitalized overnight for observation. The harvest sites may be mildly uncomfortable for 2 to 7 days after the procedure.

Hematopoietic stem cells may also be collected from the peripheral blood. However, because stem cells are not abundant in the peripheral blood, chemotherapy (for autologous transplant recipients who are providing their own stem cells for subsequent administration) or colony-stimulating factors (for healthy donors providing an allogeneic stem cell transplant product) (granulocyte colony-stimulating factor [G-CSF] or granulocyte-macrophage colony-stimulating factor [GM-CSF]) must be given before collection to drive progenitor cells into the peripheral circulation. This process is termed mobilization or priming. The chemotherapy that patients undergoing an autologous stem cell transplant receive for stem cell mobilization is also useful for tumor reduction. For both related and unrelated donors, colony-stimulating factors (CSF) alone are used to increase the number of stem cells in the peripheral blood. Protocols vary, but G-CSF or GM-CSF is given by a subcutaneous injection daily. Stem cell collections begin after 4 or 5 days of CSF injections.

Hematopoietic progenitor cells are collected from the peripheral blood by a method called leukapheresis. A commercial cell separator machine collects the progenitor cells and returns the remainder of the plasma and cellular components to the bloodstream. This is performed either through wide-bore double-lumen central catheters or large-bore antecubital angiocath intravenous catheters. The procedure takes approximately 3 to 4 hours, and the number of leukapheresis procedures required is determined by the number of stem cells harvested at each session. The goal is to collect 5×10^6 CD34-positive cells per kilogram of recipient body weight. The CD34-positive antigen is an antigen expressed on the surface of early progenitor cells.

During and immediately after apheresis and stem cell collection, the donor may have a transient hypocalcemia reaction with chills, fatigue, tingling in the lips and extremities, and vertigo resulting from the citrate infusion, which is used to prevent clotting of the blood during the procedure. The symptoms can be prevented or treated by taking an oral calcium carbonate supplement, such as Tums.

Conditioning Therapy/Preparative Regimen

A conditioning therapy or preparative regimen including total body irradiation or chemotherapy is administered for several days before stem cell infusion; it is designed to prepare the recipient to receive the transplanted stem cells. The goals of the conditioning regimen depends in part on whether the transplant is autologous or allogeneic and on the nature of the patient's underlying disease. In allogeneic transplantation, the purpose of conditioning is to eradicate any malignant disease, eliminate the bone marrow to create a space for the new donor stem cells, and provide sufficient immunosuppression to allow engraftment of the transplanted stem cells. In autologous transplantation, immunosuppression is not required because the patient is the source of the hematopoietic stem cells. However, intensive therapy is still needed to eradicate the underlying malignant disease.

The rationale for selecting the agents that are included in the preparative regimen is based on the hypothesis that increasing the total dose or dose rate will kill more tumor cells, resulting in improved response and survival rates. Typically, drugs with different (i.e., nonoverlapping) nonhematologic dose-limiting toxicities are combined in maximal doses. Alkylating agents (cyclophosphamide, carboplatin, busulfan, thiotepa, cisplatin, melphalan, carmustine), etoposide, cytarabine, and sometimes total-body irradiation are used to destroy the bone marrow and eradicate disease. The regimen is administered over 2 to 8 days. The individual drugs that may be used in combination as part of the transplant conditioning regimen may have several adverse effects (see table on page 146). The patient is then allowed 1 or 2 rest days to clear the chemotherapy from the system before the infusion of stem cells. Bone marrow aplasia occurs within days after the conditioning regimen is completed.

A reduced intensity conditioning regimen followed by allogeneic HSCT is a newer approach that may provide a treatment option for older patients and those who have undergone a prior autologous transplant or have comorbidities, such as lung, kidney, or liver disease and cannot tolerate the toxicities of a high-dose conditioning regimen. The rationale for reduced intensity conditioning regimens is that the immune-mediated graft-versus-tumor effect provided by the new immune system, rather than primarily the conditioning regimen itself, is responsible for control of the disease. Reduced intensity regimens under investigation include fludarabine, single-dose total-body irradiation ($\leq$500 cGy), cyclophosphamide, melphalan, busulfan, and a combination of potent immunosuppressive medications. Data to support the potential efficacy of a reduced intensity regimen exist for patients with Hodgkin disease, multiple myeloma, non-Hodgkin lymphoma, chronic lymphocytic leukemia, and acute leukemia and myelodysplastic syndrome (Giralt, 2005). These reduced intensity regimens are not without risk, and patients undergoing transplant after a reduced intensity conditioning regimen still experience many of the expected complications of a conventional, fully myeloablative allogeneic transplantation. The problems encountered in the early posttransplantation period, such as infection, bleeding, and regimen-related toxicities, may be reduced after non-myeloablative transplantation, but the risk of GVHD and the long-term risks of infection continue to be important. The role of strategies such as posttransplant immunotherapy and posttransplant maintenance therapy with agents such as rituximab or imatinib in improving the outcomes for patients who have received a reduced intensity allogeneic HSCT are the subject of continuing study.

Stem Cell Infusion

The infusion of stem cells is a relatively simple procedure, much like a blood transfusion. The cells are infused through a central venous catheter over 30 to 90 minutes, depending on the total volume of the product. In allogeneic HSCT, the stem cells are usually infused immediately after they are collected. Autologous stem cells are

Cancer Management

Nonhematologic Side Effects of Agents Used in Preparative Regimen/Conditioning Therapy

Therapeutic Agent	Side Effects
Antithymocyte globulin (ATG)	Mucositis, diarrhea, cardiotoxicity, fever, chills and hypersensitivity during infusion (reaction may worsen with each subsequent dose)
Busulfan	Interstitial pulmonary fibrosis, hepatic dysfunction, including veno-occlusive disease, acute cholecystitis, generalized seizures, mucositis, skin (hyperpigmentation, desquamation, acral erythema), nausea and vomiting
Carmustine (BCNU)	Hepatic, pulmonary, central nervous system, cardiac effects (arrhythmias and hypotension), nausea and vomiting
Carboplatinum	Nausea and vomiting, nephrotoxicity, liver function abnormalities including veno-occlusive disease, ototoxicity
Cisplatinum	Nausea and vomiting, neurotoxicity (peripheral neuropathy, ataxia, visual disturbances), ototoxicity, renal
Cyclophosphamide	Cardiac effects (cardiomyopathy, congestive heart failure, hemorrhagic cardiac necrosis, pericardial effusion, electrocardiographic abnormalities), interstitial pulmonary fibrosis, hemorrhagic cystitis, elevation in liver enzymes, nausea and vomiting, metabolic (syndrome of inappropriate antidiuretic hormone secretion)
Cytosine arabinoside (Ara-C)	Cerebellar toxicity, encephalopathy, seizures, conjunctivitis, skin (rash, acral erythema), nausea and vomiting, diarrhea, renal insufficiency, liver function abnormalities, pancreatitis, noncardiogenic pulmonary edema, fever, arthralgias
Etoposide	Hypersensitivity reactions, hypotension, liver function abnormalities and chemical hepatitis, renal dysfunction, nausea and vomiting, metabolic (metabolic acidosis), mucositis, stomatitis, painful skin rash on the palms, soles, and periorbital area
Fludarabine	Mucositis, diarrhea, pulmonary fibrosis, pneumonitis, hypersensitivity reaction during infusion
Ifosfamide	Hemorrhagic cystitis
Melphalan	Acute hypersensitivity, renal, mucositis, nausea and vomiting, hepatic toxicity including veno-occlusive disease
Thiotepa	Hyperpigmentation, acute erythroderma, dry desquamation, liver function abnormalities, including veno-occlusive disease, mucositis, esophagitis, dysuria, hypersensitivity reaction during infusion
Total body irradiation	Nausea, vomiting diarrhea, parotitis, xerostomia, stomatitis, erythema, pneumonitis, veno-occlusive disease

Data from Chan, 2000; Gupta-Burt & Okunieff, 1998; McAdams & Burgunder, 2004; Petros & Gilbert, 1998; Rees, Beale, & Judson, 1998; and Solimando, 1998.

cryopreserved with dimethylsulfoxide (DMSO) and must be thawed in a warm normal saline solution bath at the bedside immediately before reinfusion. Premedication with acetaminophen, hydrocortisone, and diphenhydramine is usually recommended, and patients may also receive prehydration to maintain renal perfusion. Vital signs and pulse oximetry are monitored closely before, during, and at intervals after stem cell infusion. An infusion pump should not be used to administer stem cells; normal saline solution is used to prime and flush the tubing.

Complications of stem cell infusion are rare but may include pulmonary edema, hemolysis, infection, and anaphylaxis. Infrequently, DMSO can cause an infusion reaction that may include bradycardia (rarely heart block) or hypertension, and an acute hypersensitivity reaction may occur; this is caused by excretion of DMSO. The excretion of DMSO used in cryopreserving autologous stem cells typically causes a characteristic odor or taste that may be described as "garlicky." DMSO-associated RBC hemolysis may also occur and may require vigorous hydration to prevent renal toxicity. During infusion, patients are also monitored for volume overload and for complaints suggestive of pulmonary embolism such as chest pain, dyspnea, and cough.

Early Complications of Stem Cell Transplantation

After stem cell infusion, the hematopoietic stem cells migrate to the bone marrow spaces, where they are attracted by chemotactic factors. Engraftment occurs when the transplanted progenitor cells begin to grow and manufacture new hematopoietic cells in the bone marrow. After the stem cell infusion but before complete hematopoietic cell engraftment, patients have severe pancytopenia, and the resulting complications may include infection and bleeding. Patients are also at risk for mucositis, skin toxicities, and veno-occlusive disease of the liver. Examples of early and late complications arising from autologous and allogenic stem cell transplantation can be found in the box on page 147. Nonhematologic adverse effects vary depending on the agents used for the conditioning regimen. The nonhematologic adverse effects that are associated with the agents that typically comprise stem cell transplant conditioning regimens are outlined in the table on left.

Pancytopenia. Hematopoietic growth factors (e.g., G-CSF, GM-CSF) are given to accelerate neutrophil recovery, thereby reducing the period of pancytopenia and limiting infection risk. Transfusion support with platelets and packed RBCs is also provided. All blood products (except hematopoietic stem cell grafts and donor lymphocytes) given to HSCT recipients should be leukoreduced to remove WBCs that may transmit cytomegalovirus and irradiated to 2500 cGy to prevent transfusion-associated GVHD. Most centers recommend that allogeneic stem cell recipients receive irradiated blood products for the rest of their lives, and patients should be encouraged to purchase a Medi-alert bracelet that specifies their need for irradiated blood products.

Infection. Infection is the most common posttransplantation complication owing to mucositis, the presence of central venous access devices, and severe neutropenia. In allogeneic HSCT recipients, the use of immunosuppressants

Infections After Hematopoietic Stem Cell Transplantation

PERIOD OF NEUTROPENIA (DAY 0-30)
- Gram-negative bacteria
- Gram-positive bacteria
- Herpes simplex virus
- *Candida* species
- *Aspergillus* species

PERIOD OF ACUTE GRAFT-VERSUS-HOST DISEASE (DAY 30-100)
- Gram-negative bacteria
- Gram-positive bacteria
- Cytomegalovirus
- Human polyoma virus BK
- Adenovirus
- Varicella zoster
- *Candida* species
- *Aspergillus* species
- *Pneumocystis carinii*
- *Toxoplasma gondii*

PERIOD OF CHRONIC GRAFT-VERSUS-HOST DISEASE (DAY >100)
- Encapsulated bacteria
- Varicella zoster
- Cytomegalovirus
- *Pneumocystis carinii*
- *Aspergillus* species

Early and Late Complications of Autologous and Allogeneic Stem Cell Transplantation

EARLY (OCCURRING BEFORE DAY +100)
Regimen-related toxicity
- Cystitis
- Pulmonary complications
- Renal complications
- Neurological complications

Nutritional complications
Idiopathic pneumonitis
Graft failure
Infection
- Viral
- Bacterial
- Fungal

Graft-versus-host disease
Relapse

LATE (OCCURRING AFTER DAY +100)
Regimen-related toxicity
- Cataracts
- Neurological conditions—peripheral and autonomic neuropathies
- Gonadal dysfunction
- Endocrine dysfunction

Immunodeficiency
Infection
Musculoskeletal
- Osteoporosis
- Avascular necrosis

Chronic graft-versus-host disease
Relapse of malignancy
Secondary malignancy

compounds the infection risk. Pathogens may be bacteria, fungi, viruses, and protozoa, including herpes simplex and herpes zoster viruses, cytomegalovirus, *Candida* species, *Aspergillus* species, and *Pneumocystis carinii*. Infections caused by bacteria and other organisms that commonly occur after HSCT at each phase of the posttransplant period are listed in the box on left. Until their blood counts begin to recover, patients typically receive prophylaxis for viruses and fungi. If febrile neutropenia develops, empirical treatment with broad-spectrum antimicrobials is initiated. Screening for cytomegalovirus reactivation and for invasive aspergillosis may also be conducted during periods of greatest risk (neutropenic transplant recipients, graft versus host disease flare, intensive immunosuppressive treatment) or when infection is suspected.

Strategies to limit exposure to infectious organisms are essential in transplant recipients who are neutropenic and may also be receiving immunosuppressive medications. Important nursing responsibilities include maintaining a protective environment, practicing consistent and thorough provider hand hygiene, delivering meticulous oral and skin care, monitoring vital signs frequently, and conducting a thorough review of systems and physical examination to identify potential sites (e. g., alimentary tract, skin, lungs, sinuses, intravascular access device sites) of infection. Although there is limited evidence to support their effectiveness, in some transplant centers additional protective measures include low-microbial diets, protective isolation, air filtration, gowning, and gut and skin decontamination.

Veno-Occlusive Disease of the Liver. Also called sinusoidal obstructive syndrome, veno-occlusive disease (VOD) of the liver is a potentially fatal liver complication that occurs in 15% to 20% of recipients of HSCT and carries a mortality rate of close to 50%. A complication of the conditioning regimen, the risk of VOD is increased in patients who have received total-body irradiation or busulfan as part of their conditioning and those undergoing matched unrelated allogeneic HSCT. VOD occurs when fibrous material accumulates, resulting in obstruction of small venules in the liver. Subsequently, portal hypertension, acute liver congestion, and destruction of liver cells develop, and patients with severe manifestations can have hepatorenal syndrome and multisystem failure.

Clinical manifestations of VOD usually begin during the first 2 weeks after transplantation and are characterized by hyperbilirubinemia, rapid weight gain, ascites, right upper quadrant pain, hepatomegaly, splenomegaly, and jaundice. Treatment is supportive and focuses on maintaining intravascular volume and renal perfusion while minimizing fluid accumulation (Saria & Gosselin-Acomb, 2007). Options for preventing VOD in patients who are at highest risk for development of this complication include anticoagulation with heparin, antithrombin III concentrates, defibrotide, prostaglandin E, and ursodeoxycholic acid (Actigall) (Ho et al, 2004, 2007; Imran et al, 2006; Tay et al, 2007; Wadleigh et al, 2004).

Pulmonary Complications. Pulmonary complications develop in 30% to 60% of patients after HSCT. Pulmonary complications may result from (1) infection, pulmonary edema, aspiration pneumonia, acute respiratory distress syndrome (ARDS), and septic shock and (2) from lung damage from total-body irradiation or pulmonary toxic chemotherapy agents (Saria & Gosselin-Acomb, 2007). In the early posttransplant period, before day +30, pulmonary complications may include pulmonary edema, bacterial or fungal pneumonia, pulmonary hemorrhage or diffuse alveolar hemorrhage, and ARDS associated with septic shock. Through day +100, patients remain at risk for these same complications and for viral pneumonia, *P. carinii* pneumonia, and idiopathic interstitial pneumonitis. After day +100, they may also have bronchiolitis obliterans syndrome as a result of chronic GVHD, and they remain at risk for idiopathic interstitial pneumonitis and bacterial fungal or viral pneumonias. Early detection and prompt investigation of pulmonary symptoms such as shortness of breath, cough, sputum, and fever, together with periodic pulmonary function tests and high resolution computerized tomography of the chest and, as indicated, the sinuses, and measures to limit respiratory tract infections are essential components of the pre-emptive and supportive management of pulmonary complications.

ENGRAFTMENT AND RECOVERY

Engraftment is generally defined as an absolute neutrophil count greater than 0.5×10^9/L for 3 consecutive days and a platelet count greater than 20×10^9/L achieved without transfusion support. The rate of engraftment depends on the source of the progenitor cells (faster engraftment with peripheral blood stem cells), the total progenitor cell dose, the use of colony-stimulating factors, the agents used to prevent GVHD, and the nature of any complications the patient has in the early posttransplant period.

Patients usually receive their conditioning treatment and immediate posttransplantation care in an inpatient unit. However, improved symptom management and technological advances, including the use of hematopoietic growth factors, have allowed earlier discharge from the hospital. Many autologous stem cell transplant recipients can be managed throughout their transplant course with daily outpatient visits, thereby avoiding inpatient hospitalization. The criteria for hospital discharge after HSCT are presented in the box on right.

GRAFT-VERSUS-HOST DISEASE

GVHD is a complication unique to allogeneic HSCT. GVHD results when the infused donor stem cells (graft) recognize the recipient (host) as foreign tissue. The graft then mounts an immunological response attacking the host tissues, resulting in a T-cell–mediated reaction including the skin (rash), gastrointestinal tract (enteritis), and liver (elevated liver function test results). GVHD is classified as acute or chronic. Classically, this determination has been made on the basis of the time point at which GVHD

Criteria for Hospital Discharge After Stem Cell Transplantation

Discharge from the hospital is usually permitted when the following conditions are met:

- Afebrile for at least 24 hours
- Acute posttransplant complications resolved or controlled
- Evidence of oral intake of at least 1,500 mL per day or a plan to meet patient's fluid needs through self-administration of intravenous fluid/fluid administration daily in clinic
- Nausea and vomiting controlled
- Tolerating oral medications
- Platelet count supportable with no more frequent than daily platelet product
- White blood cell count greater than 1×10^9/L
- Hematocrit of 25% supportable with no more than daily transfusion of 1 unit of packed red blood cells
- Access an appropriate transfusion-supporting clinic environment (i.e., clinic must have ready access to irradiated blood products)
- Access to a medical facility with 24-hour outpatient support (in case urgent re-evaluation or readmission is required)
- Family caregiver support
- Independent in basic activities of daily living

---

occurred after transplantation, with GVHD manifestations occurring before day +100 termed acute and those after day +100 termed chronic. There is a growing recognition that acute and chronic GVHD are best differentiated by their features, not the time point at which they occurred after transplantation. Features of acute GVHD (erythematous skin rash, liver function test abnormalities, nausea, vomiting, diarrhea, and abdominal pain) may occur after donor lymphocyte infusion, and less commonly, features of acute GVHD can occur in a patient where features of chronic GVHD are also established. Similarly, features of chronic GVHD (such as pigmentary skin changes, sclerotic skin features, bronchiolitis obliterans, keratoconjunctivitis sicca, and oral dryness) may be observed in patients before day +100. A new paradigm for identifying acute and chronic GVHD and for diagnosing and staging chronic GVHD is evolving (Filipovich et al., 2005) that includes classic acute GVHD (maculopapular rash, nausea, vomiting or diarrhea, or elevated liver function tests); persistent, recurrent, or late acute GVHD (features of acute GVHD occurring beyond 100 days, often during withdrawal of immune suppression); classic chronic GVHD without features of acute GVHD; and an overlap syndrome in which diagnostic or distinctive features of chronic GVHD and acute GVHD appear together. The figure on page 149 depicts skin and gastrointestinal tract manifestations that may occur in acute GVHD.

The incidence of GVHD is 30% to 60% in cases involving histocompatible, sibling-matched allografts, with more GVHD occurring when there is greater HLA mismatch between the donor and recipient. The mortality rate directly or indirectly related to GVHD may reach 50% (Lazarus, Vogelsang & Rowe, 1997). Risk factors other than

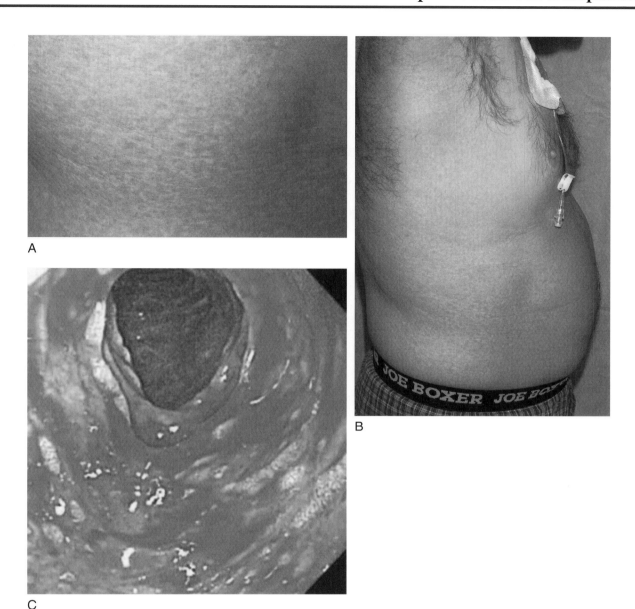

A and **B,** Acute graft-versus-host disease of the skin. **C,** Endoscopy demonstrates extensive erythema, tissue edema, and mucosal ulcerations consistent with acute graft-versus-host disease of the gastrointestinal tract (**A** and **B,** Courtesy of Dr. Edward Cowen, National Cancer Institute, Bethesda, MD. Used with permission. **C,** Courtesy of Dr. Bruce Greenwald, University of Maryland Medical Center, Baltimore, MD. Used with permission.)

histoincompatibility include sex mismatching; donor parity; older age; posttransplantation infectious complications, especially viral infections; the use of donor lymphocyte infusions post-transplantation; and the type of GVHD prophylaxis used (Socie & Cahn, 1998). GVHD is a serious complication, but it also has a beneficial effect in controlling the patient's malignancy in that immunocompetent donor cells are able to recognize the patient's malignant cells as foreign and eliminate them. This effect was originally identified by the observation that leukemic relapse was seen less often in patients with GVHD than in those without GVHD and was thus termed a "graft-versus-leukemia" effect. The absence of GVHD in autologous

transplant recipients is suspected to play a role in the higher disease relapse rates these patients experience. The infusion of donor lymphocytes (termed donor lymphocyte infusion, or DLI) is an attempt to harness the graft-versus-tumor effect to prevent or treat disease recurrence after stem cell transplantation. Research is also underway to devise strategies to induce a GVHD-like response in autologous HSCT recipients.

Acute Graft-Versus-Host Disease

Acute GVHD may occur as early as 7 to 21 days after transplantation but peaks at 30 to 40 days after transplantation. Acute GVHD targets the skin, liver, and gastrointestinal system. Skin reactions, which often occur first, include an itchy maculopapular, erythematous rash on the palms, soles, ears, face, and trunk. This may resolve or progress to generalized erythroderma and desquamation. Gastrointestinal symptoms include nausea, vomiting, anorexia, abdominal cramping, and large-volume diarrhea that is green and watery. Stool may have frank blood or be guaiac positive as a result of intestinal mucosa sloughing. An enlarged liver, right upper quadrant pain, jaundice, and elevated bilirubin and alkaline phosphatase levels may occur. The severity and extent of acute GVHD are evaluated according to a staging and grading system (see table below).

Staging and Grading System for Acute Graft-Versus-Host Disease

CLINICAL STAGING OF INDIVIDUAL ORGAN MANIFESTATIONS

Organ	Stage*	Description
Skin[†]	0	No evidence of GVHD
	+1	Maculopapular eruption over <25% of body area
	+2	Maculopapular eruption over 25%-50% of body area
	+3	Generalized erythroderma
	+4	Generalized erythroderma with bullous formation and often with desquamation
Liver	0	Bilirubin <2.0 mg/dL
	+1	Bilirubin 2.0-3.0 mg/dL
	+2	Bilirubin 3.1-6.0 mg/dL
	+3	Bilirubin 6.1-15 mg/L
	+4	Bilirubin >15 mg/dL
Gut	0	Diarrhea <500 mL/day
	+1	Diarrhea 500-999 mL/day, or persistent nausea with histologic evidence of GVHD in the stomach or duodenum
	+2	Diarrhea 1000-1499 mL/day
	+3	Diarrhea ≥1,500 mL/day
	+4	Severe abdominal pain, with or without ileus

OVERALL GRADE

Grade	Skin[‡]	Liver	Gut
0	None	None	None
I	+1 to +2	0	0
II	+1 to +3	+1 and/or	+1
III	+2 to +3	+2 to +3 and/or	+2 to +3
IV	+2 to +4	+2 to +4 and/or	+2 to +4

*Criteria for staging minimum degree of organ involvement required to confer that stage
[†]Use "rule of nines" or burn chart to determine extent of rash.
[‡]If no skin disease is present, the overall grade is the highest single organ stage
Data from Przepiorka, D., Weisdorf, D., Martin, P., Klingemann, H.G., Beatty, P., Hows, J., et al. (1995). 1994 Consensus conference on acute GVHD grading. *Bone Marrow Transplant 15*(6), 825-828.

Chronic Graft-Versus-Host Disease

Chronic GVHD usually occurs in patients who have had acute GVHD, although it can occur in the absence of acute GVHD. Among patients who survived 150 days after allogeneic stem cell transplantation, chronic GVHD was observed in 33% to 49% of HLA-identical related transplants, and in 64% of matched unrelated donor transplants (Przepiorka, Anderlini Saliba et al, 2001; Sullivan, Angura, Anasetti et al, 1991).

Risk factors for chronic GVHD include previous acute GVHD, older recipient age, and sex mismatching (female donor and male recipient). The incidence of chronic GVHD may also be higher in recipients of peripheral blood stem cells than in recipients of bone marrow–derived stem cells.

Clinical manifestations of chronic GVHD, which may be limited or extensive, may be observed in the skin, liver, eyes, oral cavity, lungs, gastrointestinal system, neuromuscular system, and a variety of other body systems. See the figure on page 151. Chronic GVHD typically occurs 100 to 400 days after transplantation, although it can begin as early as day 45 after transplantation. Some of the cutaneous manifestations of chronic GVHD are depicted in the figure. The table on pages 151-152 summarizes the clinical features, screening and evaluation, and interventions recommended for patients with chronic GVHD. It is important to note that other conditions can mimic chronic GVHD; therefore a systematic, multidisciplinary evaluation of the patient with chronic GVHD is essential (Jacobsohn, Montross, Anders & Vogelsang, 2001).

Treatment and Prophylaxis of Graft-Versus-Host Disease

Approaches to limiting and treating GVHD include optimal matching of donor and recipient, graft engineering to decrease the dose of T lymphocytes in the graft, and the administration of immunosuppressive medications. T lymphocytes play a major role in the recognition of self from nonself proteins, and depletion of the number of T lymphocytes in the graft before transplantation may decrease the incidence and severity of GVHD. Methods of T-cell depletion include physical, immunological, and pharmacological techniques. However, T lymphocytes also play a role in engraftment, and T-cell depletion carries greater risks for infection, graft failure, and disease relapse.

A variety of immunosuppressive agents, as a single agent or in combination, have been used to prevent acute GVHD. Immunosuppressive medications minimize the newly developing donor immune system's ability to recognize the host or patient as foreign and limit the immune response. Immunosuppressive drugs must often be taken for months or years after an allogeneic HSCT. Immunosuppression may be achieved with a single drug (often tacrolimus or cyclosporin A) or with a combination of drugs (methotrexate, tacrolimus, cyclosporin A, steroids, antithymocyte globulin, mycophenolate mofetil), sometimes in combination with T-cell depletion. For patients at higher risk for GVHD, for example, those undergoing matched unrelated HSCT, multidrug strategies to prevent GVHD prevention are typically needed. Many patients also derive benefit from the inclusion of topical, ocular and inhaled immunosuppressive agents, and steroid preparations formulated for topical application within the mouth (e.g. dexamethasone mouth rinses) and the gastrointestinal system, such budesonide.

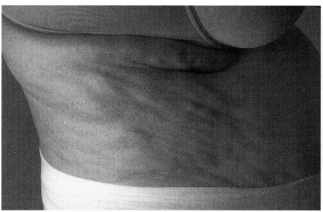
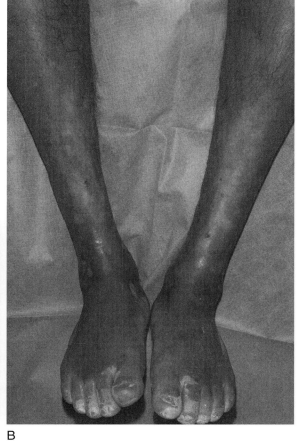

A   B

Chronic graft-versus-host disease of the skin. **A,** Superficial (movable) and deep (hide bound) sclerotic manifestations. **B,** Skin ulcerations. (Photos courtesy of Dr. Edward Cowen, National Cancer Institute, Bethesda, MD. Used with permission.)

Chronic Graft-Versus-Host Disease: Clinical Manifestations, Screening/Evaluation, Interventions

Organ/System	Clinical Manifestations	Screening Studies/Evaluation	Interventions
Dermal	Dyspigmentation, xerosis (dryness), hyperkeratosis, pruritus, scleroderma, lichenification, onychodystrophy (nail ridging/nail loss), alopecia	Clinical examination Skin biopsy—3-mm punch biopsy	Immunosuppressive therapy Psoralen and ultraviolet irradiation Topical with steroid creams, moisturizers/emollient, antibacterial ointments to prevent suprainfection Avoid sunlight exposure, use sun block lotion with a large hat that shades the face when outdoors
Oral	Lichen planus, xerostomia, ulceration	Oral biopsy	Steroid mouth rinses, oral psoralen, and ultraviolet A (PUVA), pilocarpine and anetholetrithione for xerostomia, fluoride gels/rinses Careful attention to oral hygiene; regular dental evaluations
Ocular	Keratoconjunctivitis sicca syndrome	Schirmer's test, ophthalmic evaluation	Regular ophthalmological follow-up Preservative-free tears and moisturizing lotions Temporary or permanent lacrimal duct occlusion; system specific interventions, pancreatic enzyme supplementation
Hepatic	Jaundice, abdominal pain	Liver function tests	Actigall 300 mg orally three times a day
Pulmonary	Shortness of breath, cough, dyspnea, wheezing, fatigue, hypoxia, pleural effusion	Pulmonary function studies, peak flow, arterial blood gas, high-resolution computed tomography of chest	Prevent and treat pulmonary infections Aggressively investigate changes in pulmonary function because these may represent graft-versus-host disease of lung/bronchiolitis obliterans

Continued

Chronic Graft-Versus-Host Disease: Clinical Manifestations, Screening/Evaluation, Interventions—cont'd

Organ/System	Clinical Manifestations	Screening Studies/Evaluation	Interventions
Gastrointestinal	Nausea, odynophagia, dysphagia, anorexia, early satiety, malabsorption, diarrhea, weight loss	Esophagogastroduodenoscopy, colonoscopy, nutritional assessment, fecal studies	Referral to gastroenterologist, nutrition support
Nutritional	Protein and calorie deficiency, malabsorption, dehydration, weight loss, muscle wasting	Weight, fat store measurement, Prealbumin	Nutritional monitoring, supplementation, symptom specific interventions
Genitourinary	Vaginal sicca; vaginal atrophy, stenosis, or inflammation	Pelvic examination	Efficacy of intravaginal steroid cream currently being evaluated
Immunologic	Hypogammaglobulinemia, autoimmune syndromes, recurrent infections including cytomegalovirus, herpes simplex virus, varicella-zoster virus, fungus, *Pneumocystis carinii*, and encapsulated bacteria	Quantitative immunoglobulin levels, CD4/CD8 lymphocyte subsets	Intravenous immunoglobulins, prophylactic antimicrobials for prophylaxis again *P carinii* pneumonia and encapsulated organisms, surveillance for cytomegalovirus reactivation
Musculoskeletal	Contractures, debility, muscle cramps	Performance status, formal Quality-of-life evaluation, rehabilitation needs	Physical therapy

Data from Buchsel, Leum, & Randolph, 1996; Chao, 1998; Flowers, Lee, & Vogelsang, 2003; Gold, Flowers, & Sullivan, 1998; Mitchell, 2004; and Seber & Vodelsang, 1998.

Prospective, randomized trials have demonstrated that combination therapy is superior to single-drug therapy in the prevention of acute GVHD. However, to date, research has not shown that any one prophylactic regimen is superior in preventing acute GVHD or improving overall outcome (Sullivan, 1999; Chao, 1999; Locatelli et al, 2000; Chao et al, 2000). The most widely used pharmacological regimen for the prophylaxis of acute GVHD is a combination of methotrexate and either cyclosporin A or tacrolimus. Other drugs included in some GVHD prophylaxis regimens include corticosteroids, antithymocyte globulin, daclizumab, and mycophenolate mofetil. Examples of some regimens for GVHD prophylaxis, along with the typical schedules for tapering of immunosuppression are presented in the table below.

If grade II to IV acute GVHD develops despite preventive strategies, additional immunosuppression is usually required.

Corticosteroids are the main component of therapy, along with continuation of the immunosuppressive agent used for initial prophylaxis (Deeg, 2007). High doses of methylprednisolone (1 to 20 mg/kg/day) may be added to the regimen of immunosuppression, and the dose of methylprednisolone is rapidly tapered to 1-2 mg/kg/day in divided doses. Once maximal improvement is achieved, the steroids are tapered by approximately 25% every 4 days, on the basis of patient response. Gut rest, pain control, and antimicrobial prophylaxis coupled with attention to fluid and electrolyte balance and administration of hyperalimentation, if needed, are important aspects of the supportive care of patients with acute GVHD (Jacobsohn & Vogelsang, 2007). The outcome of treatment of acute GVHD is predicted by the overall grade of acute GVHD; higher overall grades are associated with poorer outcomes. Response to treatment is another key determinant

Examples of Commonly Used Drug Regimens for Prevention of Acute Graft-Versus-Host Disease

Regimen	Dosing Schedule
Cyclosporine/steroids	Cyclosporine 3 mg/kg/day intravenous infusion from day −2, taper 10% weekly starting day +180 Methylprednisolone 0.25 mg/kg twice daily on days +7 to +14, 0.5 mg/kg twice daily on days +15 to +28, 0.4 mg/kg twice daily on days +29 to +42, 0.3 mg/kg twice daily on days +43-58, 0.25 mg/kg twice daily on days +59 to +119, and 0.1 mg/kg daily days +120-180.
Cyclosporine/methotrexate/ steroids	Cyclosporine 5 mg/kg/day intravenous infusion from day −2, taper 20% every 2 weeks starting day +84 Methotrexate 15 mg/m^2 on day +1, 10 mg/m^2 on days +3 and +6 Methylprednisolone 0.25 mg/kg twice daily on days +7 to +14, 0.5 mg/kg twice daily on days +15 to +28, 0.4 mg/kg daily on days +29 to +42, 0.3 mg/kg twice daily on days +43-58, 0.25 mg/kg twice daily on days +59 to +119, and 0.1 mg/kg daily days +120-180
Tacrolimus/minimethotrexate	Tacrolimus 0.03 mg/kg/day infusion from day −2, taper 20% every 2 weeks starting day +180 Methotrexate 5 mg/m^2 on days +1, +3, +6, and +11
Antithymocyte globulin (ATG)/cyclosporine/ methotrexate	ATG 20 mg/kg intravenously days −3, −2, and −1 Cyclosporine 5 mg/kg/day intravenous infusion from day −1, taper 10% weekly starting day +180 Methotrexate 10 mg/m^2 on days +1, +3, +6, and +11

Data from: Chao, 1998; Goker, Haznedaroglu, & Chao, 2001; Holler, 2007; Przepiorka, 2000; and Simpson, 2001.

of outcome, and mortality is greatest in patients who do not achieve a complete response to the initial treatment strategy for acute GVHD (Deeg, 2007). For patients with GVHD in whom initial therapy with high dose steroids has failed, a variety of secondary regimens, including mycophenolate mofetil, infliximab, etanercept, daclizumab, ATG, denileukin diftitox, pentostatin, rapamycin, and steroid preparations such as beclomethasone and budesonide that have a local/topical effect in the gastrointestinal tract are available (Deeg, 2007; Jacobsohn & Vogeslsang, 2004). If chronic GVHD develops, it is usually treated with a combination of steroids, cyclosporin A, tacrolimus, rapamycin, mycophenolate mofetil, rituximab, pentostatin, hydroxychloroquine, methotrexate or extracorporeal photophoresis (Akpek, Lee, Anders & Vogelsang, 2001; Alcindor et al., 2001; Arai & Vogelsang, 2000; Baird & Pavletic, 2006; Bolanos-Meade & Vogelsang, 2005; Bolanos-Meade et al., 2005; Flowers, Lee & Vogelsang, 2003; Gasova et al., 2007; Higman & Vogelsang, 2004; Holler, 2007; Jurado et al, 2007; Lee, Vogelsang & Flowers, 2003; Mitchell, 2004; Vogelsang, 2001; Wolff et al., 2004; Woltz, Castro, & Park, 2006).

The immunosuppressive agents commonly used in patients undergoing HSCT and the associated nursing implications are presented in the table on pages 154-155. Drug levels of cyclosporin A or tacrolimus should be monitored at regular intervals and dosing adjusted to maintain levels within a therapeutic range. Many drug-drug interactions are associated with cyclosporin A and tacrolimus; therefore, it is important to regularly review the patient's medication profile to identify potentially deleterious interactions (Leather, 2004). Patients should be instructed to take their immunosuppressive medications exactly as instructed and to contact their physician or nurse before starting any new medications. Because sun exposure may activate or exacerbate GVHD of the skin, patients should be advised about appropriate methods for minimizing sun exposure.

GVHD is a cause of significant morbidity after allogeneic stem cell transplantation. Supportive care measures such as infection prophylaxis and nutritional management (Charuhas, 2000; Iestra et al., 2002; Lipkin, Lenssen, & Dickson, 2005) together with coordinated multidisciplinary care are essential to improve the length and quality of life for patients with GVHD (Arai & Vogelsang, 2000; Couriel et al., 2006; Vogelsang, 2001). Continuing specialty involvement to include dentistry/oral medicine, dermatology, endocrinology, gynecology, ophthalmology, pulmonology, nutrition support, physical therapy, and occupational therapy are essential in caring for patients with acute and chronic GVHD. Chronic GVHD is a primary factor in late transplant-related morbidity, including abnormalities of growth and development in children and quality of life, functional performance status, somatic symptoms, psychological functioning, sexual satisfaction, and employment in adults (Broers et al., 2000; Harder et al., 2002). Support groups, individual and family psychotherapy, physical therapy, occupational therapy, and preventive and pre-emptive rehabilitation may help to prevent functional decline and emotional distress, thereby improving quality of life (Gillis & Donovan, 2001; Harder et al., 2002). Complicating the management is the fact that at the time that chronic GVHD develops many patients have returned to their local community and thus are at a distance from health care providers with expertise in the identification and management of the diverse manifestations of chronic GVHD.

A variety of approaches to the prevention, treatment and control of GVHD are currently undergoing development and preclinical and clinical evaluation (Alcindor et al., 2001; Bolanos-Meade & Vogelsang, 2005; Bolanos-Meade et al., 2005; Carpenter & Sanders, 2003; Cavazzana-Calvo et al., 2002; Holler, 2007; Ratanatharathorn et al., 2003; Reddy et al., 2003; Simpson, 2001, 2003). These include the application of cytokine shields to decrease the inflammatory tissue responses thought to promote acute GVHD (Hill & Ferrara, 2000), selective T-cell depletion and other graft engineering strategies (Soiffer et al., 2001), the use of new conditioning agents with potent immunosuppressive properties (Auffermann-Gretzinger et al., 2007; Shah et al., 2007; Shore et al., 2006), and modification of donor T lymphocytes through incorporation of suicide genes (Bondanza et al., 2006; Kornblau et al., 2001), or the infusion of tumor specific T-lymphocyte clones (Patterson & Korngold, 2001).

GRAFT FAILURE

Graft failure is a complete absence of engraftment after HSCT or the initial recovery of hematopoiesis with subsequent cytopenias and absent or diminished hematopoiesis occurring beyond the initial period after conditioning therapy. The overall incidence of graft failure is less than 5%, and it occurs most often in patients with aplastic anemia or those receiving unrelated donor transplants. The etiology is multifactorial and may include insufficient dose intensity of conditioning regimen, inadequate stem cell dose, insufficient posttransplant immunosuppression, posttransplant administration of medications with myelosuppressive side effects, viral infection, and folate or vitamin B_{12} deficiency (Deeg, 1998b). An important component in the evaluation is differentiating graft failure from disease recurrence or drug-induced myelosuppression. Medications with myelosuppressive side effects (such as cotrimoxazole) should be administered with caution after HSCT. Treatment of graft failure may include cytokine support and administration of additional hematopoietic stem cells, also termed a stem cell boost.

LONG-TERM COMPLICATIONS OF HEMATOPOIETIC STEM CELL TRANSPLANTATION: ASSESSMENT, PREVENTION, AND MANAGEMENT

HSCT can result in cure of the underlying malignant disease and long-term survival; however, there may be persistent sequelae and in the long term patients may have late effects of the treatment. The development of long-term

(Continued on p. 157)

Nursing Implications of Selected Immunosuppressants Used in Allogeneic Stem Cell Transplantation

Agent/Drug	Nursing Implications
Cyclosporin A (Sandimmune, Neoral)	Bioavailability differs between oral solution and capsule formulation. *Once a regimen is established, patients should be instructed not to change their formulation or brand.* Take with food. Instruct patient to notify the health care team immediately if unable to take because of gastrointestinal side effects. Monitor serum creatinine, blood urea nitrogen, potassium, magnesium, glucose, and triglyceride levels. Monitor levels carefully in patients with renal or hepatic dysfunction. Doses should be adjusted for renal dysfunction, as ordered. Avoid potassium-sparing diuretics. Replete electrolytes as indicated. Coadministration with grapefruit juice may increase cyclosporin A levels and should be avoided. Drug-drug interactions can lead to subtherapeutic or toxic cyclosporin A levels. Patients should advise their health care providers of any changes made in concurrent medications. Cyclosporin A trough levels to be drawn before administration of morning dose. Tacrolimus should be discontinued for at least 24 hours before cyclosporin A is started.
Tacrolimus (Prograf)	Take on an empty stomach. Instruct patient to notify the health care team immediately if unable to take because of gastrointestinal side effects. Monitor serum creatinine, blood urea nitrogen, potassium, magnesium, phosphorus, glucose, and triglyceride levels. Monitor levels carefully in patients with renal or hepatic dysfunction. Doses should be adjusted for renal dysfunction, as ordered. Avoid potassium-sparing diuretics. Replete electrolytes as indicated. Coadministration with grapefruit juice may increase tacrolimus levels and should be avoided. Drug-drug interactions can lead to subtherapeutic or toxic tacrolimus levels. Patients should advise their health care providers of any changes made in concurrent medications Tacrolimus trough levels to be drawn before administration of morning dose Cyclosporin A should be discontinued for at least 24 hours before tacrolimus A is started.
Corticosteroids	Consult physical therapy for proximal muscle strengthening exercise program. Monitor serum chemistries. Instruct patient in strategies to prevent or treat hyperglycemia and in diabetic self-management. Consult with diabetes educator, as indicated. Administer oral corticosteroids with food/milk to minimize gastrointestinal upset. Administer H_2 blockers or proton pump inhibitors to decrease gastric acidity. Consider need for antiviral, antibacterial, and antifungal prophylaxis. May increase tacrolimus or cyclosporin A levels. Report complaints of visual changes and consult ophthalmology. For patients on long-term steroids or otherwise at risk for or with osteopenia (e.g., patients with acute lymphoblastic leukemia, postmenopausal), ensure regular dual-energy x-ray absorptiometric scans, calcium and vitamin D supplementation, and specific treatment for osteopenia with antiresorptive agents such as alendronate (Fosamax). A tapering calendar specifying the dosage to be taken each day can help facilitate adherence in patients who are on tapering doses of steroids or an alternate-day steroid regimen.
Mycophenolate mofetil	Should be taken on an empty stomach. Monitor complete blood cell count at regular intervals and adjust dosage for pancytopenia, as ordered. Monitor liver function tests (bilirubin and serum transaminases) at regular intervals and adjust dosage for liver function abnormalities, as ordered. Monitor plasma levels of mycophenolic acid (the metabolite of mycophenolate mofetil) to guide treatment in patients with renal dysfunction. There may be decreased absorption when coadministered with magnesium oxide, aluminum- or magnesium-containing antacids, or cholestyramine.
Azathioprine	Dose reduction required when given with allopurinol. May lead to anemia and leukopenia when given with angiotensin-converting enzyme inhibitors; synergistic with other bone marrow suppressants. Use with caution in patients with hepatic or renal impairment. Teratogenic; advise patient and partner about the need for contraception.
Methotrexate	Dose and schedule for methotrexate prophylaxis for graft-versus-host disease varies by institution. A common regimen is 5-15 mg/m^2 on days 1, 3, 6, and 11 post transplant. Dose may be adjusted or held for severe mucositis and renal or liver insufficiency. Dose may need to be adjusted for hypoalbuminemia. Wait until at least 24 hours after stem cell infusion to give day +1 dose. Consider the need to monitor methotrexate levels.
Daclizumab (Zenapax)	Anaphylactoid reactions after the administration of daclizumab have not been observed; however, medications for the treatment of severe hypersensitivity reactions should be available for immediate use. No incompatibility between daclizumab and polyvinyl chloride or polyethylene bags or infusion sets has been observed. No dosage adjustment is necessary for patients with severe renal impairment.

Nursing Implications of Selected Immunosuppressants Used in Allogeneic Stem Cell Transplantation—cont'd

Agent/Drug	Nursing Implications
Infliximab (Remicade)	Monitor patient for development of infusional toxicities. Consider premedication with acetaminophen and diphenhydramine. Medications for treating hypersensitivity reactions (e.g., acetaminophen, antihistamines, corticosteroids, or epinephrine) and supplemental oxygen should be available for immediate use in the event of a reaction. Incompatible with polyvinyl chloride equipment or devices. Use glass infusion bottles and polyethylene-lined administration sets.
Antithymocyte globulin (ATGAM [equine] Thymoglobulin [rabbit])	Monitor patient closely both during and after infusion for signs of serum sickness and anaphylaxis. Consider premedication with corticosteroids, acetaminophen, and H_1 and H_2 blockers. Medications for treating hypersensitivity reactions (e.g., acetaminophen, antihistamines, corticosteroids, or epinephrine) and supplemental oxygen should be available for immediate use in the event of a reaction. Because transient and at times severe thrombocytopenia may occur after antithymocyte globulin administration in patients with platelet counts less than 100,000 per microliter, the platelet count should be evaluated 1 hour after administration and as ordered and platelets transfused as indicated.
Alemtuzumab (Campath-1)	Premedicate patient with acetaminophen and diphenhydramine. Medications for treating hypersensitivity reactions (e.g., acetaminophen, antihistamines, corticosteroids, or epinephrine) and supplemental oxygen should be available for immediate use in the event of a reaction. Consider treatment with meperidine to control infusional rigors. Administer fluid bolus as ordered to treat hypotension. Produces profound and rapid lymphopenia; patients require broad antifungal, antibacterial, antiviral, and antiprotozoal prophylaxis for at least 4 months after treatment and continuing surveillance for cytomegalovirus infection.
Rapamycin (Sirolimus)	May suppress hematopoietic recovery if used in patients who have recently undergone high-dose therapy. Oral bioavailability is variable and may be improved when administered with a high-fat meal. Like tacrolimus and cyclosporin A, it is metabolized through the cytochrome P450-3A system; anticipate drug-drug interactions.
Thalidomide (Thalomid)	Thalidomide is a potent teratogen and is contraindicated in patients who are or who are likely to become pregnant. A systematic counseling and education program, written informed consent, and participation in a confidential survey program at the start of treatment and throughout treatment is required for all patients receiving thalidomide. Both men and women who are of childbearing potential must practice protected sex while on this drug. Perform pregnancy test before initiating treatment with thalidomide. Obtain baseline electrocardiogram before treatment. Thalidomide should not be started if the absolute neutrophil count is less than 750/mm³, and therapy should be re-evaluated if the absolute neutrophil count drops below this level. Administer doses in the evening to minimize impact of drowsiness on lifestyle and safety. Teach patient to use caution when taking thalidomide with other drugs that can cause drowsiness or neuropathy. Teach patient to rise slowly from a supine position to avoid lightheadedness. Teach patient to report immediately signs or symptoms suggestive of peripheral neuropathy, including numbness or tingling in the hands or feet or the development of skin rash or skin ulcerations. These may require immediate cessation of the drug until the patient can be evaluated. Teach patient to use protective measures (e.g., sunscreens and protective clothing) against exposure to ultraviolet light or sunlight. Prevent constipation with a stool softener or mild laxative.
Methoxsoralen (Oxsoralen)	Patients who have received cytotoxic chemotherapy or radiation and who are taking methoxsoralen are at increased risk for skin cancers. Toxicity increases with concurrent use of phenothiazines, thiazides, and sulfanilamides. Instruct patient to take methoxsalen with milk or food and to divide the dose into two portions, taken approximately one-half hour apart. Severe burns may occur from sunlight or ultraviolet A exposure. Pretreatment eye examinations are indicated to evaluation for the presence of cataracts. Repeat eye examinations should be performed every 6 months while patients are undergoing psoralen ultraviolet A.

Data from Abo-Zena & Horwitz, 2002; Beauchesne, Chung, & Wasan, 2007; Bush, 1999; Cather, Abramovits, & Menter, 2001; Chan, 2000; Chao, 1998; Charuhas, 2000; Cronin et al., 2000; Gaziev et al., 2000; Goldman, 2001; Lanuza & McCabe, 2001; Lazarus, Vogelsang, & Rowe, 1997; Leather, 2004; Przepiorka et al., 1999; Saria & Gosselin-Acomb, 2007; Seeley & DeMeyer, 2002; Simpson, 2001, 2003; Solimando, 1998; and Srinivas, Meier-Kriesche, & Kaplan, 2005.

Cancer Management

Evaluation and Screening of Late Effects of Hematopoietic Stem Cell Transplantation

System/Dimension	Possible Late Effects	Evaluation/Screening
Disease status	Relapse/recurrence	Determined on the basis of the site of original disease Evaluation for minimal residual disease, as indicated
Engraftment	Graft failure/marrow dysfunction with cytopenias	Complete blood cell count with differential Bone marrow aspirate and biopsy Engraftment/chimerism studies: to detect differences between deoxyribonucleic acid of donor and recipient and thus establish engraftment: variable nucleotide tandem repeats (VNTR), short tandem repeats (STR). Cytogenetic studies may also be used to establish engraftment if the donor and recipient are of opposite sexes
Immunologic function/recovery	Disorders of B and T lymphocyte quantity and function Hypogammaglobulinemia	CD 4/CD 8 lymphocyte subsets Quantitative immunoglobulin levels Vaccination titers
Cardiopulmonary	Interstitial pneumonitis Bronchiolitis obliterans Hypertension, cardiomyopathy, pericardial damage, peripheral vascular disease	Chest x-ray Pulmonary function tests with single-breath diffusing capacity Electrocardiogram Echocardiogram History and physical examination
Neurologic	Peripheral and autonomic neuropathies Cognitive changes, shortened attention span, difficulty with concentration Leukoencephalopathy Ototoxicity	Health history Neurologic examination Neuropsychologic testing Rehabilitation medicine Audiologic testing
Gastrointestinal	Liver dysfunction Malabsorption syndromes	Liver function tests Hepatitis B serologies, hepatitis C polymerase chain reaction qualitative
Genitourinary	Renal dysfunction Radiation nephritis Hematuria, proteinuria Cancer of the bladder	Blood urea nitrogen, creatinine Urinalysis with microscopy 24-hour urine for creatine clearance, total protein, if indicated
Thyroid function	Hypothyroidism	Thyroid-stimulating hormone, tri-iodothyronine, thyroxine, free thyroxine
Gonadal function	Decreased production of gonadal hormones	Luteinizing hormone, follicle-stimulating hormone, estradiol (women) Pelvic examination Luteinizing hormone, follicle-stimulating hormone, testosterone (men)
Hypothalamic-pituitary	Abnormal pituitary gland function	Prolactin, follicle-stimulating hormone, luteinizing hormone, thyroid-stimulating hormone
Metabolic syndrome		Fasting glucose, lipid profile
Opthalmic	Cataracts	Ophthalmologic examination to include slit-lamp examination and Schirmer's test
Dental/oral cavity	Sicca syndrome Caries Periodontal disease Xerostomia Oral malignancy	Regular dental evaluations Meticulous attention to oral hygiene Fluoride gels/rinses
Musculoskeletal	Osteoporosis Avascular necrosis Myopathy	Dual-energy x-ray absorptiometry scan Magnetic resonance imaging if pain in a joint, limited range of motion, or a limp Magnetic resonance imaging, neurological examination, electromyelogram
Second malignancy	Nonmelanoma skin cancer Breast cancer Thyroid cancer	Complete physical examination with biopsy of suspicious lesions. Skin photographs may also help to monitor status. Mammogram, self-examination History and physical examination, ultrasonography, iodine 131 scan

Evaluation and Screening of Late Effects of Hematopoietic Stem Cell Transplantation—cont'd

	Acute leukemia Myelodysplastic syndrome	Complete blood cell count with differential Bone marrow aspirate and biopsy (if complete blood cell count abnormal)
	Posttransplant lymphoproliferative disorder	Computed tomographic scans if posttransplant lymphoproliferative disorder is suspected; polymerase chain reaction monitoring of Epstein-Barr viral load in first few months after allogeneic hematopoietic stem cell transplantation
	Cancer of the uterine cervix Cancer of the bladder	Gynecological examination with Papanicolaou smear Urinalysis with microscopy to detect microhematuria, urine cytology, follow-up cystoscopy
Integumentary	Increased incidence of benign and malignant nevi	Complete physical examination Skin biopsy of suspicious lesions
Psychologic/ rehabilitation quality of life	Changes in body image, roles, family relationships, lifestyle, occupation, discrimination, overcoming stigma, living with compromises, coping with symptoms	Assessment of individual adjustment, achievement of normal developmental tasks, marital stress, sexual function, body image, rehabilitation needs, symptom distress through systematic and structured evaluation

Data from Abo-Zena & Horwitz, 2002; Antin, 2002; Baker et al., 2004; Baker et al., 2007; Bhatia et al., 2005; Buchsel, Leum & Randolph, 1996; Cohen et al., 2007; Deeg, 1998a, 1998b; Deeg & Socie, 1998; Duell et al., 1997; Guise, 2006; Harder et al., 2002; Kinch et al., 2007; Nuver, Smit, Postma, Sleijfer, & Gietema, 2002; Rizzo et al., 2006; Ruccione, 1994; Sanders, 1994; Sanders, 2002; Schwartz, Hobbie, & Constine, 1994; and Wingard, Vogelsang, & Deeg, 2002.

Cancer Management

complications is multifactorial and includes the interplay of the effects of high-dose chemotherapy, total-body radiation, medication side effects, infections, acute and chronic GVHD and disease recurrence, together with the effects of prior treatment and preexisting medical conditions (Deeg, 1998a). In addition to chronic GVHD and infection, a wide range of complications may be experienced months or even years after HSCT (Moya et al., 2006).

HSCT recipients require life-long surveillance and preventive care for some of these complications, including second malignancy, cardiovascular effects, and relapse. Most transplantation centers have protocol-specific requirements for continued follow-up care, and the frequency of clinic visits is determined by the nature of the complications the patient is experiencing. The table on page 156 summarizes guidelines for screening and evaluation of the potential late effects of HSCT. Guidelines for surveillance and follow-up are available to direct long-term supportive care of HSCT recipients (Rizzo et al., 2006) and to guide recommendations for fertility preservation (Lee et al., 2006), vaccination (Ljungman et al., 2005; Singhal & Mehta, 1999), and healthy nutrition and physical activity (Doyle et al., 2006). Routine follow-up should also include the promotion of health lifestyle changes and risk reduction strategies including nutrition, exercise, safe sexual practices, colorectal screening, avoidance of sun exposure, and smoking cessation (Aziz, 2007).

BIBLIOGRAPHY

Abo-Zena, R. A., & Horwitz, M. E. (2002). Immunomodulation in stem-cell transplantation. *Current Opinion in Pharmacology, 2*, 452-457.

Akpek, G., Lee, S.M., Anders, V., et al. (2001). A high-dose pulse steroid regimen for controlling active chronic graft-versus-host disease. *Biology of Blood and Marrow Transplantation, 97*(5):1196-1201.

Alcindor, T., Gorgun, G., Miller, K. B., et al. (2001). Immunomodulatory effects of extracorporeal photochemotherapy in patients with extensive chronic graft-versus-host disease. *Blood, 98*, 1622-1625.

Antin, J. H. (2002). Clinical practice: long-term care after hematopoietic-cell transplantation in adults. *New England Journal of Medicine, 347*, 36-42.

Arai, S., & Vogelsang, G. B. (2000). Management of graft-versus-host disease. *Blood Reviews, 14*, 190-204.

Auffermann-Gretzinger, S., Eger, L., Schetelig, J., et al. (2007). Alemtuzumab depletes dendritic cells more effectively in blood than in skin: a pilot study in patients with chronic lymphocytic leukemia. *Transplantation, 83*, 1268-1272.

Aziz, N. M. (2007). Cancer survivorship research: state of knowledge, challenges and opportunities. *Acta Oncologica (Stockholm, Sweden), 46*, 417-432.

Baird, K., & Pavletic, S. Z. (2006). Chronic graft versus host disease. *Current Opinion in Hematology, 13*, 426-435.

Baker, K. S., Gurney, J. G., Ness, K. K., et al. (2004). Late effects in survivors of chronic myeloid leukemia treated with hematopoietic cell transplantation: results from the Bone Marrow Transplant Survivor Study. *Blood, 104*, 1898-1906.

Baker, K. S., Ness, K. K., Steinberger, J., et al. (2007). Diabetes, hypertension, and cardiovascular events in survivors of hematopoietic cell transplantation: a report from the bone marrow transplantation survivor study. *Blood, 109*, 1765-1772.

Baron, F., & Storb, R. (2007). Hematopoietic cell transplantation after reduced-intensity conditioning for older adults with acute myeloid leukemia in complete remission. *Current Opinion in Hematology, 14*, 145-151.

Beauchesne, P. R., Chung, N. S., & Wasan, K. M. (2007). Cyclosporine A: a review of current oral and intravenous delivery systems. *Drug Development and Industrial Pharmacy, 33*, 211-220.

Bhatia, S., Robison, L. L., Francisco, L., et al. (2005). Late mortality in survivors of autologous hematopoietic-cell transplantation: report from the Bone Marrow Transplant Survivor Study. *Blood, 105*, 4215-4222.

Bolanos-Meade, J., Jacobsohn, D. A., Margolis, J., et al. (2005). Pentostatin in steroid-refractory acute graft-versus-host disease. *Journal of Clinical Oncology, 23*, 2661-2668.

Bolanos-Meade, J., & Vogelsang, G. B. (2005). Novel strategies for steroid-refractory acute graft-versus-host disease. *Current Opinion in Hematology, 12*, 40-44.

Bondanza, A., Valtolina, V., Magnani, Z., et al. (2006). Suicide gene therapy of graft-versus-host disease induced by central memory human T lymphocytes. *Blood, 107*, 1828-1836.

Broers, S., Kaptein, A. A., Le Cessie, S., et al. (2000). Psychological functioning and quality of life following bone marrow transplantation: a 3-year follow-up study. *Journal of Psychosomatic Research, 48*, 11-21.

Brunstein, C. G., Baker, K. S., & Wagner, J. E. (2007). Umbilical cord blood transplantation for myeloid malignancies. *Current Opinion in Hematology, 14*, 162-169.

Buchsel, P. C., Leum, E. W., & Randolph, S. R. (1996). Delayed complications of bone marrow transplantation: an update. *Oncology Nursing Forum, 23*, 1267-1291.

Bush, W. W. (1999). Overview of transplantation immunology and the pharmacotherapy of adult solid organ transplant recipients: focus on immunosuppression. *AACN Clinical Issues, 10*, 253-269; quiz 304.

Carpenter, P. A., & Sanders, J. E. (2003). Steroid-refractory graft-vs.-host disease: past, present and future. *Pediatric Transplantation, 7 Suppl 3*, 19-31.

Cather, J. C., Abramovits, W., & Menter, A. (2001). Cyclosporine and tacrolimus in dermatology. *Dermatology Clinics, 19*, 119-137, ix.

Cavazzana-Calvo, M., Andre-Schmutz, I., Hacein-Bey-Abina, S., et al. (2002). Improving immune reconstitution while preventing graft-versus-host disease in allogeneic stem cell transplantation. *Seminars in Hematology, 39*, 32-40.

Chan, B. (2000). The pharmacology of peripheral blood stem cell transplantation. In P. C. Buchsel & P. M. Kaputsay (Eds.), *Stem cell transplantation: a clinical textbook* (pp. 8.3-8.24). Pittsburg, PA: Oncology Nursing Press.

Chantry, A. D., Snowden, J. A., Craddock, C., et al. (2006). Long-term outcomes of myeloablation and autologous transplantation of relapsed acute myeloid leukemia in second remission: a British Society of Blood and Marrow Transplantation registry study. *Biology of Blood and Marrow Transplantation, 12*, 1310-1317.

Chao, N. J. (1998). Graft-versus-host disease. In R. K. Burt, H. J. Deeg, S. Lothian, et al. (Eds.), *Bone marrow transplantation* (pp. 478-497). Austin, TX: Landes Bioscience.

Charuhas, P. M. (2000). Medical nutrition therapy in bone marrow transplantation. In M. P.D. & C. G. Polisen (Eds.), *The clinical guide to oncology nutrition* (pp. 90-98). Chicago: American Dietetic Association.

Cohen, J. M., Cooper, N., Chakrabarti, S., et al. (2007). EBV-related disease following haematopoietic stem cell transplantation with reduced intensity conditioning. *Leukemia & Lymphoma, 48*, 256-269.

Confer, D. L. & Miller, J. P. (2007). Optimal donor selection: beyond HLA. *Biology of Blood and Marrow Transplantation, 13*, 83-86.

Couriel, D., Carpenter, P.A., Cutler, C., et al. (2006). Ancillary therapy and supportive care of chronic graft-versus-host disease: National Institutes of Health consensus development project on criteria for clinical trials in chronic graft-versus-host disease, V: Ancillary Therapy and Supportive Care Working Group Report. *Biology of Blood and Marrow Transplantation, 12*, 375-396.

Cronin, D. C., II, Faust, T. W., Brady, L., et al. (2000). Modern immunosuppression. *Clinics in Liver Disease, 4*, 619-655, ix.

Deeg, H.J. (2007). How I treat refractory acute graft versus host disease. *Blood, 109*, 4119-4126.

Deeg, H. J. (1998a). Delayed complications. In R. K. Burt, H. J. Deeg, S. Lothian, et al. (Eds.), *Bone marrow transplantation* (pp. 515-522). Austin, TX: Landes Bioscience.

Deeg, H. J. (1998b). Graft failure. In R. K. Burt, H. J. Deeg, S. Lothian, et al. (Eds.), *Bone marrow transplantation* (pp. 309-316). Austin: Landes Bioscience.

Deeg, H. J., & Socie, G. (1998). Malignancies after hematopoietic stem cell transplantation: many questions, some answers. *Blood, 91*, 1833-1844.

Dickinson, A.M. (2007). Risk assessment in haematopoietic stem cell transplantation: pre-transplant patient and donor factors: non-HLA genetics. *Best Practice and Research Clinical Haematology, 20*(2):189-207.

Doyle, C., Kushi, L. H., Byers, T., et al. (2006). Nutrition and physical activity during and after cancer treatment: an American Cancer Society guide for informed choices. *CA: A Cancer Journal for Clinicians, 56*, 323-353.

Duell, T., van Lint, M. T., Ljungman, P., et al. (1997). Health and functional status of long-term survivors of bone marrow transplantation, EBMT Working Party on Late Effects and EULEP Study Group on Late Effects, European Group for Blood and Marrow Transplantation. *Annals of Internal Medicine, 126*, 184-192.

Filipovich, A. H., Weisdorf, D., Pavletic, S., et al. (2005). National Institutes of Health consensus development project on criteria for clinical trials in chronic graft-versus-host disease, I: diagnosis and staging working group report. *Biology of Blood and Marrow Transplantation, 11*, 945-956.

Flowers, M. E., Lee, S., & Vogelsang, G. (2003). An update on how to treat chronic GVHD. *Blood, 102*, 2312.

Gasova, Z., Spisek, R., Dolezalova, L., (2007). Extracorporeal photochemotherapy (ECP) in treatment of patients with c-GVHD and CTCL. *Transfusion and Apheresis Science, 36*, 149-158.

Gaziev, D., Galimberti, M., Lucarelli, G., (2000). Chronic graft-versus-host disease: is there an alternative to the conventional treatment? *Bone Marrow Transplantation, 25*, 689-696.

Gillis, T.A., & Donovan, E. S. (2001). Rehabilitation following bone marrow transplantation. *Cancer, 92*(4 Suppl), 998-1007.

Giralt, S. (2005). Reduced-intensity conditioning regimens for hematologic malignancies: what have we learned over the last 10 years? *Hematology The Education Program of the American Society of Hematology*, 384-389.

Goker, H., Haznedaroglu, I., & Chao, N. (2001). Acute graft-versus-host disease: pathobiology and management. *Experimental Hematology, 29*, 259-277.

Gold, P., Flowers, M., & Sullivan, K. (1998). Outpatient management of marrow and blood stem cell transplant patients. In R. K. Burt, H. J. Deeg, S. Lothian (Eds.), *Bone marrow transplantation.* (pp. 524-531). Austin, TX: Landes Bioscience.

Goldman, D. A. (2001). Thalidomide use: past history and current implications for practice. *Oncology Nursing Forum, 28*, 471-477; quiz 478-479.

Guise, T. A. (2006). Bone loss and fracture risk associated with cancer therapy. *The Oncologist, 11*, 1121-1131.

Gupta-Burt, S., & Okunieff, P. (1998). Total body irradiation. In R. K. Burt, H. J. Deeg, S. Lothian, et al. (Eds.), *Bone marrow transplantation.* Austin: Landes Bioscience.

Harder, H., Cornelissen, J. J., Van Gool, A. R., (2002). Cognitive functioning and quality of life in long-term adult survivors of bone marrow transplantation. *Cancer, 95*, 183-192.

Higman, M.A., & Vogelsang, G. B. (2004). Chronic graft versus host disease. *British Journal of Haematology, 125*, 435-454.

Hill, G. R., & Ferrara, J. L. (2000). The primacy of the gastrointestinal tract as a target organ of acute graft-versus-host disease: rationale for the use of cytokine shields in allogeneic bone marrow transplantation. *Blood, 95*, 2754-2759.

Ho, V.T., Linden, E., Revta, C., (2007). Hepatic veno-occlusive disease after hematopoietic stem cell transplantation: Review and update on the use of defibrotide. *Seminars in Thrombosis and Hemostasis, 33*(4):373-388.

Ho, V., Momtaz, P., Didas, C., (2004). Post-transplant hepatic veno-occlusive disease: Pathogenesis, diagnosis and treatment. *Reviews in Clinical and Experimental Hematology, 8*(1):E3.

Holler, E. (2007). Risk assessment in haematopoietic stem cell transplantation: GvHD prevention and treatment. *Best Practice & Research. Clinical Haematology, 20*, 281-294.

Iestra, J. A., Fibbe, W. E., Zwinderman, A. H. (2002). Body weight recovery, eating difficulties and compliance with dietary advice in the first year after stem cell transplantation: a prospective study. *Bone Marrow Transplantation, 29*, 417-424.

Imran, H., Tleyjeh, I.M., Zirakzadeh, A., et al. (2006). Use of prophylactic anticoagulation and the risk of hepatic veno-occlusive disease in patients undergoing hematopoietic stem cell transplantation: a systematic review and meta-analysis. *Bone Marrow Transplantation, 37*(7):677-686.

Jacobsohn, D.A. & Vogelsang, G.B. (2007). Acute graft versus host disease. *Orphanet Journal of Rare Diseases*, 2, 35-39.

Jacobsohn, D.A. & Vogelsang, G.B.(2004). Anti-cytokine therapy for the treatment of graft-versus-host disease. *Current Pharmaceutical Design*, 10(11):1195-1205.

Jacobsohn DA, Montross S, Anders V, et al. (2001). Clinical importance of confirming or excluding the diagnosis of chronic graft-versus-host disease. *Biology of Blood and Marrow Transplantation*,28(11):1047-1051.

Jurado, M., Vallejo, C., Perez-Simon, J.A., et al. (2007). Sirolimus as part of immunosuppressive therapy for refractory chronic graft-versus-host disease. *Biology of Blood and Marrow Transplantation*, 13(6):701-706.

Kinch, A., Oberg, G., Arvidson, J., et al. (2007). Post-transplant lymphoproliferative disease and other Epstein-Barr virus diseases in allogeneic haematopoietic stem cell transplantation after introduction of monitoring of viral load by polymerase chain reaction. *Scandinavian Journal of Infectious Diseases, 39*, 235-244.

Koreth, J., Cutler, C. S., Djulbegovic, B., et al. (2007). High-dose therapy with single autologous transplantation versus chemotherapy for newly diagnosed multiple myeloma: a systematic review and meta-analysis of randomized controlled trials. *Biology of Blood and Marrow Transplantation, 13*, 183-196.

Kornblau, S. M., Stiouf, I., Snell, V., et al. (2001). Preemptive control of graft-versus-host disease in a murine allogeneic transplant model using retrovirally transduced murine suicidal lymphocytes. *Cancer Research, 61*, 3355-3360.

Lanuza, D. M., & McCabe, M.A. (2001). Care before and after lung transplant and quality of life research. *AACN Clinical Issues, 12*, 186-201.

Lazarus, H. M., Vogelsang, G. B., & Rowe, J. M. (1997). Prevention and treatment of acute graft-versus-host disease: the old and the new: a report from the Eastern Cooperative Oncology Group (ECOG). *Bone Marrow Transplantation, 19*, 577-600.

Leather, H. L. (2004). Drug interactions in the hematopoietic stem cell transplant (HSCT) recipient: what every transplanter needs to know. *Bone Marrow Transplantation, 33*, 137-152.

Lee, S. J., Schover, L. R., Partridge, A. H., et al. (2006). American Society of Clinical Oncology recommendations on fertility preservation in cancer patients. *Journal of Clinical Oncology, 24*, 2917-2931.

Lee, S.J., Vogelsang, G., & Flowers, M.E. (2003). Chronic graft-versus-host disease. *Biology of Blood and Marrow Transplantation*, 9(4):215-33.

Lipkin, A. C., Lenssen, P., & Dickson, B. J. (2005). Nutrition issues in hematopoietic stem cell transplantation: state of the art. *Nutrition in Clinical Practice, 20*, 423-439.

Ljungman, P., Engelhard, D., de la Camara, R., et al. (2005). Vaccination of stem cell transplant recipients: recommendations of the Infectious Diseases Working Party of the EBMT. *Bone Marrow Transplantation, 35*, 737-746.

McAdams, F. W., & Burgunder, M. R. (2004). Transplant course. In S. Ezzone (Ed.), *Hematopoietic stem cell transplantation: a manual for nursing practice* (pp. 43-58). Pittsburgh: Oncology Nursing Society.

Mitchell, S.A. (2004). Graft versus host disease. In S.A. Ezzone (Ed.), *Peripheral blood stem cell transplant: guidelines for oncology nursing practice*. Pittsburg: Oncology Nursing Society Press.

Moya, R., Espigado, I., Parody, R., et al. (2006). Evaluation of readmissions in hematopoietic stem cell transplant recipients. *Transplantation Proceedings, 38*, 2591-2592.

Nademanee, A., & Forman, S. J. (2006). Role of hematopoietic stem cell transplantation for advanced-stage diffuse large cell B-cell lymphoma-B. *Seminars in Hematology, 43*, 240-250.

Nuver, J., Smit, A. J., Postma, A., et al. (2002). The metabolic syndrome in long-term cancer survivors, an important target for secondary preventive measures. *Cancer Treatment Reviews, 28*, 195-214.

Patterson, A. E., & Korngold, R. (2001). Infusion of select leukemia-reactive TCR Vbeta+ T cells provides graft-versus-leukemia responses with minimization of graft-versus-host disease following murine hematopoietic stem cell transplantation. *Biology of Blood and Marrow Transplantation, 7*, 187-196.

Petros, W. P., & Gilbert, C. J. (1998). High-dose alkylating agent pharmacology/toxicity. In R. K. Burt, H. J. Deeg, S. Lothian, et al. (Eds.), *Bone marrow transplantation* (pp. 123-130). Austin: Landes Bioscience.

Przepiorka, D. (2000). Prevention of acute graft-versus-host disease. In E. D. Ball, J. Lister & P. Law (Eds.), *Hematopoietic stem cell therapy* (pp. 452-469). New York: Churchill Livingstone.

Przepiorka, D., Devine, S., Fay, J., et al. (1999). Practical considerations in the use of tacrolimus for allogeneic marrow transplantation. *Bone Marrow Transplantation, 24*, 1053-1056.

Przepiorka, D., Anderlini, P., Saliba, R., et al. (2001). Chronic graft-versus-host disease after allogeneic blood stem cell transplantation. *Blood, 98*(6):1695-16700.

Ratanatharathorn, V., Ayash, L., Reynolds, C., et al. (2003). Treatment of chronic graft-versus-host disease with anti-CD20 chimeric monoclonal antibody. *Biology of Blood and Marrow Transplantation, 9*, 505-511.

Reddy, P., Teshima, T., Hildebrandt, G., et al. (2003). Pretreatment of donors with interleukin-18 attenuates acute graft-versus-host disease via STAT6 and preserves graft-versus-leukemia effects. *Blood, 101*, 2877-2885.

Rees, D., Beale, P., & Judson, I. (1998). Theoretical aspects of dose intensity and dose scheduling. In A. J. Barrett & J. Treleaven (Eds.), *The clinical practice of stem cell transplantation* (pp. 17-29). Oxford: Iris Medical Media.

Rizzo, J. D., Wingard, J. R., Tichelli, A., et al. (2006). Recommended screening and preventive practices for long-term survivors after hematopoietic cell transplantation: joint recommendations of the European Group for Blood and Marrow Transplantation, the Center for International Blood and Marrow Transplant Research, and the American Society of Blood and Marrow Transplantation. *Biology of Blood and Marrow Transplantation, 12*, 138-151.

Ruccione, K. S. (1994). Issues in survivorship. In C. L. Schwartz, W. Hobbie, L. S. Constine (Eds.), *Survivors of childhood cancer: assessment and management*. St. Louis: Mosby.

Sanders, J. (1994). Late effects after bone marrow transplantation. In C. L. Schwartz, W. Hobbie, L. S. Constine, et al. (Eds.), *Survivors of childhood cancer: assessment and management* (pp. 293-318). St. Louis: Mosby.

Sanders, J. E. (2002). Chronic graft-versus-host disease and late effects after hematopoietic stem cell transplantation. *International Journal of Hematology, 76 Suppl 2*, 15-28.

Saria, M. G., & Gosselin-Acomb, T. K. (2007). Hematopoietic stem cell transplantation: implications for critical care nurses. *Clinical Journal of Oncology Nursing, 11*, 53-63.

Schwartz, C. L., Hobbie, W., & Constine, L. S. (1994). Algorithms of late effects by disease. In C. L. Schwartz, W. Hobbie, L. S. Constine, et al. (Eds.). *Survivors of childhood cancer: assessment and management*. (pp. 7-19). St. Louis: Mosby.

Seber, A., & Vodelsang, G. (1998). Chronic graft-versus-host disease. In J. Barrett & J. Treleaven (Eds.). *The clinical practice of stem cell transplantation.* (pp. 620-634). Oxford: ISIS Medical Media.

Seeley, K., & DeMeyer, E. (2002). Nursing care of patients receiving Campath. *Clinical Journal of Oncology Nursing, 6,* 138-143.

Shah, A. J., Kapoor, N., Crooks, G. M., et al. (2007). The effects of Campath 1H upon graft-versus-host disease, infection, relapse, and immune reconstitution in recipients of pediatric unrelated transplants. *Biology of Blood and Marrow Transplantation, 13,* 584-593.

Shore, T., Harpel, J., Schuster, M. W., et al. (2006). A study of a reduced-intensity conditioning regimen followed by allogeneic stem cell transplantation for patients with hematologic malignancies using Campath-1H as part of a graft-versus-host disease strategy. *Biology of Blood and Marrow Transplantation, 12,* 868-875.

Simpson, D. (2001). New developments in the prophylaxis and treatment of graft versus host disease. *Expert Opinion in Pharmacotherapy, 2,* 1109-1117.

Simpson, D. (2003). T-cell depleting antibodies: new hope for induction of allograft tolerance in bone marrow transplantation? *BioDrugs, 17,* 147-154.

Singhal, S., & Mehta, J. (1999). Reimmunization after blood or marrow stem cell transplantation. *Bone Marrow Transplantation, 23,* 637-646.

Socie, G. & Cahn, J.Y. (1998). Acute graft-versus-host disease. In J. Barrett & J. Treleaven (Eds). *The clinical practice of stem cell transplantation* (p. 596-618). Oxford: Isis Medical Media.

Soiffer, R. J., Weller, E., Alyea, E. P., et al. (2001). CD6+ donor marrow T-cell depletion as the sole form of graft-versus-host disease prophylaxis in patients undergoing allogeneic bone marrow transplant from unrelated donors. *Journal of Clinical Oncology, 19,* 1152-1159.

Solimando, D. (1998). Medications. In R. K. Burt, H. J. Deeg, S. Lothian, et al. (Eds). *Bone marrow transplantation* (pp. 544-566). Austin: Landes Bioscience.

Sullivan, K.M. (1999). Graft-versus-host disease (p. 515-536). In E.D. Thomas, K.G. Blume & S.J. Forman (Eds). *Hematopoietic stem cell transplantation.* Oxford: Blackwell Science.

Sullivan KM, Agura E, Anasetti C, et al. (1991). Chronic graft-versus-host disease and other late complications of bone marrow transplantation. *Seminars in Hematology, 28*(3): 250-259.

Srinivas, T. R., Meier-Kriesche, H. U., & Kaplan, B. (2005). Pharmacokinetic principles of immunosuppressive drugs. *American Journal of Transplantation, 5,* 207-217.

Tabbara, I. A., Zimmerman, K., Morgan, C., et al. (2002). Allogeneic hematopoietic stem cell transplantation: complications and results. *Archives of Internal Medicine, 162,* 1558-1566.

Tay. J., Tinmouth, A., Fergusson, et al. (2007). Systematic review of controlled clinical trials on the use of ursodeoxycholic acid for the prevention of hepatic veno-occlusive disease in hematopoietic stem cell. *Biology of Blood and Marrow Transplantation,* 13(2):206-217.

Wadleigh, M., Ho, V., Momtaz, et al. (2003). Hepatic veno-occlusive disease: pathogenesis, diagnosis and treatment. *Current Opinion in Hematology,* 10 (6), 451-462.

Wingard, J. R., Vogelsang, G. B., & Deeg, H. J. (2002). Stem cell transplantation: supportive care and long-term complications. *Hematology (American Society of Hematology Education Program Book).* 2002; 422-444.

Wolff, D., Anders, V., Corio, et al. (2004). Oral PUVA and topical steroids for treatment of oral manifestations of chronic graft-vs.-host disease. *Photodermatology, Photoimmunology & Photomedicine, 20,* 184-190.

Woltz, P., Castro, K., & Park, B. J. (2006). Care for patients undergoing extracorporeal photopheresis to treat chronic graft-versus-host disease: review of the evidence. *Clinical Journal of Oncology Nursing, 10,* 795-802.

Yakoub-Agha, I., Mesnil, F., Kuentz, M., et al. (2006). Allogeneic marrow stem-cell transplantation from human leukocyte antigen-identical siblings versus human leukocyte antigen-allelic-matched unrelated donors (10/10) in patients with standard-risk hematologic malignancy: a prospective study from the French Society of Bone Marrow Transplantation and Cell Therapy. *Journal of Clinical Oncology, 24,* 5695-5702.

Biological Response Modifiers

Jason M. Rothaermel and Barbara Baum

HISTORICAL OVERVIEW OF BIOLOGICAL RESPONSE AND IMMUNOLOGY

Biological response modification, immunotherapy, immune system modulation, and many more terms have been used to represent the same therapeutic approach as it has developed, evolved, and begun to mature over the last several decades. For purposes of continuity, biological response modifiers will be the terminology used to represent the entire class of therapeutics and their underlying mechanism of action.

From a historical viewpoint, the study and understanding of immunology and the subsequent response of human biology succeeding a noxious event to prevent future insult have been understood for far longer than the knowledge of germ theory and of mutation and carcinogenesis (Bellanti, 1985). Dating as far back as the eleventh century, it was understood that after exposure to a virus such as smallpox, resistance to further infection would develop. The earliest active use of immunization was performed by Lady Mary Wortley Montague, who in 1721 inoculated her daughter against smallpox. (DeVita, Hellman, & Rosenberg, 1991). Early attempts at vaccination against toxins often resulted in infection and death leading to a lack of widespread belief in the technique. Later, work near the turn of the nineteenth century by Edward Jenner pioneered further work and the advancement of smallpox vaccination. Additional work done by Louis Pasteur led to a better understanding of the role and function of vaccine therapy, immunity, and the "germ theory" (Bellanti, 1985). Pasteur's work eventually led to further work in the immunology field and a better understanding of disease biology and the responses to disease that occur after an invading foreign antigen has entered the system (Bellanti, 1985).

By the early 1900s, two schools of thought emerged with regard to the immune response to foreign toxins:

1. Humoral immunity: chemical products (antibodies) produced and released by cells that destroy the specific invading toxin (antigen)
2. Cellular immunity: immunoglobins, or effector cells, detect and destroy foreign toxins (Bellanti, 1985)

Today, both schools of thought have been proven to be correct and are areas of intense research and discovery.

As a better understanding of immunology grew, theories and hypotheses as to the potential role for activation of the immune system may be beneficial in antitumor therapies. Some of the earliest of these hypotheses dates back to Paul Ehrlich and his postulations that tumors may express different cell structures and thus be recognizable to antibodies and cause increased humoral immune response (DeVita, Hellman, & Rosenberg, 1991). Unfortunately, early work in the field of tumor immunity was thwarted by the realization that antitumor activity demonstrated in mice was the result of an allogeneic rejection response to foreign "non-self" tissue as opposed to a direct antitumor immunity. This problem was later overcome by the development of various rodent models that allowed for implantation and culturing of tumor grafts without allogeneic rejection (DeVita, Hellman, & Rosenberg, 1991). These mouse and rat models are used as a staple in antitumor drug development and therapy research and as a first step in the preclinical approach of understanding a molecule's potential for further study.

By the end of the 1960s, the rodent models had shown that there were direct antitumor responses being seen in the study of these models. As such, the first human studies were undertaken to determine whether these results could be verified and replicated. The cornerstone for further investigation into biological response modification came from studies reported in 1966 by Klein and colleagues, who demonstrated that circulating antibodies associated with antigens were located on the cell surface of Burkitt's lymphoma cells (DeVita, Hellman, & Rosenberg, 1991). These results demonstrated the existence of specific tumor type–specific antigens that can potentially be targeted by the immune system for the treatment of various cancer types.

Until the 1970s the study of antibodies excreted by T lymphocytes to cause a direct tumor-specific antigen/antibody reaction for the treatment of cancer monopolized the majority of the focus and study of biological response modification. However, during this time, further understanding of the ability of certain lymphocytes to secrete other small proteins that had a direct impact on biological response and immune modulation began to be better understood (DeVita, Hellman, & Rosenberg, 2001a). This new class of proteins was termed cytokines. Cytokines are soluble glycoproteins that are typically secreted by lymphocytes and monocytes and are true hormones acting on cells in a paracrine or autocrine fashion to activate or deactivate downstream cellular function, activity, or division, among many other roles (DeVita, Hellman, & Rosenberg, 2001a).

The remainder of this section focuses on the different classes of biological response modifiers including background and development, approved indications when appropriate, administration strategies that have been studied for approval or to date, dosing schemas, side effects and other pertinent information as appropriate.

COLONY-STIMULATING FACTORS

Colony-stimulating factors comprise a family of glycoproteins that help to regulate differentiation, proliferation, and activation of cells of the hematopoietic cell lineages. Various cytokines act on different cells of the cascade at different times during the differentiation and proliferation phases of their individual cell lives. These interactions can be paracrine or autocrine in nature and can have activity that is either direct or indirect through the activation and production of downstream ligands and cytokines.

The first of the colony-stimulating factors to be discovered was erythropoietin in 1906 by Carnot and Deflandre (Metcalf & Nicola, 1995). Further purification of erythropoietin was not accomplished until 1976 by Miyake et al. Since the early 1960s, continued advancement in the bioassay field has lead to the discovery and description of some 20 additional cytokines with activity on hematopoietic cells. Initially, tissue cultured hematopoietic cells were used as bioassay platforms from which the cytokines detected would later be tested on animal models to determine target activity and utility. Today, complementary deoxyribonucleic acid (cDNA) screening is used for the detection and development of cytokines, which allows for characterization of the active molecules and determination of the receptor sites on normal cells (Metcalf & Nicola, 1995).

The term colony-stimulating factor was coined subsequent to work done in 1966 by Bradley and Metcalf and Ichikawa et al studying macrophage and granulocyte cells cultured from bone marrow. In these trials, spontaneous growth was not observed. However, when additional tissues were added to the cultures, proliferation was demonstrated, leading to the hypothesis that there were factors stimulating an increase in proliferation of the granulocytes and macrophages similar to the effect of erythropoietin on erythrocytes demonstrated years earlier (Metcalf & Nicola, 1995).

There are, at present, four colony-stimulating factors approved for use in the treatment of cancer by the U.S. Food and Drug Administration. These are (DeVita, Hellman, & Rosenberg, 2001b) as follows:

- Granulocyte colony-stimulating factor (G-CSF)
- Granulocyte-macrophage colony-stimulating factor (GM-CSF)
- Erythropoietin (EPO)
- Cytokine interleukin (IL)-11

The main purpose for use of these colony-stimulating factors is hematopoietic recovery from direct cytotoxic and radiotherapeutic insults and prevention and recovery from therapy-induced anemia, neutropenia, and thrombocytopenia. However, several additional antitumor activities associated with colony-stimulating factors have been identified and are currently being actively investigated. Uses being investigated include the antiangiogenic effects of GM-CSF alone and in combination with thalidomide or other antiangiogenesis class agents, the effect of colony-stimulating factors on the up-regulation of complement-dependent cytotoxicity, antibody-dependent cellular cytotoxicity, and the secondary release of other cytokines with antitumor properties as a response to increased circulating levels of colony-stimulating factors. Colony-stimulating factors also play an important role in the development and culturing of tumor-specific vaccine therapies and the effectiveness and utility of monoclonal antibodies.

Erythropoietins

EPO makes up a class of colony-type stimulating factor that, unlike other factors such as Flt 3 ligand and Steel factor that act directly on the pluripotent stem cell, acts in the later stages of hematopoietic development, targeting specifically the myeloid progenitor cells and erythrocytes. Erythropoietin is also unique from other colony-stimulating factors and cytokines in that it is almost exclusively secreted outside the bone marrow microenvironment by the liver and kidneys. The cDNA of the human gene for erythropoietin, 7q11-22, was cloned successfully in 1984, followed by cloning of the receptor gene on erythroid colony-forming cells in 1989.

Erythropoietin production and secretion is inversely affected by the oxygen-carrying capacity of the circulating red blood cells (DeVita, Hellman, & Rosenberg, 2001b). This negative feedback loop decreases secretion of EPO in times of high levels of oxygen-binding capacity and increases EPO secretion in times of lower oxygen-binding capacity, allowing for balance in the amount of circulating red blood cells to match the need of the body's oxygen demand without overproduction of red blood cells. In some instances overproduction of erythropoietin resulting in erythrocytosis is observed in patients noted to have primary renal tumors causing local renal hypoxic conditions or tumors that oversecrete erythropoietin intrinsically (DeVita, Hellman, & Rosenberg, 2001b).

EPO is a useful and commonly used therapeutic agent in the treatment of chemotherapy-associated anemia. Normal human serum concentrations of EPO range from 4 to 30 units/L. Recombinant EPOs have a half life of 9 to 13 hours in regard to epoetin alfa and 27 to 89 hours in regard to darbepoetin alfa (Wilkes& Barton-Burke, 2005). In healthy human subjects, EPO levels demonstrably begin to rise when hematocrit levels fall below 35%; however, in patients with chronic anemia from malignancies, serum EPO levels may remain low (DeVita, Hellman, & Rosenberg, 2001b). As a result, the administration of recombinant EPO in this instance can have a positive effect on raising the percentage of circulating erythrocytes and a subsequent impact on oxygen saturation and a qualitative impact on fatigue levels experienced by patients.

The U.S. Food and Drug Administration in 1999 approved recombinant EPO for the treatment of anemia in cancer patients after several studies using multiple dosing schemes demonstrated statistically significant decreases in necessary red blood cell transfusions among patients who received epoetin alfa (14%) versus those who received placebo (28%) between day 29 and week 16 of therapy. The effects of EPO therapy are typically not seen until between 2 and 6 weeks of therapy and measured by an increase in the hemoglobin level. Continued monitoring of serum hemoglobin levels is necessary to prevent unintended erythrocytosis (Amgen, 2004 Procrit).

Granulocyte Colony-Stimulating Factor

G-CSF is a colony-stimulating factor that regulates cell proliferation, maturation, and function in the neutrophil cell lineage of the myeloid cell line. After the human gene for G-CSF located on chromosome 17q11-21 was identified through purification of bladder and head and neck cancer cells, the gene was cloned and recombinant technology used to produce usable amounts of drug. Although G-CSF may have downstream effects on other cell lineages and the potential function of those cells under certain circumstances, its primary function is the proliferation and maturation of the neutrophil cell lineage. This becomes apparent in the setting of mice with a knockout gene for G-CSF, where the mice become severely neutropenic. Hammond et al also demonstrated the selectivity of G-CSF for neutrophils in animal models, as reflected by severe neutropenic states caused by the induction of neutralizing antiantibodies for G-CSF in those models (DeVita, Hellman, & Rosenberg, 1991; DeVita, Hellman, & Rosenberg, 2001b).

G-CSF can be secreted by a variety of cells in the body including the following (DeVita, Hellman, & Rosenberg 2001b):

- Marrow stromal cells
- Epithelial cells
- Macrophages
- Endothelial cells
- Other immune cells such as natural killer cells

G-CSF can be readily detected in circulating serum at levels of 20 to 100 mg/dL. Circulating G-CSF levels and secretion are directly affected by inflammatory response to toxins and tissue damage and are inversely affected by the total number of circulating neutrophils. In severely neutropenic subjects, detectable levels of serum G-CSF can be in excess of 2,000 mg/dL (DeVita, Hellman, & Rosenberg, 2001b).

Given the potent ability for G-CSF to up-regulate the function and proliferation of neutrophils, it is easy to see why it has made its place in the treatment of neutropenia secondary to oncologic therapies. With the production and subsequent approval of this class of drugs, patients receiving marrow-toxic chemotherapeutic regimens have a greater chance for earlier neutrophil recovery and subsequent decrease in overall risk of opportunistic, potentially life-threatening infections.

There are two main G-CSFs in use in the United States today:

- Filgrastim (Neupogen)
- Pegfilgrastim (Neulasta)

Use of these agents has reduced incidence of febrile neutropenia with a subsequent decrease in length of hospital stays.

Filgrastim is the parent molecule of this class of cytokine. Randomized clinical trials demonstrate that the use of filgrastim results in the following (Amgen, Neupogen 2004):

- A reduction in occurrence of febrile neutropenia
- A significant decrease in hospital length of stay for infection

- A decrease in overall use of antibiotics
- A reduction in the absolute neutrophil count recovery time for patients with acute myeloid leukemia (AML) undergoing induction or consolidation therapy
- A reduction in the median number of days with severe neutropenia in patients receiving myeloablative chemotherapy for bone marrow transplant
- Significant elevation of colony-forming units of granulocytes and macrophages and CD34$^+$ cells in the setting of stem cell collection and mobilization. An increase in these cells is a predictor of engraftment and time to platelet recovery after transplantation.

The pegylated formulation of filgrastim, pegfilgrastim, is a covalent conjugate of filgrastim in which a glycol molecule has been bound to filgrastim and as such results in reduced renal clearance and a resultant prolonged persistence in vivo. This molecular change results in an increase in average half-life to 15 to 80 hours with pegfilgrastim, allowing for single-dose administration after each course of chemotherapy associated with a significant risk of febrile neutropenia. (Amgen, Pegfilgrastim 2005).

Pegfilgrastim has been demonstrated through three phase III clinical trials to produce equivalent reductions in days of severe neutropenia compared with filgrastim in patients receiving chemotherapy associated with a high risk of neutropenia (Amgen, Pegfilgrastim 2005). Because of its prolonged half-life, pegfilgrastim should not be used within the 14 days leading up to the administration of chemotherapy.

Granulocyte-Macrophage Colony-Stimulating Factor

First cloned by Wong and colleagues in 1985, GM-CSF, located on chromosome 5q31, is another potent cytokine that has a direct impact on hematopoiesis as well as many other implications for the care of patients with cancer (DeVita, Hellman, & Rosenberg, 2001b). GM-CSF is excreted by a number of cell lines including the following:

- Marrow stromal cells
- Fibroblasts
- Endothelial cells
- T lymphocytes (2pp426)

The most prolific production of GM-CSF naturally occurring in the human body is that secreted by activated T lymphocytes (DeVita, Hellman, & Rosenberg, 2001b).

GM-CSF affects a diverse population of cell lineages in the hematopoietic cascade, including all myeloid cell lines, and affects myeloid dendritic cell activation proliferation and differentiation. As a result, GM-CSF increased circulating numbers of neutrophils, eosinophils, and macrophages (DeVita, Hellman, & Rosenberg, 2001b).

Pharmacokinetic studies of GM-CSF have shown a significant increase in sustained circulating levels of GM-CSF in the serum when administered by subcutaneous injection versus intravenous administration. As such, subcutaneous administration is the preferred route (DeVita, Hellman, & Rosenberg, 2001b).

GM-CSF has been and continues to be aggressively studied in the care of malignancies. It has been approved clinically for use after induction chemotherapy in AML, mobilization and after autologous peripheral blood progenitor cells, myeloid reconstitution after autologous bone marrow transplantation (BMT), myeloid reconstitution after allogeneic BMT, and in the setting of bone marrow transplant failure and engraftment delay (Berlex, 2004).

Additional clinical trials and studies to better define the future role of GM-CSF in the treatment of malignancies and treatment-related side effects are in progress. The hypotheses being clinically tested include, but are not limited to, the treatment of chemotherapy- and radiation-induced mucositis, dendritic cell activation, and tumor vaccines.

The rationale for use of GM-CSF in the treatment of mucositis comes in part by the ability of GM-CSF to activate keratinocytes and healthy well-functioning neutrophils in the epithelial lining of the gastric mucosa, including the oral pharynx. This increase in cell activation promotes healthy cell turnover and population-decreasing mucosal toxicity. A study conducted by McAleese and colleagues with a population of 29 participants demonstrated a significant reduction in radiation-related mucositis in patients being treated for laryngeal cancer with radiation therapy along with molgrastim (McAleese et al., 2006). Several other trials looking at the potential utility and benefit of cytokines and colony-stimulating factors, including GM-CSF, have been performed, demonstrating varying results (Bülttzingslöwen et al., 2006). This area needs further investigation and continues to be evaluated for optimal drug, dose, administration, and timing.

GM-CSF is a main component in the study of gene- and vaccine-based therapy for the treatment of malignancies. GM-CSF has been shown to enhance antibody response in favor of TH1, which is associated with myeloid dendritic cells and antitumor effect (Oppenheim & Fujiwara, 1996). Several clinical trials are in process to better determine the efficacy and utility of dendritic cell–based vaccine therapies. In the majority of these trials, GM-CSF is used to activate, culture, and mature naive dendritic cells for use as potent effector cells preloaded with specific tumor antibodies to elicit T-lymphocyte activation and downstream biological responses against those tumors positive for the antigen (Oppenheim & Fujiwara, 1996; Wang et al., 2006).

Interleukin-11 (Oprelvekin, Neumega)

IL-11 is a cytokine/growth factor produced by several mesenchymal cell families that has a direct effect on hematopoiesis. Cells that produce IL-11 naturally include keratinocytes, osteoblasts, fibroblasts, and bone marrow stromal cells. (DeVita, Hellman, & Rosenberg, 2001b). The predominant function of IL-11 is its direct impact on megakaryocopoiesis and thrombopoiesis and the

proliferation, maturation, and function of those cell lines. (DeVita, Hellman, & Rosenberg, 2001b; Wyeth Pharmaceuticals, 2006). As a result, there is a direct impact on thrombocytopenia as a result of the chemotherapeutic insult. IL-11 is clinically approved for the prevention of severe thrombocytopenia after myelosuppressive chemotherapy in patients with nonmyeloid malignancies and patients receiving nonmyeloablative chemotherapy regimens (Brown et al., 2001). IL-11 is expressed on gene 19q13-4-13.4 of the human genome and was first cloned by Yang and colleagues at the Genetics Institute at Case Western Reserve in the early 1990s.

In clinical studies, IL-11 has been shown to improve platelet nadir and decrease the time to platelet recovery in patients receiving chemotherapeutic regimens. Use of oprelvekin results in a decreased need for platelet transfusions (Wyeth Pharmaceuticals, 2006).

The use of IL-11 is strictly contraindicated in patients receiving myeloablative chemotherapy because of a significantly elevated occurrence of edema, conjuctival bleeding, hypotension, and tachycardia seen in this patient population. Administration of IL-11 is also associated with significant risk of allergic reaction, including anaphylaxis, and should be discontinued immediately at the first sign of a drug-related allergic response (Wyeth Pharmaceuticals, 2006).

IL-11 therapy should begin within 6 to 24 hours after chemotherapy completion. However, safety and efficacy of IL-11 has not been determined in patients undergoing chemotherapy administration associated with prolonged or delayed myelosuppression, as is the case with mitomycin-c and nitrosourea. (Wyeth Pharmaceuticals, 2006).

Keratinocyte Growth Factor (Palifermin, Kepivance)

Keratinocyte growth factor (KGF), also known as fibroblast growth factor-7, is a growth factor originating from mesenchymal cells, fibroblasts, and microvascular endothelial cells. It acts in a paracrine fashion activating epithelial cell repair and protection as a response to inflammatory cytokines and steroidal hormones (Finch & Rubin, 2006; MacDonald & Hill, 2002). In the study of KGF in myeloid malignancies, early evidence has suggested that its addition to chemotherapy can prevent gastrointestinal graft-versus-host disease by acting as a kind of cytokine protectant and reducing the generation of proinflammatory cytokines (MacDonald & Hill, 2002). In addition, KGF has been shown to help promote T-cell engraftment and reconstitution, leading to a belief that KGF may play an important role in the prevention of epithelial toxicity in the treatment of myeloid malignancies (MacDonald & Hill, 2002).

Keeping the direct effect on epithelial tissues in mind, studies have begun to look at the protective properties of KGF in the setting of chemotherapy- and radiation-induced mucositis. In patients with hematological malignancies, trials have demonstrated a direct correlation between KGF administration and a reduction in the severity and duration of oral mucositis as a result of intense chemotherapy regimens. (Finch & Rubin, 2006). In vitro and in vivo studies have shown KGF to be an important cytoprotectant through its ability to positively affect epithelial cell differentiation, proliferation, and migration as well as having beneficial effects on epithelial cell survival, repair, and detoxification after exposure to cytotoxins (Finch & Rubin, 2006). Results of a phase III trial of transplant patients with hematological malignancies receiving high-dose radiation and chemotherapy before transplantation showed a significant reduction in the incidence and duration of severe oral mucositis ($P < 0.001$) in the arm that received drugs. This has led to U.S. Food and Drug Administration approval for use of KGF in this setting.

Trials looking at the potential benefit of KGF in epithelial solid tumors are currently in progress or planned, including RTOG 0435 comparing KGF with placebo in patients with head and neck cancer undergoing chemoradiation therapy for the prevention of mucositis. A concern that has arisen with the study of KGF in epithelial malignancies is that, given the protective nature of this protein in the chemotherapy setting toward epithelial tissues, will the resultant protection cross over to the malignant cells themselves and shield them from the wanted effects of the therapies being used (Finch & Rubin, 2006; MacDonald & Hill, 2002; Oelmann et al., 2004)? Further studies are needed to determine the answer.

GENE THERAPY

The term gene therapy refers to any manipulation of the human genome with the goal or intent of producing a therapeutic effect; this broad term can be used for any manipulation including but not limited to incorporation of cytokine receptors and increasing immunization potential, addition of cytotoxics directly into tumor cell lines, or increased immunological effects of effector cells with the addition of tumor antigen genes (DeVita, Hellman, & Rosenberg, 2001b). Since its inception in the late 1980s, gene therapy has lead to many advances and a greater understanding of the potentials and limitations of manipulation of the genes responsible for tumor growth and survival. Probably the most highly publicized gene associated with malignant mutation in study today is the p53 gene. It has been noted that the absence or mutation of the p53 gene is associated to increased mutation and malignancy in the host cells with the defect.

Two approaches of gene transfer therapy have been studied to date. Limitations in technology to allow for in vivo gene therapy approaches have limited most study to be applied in the ex vivo setting, in which immune cells or tumor cells are removed from a donor and manipulated and cultured for later reintroduction to the host body (DeVita, Hellman, & Rosenberg, 2001b). When gene therapy is planned as a treatment modality, it must first be determined how the transfer will act in the long term. In certain circumstances short-term gene expression is appropriate, in which case adenoviral transfer of gene antigens is most appropriate, whereas in the setting of permanent or long-term gene expression retroviral transfer may most suitable. (DeVita, Hellman, & Rosenberg, 2001b). In addition to retroviral and adenoviral vectors being used for transfer of foreign genes into the host cell, many other transfer approaches are being studied to determine the most effective approach for various situations. Some of these transfer approaches include lentiviral vector transfer, adeno-associated viral vector transfer, pox virus vector transfer, and various nonviral transfer methods that used in large part lipids complexed to manipulated deoxyribonucleic acid strands for gene transfer (DeVita, Hellman, & Rosenberg, 2001b).

Direct modification of the immune response continues to be an area of interest and is under further study. This approach can be accomplished by either manipulation of the cells responsible for immune responses, T-cell gene manipulation, or circumventing the tumor's ability to protect itself from or hide from those cells through tumor cell manipulation. The act of manipulating the tumor cells with expressor genes to make them more recognizable to immune cells for a response can be accomplished by the induction of cytokine genes, noncytokine response genes, costimulatory signal expression genes, and genes that increase the number of T-cell receptor sites on the tumor surface. In addition, increasing the immune system response to tumor cells can be accomplished by the addition of monoclonal antibodies to targeting of T cells and increasing adaptive immune response of T cells through tumor-specific vaccine therapy.

Cytokine gene therapy refers to the act of transecting tumor cells with the genes responsible for active secretion of various immune regulating cytokines with the goal being overexpression of the cytokines in the tumor microenvironment to up-regulate attraction and activation of immune cells. Several cytokines have been studied to accomplish this end. Several trials have been completed with interleukin (IL)-2 in this arena, of which it has been shown that there is an increase in CD8[+] cells in the tumors but not CD4[+] cells, which may demonstrate the lack of need for CD4[+] helper cells with an increase in IL-2. The majority of these trials, however, have failed to demonstrate any clinical benefit in the setting of melanoma, breast, renal, and sarcoma malignancies. IL-2 has also been studied for its role in enhancing the longevity of T cells. T cells transduced with the IL-2 gene can stimulate themselves in an autocrine fashion and in doing so increase their life span and antigen specificity in an IL-2–independent state (DeVita, Hellman, & Rosenberg, 2001a; DeVita, Hellman, & Rosenberg, 2001b).

In a murine model comparative study, mice were immunized with irradiated B16 melanoma cells with a variety of cytokines to determine downstream effects on subsequent challenge with melanoma cell implantation. Of the cytokines tested in this study granulocyte-macrophage colony-stimulating factor (GM-CSF) demonstrated a significant immunization effect against later tumor rechallenge, and IL-4 and 6 demonstrated nominal protection (DeVita, Hellman, & Rosenberg, 2001b).Additional study of GM-CSF–transduced tumors has shown a correlation to increased levels of CD8[+] and CD4[+] cells and an increase in bone marrow production of effector cells. As such, trials have been undertaken in renal cell carcinoma, melanoma, and prostate cancer to determine the efficacy of GM-CSF–transduced tumor vaccines.

Several additional cytokine genes have been transduced directly into tumors and have to date failed to show a significant increase in immune response against various tumor types.

In addition, several approaches are being currently studied in the arena of gene manipulation and gene therapy at this time. Some such approaches include the transduction of the p53 gene into tumor cells to activate tumor suppression activity and transduction of oncogene suppressor genes, which can down-regulate the production or reception of molecules such as BCL-2, BCR-ABL, MYC, and MYB, which cause uncontrolled cell growth in tumors (DeVita, Hellman, & Rosenberg, 2001b). Inhibition of genes such as VEGF and PDGF are also being looked at for transduction into tumor cells for their antiangiogenic potential (DeVita, Hellman, & Rosenberg, 2001b).

Interferons

The term interferon (IFN), so named for its ability to "interfere" with viral replication, was first identified in the late 1950s by Isaacs and Lindemann. It is a naturally occurring glycoprotein making up a family of endogenous polypeptides of which three main types are involved in clinical use and investigational research at this time, interferon alfa, interferon beta, and interferon gamma. IFN is a cytokine secreted mainly by the cells of the immune system, in particular leukocytes, fibroblasts, macrophages, lymphocytes, and in some instances epithelial cells. IFN alfa and beta have both been found to arise from chromosome 9 of the human genome, whereas IFN gamma is located on chromosome 12 (Skalla, 1996). Additionally, IFN alfa and beta share a common receptor on cell surfaces, whereas IFN gamma has been shown to have two unique receptor sites (DeVita, Hellman, & Rosenberg 1991; Skalla, 1996).

Activity of IFN is seen after its binding to specific cell surface receptors. Once this has occurred, IFN produces antiproliferative effects through two main mechanisms: protein synthesis inhibition and direct cell-specific effects including overexpression of major histocompatibility complex (MHC) antigens on the cell surface to help increase auto immune response. (DeVita, Hellman, & Rosenberg, 2001a). In addition, IFN plays an essential role in anticancer therapy through its effect on immune modulation as expressed by the up-regulation of natural killer cells, a key player in antibody-dependent cellular cytotoxicity, macrophages and dendritic cells, and neutrophils and T and B cells (DeVita, Hellman, & Rosenberg, 2001a, 2001b; Roskrow & Gansbacher, 1998). The combined

activity of overexpression of MHC types I and II and up-regulation of circulating immune cells has the potential to increase the overall antitumor response in vivo.

IFN was the first of the cytokines to achieve Food and Drug Administration approval for the treatment of hairy cell leukemia (Skalla, 1996). IFN alfa 2b remains the only approved IFN for the treatment of malignancies in the United States. However, IFN beta has received approval for use in multiple sclerosis and IFN gamma is approved for use in chronic granulomatous disease. Since its approval, various forms and types of IFN have been studied in a number of clinical trials to help better understand their role in the treatment of a variety of malignancies with a large focus being the use and utility of IFN alfa 2a and 2b in the treatment of melanoma along with the use of IFN alfa in renal cell carcinoma.

To date, the highest level of efficacy seen with the use of IFNs has come from work with hematological malignancies. Study continues in the setting of solid tumors and has been extensively researched in melanoma and for its role in renal cell carcinoma. Further study of IFN use in renal cell carcinoma is needed in the advent of new antiangiogenic compounds being used for treatment of this disease. Continued investigational research of IFN is seen in multiple myeloma and other cancers. Researchers are evaluating IFN use as a single agent, in combination with other cytokines and biological response modifiers, and in biochemotherapy regimens (Skalla, 1996).

Interferon Alfa. As with all IFNs, IFN alfa demonstrates effect through direct binding with cell surface receptors through which it imposes antiproliferative activity through the inhibition of certain protein synthesis and by nonspecific immune system regulation of granulocytes and lymphocytes. As mentioned previously, IFN alfa was the first of the class of cytokines to reach Food and Drug Administration approval for its use in the treatment of hairy cell leukemia and remains the only IFN approved for the treatment of any malignant state. Since its original approval, trials in malignant melanoma, follicular lymphoma, and acquired immunodeficiency syndrome (AIDS)-related Kaposi's sarcoma have resulted in further approved indications for use.

First approved in the mid 1980s for the treatment of hairy cell leukemia as an alterative and more efficacious option than previous treatment regimens consisting of chlorambucil and splenectomy, IFN efficacy has since been surpassed by deoxycoformycin and 2-chlorodeoxyadenosine in the role of front-line therapy for this disease. IFN will continue to have a role as maintenance therapy for those patients who respond to other front line therapies as well as in the setting of recurrent disease (Schering Corporation, 2002; Skalla, 1996). IFN has also been approved for use in the treatment of chronic-phase Philadelphia chromosome–positive chronic myelogenous leukemia in patients who have had minimal prior therapy (Roche, 2005; Skalla, 1996). The cost of IFN alfa 2a can be a significant concern and trials are in progress to determine whether decreased or intermittent dosing is comparable and as efficacious as the daily regimens studied for registration.

Clinical trials to determine the potential role of high-dose IFN in AIDS-related Kaposi's sarcoma demonstrated an improved time of response to the therapy in asymptomatic patients versus those who were symptomatic. Responses were modest, resulting in an average 1- to 2-month response in the symptomatic population and 3 to 5 months in asymptomatic patients. Median survival was also demonstrated as being significantly longer in those patients who responded to IFN therapy than those who did not respond, 22.6 and 9.7 months, respectively (Schering Corporation, 2002).

Malignant melanoma, a disease in which patient survival has historically been measured in months once the disease has become metastatic, has been studied quite extensively in respect to its response to cytokine therapy, IFN in particular. In two studies of high-risk melanoma patients using IFN as an adjuvant to surgical resection, improvements were demonstrated in progression free survival and median survival but neither high- nor low-dose adjuvant IFN therapy demonstrated a demonstrable effect on overall survival (Schering Corporation, 2002).

IFN has also been used historically as an active agent in the treatment of renal cell carcinoma. IFN has been shown to have a clinically meaningful effect in approximately 10% to 15% of the patients treated; this, however, does not necessarily translate to a direct impact on overall survival in this patient subgroup. Through its inhibition of cellular proliferation and direct impact on the cells of the immune system, IFN can produce regression in measurable disease that may translate to modest median survival in small sets of patients (Boccardo, Guglielmini, & Tacchini, 2006). With the clinically significant results seen with the use of new age targeted therapies and antiangiogenic agents, IFN therapy may very well take up positioning as a salvage therapy agent or as an adjunct to other therapeutic regimens for the treatment of this disease.

Interleukins

The class of cytokines referred to as the ILs were given their name for their ability to act in a paracrine and autocrine nature on the leukocytes of the immune system, being released and affecting those cells on a variety of different levels to promote numerous functions by those cells. A vast number of ILs are being studied for their clinical potential in the treatment of malignancies. Documented are a multitude of trials studying IL1-18 with a majority of work to date being done with the use of IL-2 for its ability to mediate antitumor response through enhancing the proliferation and function of lymphokine-activated killer cells (Boccardo, Guglielmini, & Tacchini, 2006; DeVita, Hellman, & Rosenberg, 2001a).

ILs as a class play a significant role in the maintenance of hematopoiesis and response to foreign body invasion.

ILs are a key component in the biology of inflammatory response and the attraction of effector cells to the point of origin of infection. They also play an important role in the stimulation and proliferation of effector and immune cell lines during the infection process. In regard to anticancer effects, IL-1, IL-2, IL-3, IL-6, IL-7, IL-11, IL-12, and IL-16 have been clinically and preclinically proven to have the greatest potential for use.

IL-1 is considered to play a main role in inflammatory responses. IL-1 is mainly produced by macrophages in response to stimulation by toxins and other cytokines. There are two subtypes of IL-1: alpha and beta. Although IL-1 alpha and beta share the same receptor site on cell surfaces, each of these affect cells in different ways. IL-1 locally affects cells by an increase in production of the adhesion molecule, prostaglandins, and chemokines. An additional effect includes a systemic response to foreign invading toxins through the production of fever and hypotension in the host. The promise of IL-1 in cancer to date has been limited by its significant side effect profile; however, potential utility may be seen in anti-inflammatory diseases such rheumatoid arthritis and septic shock (DeVita, Hellman, & Rosenberg, 2001a).

IL-3 is secreted by activated T cells and stimulates differentiation and proliferation of pluripotent stem cells into granulocytes macrophages and megacaryocytes immune response states. The main role for clinical use of IL-3 remains as a member of a combination environment to help support cells ex vivo during cytotoxic therapy for reintroduction at a later time (DeVita, Hellman, & Rosenberg, 2001a).

IL-6 has direct effect on hematopoiesis and helps to increase immunoglobulin G antibody formation by activating B cells. IL-6 is associated with tumor cachexia and acts as a growth factor for melanoma cell lines, which may outline its role in further clinical investigation (DeVita, Hellman, & Rosenberg, 2001a).

IL-7 is an essential component in T-and B-lymphocyte formation and maturation, although it has not yet been tested clinically. Through its mechanism of action it is suggested that there may be a role for its use in the treatment of lymphoma, as a treatment against graft-versus-host disease, and for the prolongation of lymphocyte life cycles (Skalla, 1996).

IL-11 is another cytokine with a direct impact on hematopoiesis. The predominant function of IL-11 is its direct impact on megakaryocopoiesis and thrombopoiesis and the proliferation, maturation, and function of those cell lines (DeVita, Hellman, & Rosenberg 2001b; Wyeth Pharmaceuticals, 2006).

IL-12 helps promote the production of IFN and natural killer cell proliferation and differentiation. The most important role of IL-12 is its direct impact on the production of IFN by natural killer cells. Knock-out mice models have demonstrated a direct relationship between IL-12 and IFN production. In preclinical models an antitumor effect was noted in association to IL-12 administration.

Cancer Management

IL-16 is a product mainly of CD8[+] cells that elicits an attraction and subsequent activation of CD4[+] cells. It produces a chemotactic response by CD4[+] cells and promotes G0 to G1 cell cycle transition in those cells. IL-16 may potentially have a role in blast transformation in hematological malignancies (DeVita, Hellman, & Rosenberg, 2001a).

Interleukin-2. IL-2 has been the focus of the majority of clinical research in the treatment of malignancies to date, and is the only IL to receive Food and Drug Administration (FDA) approval for use in this setting. Through its ability to mediate tumor effects through up-regulation of the proliferation and differentiation of natural killer cells and T lymphocytes, much enthusiasm has been placed on IL-2 for its potential application in the treatment of several malignant processes. Il-2 has also been shown to have an impact on the activation of macrophages and B cells through a cofactor mechanism. To date, IL-2 has FDA approval for use in metastatic renal cell carcinoma and metastatic melanoma (DeVita, Hellman, & Rosenberg, 2001a; Roskrow & Gansbacher, 1998).

Through its first discovery as a growth factor able to sustain T-cell proliferation for extended periods of time ex vivo by Morgan and colleagues in 1976, IL-2 has been better described and its properties and affecting pathway better understood (DeVita, Hellman, & Rosenberg, 2001a). IL-2 demonstrates its impact as an antitumor therapy through direct stimulation of T cells and through an indirect approach by the synthesis of secondary cytokines. As such, it is recognized that IL-2 has no direct effect on tumor cells but rather plays a greater part in sustained upregulation of immune response toward tumors (DeVita, Hellman, & Rosenberg, 2001a).

During the mid 1980s, IL-2 was studied extensively in the setting of renal cell carcinoma and malignant melanoma. Trials in 1985 by Rosenberg used high-dose intravenous IL-2 to elicit an antitumor response in renal cell carcinoma. Additional phase II trials in this setting resulted in objective responses in 15% of the 255 patients participating; this included 17 complete responses, with a median survival of 16 months, leading to FDA approval of IL-2 in these diseases. No progression was demonstrated in any patients who responded for 30 months or longer in a study of 283 patients receiving high-dose IL-2 therapy. Follow-up survival data demonstrate sustained disease-free survival in 60% of the complete responders at more than 10 years after therapy (Boccardo, Guglielmini, & Tacchini, 2006; DeVita, Hellman, & Rosenberg, 1991; DeVita, Hellman, & Rosenberg, 2001a).

The primary drawbacks to treatment with high-dose IL-2 therapy come with treatment-related morbidity and mortality rates from high rates of capillary leak syndrome and hypotension and associated costs for intensive care unit administration of this regimen. Low-dose IL-2 has failed to demonstrate the level of sustained response to date as high-dose intravenous regimens but is widely used in clinical practice because it produces similar clinical response rates without the additional cost and toxicity associated (Boccardo, Guglielmini, & Tacchini, 2006; DeVita, Hellman, & Rosenberg, 1991; DeVita, Hellman, & Rosenberg 2001a; Roskrow & Gansbacher, 1998).

MONOCLONAL ANTIBODIES

Chemotherapy has long since been the standard of treatment for many patients with cancer. The 1997 introduction of the monoclonal antibody (MoAb) rituximab (Rituxan) provided advanced treatment options for many patients with non-Hodgkin lymphoma. From that initial introduction of rituximab, other MoAbs have been developed for additional malignant and nonmalignant uses. MoAbs are man-made proteins produced by B lymphocytes that target specific cell surface antigens on malignant cells (DeMeyer & Stein, 1999; Frogge, 2002). The MoAbs are cloned antibodies extracted from a single B lymphocyte cell. The structure of an antibody is in the shape of a Y. The arms of the Y are the variable region and the base is the constant region. The variable region is made up of two heavy and two light chains (Frogge, 2002). The arms of the antibody bind with the antigen. When the antibody binds with the antigen, several mechanisms of action are initiated to induce tumor cell death.

History

Kohler and Milstein developed hybridoma technology in 1975 (Sikora, 1982). Antibody-forming lymphocytes were harvested from immunized mice and fused with myeloma cells. The process produced hybrid cells that recognize a specific antigen. Hybridoma technology permitted production of large quantities of an antibody that seek out and bind with a specific antigen (DiJulio, 2001; Janeway et al., 2001). MoAbs are used alone or in combination with chemotherapy. Radioactive isotopes have been linked with MoAbs as a way to provide additional treatment options or diagnostic measures. The role of MoAbs is not restricted to oncology use. MoAbs have been developed for nonmalignant use. See the table below for a description of current MoAb use.

Current Use of Monoclonal Antibodies

Transplant Rejection	Cardiovascular Disease	Cancer	Inflammatory Disease
Daclizumab Basiliximab	Abciximab	Rituximab Trastuzumab	Omalizumab Efalizumab

www.fda.gov/cder/index.html

The original MoAbs were produced from mice. These initial mouse antibodies are called murine models. Scientific engineering led to the combination of human and mouse components within the antibody's constant and variable regions (DiJulio, 2001; Frogge, 2002). The chimeric model antibody is a combination of mouse component in the variable region and the human component in the constant region. The humanized model consists only of a small portion within the variable region, whereas the remaining variable region and all of the constant regions are composed of human components. Humanized and chimeric MoAb models can be identified by the generic name.

The generic name for a MoAb can be used to identify whether the drug is chimeric or humanized. The letter X in the generic name represents a chimeric MoAb. Rituximab is an example of a chimeric MoAb. The letter Z identifies a humanized Moab. For example, trastuzumab is the generic name for a humanized model MoAb.

Mechanism of Action

MoAbs have been developed to target specific cells. The targeting allows for normal, healthy cells to continue to function while tumor cells are killed. Mechanisms for tumor kill from MoAb use has been attributed to several mechanisms (Cheng et al., 2005; Janeway et al, 2001):

- Apoptosis
- Complement-dependent cytotoxicity cascade
- Antibody-dependent cell-mediated cytotoxicity

By targeting cell surface markers instead of killing both tumor and normal, healthy cells, systemic side effects may be reduced.

Nursing Management when Monoclonal Antibodies are used

The side effect profile for MoAbs differs from side effects associated with chemotherapy or radiation treatment. Oncology nurses must be knowledgable and prepared to manage the immediate infusion-related events along with the chronic effects (DeMeyer & Stein, 1999). The chronic effects include fatigue and flu-like symptoms. Nursing interventions and patient education instructions suggested to manage chronic effects are listed in Section Seven.

Immediate infusion-related events are common with the administration of MoAbs. The intensity of the event is associated to the specific MoAb administered and whether other treatment modalities are concomitantly used (DiJulio, 2001). In general, the destruction of tumor cells results in a group of symptoms. These symptoms are described as an infusion reaction. However, the underlying pathophysiological mechanisms for the symptoms is a cytokine-release syndrome initiated by cellular destruction along with the body's removal of antigen-antibody complexes through liver, lung, and spleen (Breslin, 2007). Symptoms include the following (Breslin, 2007; DiJulio, 2001; Kositis & Callaghan, 2000):

- Chills
- Fevers
- Rigors
- Myalgia
- Arthralgia
- Urticaria
- Nausea

- Diarrhea
- Mucosal congestion
- Hypotension
- Fatigue
- Headache
- Tachycardia
- Dyspnea

Symptoms generally occur during the first infusion and within the first 2 hours. Side effects may be mild to severe. To reduce the potential for cytokine-release syndrome, pretreatment with acetaminophen and diphenhydramine 30 to 60 minutes before infusion is recommended. Should symptoms develop during the infusion despite premedication, interrupt the infusion and administer normal saline solution. Administration of meperidine, along with additional histamine blockers, may be warranted for rigors. Most reactions will subside on their own and the infusion may be reinitiated at a slower infusion rate (Breslin, 2007; Kositis & Callaghan, 2000). Severe reactions may require supplemental oxygen, steroids, bronchodilators, and emergency medications.

Nursing knowledge of basic immune actions, MoAb type, and usual pattern of symptoms are needed to provide expertise for those receiving MoAb therapy.

Rituximab (Rituxan)

In 1997, rituximab was the first MoAb to be Food and Drug Administration (FDA) approved. The original approval was for B-cell non-Hodgkin lymphoma that has relapsed or is refractory to prior treatment. Current treatment includes as a single agent or in combination with standard chemotherapy. Rituximab is a chimeric MoAb that is specific for the CD20 surface marker on mature B cells.

One hundred sixty-six patients with unresponsive or relapsed non-Hodgkin lymphoma participated in the pivotal clinical trial. Regimens included weekly treatments of 375 mg/m^2 intravenous infusion for four doses. Forty-eight percent of the patients had tumor regression; 6% had a complete remission. Median duration of response was 11.2 months. Rituximab has been found beneficial in several types of cancer, including high-grade and intermediate-grade non-Hodgkin lymphoma, multiple myeloma, and Waldenstrom macroglobulinemia (DeVita, Hellman, & Rosenberg, 2001a).

Common side effects include nausea, fever, and chills. Less common but serious side effects include hypotension and bronchospasm. Most infusion-related side effects can be controlled with appropriate premedications and infusion rates (Rieger, 2001).

Alemtuzumab (Campath)

Alemtuzumab was approved for B-cell chronic lymphocytic leukemia (CLL) that failed other treatments. Alemtuzumab is a humanized MoAb that binds to the CD52 surface marker on B and T lymphocytes. In a multicenter, open-label study of 93 patients with B-cell CLL who failed previous treatment were evaluated after receiving alemtuzumab. This patient population has a poor prognosis and less than half survive for more than 1 year. Doses were gradually escalated to a 30-mg IV infusion three times per week for 4 to 12 weeks. Thirty-three percent overall response rates were seen. Median duration of response was 7 months.

In other trials, patients with untreated B-cell CLL were given alemtuzumab with response rates of greater than 90%. Higher response rates were seen when alemtuzumab was used in combination with fludarabine. Other T-cell malignancies, such as mycosis fungoides and Sézary syndrome, have also seen some response.

Infusion-related side effects include hypotension, rigors, fever, shortness of breath, and bronchospasm. Careful monitoring of patients is vital, along with appropriate premedications. Common side effects include infections, myelosuppression, and viral reactivation.

Trastuzumab (Herceptin)

In September 1998 the humanized MoAb trastuzumab was FDA approved for the treatment of HER-2–positive metastatic breast cancer. Human epidermal growth factor receptor 2 (HER-2) helps normal cells grow. When there are too many copies of the HER-2 gene, it can lead to increased HER-2 proteins. A proliferation of this protein may cause normal cells to turn cancerous. HER-2–positive breast cancer is an aggressive disease with a poor prognosis.

Cardiac dysfunction was the most adverse reaction. This reaction was dependent on prior exposure to anthracycline. The most common infusion-related side effects are hypotension, hypoxia, and bronchospasm.

Gemtuzumab (Mylotarg)

Gemtuzumab is the first targeted antibody-chemotherapy complex that is FDA approved. It is composed of an anti-CD33 humanized MoAb that is linked to a cytotoxic antitumor antibiotic, calicheamicin. Approximately 90% of acute myelogenous leukemia (AML) blasts are CD33 positive. Gemtuzumab is indicated for CD33 AML in patients aged 60 years or older who are not candidates for cytotoxic chemotherapy. Prognosis for these patients is dismal if they are not treated with transplant. There are several chemotherapy options for these patients; however, there is no standard of care for them.

Side effects include myelosuppression, pulmonary toxicity, elevated liver enzymes, hypersensitivity reactions, and veno-occlusive disease. Because of the addition of the cytotoxic drug calicheamicin to the antibody complex, there is a greater side effect potential than with other targeted therapies.

NON–SPECIFIC IMMUNOMODULATING AGENTS

Nonspecific immunomodulating or immune system stimulation is an approach that dates back more than a century ago to Coley and his attempts to enhance immune response by the injection of bacterial toxins to elicit tumor

regression. (DeVita, Hellman, & Rosenberg, 1991). The rationale is to enhance the natural antitumor properties of the host through increased activity and potency of the immune system to detect and eradicate "non-self" antigens. Several agents in this classification of therapy have been studied as single agent therapy with less than favorable responses (Roskrow & Gansbacher, 1998). Additional work is in progress on the use of these agents as adjuncts to other treatment modalities (Roskrow & Gansbacher, 1998).

The demonstrable clinical utility of nonspecific immune modulation has been very limited. There is a paucity in the literature as to role of nonspecific immune-modulating agents. Bacillus Calmette-Guérin (BCG) has been historically referred to for its nonspecific immunomodulatory effects as a single agent in the treatment of localized bladder cancer. The instillation of BCG vaccine into the bladder causes an inflammatory response resulting in the antitumor effect seen in superficial bladder cancers. Unfortunately, when disease has advanced to a muscle-invasive or metastatic state, BCG has little or no effect as a systemic therapeutic option. The lack of utility of BCG as a systemic adjuvant for the treatment of malignancies was supported by an article written for the *British Journal of Medicine* in 1976 in which a trial by Magrath and Ziegler demonstrated a lack of efficacy when using BCG as an immunostimulating agent for the prevention of relapse in patients who had achieved relapse from Burkitt's lymphoma after cyclophosphamide therapy. In this study an equivalent number of patients receiving BCG relapsed, as did those in the control arm (Margrath & Zeigler, 1976).

A recent review of the literature by Spelman et al. concluded that herbal medicines achieve the majority of their efficacy and subsequent nonspecific immunomodulatory effects through a direct impact on cytokine production. The cytokines most often affected were interleukin (IL)-6, IL-1, tumor necrosis factor, and interferon. It is the conclusion of the authors that there is significant evidence to support further research in the efficacy and potential role of herbal and phytotherapeutic medication for a number of disease states, including oncology (Spelman et al., 2006).

Much of the current research in nonspecific immunomodulation or stimulation is found in the form of naturally occurring herbal extracts and fungals that have immune system–activating properties. One such herb being studied in depth with demonstrated promising effects as an adjunct to chemotherapy is echinacea. Echinacea has been used for its anecdotal benefit in the anticancer setting for more than 10 years. A recent report by Miller from McGill University in Montreal, Canada, demonstrates laboratory-supported evidence for the role and rationale for the use of echinacea and its antitumor properties in the mouse model. Her work has shown an improved survival in mice, a decrease in the formation of leukemia, and increased the survival of leukemic mice when prophylactically given the drug over the life span (Miller, 2005). Echinacea contains naturally occurring alkylamides that are known to inhibit the production and secretion of many forms of prostaglandins, which are endogenous suppressors of natural killer (NK) cell proliferation. The action of echinacea in prostaglandin inhibition is similar to the action of indomethacin (Miller, 2005). An increase in circulating NK cells is seen with long-term echinacea administration and results in a nonspecific immunostimulatory effect that leads to enhanced tumor cell antigen and viral toxin recognition.

The use of echinacea in combination with low-dose cyclophosphamide and thymasim was conducted by Bauer et al. to describe the nonspecific immunostimulatory effects in advanced colorectal cancer (Lersch et al., 1992). In this category of patients with a poor prognosis, one in 15 demonstrated a partial response whereas six had stable disease. The mean survival was 4 months, with two patients surviving up to 8 months (Lersch et al., 1992). Although this is a very small, nonrandomized patient subset, it does warrant further investigation. The combination was well tolerated and did result in some modest, yet potentially meaningful, observations in a highly aggressive disease state.

Further investigation into the efficacy of immunomodulatory medications as adjunct to standard therapeutic regimens is warranted. The high level of tolerability along with the general increase in a number of cytokines and activation of the immune system cellular biology can modulate increased efficacy of other targeted therapies. Through an increase in immune response and immune sensitivity there may well be a direct impact on antibody-dependent cellular cytotoxicity as a result of increased proliferation and functioning of effector cells through increased circulating levels of immune stimulating cytokines.

VACCINES

The attempt to cure or treat cancer through means of a vaccination against its development is one of the oldest forms of immune system modulation, dating back more than 200 years. The bulk of the first cancer vaccine approaches involved physicians self-inoculating with malignant cells taken from corpses and active tumors from patients. These early approaches mainly resulted in local irritation and subsequent regional lymph node engorgement, demonstrating the adaptive immunological response to the foreign cells. Various malignancies have been studied for a vaccine-based therapeutic approach, including soft tissue sarcoma, lung, breast, head and neck, and colon cancer. However, the most highly investigated malignancies to be studied to date have been melanoma and prostate cancers (DeVita, Hellman, & Rosenberg, 1991).

Today, the traditional understanding of a true vaccination against a malignancy has evolved from that of a general population-based prophylactic approach to a more targeted approach for several reasons:

- Long-term, population-based immunizations can cause for hereditary mutations and thus increased tolerance to the vaccine over the long term.

- Vaccination against self-directed antigens may have unwanted effects resulting in an autoimmune response against healthy or nontarget tissues.
- The inability to predict and compensate for the large number of genes that might be affected by a vaccine throughout the life span of the host (DeVita, Hellman, & Rosenberg, 2001a).

The only feasible anticancer vaccine that may be used in the prophylactic setting in the future remains in the vaccination against malignancies with a natural history directly related to the infection of the host by a viral or other invading toxin (DeVita, Hellman, & Rosenberg, 2001b). This can be exemplified in the recent trials studying the efficacy of a vaccine targeted at the human papillomavirus (HPV), which has been directly related to a large majority of cervical cancers.

With these understandings, the focus has shifted to targeting specific malignant cells lines and specific antigens expressed by those malignant cell lines. Several trials in this arena have been performed with several in progress. Results have been promising to date; however, there remain no approved indications for any other cancer vaccine regimens. The goal of many antitumor vaccine approaches focuses on the ability to upregulate a specific T-cell response by exciting naive T cells by presentation to a specific tumor antigen through presentation of those antigens by precharged or loaded antigen-presenting cells. This is often accomplished through ex vivo culturing and growing of dendritic cells in a cytokine cocktail to be preloaded before reinfusion or reinjection into the host. Through this approach the dendritic cells, the most potent of the antigen-presenting cells, can present to large numbers of naive T cells and cause a downstream immune response against the specific malignant cells presenting the antigen in question. Antigens for this process can be synthetically processed proteins specific to a malignant cell line or can be derived directly from an individual's tumor cells for a more individualized specific antitumor vaccine product.

Continuing trials in both melanoma and prostate cancer are open and enrolling with results expected in the very near future.

Quadrivalent Human Papillomavirus (types 6, 11, 16, and 18) Recombinant Vaccine (Gardasil)

HPV is the cause of nearly all cervical cancers worldwide. Cervical cancer is the second leading cause of cancer deaths among women in the world, with reports in the range of 470,000 cases and 233,000 deaths annually. In the United States, there are 10,300 cases and 3,700 related deaths annually (Lowy & Schiller, 2006; Steinbrook, 2006). Gardasil is a recombinant quadrivalent vaccine prepared from virus-like particles derived from the major capsid protein of HPV types 6, 11, 16, and 18 (Merck & Company, 2006). The use of the vaccine reduces the incidence of HPV infection or development of genital warts by 90% to 100% in studies involving more than 20,000 participants.

The quadrivalent vaccine approved for use protects against types 6 and 11 HPV, which account for 90% of all infections with genital warts. Additionally, there is protection for HPV types 16 and 18. Types 16 and 18 HPV account for 70% of all cervical cancer cases. However, this vaccine does not prevent other types of HPV infections, nor does it prevent the development of HPV-related neoplasms in women exposed before vaccination. Vaccination against HPV does not take the place of regular Papanicolaou smear testing and physical examination (Koutsky et al., 2002; Lowy & Schiller, 2006). The development and approval of this vaccine is expected to have a dramatic impact on the cervical cancer–related mortality rate around the world as the cases of HPV infections reduce with time.

BIBLIOGRAPHY

Amgen. (2004). Neupogen: Filgrastim full prescribing information. Thousand Oaks, CA: Amgen.

Amgen. (2005). Neulasta: Pegfilgrastim, full prescribing information. Thousand Oaks, CA: Amgen.

Amgen. Kepivance: Palifermin, full prescribing information. Thousand Oaks, CA: Amgen.

Amgen. Procrit epoetin alfa full prescribing information. Raritan, NJ: Orthobiotech Products.

Bellanti, J.A. (1985). *Immunology III*. Philadelphia: W. B. Saunders.

Berlex. (2004). Leukine: Sargramostim, full prescribing information. Seattle, WA: Berlex.

Boccardo, F. M., Guglielmini, P., & Tacchini, L. (2006). Medical treatment of advanced renal cell carcinoma: present options and future directions. *European Association of Urology, 5*, 619-626.

Breslin, S. (2007). Cytokine-release syndrome: Overview and nursing implications. *Clinical Journal of Oncology Nursing, 11 Suppl 1*, 37-42.

Brown, K., Esper, P., Kelleher, L., et al. (2001). *Chemotherapy and biotherapy guidelines and recommendations for practice.* Pittsburgh, PA: Oncology Nursing Society.

Bültzingslöwen, I., Brennan, M.T., Spijkervet, F. K., et al. (2006). Growth factors and cytokines in the prevention and treatment of oral and gastrointestinal mucositis. *Supportive Care in Cancer, 14*, 519-527.

Cheng, J.D., Adams, G. P., Robinson, M. K., et al. (2005). Monoclonal antibodies. In V. DeVita, S. Hellman, & S. Rosenberg (Eds). *Cancer: Principles and practice of oncology* (pp. 1-44). Philadelphia: Lippincott Williams & Wilkins.

Demeyer, E., & Stein, B. (1999). Biotherapy. In C. Miaskowski & P. Buchsel (Eds.) *Oncology nursing: Assessment and clinical care* (pp. 119-141). St. Louis: Mosby.

DeVita, V.T., Hellman, S., & Rosenberg, S.A. (1991). *Biologic therapy of cancer*. Philadelphia: J. B. Lippincott.

DeVita, V. T., Hellman, S., & Rosenberg, S. A. (2001a). *Cancer principles and practice of oncology* (Volume 1, 6th ed.). Philadelphia: Lippincott Williams & Wilkins.

DeVita, V. T., Hellman, S., & Rosenberg, S. A. (2001b). *Cancer principles and practice of oncology* (Volume 2, 6th ed.). Philadelphia: Lippincott Williams & Wilkins.

DiJulio, J. E. (2001). Monoclonal antibodies: overview and use in hematologic malignancies. In P. T. Rieger (Ed.). *Biotherapy: A comprehensive overview* (pp. 283-315). Sudbury, MA: Jones & Bartlett.

Finch, P. W., & Rubin, J. S. (2006). Keratinocyte growth factor expression and activity in cancer: Implications for use in patients with solid tumors. *Journal of the National Cancer Institute, 98*, 812-824.

Frogge, M. H. (Ed.). (2002). *Teaching peers and patients about monoclonal antibodies* [monograph]. Pittsburgh, PA: Oncology Education Services.

Janeway, C. A, Travers, P., Walport, M., et al. (2001). *Immunobiology: The immune system in health and disease* (5th ed.). New York: Garland Publishing.

Kositis, C., & Callaghan, M. (2000). Rituximab: A new monoclonal antibody therapy for non-Hodgkin's lymphoma. *Oncology Nursing Forum, 27*, 51-59.

Koutsky, L.A., Ault, K.A., Wheeler, C. M., et al. (2002). A controlled trial of a human papillomavirus type 16 vaccine. *The New England Journal of Medicine, 347*, 1645-1651.

Lersch, C., Zeunner, M., Bauer, A., et al. (1992). Nonspecific immunostimulation with low doses of cyclophosphamide (LDCY), thymostimulin, and Echinacea purpurea extracts (Echanacin) in patients with far advanced colorectal cancers: preliminary results. *Cancer Investigation, 10*, 343-348.

Lowy, D. R., & Schiller, J.T. (2006). Prophylactic human papillomavirus vaccines. *The Journal of Clinical Investigation, 116*, 1167-1173.

MacDonald, K. P. A., & Hill, G. R. (2002). Keratinocyte growth factor (KGF) in hematology and oncology. *Current Pharmaceutical Design, 8*, 395-403.

Margrath, I.T., & Zeigler, J. L. (1976). Failure of BCG immunostimulation to affect the clinical course of Burkitt's lymphoma. *British Medical Journal, 1*, 615-618.

Merck & Company. (2006). Gardasil: Quadrivalent human papillomavirus (types 6, 11, 16, 18) recombinant vaccine, full prescribing information. Whitehouse Station: Merck.

Metcalf, D., & Nicola, N. A. (1995). *The hematopoietic colony stimulating factors*. Cambridge: Cambridge University Press.

Miller, S. C. (2005). Echinacea: A miracle herb against aging and cancer? Evidence in vivo in mice. *Evidence-Based Complementary and Alternative Medicine, 2*, 309-314.

Oelmann, E., Haghgu, S., Kulimova, E., et al. (2004). Influence of keratinocyte growth factor on clonal growth of epithelial tumor cells, lymphoma and leukemia cells and on sensitivity of tumor cells towards 5-fluorouracil in vitro. *International Journal of Oncology, 25*, 1001-1012.

Oppenheim, J., & Fujiwara, H. (1996). The role of cytokines in cancer. *Cytokine and Growth Factor Reviews, 7*, 279-288.

Roche. (2005). Roferon-A: Interferon alfa-2a, recombinant, full prescribing information. Nutley, NJ: Roche Pharmaceuticals.

Roskrow, M.A., & Gansbacher, B. (1998). Recent developments in gene therapy for oncology and hematology. *Critical Reviews in Oncology/Hematology, 28*, 139-151.

Schering. (2002). Interferon alfa 2b, recombinant, full prescribing information. Kenilworth, NJ: Schering.

Skalla, K. (1996). The interferons. *Seminars in Oncology Nursing, 12*, 97-105.

Spelman, K., Burns, J., Nichols, D., et al. (2006). Modulation of cytokine expression by traditional medicines: A review of herbal immunomodulators. *Alternative Medicine Review, 11*, 128-150.

Steinbrook, R. (2006). The potential of human papillomavirus vaccines. *The New England Journal of Medicine, 354*, 1109-1112.

Wang, H., Zhou, F. J., Wang, Q. J., et al. (2006). Efficacy of autologous renal tumor cell lysateloaded dendritic cell vaccine in combination with cytokine induced killer cells on advanced renal cell carcinoma—a report of ten cases. *Zheng, 25*, 625-630.

Wyeth Pharmaceuticals. (2006). Neumega: Oprelvekin, full prescribing information. Philadelphia: Wyeth Pharmaceuticals.

Biological Response Modifier Agents: Food and Drug Administration–Approved Drugs: Prescribing and Clinical Application Guidelines*

Jason M. Rothaermel and Barbara Baum

Recombinant Erythropoietin Epoetin alfa (Procrit), darbepoetin alfa (Aranesp)

DRUG CLASS

Cytokine, colony-stimulating factor

ROUTE OF ADMINISTRATION

Subcutaneous (SC) or intravenous (IV) injection

HOW TO ADMINISTER

- Recombinant erythropoietin should not be shaken before it is drawn into a syringe because vigorous shaking can denature the glycoprotein, resulting in its being made biologically inactive.
- Recombinant erythropoietin should be administered as a SQ injection and not mixed with other solutions. In the case of IV administration, recombinant erythropoietin can be directly administered by an IV or venous dialysis port.

PRETREATMENT GUIDELINES

1. Baseline complete blood cell count and hemoglobin and hematocrit to determine hematocrit value.

2. Baseline transferrin saturation should also be determined and should be >20%.
3. Serum ferritin levels should be >200 ng/mL.

USE

- Darbepoetin alfa
  ○ Indicated for the treatment of anemia in patients with nonmyeloid malignancies where anemia is due to the effect of concomitantly administered chemotherapy
- Epoetin alfa
  ○ Indicated for the treatment of anemia associated with chronic renal failure either in end-stage renal disease in patients on dialysis or not receiving dialysis
  ○ Indicated for the treatment of anemia related to therapy with zidovudine in human immunodeficiency virus–infected patients
  ○ Indicated for the treatment of anemia in patients with nonmyeloid malignancies where anemia is due to the effect of concomitantly administered chemotherapy

PHARMACOKINETICS

- Darbepoetin alfa
  ○ Peak serum level at 34 hours after SQ administration.
  ○ Half-life 49 hours (range 27-89 hours) with SQ administration
  ○ Distribution half-life of 1.4 hours and terminal half-life of 21 hours when administered parenterally
- Epoetin alfa
  ○ Elimination half-life after IV administration is 4-13 hours, approximately 20% longer in chronic renal failure.
  ○ After SQ administration, peak plasma levels are achieved within 5-24 hours.

  ○ Drug is eliminated by liver and urine with 10% unchanged drug eliminated.

USUAL DOSE AND SCHEDULE
Darbepoetin Alfa

- 2.25 mcg/kg SQ every week as a starting dose.
  ○ If <1.0 g/dL increase in hemoglobin after 6 weeks of therapy, increase dose to 4.5 mcg/kg.
  ○ If >1.0 g/dL in a 2-week period or hemoglobin exceeds 12 g/dL, reduce dose by 25%.
- If hemoglobin rises to >13 g/dL hold until hemoglobin of 12 g/dL is noted and restart at 75% original dose.

Epoetin Alfa

- 50-150 unit/kg 3 × wk
- If hematocrit does not increase by week 8, increase dose by 25-50 units/kg TIW until maximum dose of 300 units/kg 3 × wk is achieved.
- 40,000 units as a single dose SQ every week
- If hematocrit does not rise by 5%-6% in 8 weeks, increase weekly dose to 60,000 units SQ every week.
- If no response, increase to a maximum 80,000 units SQ every week.
- Interrupt therapy if hematocrit levels exceed 40%, and resume at 75% of original dose when hematocrit returns to 36%.

SIDE EFFECTS

- Fatigue
- Edema
- Nausea
- Diarrhea
- Vomiting
- Fever
- Dyspnea
- Seizures
- Hypertension
- Thrombotic events

*Please note that the information in this section is for reference purposes only. Please refer to the package inserts for complete prescribing information before administration of any medications.

Cancer Management

STORAGE

- Refrigerate: store between 36°-46° F.
- Do NOT freeze.
- Do NOT shake.

COMPATIBILITY WITH OTHER DRUGS/INTRAVENOUS FLUIDS

Recombinant erythropoietin should not be mixed with other drugs or IV fluids for administration.

PREGNANCY

Category C

SPECIAL CONSIDERATIONS

- Weekly monitoring of hemoglobin and hematocrit should be routine.
- Serum ferritin levels should be monitored while patients are being treated with recombinant erythropoietin and iron supplements given to meet the demand of increasing erythrocyte numbers.

PATIENT EDUCATION

- Reinforce proper aseptic technique with self-administration.
- Reinforce adherence to dosing guidelines.
- Reinforce iron supplementation and potential bowel regimen to prevent constipation.
- Reinforce patient contact with health care professionals for side effect management and laboratory monitoring as necessary.

Filgrastim (Neupogen), Pegfilgrastim (Neulasta)

DRUG CLASS

Cytokine, colony-stimulating factor

ROUTE OF ADMINISTRATION

Intravenous (IV) or subcutaneous (SC) infusion injection

HOW TO ADMINISTER

- **Filgrastim** can be administered by SC injection, short IV infusion (over 15-30 minutes), or continuous SQ or IV infusion.
  - Do not administer within 24 hours of chemotherapy administration.
- **Pegfilgrastim** should be administered as a single SQ injection once per cycle of chemotherapy.
  - Do not administer between 14 days before or 24 hours after any given administration of chemotherapy agents.

PRETREATMENT GUIDELINES

1. A complete blood cell count and platelet count should be obtained before the start of a chemotherapy cycle and at least twice weekly during filgrastim therapy.
2. While following baseline values, a neutrophil level should be monitored regularly while patients are receiving pegfilgrastim therapy.

USE

- Filgrastim
  - Cancer patients receiving myelosuppressive chemotherapy
  - Patients receiving induction or consolidation therapy for acute myelogenous leukemia
  - To shorten the risk and duration of neutropenia associated with bone marrow transplant
  - For mobilization of progenitor stem cells before collection for autologous transplant
- Pegfilgrastim
  - Indicated for decreasing the rate and risk of infection resulting from febrile neutropenia caused by cytotoxic chemotherapy administration in nonmyeloid malignancies

PHARMACOKINETICS

- Filgrastim
  - Serum half-life is approximately 210-230 minutes for IV and SQ administration.

- Elimination half-life is equivalent in patients with and without cancer at around 3.5 hours.
- In doses administered over 11-20 days, no evidence of drug accumulation was noted.
- Pegfilgrastim
  - Pharmacokinetics of pegfilgrastim is highly dependent on direct binding to neutrophils so is subject to the number of circulating neutrophils during drug presence.
  - Half-life ranged from 15 to 80 hours in studies of cancer patients.

USUAL DOSE AND SCHEDULE

Filgrastim. 1.5-10 mcg/kg/day, depending on the indication.

- SQ or IV infusion
- Monitor absolute neutrophil count (ANC) to determine discontinuation of filgrastim therapy when ANC >1,000 cells/mm^2.

Pegfilgrastim. 6 mg SQ to be administered once per cycle and not to overlap chemotherapy within 14 days before or 24 hours after administration

SIDE EFFECTS

- Peripheral edema
- Bone pain
- Fever
- Myalgia
- Headache
- Injection site reaction
- Splenic rupture has been reported.
- Adult respiratory distress syndrome
- Allergic reactions (wheezing, rash, urticaria, dyspnea, facial edema)
- Sickle cell disease exacerbation

STORAGE

- Store at 2°-8° C (35°-46° F).
- Avoid shaking.
- Do not freeze.
- Allow to come to room temperature for up to 24 hours before administration.

COMPATIBILITY WITH OTHER DRUGS/INTRAVENOUS FLUIDS

- **Do not mix with saline solution**. Saline solution will cause the formation of a precipitate.
- Dilution with dextrose 5% solution should be accompanied by albuminization and should be administered from polyvinyl chloride, glass, or polyolefin IV bags to prevent absorption of plastic into the fluid.
- Pegfilgrastim should not be administered by the intravenous route.

PREGNANCY

Category C

PATIENT EDUCATION

- Do not shake vial.
- Monitor for flu-like symptoms of fever, nausea and vomiting, aching, and bone pain. Possible role for analgesics to control side effects
- Monitor for infection, fever, and injection site reactions.
- Avoid large crowds and persons with infections during therapy to prevent exposure while neutropenic.
- Ensure proper administration technique and adherence to prescribed regimen.

Sargramostim (Leukine)

DRUG CLASS

Cytokine, colony-stimulating factor

ROUTE OF ADMINISTRATION

Intravenous (IV) infusion or subcutaneous (SQ) injection

PRETREATMENT GUIDELINES

- Baseline complete blood cell count (CBC) with differential, liver function panel, renal function, and weight and hydration status should be assessed before initiation of therapy with sargramostim.
- CBC should be monitored twice per week during therapy to detect excessive leukocyte production.
- Liver function tests should be monitored on a regular basis on patients with preexisting renal or hepatic dysfunction.

USE

Sargramostim has been Food and Drug Administration approved for use as follows:

- After induction chemotherapy in older patients with acute myelogenous leukemia to decrease the time to neutrophil recovery and decrease the risk of febrile neutropenia
- For mobilization of stem cells for leukapheresis collection and after transplantation of autologous cells to promote engraftment
- Myeloid reconstitution after autologous and allogeneic stem cell transplantation
- In transplant failure or engraftment delay to decrease the risk of infection from decreased neutrophil count

PHARMACOKINETICS

- IV administration: mean beta half-life in serum is measured at 60 minutes, with a peak concentration noted immediately after the completion of the infusion.
- SQ injection: mean beta half-life is 162 minutes after injection, with peak concentration measured at 1-3 hours and detectable levels out to 6 hours after injection.

USUAL DOSE AND SCHEDULE

Induction Chemotherapy in Acute Myelogenous Leukemia. 250mcg/m^2/day IV over 4 hours beginning day 4 after induction and continued until an absolute neutrophil count (ANC) of >1500 cells/mm^2 is achieved; if reconsolidation is necessary, reinitiate sargramostim according to induction guidelines.

Mobilization and After Autologous Cell Transplant. 250 mcg/m^2/day IV over 24 hours or daily as a SQ injection. Cell collection is usually performed on day 5 of sargramostim therapy.

Myeloid Reconstitution After Autologous and Allogeneic Transplant. Sargramostim therapy should be initiated no sooner than 24 hours after the last dose of chemotherapy and when ANC reaches 500 cells/mm^2 or less. At that time, 250 mcg/m^2/day by IV infusion over 2 hours should be initiated until an ANC of 1500 cells/mm^2 is attained.

Transplant Failure and Engraftment Delay. 250 mcg/m^2/day SQ for up to two courses of 14 days each followed by a third course of 500 mcg/m^2 for 14 days if engraftment has not been accomplished

SIDE EFFECTS

- First-dose reaction (rare): hypoxia, flushing, dyspnea, tachycardia (occurs at first dose of medication and not seen subsequently at following doses)
- Bone pain
- Rash
- Fever
- Chills
- Pruritus

STORAGE

- Refrigerate at 2°-8° C (36°-45° F).
- Do not freeze.
- Do not shake because this will denature the protein.

MIXING INSTRUCTIONS

- Drug compatibility information is not available.
- Sargramostim should only be mixed with normal saline solution for infusion and not mixed with other medications.
- Powder form can be reconstituted with bacteriostatic water for SQ injection.

PREGNANCY

Category C

PATIENT EDUCATION

- Instruct patient on proper injection technique: inject slowly over 1-2 minutes, do not manipulate injection site or rub after injection, ice site before and after injection, bring sargramostim to room temperature before injecting, use ⅝-inch 22-gauge needle for injection.

- Inform patient regarding first-dose reaction and advise that symptomatic support will be available. This is not a recurring event and does not constitute stopping therapy.

Oprelvekin (Neumega)

DRUG CLASS

Cytokine, colony-stimulating factor

ROUTE OF ADMINISTRATION

Subcutaneous (SQ) injection

HOW TO ADMINISTER

Administer as a SQ injection once daily to the abdomen, thigh, hip, or upper arm.

PRETREATMENT GUIDELINES

Obtain baseline complete blood cell count and platelet count before chemotherapy administration and follow platelet counts closely during oprelvekin therapy. Continue therapy until platelet count of 50 microliter is achieved.

USE

1. Prevention of severe thrombocytopenia
2. To reduce the need for platelet transfusions after myelosuppressive chemotherapy
   - *Not* indicated for use after myeloablative chemotherapy

PHARMACOKINETICS

- Peak serum concentrations of 17.4 ± 5.4 ng/mL was determined to be reached at 0.8 to 5.6 hour after a single SQ injection of 50 mcg/kg.
- Terminal half-life was determined to be 5.2 to 8.3 hours.
- Bioavailability is 80%.

USUAL DOSE AND SCHEDULE

For Patients Without Severe Renal Insufficiency: 50 mcg/kg SQ daily

For Patients With Renal Impairment (Creatinine <30 ml/min): 25 mcg/kg SQ daily

SIDE EFFECTS

- Edema
- Tachycardia
- Vasodilation
- Palpitations
- Atrial fibrillation/flutter
- Nausea and vomiting
- Oral moniliasis
- Dyspnea
- Pleural effusions

STORAGE

- Lyophilized oprelvekin and diluent should be refrigerated.
- DO NOT FREEZE
- Once mixed, product should be used within 3 hours and can be stored at room temperature during this time.

MIXING INSTRUCTIONS

- Mix one 5-mg vial with 1 mL of sterile water for injection (no preservatives).
- Direct diluent at the side of the vial during preparation, and excessive agitation should be avoided. Swirl contents gently until clear solution is noted.

COMPATIBILITY WITH OTHER DRUGS/INTRAVENOUS FLUIDS

Compatibility tests have not been fully performed.

PREGNANCY

Category C

PATIENT EDUCATION

- Inform patients of the risk for allergic or sensitivity reactions associated with oprelvekin.
- Advise patients to contact health care assistance immediately should they notice any signs of facial edema, tongue or throat swelling, lightheadedness,

shortness of breath, difficulty talking, wheezing, chest pain, confusion, loss of consciousness, flushing, or fever.

- Patients should also be made aware of the chance for lower extremity edema and dyspnea on exertion.

Palifermin (Kepivance)

DRUG CLASS

Cytokine, human keratinocyte growth factor

ROUTE OF ADMINISTRATION

Intravenous (IV) bolus injection

HOW TO ADMINISTER

Total dose of 60 mcg/kg/day should be administered as an IV bolus injection for 3 consecutive days before and 3 consecutive days after myelotoxic chemotherapy.

PRETREATMENT GUIDELINES

No specific lab abnormalities have been directly associated with the use of palifermin in clinical trials.

USE

To decrease the incidence and duration of severe oral mucositis associated with hematological malignancies requiring stem cell support after myelotoxic chemotherapy treatment

PHARMACOKINETICS

Peak concentrations after IV bolus administration decline 95% within the first 30 minutes and plateau at between 1-4 hours after injection with an elimination half-life of approximately 4 hours.

SIDE EFFECTS

- Potential for stimulation of the growth of nonhematological malignancies with the use of this medication
- Rash
- Pruritus
- Erythema

- Mouth/tongue thickness or discoloration
- Edema
- Pain
- Fever
- Altered taste

STORAGE

- Protect from light.
- Store at 2°-8° C (refrigerate).
- Use within 24 hours of mixing.

MIXING INSTRUCTIONS

- Redilute lyophilized powder with 1.2 mL of sterile water for injection.
- Gently swirl.
- Do not aggressively agitate or shake vial.
- Protect from light and keep refrigerated until use.

COMPATIBILITY WITH OTHER DRUGS/INTRAVENOUS FLUIDS

- No formal drug interaction studies have been performed.
- Palifermin binds to heparin in vitro.
- Flush IV line with normal saline solution before and after bolus to prevent any untoward mixing.

PREGNANCY

Category C

PATIENT EDUCATION

- Proper administration of this drug should be followed. The full extent of potential for development of protection against cytotoxic insult for nonhematological malignancies is not known; strict adherence to approved patient populations should be maintained.
- Care should be taken not to administer palifermin within 24 hours before or after cytotoxic chemotherapy is administered.

Interferon Alfa-2a (Roferon-A)

DRUG CLASS

Cytokine, interferon

ROUTE OF ADMINISTRATION

Subcutaneous (SQ) injection

HOW TO ADMINISTER/USUAL DOSE SCHEDULE

- Chronic myelogenous leukemia:
  - 9 million international units daily administered as SQ injection, following a dose escalation period of 3 million international units for 3 days, followed by 6 million international units for 3 days, then progression to full dose as tolerated
  - Duration of therapy has ranged from 5 to 18 months in clinical trials.
  - Optimal duration of therapy has yet to be determined.
- Hairy cell leukemia:
  - 3 million international units SQ every day for 16 to 24 weeks, followed by maintenance dosing of 3 million international units SQ three times per week

PRETREATMENT GUIDELINES

1. Appropriate baseline disease specific diagnostic testing should be performed before the initiation of therapy for determination of efficacy after the start of therapy.
2. Monthly evaluation of hematological parameters (i.e., hemoglobin, hematocrit, platelets) should be maintained during the course of therapy.
3. Liver and renal function tests should be done at baseline and throughout treatment.

USE

1. Interferon alfa-2a is approved for the treatment of hairy cell leukemia in patients 18 years of age or older.
2. It is also approved for use in patients with Philadelphia chromosome–positive chronic myelogenous leukemia with minimal prior therapies.

PHARMACOKINETICS

Peak serum concentrations after SQ injections of 36 million international units was 7.3 hours.

SIDE EFFECTS

- Suicidal ideation and behavior have been reported with interferon treatment.
- Flu-like symptoms
- Anorexia
- Fatigue
- Dyspnea on exertion
- Rash
- Pruritus
- Arrhythmias
- Headache
- Depression
- Bone marrow suppression
- Proteinuria
- Abnormal liver function test results

STORAGE

- Refrigerate.
- Do not freeze.
- Do not shake.
- Protect from light.

MIXING INSTRUCTIONS

This product is supplied in ready-to-use prefilled syringes. No mixing is required.

COMPATIBILITY WITH OTHER DRUGS AND INTRAVENOUS FLUIDS/DRUG INTERACTIONS

- Concurrent administration with interleukin-2 can potentiate renal failure.
- Interferon alfa-2a reduces the clearance of theophylline and may reduce the activity of P450 drugs.

PREGNANCY

Category C

PATIENT EDUCATION

- Patients should be made aware of the mood-altering aspect of treatment with interferon. Support and contact information should be given to patients on initiation of therapy.
- Proper self-injection techniques should be taught.
- Adherence to prescribing information should be reinforced to increase compliance with regimens.

Interferon Alfa-2b (Intron-A)

DRUG CLASS

Cytokine, interferon

ROUTE OF ADMINISTRATION

Intravenous (IV), intramuscular (IM), subcutaneous (SQ), or intralesional injection

HOW TO ADMINISTER/USUAL DOSE SCHEDULES

Hairy Cell Leukemia. 2 million international units IM three times a week for up to 6 months. Stop therapy if disease is progressive while on treatment or unacceptable toxicity is seen.

Malignant Melanoma. Induction course should consist of 20 million international units IV over 20 minutes for 5 days per week for the initial 4 weeks of therapy followed by a maintenance course of 10 million international units SQ three times a week for 48 weeks.

Follicular Lymphoma. 5 million IU SQ three times a week for up to 18 months concomitantly with an anthracycline-based cytotoxic regimen

AIDS-Related Kaposi's Sarcoma. 30 million international units/m² IM or SQ three times a week until disease progression or maximal response at 16 weeks. Dose reduce as necessary for toxicity.

PRETREATMENT GUIDELINES

1. Baseline complete blood cell count with differential, electrolytes, and liver and renal function tests
2. Patients with a history of cardiac disease should be monitored by their cardiologists while receiving therapy.

USE

1. Adults 18 years or older with hairy cell leukemia
2. As an adjunct to surgery for malignant melanoma in

patients at high risk for recurrence
3. In combination with anthracycline therapy for the treatment of aggressive follicular non-Hodgkin lymphoma
4. Treatment of acquired immunodeficiency syndrome (AIDS)–related Kaposi's sarcoma with the best results seen in asymptomatic patients

SIDE EFFECTS

- Suicidal ideation and behavior have been reported with interferon treatment.
- Flu-like symptoms
- Anorexia
- Fatigue
- Dyspnea on exertion
- Rash
- Pruritus
- Arrhythmias
- Headache
- Depression
- Bone marrow suppression
- Proteinuria
- Abnormal liver function test results

STORAGE

- Store powder, diluent, and multidose pens in refrigerator.
- Do not freeze.
- Do not agitate or shake vigorously because this may denature the product.

MIXING INSTRUCTIONS

- Mix one vial of powder with the contents of one vial of diluent (supplied 1 mL of sterile water for injection).
  - When adding diluent, inject toward the side of the vial to avoid foaming.
  - Swirl until a clear colorless or slightly yellow solution is obtained.
- IV mixing should be done immediately before infusion.
  - Mix the appropriate amount of drug in the manner mentioned above.
  - Add the appropriate dose of medication to a 100-mL bag of normal saline solution.

  - Final mixture should not exceed 10 million international units/100mL for IV infusion.

COMPATIBILITY WITH OTHER DRUGS/INTRAVENOUS FLUIDS

Mix with normal saline solution for IV administration only. Do not combine with any other drugs and flush line before and after administration.

PREGNANCY

Category C

PATIENT EDUCATION

- Patients should be made aware of mood-altering aspect of treatment with interferon. Support and contact information should be given to patients on initiation of therapy.
- Proper self-injection techniques should be taught.
- Adherence to prescribing information should be reinforced to increase compliance with regimens.

Aldesleukin (interleukin-2, Proleukine)

DRUG CLASS

Cytokine, interleukin

ROUTE OF ADMINISTRATION

Intravenous (IV) infusion over 15 minutes

HOW TO ADMINISTER/USUAL DOSE AND SCHEDULE

- Aldesleukin should be administered in 5% dextrose solution at a dose of 600,000 international units/kg as a 15-minute infusion every 8 hours for a maximum of 14 doses.
  - Following 9-day rest period repeat the second set of 15-minute infusions every 8 hours for a maximum of 28 infusions for one course.

- Evaluation for response should occur before each course every 4 weeks.
- Do not use an in-line filter when administering this medication.

PRETREATMENT GUIDELINES

Complete blood cell count with differential, blood chemistry panel, chest x-ray films

USE

- Metastatic renal cell carcinoma
- Metastatic melanoma

PHARMACOKINETICS

- Serum half-life of aldesleukin has been measured at 13 and 85 minutes after a 5-minute IV infusion.
- After rapid initial distribution the drug is primarily cleared by the kidneys with little detectable residual drug in the urine.

SIDE EFFECTS

- Cardiac arrhythmias
- Hypotension
- Mental status changes
- Abnormal renal or liver function tests
- Oliguria
- Encephalopathy
- Ascites
- Dermatitis
- Fever
- Myocardial infarction
- Nausea and vomiting
- Diarrhea
- Thrombocytopenia
- Chills
- Fatigue
- Malaise
- Asthenia
- Anorexia

STORAGE

- Aldesleukin should be refrigerated and used within 48 hours of mixing for infusion.
- Bring infusion mixture to room temperature just before infusion.

MIXING INSTRUCTIONS

- Aldesleukin should be mixed by adding 1.2 mL of sterile water for injection into the vial containing the powder by directing it at the side of the vial while gently swirling to mix the contents.
- The clear colorless mixture should be mixed with 50 mL of 5% dextrose solution for infusion.

COMPATIBILITY WITH OTHER DRUGS/INTRAVENOUS FLUIDS

- Do NOT mix with bacteriostatic water OR normal saline solution because this will cause aggregation.
- Aldesleukin should not be administered with any other medications and tubing should be flushed before and after with 5% dextrose solution.

PREGNANCY

Category C

PATIENT EDUCATION

- Patients should be advised to inform their doctors of any of the following preexisting conditions because they should not receive aldesleukin:
  - Sustained ventricular tachycardia
  - Cardiac arrhythmias not controlled with medication
  - Chest pain with electrocardiographic changes
  - Cardiac tamponade
  - Intubation for >72 hours
  - Renal failure requiring dialysis for >72 hours
  - Coma or toxic psychosis lasting >48 hours
  - Repetitive or difficult-to-manage seizures
  - Bowel ischemia/perforation
  - Gastrointestinal bleeding requiring surgery

Rituximab (Rituxan)

DRUG CLASS

Monoclonal antibody

ROUTE OF ADMINISTRATION

Intravenous (IV) infusion

HOW TO ADMINISTER

- With aseptic technique, withdraw necessary amount and dilute to final concentration of 1 to 4 mg/mL into infusion bag of 0.9% normal saline solution or 5% dextrose.
  - Gently invert to mix.
  - Solution may be stored at 2°-8° C (36°-46° F) for 24 hours.
  - Do not mix or dilute with other drugs.
- DO NOT ADMINISTER AS IV PUSH OR BOLUS.
  - Hypersensitivity reactions may occur.
  - First infusion should be administered IV at 50 mg/hr.
  - If no hypersensitivity occurs, then infusion can be escalated at 50 mg/hr increments every 30 minutes for a maximum of 400 mg/hr.
- If hypersensitivity occurs, the infusion should be slowed or stopped and then continued at one half the previous rate on resolution of symptoms.
- Subsequent infusions can be started at 100 mg/hr and increased at 100 mg/hr intervals to a maximum of 400 mg/hr.

PRETREATMENT GUIDELINES

Acetaminophen and an antihistamine should be administered before treatment.

USE

1. Low-grade or follicular CD20-positive, B-cell, relapsed or refractory non-Hodgkin lymphoma
2. First-line treatment of diffuse large B-cell non-Hodgkin lymphoma in combination with chemotherapy treatments
3. Rheumatoid arthritis in combination with methotrexate

PHARMACOKINETICS

- Peak serum half-life is proportional to dose and tumor burden.
- Rituximab was serum detectable 3 to 6 months after treatment.

USUAL DOSE AND SCHEDULE

Relapsed or Refractory, Low-Grade or Follicular, CD20-Positive B-Cell Non-Hodgkin Lymphoma. 375 mg/m^2 IV infusion per week for 4 weeks

Diffuse Large B-Cell Non-Hodgkin Lymphoma. 375 mg/m^2 IV infusion on day 1 of each cycle of chemotherapy for up to eight infusions

Rheumatoid Arthritis
1. Two doses of 1,000-mg IV infusions given 2 weeks apart
2. Also given as combination therapy with methotrexate

SIDE EFFECTS

- Infusion reactions: fever and chills/rigors, hypotension, hypertension, nausea, vomiting, pruritus, angioedema, headache, bronchospasm, rhinitis, rash, myalgia, dizziness, and asthenia
- Tumor lysis syndrome
- Severe skin reactions
- Infectious events: hepatitis B reactivation and other viral infections
- Grade 3 and 4 cytopenias
- Pulmonary events (cough, rhinitis, bronchospasm, dyspnea, and sinusitis)

STORAGE

- Do not use past expiration date.
- Protect vials from direct sunlight.
- Do not freeze.

COMPATIBILITY WITH OTHER DRUGS

Do not mix or dilute with other drugs.

PREGNANCY

Category C

SPECIAL CONSIDERATIONS

- Fatal reactions have been reported after infusions. These reactions have included hypoxia, acute respiratory distress, pulmonary infiltrates, myocardial infarction, cardiogenic shock, and ventricular fibrillation.
- Severe mucocutaneous reactions have been reported.
- Important to follow infusion instructions and monitor patients closely during and after infusions

PATIENT EDUCATION

- Provide patient with written information.
- Teach regarding potential side effects and management of side effects.
- Contact health care professional with any side effects.
- Reinforce follow-up appointments with health care professional.

Alemtuzumab (Campath)

DRUG CLASS

Monoclonal antibody

ROUTE OF ADMINISTRATION

Intravenous (IV) infusion

HOW TO ADMINISTER

- Do not shake vial before use.
  - Withdraw necessary amount from vial; aseptically inject into 100 mL 0.9% normal saline solution or 5% dextrose.
  - Gently invert to incorporate. Protect from light.
- DO NOT ADMINISTER AS AN IV PUSH OR BOLUS.

PRETREATMENT GUIDELINES

Acetaminophen and antihistamines

USE

B-cell chronic lymphocytic leukemia

PHARMACOKINETICS

Mean half-life after first dose was 11 hours and after last dose was 6 days.

USUAL DOSE AND SCHEDULE

3 mg over 2 hours IV daily until tolerated demonstrated by infusion related toxicities ≤ Grade 2
- Then the daily dose should be increased to 10 mg. Once this dose is tolerated, then final maintenance dose of 30 mg can be administered three times per week for 12 weeks.
- If dose is interrupted for 7 days or longer, then reinitiate drug at the 3 mg dosing schedule and escalate in same manner.

SIDE EFFECTS

- Infusion related:
  - Hypotension
  - Fever
  - Rigors/chills
  - Shortness of breath/bronchospasm
  - Rash
  - Immunosuppression/infection
  - Hematological toxicity

STORAGE

After dilution, use within 8 hours.

PREGNANCY

Category C

SPECIAL CONSIDERATIONS

- Weekly complete blood cell count during therapy
- Patients recently treated should not receive immunizations with live viral vaccines.

PATIENT EDUCATION

- Provide patient with written information.
- Patient education of potential side effects and management of side effects and management of side effects
- Contact health care professional with any side effects.
- Reinforce follow-up appointments with health care professional.

Gemtuzumab (Mylotarg)

DRUG CLASS

Monoclonal antibody

ROUTE OF ADMINISTRATION

Intravenous (IV) infusion

HOW TO ADMINISTER

- In-line low protein binding filter must be used during infusion.

- Do not administer other drugs through the same infusion line.
- Inject reconstituted solution into 100 mL of 0.9% normal saline solution only.

PRETREATMENT GUIDELINES

Acetaminophen and antihistamines before treatment

USE

CD33-positive acute myeloid leukemia

PHARMACOKINETICS

Total half-life approximately 41 hours

USUAL DOSE AND SCHEDULE

9 mg/m^2 IV over 2 hours
- A total of two doses should be given 14 days apart.
- Do NOT ADMINISTER AS IV PUSH OR BOLUS.

SIDE EFFECTS

- Fever
- Nausea/vomiting
- Chills
- Headache
- Dyspnea
- Hypotension/hypertension
- Hyperglycemia
- Hypoxia

STORAGE

- Light sensitive; must be protected from direct and indirect sunlight and unshielded fluorescent light
- Reconstituted vials stable for 2 hours at room temperature or refrigeration. After dilution 16 hours at room temperature

PREGNANCY

Category D

SPECIAL CONSIDERATIONS

- Monitor patient during and after infusion for potential side effects.
- Monitor complete blood cell count and blood chemistries.
- Monitor for hepatotoxicity and veno-occlusive disease.

PATIENT EDUCATION

- Provide patient with written information.

- Teach regarding potential side effects and management of side effects.
- Contact health care professional with any side effects.
- Reinforce follow-up appointments with health care professional.

Trastuzumab (Herceptin)

DRUG CLASS

Monoclonal antibody

ROUTE OF ADMINISTRATION

Intravenous (IV) infusion

HOW TO ADMINISTER

- With aseptic technique, slowly inject 20 mL of diluent into the vial. Shaking the reconstituted solution or causing excessive foaming may result in problems with dissolution and the amount withdrawn from the vial.
- Add appropriate amount into 250 mL of 0.9% normal saline.
- Dextrose solution should not be used.
- For patients with known hypersensitivity to benzyl alcohol, vial can be reconstituted with sterile water and must be used immediately.
- Do NOT ADMINISTER AS AN IV PUSH OR BOLUS.

USE

Treatment of HER-2–positive breast cancer

PHARMACOKINETICS

Loading doses of 4 mg/kg followed by weekly 2 mg/kg doses produced mean half-life of 5.8 days.

USUAL DOSE AND SCHEDULE

1. Initial loading dose of 4 mg/kg over 90 minutes. Weekly maintenance dosage is 2 mg/kg over 30 minutes if initial loading dose is tolerated.
2. May be given at 6 mg/kg over 90 minutes every 3 weeks.

3. May be administered in an outpatient setting.

SIDE EFFECTS

- Most common side effects: fever and chills, primarily seen with the first infusion
- Serious side effects include:
  - Cardiotoxicity
  - Hypersensitivity reactions including anaphylaxis
  - Exacerbation of chemotherapy-induced neutropenia
  - Pulmonary events

STORAGE

- Do not freeze reconstituted or diluted solution.
- Reconstituted vials are stable for 28 days when refrigerated, 24 hours at room temperature.

COMPATIBILITY WITH OTHER DRUGS/INTRAVENOUS FLUIDS

Do not mix or dilute with other drugs. Do not mix or administer with dextrose solutions.

PREGNANCY

Category B

SPECIAL CONSIDERATIONS

- Development of ventricular dysfunction and congestive heart failure can occur. Left ventricular function should be assessed on all patients before and during treatment.
- Severe hypersensitivity, anaphylaxis infusion reactions, and pulmonary events have been reported during and after infusions.
- Important to follow infusion instructions and monitor patients closely during and after infusions

PATIENT EDUCATION

- Provide patient with written information.
- Educate the patient about potential side effects and management of side effects. Contact health care professional with any side effects.

- Reinforce follow-up appointments with health care professional.

Quadrivalent Human Papillomavirus (Types 6, 11, 16, 18) Recombinant Vaccine (Gardasil)

DRUG CLASS
Recombinant vaccine

ROUTE OF ADMINISTRATION
Intramuscular (IM) injection

HOW TO ADMINISTER/USUAL DOSE AND SCHEDULE
- Drug should be administered as an IM injection given in three separate doses of 0.5 mL each.
- Starting dose should be followed 2 months later with the second injection and last dose at month 6 after the start date with the last 0.5 mL injection.
- The IM injection should be administered into the deltoid muscle or the high anterolateral area of the thigh.
- Subcutaneous and intradermal injections have not been studied; this drug should not be given intravenously.

PRETREATMENT GUIDELINES
1. Patients should be between 9 and 26 years of age.
2. No pretreatment laboratory tests are required for use of this medication.

USE
Indicated for use on the prevention of human papillomavirus–associated diseases including:
- Cervical cancer
- Genital warts
- Cervical adenocarcinoma in situ
- Cervical intraepithelial neoplasia grades 1, 2, and 3
- Vulvar intraepithelial neoplasia grades 2 and 3
- Vaginal intraepithelial neoplasia grades 2 and 3

SIDE EFFECTS
- Injection site reactions (pain, swelling, erythema, pruritus)
- Fever
- Dizziness
- Malaise
- Diarrhea
- Nausea and vomiting
- Arthralgia
- Insomnia

STORAGE
- Refrigerate until use.
- Protect from light.

MIXING INSTRUCTIONS
Product comes in a premeasured, prefilled single-dose syringe for IM injection. No mixing is required.

COMPATIBILITY WITH OTHER DRUGS/INTRAVENOUS FLUIDS
Concomitant administration of other vaccines is not contraindicated as long as the sites are separate form one another.

PREGNANCY
Category B

PATIENT EDUCATION
- Instruct the patient that this vaccine is not 100% reliable in all cases.
- It does not protect against all causes of cervical or other gynecological malignancies and does not protect against other sexually transmitted diseases.
- Women should be advised to maintain regular follow-up with their physicians and have routine physical examinations and Papanicolaou smears done throughout their lives.

Chemotherapy

Jimmie G. Wells and Mary Murphy

This chapter provides basic concepts and principles related to chemotherapy and the primary mechanisms of action in the treatment goals of oncology patients. In addition, standards related to safe handling, administration, patient/family education, and specific specialty populations are reviewed.

BIOLOGIC AND PHARMACOLOGICAL BASES FOR CANCER CHEMOTHERAPY

Cancer is characterized by uncontrolled abnormal cell growth, often with invasion of healthy tissues locally or throughout the body (metastasis) (Vedes & Biderman, 2001). Chemotherapy is used to prevent cancer cells from multiplying, invading, or metastasizing. Cancer spreads primarily by direct extension through the lymph nodes or the bloodstream. Unlike other cancer treatment modalities (surgery and/or radiation), chemotherapy is a systemic treatment that enables the therapy to combat primary disease sites, areas of known metastasis, and possibly microscopic spread of disease.

The biological basis of cancer chemotherapy is grounded in the understanding of cell division or the cell cycle, which is reviewed in Section One: Cancer Pathophysiology. Briefly, the cell cycle is the mechanism by which all cells divide and replicate both normal and neoplastic cells. See the figure on right for phases of the cell cycle. Generally, the cell is most vulnerable during active division. The cell cycle is the process in which the cell replicates and passes all information needed to make an identical replica of itself. Most chemotherapeutic agents are classified according to where they affect cell cycle activity and how they affect cellular function.

The goals of chemotherapy are targeted at three areas; cure, control, or palliation. Cure is the desired outcome for all patients, but the likelihood depends on several factors at the time of diagnosis and other factors throughout the planned treatment course. The extent of disease at diagnosis, functional status of the patient, physiological presentation at diagnosis, and other socioeconomic influences determine the goal of cancer treatment for each patient. Cure may be further defined as a prolonged absence of disease. The term remission, which is an absence of detectable disease, may be used instead of cure because of the likelihood of recurrence that may be seen in some cancers, such as leukemia and lymphoma. Control is the goal of most therapy when a cure is unrealistic, given disease state or type. Control is also a cautious approach to treatment outcomes. Control focuses on maintaining or improving functional status in the presence of known disease without complete elimination of disease. Chemotherapy for palliation is therapy used when cure or control is not possible because of the extent of disease. Quality of life, disease symptom management, and end of life issues/hospice are a primary focus of control as a goal.

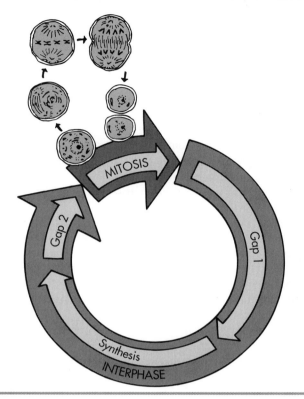

Phases of the cell cycle. (From McKance, K., & Huether, S. [1998]. *Pathophysiology: the biologic basis for disease in adults and children* [3rd ed..]. St. Louis: Mosby.)

The timing of chemotherapy in the treatment of cancer is another decision that must be made before therapy initiation. Chemotherapy may be given as adjuvant, neoadjuvant, chemopreventive, and myeloablative.

- Adjuvant therapy is given after a primary treatment (surgery, radiation); the goal is to reduce chance of recurrence by targeting remaining disease after primary treatment.
- Neoadjuvant therapy is given before another treatment with the goal of shrinking tumor before removal or decrease the likelihood of micrometastasis.
- Chemoprevention is the use of selected agents to prevent cancer from occurring in identified high-risk individuals (e.g., tamoxifen).

Myeloablation is the obliteration of bone marrow as preparation for stem cell or bone marrow transplantation (Kelleher, Polovich, & White, 2005). Chemotherapy is also used as a primary treatment to treat a tumor usually seen with minimal disease. It is very important that patient and family members are informed of treatment goals before the initiation of therapy to allow them to set realistic goals in their personal lives. The information needs to be repeated throughout the course of planned treatments.

Cancer Management

Chemotherapy is usually given as combination therapy using two or more agents together. The combinations of different agents affect the cell at different points in the cell cycle, allowing for maximum cell kill while minimizing toxicities. Principles for selection of chemotherapeutic agents for combination therapy include (1) choose drugs with single-agent activity, (2) avoid drugs with overlapping dose-limiting toxicities, (3) administer drugs at optimal dose and schedule as determined by clinical trials, (4) give chemotherapy at regular intervals, and (5) minimize the time between cycles (Tortorice, 2000). Combination therapy may also increase the range of drug activity resistance of tumor cell to single agents. In addition, combination chemotherapy may prevent or slow the development of resistance by the cancer cells and have a synergistic effect in combination with other agents (Brescia, 2003).

Tumor cells exposed to chemotherapy sometimes develop mechanisms to protect themselves against the drugs effect. Resistance is the term used to describe the process. Resistance may result from alteration in chemotherapeutic agent metabolism, alteration in cytotoxic targets, biochemical cofactor presence or absence, ability of cell to repair deoxyribonucleic acid (DNA) lesions, or decreased intracellular drug concentration. The most significant explanation of drug resistance is the P-glycoprotein efflux pump associated with overexpression of the MDR-1 gene (multidrug resistance) (Tortorice, 2000). Drug resistance may have many factors that affect response to therapy. Resistance may be inherent or acquired, single agent or multidrug, temporary or permanent. Prevention of drug resistance is another justification for combination chemotherapy (See the box below).

Biochemical Mechanisms Involved in Drug Resistance

- Impaired transport of the chemotherapeutic drug across the cell membrane
- Decreased intracellular activation of the chemotherapeutic drug
- Altered or increased amounts of the intracellular target for the chemotherapeutic drug
- Increased intracellular detoxification of the chemotherapeutic drug
- Increased efficiency of DNA repair of cellular damage caused by the chemotherapeutic drug
- The development of the multidrug resistant phenotype

From Miaskowski, C. & Viele, C. (1999). Cancer chemotherapy. In C. Miaskowski & P. Buchsel (Eds): *Oncology nursing: Assessment and clinical care*. Mosby: St. Louis, MO.

CELL CYCLE SPECIFICITY AND CHEMOTHERAPY

Chemotherapy uses knowledge of the cell cycle in the attempt to destroy or disrupt the abnormal growth of cancer cells. Most chemotherapeutic agents are classified according to where effects are produced in the cell cycle.

Cell cycle-specific agents exert effect when the cell is actively dividing (G1, S, G2, or M phases). Agents that are cell cycle specific tend to be schedule dependent because the greatest tumor kill is obtained when given in frequent divided doses or in continuous infusions to capture the cell in a specific phase. Cell cycle-nonspecific agents are effective in all cell cycle phases, including the resting phase (G0). Cell cycle-nonspecific agents also exhibit a steep dose-response curve that allows increased dosing and frequency (dose-dense/intense) with increased cell kill without extending duration of the cell exposure to the agent.

CHEMOTHERAPY CLASSIFICATIONS

Chemotherapeutic agents are classified by mechanism of action and specificity. The major classifications are listed in the box below. See the figure on page 185 for a diagram of chemotherapeutic agent mechanism of actions. Each classification contains agents that have similar characteristics and side effect profiles. Although the agents are similar, each agent must be addressed on an individual basis or in combination with finalization of a treatment plan.

Major Classification of Chemotherapeutic Drugs

Alkylating agents
Nitrosoureas
Antimetabolites
Antitumor antibiotics
Plant alkaloids
Miscellaneous agents
Hormones

From Miaskowski, C. & Viele, C. (1999). Cancer chemotherapy. In C. Miaskowski & P. Buchsel (Eds): *Oncology nursing: Assessment and clinical care*. Mosby: St. Louis, MO.

Alkylating Agents

Alkylating agents are cell cycle-nonspecific agents that bind with the DNA and protein molecules, which result in DNA strand breakage. Common toxicities include myelosuppression, hypersensitivity, renal impairment, gastrointestinal (GI) toxicities (nausea/vomiting, diarrhea, etc.), and cutaneous toxicities (alopecia, skin rashes). Side effects are dose dependent and may be cumulative. Alkylating agents are also strongly associated with secondary malignancies, which are usually different malignancies from the original disease that can occur months to years after treatment for a primary cancer. Routes of administration may include oral, intravenous, or topical, depending on the agent and treatment plan. Common alkylating agents include altretamine, busulfan, carboplatin, chlorambucil, cisplatin, cyclophosphamide, dacarbazine, ifosfamide, mechlorethamine, oxiliplatin, temozolomide, and thiotepa.

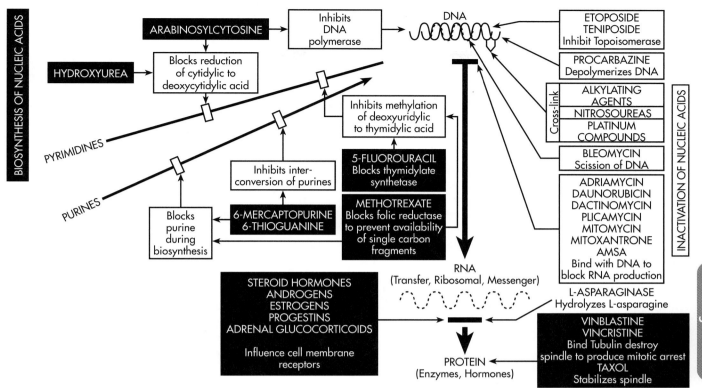

Mechanism of action of chemotherapeutic agents. (From Krakoff I. [1991]. Cancer chemotherapeutic and biologic agents. *CA: A Cancer Journal for Clinicians,* 41, 264-278.)

Nitrosoureas

Nitrosoureas are cell cycle–nonspecific agents that have the same mechanism of action and toxicities as alkylating agents with the inclusion of gonadal toxicities. They also have the ability to cross the blood-brain barrier. Nitrosoureas have a high lipid solubility that enables them free passage across membranes; therefore, they rapidly penetrate the blood-brain barrier, whereas most other agents are unable to do so (Calvo & Takimoto, 2005). Blood-brain barrier penetration allows nitrosoureas to be prominently used in the treatment of brain tumor and other central nervous system diseases. Common nitrosourea agents include carmustine, lomustine, and streptozocin.

Antimetabolites

Antimetabolites are cell cycle–specific agents that act in the S-phase of the cell cycle. Antimetabolites interfere with DNA synthesis by imitating the chemical structure of essential enzymes needed for DNA replication or by becoming incorporated into the structure of the DNA molecule. These agents are most effective against cancers that have a high growth fraction or rapidly dividing cells. Common toxicities include myelosuppression, GI toxicities (nausea/vomiting, mucositis, diarrhea), and cutaneous (rash, alopecia, photosensitivity, hyperpigmentation) toxicities. Routes of administration are based on agent and treatment plan and may include topical, oral, intravenous, intrathecal, and intramuscular. Common antimetabolites include capecitabine, cladribine, cytarabine, cytarabine liposomal, floxuridine, fludarabine, fluorouracil, gemcitabine, mercaptopurine, methotrexate, pentostatin, raltitrexed, thioguanine, trimetrexate, and uracil.

Antitumor Antibiotics

Antitumor antibiotics are cell cycle–nonspecific agents with variable sites of effect dependent on the agent used. Antitumor antibiotics are also referred to as natural products because they occur naturally or are synthesized from microorganisms and have both antimicrobial and cytotoxic activity. Antitumor antibiotics have two primary mechanisms of cell kill: free radical formation and the inhibition of topoisomerase II enzyme that results in DNA disruption and eventually cell death. Antitumor antibiotics are also known as anthracyclines. Cardiac tissues, because of a complex drug-iron complex, are especially vulnerable to anthracyclines (Tortorice, 2000). Common toxicities include myelosuppression and GI, cutaneous, and primary organ toxicities (cardiac, pulmonary). Routes of administration include intravenous, intra-arterial, or intravesical (bladder instillation). Common antitumor antibiotics include bleomycin, dactinomycin, daunorubicin, daunorubicin citrate liposomal, doxorubicin, doxorubicin liposomal, epirubicin, idarubicin, mitomycin, mitoxantrone, and valrubicin.

Plant Alkaloids

Plant alkaloids are cell cycle–specific agents that act by binding to specific cell proteins that cause mitotic arrest, causing a depletion of amino acids necessary for cell replication and apoptosis (programmed cell death). Plant alkaloids are naturally occurring alkaloids isolated from plant material or the result of synthetic and semisynthetic compounds originally extracted from plants. Common side effects include myelosuppression, GI toxicities (constipation, diarrhea), hypersensitivity reactions, and cutaneous (alopecia) and autonomic and peripheral neurological toxicities. Routes of administration are based on agent and treatment plan and include oral, intravenous, and intrathecal. Plant alkaloids include four different categories:

1. Camptothecins (irinotecan, topotecan)
2. Epipodophyllotoxins (etoposide)
3. Taxanes (paclitaxel, docetaxel)
4. Vinca alkaloids (vinblastine, vincristine, vinorelbine)

Microtubular Stabilizing Agents

A number of agents are in clinical development that target microtubules. Intact microtubules are needed for the formation of mitotic spindles in the process of cell division. This new class of chemotherapy drugs is called epothilones (Goodin, Kane, & Rubin, 2004; Petrylak & Kelly, 2004). The agents have been isolated from the mycobacterium, *Sporangium cellulosum*. The drugs work in the G2/M phase of the cell cycle to initiate apoptosis. Epothilones provide an advantage over taxanes by binding to a different site. Therefore, epothilones provide activity in cancers that have developed taxane resistance.

Epothilones have shown activity in several cancers, including breast, lymphoma, renal, prostate, and ovarian. Side effects are similar to those of taxanes. Hypersensitivity reactions have been reported in cremophor-based epothilone agents. Other side effects to monitor for are neutropenia, peripheral neuropathy, fatigue, arthralgia, myalgia, nausea/vomiting, diarrhea, and stomatitis. Several of the current agents in development are ixabepilone and patupilone (Goodin, Kane, & Rubin, 2004; Petrylak & Kelly, 2004).

Miscellaneous Agents

Miscellaneous agents are cell cycle nonspecific. They act by inhibiting protein synthesis, blocking DNA replication, or triggering mechanisms that mediate cell death. Common side effects include myelosuppression, GI toxicity, and hepatotoxicity. Routes of administration include intravenous and oral. Common miscellaneous agents include arsenic trioxide, asparaginase, bortezomib, mesylate, mitotane, pegaspargase, and procarbazine.

See the table on page 187 for classification of chemotherapeutic agents.

PATIENT AND FAMILY PREPARATION FOR CHEMOTHERAPY ADMINISTRATION

Patient and family interactions are an important dynamic and must be used to prepare for the initiation of cancer treatment. Preparation before the treatment is vital to the overall success or lack thereof to prescribed therapy. Patient and family assessment and education are critical and must be geared toward the individual needs of the patient.

Patient and Family Assessment

The nurse administrating the chemotherapy should conduct a pretreatment assessment of the patient according to the guidelines listed in the box on page 187. Along with these guidelines, the nurse should keep in mind that patients will come with a lifetime of influences that affect the response to all of the changes involved with a diagnosis of cancer and required treatment. Past experiences affect their current physical presentation at diagnosis and how they will perceive current interactions with the health care team. Preconceived ideas of cancer, cultural and ethnic background, adult learning style, educational background, socioeconomic status, past coping mechanisms, and numerous other influences will affect the needed preparation for chemotherapy. Inclusion of family, significant others, or existing support systems is critical in preparation for chemotherapy initiation.

Patient and Family Education

The education of patients and family is a continuous process that should begin at the time of diagnosis with additional teaching before the administration of chemotherapy. Principles of adult learning should be incorporated in all teaching sessions. Strongly encourage patients to bring someone with them to all sessions. This will allow patients to have needed support during a stressful and physically demanding process. The presence of a trusted individual will help to ensure understanding of information given.

Formulation of a teaching plan should incorporate knowledge of the patient's and family's primary language and level of understanding, ability to read, readiness to learn, anxiety levels, and any other potential barriers to learning (Miaskowski, 1997; Powell, 1996). The nurse should review the topics outlined in the boxes on p. 187 and provide written material to reinforce all verbal instructions.

SAFE HANDLING

One of the most prevailing issues for staff is the inherent potential for harm in the delivery of care to cancer patients. Chemotherapy agents are hazardous drugs. The term "hazardous drugs" leads one to proceed with caution in

Chemotherapy Classifications

Drug Class	Mechanism of Action	Drug Name
Alkylating agents	Cell cycle nonspecific Binds with DNA and protein molecules	Altretamine Busulfan Carboplatin Chlorambucil Cisplatin Cyclophosphamide Dacarbazine Ifosfamide mechlorethamine Oxiliplatin Temozolomide Thiotepa

Antitumor antibiotic	Cell cycle nonspecific	Bleomycin
		Dactinomycin
		Daunorubicin
		Daunorubicin
		  citrate liposomal
		Doxorubicin
		Doxorubicin
		  liposomal
		Epirubicin
		Idarubicin
		Mitomycin
		Mitoxantrone
		Valrubicin

Plant alkaloid
  Camptothecins
  Epipodophyllotoxins
  Taxanes
  Vinca alkaloids
	Cell cycle specific
	Bind to certain cell proteins to initiate mitotic arrest
		Camptothecins
		  Irinotecan
		  Topotecan
		Epipodophyllotoxins
		  Etoposide
		Taxanes
		  Paclitaxel
		  Docetaxel
		Vinca alkaloids
		  Vinblastine
		  Vincristine
		  Vinorelbine

Antimetabolites	Cell cycle specific
	Acts in the S-phase
		Cepecitabine
		Cladribine
		Cytarabine
		Cytarabine
		  liposomal
		Decitabine
		Floxuridine
		Flidarabine
		Fluorouracil
		Gemcitabine
		  mercaptopurine
		Methotrexate
		Pentostatin
		Raltitrexed
		Thioguanine
		Trimetrexate
		Uracil

Nitrosoureas	Cell cycle nonspecific Binds with DNA and protein molecules Crosses blood-brain barrier	Carmustine Lomustine Streptozocin

Microtubular stabilizer
Epothilones
	Cell cycle specific
	Acts in the G2/M-phase of the cell cycle
		Epothilones
		  Ixabepilone
		  Patupilone

Miscellaneous	Cell cycle non-specific	Arsenic trioxide Asparaginase Bortezomib mesylate Mitotane Pegaspargase Procarbazine

Guidelines for the Pretreatment Assessment of the Chemotherapy Patient

OBTAIN A COMPLETE PATIENT AND FAMILY HISTORY
1. Recent treatment, including surgery, prior chemotherapy, radiation therapy, biotherapy, or hormone therapy
2. Previous and concurrent medical illnesses
3. Previous and concurrent surgical problems
4. Laboratory data
   - Complete blood cell count with differential
   - Liver function tests: bilirubin, alkaline phosphatase, alanine aminotransferase
   - Renal function tests: serum creatine, creatine clearance, uric acid level
   - Pregnancy test for women of childbearing age with undocumented surgical sterilization (tubal ligation/hysterectomy)

OBTAIN A PSYCHOSOCIAL ASSESSMENT OF THE PATIENT AND FAMILY MEMBERS
Reactions to the diagnosis of cancer
   1. Previous experience with chemotherapy
   2. Coping styles
   3. Interpersonal resources
   4. Financial resources

From Miaskowski C & Buchsel P. (1999). *Oncology nursing assessment and clinical care.* St. Louis: Mosby.

Patient Education Regarding Chemotherapy

1. Review the treatment plan and protocol.
   - Names and actions of the drugs to be administered by the nurse
   - Names and actions of the drugs to be taken by the patient at home
   - Schedule of drug administration
   - Length of the treatment plan
2. Review the purpose or the goals (i.e., cure palliation) of the chemotherapeutic treatment.
3. Review the potential side effects of chemotherapy and self-care activities to prevent or treat the side effects.
4. Review the schedule and rationale for diagnostic tests.
5. Provide the patient and family members with information on when and how to contact the nurse or the physician.

Data from Oncology Nursing Society. (2005). *Chemotherapy and biotherapy guidelines and recommendations for practice* (2nd ed.). ONS: Pittsburgh, PA.

Patient Teaching Priorities for Chemotherapy

1. Assess willingness, readiness to learn and barriers to learning.
2. Inform patient/family about schedule of activities of chemotherapy, laboratory testing, and diagnostic tests
3. Encourage practice and repetition of newly learned skill to enhance learner's performance
4. Validate aseptic technique for medication self-administration of medication
5. Provide written material for all information given

Data from Otto, S. E. (2001). Chemotherapy. In S. E. Otto (Ed.) *Oncology nursing* (4th ed., pp. 638-671). St. Louis: Mosby.

Cancer Management

the administration of these agents. Hazardous drug handling guidelines have been available for 20 years. According to the American Society of Health System Pharmacists (ASHP), any drug that requires special handling is referred to as a hazardous drug (ASHP, 2005). Recommendations for practice have been established by the Oncology Nursing Society (ONS), the Occupational Safety and Health Administration (OSHA), and the National Institute for Occupational Safety and Health (NIOSH) for safe handling of chemotherapy. The four major goals for safe handling of chemotherapy are listed in the table below.

For a drug to be classified as a hazardous drug, one or more of the following criteria must be met: genotoxicity, carcinogenicity, teratogenicity or reproductive/fertility toxicity, and drugs that mimic existing drugs determined hazardous by the above standards (NIOSH, 2004). Drugs classified as hazardous include antineoplastic or cytotoxic agents, biological agents, antiviral agents, and immunosuppressive agents. Health care professionals involved in preparation, administration, and disposal of hazardous drugs and waste face potential work-related exposure (OSHA, 2004; OSHA, 1995). Each institution that uses hazardous drugs must have a hazardous drug safety and health plan. These plans may be better known as Material Safety Data Sheets (MSDS) or a "Right to Know" manual.

Potential routes of exposure are limited to the following: absorption through skin or mucous membranes, injection, ingestion, and inhalation (Kelleher, Polovich, & White, 2005). Recommended guidelines focus on elimination or minimizing these routes of possible exposure. Safety guidelines must be used in the storage/labeling, transportation, preparation, administration, and disposal of hazardous drugs. Environmental safety must also be a major portion of safety guidelines.

Environmental

The compounding and preparation of hazardous drugs should be done in a controlled area with access limited to authorized personnel specially trained in handling requirements. The ASHP further recommends that specific considerations for the following in the hazardous drug safety and health plan for drug preparation areas:

- Establishment of a designated hazardous drug handling area
- Use of containment devices such as biological safety cabinets
- Procedures for safe removal of contaminated waste
- Decontamination procedures

Goals, Criteria, and Recommendations for the Safe Handling of Chemotherapeutic Drugs

Goals	Criteria and Recommendations
GOAL 1 Accidental contamination of health care environment, resulting in exposure of personnel, patients, visitors, and family members to hazardous substances, is prevented by maintaining the physical integrity and security of packages of hazardous drugs.	Limited access to authorized staff Hazardous drug identification Policies for transporting hazardous drugs Storage facilities designed to prevent breakage and limit exposure from leakage
GOAL 2 The preparation of hazardous drugs does not result in contamination of the health care work environment or excessive exposure of personnel, patients, or family members to hazardous drug powders, dusts, liquids, or mists.	Written policies for drug preparation Orientation of personnel Established method of evaluation of staff adherence to policies and procedures Policies for protective apparel Proper manipulative technique for drug mixture Biological safety cabinet Procedures established for noninjectable dosage forms Procedures for accidental exposure Labeling for hazardous drug handling
GOAL 3 Procedures for administering hazardous drugs prevent the accidental exposure of patients and staff and contamination of the work environment.	Training programs for personnel Standards for safe administration Readily available protective materials
GOAL 4 The health care setting, its staff, patients, contract workers, visitors, and the outside environment are not exposed to or contaminated with hazardous drug waste materials produced in the course of using these drugs.	Written policies established and maintained Identification, containment, and segregation of hazardous drug waste materials Protocols and materials available to clean up spills Disposal in accordance with state, federal, and local regulations

From Fisher, D. S., Knopf, M. T., & Durivage, H. J. (1993). *The cancer chemotherapy handbook.* St. Louis: Mosby.

Biological safety cabinets should meet the criteria listed in the box below.

Biological Safety Cabinet

1. Provide vertical laminar air flow.
2. Eliminate exhaust through a high-efficiency particulate air filter. Ideally a biological safety cabinet should be vented to the outside (NIOSH, 2004).
3. Have blower that operates continuously (ASHP, 1990).
4. Be located in a low-traffic area to reduce interference with air flow
5. Be used by individuals trained to use techniques that reduce interference with air flow
6. Be serviced according to the manufacturer's recommendation
7. Be recertified every 6 months (ASHP, 1990)

Adapted from Oncology Nursing Society. (2005). *Chemotherapy and biotherapy guidelines and recommendations for practice* (2nd ed.). ONS: Pittsburgh, PA.

Other critical safety guidelines incorporated the use of appropriate personal protective equipment (PPE). Appropriate PPE includes the uses of gloves, gowns, respirator, and face/eye protection. The clinical setting and potential risks of exposure should determine PPE selection. PPE selection should also be guided with avoidance of latex-containing materials to avoid possible sensitivity reactions. Wear PPEs whenever there is a risk of exposure or release into the environment. See the box below for specific PPE recommendations in the use of hazardous drugs.

Appropriate Personal Protective Equipment With Hazardous Drugs

GLOVES
- Meet testing standards set by the American Society for Testing and Materials for use with hazardous drugs, designated "chemotherapy gloves"
- Inspect for defects before donning
- Powder free
- Disposable
- Double glove
- Nitrile or neoprene material (latex sensitivity)
- Change after 30-60 minutes or immediately with visible contamination or damage

GOWNS
- Disposable
- Lint free
- Low permeability fabric
- Solid front with back closure
- Long sleeves with tight cuffs
- Glove cuffs should extend over the gown cuffs.
- Gown should not be reused.
- Discard if visibly contaminated, before leaving drug preparation areas, and after handling hazardous drugs.

RESPIRATORS
- NIOSH-approved respirator mask
- Used when cleaning a hazardous drug spill
- Surgical masks **do not** provide respiratory protection.

EYE/FACE PROTECTION
- Wear whenever there is a possibility of splash
- Goggles or face shield should be available wherever hazardous drugs are prepared/mixed or administered.

Storage and Labeling

Careful attention must be paid to all potential exposure, including storage and labeling of chemotherapeutic agents. Agents should be stored in a location that permits appropriate temperature and safety inspections/regulations. Labeling should indicate the contents as a hazardous drug. Standardized instructions (MSDS sheets) on what to do in the event of accidental exposure should be readily available in all areas where hazardous drugs are stored, prepared, transported, administered, and disposed of. In the home setting, the same guidelines are to be followed and patient/family provided with extensive education.

Additional safety guidelines are listed in the box on page 190.

When chemotherapy is given in the home setting, standardized safety guidelines must be followed. Patient and family will need to be instructed in proper handling in the home. Education should include the following:
- Keep drugs out of reach of children and pets.
- Protect from puncture or breakage.
- Do not remove labels.
- Store in an area free of moisture and temperature extremes.
- Have a spill kit in the home with detailed instructions on appropriate use.
- Maintain a list of emergency contact numbers.

Transportation

Hazardous drugs should be transported in a sealed leak-proof container. Always luer-lock the end of the syringe and **NEVER** transport with needles in place. The outermost container should have a "hazardous" label. Transporters should have education on hazardous risk, safety precautions, and knowledge of spill kit use in the event of a spill or contamination.

Spill Kit

A hazardous drug spill kit should be available wherever hazardous drugs are stored, transported, prepared, or administered. All staff that work with hazardous drugs should be trained in spill cleanups. See the box on page 190 for appropriate contents of a spill kit.

Spill kits may be purchased commercially or prepared by the individual institutions as long as they meet approved guidelines.

The following are guidelines in the event of a hazardous drug spill (Kellehere, Polovich, & White, 2005):
- Post sign(s) that warns others of spill.
- Don two pairs of chemotherapy-safe gloves, disposable gown, and a face shield.
- Wear respirator.
- Contain spill with plastic-backed absorbent pad.

Hazardous Drug Safety Guidelines

1. The use of plastic-backed absorbent pad on work and delivery surfaces
2. The use of closed-system drug transfer devices
3. Use safe technique in the opening of ampule neck.
4. Avoid pressure buildup when reconstituting drugs packaged in vials if closed system not available.
5. Use tubing and syringes with luer-lock fitting.
6. Avoid overfilling syringes.
7. Prime all tubing with fluids that does not contain the hazardous drug.
8. Place a label on each container that says "Cytotoxic Drug" or similar warning.
9. Wipe outside of the container with moist gauze before placing it in a sealable bag for transport.
10. Dispose of all materials that have come in contact with hazardous drug in waste container designated for hazardous waste.
11. Remove and discard outer gloves and gown before removing inner gloves.
12. Wash hands before leaving work area.

Data from Oncology Nursing Society. (2005). *Chemotherapy and biotherapy guidelines and recommendations for practice* (2nd ed.). ONS: Pittsburgh, PA: ONS.

Contents of Spill Kit

Number	Item
1	Gowns with cuffs and back closure (made of water nonpermeable fabric)
1 pair	Shoe covers
2 pairs	Gloves
1 pair	Utility gloves
1 pair	Chemical splash goggles
1	Rebreather mask (National Institute of Occupational Safety and Health approved)
1	Disposable dust pan (to collect any broken glass)
1	Plastic scraper (to scoop materials into dust pan)
2	Plastic-backed or absorbable towels
1 each	250-mL and 1-L spill control pillows
2	Disposable sponges (one to clean up spill, one to clean up floor after removal of spill)
1	"Sharps" container
2	Large, heavy-duty waste disposal bags
1	Container of 70% alcohol for cleaning soiled area

From: Miaskowski, C. & Viele, C. (1999). Cancer Chemotherapy. In C. Miaskowski & P. Buchsel (Eds): *Oncology nursing: Assessment and clinical care.* p. 101. St. Louis, MO: Mosby.

- Pick up glass fragments by using scoop or utility gloves worn over chemotherapy gloves. Place glass in a puncture-proof container
- Place puncture-proof container inside a bag and seal. Double-bag all material and label outermost bag as hazardous waste.
- Remove PPE as previously instructed and place in disposable waste bag and seal.
- Place all items in a puncture-proof container.

Documentation of a spill should include the name of drug, approximate volume spilled, how the spill occurred, spill management procedure followed, names of personnel, patients, and others exposed, and a list of personnel notified of spill.

Waste and Disposal

Universal precautions are used when handling the blood, emesis, or excreta of a patient receiving chemotherapy and within 48 hours of chemotherapy completion. Apply protective barrier ointment to the skin of patients who are incontinent and clean skin with each diaper change. It is recommended that toilet be flushed with the lid down. Although lowering the lids in the home setting is applicable, most institutions do not have lids, so efforts must again focus on protective barriers for employees. Flushing the toilet twice has been a long-standing practice and may still be helpful with low-volume flush toilets found in home settings,. However, most institutions have high-volume flush toilets that may not require double flushing (Polovich, 2003). All linen with exposure to chemotherapy should be laundered separately in hot water. Use leak-proof disposable pads for incontinent episodes if possible. Discard all disposable items in an appropriately

labeled hazardous waste container (Kelleher, Polovich, & White, 2005).

Proper Care of Vesicants and Irritants

Although chemotherapy requires special handling to minimize exposure, special considerations must be incorporated for the patients who are receiving agents identified as vesicants or irritants.

- Vesicants are agents with the ability to cause blistering or tissue necrosis.
- Irritants are agents with the ability to cause aching, tightness, and phlebitis with or without a local inflammatory reaction but do not cause tissue necrosis.
- Extravasation is the passage of chemotherapeutic agents into tissue. Necrosis or sloughing may occur.

See the table on page 191 for a list of vesicants and irritants along with nursing considerations.

Risk factors for extravasation include the following:

- Small/fragile veins
- Poor vascular integrity
- Peripheral neuropathy
- Previous multiple venipuncture
- Limited vein selection
- Peripheral edema
- Unstable venous access because of patient condition
- Altered mental status of patient that renders him or her unable to report discomfort at intravenous (IV) site
- Site of venous access (avoid veins in hand, wrist, and antecubital fossa whenever possible)
- Device selection (avoid use of steel-tipped winged infusions) (Kelleher, Polovich, & White, 2005)

Extravasation can occur in peripherally inserted central catheters (PICC) and central access devices (CAD).

Factors related to potential extravasation in a PICC line or CAD include catheter damage, displacement, and migration.

Prevention and early detection is the primary focus to avoid extravasation. Signs and symptoms of extravasation include the following:

- Severe swelling
- Stinging, burning, or intense pain
- Blotchy redness around the needle site; not always present at the time of extravasation
- Inability to obtain blood return
- Ulceration develops within 48 to 96 hours

Nursing Actions/Considerations for Vesicants and Irritants

Agent name	Nursing Actions/Considerations
VESICANTS	
Cisplatin	Isotonic sodium thiosulfate—inject subcutaneously into affected tissue
Mechlorethamine	Isotonic sodium thiosulfate—inject subcutaneously into affected tissue
Doxorubicin	Apply ice four times daily for 24-48 hours Elevate site for 48 hours
Daunorubicin	Topical dimethylsulfoxide showed benefit in mouse experiments
Mitomycin	Protect from sunlight
Dactinomycin	Apply ice Elevate site for 48 hours
Mitoxantrone	Unknown
Epirubicin	Unknown
Vincristine	Apply warm pack 15-20 minutes at least four times daily for 24-48 hours Elevate site
Vinblastine	Apply warm pack 15-20 minutes at least four times daily for 24-48 hours Elevate site
Vindesine	Apply warm pack 15-20 minutes at least four times daily for 24-48 hours Elevate site
Vinorelbine	Apply warm pack 15-20 minutes at least four times daily for 24-48 hours Elevate site
Paclitaxel	Apply ice for 15-20 minutes at least four time daily for 24-48 hours
IRRITANTS	
Carboplatin	May cause phlebitis Local care measures unknown
Dacarbazine	May cause phlebitis Protect from light
Ifosfamide	May cause phlebitis Local care measures unknown
Oxiliplatin	Consider high dose of dexamethasone
Carmustine	May cause phlebitis Local care measures unknown
Daunorubicin citrate liposomal	May cause pain or burning at IV site Little known information
Doxorubicin liposomal	May produce redness and tissue edema
Bleomycin	May cause irritation to tissue Little information is known
Etoposide	Apply warm pack only if large amount of concentrated solution extravasates
Teniposide	Apply warm pack only if large amount of concentrated solution extravasates

Data from Oncology Nursing Society. (2005). *Chemotherapy and biotherapy guidelines and recommendations for practice* (2nd ed.). Pittsburgh, PA: ONS.

Nurses must be knowledgeable of which agents can cause this damage, be aware of the warning symptoms, and be familiar with agents that may cause extravasation. In the event extravasation does occur, nursing management is critical to patient outcome. Initial management includes the following measures:

- Stop infusion.
- Disconnect IV tubing from site or device. Do not remove device or catheter.
- Attempt to aspirate residual drug from device with small (1-3 mL) syringe.
- Notify physician.
- Apply hot or cold compress as indicated.
- Initiate antidote, if applicable.

After extravasation, the following measures should be taken:

- Photograph the extravasation site and repeat weekly if appropriate.
- Instruct patient to rest and elevate extremity for 48 hours.
- Give written instructions regarding what symptoms to report immediately.
- Arrange for return appointment.
- Consult plastic surgeon, if applicable.

Extravasation is a serious matter that causes added pain, discomfort, wound healing issues, and treatment delays. By following administration guidelines, nurses can limit the possibility of an extravasation.

ROUTES OF ADMINISTRATION

Armed with knowledge of the characteristics of the different chemotherapeutic agents to be given, the next decision is route of administration selection. Chemotherapeutic agents are administered by multiple routes to achieve systemic or regional delivery of the agents.

The goal of systemic therapy is to attain a drug concentration that is sufficient to achieve a therapeutic toxic effect in the presumed or known metastatic disease without causing excessive toxicity to normal tissue. Regional chemotherapy is directed toward the goal of delivering the agent directly into the blood supply of the tumor or the cavity/area in which the tumor is located. Regional administration of chemotherapy often allows for higher concentrations of the drug to be delivered to the area of the tumor with fewer systemic side effects.

The major routes used for systemic administration include oral, intravenous, subcutaneous, and intramuscular. Regional routes include intrathecal, intra-arterial, and intracavity. Once the route of administration has been identified, appropriate patient/family and staff education must occur.

Education should include the identified route of administration, potential complications of identified route, and the possible use of vascular access device. With administration routes that may be used in the home (oral, subcutaneous [SQ]/intramuscular [IM], IV) setting, special attention should be given to instructions on keeping agents out of the reach of small children and pets, proper storage without temperature extremes, and the use of spill kits.

Oral

The use of oral chemotherapeutic agents has escalated in the last few years. Advantages with oral chemotherapeutic agents include ease of use, portability, and patient independence. Several factors need to be evaluated prior to initiating oral therapy. Factors include the following:

1. Availability of the drug in an oral formulation
2. Functional status of the gastrointestinal tract
3. Presence of nausea, vomiting, or dysphasia
4. Patient's level of consciousness
5. Patient's willingness and ability to adhere with the dosing schedule
6. Cost and reimbursement issues for oral preparations

Although it may seem deceptively simple to administer oral preparations, oral agents require special consideration and planning. Extensive patient/family and staff education should occur. Teaching should include the name, dose, and time agent should be taken, known, or anticipated side effects, established prophylaxis for known side effect, appropriate physician or nurse notification, and safe handling issues as well. To ensure compliance with the administration schedule, assess the following factors: a caregiver(s) presence in the home, living conditions (plumbing, electricity, etc.), access to emergency assistance, and whether the patient will need nursing follow-up in the home. Patients may also benefit from some form of organized delivery system (pill box) and a daily diary. A diary will allow consistent documentation of agent administration, side effect occurrence, and barriers to agent being administered. It will also serve as an incentive to maintain scheduled dosing of medication.

Subcutaneous and Intramuscular

Similar to the oral agents, administration of chemotherapy by SQ or IM routes continues to allow a high degree of patient independence. Although SQ or IM delivery methods cause some discomfort at the site of injection, it is usually short term and fairly well tolerated. Patient and family education on self-injection, disposal of sharps, and site rotation and monitoring should be incorporated in the teaching plan along with safe handling in the preparation, administration, and disposal of waste in the home setting. Although the advantages are similar to those of oral preparations, the disadvantages vary greatly. Disadvantages include pain/discomfort at site of injection, possible infection of injection sites, and bleeding.

Topical

Although the route of topical application of chemotherapy is not frequently used, it remains an option. Careful guidelines should be adhered to with the application of topical chemotherapy. Strict adherence to wearing PPE is critical along with environmental control during application and disposal of waste.

Intravenous

Administration of chemotherapy by the IV route is the most common route used in most patient care settings (Camp-Sorrell, 2004). Methods of administration include the following:

- Push—administered through syringe directly into vein
- Free-flow with a direct push—agent administered with syringe into the side port of a free-flowing IV
- Piggyback—use of secondary bag/bottle and tubing connected to a primary infusion of IV fluids
- Continuous infusion—usually given over 12 hours up to 5 to 7 days

The choice of IV method of administration depends on several factors, including the venous status of patient, vesicant/irritant potential of agent, and patient preference. In the use of peripheral site of administration, several factors must be incorporated. The patient's age and vein status, the drugs infused, and the expected period of infusion determine selection of the appropriate site and equipment. Select the shortest catheter with the smallest gauge appropriate for the type and duration of the infusion. See the box on page 193 for vein selection guidelines and the table on page 193 for issues and arguments for and against chemotherapy administration practices.

Other options for IV administration include the use of central venous catheters or central venous access devices (VAD). Types of devices include percutaneous subclavian catheters (Hickman, Groshon, Broviac, etc.), peripherally inserted central catheters (PICC), and implanted devices/ports (chemoport, passport, infusa port, etc.). With all of these devices, proper placement must initially be verified by radiographic study. Thereafter, placement is verified by aspirating for a blood return before each use. Follow manufacturer or institutional guidelines for care, maintenance, and use of central access devices. Infection prevention should be a primary focus of VAD use with their direct entry/access to the vascular system (Otto, 2001).

Intrathecal

Intrathecal (IT) chemotherapy is the direct installation of chemotherapy into the central nervous system (CNS) by lumbar puncture or through an implanted intraventricular device (e.g., Ommaya reservoir). This method allows therapy to bypass the blood-brain barrier issues with direct entry into the CNS. There is more consistent drug concentration in the cerebrospinal fluid with IT administration. Delivery requires multiple invasive procedures (lumbar punctures) or surgery for device implantation. Therapy administration requires a physician, specially trained registered nurse, or a nurse practitioner to access and administer chemotherapy by the IT route. Patients should be monitored for headache or other signs of increased intracranial pressure.

Peripheral Vein Selection

EXISTING INTRAVENOUS SITE
- Do not use site greater than 24 hours old.
- Assess site for inflammation/infiltration; if present, choose alternate site.
- Assess for blood return and patency.

NEW INTRAVENOUS SITE
- Select vein that is smooth and pliable.
- Avoid small, fragile, injured, or sclerosed veins.
- Avoid extremity with altered venous return or lymphedema.
- Avoid lower extremities.
- Avoid veins in the wrist, hand, or antecubital areas.

Adapted from Oncology Nursing Society. (2005). Chemotherapy and biotherapy guidelines and recommendations for practice (2nd ed.). Pittsburgh, PA: ONS.

Intra-Arterial

Intra-arterial chemotherapy involves cannulation of the artery that provides a tumor's blood supply or directly into an organ by way of an artery. The primary use of this route is the hepatic artery for the management of liver metastasis (Goodman, 2000). For consistent delivery of chemotherapy, the drug is delivered via an implanted pump. The pump is used once correct placement is verified. Using a noncoring needle, the pump is accessed and filled with either chemotherapy or heparinized sterile saline solution. Nursing considerations involve monitoring for drug side effects and potential pump complications, such as infections, occlusion, extravasation, and malfunction.

Intracavity

Intracavity is the direct instillation of chemotherapy into a body cavity. Examples include intrapleural (lung),

Controversial Issues and Arguments For and Against Vesicant Chemotherapy Administration Practices

Controversial Practices	For	Against
Vesicant first	Vascular integrity decreases over time Initially, practitioner's assessment skills more accurate Patient may become more sedated from antiemetic and less able to report burning, pain at infusion site	Vesicant is irritating, compromising integrity of vein Nonvesicants are less irritating to veins Venous spasm may occur early during injection, altering assessment of patency
Side arm administration	Free-running IV lines allow for maximal dilution of drugs that could be potentially irritating	
Direct push administration	Integrity of vein can be assessed more easily, and the early signs of extravasation can be noted more easily	
Use of antecubital fossa	Larger veins permit more rapid infusion/administration of drug Larger veins permit potentially irritating chemotherapeutic agents to reach the general circulation sooner with less irritation to small veins	Arm mobility is restricted with needle in place The risk of extravasation is increased because of patient mobility (e.g., coughing, vomiting) Infiltration could require extensive reconstruction efforts with limited arm use during the healing process, resulting in increased morbidity and decreased function Because of the subcutaneous tissues, early infiltration is more difficult to assess
Large-gauge needles (e.g., 19 and 21 scalp vein needles)	Potentially irritating chemotherapeutic agents can reach the general circulation sooner, with reduced irritation to the peripheral veins Drug administration time is decreased, which reduces the patient's exposure to a potentially stressful environment	
Small-gauge needles (e.g., 23 and 25 scalp vein needles)	Smaller-gauge needles are less likely to puncture the wall of a small vein Scar tissue may be formed with needle insertion; small-gauge needles cause less scar tissue formation The patient may have less pain during the insertion of a smaller needle Increased blood flow around a smaller-bore needle increases dilution of the chemotherapeutic agent Mechanical phlebitis may be minimized with a smaller bore needle Potential episodes of nausea and vomiting may be decreased by slow infusion of the chemotherapeutic agents	

From Powell, L. L. (1996). *Cancer chemotherapy guidelines and recommendations for practice*, Pittsburgh, PA: Oncology Nursing Press.

intraperitoneal (abdomen), and intravesicular (bladder). This route allows direct exposure of known area of disease to chemotherapy. Side effects of this route are directly related to the cavity receiving instillation. The intrapleural instillation is usually geared at sclerosing the pleural lining to prevent reoccurrence of effusions and requires placement of a thoracotomy (chest) tube. The intraperitoneal route requires instillation into a peritoneal catheter or intraperitoneal port. The intravesicular route requires the placement of a Foley catheter. Each of these methods carries the risk of infection along with other site-specific complication. Special attention must be given to PPE (including face shield) with the use of this route (Kelleher, Polovich, & White, 2005).

ADMINISTRATION IN SPECIALTY POPULATIONS

There are identified specialty populations in the treatment of cancer in adult populations. Although cancer is a difficult prospect in the best of situations, the addition of special-needs populations requires increased knowledge from treatment providers. Cancer during pregnancy and in the elderly will be reviewed with appropriate interventions discussed.

Pregnancy

Cancer is the second leading cause of death during the reproductive years. The most common cancers associated with pregnancy are lymphoma, leukemia, malignant melanoma, and cancers of the breast, cervix, ovary, and colorectum. A diagnosis of cancer during pregnancy is a devastating time for expectant mothers and family members. Not only must they consider the mother's health, but also the health of the unborn fetus cannot be ignored.

Chemotherapy has been administered before and concurrent with pregnancy. The decision to initiate chemotherapy during the first trimester usually results in a therapeutic abortion before the initiation of therapy. Chemotherapy may be given in the second and third trimesters of pregnancy with careful monitoring of mother and fetus and careful selection of the agent used. When to proceed with chemotherapy is ultimately the mother's choice. The options are to delay treatment until the fetus is viable or near term or to proceed with therapy during pregnancy (Goodman, 2000). Nursing interventions include incorporation of standardized education and emotional support for patient and family in a nonjudgmental, professional manner.

Elderly

It is estimated that by 2030 approximately 70 million people will be 65 to 85 years of age or older. Age is the most important factor in determining cancer risk. More than 50% of all cancers occur in persons over the age of 65 years (Phillips, Brown, & Belcher; 2004). Physiological changes are a part of the normal aging process the body goes through. The physiological changes that occur with biological aging are important to consider when combined

with a cancer diagnosis and planning treatment for the elderly (Repetto, 2003). These changes will affect decisions of treatment to be made for some elderly, but not all. Physiological status and not chronological age should dictate treatment options. Myths and misconceptions held by both the elderly and the public in general are obstacles to prevention, early detection, diagnosis, and treatment of cancer in this group. Some of these misconceptions include poor health as a natural part of aging, the question of dementia and self-care issues, multiple comorbidities eliminate the possibility of chemotherapy, and so forth. Other issues that factually affect treatment options include impaired immune system, inadequate nutritional status, obesity, polypharmacy, poor/limited support systems, and limited financial resources. Although consideration of these issues must be incorporated into the plan of care for the elderly, it does not eliminate the possibility of productive treatment for a cancer diagnosis. Treatment plans should be individualized to meet the individual needs of the elderly. The elderly will require close, careful monitoring and the addition of supportive care while receiving chemotherapy (Hood & Musenski, 2003).

Palliative Chemotherapy

- Palliative care is defined as the active total care of patients whose disease is not responsive to curative treatment (World Health Organization, 1990, NCCN, 2003).
- Palliative chemotherapy is defined as the use of antitumor therapy for control of symptoms that are directly or indirectly due to the malignancy (Prommer, 2004).

Criteria

- Review patient and caregiver wishes for further treatment.
- Evaluate the patient's performance status and comorbid conditions that may affect treatment tolerance.
- Determine the response rate and symptom management potential related to toxicity and quality of life.
- Consider outcomes to the expected clinical prognosis.

Common Palliative Symptom Improvement

- Pain
- Shortness of breath
- Bowel obstruction
- Nausea/vomiting (Weissman, 2000)

Clinical Diagnosis

- All cancers are appropriate for palliative chemotherapy.
- Common palliative chemotherapy treatment diagnoses:

○ Breast
○ Colon
○ Lung
○ Pancreas
○ Prostate
○ GI

Common Types of Palliative Drugs
• Gemzar
• Temozolomide
• Tarceva
• 5-Fluorouracil/Xeloda/oxaliplatin
• Hormonal breast and prostate therapy
• Carboplatin
• Cisplatin
• Methotrexate
• Taxol, Taxotere

Response to Palliation. Evaluated after two or three cycles of treatment

Measurement Criteria
• Patient's wishes for continuing treatment
• Tumor markers
• Performance status
• Weight loss
• Toxicity to treatment
• Computed tomographic scan, magnetic resonance imaging, positron emission tomographic scan, routine laboratory tests

Common Response Rate. 15%-20% (months to 1 year) (Weissman & Von Guter, 2003)

Controversies and Concerns
• Palliative chemotherapy may be offered to avoid the conversation of disease progression.
• Offering false hope versus not being able to stop treatment
• Ease of oral chemotherapy administration may promote increased use of inappropriate use of therapy.
• Demanding families who pressure for aggressive care
• Clinical trial options

Nursing Considerations
• Encourage open communication with oncologist.
• Monitor risk versus benefit of therapy.
• Offer resources and support if therapy fails (Brescia, 2003)

REFERENCES

American Society of Hospital Pharmacists. (2005). ASHP guidelines on handling hazardous drugs. *American Journal of Hospital Pharmacists, 47,* 1033-1049.

Brescia, F. J. (2003). Cancer. In G. S. Taylor & J. E. Kurent (Eds.). *A clinician's guide to palliative care* (pp. 140-152). Malden, MA: Blackwell.

Calvo, E., & Takimoto, C.H. (2005). Principles of oncologic pharmacotherapy. In R. Pazdur, W. Hoskins, L. Coia, et al. (Eds.). *Cancer management: a multidisciplinary approach—medical, surgical & radiation oncology* (9th ed., pp. 23-42). CMP Healthcare Media, Manhasset, NY.

Camp-Sorrell.(Ed.).(2004). *Access device guidelines: Recommendations for nursing practice and education.* Pittsburgh, PA: Oncology Nursing Society.

Chu, E., & DeVita, V.T. (2001). Principles of cancer management: chemotherapy. In V. T. DeVita, S. Hellman, & S. A. Rosenberg (Eds.). *Cancer: principles and practice of oncology* (6th ed., pp. 289-306). Philadelphia: Lippincott Williams & Wilkins.

Davis, M. P. (2005). Integrating palliative medicine into an oncology practice. *American Journal of Hospice and Palliative Care, 22,* 447-452.

Fisher, D. S., Knopf, M. T., & Durivage, H. J. (1993). *The cancer chemotherapy handbook.* St. Louis: Mosby.

Goodin, S., Kane, M., & Rubin, E. (2004). Epothilones: mechanism of action and biologic activity. *Journal of Clinical Oncology, 22,* 2015-2025.

Goodman, M. (2000). Chemotherapy: principles of administration. In C. H. Yarbro, M. H. Frogge, M. Goodman, et al. (Eds.). *Cancer nursing: principles and practice* (5th ed., pp. 385-423). Sudbury, MA: Jones & Bartlett.

Hood, L. E., & Mucenski, J. (2003). *Management of elderly patients with cancer: treatment of chemotherapy-induced neutropenia and anemia. An independent study program accredited for nurses and pharmacists.* Chicago: Discovery International.

Kelleher, L. O., Polovich, M., & White, J. M. (Eds.). (2005). *Chemotherapy and biotherapy guidelines & recommendations for practice* (2nd ed.). Pittsburgh, PA: Oncology Nursing Society.

Miaskowski, C. & Viele, C. (1999). Cancer chemotherapy. In C. Miaskowski & P. Buchsel (Eds): *Oncology nursing: Assessment and clinical care.* pp. 83-106. Mosby: St. Louis, MO.

National Comprehensive Cancer Network. (2003). *Advanced and cancer palliative care treatment guidelines version 1.* Retrieved on October 17, 2007 from http://www.nccn.org/patients/patient_gls/_english/pdf/NCCN%20Palliative%20Care%20Guidelines.pdf.

National Institute for Occupational Safety and Health. (2004). *Preventing occupational exposure to antineoplastic and other hazardous drugs in health care settings.* Retrieved August 29, 2006, from http://www.cdc.gov/noish/docs/2004-165/.

Occupational Safety and Health Administration. (1995). *Controlling occupational exposure to hazardous drugs (OSHA) instructions (CPL 2-2.20B).* Washington, DC: The Administration. Occupational Safety and Health Administration. (2004).

Controlling occupational exposure to hazardous drugs (OSHA) technical manual (Section VI: Chapter 2). Washington, DC: U.S. Government Printing Office. Retrieved August 29, 2006, from http://www.osha.gov/dts/osta/otm/otm_vi/otm_vi_2.html.

Otto, S. E. (2001). Chemotherapy. In S. E. Otto (Ed.) *Oncology nursing* (4th ed., pp. 638-671). St. Louis: Mosby.

Petrylak, D., & Kelly, W. (2004). *Chemotherapeutic options in prostate cancer.* Retrieved February 25, 2007, from http://www.medscape.com/viewprogram/3444.

Phillips, J., Brown, S.,, & Belcher, A. (2004). Culturally Competent Care. In C. Varricchio, P. Pierce, P. Hinds, et al. (Eds.). *A Cancer Sourcebook for Nurses.* Atlantic, GA: American Cancer Society.

Cancer Management

Polovich, M. (Ed). (2003). *Safe handling of hazardous drugs.* Pittsburg, PA: Oncology Nursing Society.

Powell, L. L. (1996). *Cancer chemotherapy guidelines and recommendations for practice,* Pittsburgh, PA: Oncology Nursing Press.

Prommer, E. (2004). Guidelines for use of palliative chemotherapy. *American Academy of Hospice and Palliative Medicine Bulletin, 5,* 1-5.

Repetto, L. (2003). Greater risks of chemotherapy toxicity in elderly patients with cancer. *Journal of Supportive Oncology, 1* (4 suppl. 2), 18-24.

Vedes, D., Biderman, A. (Ed.). (2005). *Taber's Cyclopedic Medical Dictionary.* Philadelphia: F.A Davis Company.

Tortorice, P. V. (2000). Chemotherapy: principles of therapy. In C. H. Yarbro, M. H. Frogge, M. Goodman, et al. (Eds.). *Cancer nursing: principles and practice* (5th ed., pp. 352-382). Sudbury, MA: Jones & Bartlett.

Weissman, D. (2000). *Fast facts and Concepts #14.* palliative chemotherapy end of life education resource center. Retrieved September 4, 2006 from www.eperc.mcw.edu.

Weissman, D. E., & Von Gunten, C. F. (2003). *Facts and concepts #99, chemotherapy: response and survival data.* End of Life Education Resource Center. Retrieved September 4, 2006 from www.eperc.mcw.edu.

World Health Organization. (1990). *Cancer pain relief and palliative care: a report of a WHO Expert Committee* (Technical Report No. 804). Geneva: World Health Organization.

Chemotherapeutic Agents

5-Fluorouracil (Fluorouracil, 5-FU)

Christa Braun-Inglis

DRUG CLASS

- Antimetabolite

ROUTE OF ADMINISTRATION

- Intravenous bolus
- Continuous infusion
- Hepatic artery infusion
- Topical

HOW TO ADMINISTER

- Given as an intravenous (IV) push injection, over 1-3 minutes, bolus infusion over 5-15 minutes, or as a continuous infusion

PRETREATMENT GUIDELINES

- Complete blood cell count
- Chemistry profile with liver functions. Hold dose for total bilirubin > 5mg/dL

USE

- Anal cancer
- Breast cancer
- Colorectal cancer
- Esophageal cancer
- Gastric cancer
- Head and neck cancer
- Pancreatic cancer
- Basal cell carcinoma (topical use only)
- Hepatoma
- Ovarian cancer

PHARMACOKINETICS

- 5-Fluorouracil is metabolized intracellularly to become cytoxic. It is excreted mainly by the kidneys and lungs.
- Terminal half-life is 10 to 20 minutes with prolonged half-lives of active metabolites

USUAL DOSE AND SCHEDULE
Single Agent

- 425-450 mg/m^2 IV bolus on days 1-5 every 28 days
- 500-600 mg/m^2 IV bolus every week for 6 weeks every 8 weeks
- 2,400-2,600 mg/m^2 IV weekly by continuous infusion

Combination Therapy

- 800-1,000 mg/m^2/day IV continuous infusion days 1-4 every 21-28 days
- 1,000 mg/m^2/day IV continuous infusion days 1-5 every day for 21-28 days
- 200-400 mg/m^2/day IV protracted continuous infusion

SIDE EFFECTS

- Myelosuppression, worse with bolus administration
- Mucositis, worse with continuous infusion
- Diarrhea, worse with continuous infusion
- Hand-foot syndrome
- Neurologic toxicity
- Cardiac symptoms (rare)
- Blepharitis
- Skin sensitivity
- Metallic taste
- Alopecia (depending on type of administration)
- Rash and dry skin
- Photosensitivity

NADIR

- 10-14 days with recovery in 14-21 days

STORAGE
Unopened Vials

- Intact vials should be stored at controlled room temperature and protected from light.

MIXING INSTRUCTIONS

- 5-Fluorouracil is available in 10- and 20-mL single-use vials and in 50- and 100-mL bulk pharmacy vials; each milliliter contains 50 mg of the drug. No dilution is required; however, it can be added to 0.9% sodium chloride or 5% dextrose.

PRODUCT STABILITY

- Once solution is mixed in standard 0.9% normal saline solution (NS) or 5% dextrose, 5-Fluorouracil is stable for at least 72 hours. Many preparations are on pumps for 5 to 7 days.

COMPATABILITY WITH OTHER DRUGS/INTRAVENOUS FLUIDS

- Compatible with 0.9% normal saline solution (NS) and 5% dextrose

DRUG INTERACTIONS

- When given with cimetidine, the pharmacological effects of 5-Fluorouracil are increased.
- When given with thiazide diuretics, there is an increased risk of myelosuppression.
- Leucovorin causes increased 5-Fluorouracil toxicity and efficacy, must administer leucovorin before fluorouracil for this effect.

PREGNANCY

Category D

SPECIAL CONSIDERATIONS

- Contraindicated in patients with bone marrow depression, poor nutritional status, infection, active ischemic heart disease, or history of myocardial infarction within 6 months
- Monitor patients closely for mucositis and gastrointestinal toxicity.
- Patients who have grade 3 or 4 myelosuppression, gastrointestinal toxicity, or neurological toxicities may have an underlying deficiency of dihydropyrimidine dehydrogenase.
- Vitamin B$_6$ may help to prevent the recurrence of hand-foot syndrome.

Cancer Management

PATIENT EDUCATION

- Instruct patient to perform meticulous oral care.
- Teach patient to report diarrhea and instruct on antidiarrheal regimen.

BIBLIOGRAPHY

Chu, E., Mota, A., Bromberg, M., et al. (2003). Chemotherapeutic and biologic drugs. In E. Chu & V. T. DeVita (Eds.). *Cancer chemotherapy drug manual 2005* (pp. 181-188). Sudbury, MA: Jones & Bartlett.

Takimoto, C. H., & Calvo, E. (2005). Principles of oncologic pharmacotherapy. In R. Pazdur, L. R. Coia, W. J. Hoskins, et al. (Eds.). *Cancer management: multidisciplinary approach* (pp. 11-22). Lawrence, KS: CMP Healthcare Media.

Trissel, L. A. (2005). *Handbook on injectable drugs* (13th ed.) (pp 672-674). Bethesda, MD: American Society of Health-Systems Pharmacist.

Wilkes, G. M., & Barton-Burke, M. (2005). *2005 Oncology nursing drug handbook* (pp. 168-170). Sudbury, MA: Jones & Bartlett.

Altretamine (Hexalen)

Carol S. Blecher

DRUG CLASS

- Alkylating agent—nonclassic alkylator

ROUTE OF ADMINISTRATION

- Oral

HOW TO ADMINISTER

- Orally after meals to reduce stomach upset
- Take missed dose as soon as possible unless it is almost time for the next dose.

PRETREATMENT GUIDELINES

- Complete blood cell count with differential before therapy is initiated, at the beginning of each subsequent cycle, and at periodic intervals during therapy
- Liver function studies (LFTs) before therapy is initiated, at the beginning of each subsequent cycle, and at periodic intervals during therapy
- Neurological examinations

USE

- Ovarian cancer

Off-Label Uses:

- Colon carcinoma
- Cervical carcinoma
- Endometrial carcinoma
- Lung cancer
- Non-Hodgkin lymphoma

PHARMACOKINETICS

- Well absorbed orally
- Rapidly metabolized in the liver
- Peak plasma levels reached between 0.5 and 3 hours
- Half-life of elimination is 4.7 to 10 hours
- Eliminated in the urine 90% within 72 hours
- Less than 1% eliminated unchanged

USUAL DOSE AND SCHEDULE
Single-Agent Therapy

- 260 mg/m^2/day in four doses for 14-21 days every 28 days
- 4-12 mg/kg/day in four doses for 14-21 days every 28 days

Combination Therapy

- 150 mg/m^2/day in four doses for 14 days every 28 day cycle

SIDE EFFECTS

- Neurological toxicity, both peripheral and central
- Nausea
- Vomiting
- Myelosuppression
- Hypersensitivity
- Skin rash
- Elevation of LFTs
- Flu-like syndrome
- Abdominal cramps
- Diarrhea

NADIR

- 14-21 days after the start of therapy with usual recovery within 28 days

STORAGE

- Store in tightly sealed bottles at controlled room temperatures (15°-30° C; 59°-86° F).
- Avoid excess heat and moisture.

MIXING INSTRUCTIONS

- No preparation or admixture necessary
- Available as a 50-mg gelatin capsule

PRODUCT STABILITY

- Intact capsules are stable for 2 years.

DRUG INTERACTIONS

- Concomitant use with monoamine oxidase inhibitors listed below may cause severe orthostatic hypotension:
  - Phenelzine (Nardil, Parke-Davis, Morris Plains, NJ)
  - Tranylcypromine (Parnate, GlaxoSmithKline, Research Triangle Park, NC)
  - Selegiline (Eldepryl, Somerset Pharmaceuticals, Tampa, FL)
  - Procarbazine (Matulane, Sigma-Tau Pharmaceuticals, Gaithersburg, MD)
- Phenobarbital increases the metabolism of altretamine, with a potential for decreased effect of altretamine.
- Cimetidine inhibits drug metabolism, increasing the half-life and toxicity of altretamine.
- Concomitant use of tricyclic antidepressants may cause severe dizziness and syncopal episodes.

PREGNANCY

Category D

- It is unknown whether altretamine is excreted in human milk. Breast-feeding is not recommended while taking altretamine.

SPECIAL CONSIDERATIONS

- Take after meals to reduce stomach upset.
- Moderately emetogenic, premedicate with a 5-hydroxytryptamine-3 receptor antagonist and dexamethasone.

PATIENT EDUCATION

- After stopping treatment with altretamine, do not receive any immunizations without the approval of your oncologist.
- Immediately report any feelings of anxiety, clumsiness, confusion, dizziness, numbness, or weakness in arms or legs.
- Explore sexual issues with the patient and discuss the impact of chemotherapy.

BIBLIOGRAPHY

Gullatte, M. M. (2001). *A cancer chemotherapy handbook* (pp. 76-78). Pittsburgh, PA: Oncology Nursing Press.

Huntsman Online Patient Education Guide. (2006). *Altretamine*. Retrieved May 14, 2006, from http://www.hopeguide.org-altretamine.

Medline Plus. (1999). *Altretamine*. Retrieved April 29, 2006, from http://www.nlm.nih.gov/medlineplus/druginfo/uspdi/202634.html.

Medline Plus. (2003). *Altretamine*. Retrieved April 29, 2006, from http://www.nlm.nih.gov/medlineplus/drugi nfo/medmaster/a601200.html.

Polovich, M., White, J. M., & Kelleher, L. O. (2005). *Chemotherapy and biotherapy guidelines and recommendations for practice* (p. 20). Pittsburgh, PA: Oncology Nursing Press.

Wilkes, G. M., & Barton-Burke, M. (2005). *Oncology nursing drug handbook* (pp. 47-48). Sudbury, MA: Jones & Bartlett.

Amifostine for Injection (Ethyol, WR-2721)

Carol S. Blecher

DRUG CLASS

- Cytoprotectant; free radical scavenger; miscellaneous classification

ROUTE OF ADMINISTRATION

- Parenteral injection

HOW TO ADMINISTER

- Intravenous (IV) infusion. Infusion duration is dose dependent.

Off-Label Administration

- Subcutaneous

PRETREATMENT GUIDELINES

- Hydration
- Premedicate with a 5-HT3 antagonist and dexamethasone.
- Blood pressure monitoring before treatment (NOTE: Blood pressure must also be monitored at 5-minute intervals during treatment and after treatment.)
- Patient should be placed in a supine position during treatment.
- Serum calcium and magnesium levels before treatment and periodically during therapy

USE

- To reduce the cumulative renal toxicity associated with cisplatin in patients with advanced ovarian carcinoma and non–small cell lung carcinoma
- To reduce the incidence of xerostomia in patients with head and neck carcinoma undergoing radiation therapy

Off-Label Uses

- To reduce neutropenia and thrombocytopenia and prevent cisplatin-related neurotoxicities and ototoxicities
- To reduce paclitaxel-induced neurotoxicity
- To reduce radiation-induced mucositis
- Myelodysplastic syndrome

PHARMACOKINETICS

- Metabolized well by the IV route (NOTE: Recent studies demonstrate good absorption subcutaneously.)
- Rapidly metabolized in the tissues to an active free thiol metabolite
- Half-life of elimination is 9 minutes
- Small amounts of amifostine and the subsequent metabolites are excreted in the urine.
- Prodrug dephosphorylated by alkaline phosphatase in tissues to an active free thiol metabolite preferentially taken up in normal cells. Protectant effect mediated by scavenging of free radicals, competition with oxygen, promotion of damage repair, and a protectant effect of normal tissue

USUAL DOSE AND SCHEDULE
For Reduction of Cumulative Renal Toxicity of Cisplatin

- 740-910 mg/m^2 IV once daily as an IV infusion over 5 to 15 minutes 30 minutes before beginning chemotherapy

For Xerostomia Reduction

- 200 mg/m^2 IV over 3 minutes 15-30 minutes before radiation
  Note: Recent studies demonstrate good absorption subcutaneously and amifostine has been administered in this manner in an off-label use.

Myelodysplastic Syndrome

- 200 mg/m^2 IV 3 days per week for 3 weeks, then 2 weeks off; recycle every 5 weeks. Evaluate response after two cycles.

SIDE EFFECTS

- Nausea and vomiting
- Hypotension
- Flushing/feeling of warmth
- Fever
- Dizziness, faintness, or lightheadedness
- Somnolence
- Blurred vision
- Confusion
- Chills
- Hiccups
- Sneezing
- Hypocalcemia
- Hypomagnesemia
- Allergic reactions ranging from skin rash to rigors
- Rare anaphylaxis
- Rare reports of seizures

STORAGE

- Store 10-mL single-dose glass vials at room temperatures (15°-30° C; 59°-86° F)

MIXING INSTRUCTIONS

- Reconstitute with 9.7 mL of sterile 0.9% normal saline solution
- Further dilute in 50 mL of sterile 0.9% normal saline solution

PRODUCT STABILITY

- Stable at dilutions of 5 to 40 mg/mL for 5 hours at room temperature and for 24 hours when refrigerated

COMPATIBILITY WITH OTHER DRUGS/INTRAVENOUS FLUIDS

- Use only with 0.9% normal saline solution.

DRUG INTERACTIONS

- Amantadine
- Antidepressants
- Antihypertensives
- Antipsychotics
- Optic beta-adrenergic blocking agents (e.g., betaxolol, carteolol, levobunolol, metipranolol, and timolol)
- Bromocriptine
- Deferoxamine
- Diuretics
- Levodopa
- Nabilone
- Narcotic pain medication
- Nimodipine
- Pentamidine
- Pimozide
- Promethazine
- Trimeprazine
- Use with caution when used with other drugs that can lower blood pressure due to added hypotensive or orthostatic hypotension effect

PREGNANCY

Category C

- Amifostine has not been studied in pregnant women. In animal studies large doses cause toxic or harmful effects in the fetus.

SPECIAL CONSIDERATIONS

- Stop antihypertension medication.
- Ensure adequate hydration.
- Premedicate with a 5-hydroxytryptamine-3 antagonist and dexamethasone.
- Longer infusions and larger doses cause greater hypotension. Mean onset of hypotension is 14 minutes with a mean duration of 6 minutes with a 15 minute infusion.

PATIENT EDUCATION

- Move slowly when you sit or stand up if you feel dizzy or lightheaded.
- Drink extra fluids before you get amifostine so your blood pressure will not get too low.
- Do not take your blood pressure medicine for a day before you get amifostine.
- Ask your doctor before restarting your blood pressure medicine.

BIBLIOGRAPHY

Gullatte, M. M. (2001). *A cancer chemotherapy handbook* (pp. 79-81). Pittsburgh, PA: Oncology Nursing Press.

Huntsman Online Patient Education Guide. (2006). *Amifostine*. Retrieved May 14, 2006, from http://www.hopeguide.org-amifostine.

Medline Plus. (2003). *Amifostine*. Retrieved April 29, 2006, from http://www.nlm.nih.gov/medlineplus/druginfo/medmaster/a696014.html.

Medline Plus. (2005). *Amifostine*. Retrieved April 29, 2006, from http://www.nlm.nih.gov/medlineplus/druginfo/uspdi/203557.html.

Polovich, M., White, J. M., & Kelleher, L. O. (2005). *Chemotherapy and biotherapy guidelines and recommendations for practice* (p. 190). Pittsburgh, PA: Oncology Nursing Press.

Wilkes, G. M., & Barton-Burke, M. (2005). *Oncology nursing drug handbook* (p. 386). Sudbury, MA: Jones & Bartlett.

Arsenic Trioxide (Trisenox)

Carol S. Blecher

DRUG CLASS

- Miscellaneous
- Degrades the fusion protein promyelocytic leukemia–retinoic acid receptor alpha

ROUTE OF ADMINISTRATION

- Intravenous (IV) infusion

HOW TO ADMINISTER

- IV infusion over 1-2 hours

PRETREATMENT GUIDELINES

- Electrocardiogram (ECG)
- Complete blood cell count with differential
- Electrolytes
- Renal function studies
- Prothrombin time and international normalized ratio
- Liver function tests: aspartate aminotransferase and alanine aminotransferase
- Pregnancy testing

USE

- Acute promyelocytic leukemia (APL)

Off-Label Uses

- Myelodysplastic syndrome
- Multiple myeloma

PHARMACOKINETICS

- Arsenic trioxide undergoes reduction and methylation in the liver.
- Drug is stored in the liver, kidney, heart, lung, nail, and hair.
- Trivalent form is excreted in the urine.

USUAL DOSE AND SCHEDULE

Acute Promyelocytic Leukemia (APL)

- Induction—0.15 mg/kg/day until bone marrow remission, not to exceed 60 doses
- Consolidation—6 weeks after induction 0.15mg/kg/day for 25 doses over a period of 5 weeks

Myelodysplastic Syndrome

- Loading dose—0.30 mg/kg/day for 5 days followed by a maintenance dose of 0.25 mg/kg/day for 2 days a week until disease progression

Multiple Myeloma

- 0.15 mg/kg/day daily for 30 days by infusion over 2 hours

SIDE EFFECTS

- Hematological—leukocytosis, anemia, thrombocytopenia, neutropenia, and disseminated intravascular coagulation

- Gastrointestinal (GI) abnormalities—nausea, vomiting, diarrhea, constipation, anorexia, abdominal pain, dyspepsia, sore throat, GI hemorrhage, and fecal incontinence
- Musculoskeletal—arthralgias, myalgias, bone pain, neck and back pain
- Neurological—dizziness, headache, insomnia, tremor, anxiety, depression, agitation, paresthesias, somnolence, convulsions, and coma
- Dermatological—dermatitis, pruritus, petechiae, erythema, dry skin, hyperpigmentation, urticaria, pallor, flushing, eye irritation
- Respiratory events—cough, dyspnea, rales, wheezing
- APL differentiation syndrome characterized by fever, weight gain, dyspnea, and pulmonary or pleural infiltrates
- Cardiovascular—QT prolongation and other ECG abnormalities, tachycardia, palpitations, edema, and hypotension or hypertension
- Miscellaneous—fatigue and weakness, rigors, injection site pain, hypersensitivity, dry mouth, hypokalemia or hyperkalemia, hypomagnesemia, hypocalcemia, hyperglycemia, increased hepatic transaminases, infections, blurred vision, renal impairment/failure, and earache

NADIR

- 14-21 days

STORAGE

- Store 10-mL single-dose glass vials at room temperatures (15°-30° C; 59°-86° F)

MIXING INSTRUCTIONS

- Further dilute in 100 to 500 mL of dextrose injection or 0.9% sodium chloride

PRODUCT STABILITY

- Diluted solutions are stable for 24 hours at room temperature and 48 hours under refrigeration

COMPATABILITY WITH OTHER DRUGS/INTRAVENOUS FLUIDS

- Do not mix with other medications.

DRUG INTERACTIONS

- Amphotericin B
- Antiarrhythmics: adenosine, amiodarone, atenolol, digoxin, digitoxin, diltiazem, metoprolol, nadolol, propranolol, quinidine, verapamil
- Antifungals: fluconazole, ketoconazole
- Antihistamines
- Fluoroquinolones: ciprofloxacin, enoxacin, levofloxacin, lomefloxacin
- Diuretics: especially those that are potassium-depleting: bumetanide, furosemide, thiazide diuretics
- Tricyclic antidepressants: amitriptyline, desipramine, doxepin, imipramine, nortriptyline
- Thioridazine

PREGNANCY

Category C

- Arsenic trioxide is a human carcinogen. It has not been studied in pregnancy in humans, but studies in mice and rats have resulted in birth defects and other problems, including miscarriage.

SPECIAL CONSIDERATIONS

- Causes APL differentiation syndrome, which can be fatal.
- High-dose steroids (dexamethasone 10 mg IV twice daily) should be instituted for at least 3 days or until the symptoms abate.
- Causes QT interval prolongation and complete A-V block. Monitor patient for concomitant use of medications that prolong QT interval, previous history of torsades de pointes, preexisting QT prolongation, congestive heart failure, use of potassium-wasting diuretics, concurrent administration of amphotericin B.

PATIENT EDUCATION

- Avoid people with infections.

- Monitor for bruising, bleeding, pinpoint red spots on the skin.
- Avoid contact sports where bruising or injury can occur.
- Use care when handling sharp objects.
- Explore sexual issues with the patient and discuss the impact of chemotherapy.

BIBLIOGRAPHY

Gullatte, M. M. (2001). *A Cancer chemotherapy handbook* (pp. 81-83). Pittsburgh, PA: Oncology Nursing Press.

Medline Plus. (2005). *Arsenic trioxide.* Retrieved April 29, 2006, from http://www.nlm.nih.gov/medlineplus/druginfo/uspdi/500241.html.

Munshi, N. C. (2001). Arsenic trioxide: an emerging therapy for multiple myeloma. *The Oncologist,* 6 Suppl 2, 17-21.

Polovich, M., White, J. M., & Kelleher, L. O. (2005). *Chemotherapy and biotherapy guidelines and recommendations for practice* (p. 30). Pittsburgh, PA: Oncology Nursing Press.

Wilkes, G. M., & Barton-Burke, M. (2005). *Oncology nursing drug handbook* (pp. 57-64). Sudbury, MA: Jones & Bartlett.

Asparaginase (Elspar)

Carol S. Blecher

DRUG CLASS

- Miscellaneous—enzyme

ROUTE OF ADMINISTRATION

- Intramuscular (IM)
- Intravenous (IV)
- Subcutaneously

HOW TO ADMINISTER

- IV infusion over at least 30 minutes
- IM injections—volume should not exceed 2 mL. If greater than 2 mL is needed, the dose should be split between two injection sites.
- Intradermal test dose is recommended.

PRETREATMENT GUIDELINES

- Intradermal test dose before first dose and if there has been the lapse of 1 week between doses
- Complete blood cell count with differential
- Chemistries with: glucose, uric acid, renal function studies, liver function tests, and serum amylase
- Prothrombin time
- Fibrinogen

USE
Primary Use

- Acute lymphocytic leukemia (ALL)

Other Uses

- Acute myelogenous leukemia
- Chronic myelogenous leukemia
- Lymphoma
- Soft tissue sarcoma

PHARMACOKINETICS

- Asparaginase hydrolyzes serum asparagines into aspartate, depriving leukemia cells of the amino acid needed for protein synthesis.
- The drug is cell cycle specific in the G1 postmitotic phase.
- Half-life is 8-30 hours.
- Metabolism is independent of renal and hepatic function. Only trace amounts are excreted in the urine.
- Drug does not cross the blood-brain barrier.

USUAL DOSE AND SCHEDULE
Single Agent

- (ALL) 200 international units/kg IV daily for 28 days

Combination Therapy

- 1,000-6,000 international units/m^2 given in various schedules from daily to every third day. Higher doses given less frequently are also used.

SIDE EFFECTS

- Hypersensitivity/anaphylaxis including respiratory distress, hypotension, laryngeal constriction, diaphoresis, bronchospasms, loss of consciousness, or death can occur in 10%-40% of patients. Hypersensitivity is more common when asparaginase is given IV and when previous cumulative doses exceed 6000 – 12,000 international units/m^2. Intradermal test dose is recommended. If hypersensitivity reaction occurs with asparaginase product, obtain Erwinia L-asparaginase (from E. coli) or pegaspargase and use with caution.
- Coagulation defects such as disseminated intravascular coagulation and prolongation of factors V, VII, VIII, and IX and prothrombin and fibrinogen.
- Pancreatitis is uncommon but may occur.
- Hepatotoxicity with elevated aspartate aminotransferase, alanine aminotransferase, alkaline phosphatase, and bilirubin
- Hyperglycemia with glucosuria, polyuria, and diabetic ketoacidosis
- Neurotoxicity manifested as depression, fatigue, coma, confusion, agitation, hallucinations, or a parkinson-like syndrome
- Renal insufficiency, nausea and vomiting, myelosuppression, skin rash, urticaria, arthralgia, fever, and chills

STORAGE
Unreconstituted Powder

- White lyophilized powder in 10-mL vials should be stored under refrigeration.

Reconstituted Solution

- Reconstituted solutions are stable for 8 hours at room temperature.

MIXING INSTRUCTIONS
Intravenous Administration

- Powder should be reconstituted with 5 mL of sterile water for injection or sodium chloride for injection without preservative. Do not shake vigorously.
- It may be further diluted in 50-250 mL of normal saline solution or 5% dextrose in water.

Intramuscular Administration

- Reconstitute 10,000-unit vial with 2 mL of sodium chloride for injection.

PRODUCT STABILITY

- Diluted solutions are stable for 8 hours at room temperature.
- Solutions that become cloudy should be discarded.

COMPATABILITY WITH OTHER DRUGS/INTRAVENOUS FLUIDS

- Compatible with sterile water, normal saline solution, and 5% dextrose in water

DRUG INTERACTIONS

- Asparaginase used concomitantly with methotrexate can diminish the antineoplastic effects of the methotrexate.
- Increased likelihood of hyperglycemia if given concomitantly with prednisone.
- Neurotoxicities associated with vincristine can be increased if asparaginase is administered before the vincristine.
- Asparaginase has the potential for affecting liver function and can increase the toxicities of other drugs metabolized by the liver, such as probenecid (Benemid) or sulfinpyrazone (Anturane)

PREGNANCY
Category C

- In mice and rats, asparaginase has been shown to retard the weight gain of both mothers and fetus.
- In studies with rabbits, there were embryotoxicities and gross abnormalities.
- There are no studies in pregnant women.
- It is not known whether this drug is secreted in human milk.

SPECIAL CONSIDERATIONS
Intradermal Test Dose

- Administer 2 International Units of asparaginase. Skin test should be observed for 1 hour for reaction. A negative skin test does not ensure that there will be no reaction when full-dose therapy is administered. Be prepared to treat anaphylaxis with each administration.

- Monitor fibrinogen: if the fibrinogen level is below 100 mg/dL, hold the dose and obtain order for fresh-frozen plasma.

PATIENT EDUCATION

- Instruct patient regarding potential for hypersensitivity reaction.
- Teach patient about the potential for excess bleeding and blood clotting and instruct patient to report any unusual symptoms.
- Educate patient about the potential for hyperglycemia and instruct them to report increased thirst, urination, and appetite.
- Instruct patient about potential central nervous system toxicities and to report any unusual symptoms.
- Explore sexual issues with the patient and discuss the impact of chemotherapy.

BIBLIOGRAPHY

Gullatte, M. M. (2001). *A cancer chemotherapy handbook* (pp. 83-86). Pittsburgh, PA: Oncology Nursing Press.

Medline Plus. (1998). *Asparaginase.* Retrieved April 29, 2006, from http://www.nlm.nih.gov/medlineplus/drugi nfo/uspdi/202072.html.

Medline Plus. (2003). *Asparaginase.* Retrieved April 29, 2006, from http://www.nlm.nih.gov/medlinep lus/druginfo/medmaster/a682046. html.

Polovich, M., White, J. M., & Kelleher, L. O. (2005). *Chemotherapy and biotherapy guidelines and recommendations for practice* (p. 30). Pittsburgh, PA: Oncology Nursing Press.

Wilkes, G. M., & Barton-Burke, M. (2005). *Oncology nursing drug handbook* (pp. 57-64). Sudbury, MA: Jones & Bartlett.

Azacitidine (Vidaza)

Joyce Marrs

DRUG CLASS

- Antimetabolite

ROUTE OF ADMINISTRATION

- Intravenous (IV)
- Subcutaneous (SQ)

HOW TO ADMINISTER

- IV dose is administered over 10 to 40 minutes.
- Dose must be given within 1 hour of drug reconstitution.

PRETREATMENT GUIDELINES

- Measure complete blood cell count with differential.
- Measure liver and renal functions.

USE

- Myelodysplastic syndrome

PHARMACOKINETICS

- After SQ administration, mean half-life is 41 minutes.
- Drug is primarily excreted renally.

USUAL DOSE AND SCHEDULE

- Administer 75 mg/m^2 IV or SQ daily for 7 days. Repeat cycle every 4 weeks.
- Dose may be increased to 100 mg/m^2 if two treatment cycles fail to obtain desired response and no toxicities other than nausea and vomiting have developed.
- A minimum of four treatment cycles is recommended.
- Treatment may be continued as long as benefit is observed.

SIDE EFFECTS

- Nausea and vomiting
- Anemia
- Neutropenia
- Thrombocytopenia
- Injection site irritation
- Fatigue
- Fever
- Constipation
- Bruising

- Rigors
- Hypokalemia with IV administration

NADIR

- White blood cell nadir occurs between 14 and 17 days and lasts about 2 weeks with a 14-day recovery period.

STORAGE

- Unreconstituted vial is stored at 25° C (77° F) with a temperature range of 15°-30° C (59°-86° F) allowed.

MIXING INSTRUCTIONS
Intravenous Administration

- Add 10 mL of sterile water to vial and mix with a shaking and rolling motion until clear.
- Reconstituted solution will yield 10 mg/mL.
- Withdraw appropriate dose and add to 50-100 mL of normal saline solution or lactated Ringer's IV solution.

Subcutaneous Administration

- Add 4 mL of sterile water to 100-mg vial and mix.
- Reconstituted solution will yield 25 mg/mL; mixture will be cloudy.
- Before injection, shake and roll syringe to resuspend drug.

PRODUCT STABILITY

- Drug must be administered within 1 hour of mixing.
- Drug mixed for SQ administration may be stored in refrigerator for up to 8 hours and should be brought to room temperature no longer than 30 minutes before administration.

COMPATABILITY WITH OTHER DRUGS/INTRAVENOUS FLUIDS

- Drug is not compatible with 5% dextrose in water (D5W), Hespan, or fluids that contain bicarbonate.

DRUG INTERACTIONS

- Unknown; studies have not been conducted to evaluate for interactions.

Cancer Management

PREGNANCY
Category D

SPECIAL CONSIDERATIONS
- Monitor patients with liver failure closely.
- Rare instances of hepatic coma and death have been reported.

PATIENT EDUCATION
- Instruct patient to monitor for infection or bleeding.
- Instruct patient in use of antiemetics and measures used to control or limit nausea.
- Patients may have diarrhea or constipation; instruct in symptom management measures and when to notify physician.

BIBLIOGRAPHY
Pharmion. (2007). *Vidaza prescribing information*. Retrieved March 20, 2007, from http://www.vidaza.com/corporateweb/vidazaus/homeb.nsf/AttachmentsByTitle/FullPrescribingInformation/$FILE/FullPrescribingInformationforVidaza.pdf.

Wilkes, G. M., & Barton-Burke, M. (2007). *Oncology nursing drug handbook* (pp. 70-73). Sudbury, MA: Jones & Bartlett.

Bacillus Calmette-Guérin (BCG, TheraCys, TICE BCG)

Carol S. Blecher

DRUG CLASS
- Biological response modifier; a vaccine prepared from a live attenuated virus

ROUTE OF ADMINISTRATION
- Intravesical—into the bladder

HOW TO ADMINISTER
- The solution is instilled into the bladder after the bladder has been emptied and allowed to remain in the bladder for 1-2 hours.
- The patient is to lie on each side and in the prone and supine positions for 15 minutes each; then the patient can get up while still retaining the solution for the second hour.
- After 2 hours the patient may empty their bladder, voiding in a seated position.

PRETREATMENT GUIDELINES
- Purified protein derivative skin test
- Complete blood cell count with differential
- Routine urinalysis

USE
- Treatment and prophylaxis of carcinoma in situ of the bladder
- Prophylaxis of primary or recurrent stage Ta and/or T1 papillary tumors after transurethral resection
- Superficial transitional cell carcinoma of the bladder

PHARMACOKINETICS
- Induces a granulomatous reaction at the local site of administration
- Induces a variety of cytokines into the urine of patients with transitional cell carcinoma of the bladder. Some of these cytokines have antiangiogenic activity.
- May induce a cytokine-mediated antiangiogenic environment in addition to a cellular immune response.

USUAL DOSE AND SCHEDULE
- One vial of $1\text{-}8 \times 10^8$ colony-forming units of Bacillus Calmette-Guérin in 50 mL of preservative-free saline solution is given weekly for 6 consecutive weeks and then monthly for 1 year.
- The 6-week schedule may be repeated once.
- Begin no sooner than 2 weeks after tumor resection.

SIDE EFFECTS
- Dysuria, bladder irritability, burning, especially on first urination
- Urinary problems, such as continuing pain and burning
- Urinary urgency, urinary frequency, cramps/pain
- Blood or blood clots in the urine
- Flu-like symptoms including malaise, fever, chills, rigors, and joint pain
- Infections with fevers
- Nausea/vomiting
- Increased fatigue
- Frequent or persistent coughing
- Myalgias/arthralgias
- Anemia, thrombocytopenia, leukopenia

STORAGE
Unreconstituted Powder
- White lyophilized powder in vials should be stored under refrigeration.

Reconstituted Powder or Solution
- Reconstituted solutions are stable for 2 hours at room temperature.

MIXING INSTRUCTIONS
- Preparation should be performed by using aseptic technique. To avoid cross-contamination, parenteral drugs should not be prepared in the same area as Bacillus Calmette-Guérin.
- Wear gloves and a mask when preparing Bacillus Calmette-Guérin.
- Please check guidelines for specific brand. The mixing instructions will vary depending on which product is used. Usual instruction is to draw 1 mL of sterile preservative-free saline solution into a small syringe and add to one vial of Bacillus Calmette-Guérin to resuspend. Swirl until a homogenous suspension is obtained. Add to the top end of a catheter-tipped syringe that contains 49 mL of saline solution to bring the total volume to 50 mL.
- Use immediately after preparation.

PRODUCT STABILITY
- Diluted solutions are stable for 2 hours at room temperature.

COMPATABILITY WITH OTHER DRUGS/INTRAVENOUS FLUIDS

- Compatible with sterile water and normal saline solution

DRUG INTERACTIONS

- Quinolone antibiotics
  - Trovafloxacin
  - Ciprofloxacin
  - Sparfloxacin
  - Levofloxacin
  - Lomefloxacin
  - Norfloxacin
  - Ofloxacin
- Doxycycline antibiotics
  - Periostat
  - Atridox
  - Vibramycin Ca
  - Doryx
  - Doxycycline
  - Vibra Tabs
  - Monodox
- Gentamicin
  - Garamycin
  - Genoptic
  - Gentacidin
  - Gentak
- Other
  - Amphotericin B
  - Antineoplastics
  - Antithyroid agents
  - Azathioprine
  - Chloromycetin
  - Colchicine
  - Corticosteroids
  - Cyclosporine
  - Flucytosine
  - Ganciclovir
  - Interferon
  - Zidovudine

PREGNANCY

Category C

- There are no studies in pregnant women.
- It is not known whether this drug is secreted in human milk.

SPECIAL CONSIDERATIONS

- Should not be used in individuals with concurrent infections
- Should not be used within 7-14 days of transurethral resection, biopsy, or traumatic catheterization
- Should not be used in patients who are immunosuppressed
- Should not be administered to individuals with active tuberculosis
- Bacillus Calmette-Guérin is capable of dissemination when administered intravesically and serious infections have been reported.

PATIENT EDUCATION

- Limit fluids for 8-12 hours before treatment and do not drink for 4 hours before treatment.
- The medication will be instilled into the bladder through a catheter, which will be removed immediately after the medication has been instilled.
- The medication must be retained in the bladder for about 2 hours.
- After the 2 hours you must urinate in a sitting position; it is important to fully empty your bladder.
- After urinating, pour 2 cups of bleach into the toilet bowl and allow it to sit for 15 to 20 minutes before flushing; repeat for 6 hours after each treatment.
- Clean hands and genital area with soap and water after each voiding.
- Handle voided urine as infectious waste.
- Drink plenty of fluids after the treatment.

BIBLIOGRAPHY

Bladder cancer WebCafe. (2002). *BCG*. Retrieved June 25, 2006, from http://blcwecafe.org/bcg.asp.

Cancer Information from Cancer-Consultants.com. (2004). *Stage 1 bladder cancer*. Retrieved June 25, 2006, from http://patient.cancerconsultants.com/print_tmpv.aspx/id=603,

Medline Plus. (2000). *Bacillus Calmette-Guerin*. Retrieved April 29, 2006, from http://www.nlm.nih.gov/medlineplus/druginfo/uspdi/202079.html.

Polovich, M., White, J. M., & Kelleher, L. O. (2005). *Chemotherapy and biotherapy guidelines and recommendations for practice* (p. 30). Pittsburgh, PA: Oncology Nursing Press.

RxList. (2006). *Bacillus of Calmette and Guerin*. Retrieved June 25, 2006, from http://www.rxlist.com/cgi/generic2/bcg.htm.

Bexarotene (Targretin)

Carol S. Blecher

DRUG CLASS

- Miscellaneous—retinoid

ROUTE OF ADMINISTRATION

- Oral
- Topical

HOW TO ADMINISTER

- Orally as a single daily dose
- Topically, drug is applied once every other day for the first week and then increased on a weekly basis to two, three, and four times daily.

PRETREATMENT GUIDELINES
Capsules

- Complete blood cell count with differential
- Liver function tests
- Thyroid function studies
- Lipid studies

Gel

- Monitor for dermal toxicities.

USE

- Cutaneous T-cell lymphoma refractory to one prior systemic chemotherapy

PHARMACOKINETICS

- Bexarotene is highly plasma protein bound.
- Maximum plasma concentrations are reached at approximately 2 hours after oral administration. Half-life is about 7 hours.
- Administration after a fat-containing meal increases plasma concentrations.
- After topical therapy, plasma concentrations are generally low but increase with the increasing amount of body surface area being treated.

USUAL DOSE AND SCHEDULE
Oral

- 300 mg/m^2/day taken as a single daily dose. The dose should be

Cancer Management

taken with or immediately after a fat-containing meal.

Topical

- Apply to the lesions once every other day for the first week. Increase in frequency weekly to a final frequency of two to four times daily.

SIDE EFFECTS
Capsules
Acute/potentially fatal
- Acute pancreatitis
- Subdural hematomas
- Liver failure

Serious
- Asthenias
- Headaches
- Hyperlipidemia
- Hypercholesterolemia
- Leukopenia
- Gastrointestinal symptoms including anorexia, diarrhea, vomiting and pancreatitis

Others
- Peripheral edema
- Rash, dry skin, pruritus, alopecia, exfoliative dermatitis
- Hypothyroidism
- Leukopenia, anemia, infection
- Insomnia
- Flu-like syndrome: chills, fever, back pain
- Increased lactate dehydrogenase levels

STORAGE

- Capsules should be stored at 36°-77° F.
- Gel should be stored at room temperature.
- Avoid high temperatures, humidity, and protect from light when storing both capsules and gel.

MIXING INSTRUCTIONS

- No mixing necessary

PRODUCT STABILITY

- See packaging

COMPATABILITY WITH OTHER DRUGS/INTRAVENOUS FLUIDS

- No compatibility studies have been performed with the gel formulation.

DRUG INTERACTIONS
Gel

- Insect repellants containing DEET and vitamin A supplements

Capsules

- Anticonvulsants
- Oral antidiabetics
- Antiinfectives
- Antipsychotics
- Captopril
- Enalapril
- Gold salts
- Lisinopril
- Procainamide
- Promethazine
- Tricyclic antidepressants
- Interferons
- Antithyroid medication
- Phenobarbital
- Phenytoin
- Grapefruit juice
- Rifampin
- Erythromycin
- Gemfibrozil
- Vitamin A supplements

PREGNANCY

Category X; causes birth defects in rats
- There are no studies in pregnant women, but bexarotene should not be taken during pregnancy and a pregnancy test should be performed before this medication is started and once a month while on therapy.
- It is not known whether this drug is secreted in human milk, but lactation is contraindicated.

SPECIAL CONSIDERATIONS

- Capsules should be taken with or immediately after a meal.
- Gel should be applied in sufficient quantities to fully cover the lesion generously and allow drying before covering with clothing.
- Avoid gel contact with normal healthy skin and mucous membranes.

- Occlusive dressings should not be used.
- Retinoids have been associated with photosensitivity reactions; exposure to sunlight and ultraviolet light should be limited.

PATIENT EDUCATION
Gel

- Avoid sunlight, especially between 10 AM and 3 PM.
- Wear protective clothing, a hat, and sunglasses and apply a sun block with a sun protection factor (SPF) of 15 or better.
- Do not use sunlamps or tanning beds.

Capsules

- Must use two forms of birth control. The drug should be stopped immediately if patient becomes pregnant while taking.
- Avoid people with infections.
- Monitor for bleeding.
- Avoid contact sports.
- Avoid sunlight, especially between 10 AM and 3 PM.
- Wear protective clothing, a hat, and sunglasses and apply a sun block with SPF of 15 or better.
- Do not use sunlamps or tanning beds.

BIBLIOGRAPHY

Gullatte, M. M. (2001). *A cancer chemotherapy handbook* (pp. 86-89). Pittsburgh, PA: Oncology Nursing Press.

Medline Plus. (2003). *Bexarotene (systemic)*. Retrieved April 29, 2006, from http://www.nlm.nih.gov/medlineplus/druginfo/uspdi/500095.html.

Medline Plus. (2003). *Bexarotene (topical)*. Retrieved April 29, 2006, from http://www.nlm.nih.gov/medlineplus/drug info/uspdi/500313.html.

Wilkes, G. M., & Barton-Burke, M. (2005). *Oncology nursing drug handbook* (pp. 57-64). Sudbury, MA: Jones & Bartlett.

Bleomycin (Blenoxane)

Carol S. Blecher

DRUG CLASS

- Antitumor antibiotic

ROUTE OF ADMINISTRATION

- Intravenous (IV)
- Intramuscular (IM)
- Subcutaneous (SQ)
- Intracavitary

HOW TO ADMINISTER

- IV slow push. Do not exceed 1 unit per minute.
- Intrapleural through a chest tube
- IM or SQ routes may cause burning pain at the injection site.

PRETREATMENT GUIDELINES

- Pulmonary function studies before initiation of therapy and then monthly to every 2 months during treatment
- Chest x-ray film before treatment and at regular intervals during treatment
- Renal function tests, creatinine clearance (actual or calculated), or serum creatinine before the initiation of therapy and before each subsequent dose
- Test dose of 1-2 units IV, IM, or SQ should be administered before the first dose, especially in patients with lymphoma.

USE

- Malignant pleural effusion
- Hodgkin disease
- Non-Hodgkin lymphoma
- Testicular cancer
- Penile cancer
- Squamous cell carcinomas of the head and neck
- Cervical and vulvar cancer
- Melanoma

Off-Label Uses

- Kaposi's sarcoma
- Soft tissue and osteosarcomas
- Mycosis fungoides
- Bladder cancer
- Esophageal cancer
- Endometrial cancer
- Ovarian cancer
- Skin carcinomas

PHARMACOKINETICS

- IM and intraperitoneal absorption is 30% less than that of the serum levels produced by IV administration.
- SQ route produces serum concentration equal to that of IV administration.
- Half-life is dependent on renal function. Normally 3 to 5 hours, but can be as much as 30 hours in patients with severe renal problems.
- Drug concentrates in the skin, kidneys, lung, and heart.
- 50%-70% of the drug is excreted in the urine as active drug.

USUAL DOSE AND SCHEDULE

- IM, SQ, or IV: 10-20 units/m^2 once or twice weekly
- Do not exceed 30 units per dose or 400-500 units total lifetime dose.
- Intrapleural dose is normally 60 units in 100 mL of normal saline solution.
- If creatinine clearance 10-50 mL/min: administer 75% of normal dose.
- If creatinine clearance <10mL/min: administer 50% of normal dose.

SIDE EFFECTS
Acute and Potentially Life Threatening

- Pulmonary toxicity: interstitial pneumonitis that can potentially advance and become pulmonary fibrosis that will ultimately cause death.
- Hypersensitivity or anaphylactic reactions—rare

Other Side Effects

- Fever and chills usually occurring 4-10 hours after administration and lasting for 4-12 hours
- Dermatologic toxicities including hyperpigmentation, thickening of the nail beds, alopecia, skin erythema, rash, edema, photosensitivity, and mild stomatitis
- Nausea and vomiting—generally mild
- Renal toxicity
- Hepatotoxicity

NADIR

- Rare. Incidence of myelosuppression < 1%. If this occurs, will peak at 14 days, onset beginning day 7, and recovery occurring within 21 days.

STORAGE

- Vials should be stored under refrigeration at 2°-8° C (36°-46° F)

MIXING INSTRUCTIONS
IM or SQ Administration Route

- Reconstitute with sterile water, sodium chloride, or bacteriostatic water using 1-5 mL for a 15 unit dose vial and 2-10 mL with the 30 unit dose vial.

Solutions

- For IV administration, reconstitute the 15 unit vial with 5 mL of sodium chloride and the 30 unit vial with 10 mL of sodium chloride.
- For intrapleural administration, a standard dose of 60 units is typically used mixed with 50-100 mL of sodium chloride.
  Note: Bleomycin should not be reconstituted or diluted with dextrose-containing solutions because it may cause a loss of potency.

PRODUCT STABILITY

- Reconstituted solutions are stable for 24 hours at room temperature and for 14 days under refrigeration.

COMPATIBILITY WITH OTHER DRUGS/INTRAVENOUS FLUIDS

- Bleomycin should not be reconstituted or diluted with dextrose-containing solutions because it may cause a loss of potency.
- Bleomycin is incompatible with solutions containing divalent and

Cancer Management

trivalent cations because of chelation.

- Bleomycin is also inactivated by hydrogen peroxide.

DRUG INTERACTIONS

- Cisplatin causes delayed bleomycin elimination and an increase in toxicity.
- Digoxin given concomitantly with bleomycin causes a decrease in the plasma levels of digoxin and increases the renal excretion of digoxin.
- Monitor phenytoin levels when given concomitantly with bleomycin because the phamacologic effects of the phenytoin may be decreased.

PREGNANCY

Category D
- There are no studies in pregnant women, but bleomycin may cause birth defects if either the male or female is taking the drug at time of conception or if it used during pregnancy. Sterility has not been reported with bleomycin, but this does not eliminate the possibility.
- It is not known whether this drug is secreted in human milk.

SPECIAL CONSIDERATIONS

- Patients should be monitored for signs and symptoms of pulmonary toxicity, including shortness of breath or dyspnea on exertion.
- Monitor complete blood cell count with differential before each dose of bleomycin.
- Administer acetaminophen 650 mg every 4 to 6 hours for four doses to prevent/treat bleomycin-induced febrile episodes.
- Use of oxygen concentrations (>30%) in animals previously treated with bleomycin has been reported to promote pulmonary toxicity. Although this is controversial, supplemental oxygen should be used judiciously in people who have received bleomycin.

PATIENT EDUCATION

- There is a life-long necessity for reporting previous use of bleomycin when the need for anesthesia occurs.
- Loss of appetite may occur along with nausea or vomiting.
- Taking acetaminophen on a regular basis will decrease the severity of fever or chills.
- Report any change in respiratory status such as difficulty breathing, wheezing, air hunger, increased secretions, and difficulty expectorating secretions.
- Promptly report any burning or stinging at injection site.

BIBLIOGRAPHY

Gullatte, M. M. (2001). *A cancer chemotherapy handbook* (pp. 89-91). Pittsburgh, PA: Oncology Nursing Press.

Medline Plus. (1998). *Bleomycin (systemic)*. Retrieved April 29, 2006, from http://www.nlm.nih.gov/medline-plus/drug info/uspdi/202093.html.

Medline Plus. (2003). *Bleomycin*. Retrieved April 29, 2006, from http://www.nlm.nih.gov/medline-plus/medmaster/a682125.html.

Pharmacy Services. (2002). *Bleomycin*. Retrieved November 25, 2006, from www.musc.edu/pharmacyservices/Drugs/B/Bleomycin.htm.

Polovich, M., White, J. M., & Kelleher, L. O. (2005). *Chemotherapy and biotherapy guidelines and recommendations for practice* (p. 26). Pittsburgh, PA: Oncology Nursing Press.

Wilkes, G. M., & Barton-Burke, M. (2005). *2005 Oncology nursing drug handbook* (p. 72-75). Sudbury, MA: Jones & Bartlett.

Bortezomib (Velcade)

Joyce Marrs

DRUG CLASS

- Proteasome inhibitor

ROUTE OF ADMINISTRATION

- Intravenous (IV)

HOW TO ADMINISTER

- IV push over 3-5 seconds

PRETREATMENT GUIDELINES

- Measure complete blood cell count with differential; electrolytes; kidney and hepatic functions.
- Verify that serum sodium level is above 130 mg/dL.
- Assess for presence and degree of peripheral neuropathy.
- Administer antiemetics as ordered.

USE

- Multiple myeloma that has progressed after at least one prior therapy
- Mantle cell lymphoma

PHARMACOKINETICS

- Half-life is 9-15 hours.
- Drug is metabolized through the cytochrome P450 enzyme pathway.

USUAL DOSE AND SCHEDULE

- Administer 1.3 mg/m^2 IV twice a week for 2 weeks: days 1, 4, 8, and 11.
- Repeat every 21 days.

SIDE EFFECTS

- Nausea and vomiting
- Peripheral neuropathy
- Orthostatic hypotension
- Thrombocytopenia
- Neutropenia
- Constipation
- Diarrhea
- Dehydration
- Decreased appetite
- Fatigue
- Weakness

- Fever
- Headache
- Insomnia
- Arthralgias
- Edema
- Dyspnea
- Dizziness
- Pruritus
- Blurred vision

NADIR

- Platelet count and neutrophils were lowest at day 11 with recovery by day 21.
- No evidence of cumulative effect

STORAGE

- Store at room temperature.

MIXING INSTRUCTIONS

- Mix with 3.5 mL of normal saline solution.
- The reconstituted solution should be clear and colorless.

PRODUCT STABILITY

- Stable up to 8 hours at room temperature

COMPATIBILITY WITH OTHER DRUGS/INTRAVENOUS FLUIDS

- Compatible with normal saline solution

DRUG INTERACTIONS

- Unknown; studies have not been conducted to evaluate for interactions.

PREGNANCY

Category D

SPECIAL CONSIDERATIONS

- Peripheral neuropathy: may develop or worsen during treatment. Symptoms may improve or resolve with discontinuation of drug.
- Dose adjustment for peripheral neuropathy toxicity:
  - Reduce dose at grade 1 with pain or grade 2 without pain. Reinstitute at 1 mg/m².
  - Hold drug for grade 2 with pain or any grade 3. Drug may then be reinstituted at 0.7 mg/m²

and once weekly treatment when toxicity resolves.
  - Discontinue drug for grade 4 toxicity.
- Orthostatic hypotension may require intervention such as IV hydration, adjustment of hypertensive medications, or initiation of mineralocortico-steroids or sympathomimetics.
- Congestive heart failure may develop or worsen during treatment. Monitor cardiac status.
- Rare reports of pulmonary disorders such as pneumonitis, interstitial pneumonia, lung infiltrates, and acute respiratory distress syndrome.
- Rare occurrences of reversible posterior leukoencephalopathy syndrome (RPLS) have been reported. RPLS is a rare neurological disorder characterized by seizure, headache, confusion, blindness, lethargy, and other neurological manifestations.
- Monitor for tumor lysis syndrome.
- Hold dose for platelet count less than 25,000/mcL.
- Drug should be held for grade 3 nonhematologic or grade 4 hematological toxicities.

PATIENT EDUCATION

- Advise patient concerning safety issues surrounding peripheral neuropathy.
- Patient should be cautioned to avoid driving or operating heavy machinery if hypotension, dizziness, fatigue, syncope, or peripheral neuropathy occurs.
- Patient should be instructed in ways to prevent dehydration that can be related to nausea, vomiting, or diarrhea.
- Patients with diabetes should closely monitor blood sugar levels.
- Instruct patients to notify physician for a temperature above 100.4° F.

BIBLIOGRAPHY

Chu, E., Mota, A., Bromberg, M., D., et al. (2006). Bortezomib. In E. Chu & V. DeVita (Eds.). *Physicians' cancer chemotherapy*

drug manual 2006 (pp. 71-73). Sudbury, MA: Jones & Bartlett.
Velcade: prescribing information. (2006). Retrieved March 30, 2007, from http://www.millennium.com/produ cts/velcade/full_prescrib_velcade.pdf.
Wilkes, G. M., & Barton-Burke, M. (2006). *Oncology nursing drug handbook* (pp. 483-488). Sudbury, MA: Jones & Bartlett.

Busulfan (Myleran)

Carol S. Blecher

DRUG CLASS

- Alkylating agent, nitrogen mustard derivative

ROUTE OF ADMINISTRATION

- Intravenous (IV)
- Oral

HOW TO ADMINISTER

- Oral formulation should be administered on an empty stomach to decrease the risk of nausea and vomiting.
- IV formulation should be administered through a central venous catheter over 2 hours.

PRETREATMENT GUIDELINES

- Liver function studies including alanine aminotransferase, aspartate aminotransferase, alkaline phosphatase, total bilirubin, and lactate dehydrogenase
- Complete blood cell count with differential and platelet count before initiation of therapy and then before each subsequent dose
- Pulmonary function studies are recommended if pulmonary toxicities are a potential.
- Uric acid level
- Renal function studies before initiation of therapy and then before each subsequent dose

USE

- Chronic myelogenous leukemia
- Bone marrow transplant preparation in combination with cyclophosphamide

Off-Label Uses

- Acute myelogenous leukemia and brain tumors
- May also be used for polycythemia vera and myeloid metaplasia

PHARMACOKINETICS
Oral Preparation

- Well absorbed
- The metabolites are excreted in the urine.
- Peak plasma concentrations are reached within 4 hours of oral administration and within 5 minutes of IV administration.
- The oral preparation has a half-life of approximately 3 hours.
- The drug crosses the blood-brain barrier resulting in cerebral spinal fluid levels similar to those in plasma.

Intravenous Busulfan

- Has not been studied regarding distribution, metabolism, and elimination

USUAL DOSE AND SCHEDULE

- Oral adult dosage for chronic myelogenous leukemia
  ○ Induction is 4-8 mg/day until white blood cell count falls below 15,000.
- Maintenance dosage
  ○ Ranges from 2 mg/week to 4 mg/day
- Bone marrow transplant dosage
  ○ Ranges from 8-16 mg/kg administered as 0.8 to 1 mg/kg every 6 hours for a total of 16 doses
  ○ It is administered through a central venous catheter over 2 hours.
  ○ IV Busulfan should be dosed on the basis of ideal body weight or actual body weight, whichever is less. Obese patients must be dosed on the basis of adjusted body weight.

SIDE EFFECTS
Acute and Potentially Life Threatening

- Pulmonary toxicity, manifested by bronchopulmonary dysplasia that can progress to pulmonary fibrosis
- Seizures may occur with high–dose bone marrow transplant regimens and phenytoin should be started before the administration of high dose busulfan.
- High-dose busulfan may also be associated with venoocclusive disease and hyperbilirubinemia.

Other Side Effects

- Severe bone marrow suppression that may cause bone marrow fibrosis or aplasia
- Skin hyperpigmentation, urticaria, erythema, alopecia, ovarian suppression, amenorrhea, sterility, nausea/vomiting, loss of appetite, diarrhea, confusion, blurred vision, weakness, fatigue, elevated liver enzymes, hyperuricemia, uric acid nephropathy, mucositis

NADIR

- Begins on days 7-10, lasts 14-21 days from onset, and recovery occurs within 28 days

STORAGE
Tablets

- Can be stored in a dry place at room temperature

Ampules

- Stored under refrigeration and can be used until the date indicated on the ampule.

MIXING INSTRUCTIONS

- IV busulfan can be diluted with 10 times the volume of the busulfan of 0.9% saline solution or 5% dextrose injection.
- Final concentration should be > 0.5 mg/mL.
- The diluted busulfan is to be added to an IV solution and mixed by inverting the solution a number of times.

PRODUCT STABILITY

- Reconstituted solutions that have been diluted in normal saline solution (NS) or 5% dextrose in water (D5W) are stable for 8 hours at room temperature and up to 12 hours if refrigerated.
- Infusions kept at room temperature must be completed within 8 hours of admixture, whereas refrigerated solutions must be completely infused within 12 hours of admixture.

COMPATIBILITY WITH OTHER DRUGS/INTRAVENOUS FLUIDS

- Compatible with NS and 5% D5W only

DRUG INTERACTIONS

- Acetaminophen, when administered before or concurrently with busulfan, causes a reduction in busulfan clearance.
- CYP3A4 inhibitors may increase the levels of busulfan.
- Use of concurrent itraconazole causes a 25% reduction in busulfan clearance.
- Concomitant phenytoin or other CYP3A4 inducers may increase busulfan clearance and decrease the levels/effect of busulfan.
- Long-term addition of thioguanine to busulfan therapy can result in esophageal varices and hepatotoxicity.

PREGNANCY
Category D

- Drug may be hazardous to the fetus.

SPECIAL CONSIDERATIONS

- Dosage of oral busulfan needs to be adjusted on the basis of clinical response and degree of bone marrow suppression.

PATIENT EDUCATION

- Take pills by mouth with chilled liquids and drink at least 2 to 3 quarts of fluid every 24 hours, unless you are instructed otherwise. The increased fluids will help to increase urination and prevent kidney problems.

- The pills should be taken at the same time each day with the prescribed antiemetics.
- Do not double the dose if a dose is missed.
- You may be at risk of infection, so try to avoid crowds or people with colds and immediately report fever or any other signs of infection to your health care provider.
- To help treat/prevent mouth sores, use a soft toothbrush and rinse three times a day with $1/2$ to 1 teaspoon of salt mixed with 8 ounces of water.
- Use an electric razor and a soft toothbrush to minimize potential for bleeding. Avoid contact sports or activities that could cause injury.
- To reduce nausea, take antinausea medications as prescribed by your doctor and eat small, frequent meals.
- Avoid sun exposure. Wear sun protection factor (SPF) 15 (or higher) sunblock and protective clothing.
- If you experience symptoms or side effects, be sure to discuss them with your health care team.

BIBLIOGRAPHY

Gullatte, M. M. (2001). *A cancer chemotherapy handbook* (pp. 92-94). Pittsburgh, PA: Oncology Nursing Press.

Medical University of South Carolina, Garrison K. L., coordinator. *Busulfan*. Retrieved November 25, 2006, from http://www.musc.edu/pharmacyservices/Drugs/B/Busulfan.doc.

Medline Plus. (2003). *Busulfan*. Retrieved April 29, 2006, from http://www.nlm.nih.gov/medlineplus/druginfo/medmaster/a682248.html.

Medline Plus. (2005). *Busulfan (systemic)*. Retrieved April 29, 2006, from http://www.nlm.nih.gov/medlineplus/drug info/uspdi/202101.html.

Polovich, M., White, J. M., & Kelleher, L. O. (2005). *Chemotherapy and biotherapy guidelines and recommendations for practice* (p. 20). Pittsburgh, PA: Oncology Nursing Press.

Wilkes, G.M., & Barton-Burke, M. (2005). *Oncology nursing drug handbook* (pp.75-83). Sudbury, MA: Jones & Bartlett.

Capecitabine (Xeloda)

Carol S. Blecher

DRUG CLASS

- Antimetabolite
- Fluoropyrimidine carbamate

ROUTE OF ADMINISTRATION

- Oral

HOW TO ADMINISTER

- This drug should be taken within $1/2$ hour after a meal.
- The pills should be taken with water.
- Missed doses should be skipped.

PRETREATMENT GUIDELINES

- Tests should be performed before the start of therapy and at periodic intervals during treatment, usually before each subsequent cycle of treatment.
  - Liver function studies: aspartate aminotransferase, alanine aminotransferase, alkaline phosphatase, total bilirubin, and lactate dehydrogenase
  - Complete blood cell count with differential and platelet count, creatinine

USE

- Metastatic breast cancer that is resistant to paclitaxel and anthracycline therapy or when anthracycline therapy is not indicated
- Metastatic colorectal carcinoma
- Adjuvant colorectal carcinoma

Off-Label Uses

- All settings in which 5-fluorouracil (5-FU) therapy is used

PHARMACOKINETICS

- Capecitabine is converted to 5-FU in the liver and tissues. 5-FU is further metabolized in normal and tumor cells.
- The half-life of capecitabine is approximately 45 minutes and it is excreted in the urine.

USUAL DOSE AND SCHEDULE

- Usual dose is 2,500 mg/m²/day administered in two divided doses 12 hours apart. The dose is administered for 2 weeks followed by a 1-week rest period. This cycle is repeated every 3 weeks.
- Dose should be adjusted in patients who have a renal dysfunction.
  - Creatinine clearance 30-50mL/min—reduce normal dose by 25%
  - Creatinine clearance <30mL/min—do not use

SIDE EFFECTS

- Acute and potentially life threatening: severe diarrhea and necrotizing enterocolitis
- Other side effects: stomatitis, hand-and-foot syndrome (palmar plantar erythrodysesthesia), skin rash or itching, changes in fingernails or toenails, photosensitivity, radiation recall syndrome, nausea/vomiting, anorexia, abdominal pain, myelosuppression, headache, dizziness, insomnia, fatigue, myalgias, elevated bilirubin, hepatitis, edema, cardiac toxicity including ischemia, arrhythmias, congestive heart failure, myocardial infarction, and tachycardia

NADIR

- Nadir is observed between 9 and 14 days after first course; maximal depression may be delayed for as long as 20 days. By day 30, count usually returns to normal range.

STORAGE

- Tablets should be stored in tightly sealed bottles at room temperature (15°-30° C [59°-86° F).

DRUG INTERACTIONS

NOTE: Capecitabine is **contraindicated** in those individuals who have demonstrated prior hypersensitivity to 5-FU.

- Capecitabine may interact with warfarin and increase bleeding risk. It is recommended to watch coagulation levels (international normalized ratio) closely and to adjust warfarin doses appropriately.

- Capecitabine may inhibit cytochrome CYP2C9 enzyme, therefore resulting in an increase in phenytoin levels. Monitor phenytoin levels in patients taking both medications.
- Antacids can cause an increase in capecitabine blood concentrations
- Leucovorin can increase both the therapeutic and toxic effects of the fluorouracil.

PREGNANCY

Category D
- Women of childbearing potential are advised to avoid becoming pregnant while using capecitabine.
- Significant amounts of capecitabine may be excreted into the breast milk. It is recommended to discontinue nursing while using capecitabine.

SPECIAL CONSIDERATIONS

- Capecitabine should be taken with water within 30 minutes after a meal.
- Swallow whole, do not crush or chew.
- Missed doses should be omitted and doses should not be doubled up.
- Nausea/vomiting, diarrhea, and stomatitis should be treated symptomatically.
- Capecitabine should be discontinued for National Cancer Institute toxicities that are grade 2 or greater.
- When toxicities are resolved, dose adjustment should be considered before drug is restarted.

PATIENT EDUCATION

- This drug should be taken within $\frac{1}{2}$ hour after a meal.
- The pills should be taken with water.
- The pills should be taken at the same time each day with the prescribed antiemetics.

- Do not double the dose if a dose is missed.
- Diarrhea may be treated with loperamide (Imodium AD), but if diarrhea persists notify the health care team.
- Call your health care team if you experience redness or swelling along with numbness and tingling of your hands or feet.
- You may be at risk of infection, so try to avoid crowds or people with colds.
- It is important to report fever or any other signs of infection immediately to your health care provider.
- To help treat/prevent mouth sores, use a soft toothbrush and rinse three times a day with $\frac{1}{2}$ to 1 teaspoon of salt mixed with 8 ounces of water.
- Use an electric razor and a soft toothbrush to minimize potential for bleeding. Avoid contact sports or activities that could cause injury.
- To reduce nausea, take antinausea medications as prescribed by your doctor and eat small, frequent meals.
- Avoid sun exposure. Wear sun protection factor (SPF)15 (or higher) sunblock and protective clothing.
- If you experience any symptoms or side effects, be sure to discuss them with your health care team.

BIBLIOGRAPHY

Capecitabine. (No Date). Retrieved November 25, 2006, from www.mrsci. com/Chemotherapeutic-Agents/ Capecitabine.php.

Gullatte, M. M. (2001). *A cancer chemotherapy handbook* (pp. 94-97). Pittsburgh, PA: Oncology Nursing Press.

Karch, A. M. (2000). *Focus on nursing pharmacology (LWW): capecitabine*. Retrieved November 25, 2006, from http://www.mubabol.ac.ir/pdlm/Clas/ Sources/NursingPharmacology/mg/ca pecitabine.htm.

Medline Plus. (2003). *Capecitabine*. Retrieved April 29, 2006, from http:// www.nlm.nih.gov/medlineplus/drug- info/medmaster/a699003.html.

Medline Plus. (2005). *Capecitabine (systemic)*. Retrieved April 29, 2006, from http://www.nlm.nih.gov/medlineplus/ drug info/uspdi/203548.html.

Polovich, M., White, J. M., & Kelleher, L. O. (2005). *Chemotherapy and biotherapy guidelines and recommendations for practice* (p. 23). Pittsburgh, PA: Oncology Nursing Press.

Wilkes, G. M., & Barton-Burke, M. (2005). *Oncology nursing drug handbook* (pp. 83-86). Sudbury, MA: Jones & Bartlett.

Carboplatin (Paraplatin)

Carol S. Blecher

DRUG CLASS

- Alkylating agent, heavy metal compound
- Second-generation platinol

ROUTE OF ADMINISTRATION

- Intravenous (IV)
- Intraperitoneal in patients with advanced ovarian cancer

HOW TO ADMINISTER

- IV: do not use aluminum needles for mixing or administration.
- Drug is administered IV over 15 minutes to 1 hour.
- Can also be administered over 24 hours

PRETREATMENT GUIDELINES

- Tests should be performed before the start of therapy and at periodic intervals during treatment, usually before each subsequent cycle of treatment and at periodic intervals during treatment.
  - ○ Complete blood cell count with differential and platelet counts
  - ○ Liver function tests: alanine aminotransferase, aspartate aminotransferase, alkaline phosphatase, total bilirubin, and lactate dehydrogenase
  - ○ Renal function tests: creatinine clearance actual or calculated and or serum creatinine

USE

- Ovarian carcinoma
- Non–small cell lung cancer

- Testicular cancer
- Cervical cancer
- Head and neck cancer
- Wilms' tumor
- Brain tumors
- Bladder cancer
- Cancer of the fallopian tube or lining of the abdomen (spreading from the ovary)
- Retinoblastoma
- Breast cancer
- Melanoma

Off-Label Uses

- Small cell lung cancer
- Cancer of the breast
- Cancer of the esophagus, including the junction between the esophagus and stomach
- Cancers of the lymphatic system
- Cancer of the endometrium
- Cancer of unknown origin
- Malignant melanoma
- Bone marrow transplant conditioning

PHARMACOKINETICS

- Terminal half-life is about 2.5 to 6 hours in normal renal function.
- Initial half-life is 1 to 2 hours.
- Distribution is to the liver, kidney, and large and small bowel. 90% is bound in plasma protein.
- The drug is excreted renally and 70% is excreted unchanged.

USUAL DOSE AND SCHEDULE
Single Agent

- 350-400 mg/m^2 IV every 4 weeks

Common Dosing

- Area under the curve (AUC) dosing is commonly used by the Calvert formula for predictable pharmacokinetics.
- AUC of two weekly or AUC of six administered every 3 weeks

SIDE EFFECTS
Acute and Potentially Life Threatening

- Hypersensitivity reactions, most frequently seen after the seventh or eighth cycle of treatment

- Mild to moderate nausea and vomiting, which generally occurs within 6-24 hours after administration
- Myelosuppression

Other Side Effects

- Alopecia (mild)
- Skin rash
- Urticaria
- Pruritus
- Anorexia
- Diarrhea
- Constipation
- Weight loss
- Mild paresthesias
- Peripheral neuropathies
- Emboli
- Strokes
- Heart failure
- Elevated aspartate aminotransferase/alanine aminotransferase
- Electrolyte abnormalities
- Bronchospasms
- Hematuria
- Renal dysfunction
- Ototoxicity

NADIR

- Nadir occurs between days 14 and 21 with recovery within 4-6 weeks. Platelet nadir occurring between days 14-21 and recovery by day 28. White blood cell nadir usually occurs on about day 21 with recovery by week 5 or 6.

STORAGE

- This product is light sensitive. Vials should be stored at room temperature.

MIXING INSTRUCTIONS

- Carboplatin can be reconstituted with sterile water, normal saline solution (NS), or 5% dextrose in water (D5W) to a concentration of 10 mg/mL.
- The drug is then further diluted in D5W or NS for infusion.

PRODUCT STABILITY

- After reconstitution, carboplatin is stable at room temperature for 8 hours.

COMPATIBILITY WITH OTHER DRUGS/INTRAVENOUS FLUIDS

- Incompatible with aluminum

DRUG INTERACTIONS

- Use with any product containing aluminum will cause a loss of potency and the carboplatin will form a precipitate.
- Serum phenytoin levels must be monitored because carboplatin reduces the serum concentration of phenytoin and reduces its efficacy.
- Carboplatin administered concomitantly with aminoglycosides or other nephrotoxic drugs may enhance nephrotoxicity.

PREGNANCY

Category D

- This drug may cause birth defects or miscarriages.
- Crosses placenta; may pass into breast milk

SPECIAL CONSIDERATIONS

- Carboplatin is an irritant.
- Incompatible with aluminum. Use of aluminum needles causes a black precipitate.
- Monitor hydration and emetic control.
- Monitor closely for hypersensitivity reactions, which are most frequently seen after the seventh or eighth cycle of treatment.

PATIENT EDUCATION

- Patients may be at risk of infection, so advise them to avoid crowds or people with colds.
- It is important to report fever or any other signs of infection immediately to health care providers.
- Adequate hydration is important during treatment with carboplatin. Administration of intravenous fluids may be prescribed or additional fluid intake by mouth may be recommended during treatment.

Cancer Management

- If patients have an allergic reaction (including difficulty breathing; closing of the throat; swelling of the lips, tongue, or face; or hives) they should notify a member of the health care team immediately.
- Advise patients to inform the health care team if they experience blurred vision, altered color perception, temporary blindness, and other visual problems.
- Use an electric razor and a soft toothbrush to minimize potential for bleeding. Avoid contact sports or activities that could cause injury.
- To reduce nausea, take antinausea medications as prescribed, and eat small, frequent meals.
- If patients have hearing loss or ringing in the ears, they should talk to the physician.

BIBLIOGRAPHY

Bristol-Myers Squibb. (2005). *Carboplatin.* Retrieved November 25, 2006, from www.paraplatin.com.

Gullatte, M. M. (2001). *A cancer chemotherapy handbook* (pp. 97-99). Pittsburgh, PA: Oncology Nursing Press.

Medline Plus. (2003). *Carboplatin..* Retrieved April 29, 2006, from http://www.nlm.nih.gov/medlineplus/druginfo/medmaster/a695017.html.

Micromedex. (2004). *Carboplatin..* Retrieved November 25, 2006, from www.drugs.com/cons/Carboplatin.html.

Polovich, M., White, J. M., & Kelleher, L. O. (2005) *Chemotherapy and biotherapy guidelines and recommendations for practice* (p. 20). Pittsburgh, PA: Oncology Nursing Press.

Wilkes, G. M., & Barton-Burke, M. (2005) *2005 Oncology nursing drug handbook* (pp. 86-89). Sudbury, MA: Jones & Bartlett.

Carmustine (BCNU, Gliadel Wafer)

Carol S. Blecher

DRUG CLASS

- Nitrosurea

ROUTE OF ADMINISTRATION

- Intravenous (IV)
- Intraarterial
- Topical
- Intratumoral

HOW TO ADMINISTER

- Administered IV in 100 mL or more over 15-45 minutes using glass or non-PVC containing infusion bags and administration sets. Longer infusion times (1-2 hours) are recommended to alleviate venous pain and irritation.
- Wafer is implanted into the tumor bed after the removal of the tumor.
- Topical solution may be painted on the lesions daily for 14 days after showering.

PRETREATMENT GUIDELINES

- Tests should be performed before the start of therapy and at periodic intervals during treatment, usually before each subsequent cycle of treatment.
  - Liver function studies: aspartate aminotransferase, alanine aminotransferase, alkaline phosphatase, total bilirubin, and lactate dehydrogenase
  - Complete blood cell count with differential and platelet count
  - Renal function tests: creatinine clearance actual or calculated or serum creatinine
  - Pulmonary function studies before beginning therapy and at frequent intervals

USE

- Hodgkin disease
- Non-Hodgkin lymphoma
- Central nervous system tumors
- Multiple myeloma
- Malignant melanoma
- Bone marrow transplant

Off-Label Uses

- Ewing's sarcoma
- Mycosis fungoides
- Cancers of the breast, colon, rectum, liver, and stomach

PHARMACOKINETICS

- Carmustine is a highly lipid soluble. It is distributed rapidly into the tissues and crosses the blood-brain barrier.
- Carmustine is metabolized by the liver.
- Parent drug has a short half-life, but the active metabolites have a half life of 67 hours.
- About 70% of the drug and its metabolites are excreted through the kidneys.

USUAL DOSE AND SCHEDULE

- Usual IV dose is 150-200 mg/m^2 as a single dose or as divided doses over 2 days every 6 to 8 weeks.
- Recommended maximum cumulative dose of 1400 mg/m^2.
- Doses up to 300-900 mg/m^2 have been used in high-dose chemotherapy before transplant.
- Implantation: up to 8 wafers used in resection cavity or less as space permits.

SIDE EFFECTS
Acute and Potentially Life Threatening

- Pulmonary toxicity usually occurring 9-10 years after treatment manifested as interstitial pneumonia and fibrosis, which may be progressive and fatal.
- Renal toxicity and failure is usually associated with high cumulative doses or prolonged therapy.

Other Side Effects

- Facial flushing with rapid infusion
- Alopecia
- Hyperpigmentation
- Severe nausea and vomiting
- Diarrhea
- Elevated liver enzymes
- Severe myelosuppression
- Phlebitis along vein during infusion
- Hypotension
- Dizziness
- Ataxia
- Seizures
- Blindness
- Retinal toxicity (with intracranial use)
- Secondary malignancies

NADIR

- Nadir is delayed with onset at 7 to 14 days. Nadir is usually at 21 to 35 days with recovery within 42 to 56 days.

STORAGE

- Vials should be stored under refrigeration.
- Vials are stable at room temperature for 7 days.
- The vials should not be exposed to heat because the powder may become oily.

MIXING INSTRUCTIONS

- The lyophilized powder is reconstituted with 3 mL of sterile diluent (dehydrated alcohol solution) supplied by the manufacturer. It is then to be further diluted with 27 mL of sterile water for injection.

PRODUCT STABILITY

- Reconstituted solution is stable for 8 hours at room temperature and 24 hours under refrigeration.
- Solutions that have been further diluted with normal saline solution or 5% dextrose in water (D5W) are stable for 8 hours at room temperature and for 48 hours if refrigerated and protected from light in glass or other manufacturer-approved container.

COMPATIBILITY WITH OTHER DRUGS/INTRAVENOUS FLUIDS

- Incompatible with polyvinyl chloride–containing infusion bags and with sodium bicarbonate.
- Compatible with cisplatin when mixed at a concentration of carmustine 1.5 mg/mL and cisplatin 0.86 mg/mL. This solution is stable at room temperature for 4 hours when mixed in a glass container

DRUG INTERACTIONS

- Use with cimetidine may increase the toxicities of carmustine.
- Concomitant use of amphotericin can enhance the cellular uptake of carmustine.

- When administered with etoposide, severe hepatic dysfunction, hyperbilirubinemia, ascites, and thrombocytopenias can develop.
- Carmustine may decrease the effectiveness of phenytoin.

PREGNANCY

Category D

- Women of childbearing potential are advised to avoid becoming pregnant while using carmustine.

SPECIAL CONSIDERATIONS

- Reconstituted and diluted solutions must be protected from light.
- Application of ice may ease pain/burning on administration.
- Myelosuppression is delayed and prolonged, so doses should not be repeated before 6-week intervals.
- Recommended cumulative dose of 1400 mg/m^2 because of potential for pulmonary toxicity

PATIENT EDUCATION

- Patients may be at risk of infection, so advise them to try to avoid crowds or people with colds.
- It is important to report fever or any other signs of infection immediately to health care providers.
- Use an electric razor and a soft toothbrush to minimize potential for bleeding. Avoid contact sports or activities that could cause injury.
- To reduce nausea, take antinausea medications as prescribed and eat small, frequent meals.
- Advise patients to discuss any symptoms or side effects with the health care team.

BIBLIOGRAPHY

Gullatte, M. M. (2001). *A cancer chemotherapy handbook* (pp. 99-102). Pittsburgh, PA: Oncology Nursing Press.
Medline Plus. (1997). *Carmustine (implantation—local)*. Retrieved April 29, 2006, from http://www.nlm.nih.gov/medlineplus/druginfo/uspdi/203660.html.

Medline Plus. (1997). *Carmustine (systemic)*. Retrieved April 29, 2006, from http://www.nlm.nih.gov/medlineplus/drug info/uspdi/202117.html.
Medline Plus. (2003). *Carmustine*. Retrieved April 29, 2006, from http://www.nlm.nih.gov/medlineplus/drug-info/medmaster/a682060.html.
Polovich, M., White, J. M., & Kelleher, L. O. (2005). *Chemotherapy and biotherapy guidelines and recommendations for practice* (p. 32). Pittsburgh, PA: Oncology Nursing Press.
Wilkes, G. M., & Barton-Burke, M. (2005). *2005 Oncology nursing drug handbook* (pp. 89-92). Sudbury, MA: Jones & Bartlett.

Chlorambucil (Leukeran)

Carol S. Blecher

DRUG CLASS

- Alkylating agent, nitrogen mustard derivative

ROUTE OF ADMINISTRATION

- Oral

HOW TO ADMINISTER

- Oral formulation should be administered on an empty stomach because food may decrease the oral bioavailability of the chlorambucil.

PRETREATMENT GUIDELINES

- Complete blood cell count with differential and platelet counts before the initiation of therapy and then before each subsequent dose
- Uric acid level before the initiation of therapy and at periodic intervals during therapy
- Liver function studies: alanine aminotransferase, aspartate aminotransferase, alkaline phosphatase, total bilirubin, and lactate dehydrogenase before the initiation of therapy and at periodic intervals during therapy

USE

- Chronic lymphocytic leukemia (CLL)

- Malignant lymphomas—giant follicular lymphoma, lymphosarcoma, and advanced Hodgkin disease

Off-Label Uses

- Waldenstrom's macroglobulinemia
- Polycythemia vera
- Trophoblastic neoplasms
- Ovarian carcinoma
- Breast carcinoma
- Testicular carcinoma
- Choriocarcinoma
- Multiple myeloma
- Nephritic syndrome

PHARMACOKINETICS

- Chlorambucil is well absorbed orally with peak plasma concentrations reached within 1 hour of administration. It is bound extensively to plasma proteins and is metabolized almost entirely in the liver.

USUAL DOSE AND SCHEDULE

- Normal dose is 0.1 to 0.2 mg/kg daily for 3 to 6 weeks. The average dose is between 4 and 10 mg per day. Dose adjustments are based on patient response and doses are decreased when there is a decrease in the white blood cell count (WBC).
- In CLL, alternating dosing schedules may be used. These may be intermittent, biweekly, or monthly schedules.

SIDE EFFECTS
Acute and Potentially Life Threatening

- Pulmonary fibrosis may occur with long-term use.
- Focal or generalized seizures may occur.
- Skin rash can progress to erythema multiforme, epidermal necrolysis, and Stevens-Johnson syndrome.

Other Side Effects

- Myelosuppression, especially leukopenia, lymphopenia, and thrombocytopenia
- Nausea, vomiting, anorexia, diarrhea

- Hyperuricemia
- Neurotoxicity manifested as confusion, agitation, and weakness
- Ovarian or sperm suppression
- Secondary malignancies

NADIR

- Nadir is at about 14 days, with onset beginning around day 7, and recovery occurs within 28 days, although some patients may have recovery delayed for 6 to 8 weeks.

STORAGE

- Tablets can be stored in a dry place at room temperature.

DRUG INTERACTIONS

- Simultaneous use of barbiturates may increase the toxicity of chlorambucil as a result of hepatic drug activation.
- Tricyclic antidepressants, monoamine oxidase (MAO) inhibitors, and phenothiazides can increase the potential for chlorambucil-induced seizures.

PREGNANCY

Category D

- Chlorambucil may be hazardous to the fetus because it crosses the placenta.
- Breast-feeding is not recommended because of the potential secretion of chlorambucil into breast milk.

SPECIAL CONSIDERATIONS

- Administer with caution within 4 weeks of radiation therapy, chemotherapy, or if bone marrow is severely depressed. Full doses should not be given during this period because of the potential for severe bone marrow toxicity.

PATIENT EDUCATION

- Take pills by mouth on an empty stomach.
- Increase fluid intake to 2 liters per day.
- The pills should be taken at the same time each day.
- If a dose is missed and the medication is ordered daily, take when remembered later that day.

If ordered more frequently, take as soon as possible unless almost time for next dose.
- Do not double dose.
- Patients may be at risk of infection. Advise patients to try to avoid crowds or people with colds and to report fever or any other signs of infection (fever, sore throat, chills, cough, hoarseness, lower back or side pain, difficult or painful urination) immediately to the health care provider.
- To help treat/prevent mouth sores, use a soft toothbrush and rinse three times a day with $\frac{1}{2}$ to 1 teaspoon of salt mixed with 8 ounces of water. Monitor oral cavity by inspecting the oral mucosa at least daily for redness and ulceration
- Instruct patient to report unusual bleeding or bruising. Advise patient of thrombocytopenia precautions (use soft toothbrush, electric razor, and avoid falls; do not drink alcoholic beverages or take medication containing aspirin or nonsteroidal anti-inflammatory drugs [NSAIDs] because they may precipitate gastric bleeding).
- To reduce nausea, take antinausea medications as prescribed and eat small, frequent meals.
- Instruct patient not to receive any vaccinations without advice of health care professional.
- Advise patients to discuss any symptoms or side effects with the health care team.

BIBLIOGRAPHY

Chlorambucil. (2007). In *Davis's drug guide for nurses*. Retrieved November 25, 2006, from http://www.drugg uide.com/monograph_library/addit ional_monographs/chlorambucil.htm.

Gullatte, M. M. (2001). *A cancer chemotherapy handbook* (pp. 102-103). Pittsburgh, PA: Oncology Nursing Press.

Medline Plus. (2003). *Chlorambucil*. (2003). Retrieved April 29, 2006, from http://www.nlm.nih.gov/medlineplus/druginfo/medmaster/a682899.html.

Medline Plus. (2005). *Chlorambucil (Systemic)*. Retrieved April 29, 2006, from http://www.nlm.nih.gov/medline plus/drug info/uspdi/202124.html.

Polovich, M., White, J. M., & Kelleher, L. O. (2005). *Chemotherapy and biotherapy guidelines and recommendations for practice* (p. 20). Pittsburgh, PA: Oncology Nursing Press.

Wilkes, G. M., & Barton-Burke, M. (2005). *2005 Oncology nursing drug handbook* (pp.93-95). Sudbury, MA: Jones 7 Bartlett.

Cisplatin (Platinol)

Carol S. Blecher

DRUG CLASS

- Alkylating agent, heavy metal compound

ROUTE OF ADMINISTRATION

- Intravenous (IV)
- Intraperitoneal

HOW TO ADMINISTER

- IV infusion rate is up to 1 mg/min.
- Intraperitoneal dose is administered in 2 L of normal saline solution infused over 10-15 minutes with a dwell time of 4 hours.

PRETREATMENT GUIDELINES

- Complete blood cell count (CBC) with differential and platelet counts before the initiation of therapy and then before each subsequent dose
- Liver function studies: alanine aminotransferase (ALT), aspartate aminotransferase (AST), alkaline phosphatase, total bilirubin, and lactate dehydrogenase (LDH) before the initiation of therapy and at periodic intervals during therapy
- Renal function studies: creatinine clearance or serum creatinine before the initiation of therapy and then before each subsequent dose
- Neurological function
- Auditory examination
- Intake and output

USE

- Lung, bladder, ovarian, testicular, cervical, prostate, and head and neck carcinomas
- Multiple myeloma
- Hodgkin disease
- Non-Hodgkin lymphoma
- Leukemia
- Wilms' tumor
- Brain tumors

Off-Label Use

- Endometrial carcinoma
- Breast cancer
- Gastric cancer
- Mesothelioma

PHARMACOKINETICS

- Cisplatin is 50%-100% absorbed systemically. 90% of the drug is protein bound.
- The drug seems to concentrate in the liver and kidneys.
- Plasma decay is biphasic. The initial phase is rapid with a half-life of 25-49 minutes, which is followed by a prolonged elimination phase with a half-life of 2-4 days. It is eliminated unchanged in the urine.

USUAL DOSE AND SCHEDULE

- When administering as single-agent therapy, typical doses and schedules are 50-100 mg/m^2 as a single IV infusion every 3 to 4 weeks over 6-8 hours or slow IV infusion of 15-20 mg/m^2 for 5 days every 3 to 4 weeks.
- Cisplatin may be used as a radiation sensitizer at a dose of 25 mg/m^2 weekly concurrently with radiation therapy.

SIDE EFFECTS
Acute and Potentially Life Threatening

- Nausea and vomiting are severe with cisplatin and begin within 1-4 hours after the start of treatment. Delayed nausea and vomiting occur up to 96 hours (4 days) after treatment.
- Acute renal failure may occur. Cisplatin is severely nephrotoxic.
- Peripheral neuropathies, both motor and sensory, are dose and duration related, progressive with continued therapy.
- Ototoxicity occurring in 10%-30% of patients is manifested by high-frequency hearing loss.

Other Side Effects

- Postural hypotension
- Hypertension
- Bradycardia
- ST-T wave changes
- Bundle branch block atrial fibrillation
- Hypomagnesemia
- Hypocalcemia
- Hypokalemia
- Anorexia
- Constipation and diarrhea
- Papilledema
- Tonic/clonic seizures
- Pulmonary fibrosis

NADIR

- Nadir is at about 18 days with a range between 14 and 21 days. Onset begins on day 14 and recovery occurs within 21-39 days.

STORAGE

- Aqueous solution vials are stable at room temperature. Powder vials are also stable at room temperature. Once reconstituted, drug is stable for 20 hours. Product should be protected from light.

MIXING INSTRUCTIONS

- Product should be mixed with sterile water for injection at a concentration of 1 mg/mL and further dilute in 0.9% NaCl.

PRODUCT STABILITY

- The product is stable at room temperature for 20 hours.
- Do not refrigerate.

COMPATIBILITY WITH OTHER DRUGS/INTRAVENOUS FLUIDS

- Incompatible with aluminum; use only stainless steel.
- Do not mix with dextrose 5%, dextrose 5% and water, or other chloride-lacking solutions.

Cancer Management

DRUG INTERACTIONS

- Aluminum and cisplatin will form a precipitate and the cisplatin will lose efficacy.
- Cisplatin should be used cautiously when using other drugs that cause renal failure such as the aminoglycosides.
- Loop diuretics may increase the potential of cisplatin to cause ototoxicity, especially in the presence of renal impairment.
- Cisplatin may alter the renal elimination of bleomycin and methotrexate and enhance their toxicity.
- Phenytoin serum concentrations may be decreased when administered concomitantly with cisplatin.
- Administer cisplatin after docetaxel or paclitaxel to prevent myelosuppression.

PREGNANCY

Category D
- Cisplatin may be hazardous to the fetus because it crosses the placenta.
- Breast-feeding is not recommended because of the potential secretion of cisplatin into breast milk.

SPECIAL CONSIDERATIONS

- Avoid the use of IV sets and needles containing aluminum.
- Hearing loss and peripheral neuropathies occur with prolonged high-dose therapy.
- Hypersensitivity reactions may occur.
- Pre-treatment hydration with 1-2 liters of fluid is recommended for preventing nephrotoxicity. Mannitol is used to achieve osmotic diuresis.
- Magnesium and potassium levels must be monitored.

PATIENT EDUCATION

- Increase fluid intake to 2 liters per day.
- Nausea may be severe. Have antiemetic medications available and instruct the patient to take antinausea medications regularly to prevent nausea and vomiting. Try to eat small, frequent meals.
- Patients may be at risk of infection; advise them to avoid crowds or people with colds and report fever or any other signs of infection (fever, sore throat, chills, cough, hoarseness, lower back or side pain, difficult or painful urination) immediately to the health care provider.
- To help treat/prevent mouth sores, use a soft toothbrush and rinse three times a day with $1/2$ to 1 teaspoon of salt mixed with 8 ounces of water. Monitor oral cavity by inspecting the oral mucosa at least daily for redness and ulceration.
- Instruct patient to report unusual bleeding or bruising. Advise patient of thrombocytopenia precautions (use soft toothbrush, electric razor, and avoid falls; do not drink alcoholic beverages or take medication containing aspirin or nonsteroidal anti-inflammatory drugs [NSAIDs] because they may precipitate gastric bleeding).
- Advise patients to discuss any symptoms or side effects with the health care team.

BIBLIOGRAPHY

Cisplatin data sheet. (2006). Retrieved November 25, 2006, from http://www.medsafe.gov.nz/Profs/Datasheet/c/Cisplatininj.htm.

Gullatte, M. M. (2001). *A cancer chemotherapy handbook* (pp. 103-105). Pittsburgh, PA: Oncology Nursing Press.

Medline Plus. (2002). *Cisplatin (systemic)*. Retrieved April 29, 2006, from http://www.nlm.nih.gov/medlineplus/drug info/uspdi/202143.html.

Medline Plus. (2003). *Cisplatin*. Retrieved April 29, 2006, from http://www.nlm.nih.gov/medlineplus/druginfo/medmaster/a684036.html.

Polovich, M., White, J. M., & Kelleher, L. O. (2005). *Chemotherapy and biotherapy guidelines and recommendations for practice* (p. 20). Pittsburgh, PA: Oncology Nursing Press.

Wilkes, G. M., & Barton-Burke, M. (2005). *2005 Oncology nursing drug handbook* (pp. 95-100). Sudbury, MA: Jones & Bartlett.

Cladribine (Leustatin 2-CDA)

Carol S. Blecher

DRUG CLASS

- Antimetabolite, purine nucleoside analog

ROUTE OF ADMINISTRATION

- Intravenous (IV)

HOW TO ADMINISTER

- IV continuous infusion over 7 days

PRETREATMENT GUIDELINES

- Complete blood cell count (CBC) with differential and platelet counts before the initiation of therapy and then before each subsequent dose
- Uric acid
- CD4 and CD8 counts should be monitored before the start of therapy and at intervals during and after therapy.

USE

- Hairy cell leukemia

Off-Label Uses

- Non-Hodgkin lymphoma
- Chronic lymphocytic leukemia (CLL)
- Waldenstrom's macroglobulinemia

PHARMACOKINETICS

- Cladribine is rapidly distributed and has an elimination half-life of 7 hours.
- This drug crosses the blood-brain barrier and it can be detected in the central nervous system (CNS).

USUAL DOSE AND SCHEDULE

- Usual dosing for patients with hairy cell leukemia is 0.09 to 0.1 mg/kg/day for 7 days or 4 mg/m^2/day as a continuous infusion.
- Other regimens have dosed cladribine at 0.1 mg to 0.3 mg/kg/day for 7 days with doses not to exceed 0.3 mg per day.

- Cladribine is administered by infusion through a vein. The infusion may be over 1-2 hours on consecutive days or may be a continuous infusion over several days.

SIDE EFFECTS
Acute and Potentially Life Threatening
- Myelosuppression and immunosuppression
- Tumor lysis syndrome

Other Side Effects
- Dermatological, rash, pruritus, and erythema
- Nausea and vomiting
- Abdominal pain and constipation
- Headache
- Insomnia
- Fatigue and dizziness
- Fever
- Arthralgias
- Myalgias
- Pain and erythema at the injection site
- Neurotoxicity
- Hypersensitivity reaction
- Shortness of breath
- Tachycardia.

NADIR
- Nadir occurs between 14 and 21 days and recovery occurs within 4-8 weeks.

STORAGE
- The intact vials should be refrigerated at 2°-8° C (36°-46° F).
- Vial must be protected from light.

MIXING INSTRUCTIONS
- Dilute before administration. Twenty-four-hour solutions should be diluted in 500 mL of sodium chloride for injection. Seven-day solutions should be mixed with use of a 0.22 micron hydrophilic filter in 0.9% normal saline solution (NS) for a total volume of 100 mL.

PRODUCT STABILITY
- The 24-hour product is stable at room temperature for 24 hours

and the 7-day product is stable at room temperature for 7 days.
- Once the cladribine has been diluted, it must be administered promptly; it may be stored in the refrigerator for a maximum of 8 hours before the start of the infusion.

COMPATIBILITY WITH OTHER DRUGS/INTRAVENOUS FLUIDS
- Incompatible with 5% dextrose in water (D5W)
- Cladribine should not be administered concomitantly with other IV drugs or additives. It should also not be infused simultaneously by the same IV line because compatibility testing has not been performed.

DRUG INTERACTIONS
- No known drug interactions

PREGNANCY
Category D
- Cladribine may be hazardous to the fetus.
- Breast-feeding is not recommended while taking cladribine.

SPECIAL CONSIDERATIONS
- If fever occurs, the patient must be evaluated for infection.
  NOTE: The patient will be considered immunosuppressed for up to 1 year after taking cladribine.

PATIENT EDUCATION
- Do not receive any kind of immunization or vaccination without a doctor's approval while taking cladribine.
- To reduce nausea, take antinausea medications as prescribed and eat small amounts of food frequently.
- Drink at least 2 to 3 quarts of fluid every 24 hours, unless instructed otherwise.
- Patients may be at risk of infection, so they should try to avoid crowds or people with colds and report fever or any other signs of infection immediately to the health care provider.

- Patients should wash their hands often.
- Use an electric razor and a soft toothbrush to minimize bleeding.
- Avoid contact sports or activities that could cause injury.
- In general, drinking alcoholic beverages should be kept to a minimum or avoided completely. Patients should discuss this with their doctors.
- Avoid sun exposure. Wear sun protection factor (SPF) 15 (or higher) sunblock and protective clothing.
- Get plenty of rest.
- Maintain good nutrition.
- Advise patients to discuss symptoms or side effects with the health care team.

BIBLIOGRAPHY
Chemocare.com. (2005). *Cladribine*. Retrieved November 25, 2006, from http://www.chemocare.com/BIO/cladribine.asp.

Gullatte, M. M. (2001). *A cancer chemotherapy handbook* (pp. 106-108). Pittsburgh, PA: Oncology Nursing Press.

Medline Plus. (2002). *Cladribine (systemic)*. Retrieved April 29, 2006 from http://www.nlm.nih.gov/medlineplus/drug info/uspdi/202699.html.

Medline Plus. (2003). *Cladribine*. Retrieved April 29, 2006, from http://www.nlm.nih.gov/medlineplus/druginfo/medmaster/a693015.html.

Polovich, M., White, J. M., & Kelleher, L. O. (2005). *Chemotherapy and biotherapy guidelines and recommendations for practice* (p. 20). Pittsburgh, PA: Oncology Nursing Press.

Wilkes, G. M., & Barton-Burke, M. (2005). *2005 Oncology nursing drug handbook* (pp. 95-100). Sudbury, MA: Jones & Bartlett.

Cancer Management

Cyclophosphamide (Cytoxan, Neosar, Endoxan)

Carol S. Blecher

DRUG CLASS

- Alkylating agent, nitrogen mustard derivative

ROUTE OF ADMINISTRATION

- Intravenous (IV)
- Intraperitoneal
- Oral

HOW TO ADMINISTER

- IV slow push through the side arm of a free-flowing IV of 5% dextrose in water (D5W)
- IV infusion over 30 minutes to 3 hours diluted in either D5W or normal saline solution
- Intraperitoneal dose should be warmed prior to infusion.
- Oral doses should be taken in the morning with food to decrease nausea.

PRETREATMENT GUIDELINES

- Complete blood cell count (CBC) with differential and platelet counts before the initiation of therapy and then before each subsequent dose
- Liver function studies: alanine aminotransferase (ALT), aspartate aminotransferase (AST), alkaline phosphatase, total bilirubin, and lactate dehydrogenase (LDH) before the initiation of therapy and at periodic intervals during therapy
- Renal function studies: creatinine clearance or serum creatinine before the initiation of therapy and then before each subsequent dose
- Serum chemistry profile before initiation of therapy and at periodic intervals during therapy
- Urinalysis should be performed if hemorrhagic cystitis is suspected.

USE

- Acute myelogenous leukemia (AML)
- Acute lymphocytic leukemia (ALL)
- Chronic myelogenous leukemia (CML)
- Chronic lymphocytic leukemia (CLL)
- Hodgkin disease
- Non-Hodgkin lymphoma
- Breast carcinoma
- Ovarian carcinoma
- Multiple myeloma
- Neuroblastoma
- Retinoblastoma
- Mycosis fungoides.

Off-Label Uses

- Bronchogenic carcinoma
- Small cell lung cancer
- Bone marrow transplant

PHARMACOKINETICS

- About one half of the drug is bound to the plasma proteins.
- Cyclophosphamide crosses the blood-brain barrier.
- It is a prodrug metabolized by the liver to several active metabolites and excreted in the urine.
- The half-life of cyclophosphamide is between 4 and 6.5 hours. When it is administered orally, 75%-90% of the drug is absorbed through the gastrointestinal (GI) tract.

USUAL DOSE AND SCHEDULE
Cyclophosphamide

- 400 mg/m² IV for 5 days
- 100 mg/m² orally for 14 days
- 500-1,500 mg/m² IV every 3 to 4 weeks

High-Dose Cyclophosphamide with Bone Marrow Transplant

- 1.8 to 7 g/m² used in combination with other cytotoxic agents

SIDE EFFECTS
Acute and Potentially Life Threatening

- Very emetogenic in high-dose protocols
- Acute hemorrhagic cystitis may be severe or fatal. Mesna may be necessary as a bladder protectant.

- High-dose cyclophosphamide can cause cardiac toxicity manifested by congestive heart failure (CHF) or cardiac necrosis.

Other Side Effects

- Alopecia
- Rash
- Hives
- Pruritus
- Nausea
- Vomiting
- Diarrhea
- Myelosuppression
- Headache and dizziness
- Pulmonary fibrosis
- Pneumonitis
- Myxedema
- Facial flushing
- Congestion
- SIADH

NADIR

- Nadir occurs on or about days 7 to 14 with recovery within 4-5 weeks.

STORAGE

- Vials and tablets should be stored at 25° F (77° F).

MIXING INSTRUCTIONS

- Drug should be reconstituted with sterile or bacteriostatic water. Further dilution may be in D5W or normal saline (NS) solution.

PRODUCT STABILITY

- The product is stable for 24 hours at room temperature and for 6 days when refrigerated.

COMPATIBILITY WITH OTHER DRUGS/INTRAVENOUS FLUIDS

- Compatible with D5W and NS for infusion.

DRUG INTERACTIONS

- When administered with corticosteroids, the metabolism of cyclophosphamide may be inhibited.
- If administered in conjunction with succinylcholine, there is an increased potential for respiratory distress.

- Barbiturates and phenytoin increase cyclophosphamide metabolism.
- Cyclophosphamide potentiates the toxicity of doxorubicin, increasing its cardiotoxic effects.
- Cyclophosphamide increases the effects of anticoagulants.
- Cyclophosphamide decreases digoxin serum levels.
- Cyclophosphamide decreases the antimicrobial effects of quinolone antibiotics.

PREGNANCY

Category D
- Cyclophosphamide may be hazardous to the fetus.
- Breast-feeding is not recommended while taking cyclophosphamide.

SPECIAL CONSIDERATIONS

- Hydrate vigorously before and after cyclophosphamide infusion to prevent or minimize hemorrhagic cystitis.
- Force fluids to 4 L per day when administering oral cyclophosphamide.
- Cyclophosphamide should be taken early in the day to avoid metabolites remaining in the bladder for long periods of time.
- The oral formulation should be administered with food.

PATIENT EDUCATION

- While being treated with cyclophosphamide, patients should drink 3 or 4 liters of fluid a day to help prevent bladder problems. The extra fluid will dilute urine and make patients urinate frequently, thus minimizing the cyclophosphamide byproducts' contact with the bladder.
- Patients should not take missed doses. They should go back to the regular schedule and contact their doctor. Do not take two doses at once.
- To reduce nausea, take antinausea medications as prescribed and eat small amounts of food frequently.

- Patients may be at risk of infection, so advise them to try to avoid crowds or people with colds and report fever or any other signs of infection immediately to the health care provider.
- Patients should wash their hands often.
- Use an electric razor and a soft toothbrush to minimize bleeding.
- Avoid contact sports or activities that could cause injury. Cyclophosphamide may cause mouth sores. Avoid spicy foods and do not use mouthwash because it may contain alcohol and worsen mouth pain. Health care providers may provide suggestions on caring for the patient's mouth or managing mouth sores, and these directions should be followed carefully.
- Cyclophosphamide may cause skin to darken slightly. Ridges may form on fingernails and toenails.
- Patients should be advised to discuss symptoms and side effects with the health care team.

BIBLIOGRAPHY

Chemotherapy Resource Area. (2006). *Cyclophosphamide*. Retrieved November 25, 2006, from http://www.ons.org/patiented/treatment/patientmeds/cyclophosphamide/shtml.
Gullatte, M. M. (2001). *A cancer chemotherapy handbook* (pp. 108-109). Pittsburgh, PA: Oncology Nursing Press.
Medline Plus. (2002). *Cyclophosphamide (systemic)*. Retrieved April 29, 2006, from http://www.nlm.nih.gov/medlineplus/drug info/uspdi/202174.html.
Medline Plus. (2003). *Cyclophosphamide*. Retrieved April 29, 2006, from http://www.nlm.nih.gov/medlineplus/drug info/medmaster/a682080.html.
Polovich, M., White, J. M., & Kelleher, L. O. (2005). *Chemotherapy and biotherapy guidelines and recommendations for practice* (p. 21). Pittsburgh, PA: Oncology Nursing Press.
Wilkes, G. M., & Barton-Burke, M. (2005). *2005 Oncology nursing drug handbook* (pp. 103-107). Sudbury, MA: Jones & Bartlett.

Cytarabine (Cytosine arabinoside, ARA-C, Cytosar-U, DepoCyt)

Carol S. Blecher

DRUG CLASS

- Antimetabolite, pyrimidine analog

ROUTE OF ADMINISTRATION

- Intravenous (IV)
- Subcutaneous (SQ)
- Intrathecal

HOW TO ADMINISTER

- IV by infusion over 1 to 24 hours.
- Bolus doses may be administered intramuscularly, SQ, or intrathecally.

PRETREATMENT GUIDELINES

- Complete blood cell count (CBC) with differential and platelet counts before the initiation of therapy and then before each subsequent dose
- Liver function studies, alanine aminotransferase (ALT), aspartate aminotransferase (AST), alkaline phosphatase, total bilirubin, and lactate dehydrogenase (LDH) before the initiation of therapy and at periodic intervals during therapy
- Renal function studies, creatinine clearance, or serum creatinine before the initiation of therapy and then before each subsequent dose
- Uric acid

USE

- Acute nonlymphocytic leukemia (ANLL)
- Acute myelogenous leukemia (AML)
- Acute lymphocytic leukemia (ALL)
- Chronic myelogenous leukemia (CML)
- Hodgkin disease
- Non Hodgkin lymphoma

Cancer Management

- Central nervous system (CNS) leukemia

Off-Label Uses
- Carcinomatous meningitis
- Myelodysplastic syndrome (MDS)

PHARMACOKINETICS
- This drug undergoes rapid deamination in blood and tissues, especially the liver, but minimally in the cerebrospinal fluid (CSF).
- Excretion is in the urine with less than 10% of the drug unchanged.
- Half-life is biphasic with the alpha phase being 10 minutes and the beta phase lasting 1 to 3 hours.
- Cytarabine preparation has a terminal half-life of 100-263 hours.

USUAL DOSE AND SCHEDULE
- Doses for ANLL are 60-200 mg/m^2/day continuous infusion for 5-10 days or 100 mg/m^2/day every 12 hours on days 1-7.
- IV or SQ dose of 100 mg/m^2/day twice daily for 5 days every 28 days. Another SQ protocol is the use of 10 mg/m^2 every 12 hours for 15-21 days.
- High-dose therapy is 1-3 g/m^2/day every 12 hours to infuse over 3 hours for 2-6 days.

SIDE EFFECTS
Acute and Potentially Life Threatening
High-dose therapy associated with severe and potentially fatal toxicity, including:
- Reversible corneal toxicity and hemorrhagic conjunctivitis (prevented or reduced by prophylactic administration of a local corticosteroid eye drop)
- Cerebral dysfunction (confusion, tiredness, memory loss, seizures)
- Cerebellar dysfunction (trouble in speaking, standing, or walking; tremors)
- Gastrointestinal ulceration
- Peritonitis, sepsis, and liver abscess
- Pulmonary edema
- Hepatic damage with hyperbilirubinemia
- Bowel necrosis
- Necrotizing colitis
- Skin rash leading to desquamation
- Fatal cardiomyopathy
- A potentially fatal syndrome of sudden respiratory distress progressing to pulmonary edema and cardiomegaly
- Peripheral motor and sensory neuropathies
- Capillary leak syndrome may occur.

Other Side Effects
- Rash
- Hives
- Pruritus
- Nausea
- Vomiting
- Diarrhea
- Stomatitis
- Myelosuppression
- Headache and dizziness

NADIR
- Nadir begins at about 5 days, dropping to the lowest levels on days 5-15 days after treatment with recovery within 21-28 days.

STORAGE
- Vials should be stored at 20°-25° F (68°-77° F).

MIXING INSTRUCTIONS
- Drug should be reconstituted with bacteriostatic water with benzyl alcohol for IV, IM and SQ use.
- High-dose and intrathecal preparations should not be reconstituted with bacteriostatic water with benzyl alcohol.
- Further dilution may be in 5% dextrose in water (D5W) or normal saline solution (NS).

PRODUCT STABILITY
- The product is stable for 48 hours at room temperature and for 7 days when refrigerated.

COMPATIBILITY WITH OTHER DRUGS/INTRAVENOUS FLUIDS
- Compatible with D5W and NS for infusion

DRUG INTERACTIONS
- Use of gentamicin with cytarabine may decrease the effectiveness of the gentamicin.
- When cytarabine is used with flucytosine, there is a decreased efficacy of the flucytosine.
- Digoxin levels must be carefully monitored because the use of digoxin with cytarabine decreases the plasma level of the digoxin.
- Cytarabine may have a synergistic cytotoxic effect when administered following methotrexate.
- There have been reports of a potential increase in cardiotoxicity when high-dose cytarabine is used in conjunction with cyclophosphamide in the transplant setting.

PREGNANCY
Category D
- Cytarabine may be hazardous to the fetus.
- Breast-feeding is not recommended while taking cytarabine.

SPECIAL CONSIDERATIONS
- Administer corticosteroid eye drops to prevent conjunctivitis.

PATIENT EDUCATION
- To reduce nausea, take antinausea medications as prescribed and eat small amounts of food frequently.
- Patients may be at risk of infection, so advise them to try to avoid crowds or people with colds and to report fever or any other signs of infection immediately to the health care provider.
- Patients should wash their hands often.
- Patients should check with the doctor immediately if they notice any unusual bleeding or bruising; black, tarry stools; blood in urine or stools; or pinpoint red spots on the skin.
- Use an electric razor and a soft toothbrush to minimize bleeding.
- Avoid contact sports or activities that could cause injury.

- Patients should not have any immunizations (vaccinations) without a doctor's approval. Cytarabine may lower the body's resistance, and there is a chance they might get the infection the immunization is meant to prevent. In addition, other persons living in the patient's household should not take oral polio vaccine because there is a chance they could pass the polio virus on to the patient. Patients should avoid persons who have recently taken the oral polio vaccine.
- Advise patients to discuss symptoms and side effects with the health care team.

BIBLIOGRAPHY

Drugs.com. (2004). *Cytarabine.* Retrieved November 25, 2006, from http://www.drugs.com/cons/cytarabine.html.

Gullatte, M. M. (2001). *A cancer chemotherapy handbook* (pp. 110-114). Pittsburgh, PA: Oncology Nursing Press.

Medline Plus. (1999). *Cytarabine, liposomal (intrathecal).* Retrieved April 29, 2006, from http://www.nlm.nih.gov/medlineplus/drug info/uspdi/500008.html.

Medline Plus. (2003). *Cytarabine.* Retrieved April 29, 2006, from http://www.nlm.nih.gov/medlineplus/druginfo/medmaster/a682222.html.

Medline Plus. (2004). *Cytarabine (systemic).* Retrieved April 29, 2006, from http://www.nlm.nih.gov/medlineplus/drug info/uspdi/202177.html.

Polovich, M., White, J. M., & Kelleher, L. O. (2005). *Chemotherapy and biotherapy guidelines and recommendations for practice* (p. 23-24). Pittsburgh, PA: Oncology Nursing Press.

Wilkes, G. M., & Barton-Burke, M. (2005). *2005 Oncology nursing drug handbook* (pp. 107-113). Sudbury, MA: Jones & Bartlett.

Dacarbazine (DTIC-Dome)

Christa Braun-Inglis

DRUG CLASS

- Alkylating agent

ROUTE OF ADMINISTRATION

- Intravenous (IV) route by short infusion or by continuous infusion

HOW TO ADMINISTER

- Administer over 30-60 minutes.

PRETREATMENT GUIDELINES

- Liver function studies
- Complete blood cell count (CBC) with each treatment
- Potential for severe nausea and vomiting; premedicate with antiemetics

USE

- Melanoma
- Hodgkin disease
- Soft tissue sarcomas
- Neuroblastoma

PHARMACOKINETICS

- Initial half-life is 19 minutes.
- Terminal half-life is 5 hours.
- Metabolized in the liver and excreted by the kidney
- In a patient with renal and hepatic dysfunction, the half-lives were lengthened to 55 minutes and 7.2 hours, respectively.

USUAL DOSE AND SCHEDULE
Single Agent

- 250 mg/m^2 days 1-5 every 28 days

Combination Therapy

- 375 mg/m^2 days 1 and 15 every 28 days
- 750 mg/m^2 day 1 every 21 days
- 220 mg/m^2 days 1-3, days 22-24 every 6 weeks

Continuous Infusion

- 250 mg/m^2 days 1-4 every 21 days
- 300 mg/m^2 days 1-3 every 21 days

SIDE EFFECTS
Vesicant

- Nausea
- Vomiting
- Anorexia
- Flu-like syndrome
- Myelosuppression
- Fatigue
- Mucositis
- Diarrhea
- Liver necrosis
- Hypersensitivity
- Hair loss
- Photosensitivity

NADIR

- 21-25 days with usual recovery by 35 days

STORAGE

- Intact vials of dacarbazine should be stored at 2°-8° C and protected from light.

MIXING INSTRUCTIONS

- Reconstitute 100-mg vials with 9.9 mL of sterile water, 200-mg vials with 19.8 mL; may be mixed in up to 500 mL of 5% dextrose in water (D5W) or 0.9% normal saline solution (NS).

PRODUCT STABILITY

- Stable for 8 hours at room temperature and in light and for 72 hours when refrigerated
- Drug decomposition is denoted by a change in color from yellow to pink.
- Studies have shown stability for up to 24 hours at room temperature.

COMPATIBILITY WITH OTHER DRUGS/INTRAVENOUS FLUIDS

- Dacarbazine is compatible with 0.9% NS.
- Dacarbazine is incompatible with heparin, lidocaine, and hydrocortisone.

DRUG INTERACTIONS

- Decreased levels/effect of dacarbazine when administered with phenytoin, rifampin, carbamazepine, or phenobarbital because these drugs induce

Cancer Management

dacarbazine metabolism by the P450 system.

- Increased levels/effects of dacarbazine when administered with amiodarone, ciprofloxacin, norfloxacin, ofloxacin, fluvoxamine, azole antifungals, and isoniazid.

PREGNANCY

Category C

SPECIAL CONSIDERATIONS
Vesicant

- Follow proper procedure for extravasation.
- Apply ice to affected area for 15 minutes, four times per day for 48 hours.
- When dacarbazine is leaked into tissue, cells die, causing the drug to be further released into adjacent cells. This causes progressive necrosis. Patient may require plastic surgery for skin grafting.

Highly Emetogenic Agent

- Premedicate aggressively.

Photosensitivity

- Patients should avoid sun exposure for several days after dacarbazine therapy.

PATIENT EDUCATION

- Patient should notify nurse if any pain, stinging, or burning occurs while dacarbazine is being administered.
- Instruct patient to stay out of the sun for several days after receiving drug.
- Instruct patient on antiemetic regimen.

BIBLIOGRAPHY

Chu, E., Mota, A., Bromberg, M., et al. (2003). Chemotherapeutic and biologic drugs. In E. Chu & V. T. DeVita (Eds.). *Cancer chemotherapy drug manual 2004* (pp. 104-106). Sudbury, MA: Jones & Bartlett.

Rx List. (2004). *Dacarbazine*. Retrieved January 17, 2006, from http://www.rxlist.com/cgi/generic2/dacarbazine.html.

Takimoto, C. H., & Calvo, E. (2005). Principles of oncologic pharmacotherapy. In R. Pazdur, L. R. Coia, W. J. Hoskins, et al. (Eds.), *Cancer management: Multidisciplinary approach* (pp. 11-22). Lawrence, KS: CMP Healthcare Media.

Trissel, L. A. (2005). *Handbook on injectable drugs* (13th ed., p. 428). Bethesda, MA: American Society of Health-Systems Pharmacists.

Wilkes, G. M., & Barton-Burke, M. (2005). *2005 Oncology nursing drug handbook* (pp. 113-116). Sudbury, MA: Jones & Bartlett.

Dactinomycin-D (Cosmegen)

Christa Braun-Inglis

DRUG CLASS

- Antitumor antibiotic

ROUTE OF ADMINISTRATION

- Intravenous (IV) route by IV push

HOW TO ADMINISTER

- Slow IV push over 10-15 minutes

PRETREATMENT GUIDELINES

- Assess patient for current herpes zoster or chickenpox.
- Baseline complete blood cell count (CBC) and liver function tests (LFTs), serum calcium

USE

- Testicular cancer
- Ewing's sarcoma
- Wilms' tumor
- Rhabdomyosarcoma
- Gestational trophoblastic tumors
- Choriocarcinoma

PHARMACOKINETICS

- Minimally metabolized
- Does not cross the blood-brain barrier
- Terminal plasma half-life 36 hours

USUAL DOSE AND SCHEDULE
Combination Therapy

- 0.4-0.45 mg/m² days 1-5 every 2-3 weeks (adults)
- 0.010-0.015 mg/kg IV days 1-5 every 21 days (children)
- 2 mg/m² day 1 every 21-28 days

SIDE EFFECTS
Vesicant

- Mucositis
- Myelosuppression
- Anorexia
- Nausea
- Vomiting
- Diarrhea
- Alopecia
- Hyperpigmentation
- Photosensitivity
- Radiation recall
- Allergic reaction
- Increased values on LFTs

NADIR

- 8-14 days after administration

STORAGE

- Store at 25° C (77° F), with variations in temperature permitted from 15°-30° C (59°-86° F).
- Protect from light and humidity.

MIXING INSTRUCTIONS

- Reconstitute 0.5 mg vials with 1.1 mL of sterile water to yield a gold-colored solution containing 0.5 mg/mL dactinomycin.
- Use preservative-free water; otherwise precipitate may develop.

PRODUCT STABILITY

- The solution maintains cytotoxicity for 24 hours either at 4° C (39° F) or room temperature.

COMPATIBILITY WITH OTHER DRUGS/INTRAVENOUS FLUIDS

- Dactinomycin is compatible with 0.9% normal saline solution.

DRUG INTERACTIONS

- None known

PREGNANCY

Category D

SPECIAL CONSIDERATIONS
Vesicant

- Follow proper procedure for extravasation.
- Apply ice to affected area for 15 minutes, four times per day for 48 hours.

- When dactinomycin is leaked into tissue, cells die, causing the drug to be further released into adjacent cells. This causes progressive necrosis. Patient may require plastic surgery for skin grafting.

Highly Emetogenic Agent

- Use aggressive antiemetics as premedication.

Chickenpox/Herpes Zoster

- Contraindicated in patients infected with chickenpox or herpes zoster because generalized infection may result in death

Radiation Recall

- Use with caution in patients either previously treated with radiation or with concurrent radiation.

Dosage

- Dosage is usually expressed in micrograms although many regimens list the dose in milligrams.

PATIENT EDUCATION

- Patient should notify nurse if any pain, stinging, or burning occurs while dacarbazine is being administered.
- Instruct patient to stay out of the sun for several days after receiving drug.
- Instruct patient on antiemetic regimen.

BIBLIOGRAPHY

Chu, E., Mota, A., Bromberg, M., et al. (2003). Chemotherapeutic and biologic drugs. In E. Chu & V. T. DeVita (Eds.). *Cancer chemotherapy drug manual 2004* (pp. 107-109). Sudbury, MA: Jones & Bartlett.

Rx List. (2004). *Dactinomycin*. Retrieved January 17, 2006, from http://www.rxlist.com/cgi/generic2/dactinomycin_wcp.htm.

Takimoto, C. H., & Calvo, E. (2005). Principles of oncologic pharmacotherapy. In R. Pazdur, L. R. Coia, W. J. Hoskins, et al. (Eds.). *Cancer management: Multidisciplinary approach* (pp. 11-22). Lawrence, KS: CMP Healthcare Media.

Trissel, L. A. (2005). *Handbook on injectable drugs* (13th ed.) (pp. 431-432). Bethesda, MD: American Society of Health-Systems Pharmacists.

Wilkes, G. M., & Barton-Burke, M. (2005). *2005 Oncology nursing drug handbook* (pp. 116-118). Sudbury, MA: Jones & Bartlett.

Daunorubicin (Cerubidine, Daunomycin HCl, Rubidomycin)

Christa Braun-Inglis

DRUG CLASS

- Anthracycline antibiotic

ROUTE OF ADMINISTRATION

- Short intravenous (IV) infusion or by IV push through rapidly infusing IV solution.
- Drug is not to be given intramuscularly or subcutaneously.

HOW TO ADMINISTER

- Administer drug IV push over 2-3 minutes or IV piggyback over 15-30 minutes.
- Administer into large vein.

PRETREATMENT GUIDELINES

- Liver function studies
  - For total bilirubin 1.2–3 mg/dL: decrease normal dose by 50%.
  - For total bilirubin 3.1–5 mg/dL: decrease normal dose by 75%.
  - For total bilirubin >5 mg/dL: do not give dose.
- Renal function studies
- Baseline echocardiogram or multiple gated acquisition (MUGA) scan to evaluate cardiac function

USE

- Acute myelogenous leukemia (AML)
- Acute lymphocytic leukemia (ALL)

PHARMACOKINETICS

- Initial half-life 45 minutes
- Terminal phase is 18.5 hours.

- Metabolized in the liver and excreted by both the biliary system and kidneys

USUAL DOSE AND SCHEDULE
Combination Therapy

- Adults: 30-60 mg/m^2 IV days 1-5 for induction therapy only
- Pediatric: 25 mg/m^2 IV day 1 weekly

SIDE EFFECTS
Vesicant

- Nausea
- Vomiting
- Alopecia
- Mucositis
- Rash
- Myelosuppression
- Cardiotoxicity
- Radiation recall

NADIR

- 10-14 days with recovery in 21-28 days.

STORAGE
Unreconstituted Powder

- Intact vials of daunorubicin should be stored at controlled room temperature and protected from light.

Reconstituted Powder or Solution

- May be stored at room temperature or refrigerated; see stability information

MIXING INSTRUCTIONS

- Reconstitute 20-mg vials with 4 mL of sterile water to yield a solution containing 5 mg/mL of daunorubicin.
- Product will appear orange-red in color.

PRODUCT STABILITY

- Stable for 24 hours at controlled room temperature and for 48 hours under refrigeration

COMPATABILITY WITH OTHER DRUGS/INTRAVENOUS FLUIDS

- Daunorubicin is compatible with 0.9% normal saline solution or 5% dextrose in water (D5W).

DRUG INTERACTIONS

- Daunorubicin is incompatible with dexamethasone and heparin because precipitate will form.

PREGNANCY

Category D

- Breast-feeding is not recommended while receiving daunorubicin.

SPECIAL CONSIDERATIONS
Vesicant

- Follow proper procedure for extravasation.
- Apply ice to area of extravasation for 15 minutes, four times a day, for 3 days.
- When daunorubicin is leaked into tissue, cells die, causing daunorubicin to be further released into adjacent cells, thus causing progressive tissue necrosis. Patient may require a plastic surgeon consult and skin grafting.
- Few evidence-based guidelines exist for extravasation management; therefore, proper procedure continues to be controversial.
- Cardiotoxicity may develop during treatment or months to years after treatment. Monitor patient's total cumulative dose. Risk for development of cardiotoxicity rises when total cumulative dose is more than 550 mg/m². Cumulative doses which exceed 550 mg/m², or 400 mg/m² in patients who have received previous anthracycline, mitoxantrone, or radiation of the cardiac region, should be given with extreme caution.

PATIENT EDUCATION

- Patient should notify nurse if any pain, burning, or stinging occurs while medication is being administered.
- Instruct patient that urine may have a red-orange discoloration for 1-3 days. If the discoloration occurs longer than 72 hours, contact physician.

BIBLIOGRAPHY

Chu, E., Mota, A., Bromberg, M., et al. (2003). Chemotherapeutic and biologic drugs. In E. Chu, & V. T. DeVita (Eds.). *Cancer chemotherapy drug manual 2004* (pp. 104-106). Sudbury, MA: Jones & Bartlett.

Rx List. (2004). *Daunorubicin*. Retrieved March 4, 2006, from http://www.rxlist.com/cgi/generic2/daunorubicin_wcp.htm.

Takimoto, C. H., & Calvo, E. (2005). Principles of oncologic pharmacotherapy. In R. Pazdur, L. R. Coia, W. J. Hoskins, et al. (Eds.). *Cancer management: multidisciplinary approach* (pp. 11-22). Lawrence, KS: CMP Healthcare Media.

Trissel, L.A. (2005). *Handbook on injectable drugs* (13th ed., p. 434). Bethesda, MD: American Society of Health-Systems Pharmacists.

Wickham, R., Engelking, C., Sauerland, C., et al. (2006). Vesicant extravasation part II: evidenced-based management and continuing controversies. *Oncology Nursing Forum, 33*, 1145-1149.

Wilkes, G. M., & Barton-Burke, M. (2005). *2005 Oncology nursing drug handbook* (pp. 123-126). Sudbury, MA: Jones & Bartlett.

Daunorubicin Liposome (DaunoXome®)

Christa Braun-Inglis

DRUG CLASS

- Anthracycline antibiotic

ROUTE OF ADMINISTRATION

- Intravenous infusion
- Drug is not to be given intramuscularly or subcutaneously.

HOW TO ADMINISTER

- Drug is administered over 60 minutes.

PRETREATMENT GUIDELINES

- Liver function studies for total bilirubin 1.2-3 mg/dL, decrease normal dose by 50%, for total bilirubin 3.1-5 mg/dL, decrease normal dose by 75%, for total bilirubin >5 mg/dL, do not give the dose.
- Renal function studies for serum creatinine >3 mg/dL, administer 50% of the normal dose.
- Baseline echocardiogram or MUGA scan to evaluate cardiac function

USE

- HIV-associated Kaposi's sarcoma

PHARMACOKINETICS

- Elimination half-life is 4.5 hours
- Metabolized in the liver

USUAL DOSE AND SCHEDULE
Combination Therapy

- Adults: 20-40 mg/m² IV, repeat every 14 days

SIDE EFFECTS

- Nausea/vomiting (mild)
- Mucositis
- Diarrhea
- Hyperpigmentation
- Myelosuppression-dose limiting toxicity leukopenia
- Cardiotoxicity
- Infusion related reaction
- Fatigue

NADIR

- 10-14 days with recovery in 21-28 days

STORAGE
Unreconstituted Vials

- Intact vials of daunorubicin liposome should be refrigerated at 2°-8° C (36°-46° F) and protected from light.

Reconstituted Solution

- May be stored refrigerated at 2°-6° C (36°-42° F) for 6 hours

MIXING INSTRUCTIONS

- Visually inspect for particulate matter and discoloration; prior to mixing, drug appears as a translucent dispersion of liposomes that scatters light. It should not appear opaque or have any precipitate.
- Withdraw calculated volume of drug and add to an equal volume of 5% dextrose to deliver a 1:1, or 1 mg/mL solution.
- Product will appear orange-red in color.

PRODUCT STABILITY

- Administer immediately or stored refrigerated at 2°-6° C (36°-42° F) for 6 hours.

COMPATABILITY WITH OTHER DRUGS/IV FLUIDS

- Daunorubicin liposome is compatible with 5% dextrose only.

DRUG INTERACTIONS

- None known

PREGNANCY

Category D

SPECIAL CONSIDERATIONS

Infusion Reaction

- Patients may develop back pain, flushing, and chest tightness during the first 5 minutes of the infusion. Infusion should be discontinued until symptoms resolve and then resumed at a slower rate.

Cardiotoxicity

- May develop during treatment
- May develop months to years following treatment
- Monitor patient's total cumulative dose. The risk for developing cardiotoxicity increases when total cumulative dose is over 320 mg/m^2.

PATIENT EDUCATION

- Patients should report any infusion-related reaction.
- Patients should report dyspnea, palpitations, or swelling of the extremities.
- Patients should report fatigue and activity intolerance.

BIBLIOGRAPHY

Chu, E., Mota, A., Bromberg, M., et al. (2003). Chemotherapeutic and biologic drugs. In E. Chu & V. T. DeVita (Eds.), *Cancer chemotherapy drug manual 2004* (pp. 118-121). Sudbury, MA: Jones & Bartlett Publishers.

Takimoto, C. H. & Calvo, E. (2005). Principles of oncologic pharmacotherapy. In R. Pazdur, L. R. Coia, W. J. Hoskins, et al (Eds.), *Cancer management: multidisciplinary approach* (pp. 11-22). Lawrence, KS: CMP Healthcare Media.

Trissel, L. A. (2005). *Handbook on injectable drugs* (13th Ed.) (p 434). Bethesda, MD: American Society of Health-Systems Pharmacists.

Wilkes, G. M. & Barton-Burke, M. (2005). *2005 Oncology nursing drug handbook* (pp. 119-122). Sudbury, MA: Jones & Bartlett Publishers.

Decitabine (Dacogen®)

Joyce Marrs

DRUG CLASS

- Antimetabolite, DNA methylating agent

ROUTE OF ADMINISTRATION

- Intravenous infusion

HOW TO ADMINISTER

- Administer over 3 hours

PRETREATMENT GUIDELINES

- Measure creatinine, AST, and bilirubin levels before therapy. In clinical trials, patients were excluded if creatinine >2.0 mg/dL, AST >2 times the upper limit of normal, and bilirubin >1.5 mg/dL.

USE

- FDA approved for use in patients with myelodysplastic syndrome

PHARMACOKINETICS

- Half-life is 1 hour

USUAL DOSE AND SCHEDULE

- 15 mg/m^2 administered over 3 hours every 8 hours for 3 consecutive days every 6 weeks

SIDE EFFECTS
Common

- Neutropenia
- Thrombocytopenia
- Anemia
- Fatigue
- Fever
- Petechiae
- Nausea
- Cough
- Constipation
- Diarrhea
- Hyperglycemia

Less Common

- Headache
- Insomnia
- Edema
- Hypomagnesemia
- Low albumin
- Rash
- Dizziness
- Cardiac murmur
- Anorexia

NADIR

- Myelosuppression is a common effect. WBC nadir occurs at day 19 with recovery at 45 days. Platelet count nadir occurs at days 14-15 with recovery between 20-28 days. Monitor CBC for recovery.

STORAGE

- Store vials at 25° C (77° F)

MIXING INSTRUCTIONS

- Each 50-mg vial should be mixed with 10 mL of sterile water for injection. Dilute further in normal saline, D5, or lactated Ringer's solution to a final concentration of 0.1-1 mg/mL.

PRODUCT STABILITY

- Use within 15 minutes of reconstitution. If unable to use within 15 minutes, prepare solution using cold solution and store for up to 7 hours at 2°-8° C (36°-46° F).

DRUG INTERACTIONS

- Drug interaction studies have not been conducted.
- Decitabine does not appear to use the cytochrome P450 pathway for metabolism.

PREGNANCY

Category D

- May cause harm to the fetus if administered to a pregnant woman. Pregnancy should be avoided while on therapy. If the patient becomes pregnant while receiving decitabine, she should be advised as to the potential harm to the fetus.
- Men should avoid conception during treatment and for 2 months following completion of therapy.

SPECIAL CONSIDERATIONS

- Safety and effectiveness in the pediatric setting has not been established.
- Patients should be treated for a minimum of 4 cycles. Therapy may continue as long as beneficial.

PATIENT EDUCATION

- Patients should avoid dehydration by drinking 6 to 8 glasses of water daily.
- Monitor for and report any signs of bleeding.
- Monitor for change in bowel habits. Patients may have either constipation or diarrhea.
- If nauseated, patients should eat light, non-greasy, or non-spicy meals. Use anti-emetics as prescribed.
- Due to the incidence of febrile neutropenia, patients should monitor for fevers and call if temperature is ≥100.4° F.

BIBLIOGRAPHY

MGI Pharma. (2006). *Dacogen™, decitabine injection*. Bloomington, MI: MGI Pharma.

Dexrazoxane (Zinecard®)

Christa Braun-Inglis

DRUG CLASS

- Cardioprotectant, iron-chelating agent

ROUTE OF ADMINISTRATION

- IV push or piggyback

HOW TO ADMINISTER

- Administer drug within 30 minutes before cardiotoxic anthracyclines, such as doxorubicin and daunorubicin.

PRETREATMENT GUIDELINES

- Baseline liver, renal function studies, CBC

USE

- Cardiac protection for patients receiving doxorubicin and/or other anthracyclines

- FDA approved to prevent and/or reduce cardiotoxicity in women with metastatic breast cancer who have received a total cumulative dose of doxorubicin 300 mg/m^2 and who would benefit from continuing therapy
- Dexrazoxane is not recommended with adjuvant chemotherapy.

PHARMACOKINETICS

- Plasma elimination half-life is 2-3 hours

USUAL DOSE AND SCHEDULE

- 10:1 ratio of dexrazoxane to doxorubicin (i.e., 600 mg/m^2 of dexrazoxane to 60 mg/m^2 doxorubicin)

SIDE EFFECTS

- Enhanced bone marrow suppression
- Elevated renal and liver function studies
- Pain at injection site

NADIR

- Does not affect CBC indices

STORAGE
Unreconstituted Vials

- Available in 250 or 500 mg vials; lyophilized powder stored at room temperature

Reconstituted Solution

- Stable at room temperature or refrigerated at 2°-6° C (36°-42° F) for 6 hours

MIXING INSTRUCTIONS

- Reconstitute drug with provided diluent; drug may be further diluted in 0.9% sodium chloride or 5% dextrose to a concentration of 1.3-5 mg/mL.

PRODUCT STABILITY

- Stable at room temperature or refrigerated at 2°-6° C (36°-42° F) for 6 hours.

COMPATABILITY WITH OTHER DRUGS/IV FLUIDS

- 0.9 % Sodium chloride or 5% dextrose

DRUG INTERACTIONS

- None known

PREGNANCY

Category C
- Breast feeding should be avoided.

SPECIAL CONSIDERATIONS

- Dexrazoxane should not be used at the start of doxorubicin therapy because there is evidence to suggest that it may interfere with anti-tumor efficacy.
- Monitor cardiac function studies before and periodically during therapy.
- Sequencing of drugs is important; dexrazone should be administered 30 minutes before doxorubicin or daunorubicin.

PATIENT EDUCATION

- Patient should report any infusion-related reaction.
- Patient should report dyspnea, palpitations, or swelling of the extremities.
- Patient should report fatigue and activity intolerance.

BIBLIOGRAPHY

Chu, E., Mota, A., Bromberg, M., et al. (2003). Chemotherapeutic and biologic drugs. In E. Chu & V. T. DeVita (Eds.), *Cancer chemotherapy drug manual 2004* (pp. 125-127). Sudbury, MA: Jones & Bartlett.

Trissel, L. A. (2005). *Handbook on injectable drugs* (13th Ed.; p. 454). Bethesda, MD: American Society of Health-Systems Pharmacists.

Wilkes, G. M. & Barton-Burke, M. (2005). *2005 Oncology nursing drug handbook* (pp. 389-391). Sudbury, MA: Jones & Bartlett.

Docetaxel (Taxotere®)

Christa Braun-Inglis

DRUG CLASS

- Taxane, antimicrotubule agent

ROUTE OF ADMINISTRATION

- Intravenous infusion
- Drug is not to be given intramuscularly or subcutaneously.

HOW TO ADMINISTER

- Drug is administered over 60 minutes.

PRETREATMENT GUIDELINES

- CBC and baseline liver function studies; if abnormal, discuss with MD. Do not administer docetaxel if total bilirubin ≥ULN or AST/ALT >1.5 times ULN and alkaline phosphate >2.5 times ULN.

USE

- Breast
- Non-small cell lung
- Prostate
- Gastric

Off-Label Uses

- Ovarian
- Pancreatic
- Head and neck
- Esophagus
- Sarcoma
- Uterine
- Bladder

PHARMACOKINETICS

- Plasma elimination is 3-fold with a terminal half-life of 10-18 hours.
- Extensively metabolized by the hepatic P450 microsomal system; see drug interaction section for more information.
- About 75% of drug is eliminated in the stool.
- Renal clearance is relatively low at about 10%.

USUAL DOSE AND SCHEDULE
Single Agent

- 75-100 mg/m^2 every 21 days
- 35-40 mg/m^2 IV weekly

Combination Therapy

- 60-100 mg/m^2 IV every 21 days
- 35-40 mg/m^2 IV weekly

SIDE EFFECTS

- **Irritant, potential vesicant**
- Fatigue
- Myelosuppression
- Hypersensitivity reaction
- Fluid retention syndrome
- Rash
- Nail changes
- Alopecia
- Mucositis
- Peripheral neuropathy
- Hyperlacrimation secondary to ductal stenosis, which can be treated with stent placement. Patient needs referral to ophthalmologist.

NADIR

- 7-10 days with recovery in 14-21 days

STORAGE
Unreconstituted Vials

- Unopened vials require protection from bright light.
- May be stored at room temperature or refrigerated.

MIXING INSTRUCTIONS

- Allow refrigerated vials to stand at least 5 minutes at room temperature before reconstitution.
- Vials available as 80-mg or 20-mg concentrate as single dose blister packs with diluent; do not reuse single dose vials. Once diluent added to concentrate, resulting concentration is docetaxel 10 mg/mL—must be further diluted.
- Gently invert repeatedly. Do not shake initial diluted solution.
- Withdraw ordered dose and further dilute in appropriate volume of 5% dextrose or 0.9% sodium chloride to a final concentration of 0.3-0.74 mg/mL.
- Thoroughly mix by manual rotation.

PRODUCT STABILITY

- Reconstituted solution is good for 8 hours at room temperature or refrigerated.

COMPATABILITY WITH OTHER DRUGS/IV FLUIDS

- Docetaxel is compatible 5% dextrose or 0.9% sodium chloride.

DRUG INTERACTIONS

- Radiosensitizing effect
- CYP3A4 inhibitors such as, ketoconazole, erythromycin, cyclosporine, terfeneradine, nifedipine can inhibit docetaxel metabolism.
- CYP3A4 inducers such as phenytoin, carbamazepine, phenobarbital, and St. John's Wort may decrease serum level of docetaxel. Infuse docetaxel prior to platinum compounds to decrease toxicity.

PREGNANCY

Category D

SPECIAL CONSIDERATIONS

- Patients should receive steroid premedication to decrease the incidence and severity of hypersensitivity reactions and fluid retention.
- Assess baseline vital signs and mental status before drug administration.
- Monitor vital signs every 15 minutes and stay with patient during 15 minutes of infusion with first and second dose.
- During first and second treatments, closely monitor patients for hypersensitivity reaction.
- Use only glass, polypropylene bottles, or polypropylene bags or polyolefin plastic bags for drug administration.
- Administer through polyethylene-lined administration sets.
- Contraindicated in patients with severe hypersensitivity reactions to docetaxel or other drugs formulated with polysorbate 80.
- Docetaxel should be used with caution in patients with abnormal liver function.
- Administer slowly with a rapidly flowing IV due to vesicant potential.
- Flush peripheral line before removal to reduce the potential for leakage of drug into the skin.

PATIENT EDUCATION

- Patient should report any symptoms related to infusion reaction, such as fever, chills, throat irritation, lightheadedness, facial flushing, chest tightness, or dyspnea.
- Teach patient to take prescribed steroids to avoid fluid retention.
- Teach patient self-care measures to minimize infection.
- Teach patient fatigue prevention strategies.

BIBLIOGRAPHY

Chu, E., Mota, A., Bromberg, M., et al. (2003). Chemotherapeutic and biologic drugs. In E. Chu & V. T. DeVita (Eds.), *Cancer chemotherapy drug manual 2004* (pp. 128-132). Sudbury, MA: Jones & Bartlett.

Takimoto, C. H. & Calvo, E. (2005). Principles of oncologic pharmacotherapy. In R. Pazdur, L. R. Coia, W. J. Hoskins, et al (Eds.), *Cancer management: multidisciplinary approach* (pp. 11-22). Lawrence, KS: CMP Healthcare Media.

Taxotere. (2005). Retrieved March 12, 2006, from ttp://www.taxotere.com/professional/home.do

Trissel, L. A. (2005). *Handbook on injectable drugs* (13th ed.; pp. 504-505). Bethesda, MD: American Society of Health-Systems Pharmacists.

Wilkes, G. M. & Barton-Burke, M. (2005). *2005 Oncology nursing drug handbook* (pp. 128-135). Sudbury, MA: Jones & Bartlett.

Doxorubicin HCL (Adriamycin®)

Christa Braun-Inglis

DRUG CLASS

- Anthracycline antibiotic

ROUTE OF ADMINISTRATION

- Slow IV push or continuous infusion
- Drug is not to be administered intramuscularly or subcutaneously.

HOW TO ADMINISTER

- Administer drug at a maximum rate of 4 mg/min, if administering via IV push (preferably into the tubing or running IV solution of 0.9% sodium chloride or 5% dextrose); check for blood return every 2-3 mL.
- Administer into a large vein if administered peripherally.
- Avoid use of a vein over joints or in an extremity in which lymphedema is present.
- Must administer via a central line if given by continuous infusion.

PRETREATMENT GUIDELINES

- Liver function studies—If ALT/AST is 2-3 times ULN, administer 75% of normal dose. If ALT/AST >3 times ULN or total bilirubin 1.2-3 mg/dL, administer 50% of normal dose. If total bilirubin 3.1-5 mg/dL, administer 25% of normal dose. If total bilirubin >5 mg/dL, hold the dose.
- Renal function studies
- Baseline echocardiogram or MUGA scan to evaluate cardiac funtion. Generally not given for left ventricular ejection fraction <40%.

USE

- Breast cancer
- Lymphoma (Hodgkin and non-Hodgkin)
- ALL
- AML
- Bladder cancer
- Thyroid cancer
- Hepatocellular cancer
- Neuroblastoma
- Pancreatic cancer
- Soft tissue sarcoma
- Small cell lung cancer
- Gastric gancer
- Wilms' tumor
- Thymoma

PHARMACOKINETICS

- Initial half-life is 1-3 hours
- Terminal half-life is 20-48 hours
- Metabolized in the liver
- Excreted primarily via the biliary system
- Less than 10% is excreted by the kidneys.

USUAL DOSE AND SCHEDULE
Single Agent

- 60-75 mg/m^2 every 21 days
- 15-20 mg/m^2 once a week

Combination Therapy

- 40-60 mg/m^2 every 21 to 28 days

Dose Dense Therapy

- 60 mg/m^2 every 14 days with hematopoietic growth factor support

Continuous Infusion

- 60-90 mg/m^2 over 96 hours

SIDE EFFECTS
Vesicant

- Nausea/vomiting
- Anorexia
- Mucositis
- Diarrhea
- Alopecia
- Myelosuppression
- Cardiotoxicity
- Infusion-related reaction
- Fatigue
- Hyperpigmentation
- Birth defects
- Radiation recall

NADIR

- 10-14 days with recovery in 15-21 days

STORAGE
Unreconstituted Vials

- Intact vials of doxorubicin should be stored in their cartons until use; kept at room temperature and protected from light.

MIXING INSTRUCTIONS

- Reconstitution of the lyophilized products should be performed with 0.9% sodium chloride.
- Add 5, 10, or 25 ml of 0.9% sodium chloride to the 10, 20, or 50 vial, respectively.
- The 150 mL multi-dose vial is to be reconstituted with 75 mL of 0.9% sodium chloride.
- Once the diluents are added, the vial is to be shaken and drug will dissolve yielding a 2 mg/mL orange-red solution.
- The drug is also available in a ready to use multi-dose vial containing 2 mg/mL solution.

PRODUCT STABILITY

- Reconstituted product is stable for 7 days at room temperature and 15 days under refrigeration; other studies have shown the product is good for up to 43 days when refrigerated.

COMPATIBILITY WITH OTHER DRUGS/IV FLUIDS

- Doxorubicin is compatible with 0.9% normal saline or 5% dextrose water.
- Doxorubicin will precipitate when given with fluorouracil, heparin, or dexamethasone.

DRUG INTERACTIONS

- Cyclosporine may increase doxorubicin levels/effects and precipitate seizures or induce coma. 6-mercaptopurine, streptozocin, dactinomycin, verapamil and radiation may enhance doxorubicin toxicity.

- Paclitaxel may enhance doxorubicin toxicity if administered prior to doxorubicin.
- Phenobarbital will increase the rate of doxorubicin elimination.
- When given with mitomycin or cyclophosphamide, there is an increased risk of cardiotoxicity.
- Phenytoin levels may decrease when doxorubicin is administered.
- Administration of live vaccines while on doxorubicin is contraindicated due to compromised immune function.

PREGNANCY
Category D

SPECIAL CONSIDERATIONS
Infusion Reaction
- Patients may develop back pain, flushing, and chest tightness during the first 5 minutes of the infusion.
- Infusion should be discontinued until symptoms resolve and then resumed at a slower rate

Cardiotoxicity
- May develop during treatment.
- May develop months to years following treatment.
- Monitor patient's lifetime cumulative dose. Risk for developing cardiotoxicity increases when total cumulative dose is over 550 mg/m^2.

Vesicant
- Follow proper procedure for extravasation.
- Apply ice to area of extravasation for 15 minutes, 4 times a day, for 3 days.
- When doxorubicin is leaked into tissue, cells die causing doxorubicin to be further released into adjacent cells, thus causing progressive necrosis. Patient may require a plastic surgeon consult and skin grafting.*

---

*Little evidence-based guidelines exist for extravasation management; therefore proper procedure continues to be controversial.

Liver dysfunction
- Use with caution in patients with abnormal liver function.
- Dose reduction is required in the setting of liver dysfunction.

Patient Education
- Patient should notify nurse if any pain, stinging, or burning occurs while medication is administered.
- Instruct patient that urine may have a red-orange discoloration for 1-3 days. If the discoloration occurs longer than 72 hours, contact physician.
- Patient should report any infusion-related reaction.
- Patient should report dyspnea, palpitations, or swelling of the extremities.

BIBLIOGRAPHY

Chu, E., Mota, A., Bromberg, M., et al. (2003). Chemotherapeutic and biologic drugs. In E. Chu & V. T. DeVita (Eds.), *Cancer chemotherapy drug manual 2004, CD-ROM*. Sudbury, MA: Jones & Bartlett. Available at D:\Chapter02\doxorubicin.html

Takimoto, C. H. & Calvo, E. (2005). Principles of oncologic pharmacotherapy. In R. Pazdur, L. R. Coia, W. J. Hoskins, et al (Eds.). *Cancer Management: Multidisciplinary Approach* (pp. 11-22). CMP Healthcare Media, KS: Lawrence.

Trissel, L. A. (2005). *Handbook on injectable drugs* (13th Ed.) (pp. 525-527). Bethesda, MD: American Society of Health-Systems Pharmacists.

Wickham, R., Engelking, C., Sauerland, C., et al (2006). Vesicant extravasation part II: evidenced-based management and continuing controversies. *Oncology Nursing Forum, 33*, 1145-1149.

Wilkes, G. M. & Barton-Burke, M. (2005). *2005 Oncology nursing drug handbook* (pp. 136-139). Sudbury, MA: Jones & Bartlett.

Doxorubicin Hydrochloride Liposome (Doxil)

Christa Braun-Inglis

DRUG CLASS
- Anthracycline antibiotic

ROUTE OF ADMINISTRATION
- By short intravenous (IV) infusion

HOW TO ADMINISTER
- Begin infusion at a rate 1 mg/min to minimize risk of reaction; if no reaction after 30 minutes, may increase rate and administer over 1 hour
- Do not administer intramuscularly (IM) or subcutaneously (SQ).
- Do not use an in-line filter.

PRETREATMENT GUIDELINES
- Baseline echocardiogram or multiple gated acquisition (MUGA) scan to evaluate cardiac function
- Liver function tests
  - ALT/AST >2-3 times ULN, administer 75% of normal dose
  - ALT/AST >3 times ULN or total bilirubin 1.2 – mg/dL, administer 50% of normal dose
  - Total bilirubin >5 mg/dL, do not administer

USE
- Ovarian cancer
- Breast cancer
- Non-Hodgkin lymphoma
- Multiple myeloma
- Kaposi's sarcoma

PHARMACOKINETICS
- Terminal half-life is 55 hours.

USUAL DOSE AND SCHEDULE
Single Agent
- 40-50 mg/m^2 IV every 4 weeks
- 20 mg/m^2 IV every 3 weeks

Combination Therapy
- 15 mg/m^2 days 1 and 8 every 21 days
- 40 mg/m^2 day 1 every 4 weeks

SIDE EFFECTS
Irritant
- Nausea/vomiting (mild)
- Anorexia
- Mucositis/stomatitis
- Diarrhea
- Alopecia
- Myelosuppression
- Cardiotoxicity
- Infusion-related reaction
- Fatigue
- Hyperpigmentation

- Hand-foot syndrome
- Radiation recall

NADIR

- 10-14 days with recovery in 21 days.

STORAGE
Unreconstituted Vials

- Intact vials of doxorubicin should be stored in their cartons until use, kept at room temperature, and protected from light.

MIXING INSTRUCTIONS

- Drug comes as 2 mg/mL concentration. Further dilute drug in 250 mL of 5% dextrose for doses up to 90 mg and in 500 mL for doses greater than 90 mg.

PRODUCT STABILITY

- Reconstituted product is stable for 24 hours under refrigeration.

COMPATABILITY WITH OTHER DRUGS/INTRAVENOUS FLUIDS

- Doxorubicin is compatible with 5% dextrose only.

DRUG INTERACTIONS

- Liposomal doxorubicin may interact with drugs known to interact with the conventional formulation of doxorubicin.
- May potentiate cardiac toxicity in patients treated with cyclophosphamide
- May potentiate hemorrhagic cystitis in patients treated with cyclophosphamide
- May increase hepatotoxicity in patients treated with 6-mercaptopurine
- Doxorubicin toxicity may increase when given with mercaptopurine, cyclosporine, dactinomycin, streptozocin and verapamil.
- Increased plasma clearance of doxorubicin when given concurrently with barbiturates and phenytoin
- Decreases the effectiveness of digoxin, zidovudine and quinolone antibiotics.

PREGNANCY
Category D

SPECIAL CONSIDERATIONS
Infusion Reaction

- Patients may have back pain, flushing, and chest tightness during the first 5 minutes of the infusion. Infusion should be discontinued until symptoms resolve and then resumed at a slower rate.

Cardiotoxicity

- Acute form presents within the first 2-3 days as arrhythmias or conduction abnormalities, electrocardiographic (ECG) changes, pericarditis, or myocarditis.
- Usually transient and asymptomatic
- Not dose related
- Chronic form results in a dose-dependent dilated cardiomyopathy associated with congestive heart failure; exact cumulative dose is unknown, cumulative doses that exceed 550 mg/m^2, or 400 mg/m^2 in patients who have received previous anthracycline, mitoxantrone, or radiation of the cardiac region, should be given with extreme caution. Baseline and periodic echocardiograms or MUGA scans are recommended.
- Refer to package insert for specific dose modification guidelines for hand-foot syndrome, stomatitis, and hematologic toxicity.
- Do not substitute doxorubicin liposomal for doxorubicin on a mg-per-mg basis.

PATIENT EDUCATION

- Patients should be instructed to follow these guidelines for at least a day before and 3 to 5 days after treatment to avoid hand-foot syndrome:
  ○ Avoid heat, direct sunlight, and hot water.
  ○ Wear loose clothing.
  ○ Wear comfortable, well-ventilated, low-heeled shoes.
  ○ Wear sunblock (sun protection factor [SPF] 15 or higher) every day on all exposed skin.
  ○ Take cool, short showers or baths.
  ○ Don't put pressure on the skin, such as kneeling, leaning on the

elbows, wearing tight jewelry or clothing, chopping hard foods, or engaging in excessive exercise.

- Instruct patient to report any infusion-related reaction.
- Instruct patient to report fatigue and activity intolerance.

BIBLIOGRAPHY

Chu, E., Mota, A., Bromberg, M., et al. (2003). Chemotherapeutic and biologic drugs. In E. Chu & V. T. DeVita (Eds.). *Cancer chemotherapy drug manual 2004* (pp. 118-121). Sudbury, MA: Jones & Bartlett.

Doxil: preparing for infusion. (2004). Retrieved April 4, 2006, from http://www.doxil.com/02_treatment/03_infusions.html.

Trissel, L. A. (2005). *Handbook on injectable drugs* (13th ed., p 434). Bethesda, MD: American Society of Health-Systems Pharmacists.

Wilkes, G. M., & Barton-Burke, M. (2005). *2005 Oncology nursing drug handbook* (pp. 139-144). Sudbury, MA: Jones & Bartlett.

Epirubicin Hydrochloride (Ellence)

Christa Braun-Inglis

DRUG CLASS

- Anthracycline antibiotic

ROUTE OF ADMINISTRATION

- By intravenous (IV) push over 3-5 minutes

HOW TO ADMINISTER

- Administer into a freely running IV infusion of sodium chloride 0.9% or dextrose 5% in water.

PRETREATMENT GUIDELINES

- Baseline echocardiogram or multiple gated acquisition (MUGA) scan to evaluate cardiac function
- Liver function tests
  ○ For total bilirubin 1.2–3 mg/dL or AST 2-4 times ULN, decrease normal dose by 50%

○ For total bilirubin 3.1–5 mg/dL or AST >4 times ULN, decrease normal dose by 75%.
○ For total bilirubin >5 mg/dL, do not give the dose
- Renal function tests

USE
- Breast cancer
- Gastric cancer

PHARMACOKINETICS
- Half-life is approximately 30-38 hours for the parent compound and 20-31 hours for the metabolite.

USUAL DOSE AND SCHEDULE
Single Agent
- In heavily pretreated patients, consider starting at lower dose of 75-90 mg/m² IV every 3 weeks.
- Alternative schedule is 12-25 mg/m² IV on a weekly basis.

Combination Therapy
- 100-120 mg/m² IV every 3 weeks or may be divided equally and given on days 1 and 8

SIDE EFFECTS
Vesicant
- Nausea/vomiting (mild)
- Anorexia
- Mucositis
- Diarrhea
- Alopecia
- Myelosuppression
- Cardiotoxicity
- Infusion-related reaction
- Hyperpigmentation
- Radiation recall

NADIR
- 10-14 days with recovery in 21 days

STORAGE
- Intact vials of epirubicin hydrochloride should be stored under refrigeration at 2°-8° C and protected from freezing and exposure to light.

MIXING INSTRUCTIONS
- Available as a ready-to-use, preservative-free solution in single-use vials of 50 mg/25 mL and 200 mg/100 mL for IV use

PRODUCT STABILITY
- Use product within 24 hours of penetration of rubber stopper.
- Discard any unused drug.

COMPATABILITY WITH OTHER DRUGS/INTRAVENOUS FLUIDS
- Epirubicin is compatible with both sodium chloride 0.9% and dextrose 5% water.

DRUG INTERACTION
- Heparin: if mixed with epirubicin, a precipitate will form.
- 5-Fluorouracil (5-FU), cyclophosphamide: increased risk of myelosuppression when epirubicin is used in combination with either of these drugs
- Cimetidine should be discontinued when starting epirubicin. It significantly increases the area under the curve (AUC) of epirubicin.
- Use cautiously with cardioactive drugs such as calcium channel blockers; may increase the risk of congestive heart failure

PREGNANCY
Category D

SPECIAL CONSIDERATIONS
Liver Dysfunction
- Use with caution in patients with abnormal liver function. Dose modification should be considered in patients with liver dysfunction.

Renal Impairment
- Use with caution in patients with severe renal impairment. When serum creatinine level >5 mg/dL, reduce dose by at least 50%.

Vesicant
- Follow proper procedure for extravasation. Apply ice to area of extravasation for 15 minutes, four times a day, for 3 days.*

---

*Few evidence-based guidelines exist for extravasation management; therefore, the proper procedure continues to be controversial.

- When epirubicin is leaked into tissue, cells die, causing drug to be further released into adjacent cells, thus causing progressive necrosis. Patient may require a plastic surgeon consultation and skin grafting.

Cardiotoxicity
- May develop during treatment; baseline echocardiogram or MUGA scan is recommended
- Risk of cardiotoxicity is higher in elderly patients >70 years of age, in patients with history of hypertension or preexisting heart disease, in patients previously treated with anthracyclines or mitoxantrone, or in patients with prior radiation therapy to the chest.
- Cumulative doses of 900 mg/m² are associated with increased risk for cardiotoxicity; lower cumulative doses pose cardiac risk if patient has received previous anthracycline therapy. Cumulative doses which exceed 900 mg/m² should be given with extreme caution.

PATIENT EDUCATION
- Patient should notify the nurse if there is any pain, burning, or stinging while medication is being administered.
- Instruct patient that urine may have a red-orange discoloration for 1-3 days. If the discoloration occurs longer than 72 hours, contact physician.

BIBLIOGRAPHY
Chu, E., Mota, A., Bromberg, M., et al. (2003). Chemotherapeutic and biologic drugs. In E. Chu & V. T. DeVita (Eds.). *Cancer chemotherapy drug manual 2004* (CD-ROM). Sudbury, MA: Jones & Bartlett.

Trissel, L. A. (2005). *Handbook on injectable drugs* (13th ed., pp.570-571). Bethesda, MD: American Society of Health-Systems Pharmacists.

Wickham, R., Engelking, C., Sauerland, C., et al. (2006). Vesicant extravasation part II: evidenced-based management and continuing controversies. *Oncology Nursing Forum, 33*, 1145-1149.

Wilkes, G. M., & Barton-Burke, M. (2005). *2005 Oncology nursing drug handbook* (pp. 147-151). Sudbury, MA: Jones & Bartlett.

Estramustine (Emcyt)

Christa Braun-Inglis

DRUG CLASS

- Antimicrotubule agent

ROUTE OF ADMINISTRATION

- By mouth
- Intravenous (IV) use is under investigation.

HOW TO ADMINISTER

- Given orally three times a day in three to four divided doses, 1 hour before or 2 hours after meals

PRETREATMENT GUIDELINES

- Complete blood cell count (CBC)
- Liver function tests

USE

- Hormone refractory prostate cancer

PHARMACOKINETICS

- Highly bioavailable by the oral route; approximately 75% of the oral dose is absorbed.
- Drug is primarily metabolized by the liver and excreted in the urine.
- Prolonged half-life is 20-24 hours.

USUAL DOSE AND SCHEDULE
Single Agent

- 14 mg/kg/day orally in three to four divided doses

Combination Therapy

- 15 mg/kg/d in four divided doses days 1-21, repeated every 28 days
- 420 mg three times daily (for 4 doses), then 280 mg three times daily (for next five doses) days 1-3 and 8-10; repeat every 21 days
- 600 mg/m²/day orally days 1-42, repeated every 8 weeks

SIDE EFFECTS

- Nausea and vomiting
- Gynecomastia
- Breast tenderness
- Decreased libido
- Dyspnea
- Diarrhea
- Thromboembolism
- Skin rash
- Cardiac ischemia, congestive heart failure (CHF), edema

NADIR

- Myelosuppression is rare.

STORAGE

- Store in refrigerator; may be stored at room temperature for 24-48 hours.

DRUG INTERACTIONS

- Milk products and calcium-rich foods may impair absorption of estramustine

PREGNANCY

Category D

SPECIAL CONSIDERATIONS

- Contraindicated in patients with active thrombophlebitis or thromboembolic disorders
- Patients are often given anticoagulation medication when on estramustine to decrease risk of thromboembolism.
- Contraindicated in patients with known sensitivity to estradiol or nitrogen mustard
- Contraindicated in patients with peptic ulcer disease, severe liver disease, or cardiac disease

PATIENT EDUCATION

- Instruct patient that milk, milk products, and calcium-rich foods may impair absorption of drug.
- Teach patient to take drug 1 hour before or 2 hours after meals.

BIBLIOGRAPHY

Chu, E., Mota, A., Bromberg, M., et al. (2005). Chemotherapeutic and biologic drugs. In E. Chu & V. T. DeVita (Eds.). *Cancer chemotherapy drug manual 2006* (pp. 462-463). Sudbury, MA: Jones & Bartlett.

Hudes, G. (1997). Phase II trial of 96-hour paclitaxel plus oral estramustine phosphate in metastatic hormone refractory prostate cancer. *Journal of Clinical Oncology, 15*, 3156-3163.

Takimoto, C. H., & Calvo, E. (2005). Principles of oncologic pharmacotherapy. In R. Pazdur, L.R. Coia, W.J. Hoskins, et al. (Eds.). *Cancer management: multidisciplinary approach* (pp. 11-22). Lawrence, KS: CMP Healthcare Media.

Wilkes, G. M., & Barton-Burke, M. (2005). *2005 Oncology nursing drug handbook* (pp. 152-154). Sudbury, MA: Jones & Bartlett.

Etoposide (VP-16, VePesid)

Christa Braun-Inglis

DRUG CLASS

- Plant alkaloid

ROUTE OF ADMINISTRATION

- By intravenous (IV) infusion or by mouth.

HOW TO ADMINISTER

- Administer drug over 30-60 minutes to minimize risk of hypotension and bronchospasm; may want to administer test dose in certain instances. May also be administered as a 24-hour IV infusion.
- Oral administration: may be given as a single dose up to 400 mg, otherwise divide into two to four doses.

PRETREATMENT GUIDELINES

- Complete blood cell count (CBC) and baseline liver function studies; if results are abnormal, discuss with physician.
  - If total bilirubin 1.5-3 mg/dL or AST 60-180 units, give 50% of normal dose.
  - If total bilirubin 3-5 mg/dL or AST >180 units, give 25% of normal dose.
  - If total bilirubin >5 mg/dL, hold dose.
  - If CrCl 15-50 mL/min, administer 75% of the normal dose
  - If CrCl <15mL/min, consider further dose reduction

USE

- Non–small cell lung cancer
- Small cell lung cancer
- Testicular cancer
- Non-Hodgkin lymphoma
- Gastric cancer
- Kaposi's sarcoma
- High dose for bone marrow transplantation

PHARMACOKINETICS

- Rapidly excreted through the urine and to a lesser extent in the bile; the elimination half-life ranges from 3-10 hours.

USUAL DOSE AND SCHEDULE
Single Agent

- 50 mg/m^2 orally daily for 21 days

Combination Therapy

- 50-100 mg/m^2 IV daily for 5 days every 21-28 days
- 75-200 mg/m^2 IV daily for 3 days every 21-28 days

High Dose

- 750-2,400 mg/m^2 IV or 10-60 mg/kg for one dose in combination with other agents and radiation

SIDE EFFECTS

- Fatigue
- Myelosuppression
- Hypersensitivity reaction
- Rash
- Alopecia
- Mucositis
- Peripheral neuropathy (rare and mild)
- Nausea and vomiting (mild)
- Radiation recall
- Anorexia
- Arrhythmias (rare)

NADIR

- 10-14 days with recovery in 21 days

STORAGE
Unreconstituted Vials

- Unopened vials are stable at room temperature for 24 months. Not affected by exposure to normal fluorescent light

Capsules

- Available in 50- or 100-mg capsules; storage in a refrigerator is recommended.

MIXING INSTRUCTIONS

- Vials available as 100 mg, reconstituted with 5 or 10 mL of normal saline solution (NS), sterile water, bacteriostatic sterile water, or bacteriostatic NS with benzyl alcohol to 20 mg/mL or 10 mg/mL, respectively. Also available as a 20 mg/ml solution for injection.
- Further dilute with NS or 5% dextrose in water (D5W) to yield a 0.1 – 0.4 mg/mL final concentration.

PRODUCT STABILITY

- Reconstituted solution is good for 96 hours in glass or 46 hours in plastic containers at room temperature.

COMPATABILITY WITH OTHER DRUGS/IV FLUIDS

- Etoposide is compatible with D5W or 0.9% sodium chloride.

DRUG INTERACTIONS

- Enhances warfarin action by increasing prothrombin time (PT); need to monitor patients on warfarin closely
- Increased toxicity of methotrexate when given concurrently
- Increased cytotoxicity when given concurrently with cyclosporine
- CYP3A4 inhibitors can increase etoposide effects/levels— including azole antifungals, clarithromycin, doxycycline, protease inhibitors and verapamil
- CYP3A4 inhibitors can increase etoposide effects/levels— including azole antifungals, clarithromycin, doxycycline, protease inhibitors and verapamil

PREGNANCY

Category D

SPECIAL CONSIDERATIONS

- Assess baseline vital signs and mental status before drug administration.
- During first treatment, closely monitor patients for hypersensitivity reaction.
- Administer drug over 45-60 minutes to avoid risk of hypotension. If patient's blood pressure drops, immediately stop the infusion and administer IV fluids. Rate of administration must be reduced on restarting therapy.
- Use with caution in patients with abnormal liver function. Dose reduction is recommended in this setting.
- Use with caution in patients with impaired renal function. Baseline creatinine clearance should be obtained and renal status should be monitored during therapy. Dose reduction is recommended in patients with renal dysfunction.

PATIENT EDUCATION

- Instruct patient to report any chest tightness, dizziness, or lightheadedness.
- Teach patient about possible reproductive issues and need for contraception as appropriate.

BIBLIOGRAPHY

Chu, E., Mota, A., Bromberg, M., et al. (2003). Chemotherapeutic and biologic drugs. In E. Chu & V. T. DeVita (Eds.). *Cancer chemotherapy drug manual 2005* (pp. 160-163). Sudbury, MA: Jones & Bartlett.

Takimoto, C.H., & Calvo, E. (2005). Principles of oncologic pharmacotherapy. In R. Pazdur, L. R. Coia, W. J. Hoskins, et al. (Eds.). *Cancer management: Multidisciplinary approach* (pp. 11-22). Lawrence, KS: CMP Healthcare Media.

Trissel, L. A. (2005). *Handbook on injectable drugs* (13th ed., pp 590-596). Bethesda, MD: American Society of Health-Systems Pharmacists.

Wilkes, G. M., & Barton-Burke, M. (2005). *2005 Oncology nursing drug handbook* (pp. 156-160). Sudbury, MA: Jones & Bartlett.

Cancer Management

Floxuridine (5-Fluoro-deoxyuridine, FUDR)

Christa Braun-Inglis

DRUG CLASS

- Antimetabolite

ROUTE OF ADMINISTRATION

- By intrahepatic arterial infusion

HOW TO ADMINISTER

- Administer drug over 7-14 days by intrahepatic arterial infusion.

PRETREATMENT GUIDELINES

- Complete blood cell count (CBC) and baseline liver function studies; if results are abnormal, discuss with physician.

USE

- Metastatic colon cancer (disease to liver)
- Metastatic gastric cancer (disease to liver)

PHARMACOKINETICS

- Terminal half-life is 20 hours.

USUAL DOSE AND SCHEDULE
Single Agent

- 0.1-0.6 mg/kg/day intraarterially for 7-14 days by the hepatic artery

SIDE EFFECTS

- Hepatotoxicity
- Myelosuppression
- Mucositis
- Diarrhea
- Mild nausea and vomiting
- Peptic ulcer
- Palmar-plantar erythrodysesthesia (hand-foot syndrome)
- Neurological toxicity
- Blepharitis
- Rash
- Rare cardiac ischemia (in patient's with preexisting coronary artery disease [CAD])
- Catheter-related complications

NADIR

- 7-10 days with recovery in 14-17 days

STORAGE
Reconstituted Solution

- Store under refrigeration at 2°-8° C.

MIXING INSTRUCTIONS

- Vials available as 500 mg lyophilized powder; reconstitute with 5 mL of sterile water to yield a 100 mg/mL concentration. Further dilute with normal saline solution (NS) or 5% dextrose in water (D5W) to yield a 0.5 mg/mL concentration.

PRODUCT STABILITY

- Reconstituted solution is good for 2 weeks under refrigeration.

COMPATABILITY WITH OTHER DRUGS/INTRAVENOUS FLUIDS

- Floxuridine is compatible with 0.9% NS or 5% lD5W.

DRUG INTERACTIONS

- Leucovorin enhances toxicity and antitumor activity of floxuridine when given first in sequence.
- Pentostatin and floxuridine administered together has resulted in fatal pulmonary toxicity.
- Thymidine will rescue against toxic effects of floxuridine.

PREGNANCY
Category D

SPECIAL CONSIDERATIONS

- Hepatoxicity is dose-limiting toxicity. Patient will typically have abdominal pain, elevated alkaline phosphatase, liver transaminase, and bilirubin.
- Contraindicated in patient with poor performance status
- Patients should be placed on H_2 blocker, such as ranitidine, to prevent against peptic ulcer disease while on therapy.

PATIENT EDUCATION

- Instruct patient on the importance of taking H_2 blocker routinely to prevent against peptic ulcer disease.
- Teach patient to report symptoms of new or increased abdominal pain.

BIBLIOGRAPHY

Chu, E., Mota, A., Bromberg, M., et al. (2003). Chemotherapeutic and biologic drugs. In E. Chu & V. T. DeVita (Eds.). *Cancer chemotherapy drug manual 2005* (pp. 173-176). Sudbury, MA: Jones & Bartlett.

Takimoto, C. H., & Calvo, E. (2005). Principles of oncologic pharmacotherapy. In R. Pazdur, L. R. Coia, W. J. Hoskins, et al. (Eds.). *Cancer management: Multidisciplinary approach* (pp. 11-22). Lawrence, KS: CMP Healthcare Media.

Trissel, L. A. (2005). *Handbook on injectable drugs* (13th ed., pp. 656-658). Bethesda, MD: American Society of Health-Systems Pharmacists.

Wilkes, G. M., & Barton-Burke, M. (2005). *2005 Oncology nursing drug handbook* (pp. 163-165). Sudbury, MA: Jones & Bartlett.

Fludarabine (Fludara)

Christa Braun-Inglis

DRUG CLASS

- Antimetabolite (purine analog)

ROUTE OF ADMINISTRATION

- By intravenous (IV) infusion

HOW TO ADMINISTER

- Administer drug over 30 minutes.

PRETREATMENT GUIDELINES

- Complete blood cell count (CBC), baseline renal and liver function studies; if results are abnormal, discuss with physician.
- Usual dose adjustments
- CrCl 30-70 mL/min, administer 80% of the dose
- CrCl <30 mL/min, hold the dose

USE

- Chronic lymphocytic leukemia
- Non-Hodgkin lymphoma (low grade)

Off-Label Uses

- Cutaneous T-cell lymphoma
- Bone marrow transplant

PHARMACOKINETICS

- Considered a prodrug; after administration, it is rapidly dephosphorylated to 2-fluoro-ara-adenosine.
- Terminal half-life is 9 hours.

USUAL DOSE AND SCHEDULE

- 25 mg/m^2 IV daily for 5 days every 28 days

SIDE EFFECTS

- Myelosuppression
- Immunosuppression (decreased CD4$^+$ and CD8$_+$ T cells)
- Peripheral neuropathy (rare and mild)
- Nausea and vomiting (mild)
- Somnolence, fatigue
- Fever
- Hypersensitivity with maculopapular skin rash, erythema, and pruritus
- Central nervous system (CNS) effects: severe neurologic effects associated with higher doses
- Pulmonary toxicity
- Transient increase in liver function tests

NADIR

- 10-13 days with recovery in 5-7 weeks

STORAGE
Unopened Vials

- Intact vials should be stored under refrigeration.

MIXING INSTRUCTIONS

- Drug available in 50-mg vials as a white, lyophilized cake; add 2 mL of sterile water to yield a 25 mg/mL concentration. Further dilute in 100 mL of normal saline solution (NS) or 5% dextrose in water (D5W).

PRODUCT STABILITY

- Reconstituted solution is good for 8 hours only.

COMPATABILITY WITH OTHER DRUGS/INTRAVENOUS FLUIDS

- Compatible with 0.9% NS and 5% dextrose
- Incompatible with acyclovir and amphotericin B

DRUG INTERACTIONS

- Fludarabine may enhance the antitumor activity of cytarabine, cyclophosphamide, cisplatin, and mitoxantrone.
- Fatal pulmonary toxicity when used in combination with pentostatin

PREGNANCY

Category D

SPECIAL CONSIDERATIONS

- Use with caution in patients with abnormal renal function; dose may need to be adjusted in proportion to creatinine clearance.
- Use with caution in the elderly and in those with bone marrow impairment or increased risk of myelosuppression.
- Monitor for signs and symptoms of infection. Patients are at increased risk of opportunistic infections. Patients should be placed on co-trimoxazole prophylaxis. Monitor for signs and symptoms of tumor lysis syndrome (TLS). Allopurinol may be given to prevent TLS.
- Use irradiated blood products in patients requiring transfusions because, although rare, fludarabine can cause graft-versus-host disease.

PATIENT EDUCATION

- Instruct patient to monitor for signs and symptoms of infection.
- Teach patient self-care measure to minimize risk of infection.

BIBLIOGRAPHY

Chu, E., Mota, A., Bromberg, M., et al. (2003). Chemotherapeutic and biologic drugs. In E. Chu & V. T. DeVita (Eds.). *Cancer chemotherapy drug manual 2005* (pp. 177-180). Sudbury, MA: Jones & Bartlett.

Takimoto, C. H., & Calvo, E. (2005). Principles of oncologic pharmacotherapy. In R. Pazdur, L. R. Coia, W. J. Hoskins, et al. (Eds.). *Cancer management: Multidisciplinary approach* (pp. 11-22). Lawrence, KS: CMP Healthcare Media.

Trissel, L. A. (2005). *Handbook on injectable drugs* (13th ed) (pp 665-667). Bethesda, MD: American Society of Health-Systems Pharmacists.

Wilkes, G. M., & Barton-Burke, M. (2005). *2005 Oncology nursing drug handbook* (pp. 165-168). Sudbury, MA: Jones & Bartlett.

Gemcitabine (Gemzar)

Christa Braun-Inglis

DRUG CLASS

- Antimetabolite

ROUTE OF ADMINISTRATION

- By intravenous (IV) bolus

HOW TO ADMINISTER

- Administer drug over 30 minutes. Infusion times lasting longer than 60 minutes may enhance toxicity.

PRETREATMENT GUIDELINES

- Complete blood cell count (CBC), baseline renal and liver function studies; if results are abnormal, discuss with physician.

USE

- Breast cancer
- Non–small cell lung cancer
- Pancreatic cancer

Off-Label Uses

- Soft tissue sarcoma
- Non-Hodgkin lymphoma
- Bladder cancer
- Ovarian cancer
- Hodgkin disease

PHARMACOKINETICS

- Hepatic activation to active metabolites.

Cancer Management

- With infusions <70 minutes, half-life ranges from 30-90 minutes; whereas with infusions >70 minutes, half-life is 4-10 hours.

USUAL DOSE AND SCHEDULE
Single Agent

- 1,000 mg/m^2 IV weekly × 7 followed by 1 week rest, then given:
  - 1,000 mg/m^2 IV days 1, 8, and 15; repeat cycle every 28 days

Combination Therapy

- 1,000 mg/m^2 days 1, 8, and 15; repeat cycle every 28 days
- 1,250 mg/m^2 days 1 and 8; repeat cycle every 21 days

SIDE EFFECTS

- Myelosuppression (thrombocytopenia; dose-limiting toxicity)
- Nausea and vomiting (mild)
- Fever, flu-like syndrome
- Maculopapular skin rash
- Pulmonary toxicity
- Transient increase in liver function tests

NADIR

- 10-14 days with recovery in 21 days

STORAGE
Unopened Vials

- Intact vials should be stored at controlled room temperature.

MIXING INSTRUCTIONS

- Drug is available in 200 mg and 1 g vials as a lyophilized powder. Reconstitute 200-mg vial with 5 mL of normal saline solution (NS) and 1-g vial with 25 mL of NS to yield 38 mg/mL solution. Shake vial to dissolve powder. Further dilute in 50-100 mL of NS.

PRODUCT STABILITY

- Reconstituted solution is good for 24 hours at room temperature.
- DO NOT REFRIGERATE.

COMPATABILITY WITH OTHER DRUGS/INTRAVENOUS FLUIDS

- Compatible with 0.9% NS and 5% dextrose
- Incompatible with acyclovir and amphotericin B

DRUG INTERACTIONS

- Gemcitabine enhances the cytotoxity of cisplatin.
- Gemcitabine cytotoxicity may be enhanced by the presence of etoposide.
- Gemcitabine is a potent radiosensitizer.

PREGNANCY

Category D

SPECIAL CONSIDERATIONS

- Monitor CBC on a regular basis during therapy. Dose reduction may be recommended on the basis of the degree of myelosuppression.
- Use with caution in patients with moderate to severe liver dysfunction; dose modification should be considered in this setting.
- Use with caution in the elderly and in those with bone marrow impairment, increased risk of myelosuppression.
- Prolonged infusion time increases risk of toxicity.
- Use with caution in women and the elderly because drug clearance is decreased.

PATIENT EDUCATION

- Instruct patient to monitor for signs and symptoms of infection, bleeding.
- Teach patient self-care measures to minimize risk of infection.

BIBLIOGRAPHY

Chu, E., Mota, A., Bromberg, M., et al. (2003). Chemotherapeutic and biologic drugs. In E. Chu & V. T. DeVita (Eds.). *Cancer chemotherapy drug manual 2005* (pp. 196-198). Sudbury, MA: Jones & Bartlett.

Takimoto, C. H., & Calvo, E. (2005). Principles of oncologic pharmacotherapy. In R. Pazdur, L. R. Coia, W. J. Hoskins,

et al. (Eds.). *Cancer management: Multidisciplinary approach* (pp. 11-22). Lawrence, KS: CMP Healthcare Media.

Trissel, L. A. (2005). *Handbook on injectable drugs* (13th ed., pp 714-721). Bethesda, MD. American Society of Health-Systems Pharmacists.

Wilkes, G. M., & Barton-Burke, M. (2005). *2005 Oncology nursing drug handbook* (pp. 174-178). Sudbury, MA: Jones & Bartlett.

Hydroxyurea (Droxia, Hydrea)

Barbara Holmes Gobel and Deborah Mast

DRUG CLASS

- Antimetabolite, miscellaneous

ROUTES OF ADMINISTRATION

- Oral (capsules or tablets, depending on manufacturer)
- Intravenous (IV): *IV form not available in the United States*
- High-dose continuous IV infusion (investigational): *IV form not available in the United States*

HOW TO ADMINISTER

- Administer orally.
- Contents of capsules can be emptied into a glass of water for immediate ingestion, if capsules are unable to be swallowed.

PRETREATMENT GUIDELINES

- Baseline leukocyte count and platelet count; hold therapy if leukocyte count is <2500/mm^3 or platelet count is <100,000/mm^3.
- May need to pretreat with allopurinol to minimize risk of tumor lysis syndrome
- Baseline uric acid to evaluate for tumor lysis syndrome
- Baseline evaluation of renal status; blood urea nitrogen (BUN), creatinine
- Renal dysfunction dose modification: reduce dose by 50% if creatinine clearance is 10-50 mL/min; reduce dose by 80% if creatinine clearance is <10 mL/min.

USE

- Chronic myelogenous leukemia in chronic phase
- Head and neck cancer (used as a radiosensitizer)
- Malignant melanoma
- Ovarian cancer (recurrent, metastatic, or inoperable)
- Sickle cell disease

Off-Label Uses

- Acute myelogenous leukemia
- Astrocytoma and malignant glioma (radiosensitizer)
- Human immunodeficiency virus infection
- Lung cancer (radiosensitizer)
- Polycythemia vera
- Psoriasis
- Thrombocytosis

PHARMACOKINETICS

- Rapidly absorbed from the gastrointestinal (GI) tract after oral administration, peak serum concentrations within 60 to 120 minutes
- Drug enters all body compartments including central nervous system (CNS) and genital tract
- Plasma half-life is 3.5 to 4.5 hours.
- About 50% of the drug is metabolized by the liver to inactive compounds and the other 50% of the drug is excreted as unchanged drug by the kidneys.
- Drug crosses the blood-brain barrier.

USUAL DOSE AND SCHEDULE
Chronic Myelogenous Leukemia

- Oral: 20 to 30 mg/kg daily

Control of Hyperleukocytosis

- Oral: initial doses up to 50 mg/kg daily may be used.

Head and Neck Cancer

- Oral: 80 mg/kg every third day in combination with radiation therapy, starting 7 days before radiation and continuing during and after radiation therapy

Malignant Melanoma

- Oral: 20 to 80 mg/kg daily in one to three divided doses

Ovarian Cancer

- Oral: 80 mg/kg every third day or 20 to 30 mg/kg/day. If given concurrently with radiation therapy, administer 80 mg/kg every third day.

SIDE EFFECTS

- Acral erythema
- Alopecia (rare)
- Anemia
- Constipation (rare)
- Diarrhea (rare)
- Dizziness (rare)
- Drowsiness (rare)
- Disorientation (rare)
- Dysuria
- Facial erythema (rare)
- Flu-like syndrome (fever, chills, malaise)
- Hallucinations
- Hepatic failure (rare); transient elevation of hepatic aminotransferase levels
- Hyperpigmentation
- Hyperuricemia
- Infertility
- Leukopenia
- Maculopapular rash
- Mucositis (rare)
- Nausea/vomiting
- Neutropenia
- Peripheral neuropathy
- Pruritus
- Seizures (rare)
- Thrombocytopenia

NADIR

- Hydroxyurea can dramatically lower the white blood cell count (WBC) in a short period of time (24 to 48 hours). Nadir at 10 days with recovery 7 days after stopping drug.

STORAGE

- Store capsules at 25° C (77° F); excursions permitted to 15°-30° C (59°-86° F)
- Keep tightly closed.

MIXING INSTRUCTIONS

- None. Hydroxyurea is available from drug manufacturers as 500-mg capsules or in 200-, 300-, or 400-mg tablets.

- An injectable form is available from the National Cancer Institute (NCI) as a 2,000-mg vial.

DRUG INTERACTIONS

- Cytarabine is potentiated by the activity of hydroxyurea.
- Administration of additional myelosuppressive agents may lead to additive effects of immunosuppression.
- Administration of live vaccines while on hydroxyurea is contraindicated because of compromised immune function.
- Anticoagulants, nonsteroidal anti-inflammatory drugs (NSAIDs), platelet inhibitors, strontium 89 chloride, and thrombolytic agents can cause increased risk of bleeding in patients receiving hydroxyurea.
- Sargramostim and filgrastim should not be used 24 hours before or after treatment.
- The combined use of hydroxyurea and didanosine (ddI) with or without stavudine (d4T) is associated with an increased incidence of pancreatitis and peripheral neuropathy.

PREGNANCY
Category D

SPECIAL CONSIDERATIONS

- Patients and caregivers should be instructed to wear disposable gloves when handling bottles or the capsules to minimize the risk of exposure to the drug, followed by washing of hands before and after contact with the drug.
- Breast-feeding during treatment with hydroxyurea is not recommended because it passes into breast milk.
- Hydroxyurea can dramatically lower the WBC in a short period of time (24 to 48 hours).
- Radiation recall may occur with the use of hydroxyurea.
- Mucosal reactions may be severe when hydroxyurea is used in combination with radiation therapy.

Cancer Management

- Dose modification on the basis of renal function (see Pretreatment Guidelines), absolute neutrophil count and platelet count.

PATIENT EDUCATION

- Hydroxyurea capsules should be taken by mouth.
- If patient has difficulty swallowing the capsule, it can be carefully opened and emptied into a glass of water. (Some of the medication may not dissolve in the water.) Patient should drink the liquid at once and thoroughly rinse the glass after use.
- Hydroxyurea is to be handled with care. Patient and caregivers should wear gloves when handling the medication bottle or the capsules. Patient should wash hands before and after handling the medication bottle or capsules.
- Patients should be instructed to call the health care provider if they vomit after taking a dose.
- Monitor for signs of low platelet count (easy bruising, petechiae, black tarry stool, or bloody stool).
- Monitor for signs of infection (temperature, redness, tenderness or pus at the insertion site of central lines or drains).

BIBIOGRAPHY

Clinical Pharmacology. (2006). *Hydroxyurea*. Retrieved June 19, 2006, from http://cpip.gsm.com/ (subscription required).

Fischer, D. S., Knobf, M. T., Durivage, H. J., et al. (2003). *The cancer chemotherapy handbook* (6th ed., pp. 139-140). St. Louis: Mosby.

Goodman, M. (2004). Skin and nail bed changes. In C. H. Yarbro, M. H. Frogge & M. Goodman (Eds.). *Cancer symptom management* (3rd ed., pp. 319-330). Sudbury, MA: Jones & Bartlett.

Rx List. (2004). *Hydroxyurea*. Retrieved May 15, 2006, from http://www.rxlist.com/cgi/generic/hydroxyurea.htm.

Wilkes, G. M., & Barton-Burke, M. (2005). *2005 Oncology nursing drug handbook*. Sudbury, MA: Jones & Bartlett.

Idarubicin (Idamycin PFS, Idamycin)

Barbara Holmes Gobel and Deborah Mast

DRUG CLASS

- Anthracycline antitumor antibiotic

ROUTES OF ADMINISTRATION

- Intravenous (IV) route by IV push
- Idarubicin is a vesicant; this drug is not to be administered intramuscularly (IM) or subcutaneously (SQ).

HOW TO ADMINISTER

- Administer as an IV injection over 10 to 15 minutes in the sidearm of a freely running IV.
- Follow extravasation precautions.
- Administer into a large vein.

PRETREATMENT GUIDELINES

- Pretreat for nausea and vomiting.
- Baseline leukocyte and platelet count: hold or reduce therapy if leukocyte count is <2500/mm³ or platelet count is <100,000/mm³.
- Multiple gated acquisition (MUGA) scan or two-dimensional echogram to assess for baseline ejection fraction
- Baseline evaluation of renal status: blood urea nitrogen (BUN), creatinine
- Serum bilirubin
  - For total bilirubin between 1.2-3 mg/dL or AST 2-4 times the upper limits of normal (ULN), decrease normal dose by 50%.
  - For total bilirubin between 3.1-5 mg/dL or AST >4 times ULN, decrease normal dose by 75%.
  - Hold dose if serum bilirubin is >5 mg/dL

USE

- Acute myelogenous leukemia

Off-Label Uses

- Acute lymphocytic leukemia

- Breast cancer
- Chronic myelogenous leukemia
- Non-Hodgkin lymphoma

PHARMACOKINETICS

- Cell cycle phase specific, specific for the S phase
- Metabolized primarily by the liver to several metabolites, including idarubicinol
- Drug penetrates into the cerebrospinal fluid.
- Excreted primarily in the bile (25%) and the urine (2% to 3%)
- Elimination half-life is 13 to 26 hours for idarubicin and 38 to 63 hours for idarubicinol.

USUAL DOSE AND SCHEDULE

- Acute myelogenous leukemia (for induction therapy or postremission therapy in combination with cytarabine): 8 to 12 mg/m²/day for 3 days combined with cytarabine
- Reduce dose for serum bilirubin between 2.5 to 5 mg/dL and hold dose if serum bilirubin is >5 mg/dL.
- Dosage adjustment (75% of normal dose) recommended for serum creatinine >2 mg/dL.
- Proposed maximum lifetime dosage of idarubicin is 150 mg/m².

SIDE EFFECTS

- Alopecia—often partial
- Anemia
- Bleeding
- Bradycardia
- Cardiomyopathy
- Diarrhea
- Elevated hepatic enzymes (usually transient)
- Gonadal dysfunction (temporary or permanent)
- Heart failure
- Leukopenia
- Myocardial infarction
- Nausea and vomiting
- Neutropenia
- QT prolongation
- Radiation recall reaction
- Skin necrosis (potential) with extravasation
- ST-T wave changes

- Stomatitis
- Supraventricular tachycardia (SVT)
- Thrombocytopenia
- Urine discoloration (red)
- Ventricular tachycardia

NADIR

- 10-15 days with recovery in 21-18 days

STORAGE

- Idarubicin powder for injection is stored at room temperature and is protected from light.
- Idarubicin PFS (preservative-free solution) is stored in the refrigerator and is protected from light.

MIXING INSTRUCTIONS

- Reconstitute 5, 10, or 20 mg of idarubicin with 5, 10, or 20 mL, respectively, of nonbacteriostatic water for injection to yield a 1 mg/mL solution.
- Vial contents are under pressure; thus, needle should be inserted carefully into vial.

Product Stability

- Reconstituted solution is stable for 72 hours at room temperature and 1 week under refrigeration.

COMPATIBILITY WITH OTHER DRUGS/INTRAVENOUS FLUIDS

- Cytarabine, at the "Y" site

DRUG INTERACTIONS

- Administration of additional myelosuppressive agents may lead to additive effects of immunosuppression.
- Administration of live vaccines while on idarubicin is contraindicated because of compromised immune function.
- Administration of idarubicin to patients who have received their maximum cumulative doses of other anthracyclines (e.g., daunorubicin, doxorubicin, or epirubicin) is not recommended because of the increased risk of cardiotoxicity.

- Patients who have received mitoxantrone therapy may also have increased cardiotoxicity.
- Cyclophosphamide may potentiate anthracycline-induced cardiotoxicity.
- Anticoagulants, nonsteroidal anti-inflammatory drugs (NSAIDs), platelet inhibitors, strontium 89 chloride, and thrombolytic agents can cause increased risk of bleeding in patients receiving idarubicin.
- Idarubicin is deactivated on prolonged contact with alkaline solutions.
- Incompatible with heparin; causes a precipitant
- Sargramostim and filgrastim should not be used 24 hours before or after treatment.

PREGNANCY

Category D
- Breast-feeding during therapy with idarubicin is not recommended because there are reports of drug distribution into breast milk.

SPECIAL CONSIDERATIONS
Vesicant

- Follow proper procedure for extravasation.
- Apply ice to area of extravasation for 15 minutes, four times a day, for 3 days.
- Plastic surgery consultation may be necessary because of progressive skin necrosis.
- IM and SQ administration of idarubicin are contraindicated because of the potential for severe skin and tissue necrosis.

Cardiomyopathy

- Acute cardiotoxicity can occur during treatment, although incidence is rare.
- Acute electrocardiographic (ECG) changes during anthracycline treatment are usually transient and include ST-T wave changes, QT prolongation, and changes in QRS voltage.
- Cardiac status should be assessed before therapy with

anthracyclines; patients with a left ventricular ejection fraction of <50% are not considered candidates for anthracycline therapy.
- Monitor patient's total cumulative dose. Proposed lifetime maximum dose of idarubicin is 150 mg/m^2.

Urine Discoloration

- Urine may turn red-orange after idarubicin is administered.
- Discoloration may last for up to 1 to 3 days.

Radiation Recall

- Idarubicin may potentiate a radiation recall reaction, similar to other anthracyclines.
- Skin reactions occur in fields of previous radiation therapy and include erythema, desquamation of the skin, and rarely, tissue necrosis.

PATIENT EDUCATION

- Hair loss may occur, although it may be partial.
- Monitor for signs of low platelet count (easy bruising, petechiae, black tarry stool, or bloody stool).
- Monitor for signs of infection (temperature, redness, tenderness or pus at the insertion site of central lines or drains).
- Patient should notify nurse if any pain, stinging, or burning occurs while medication is being administered.
- Instruct patient that urine may have a red-orange discoloration for 1 to 3 days, and if the discoloration lasts longer than 72 hours, contact health care professional.
- Instruct patients that cardiotoxicity is a possible side effect of idarubicin.
- Instruct patients about signs and symptoms of congestive heart failure (CHF) and when to report to the health care professional.

BIBLIOGRAPHY

Clinical Pharmacology. (2006). *Idarubicin*. Retrieved June, 30, 2006, from http://cpip.gsm.com/ (subscription required).

Fischer, D. S., Knobf, M. T., Durivage, H. J., et al. (2003). *The cancer chemotherapy handbook* (6th ed., pp. 140-141). St. Louis: Mosby.

Idamycin (idarubicin). (2000). Princeton, NJ: Mead Johnson Oncology Products.

Polovich, M., White, J. M., & Kelleher, L. O. (2005). *Chemotherapy and biotherapy guidelines and recommendations for practice* (2nd ed.). Pittsburgh, PA: Oncology Nursing Service.

Shan, K., Lincoff, M., & Young, J. B. (1996). Anthracycline-induced cardiotoxicity. *Annals of Internal Medicine, 125,* 47-58.

Wilkes, G. M., & Barton-Burke, M. (2005). *2005 Oncology nursing drug handbook* (pp. 184-186). Sudbury, MA: Jones & Bartlett.

Ifosfamide (Ifex)

Barbara Holmes Gobel and Deborah Mast

DRUG CLASS

- Alkylating agent

ROUTE OF ADMINISTRATION

- Intravenous (IV)

HOW TO ADMINISTER

- Administer IV in 50-1000 mL of normal saline solution over 30 minutes or longer (may be given as a continuous infusion).
- To prevent hemorrhagic cystitis from ifosfamide, it is recommended that patients receive aggressive concomitant hydration (1,500 to 2,000 mL/day) and uroprotective therapy with mesna.

PRETREATMENT GUIDELINES

- Renal evaluation: blood urea nitrogen (BUN), serum creatinine, and creatinine clearance before each dose with corresponding dosage changes:
  - Creatinine clearance (CrCl) >60 mL/min: no change
  - CrCl 31-60 mL/min: reduce dose by 25%
  - CrCl 10-30 mL/min: reduce dose by 50%
  - CrCl <10 mL/min: omit dose
- White blood cell count: >2,500
- Platelet count: >100,000
- Hemoglobin: >10 mg/dL
- Urinalysis to monitor for hematuria
- Pretreat for nausea and vomiting

USE

- Testicular cancer: ifosfamide has been designated as an orphan drug by the Food and Drug Administration (FDA) for the treatment of testicular cancer. Ifosfamide is used as a third-line chemotherapeutic agent for the treatment of germ cell testicular cancer.

Off-Label Uses

- Bladder cancer
- Breast cancer
- Cervical cancer
- Desmoid tumor
- Ewing's sarcoma
- Lung cancer
- Hodgkin lymphoma
- Non-Hodgkin lymphoma
- Osteogenic sarcoma
- Pancreatic cancer
- Rhabdomyosarcoma
- Soft tissue sarcoma

PHARMACOKINETICS

- Ifosfamide is activated and metabolized by the liver. Only about 50% of the drug is metabolized, with much of the drug excreted as unchanged drug in the urine.
- The metabolite chloroacetaldehyde is chemically related to chloral hydrate and explains some of the neurotoxic effects of ifosfamide. The clearance of this metabolite is slowed in patients with renal dysfunction.
- Terminal half-life of 7 to 15 hours (dose dependent)

USUAL DOSE AND SCHEDULE

- Testicular cancer: 1,200 to 2,000 mg/m^2/day for 5 consecutive days, repeated every 3 weeks after hematological recovery
- Ifosfamide is given in various salvage regimens after BEP (bleomycin, etoposide, cisplatin) therapy including VEIP (vinblastine, ifosfamide, cisplatin) and with paclitaxel and cisplatin.
- Ifosfamide is given in combination with mesna to decrease bladder toxicity.

SIDE EFFECTS

- Alopecia
- Anemia
- Confusion
- Dizziness
- Drowsiness
- Dysuria
- Elevated hepatic enzymes (mild, transient, uncommon)
- Hallucinations
- Hematuria
- Hemorrhagic cystitis (dose and schedule related [more common with single high-dose regimens than with multiple-dose regimens])
- Hyponatremia
- Hypokalemia
- Leukopenia
- Nausea and vomiting
- Neutropenia
- Psychosis
- Renal failure (unspecified)
- Seizures
- Somnolence
- Thrombocytopenia

NADIR

- Leukopenia: 7 to 10 days after treatment. Thrombocytopenia and anemia occur less frequently.

STORAGE
Unreconstituted

- Unreconstituted vials are stored at room temperature. (Ifosfamide liquefies at temperatures above 35° C.)

Reconstituted

- Reconstituted ifosfamide and ifosfamide further diluted are stable for 7 days at room temperature and for 6 weeks with refrigeration.
- When ifosfamide is reconstituted to a solution of 10 to 80 mg/mL in normal saline solution, this solution is stable for at least 8 days in portable pump infusion cassettes.

MIXING INSTRUCTIONS

- Reconstitute 1,000- and 3,000-mg vials with 20 and 60 mL, respectively, of sterile water or bacteriostatic water containing parabens or benzyl alcohol to a concentration of 50 mg/mL.
- Solutions of ifosfamide may be further diluted to yield a concentration of 0.6 to 20 mg/mL in 5% dextrose, 5% dextrose and Ringer's injection, 5% dextrose and normal saline solution, lactated Ringer's solution, 0.45% sodium chloride, normal saline solution, or $\frac{1}{6}$ molar sodium lactate solution.

Product Stability

- Reconstituted ifosfamide and ifosfamide further diluted are stable for 7 days at room temperature and for 6 weeks with refrigeration.
- When ifosfamide is reconstituted to a solution of 10 to 80 mg/mL in normal saline solution, this solution is stable for at least 8 days in portable pump infusion cassettes.

COMPATIBILITY WITH OTHER DRUGS/INTRAVENOUS FLUIDS

- Bacteriostatic water for injection
- Carboplatin
- Cisplatin
- Dextrose 5% in Ringer's solution
- Dextrose 5% in sodium chloride 0.9%
- Dextrose 5% in water
- Doxorubicin
- Epirubicin
- Etoposide
- Gemcitabine
- Granisetron
- Mesna
- Ondansetron hydrochloride
- Paclitaxel
- Palonosetron
- Ringer's lactated solution
- Sodium chloride 0.45%
- Sodium chloride 0.9%
- Sodium lactate M/6
- Sterile water for injection

DRUG INTERACTIONS

- Administration of additional myelosuppressive agents may lead to additive effects of immunosuppression.
- Administration of live vaccines while on ifosfamide is contraindicated because of compromised immune function.
- Anticoagulants, nonsteroidal anti-inflammatory drugs (NSAIDs), platelet inhibitors, strontium 89 chloride, and thrombolytic agents can cause increased risk of bleeding in patients receiving ifosfamide.
- Phenobarbital, phenytoin, carbamazepine, and other CYP3A4 inducers may accelerate the conversion of ifosfamide to its active metabolites, thus increasing the clinical or neurotoxic effects of ifosfamide.
- Azole antifungals, clarithromycin, erythromycin, doxycycline, protease inhibitors, verapamil, St. John's Wort and other CYP3A4 inhibitors may inhibit the conversion of ifosfamide to its active metabolites, thus decreasing the clinical and/or neurotoxic effects of ifosfamide.
- Nalidixic acid is contraindicated because of reports of serious gastrointestinal toxicity, such as hemorrhagic ulcerative colitis.
- Patients who are receiving ifosfamide and have received cisplatin in the past may have delayed renal clearance and additive nephrotoxicity and neurotoxicity.
- Nephrotoxic agents such as aminoglycosides, amphotericin B, bacitracin injection, cisplatin, cyclosporine, foscarnet, loop diuretics, NSAIDs, pentamidine, polymyxin B injection, salicylates, streptozocin, tacrolimus, and IV vancomycin, may all increase the nephrotoxicity of ifosfamide.
- Sargramostim and filgrastim should not be used 24 hours before or after treatment.

PREGNANCY

Category D

- Breast-feeding is not recommended during treatment with ifosfamide.

SPECIAL CONSIDERATIONS
Neurologic Toxicity

- Neurologic toxicity is increased by concurrent use of barbiturates.
- Neurologic toxicities occur more frequently when ifosfamide is given over a 1-day period versus over a 5-day period, in patients with impaired renal function, in patients with hypoalbuminemia, and when sedatives are given concomitantly.
- Methylene blue (50 mg of a 1% to 2% solution) has been used as an effective treatment for ifosfamide-induced neurotoxicity. If needed, the dose of methylene blue can be repeated three to four times per day with subsequent dosing of ifosfamide.

Renal and Bladder Considerations

- Therapy requires the concurrent administration of mesna as a uroprotectant. Mesna should be given with the ifosfamide. Regimens differ according to the timing and scheduling of the mesna.
- Prehydration and posthydration of the patient is also required to minimize bladder toxicity. Patient may require catherization and continuous bladder irrigation.
- Renal and bladder dysfunction are dose-limiting toxicities.

Myelosuppression

- Major dose-limiting toxicity
- Leukopenia is the most common of the hematologic toxicities; thrombocytopenia and anemia occur less frequently.

PATIENT EDUCATION

- Hair loss
- This drug can cause nausea and vomiting; an antiemetic should be taken before treatment.
- Observe for signs of low platelets (easy bruising, petechiae, black tarry stool, or bloody stool).

- Observe for signs of infection (fever, redness, tenderness or pus at the insertion site of central lines or drains).
- Observe for signs of anemia (fatigue, shortness of breath).
- Avoid exposure to infections or infected persons.
- This drug can cause bleeding in the urine; patients should notify the health care professional if they have bleeding in the urine, painful urination, or urinary frequency.
- This drug can cause dizziness, drowsiness, confusion, and hallucinations. Patients should be instructed to notify the health care professional if any of these symptoms occur.

BIBLIOGRAPHY

Aeschlimann, C., Kupfer, A., Schefer, H., et al. (1998). Comparative pharmacokinetics of oral and intravenous ifosfamide/mesna/methylene blue therapy. *Drug Metabolism Disposition, 26,* 883-890.

Camp-Sorrell, D. (2005). Chemotherapy toxicities and management. In C. H. Yarbro, M. H. Frogge & M. Goodman (Eds.). *Cancer nursing principles and practice* (6th ed., pp. 412-457). Sudbury, MA: Jones & Bartlett.

Clinical Pharmacology. (2006). *Ifosfamide.* Retrieved June 19, 2006, from http://cpip.gsm.com/ (subscription required).

Fischer, D. S., Knobf, M. T., Durivage, H. J., et al. (2003). *The cancer chemotherapy handbook* (6th ed.). St. Louis: Mosby.

Kintzel, P. E., & Dorr, R. T. (1995). Antitumor treatment-anticancer drug renal toxicity and elimination: dosing guidelines for altered renal function. *Cancer Treatment Review, 21,* 33-64.

Rx List. (2004). *Ifosfamide.* Retrieved June 15, 2006, from http://www.rxlist.com/cgi/generic/ifosfamide.htm.

Wilkes, G.M., & Barton-Burke, M. (2005). *2005 Oncology nursing drug handbook.* Sudbury, MA: Jones & Bartlett.

Irinotecan (Camptosar)

Barbara Holmes Gobel and Deborah Mast

DRUG CLASS

- Topoisomerase I inhibitor

ROUTE OF ADMINISTRATION

- Intravenous (IV)

HOW TO ADMINISTER

- Administer IV over 60 to 90 minutes or longer.

PRETREATMENT GUIDELINES

- Premedicate for nausea and vomiting.
- Liver evaluation: contraindicated for serum bilirubin >2 mg/dL or serum aminotransferases more than three times the upper limit of normal in patients without liver metastasis or serum aminotransferases more than five times the upper limit of normal in patients with liver metastasis (on the basis of clinical trials)
- White blood cell count and absolute neutrophil count (>1,500/mm^2)
- Platelet count >100,000/mm^2
- Assess for treatment-related diarrhea: should be fully resolved before next cycle.
- In patients known to be homozygous for the UGT1A1*28: reduction of starting dose by one level of irinotecan should be considered.

USE

- Colorectal cancer: irinotecan is used for the treatment of metastatic colorectal cancer. It is approved for the first-line treatment of colorectal cancer in combination with 5-fluorouracil (5-FU) and leucovorin and as a single agent for colorectal cancer recurring or progressing after treatment with 5-FU.

Off-Label Uses

- Cervical cancer
- Gastric cancer
- Lung cancer
- Malignant glioma
- Ovarian cancer
- Pancreatic cancer

PHARMACOKINETICS

- Irinotecan is metabolized by the liver to its active metabolite, SN-38. Individuals with a homozygous UGT1A1*28 allele (about 10% of the North American population) have a decreased ability to form the SN-38 and are at increased risk for neutropenia.
- Plasma protein binding (primarily to albumin) is 30%-68% for irinotecan and 95% for SN-38.
- Excretion of irinotecan and its metabolites is primarily through the bile and feces (5%-39%) and the kidneys (11%-20%).
- Mean terminal half-life is 6-12 hours for irinotecan and 10-20 hours for SN-8.

USUAL DOSE AND SCHEDULE
IFL (Salz Regimen)

- Metastatic colorectal cancer: irinotecan 125 mg/m^2 IV over 90 minutes followed by Leucovorin (20 mg/m^2 IV bolus) and 5-FU (500 mg/m^2 IV bolus) on days 1, 8, 15, and 22, followed by a 2-week rest period, or when toxicity has recovered to National Cancer Institute (NCI) grade 1 or less.
- Recurrent colorectal cancers: irinotecan 125 mg/m^2 over 90 minutes weekly for 4 weeks, followed by a 2-week rest period. This 6-week cycle is then repeated. There may be a dose increase up to 150 mg/m^2 as tolerated.
- Recurrent colorectal cancers: irinotecan 350 mg/m^2; irinotecan 300 mg/m^2 in patients who are >70 years old, have received prior pelvic/abdominal radiotherapy, or those with performance status of 2. Dose given every 3 weeks.

Douillard Regimen

- Metastatic colorectal cancers
  - Day 1—irinotecan 180 mg/m^2 over 90 minutes given concomitantly with leucovorin

200 mg/m^2 over 2 hours, followed by 5-FU 400 mg/m^2 IV bolus, then 5-FU 600 mg/m^2 given as a 22-hour IV continuous infusion.

○ Day 2—leucovorin 200 mg/m^2 IV over 2 hours, then 5-FU 400 mg/m^2 IV bolus, then 5-FU 600 mg/m^2 over 22 hours as a continuous infusion.

○ Repeat cycle every 2 weeks.

SIDE EFFECTS

- Abdominal pain
- Alopecia
- Anemia
- Anorexia
- Bradycardia
- Dizziness
- Dyspnea (rare)
- Eosinophilia
- Constipation
- Diarrhea—can be dose limiting and severe
- Elevated liver enzymes
- Fatigue
- Fever
- Headache
- Insomnia
- Lacrimation
- Mucositis (rare)
- Nausea and vomiting
- Neutropenia—can be dose limiting
- Pulmonary infiltrates (rare)
- Salivation
- Thrombocytopenia

NADIR

- Granulocytopenia: 6 to 9 days

STORAGE

- Store unopened vials as room temperature and protect from light.

MIXING INSTRUCTIONS

- Dilute and mix drug in 250 to 500 mL of 5% dextrose (preferred) or normal saline solution to a concentration of 0.12 to 2.8 mg/mL.

Product Stability

- Diluted drug is stable for 24 hours at room temperature. If the drug is diluted in 5% dextrose, the drug is stable at refrigerated temperatures (2°-8° C [36°-46° F]) for 48 hours.

COMPATIBILITY WITH OTHER DRUGS/INTRAVENOUS FLUIDS

- Dextrose 5% in water
- Palonosetron
- Sodium chloride 0.9%

DRUG INTERACTIONS

- Administration of additional myelosuppressive agents may lead to additive effects of immunosuppression.
- Administration of live vaccines while on irinotecan is contraindicated because of compromised immune function.
- Anticoagulants, nonsteroidal anti-inflammatory drugs (NSAIDs), platelet inhibitors, strontium 89 chloride, and thrombolytic agents can cause increased risk of bleeding in patients receiving irinotecan.
- Increased prothrombin times are seen in patients taking concomitant warfarin.
- Laxatives or laxative-like agents must be avoided because they may exacerbate the diarrhea seen with irinotecan.
- Metoclopramide should be avoided; it can increase diarrhea when used in combination with irinotecan.
- Phenobarbital and phenytoin (inducers of cytochrome P450 3A4) will increase the elimination of irinotecan. Higher doses of irinotecan are needed to achieve the same therapeutic effect in patients receiving these medications.
- Desipramine, paroxetine, sertraline, azole antifungals, clarithromycin, erythromycin, doxycycline, protease inhibitors, verapamil and other CYP2B6 or CYP3A4 inhibitors may increase the levels/effects of irinotecan.
- Discontinue ketoconazole at least 1 week prior to irinotecan, concurrent use is contraindicated.
- Sargramostim and filgrastim should not be used 24 hours before or after treatment.

- St. John's wort significantly decreases the levels of irinotecan. It is recommended to discontinue the use of St. John's wort at least 2 weeks before treatment with irinotecan.

PREGNANCY

Category D

SPECIAL CONSIDERATIONS
Diarrhea

- Diarrhea associated with irinotecan is dose limiting and occasionally severe.
  ○ Early-onset diarrhea begins within 24 hours of irinotecan administration; administration of atropine 0.25 to 1 mg SQ/IV may alleviate this side effect.
  ○ Late-onset diarrhea begins 24 hours after an irinotecan infusion.
- Loperamide should be initiated at first sign of diarrhea. The recommended loperamide dose is 4 mg at first sign of diarrhea, followed by 2 mg every 2 hours (or 4 mg every 4 hours at night) until there are no signs of diarrhea for at least 12 hours.
- Patients should receive self-care instructions on the management of diarrhea.
- Patients should be taught to avoid taking any laxatives while receiving irinotecan.

Myelosuppression

- Major dose-limiting toxicity
- Neutropenia is the most common of the hematological toxicities; thrombocytopenia and anemia occur less frequently.
- Patients must have weekly assessment for toxicity.
- Dose reductions or holding of dose should be done for neutropenia and diarrhea.
- Premedicate for nausea and vomiting.
- Irinotecan is contraindicated in patients with serum bilirubin >2.0 mg/dL.

PATIENT EDUCATION

- Hair loss is likely to occur.
- Teach patient to report diarrhea, sweating, and abdominal cramping to the health care professional after the irinotecan infusion.
- Teach patient self-management of diarrhea including diet, medication management, fluid management, and avoidance of laxatives.
  - Diet teaching should include drinking 8-10 glasses of fluid a day, eating small meals throughout the day, eating primarily bland, low-fiber foods, avoiding fatty and spicy foods.
  - Patients should be taught to avoid taking all laxatives while receiving irinotecan.
- This drug can cause nausea and vomiting; an antiemetic should be taken before treatment.
- Observe for signs of low platelets (easy bruising, petechiae, black tarry stool, or bloody stool).
- Observe for signs of infection (fever, redness, tenderness or pus at the insertion site of central lines or drains). Avoid exposure to infections or infected persons.
- Observe for signs of anemia (fatigue, shortness of breath).

BIBLIOGRAPHY

Abigerges, D., Chabot, C. C., Armaund, J. P., et al. (1995). Phase I and pharmacologic studies of the camptothecin analog irinotecan administered every 3 weeks in cancer patients. *Journal of Clinical Oncology, 13,* 210-221.

Camptosar. (2002). Kalamazoo, MI: Pharmacia & Upjohn.

Clinical Pharmacology. (2006). *Irinotecan.* Retrieved June 19, 2006, from http://cpip.gsm.com/ (subscription required).

Fischer, D. S., Knobf, M. T., Durivage, H . J., et al. (2003). *The cancer chemotherapy handbook* (6th ed.) (pp. 146-147). St. Louis: Mosby.

Leslie, K. K. (2002). Chemotherapy and pregnancy. *Clinical Obstetrics and Gynecology, 45,* 153-164.

Wilkes, G. M., & Barton-Burke, M. (2005). *2005 Oncology nursing drug handbook* (pp. 191-196). Sudbury, MA: Jones & Bartlett.

Isotretinoin (Accutane, Amnesteem, Claravis, Sotret)

Barbara Holmes Gobel and Deborah Mast

DRUG CLASS

- Dermatologic
- Retinoid (derivative of vitamin A)

ROUTE OF ADMINISTRATION

- Oral, as a single daily dose

HOW TO ADMINISTER

- Administer drug orally with food, high fat meal preferable, to maximize gastrointestinal (GI) absorption.
- Do not crush or open capsules.

PRETREATMENT GUIDELINES

- All prescribers, pharmacists, and patients must comply with the conditions of the iPLEDGE program when prescribing, dispensing, or receiving isotretinoin.
  - *Prescribers* must register the patients into the iPLEDGE program through the Internet or the telephone and provide monthly confirmation that the patient has received counseling and education.
  - *Pharmacists* may only dispense isotretinoin from an iPLEDGE-registered pharmacy. Medication guides are to be given to every patient with every prescription.
  - *Patients* must sign a consent form before starting isotretinoin therapy. Sexually active patients are taught to use two forms of contraception for 1 month before starting therapy, during therapy, and for 1 month after therapy is complete.
  - Baseline and periodic complete blood count (CBC), chemistry

profile, liver function, and lipid panel is recommended.

USE

- Acne vulgaris
- Cystic acne

Off-Label Uses

- Isotretinoin is undergoing studies to evaluate its effectiveness as a chemoprevention drug for the following cancers:
  - Cervical cancer
  - Chronic myelogenous leukemia
  - Cutaneous T-cell lymphoma
  - Head and neck cancer
  - Melanoma
  - Myelodysplastic syndrome
  - Neuroblastoma
  - Squamous cell cancer of the skin

PHARMACOKINETICS

- Natural retinoic acid metabolite
- Metabolized in the liver
- Absorption of isotretinoin after an oral dose is incomplete, but bioavailability can be enhanced through administration with food or milk. Foods high in cholesterol should be avoided to reduce the risk of hypertriglyceridemia.
- Peak plasma levels occur in approximately 3 hours.
- Drug is totally bound to plasma albumin.
- Elimination is through the urine and feces.
- Elimination half-life of 10 to 20 hours.

USUAL DOSE AND SCHEDULE
Chemoprevention Treatment

- 0.5 to 2 mg/kg/day for 3 months or longer (oral leukoplakia)
- 2.5 to 4 mg/kg/day for 8 weeks
- 20 to 125 mg/m^2 for up to 6 months (myelodysplastic syndrome)

SIDE EFFECTS

- Abdominal pain
- Anaphylactoid reactions
- Anemia—rare
- Arthralgia
- Bone pain
- Chelitis

- Conjunctivitis
- Elevated liver enzymes
- Elevated sedimentation rate
- Glossitis
- Hypertriglyceridemia
- Pancreatitis
- Inflammatory bowel disease
- Myalgia
- Nausea and vomiting
- Photosensitivity
- Pruritus
- Pseudotumor cerebri
- Psychiatric disorder
- Teratogenesis
- Thrombocytopenia—rare
- Thrombocythemia—rare
- Transient elevations of liver enzymes/hyperbilirubinemia
- Skin fragility
- Stomatitis
- Visual disturbances
- Xerostomia

STORAGE

- Stored at room temperature, protected from light

MIXING INSTRUCTIONS

- Drug is manufactured as 10-, 20-, and 40-mg capsules.

DRUG INTERACTIONS

- Vitamin A–containing supplements given concomitantly with isotretinoin may increase toxicity and should be avoided.
- Anticoagulation effects of warfarin may be decreased with concomitant use of isotretinoin.
- Isotretinoin should be administered at least 1 hour before or 4 to 6 hours after cholestyramine or colestipol to minimize drug interactions (may decrease the oral bioavailability of isotretinoin).
- Isotretinoin given concomitantly with carbamazepine may decrease serum carbamazepine levels.
- Tetracycline or minocycline given concomitantly with isotretinoin has resulted in papilledema or pseudotumor cerebri (benign intracranial hypertension).
- Isotretinoin given concomitantly with alcohol may cause disulfiram-like reactions.

PREGNANCY

Category X

SPECIAL CONSIDERATIONS
Oral Bioavailability

- Drug must be taken with food or milk to increase the oral bioavailability.
- Do not crush or open capsules.

Teratogenicity

- There is a high risk of birth defects in patients who take isotretinoin in any dosage for any amount of time. Because of this risk, the iPLEDGE program has been developed to prevent isotretinoin exposure during pregnancy.

PATIENT EDUCATION

- Patients must participate in the iPLEDGE program and sign a consent form to be able to receive isotretinoin.
- The isotretinoin therapy should not be started until negative results from two urine or serum pregnancy tests are confirmed in women of childbearing potential, and monthly pregnancy testing during therapy is required.
- Women who become sexually active during treatment should be counseled to use two effective forms of birth control for at least 1 month before, during, and for 1 month after discontinuation of therapy.
- Women must sign another patient information/consent form about isotretinoin and birth defects.
- Breast-feeding is not recommended during isotretinoin therapy.
- Blood donation must be avoided during and for 1 month after completion of isotretinoin therapy.
- Isotretinoin should be taken with food or milk.
- Isotretinoin capsules should not be shared with anyone else because of the risk of birth defects.
- If patients wear contact lenses, their eyes may feel uncomfortable.

Patients should be instructed to contact the eye doctor if their eyes get dry.

BIBLIOGRAPHY

Clinical Pharmacology. (2006). *Isotretinoin*. Retrieved July, 10, 2006, from http://cpip.gsm.com/ (subscription required).

Fischer, D. S., Knobf, M. T., Durivage, H. J., et al. (2003). *The cancer chemotherapy handbook* (6th ed.) (pp. 140-150). St. Louis: Mosby.

Freemantle, S. J., Dragnev, K. H., & Dmitrovsky, E. (2006). The retinoic acid paradox in cancer chemoprevention. *Journal of the National Cancer Institute, 98,* 426-427.

Khuri, J. R., Lee, J. J., Lippman, S. M., et al. (2006). Randomized phase III trial of low-dose isotretinoin for prevention of second primary tumors in stage I and II head and neck cancer patients. *Journal of the National Cancer Institute, 98,* 441-450.

Leucovorin Calcium (Folinic Acid, Citrovorum Factor)

Barbara Holmes Gobel and Deborah Mast

DRUG CLASS

- Water-soluble vitamin in the folate group (folinic acid)

ROUTE OF ADMINISTRATION

- Oral
- Parenteral—intravenous (IV), intramuscular (IM)

HOW TO ADMINISTER
Oral Administration

- Oral doses >25 mg should not be given because of decreased absorption.
- Do not give oral leucovorin rescue therapy if the patient is unable to tolerate oral medication, if the patient is vomiting, or if the patient has diarrhea or mucositis.

Parenteral Administration

- May give drug IM, by IV push and IV infusion in 50 mL or more of 5% dextrose or normal saline solution over a period of several minutes or longer

- IV leucovorin is incompatible with fluorouracil; thus these agents cannot be administered simultaneously.
- Do **not** give agent intrathecally.
- Do not use preparations containing benzyl alcohol for doses >10 mg/m².

PRETREATMENT GUIDELINES

- When given as a rescue dose for methotrexate, agent must be given on time.
- Potential for nausea and vomiting; can be given with antacids, milk, or juice

USE

- Fluorouracil therapy—potentiates the action of fluorouracil in the treatment of advanced colorectal cancer
- Macrocytic anemia
- Megaloblastic anemia
- Methotrexate toxicity prophylaxis—"methotrexate rescue" (Methotrexate has been identified as an orphan drug by the Food and Drug Administration [FDA] for this indication.)
- Counteract the effects of folic acid antagonists (e.g., trimethoprim or pyrimethamine)

PHARMACOKINETICS

- Leucovorin may be given orally or parenterally by the IV, IM, or intraperitoneal routes.
- Leucovorin is rapidly absorbed by active transport after oral administration.
- Peak serum concentrations occur approximately 1.7 to 2.5 hours after an oral dose.
- Leucovorin is converted to its primary active metabolite, 5-methyletrahydrofolate (MTHF), in the gastrointestinal (GI) tract. In the presence of this metabolite, the active form of fluorouracil binds more tightly to the target enzyme.
- The kidneys excrete both leucovorin and MTHF; 50% of the single dose is excreted in 6 hours

in the urine (80%-90% of the dose) and the stool (8% of the dose)
- Leucovorin and MTHF rapidly enter the cerebrospinal fluid (CSF). After intrathecal administration of methotrexate, only low doses of leucovorin should be given.

USUAL DOSE AND SCHEDULE

- When used to potentiate the action of fluorouracil: doses ranging from 20 to 500 mg/m² orally or IV are used. High-dose oral therapy (500 mg/m²) is usually given in 125 mg/m² increments of four doses.
- Rescue agent for methotrexate: various regimens have been used on the basis of methotrexate dose; most commonly used doses include 10 to 25 mg/m² orally or IV every 6 hours for six to eight doses (beginning 6 to and no later than 24 hours after methotrexate). Dose adjustments are made on the basis of methotrexate serum levels and serum creatinine levels. Continue until serum methotrexate levels are < 0.05 micromole/L.
- Intrathecal dosing of methotrexate: smaller doses of leucovorin may be given orally or intravenous immediately after dosing of intrathecal methotrexate. Intrathecal dosing of leucovorin is contraindicated.
- Counteracting the effects of trimethoprim or pyrimethamine-induced myelosuppression: 5 to 15 mg daily of oral or IM dose

SIDE EFFECTS

- Hypersensitivity reactions
- Nausea and vomiting
- Seizures
- Skin rash
- Syncope
- Thrombocytosis
- May potentiate the toxic effects of fluoropyrimidine therapy, resulting in increased hematological and GI side effects (e.g., diarrhea and stomatitis)

NADIR

- None; leucovorin is not cytotoxic.

STORAGE

- Store at room temperature between 15° and 25° C (59° and 77° F).
- Protect from light and moisture.

MIXING INSTRUCTIONS
Vials of Leucovorin

- 50- or 100-mg vial: add 5 or 10 mL of bacteriostatic water or sterile water, respectively, for injection to produce a concentration of 10 mg/mL.
- 350-mg vial: add 17 mL of bacteriostatic or sterile water for injection to produce a concentration of 20 mg/mL.

PRODUCT STABILITY

- If reconstituted with sterile water, the injection must be used immediately.
- If reconstituted with bacteriostatic water, the solution is stable for 7 days at room temperature.

Ampules of Leucovorin

- No reconstitution is needed for commercial ampules when used for IM administration of leucovorin. Use 3 or 5 mg/mL commercial ampules for IM injection.

Intermittent IV Infusion

- Further dilute reconstituted solution with 100 to 500 mL of 5% dextrose in water (D5W), 10% dextrose in water (D10W), Ringer's, or lactated Ringer's solution.
- The diluted solution is stable for 24 hours.

COMPATIBILITY WITH OTHER DRUGS/INTRAVENOUS FLUIDS

- Bacteriostatic water
- Dextrose 10% in sodium chloride
- D10W
- Dextrose 5% in sodium chloride
- D5W
- Furosemide
- Heparin sodium
- Sodium chloride
- Fluorouracil—incompatible

DRUG INTERACTIONS

- 5-Fluorouracil (5-FU)—potentiation, which can be therapeutically advantageous but can also potentiate the adverse effects associated with 5-FU.
- Phenytoin, phenobarbital, primidone, or other barbiturates may have decreased anticonvulsant action (when leucovorin is given in large doses [e.g., >500 mg/m² of oral therapy]).

PREGNANCY

Category C
- It is not known whether leucovorin is excreted into breast milk; thus it is recommended that leucovorin be used with caution in breast-feeding women.

SPECIAL CONSIDERATIONS

- Leucovorin given as a methotrexate "rescue" must be given on schedule to avoid methotrexate toxicity.
- When using leucovorin for an IM injection, inject deeply into a large muscle.
- When using leucovorin for a direct IV injection, the rate should not exceed 160 mg/min.
- Intrathecal administration of leucovorin is contraindicated.
- Oral administration of leucovorin should only be given to patients who tolerate oral medications, who are not vomiting, and who do not have diarrhea.
- A preservative-free diluent should be used for reconstitution for doses >10 mg/m² or in neonates because of the benzyl alcohol found in certain diluents.
- Patients should be monitored closely when patients receiving leucovorin are also taking anticonvulsants. Anticonvulsant therapy may need to be increased.

PATIENT EDUCATION

- All oral doses must be taken at the time prescribed by the nurse or the physician, if the leucovorin is given as a "methotrexate rescue."
- Leucovorin may be given by injection into a muscle or by a slow injection into a vein. It is given in a hospital or a clinic setting by a health care professional.
- Patients should notify their health care providers if they are taking any barbiturate medications for inducing sleep or treating seizures. Leucovorin can decrease the activity of barbiturate medications.
- If the leucovorin is given with 5-FU, patients may experience more side effects from the 5-FU, such as mouth sores or diarrhea. Patients should notify their health care providers know if these side effects do not get better or get worse.

BIBLIOGRAPHY

Clinical Pharmacology. (2006). *Leucovorin.* Retrieved May 31, 2006, from http://cpip.gsm.com/ (subscription required).

Fischer, D. S., Knobf, M. T., Durivage, H. J., et al. (2003). *The cancer chemotherapy handbook* (6th ed., pp. 154-155). St. Louis: Mosby

Polovich, M., White, J. M., & Kelleher, L. O. (2005). *Chemotherapy and biotherapy guidelines and recommendations for practice* (2nd ed., pp. 120-121). Pittsburgh, PA: Oncology Nursing Service.

Rx List. (2004). *Leucovorin calcium.* Retrieved May 31, 2006, from http://www.rxlist.com/cgi/generic/leucovorincalcium.htm.

Wilkes, G. M., & Barton-Burke, M. (2005). *2005 Oncology nursing drug handbook* (pp. 373-374). Sudbury, MA: Jones & Bartlett.

Lomustine (CCNU, CeeNU)

Barbara Holmes Gobel and Deborah Mast

DRUG CLASS

- Alkylating agent (nitrosourea)

ROUTE OF ADMINISTRATION

- Oral

HOW TO ADMINISTER

- Administer on an empty stomach 1 hour before meals or 2 hours after a meal (this may help to reduce the associated nausea and vomiting).

PRETREATMENT GUIDELINES

- Pretreat for nausea and vomiting because lomustine is a highly emetogenic agent.
- Neutrophil count (may cause severe myelosuppression)
- Platelet count (may cause severe myelosuppression)
- Hemoglobin/hematocrit (may cause severe myelosuppression)
- Renal function
  - CrCl 10-50 mL/min, administer 75% of the normal dose.
  - CrCl <10 mL/min, administer 50% of the normal dose

  Note: Patients with aggressive Hodgkin disease may require treatment with lomustine despite severe bone marrow suppression.

USE

- Brain cancers
- Hodgkin disease
- Non-Hodgkin lymphoma

Off-Label Uses

- Malignant melanoma

PHARMACOKINETICS

- Cell cycle–phase nonspecific
- Half-life is 16 hours to 2 days.
- Drug is converted into metabolites by first-pass metabolism in the liver.
- Metabolites are eliminated slowly in the urine.

- Drug is administered orally and is rapidly absorbed from the gastrointestinal (GI) tract, with nearly complete oral absorption in 30 minutes.
- Drug crosses the blood-brain barrier effectively because of high lipid solubility.

USUAL DOSE AND SCHEDULE
Single Agent

- 130 mg/m² orally every 6 weeks
- 100 mg/m² initial dose for patients with compromised bone marrow function
- Dosing for subsequent cycles based upon WBC and platelet nadir from previous cycles, refer to package insert for specific dosing guidelines

Combination Therapy

- 75 to 100 mg/m² every 6 weeks
  Note: Repeat dosages should not be given until bone marrow recovery has occurred. Recovery is defined as WBC > 4000 and platelets >100,000.
- Drug manufactured as capsules
- 100 mg capsules = green/green
- 40 mg capsules = green/white
- 10 mg capsules = white

SIDE EFFECTS

- Alopecia
- Anorexia
- Confusion
- Hepatotoxicity (reversible)
- Lethargy
- Myelosuppression (can be delayed and cumulative)
- Nausea and vomiting
- Pulmonary fibrosis/pulmonary infiltrates
- Renal toxicity (progressive azotemia, decrease in kidney size, and renal failure)
- Stomatitis
- Visual impairment

NADIR

- Platelets: days 26 to 34, lasting 1 to 2 weeks.
- Neutrophils: days 41 to 46, lasting 9 to 14 days. Recovery takes 6 to 8 weeks.
- Bone marrow suppression is a dose-limiting toxicity.

STORAGE

- Store at room temperature (below 40° C/104° F).
- Protect from heat and humidity.
- Keep container of drug tightly closed.

COMPATIBILITY WITH OTHER DRUGS/INTRAVENOUS FLUIDS

- To be taken on an empty stomach with no other medications

DRUG INTERACTIONS

- Alcohol should be avoided during use of lomustine.
- Alkylating agents or other immunosuppressive agents may increase bone marrow toxicity.
- Anticoagulants, nonsteroidal anti-inflammatory drugs (NSAIDs), platelet inhibitors, strontium 89 chloride, and thrombolytic agents can cause increased risk of bleeding in patients receiving lomustine.
- CYP2D6 inhibitors, including cimetidine, paroxetine, fluoxetine, quinidine and others, may inhibit lomustine metabolism, resulting in an increase in lomustine levels/effects, including increased bone marrow toxicity.
- Nalidixic acid
- Phenobarbital decreases lomustine's antineoplastic activity.
- Sargramostim and filgrastim should not be used 24 hours before or after treatment.

PREGNANCY

Category D

- Breast-feeding while receiving lomustine is not recommended because of the carcinogenic, teratogenic, and mutagenic effects of this agent.

SPECIAL CONSIDERATIONS

- Lomustine should be dispensed one dose at a time to minimize overdosage.
- Agent should be taken on an empty stomach to minimize the problem of nausea and vomiting; may require antiemetic therapy.

PATIENT EDUCATION

- Agent can cause a loss of appetite; anorexia may last several days.
- Agent can cause nausea and vomiting; thus it should be taken on an empty stomach and patient should be instructed to take an antiemetic.
- Monitor for signs of low platelet count (easy bruising, petechiae, black tarry stool, or bloody stool).
- Monitor for signs of infection (temperature, redness, tenderness or pus at the insertion site of central lines or drains).

BIBLIOGRAPHY

Belford, K. (2005). Central nervous system cancers. In C. H. Yarbro, M. H. Frogge, & M. Goodman (Eds.). *Cancer nursing principles and practice* (6th ed., pp. 1089-1136). Sudbury, MA: Jones & Bartlett.

Buckner, J. C., Gesme, D., O'Fallon, J. R., et al. (2003). Phase II trial of procarbazine, lomustine, and vincristine as initial therapy for patients with low-grade oligodendroglioma or oligoastrocytoma: efficacy and associations with chromosome abnormalities. *Journal of Clinical Oncology, 21*, 251-255.

Clinical Pharmacology. (2006). *Lomustine*. Retrieved May 1, 2006, from http://cpip.gsm.com/ (subscription required).

Fischer, D. S., Knobf, M. T., Durivage, H. J., et al. (2003). *The cancer chemotherapy handbook* (6th ed.) (pp. 157-158). St. Louis: Mosby.

Rx List. (2004). *Lomustine*. Retrieved May 15, 2006, from http://www.rxlist.com/cgi/generic/lomustine.htm.

Wilkes, G. M., & Barton-Burke, M. (2005). *2005 Oncology nursing drug handbook* (pp. 204-205). Sudbury, MA: Jones & Bartlett.

Mechlorethamine Hydrochloride (Nitrogen Mustard, Mustargen)

Barbara Holmes Gobel and Deborah Mast

DRUG CLASS

- Alkylating agent (first alkylating agent introduced for cancer therapy)

ROUTE OF ADMINISTRATION

- Intravenous (IV)
- Intracavitary
- Topical

HOW TO ADMINISTER
Intravenous

- Inject the agent through the sidearm of a freely flowing IV infusion to reduce the risk of severe local reactions from extravasation or high concentrations of the drug.
- Administer the agent over 3 to 5 minutes, followed by a flush of running IV infusion or 5 to 10 mL of the IV solution.
- The infusion site should be monitored closely for signs of extravasation such as redness, swelling, erythema, induration, and sloughing. Because the agent is a severe vesicant, caution should be taken to avoid contact with the skin.
- The agent should be administered shortly after admixture because it decomposes on standing.

Intracavitary

- The reconstituted agent should be further diluted in up to 100 mL of normal saline solution before administration.
- Administration of this drug is done after fluid has been removed from the intracavitary space (e.g., intrapleural, intrapericardial, intraperitoneal) to facilitate contact of the agent with the membranes of the intracavitary space.
- The drug should be injected slowly with frequent aspiration to ensure a free flow of fluid.
- Once the agent has been injected, the position of the patient should be changed every 5 to 10 minutes for 1 hour to evenly distribute the drug throughout the body cavity.

Topical*

- Use protective gloves to apply the solution to the entire body surface.
- There should be minimal drug applied to the peritoneum and the axillary, inguinal, and inframammary areas.

PRETREATMENT GUIDELINES

- Pretreat for nausea and vomiting 30 to 45 minutes before administration because mechlorethamine is highly emetogenic.
- Neutrophil count
- Platelet count
- Chemistry profile and uric acid
- A good vein with a brisk blood return should be identified for peripheral administration.

USE

- Hodgkin disease (major role of this drug)
- Non-Hodgkin lymphoma
- Bronchogenic carcinoma
- Chronic lymphocytic leukemia
- Chronic myelogenous leukemia
- Lymphosarcoma
- Malignant pericardial, peritoneal, and pleural effusions
- Polycythemia vera

Off-Label Uses

- Mycosis fungoides
- Cutaneous T-cell lymphoma
- Skin cancer

PHARMACOKINETICS

- Cell cycle–phase nonspecific
- After IV administration, mechlorethamine has a short half-life and is undetected in the blood within a few minutes. The drug is rapidly inactivated by body fluids. Metabolites of the drug are excreted in the urine within 24 hours.
- Cytotoxic activity occurs as a result of interstrand and intrastrand cross-linkages of deoxyribonucleic acid (DNA) and ribonucleic acid (RNA), causing miscoding, breakage, and failure of replication.

USUAL DOSE AND SCHEDULE
Intravenous Dosage

- Hodgkin disease or non-Hodgkin lymphoma: 0.2 mg/kg or 6 mg/m^2 given as a single dose on day 1 or on day 1 and 8 of a regimen
- Chronic myelogenous leukemia: 0.4 mg/m^2 as a single IV dose monthly or as necessary to lower the white blood cell count
- Lung cancer: 6 mg/m^2 every 2 weeks with doxorubicin and methotrexate and every 4 weeks with doxorubicin, methotrexate, fluorouracil, hydroxyurea, and procarbazine
- Polycythemia vera: 0.4 mg/kg or 6 mg/m^2 as a single IV dose monthly or more often as necessary to lower the red blood cell count

Intracavitary Dosage

- Intracavitary administration for malignant effusions: 0.2-0.4 mg/kg as a single intracavitary injection

Topical Dosage*

- Mycosis fungoides/cutaneous T-cell lymphoma: solution/ointment is applied to entire skin surface, covering all lesions, one to four times a day for 6 to 12 months or until lesions disappear. Maintenance therapy is every 2 to

---

Not approved by the Food and Drug Administration (FDA) and not commercially available; topical form will need to be compounded by a pharmacist.

Not approved by the FDA.

7 days and should be continued for 3 years without recurrence.

SIDE EFFECTS

- Alopecia
- Amyloidosis
- Amenorrhea
- Deafness
- Herpes zoster reactivation
- Hyperkalemia
- Hyperphosphatemia
- Hyperuricemia
- Hypocalcemia
- Infertility
- Myelosuppression (can be severe)
- Nausea and vomiting (can be severe)
- Petechiae
- Secondary malignancies
- Subcutaneous hemorrhages
- Tinnitus
- Vesicant

NADIR

- Occurs in 7 to 14 days, recovery generally occurs in 21 days

STORAGE

- Store unreconstituted powder at room temperature.

MIXING INSTRUCTIONS

- Reconstitute 10 mg of powder with 10 mL of normal saline solution or sterile water at a concentration of 1 mg/1 mL.
- Shake the vial several times for complete dissolution of the drug, keeping the needle in the rubber stopper (minimizes risk of skin contact).
- Further dilute the reconstituted solution in 100 mL of normal saline solution for intracavitary administration.

Product Stability

- 60 minutes for the reconstituted solution
- Ointment (10 mg/dL) has a 3-month expiration date.

COMPATIBILITY WITH OTHER DRUGS/INTRAVENOUS FLUIDS

- Granisetron
- Ondansetron
- Sterile water

DRUG INTERACTIONS

- Anticoagulants, nonsteroidal anti-inflammatory drugs (NSAIDs), platelet inhibitors, strontium 89 chloride, and thrombolytic agents can cause increased risk of bleeding in patients receiving mechlorethamine.
- The activity of succinylcholine may be prolonged, which may lead to increased respiratory depression from succinylcholine.
- Sargramostim and filgrastim should not be used 24 hours before or 24 hours after treatment.
- Nalidixic acid may cause serious gastrointestinal toxicity such as hemorrhagic ulcerative colitis or intestinal necrosis.

PREGNANCY

Category D

- Mechlorethamine has the potential to cause teratogenesis and carcinogenesis.
- Contraindicated in lactating women

SPECIAL CONSIDERATIONS
Vesicant

- Antidote is sodium thiosulfate.
- Infiltrate area of extravasation with sodium thiosulfate subcutaneously (dilute 4 mL of sodium thiosulfate [10% solution] with 6 mL of sterile water).
- Follow institutional guidelines for extravasation of medication.

Severe Nausea and Vomiting

- Patient should be premedicated with antiemetics.

Tumor Lysis Syndrome

- Mechlorethamine may cause tumor lysis syndrome, manifested by hyperkalemia, hyperuricemia, hyperphosphatemia, and hypocalcemia.

PATIENT EDUCATION

- Hair loss
- Significant nausea and vomiting, which requires premedication with antiemetics
- Potent myelosuppressive agent

- Observe for signs of low platelets (easy bruising, petechiae, black tarry stool, or bloody stool).
- Observe for signs of infection (fever, redness, tenderness or pus at the insertion site of central lines or drains).
- Avoid exposure to infections or infected persons.
- May cause gonadal suppression during therapy, which may cause amenorrhea or azoospermia. May cause infertility
- Birth control during therapy is encouraged.
- Fatigue may occur from treatment or from low hemoglobin levels.

BIBLIOGRAPHY

Camp-Sorrell, D. (2005). Chemotherapy toxicities and management. In C.H. Yarbro, M.H. Frogge, & M. Goodman (Eds.). *Cancer nursing principles and practice* (6th ed., pp. 412-457). Sudbury, MA: Jones & Bartlett.

Clinical Pharmacology. (2006). *Mechlorethamine*. Retrieved May 1, 2006, from http://cpip.gsm.com/ (subscription required).

Fischer, D. S., Knobf, M. T., Durivage, H. J., et al. (2003). *The cancer chemotherapy handbook* (6th ed., pp. 158-160). St. Louis: Mosby.

Rx List. (2004). *Mechlorethamine*. Retrieved May 5, 2006, from http://www.rxlist.com/cgi/generic/methlorethamine.htm.

Wilkes, G. M., & Barton-Burke, M. (2005). *2005 Oncology nursing drug handbook* (pp. 206-209). Sudbury, MA: Jones & Bartlett.

Melphalan (Alkeran)

Barbara Holmes Gobel and Deborah Mast

DRUG CLASS

- Alkylating agent

ROUTE OF ADMINISTRATION

- Oral
- Intravenous (IV)

HOW TO ADMINISTER
Oral Administration

- Food interferes with absorption. Administer orally on an empty stomach (i.e., at least 1 hour before or 2 hours after a meal).

Intravenous Administration

- Time between reconstitution and administration should be kept to a minimum because the melphalan solution is unstable.
- Infuse dose over 15-20 minutes. Administration should be complete within 60 minutes of reconstitution.
- Administer into a large vein because the drug is a vesicant.
- Use vesicant precautions during administration.

PRETREATMENT GUIDELINES

- Neutrophil count >3,000/mm^3
- Platelet count >100,000mm^3
- Renal function: the manufacturer suggests that the dosage of melphalan should be reduced in patients with renal impairment.
  - CrCl 10-50mL/min, administer 75% of normal dose.
  - CrCl < 10mL/min OR BUN >30mg/dL, administer 50% of normal dose

Note: Patients with aggressive leukemia or lymphoma may require treatment with melphalan despite severe bone marrow suppression.

USES

- Multiple myeloma
- Ovarian cancer
- Stem cell transplant preparation

Off-Label Uses

- Sarcoma
- Testicular cancer
- Melanoma
- Breast cancer
- Neuroblastoma

PHARMACOKINETICS

- Terminal elimination half-life is 90 minutes.
- Absorbed incompletely from the gastrointestinal (GI) tract after oral administration.
- 80%-90% bound to plasma proteins over time
- Eliminated as unchanged drug, and its metabolites are excreted by the kidneys

USUAL DOSE AND SCHEDULE

- Multiple myeloma: 150 mcg/kg/day orally for 7 days every 4 weeks
- Ovarian cancer: 10 mg/day orally for 5 days; repeat every 6 weeks for up to six cycles on the basis of treatment-related toxicities
- Preparative regimens for stem cell transplantation: 140 to 280 mg/m^2 IV on 1 day or divided over 2 days before stem cell transplantation

SIDE EFFECTS

- Nausea
- Vomiting
- Irritant
- Mucositis (melphalan dosages above 200 mg/m^2 have been associated with unacceptable rate of grade 4 mucositis)
- Hypersensitivity reactions
- Myelosuppression (may be delayed and last 4 to 6 weeks)
- Sterility

NADIR

- Myelosuppression may be delayed and last 4 to 6 weeks.

STORAGE
Unreconstituted Powder

- Store unopened vials at 15°-30° C (59°-86° F).
- Protect from light.

Reconstituted Powder

- Do not refrigerate because a precipitate will form.
- Administer within 60 minutes (1% of the labeled dose hydrolyzes every 10 minutes after dilution with normal saline solution [NS]).

MIXING INSTRUCTIONS

- Reconstitute 50 mg with 10 mL of the diluent provided by the manufacturer to give a solution containing 5 mg/mL; then shake vial vigorously until solution is clear.
- Immediately dilute reconstituted solution with NS to a concentration no greater than 0.45 mg/mL.

- Once reconstituted, a precipitate will form if stored at 5° C; do not refrigerate reconstituted product.

Product Stability

- 60 minutes

COMPATIBILITY WITH OTHER DRUGS/INTRAVENOUS FLUIDS

- Heparin sodium
- Potassium chloride
- Sodium bicarbonate

DRUG INTERACTIONS

- Anticoagulants can cause increased risk of bleeding.
- May reduce threshold for carmustine lung toxicity
- Cimetidine and other histamine 2 receptors can decrease bioavailability.
- Cisplatin can delay renal clearance.
- Corticosteroids may enhance the antitumor effects of melphalan.
- Cyclosporine can cause increased nephrotoxicity.
- Filgrastim and sargramostim should not be used 24 hours before or after treatment.
- Nonsteroidal anti-inflammatory drugs (NSAIDs) can cause increased risk of bleeding.
- Interferon can cause reduced levels of melphalan.

PREGNANCY

Category D

- Melphalan is a known teratogen and has embryocidal effects in animals.

SPECIAL CONSIDERATIONS

- Vesicant; follow institutional guidelines for extravasation of medication.
- Dosage should be modified depending on clinical response and degree of renal impairment.
- Oral dose should be taken 1 hour before or 2 hours after a meal.

PATIENT EDUCATION

- Oral dose should be taken on an empty stomach.

Cancer Management

- If you miss a dose, do not double the dose; check with the prescriber.
- Monitor for signs of low platelets (easy bruising, petechiae, back tarry stool, or bloody stool).
- Monitor for signs of infection (temperature, redness, tenderness, or pus at the insertion site of central lines or drains).
- Hair loss

BIBLIOGRAPHY

Cancer Care Ontario. (2007). *Melphalan.* Retrieved March 28, 2006, from http://www.cancercare.on.ca/pdfdrugs/melphala.pdf.

Carlson, K. (2005). Melphalan 200 mg/m² with blood stem cell support as first-line myeloma therapy: impact of glomerular filtration rate on engraftment, transplantation-related toxicity and survival. *Bone Marrow Transplantation, 35*, 985-990.

Cleri, L., & Haywood, R. (1995). *Oncology: pocket guide to chemotherapy* (Revised edition., pp. 151-154). Philadelphia: Elsevier Science.

Clinical Pharmacology. (2006). *Melphalan.* Retrieved March 28, 2006, from http://cpip.gsm.com (subscription required).

Hasan, J. (2003). Oral melphalan as a treatment for platinum-resistant ovarian cancer. *British Journal of Cancer, 88*, 1828.

Medline Plus. (2003). *Melphalan.* Retrieved March 28, 2006, from http://www.nlm.nih.gov/medlineplus/druginfo/medmaster/a682220.html.

Polovich, M., White, J. M., & Kelleher, L. O. (2005). *Chemotherapy and biotherapy guidelines and recommendations for practice* (2nd ed., pp.22, 53). Pittsburgh: Oncology Nursing Service.

Spencer, A., Horvath, N., Gibson, J., et al. (2005). Prospective randomized trial of amifostine cytoprotection in myeloma patients undergoing high-dose melphalan conditioned autologous stem cell transplantation. *Bone Marrow Transplantation, 35*, 971-977.

Spratto, G. R., & Woods, A. L. (Eds.). (2003). *2003 PDR nurse's drug handbook* (pp. 925-926). Clifton Park, NY: Delmar Learning.

Mercaptopurine (6-MP, Purinethol)

Barbara Holmes Gobel and Deborah Mast

DRUG CLASS

- Antimetabolite

ROUTE OF ADMINISTRATION

- Oral

Off Label

- Intravenous (IV)

HOW TO ADMINISTER

- Administer orally; tablets may be crushed.
- Should not be administered with meals

PRETREATMENT GUIDELINES

1. Hepatic function. Consider dose reduction in patients with hepatic impairment, but no quantitative dosage recommendations are available.
2. Renal function. Dosage should be modified depending on clinical response and degree of renal impairment. The following guidelines have been suggested:
   - Creatinine clearance (CrCl) 50-80 mL/min: modify dosage interval to every 24-36 hours
   - CrCl 10-50 mL/min: modify dosage interval to every 48 hours
   - CrCl <10 mL/min: no quantitative dosage recommandations are avalable
3. Patients with genetic deficiency of thiopurine methyltransferase (TPMT) may be sensitive to myelosuppressive effects.

USE

- Acute lymphocytic leukemia

Off-Label Uses

- Acute myelogenous leukemia
- Chronic myelogenous leukemia

PHARMACOKINETICS

- Half-life is about 1-1.5 hours.
- Inactivated by oxidation of xanthine oxidase to 6-thiouric acid
- Hepatic metabolism of mercaptopurine to inactive metabolites
- After 24 hours, >50% of dose can be recovered in the urine as intact drug and metabolites.
- Oral dose is incomplete and variable; approximately 50% of oral dose is absorbed.

USUAL DOSE AND SCHEDULE
Acute Lymphocytic Leukemia

- Adults: 2.5-5 mg/kg/day by mouth once daily or 80-100 mg/m²/day by mouth once daily. Maintenance dosages are 1.5-2.5 mg/kg/day by mouth once daily.
- Children, aged 5 years and over: for induction, 2.5-5 mg/kg/day by mouth once daily. Maintenance dosages are 1.5-2.5 mg/kg/day by mouth once daily or 70-100 mg/m²/day by mouth once daily.

Acute Myelogenous Leukemia*

- Adults and children: 2.5 mg/kg/day orally once daily. If after 4 weeks at this dose, there is no clinical improvement and no definite evidence of leukocyte or platelet depression, the dose may be increased to 5 mg/kg/day orally once daily.

Chronic Myelogenous Leukemia*

- For chronic phase in adults: 60 to 75 mg/m²/day orally
- For blast crisis in adults: 100 mg/m² orally every 12 hours for 5-7 days

SIDE EFFECTS

- Hepatotoxicity
- Mild diarrhea
- Skin rashes
- Fever
- Hyperpigmentation
- Alopecia

---

*Not approved by the Food and Drug Administration (FDA).

- Bone marrow toxicity—anemia, leukopenia, thrombocytopenia

NADIR

- Neutropenia nadir day 16 (range: 11-23 days)
- Thrombocytopenia nadir day 15 (range: 12-21 days)

STORAGE

- Store oral doses in an air-tight container at room temperature, 68°-77° F (20°-25° C).
- Keep away from heat, moisture, and direct light.

MIXING INSTRUCTIONS

- IV form not available in United States
- Dilute 500-mg vials with 49.8 mL of sterile water, with final concentration of 10 mg/mL.
- Reconstituted solution should be further diluted in normal saline solution or dextrose 5% to a final concentration of 1-12 mg/mL before IV administration.

Product Stability

- Stable for 4 hours after dilution when refrigerated

COMPATIBILITY WITH OTHER DRUGS/INTRAVENOUS FLUIDS

- Dextrose 5%
- Normal saline solution
- IV formula not available in United States

DRUG INTERACTIONS

- Allopurinol can increase toxicity of mercaptopurine. Mercaptopurine should be reduced to one third to one fourth of usual dose when given concurrently with allopurinol.
- Captopril can increase toxicity of mercaptopurine.
- Increased hepatotoxicity when mercaptopurine given with doxorubicin.
- Olsalazine, mesalamine and sulfasalazine may increase levels/effects of mercaptopurine
- Sulfamethoxazole (SMX), trimethoprim (TMP): SMX-TMP

can enhance bone marrow suppression.
- Mercaptopurine inhibits the anticoagulation effect of warfarin; monitor PT/INR closely.

PREGNANCY

Category D
- Has teratogenic effects and should not be used during pregnancy
- Breast-feeding should be avoided.

SPECIAL CONSIDERATIONS

- Mercaptopurine has been given as continuous IV infusion for 12-24 hours or as a slow IV push (off label). IV formula not available in United States.
- Individuals with homozygous thiopurine methyltransferase (TPMT) deficiency are unusually sensitive to the myelosuppressive effects of mercaptopurine and prone to the development of rapid bone marrow suppression after initiation of treatment.
- Monitor serum aminotransferases, alkaline phosphatase, and bilirubin levels.

PATIENT EDUCATION

- Increased risk of infection after therapy
- Increased risk of bleeding after therapy
- Nausea, vomiting, or loss of appetite can occur.
- Darkening of fingernail or toenails may occur.
- Reddening or darkening of skin on soles or palms can occur.
- If patients miss a dose, they should not increase their normal dose to make up for the missed dose. Advise patients to report the missed dose to the care provider and return to their regular schedule.

BIBLIOGRAPHY

Bostrom, B. C., Sensel, M. R., Sather, H. N., et al. (2003). Dexamethasone versus prednisone and daily oral versus weekly intravenous mercaptopurine for patients with standard-risk acute lymphoblastic leukemia: a report from Children's Cancer Group. *Blood, 101,* 3809-3817.

Clinical Pharmacology. (2006). *Mercaptopurine.* Retrieved May 3, 2006, from http://cpip.gsm.com/ (subscription required).

Huntsman Cancer Institute. (2006). *Mercaptopurine.* Retrieved May 3, 2006, from http://www.hci.utah. edu/patientdocs/hci/drugs/mercaptopurine. htm.

Medline Plus. (2006). *Mercaptopurine..* Retrieved May 1, 2006, from http://www. nlm.nih.gov/medlineplus/druginfo/ uspdi/202350.html.

Springhouse. *2001 Physician's drug handbook* (9th ed., pp.647-648). Springhouse, PA: Springhouse Publishing.

University of North Carolina School of Medicine. (1998). *Clinically significant drug interactions.* Retrieved May 3, 2006, from http://www.med.unc. edu/medicine/edursrc/drug_int.htm.

Wilkes, G., & Barton-Burke, M. (2005). *2005 Oncology nursing drug handbook* (pp. 215-216). Sudbury, MA: Jones & Bartlett.

Mesna (Mesnex)

Barbara Holmes Gobel and Deborah Mast

DRUG CLASS

- Chemotherapy protectant (uroprotectant)

ROUTE OF ADMINISTRATION

- Oral
- Intravenous (IV)

HOW TO ADMINISTER
Oral Administration

- Oral dose may be given without regard to meals.
- Mesna injection may be diluted 1:1 to 1:10 in carbonated cola drink or chilled fruit juice such as apple, grape, tomato, or orange for oral administration. Plain or chocolate milk may be used. Because of the sulfur odor of mesna injection, more dilute solutions may be better tolerated.
- Oral dosage form available in 400 mg tablet

Intravenous Administration

- May be given as rapid IV infusion or bolus

- May be given as continuous IV infusion

PRETREATMENT GUIDELINES

- Emesis control for patients taking oral doses
- Use with caution in infants.
- Baseline blood urea nitrogen (BUN) and creatinine

USE

- Prophylaxis of ifosfamide-induced hemorrhagic cystitis
- Prophylaxis of high-dose cyclophosphamide-induced hemorrhagic cystitis

PHARMACOKINETICS

- Initial half-life of 10.2 minutes after IV administration
- Half-life ranges from 1.2-8.3 hours after administration of IV plus oral doses.
- Filtered by the glomeruli, reabsorbed by the proximal tubule, and then secreted back in the tubule of the kidney

USUAL DOSE AND SCHEDULE
Ifosfamide

- Given with every dose
- Given by IV short infusion, mesna should equal 60% of the total daily dose and be administered 15 minutes before and at 4 and 8 hours after each infusion of ifosfamide.
- Given standard-dose by continuous infusion, mesna can be administered with ifosfamide, as a continuous infusion at 60%-100% of the ifosfamide dose, after a loading dose of 20% of the total daily ifosfamide dose. Continuous infusion mesna should be given for 12-24 hours after ifosfamide is completed.
- Oral dosing: 100% of the ifosfamide dose, given as 20% of the dose at hour 0, then 40% of the dose at 2 and 6 hours after the start of ifosfamide.

Cyclophosphamide

- Given with every dose of high-dose cyclophosphamide (at least 120 mg/kg)

- Given as short infusion, mesna should be at least 40% of the total cyclophosphamide dose. Doses of 60%-120% have been administered, but efficacy has not been established. Administer 15 minutes before and at 4 and 8 hours after the cyclophosphamide dose.

SIDE EFFECTS

- Nausea
- Diarrhea
- Vomiting
- Headache
- Hypotension
- Abdominal pain
- Taste alteration
- Injection site reactions

STORAGE
Unreconstituted Powder

- Store at controlled room temperature 15°-30° C (59°-86° F).

Reconstituted Powder

- Multidose reconstituted vials may be stored and used for up to 8 days.
- Dilute solutions are chemically and physically stable for 24 hours at room temperature, 68°-77° F (20°-25° C).

MIXING INSTRUCTIONS

- Injection should be diluted to final concentration of 20 mg/mL.
- May be admixed with cyclophosphamide and ifosfamide

Product Stability

- Diluted solutions are stable for 24 hours at room temperature.

COMPATIBILITY WITH OTHER DRUGS/INTRAVENOUS FLUIDS

- Cyclophosphamide
- Dextrose 5%
- Ifosfamide
- Sodium bicarbonate
- Sodium chloride 0.9%

DRUG INTERACTIONS

- Cisplatin and carboplatin can be deactivated when given with mesna because mesna provides sulfhydryl groups that bind to and deactivate cisplatin and carboplatin if these drugs are given simultaneously.

PREGNANCY
Category B

- No controlled studies of mesna have been performed in pregnant women.
- Mesna should be used in women who are pregnant or breast-feeding only if the benefit outweighs the risk.

SPECIAL CONSIDERATIONS

- Contraindicated in patients with hypersensitivity to thiol compounds
- Contains benzyl alcohol as a preservative, which has been associated with a fatal gasping syndrome in neonates; use caution in infants.
- Patients with benzyl alcohol hypersensitivity may be at increased risk for hypersensitivity during treatment with mesna.

PATIENT EDUCATION

- Increase oral intake 12-24 hours before scheduled treatment.
- Increase oral intake to 2 to 3 liters/day.
- Administer final oral dose of cyclophosphamide before 4 PM to allow drug to pass through the bladder before bedtime.
- Frequent voiding, both day and night
- Instruct patient to visually observe urine and look for any signs of bleeding.
- If vomiting occurs within 2 hours of oral mesna dose, the dose should be repeated and prescriber notified.

BIBLIOGRAPHY

Baxter. (2002). *Mesnex*. Retrieved April 5, 2006, from http://www.baxter.com/ products/oncology/chemoprotectant/ mesnex_pi.pdf.

Clinical Pharmacology. (2006). *Mesna*. Retrieved March 9, 2006, from http:// cpip.gsm.com (subscription required).

Polovich, M., White, J. M., & Kelleher, L. O. (2005). *Chemotherapy and biotherapy guidelines and recommendations for practice* (2nd ed., pp 181-182). Pittsburgh, PA: Oncology Nursing Service.

Rx List. (2006). *Mesna*. Retrieved April 5, 2006, from http://www.rxlist.com/cgi/generic2/mesna_ad.htm.

U.S. Food and Drug Administration. (2002). *Mesna*. Retrieved May 18, 2006, http://www.accessdata.fda.gov/scripts/cder/onctools/prepare.cfm?GN=mesna.

Methotrexate (Rheumatrex)

Barbara Holmes Gobel and Deborah Mast

DRUG CLASS

- Antimetabolite

ROUTE OF ADMINISTRATION

- Oral
- Intrathecal
- Intravenous (IV)
- Intramuscular (IM)

HOW TO ADMINISTER
Oral Administration

- Preferred for low-dose therapy
- Absorption is dose dependent.
- Given 1 hour before or 2 hours after meals to increase absorption

Intrathecal

- Use preservative-free solutions only for administration.
- Withdraw an amount of cerebrospinal fluid (CSF) equivalent to the volume of methotrexate injection to be administered.
- Allow CSF to flow into the syringe and mix with the drug; inject intrathecally over 15-20 seconds with the bevel of the needle directed upward.

Intravenous

- Direct IV injection: inject at a rate of 10 mg/min through a free-flowing compatible IV infusion.
- Intermittent or continuous infusion: dilute solution with 5% dextrose in normal saline solution (D5NS), 5% dextrose in water (D5W), or normal saline

solution (NS); check vein patency by flushing with 5-10 mL of D5W or NS. Infuse at rate prescribed. After infusion, flush the IV tubing.

Intramuscular

- Inject deeply into a large muscle.

PRETREATMENT GUIDELINES

- Liver function
- For parenteral administration of intermediate- or high-dose methotrexate (500 mg/m^2 over <4 hours or >1 g/m^2 over >4 hours):
  - White blood cell count >1,500/mm^3
  - Neutrophil count >200/mm^3
  - Platelet count >75,000/mm^2
  - Serum bilirubin <1.2 mg/dL
  - Normal creatinine level
  - Hydrate with alkalinized IV fluids using sodium bicarbonate over 4-6 hours before initiation of methotrexate infusion.
- Renal function:
  - When CrCl is between 61-80mL/min, administer 75% of normal dose
  - When CrCl is between 51-60mL/min, administer 70% of the normal dose
  - When CrCl is between 10-50mL/min, administer 30-50% of the normal dose although dose is generally held at this level
  - When CrCl <10mL/min, avoid use

USE

- Lung cancer
- Breast cancer
- Osteogenic sarcoma
- Head and neck caner
- Non-Hodgkin lymphoma
- Acute lymphocytic leukemia
- Cutaneous T-cell lymphoma (mycosis fungoides)
- Gestational trophoblastic carcinomas (choriocarcinoma, chorioadenoma destruens, and hydatidiform mole)
- Rheumatoid arthritis

Off-Label Uses

- Bladder cancer
- Desmoid tumor

- Burkitt's lymphoma
- Carcinomatous meningitis
- Graft-versus-host-disease (GVHD) prophylaxis

PHARMACOKINETICS

- Initial half-life is 3.5 hours, primarily through renal clearance.
- Terminal half-life is about 10-12 hours and reflects enteric hepatic circulation.
- Blocks the enzyme dihydrofolate reductase (DHFR), which inhibits the conversion of folic acid to tetrahydrofolic acid, which results in the arrest of deoxyribonucleic acid (DNA), ribonucleic acid (RNA), and protein synthesis

USUAL DOSE AND SCHEDULE
Lung Cancer

- Adults, IV dose: many regimens exist; common combinations include methotrexate 20 mg/m^2 IV as a single dose with cisplatin, doxorubicin, and cyclophosphamide, every 28 days; methotrexate 40 mg/m^2 IV for one dose with etoposide and cisplatin; and methotrexate 100 mg/m^2 for one dose along with cyclophosphamide, vincristine, and doxorubicin.
- Adults, oral dose: 10 mg/m^2 orally twice weekly for 4 doses every 3 weeks in combination with lomustine and cyclophosphamide

Breast Cancer

- Adults and children, IV dose: 40-60 mg/m^2 IV every 21-28 days along with cyclophosphamide and fluorouracil (CMF regimen)

Osteogenic Sarcoma*

- Adults and children, IV dose: 12 g/m^2 IV every 2 weeks. If this does not produce peak serum methotrexate concentration of 1,000 micromolar at the end of the methotrexate infusion, the dose may increased to 15 g/m^2

---

*Has been designated an orphan drug by the Food and Drug Administration (FDA).

IV in subsequent treatments. These doses require leucovorin rescue dosing.

Head and Neck Cancer

- Adults and children, IV dose: 40 mg/m² IV on days 1 and 15, every 21 days alone or in combination with bleomycin and cisplatin
- Adults, oral dose: doses of 25-50 mg/m² orally once every 7 days have been used.
- Children, oral dose: 7.5-30 mg/m² PO every 7-14 days

Non-Hodgkin Lymphoma

- Adults and children, IV dose: two common regimens are methotrexate 200 mg/m² IV days 8 and 15 every 21 days in combination with bleomycin, doxorubicin, cyclophosphamide, vincristine, and dexamethasone and methotrexate 120 mg/m² IV on day 8 every 28 days in combination with cyclophosphamide, doxorubicin, etoposide, prednisone, cytarabine, bleomycin, and vincristine
- Children, IV dose: 200 to 500 mg/m² IV every 28 days, in combination with other chemotherapeutic agents

Acute Lymphocytic Leukemia

- Adults and children, oral or IM dose: 3.3 mg/m² orally or IM daily for 4-6 weeks or until remission occurs, followed by maintenance therapy with 20-30 mg/m² orally or IM twice weekly
- Adults and children, IV dose: 3.3 mg/m² IV daily for 4-6 weeks or until remission occurs; followed by 2.5 mg/kg IV every 14 days or 30 mg/m² as maintenance therapy

Cutaneous T-Cell Lymphoma (Mycosis Fungoides)

- Adults, in early stages, oral dose: 5-50 mg orally once weekly. Dose adjustment on the basis of patient response and toxicity. Doses of 15-37.5 mg PO twice weekly have been used.

- Adults, in early stages, IV dose: 50 mg IM/IV once weekly. Dose adjustment on the basis of patient response and toxicity. Doses of 15-37.5 mg twice weekly have been used.
- Adults, advanced disease: combination regimens including high-dose methotrexate IV with leucovorin have been used.

Gestational Trophoblastic Carcinomas (Choriocarcinoma, Chorioadenoma Destruens, and Hydatidiform Mole)

- Adults, oral or IM dose: 15-30 mg orally or IM once daily for 5 days. Repeat after 1 or more weeks, depending on the response or toxicity.

SIDE EFFECTS

- Fever
- Fatigue
- Diarrhea
- Vomiting
- Dizziness
- Stomatitis
- Drowsiness
- Renal failure
- Hepatotoxicity
- Mental status changes
- Nausea (more common with high dose)

NADIR

- 7-9 days after drug administration

STORAGE
Unreconstituted Powder

- Store between 59° and 77° F; avoid light.

Reconstituted Powder or Solution

- Store between 59° and 77° F; avoid light.

MIXING INSTRUCTIONS

- IV administration: reconstitute immediately before use with appropriate sterile, preservative-free medium such as 5% dextrose or sodium chloride injection. Reconstitute 20-mg vial to concentration no greater than 25 mg/mL. The 1-g vial should be

reconstituted with 19.4 mL to concentration of 50 mg/mL. When high-dose methotrexate is administered, total dose is diluted in 5% dextrose solution.
- Intrathecal administration: reconstitute with preservative-free medium such as 0.9% sodium chloride injection. Concentration should be 1 mg/mL.

COMPATIBILITY WITH OTHER DRUGS/INTRAVENOUS FLUIDS

- Sodium bicarbonate
- D5W
- 0.9% Sodium chloride

DRUG INTERACTIONS

- Nonsteroidal anti-inflammatory drugs can decrease the clearance of methotrexate.
- Salicylates can impair the renal secretion of methotrexate.
- Sulfamethoxazole-trimethoprim (SMX-TMP) can increase bone marrow suppression.
- Penicillins may reduce the renal clearance of methotrexate.
- Phenytoin can cause methotrexate-induced toxicity.
- Oral antibiotics such as tetracyclines, chloramphenicol, and nonabsorbable broad-spectrum antibiotics can suppress metabolism.
- Vitamin C (ascorbic acid) acidifies the urine and may increase methotrexate toxicity.

PREGNANCY

Category X

SPECIAL CONSIDERATIONS

- Guidelines for parenteral administration of intermediate- or high-dose methotrexate:
  - Hydrate with 1 L/m² of IV fluids before therapy.
  - Hydration continues at 125 mL/hr during the methotrexate infusion and for 2 days after the infusion is complete.
  - Urine should be alkalinized using sodium bicarbonate to maintain urine pH >7; oral or IV

sodium bicarbonate can be administered.

- ○ Serum creatinine and methotrexate serum levels should be done 24 hours after starting methotrexate and at least daily until the methotrexate level is below 0.05 micromolar.
- "MTX" is an error-prone abbreviation and should be written out as "methotrexate".
- Methotrexate distributes into the third space fluids such as ascites, pleural effusions, edema; results in a long terminal half-life requiring longer leucovorin rescue.

PATIENT EDUCATION

- Avoid alcohol while on methotrexate treatment.
- If taken orally, take 1 hour before or 2 hours after meals to increase absorption.
- Patients should be instructed to notify the prescriber immediately if they have yellowing eyes or skin, decrease in the amount of urine, darker urine, chest pain, mental status or mood changes, or black stools.

BIBLIOGRAPHY

Clinical Pharmacology. (2006). *Methotrexate*. Retrieved May 25, 2006, from http://cpip.gsm.com (subscription required).

Drug facts and comparisons 2004 (58th ed.). St. Louis: JB Lippincott.

Medicine Net. (2001). *Methotrexate*. Retrieved May 25, 2006, from http://www.medicinenet.com/methotrexate/article.htm.

Rx List. (2006). *Methotrexate—oral*. Retrieved May, 25, 2006, from http://www.rxlist.com/drugs/drug-20913-Trexall+Oral.aspx?drugid=20913&drugname=Trexall+Oral.

Springhouse. (2001). *2001 Physician's drug handbook* (9th ed., pp. 664-666). Springhouse, PA: Springhouse Publishing.

Wilkes, G., & Barton-Burke, M. (2005). *2005 Oncology nursing drug handbook* (pp. 216-220). Sudbury, MA: Jones & Bartlett.

Mitomycin (Mutamycin)

Barbara Holmes Gobel and Deborah Mast

DRUG CLASS

- Antitumor antibiotic

ROUTE OF ADMINISTRATION

- Intravenous (IV)

Off-Label

- Intravesical
- Intra-arterial

HOW TO ADMINISTER

- Administer in a large vein over 5 to 10 minutes.
- Monitor for signs of extravasation because mitomycin is a vesicant.
- Administer through side arm of a running IV to avoid extravasation.

PRETREATMENT GUIDELINES

- White blood cell count >4,000/mm^3
- Platelet count >100,000/mm^3
- Serum creatinine <1.7 mg/dL

USE

- Gastric cancer
- Pancreatic caner

Off-Label Uses

- Lung cancer
- Breast cancer
- Mesothelioma
- Bladder cancer
- Cervical cancer
- Desmoid tumor
- Colorectal cancer
- Bone marrow ablation
- Head and neck cancer
- Hepatocellular cancer
- Stem cell transplant preparation

PHARMOCOKINETICS

- Initial half-life is 2-10 minutes.
- Elimination half-life is 25-90 minutes.
- Metabolism occurs primarily in the liver.
- 1%-20% of a dose is recovered in the urine.

USUAL DOSE AND SCHEDULE
Gastric Cancer

- Adults, IV dose: 5-20 mg/m^2 IV every 6-8 weeks in combination with other chemotherapeutic agents

Pancreatic Cancer

- Adults, IV dose: 5-20 mg/m^2 IV every 6-8 weeks in combination with other chemotherapeutic agents

SIDE EFFECTS
Vesicant

- Alopecia
- Mucositis
- Pulmonary toxicity (rare)
- Hemolytic uremic syndrome (rare)
- Cumulative bone marrow suppression
- Congestive heart failure

NADIR

- 4-6 weeks after drug administration

STORAGE
Unreconstituted Powder

- Store at room temperature between 59° and 86° F (15° and 30° C).

Reconstituted Powder

- Solution is stable for 1 week at room temperature or 14 days under refrigeration.

MIXING INSTRUCTIONS

- Reconstitute mitomycin with sterile water for injection to give an IV solution containing 0.5 mg/mL mitomycin.
- Shake vial to dissolve the powder.
- If powder does not dissolve immediately, let stand at room temperature until completely dissolved.

COMPATIBILITY WITH OTHER DRUGS/INTRAVENOUS FLUIDS

- Fluorouracil
- Methotrexate
- Doxorubicin
- Ondansetron
- 0.9% Sodium chloride

Cancer Management

DRUG INTERACTIONS

- Vinca alkaloids can cause shortness of breath and bronchospasm after administration in patients who have had previous or simultaneous doses of mitomycin.
- Vinca alkaloids or doxorubicin may enhance cardiac toxicity when co-administered with mitomycin.
- Anticoagulants, nonsteroidal anti-inflammatory drugs (NSAIDs), platelet inhibitors, and antithrombocytic agents may increase risk of bleeding.

PREGNANCY

Category D

SPECIAL CONSIDERATIONS

- Vesicant
- Concurrent use with other immune suppressive medication can increase bone marrow suppression.
- Bone marrow toxicity is delayed and cumulative.

PATIENT EDUCATION

- Notify prescriber of signs and symptoms of infection.
- Notify prescriber of signs and symptoms of bleeding.
- Notify prescriber of pain at infusion site post infusion.
- Notify prescriber of nonproductive cough, coughing up blood, or shortness of breath.

BIBLIOGRAPHY

Clinical Pharmacology. (2006). *Mitomycin.* Retrieved May 25, 2006, from http://cpip. gsm.com/ (subscription required).

Medicine Net. (2005). *Mitomycin.* Retrieved May 25, 2006, from http://www.medic inenet.com/mitomycininjection/article. htm.

Rx List. (2006). *Mutamycin.* Retrieved May, 25, 2006, from http://www.rxlist. com/cgi/generic3/mitomycin_wcp.htm.

Wilkes, G., & Barton-Burke, M. (2005). *2005 Oncology nursing drug handbook* (pp. 223-226). Sudbury, MA: Jones & Bartlett.

Mitotane (Lysodren)

Barbara Holmes Gobel and Deborah Mast

DRUG CLASS

- Hormones and hormone modifiers

ROUTE OF ADMINISTRATION

- Oral: available dosage form— 500 mg tablet

HOW TO ADMINISTER

- Swallow the tablet with a drink of water.
- Daily dose is divided into three or four doses.

PRETREATMENT GUIDELINES

- Liver function tests
- No evidence of active infection

USE

- Adrenocortical cancer, functional and nonfunctional

PHARMACOKINETICS

- Approximately 30%-40% of an oral dose is absorbed across the gastrointestinal (GI) tract after administration.
- Drug distributes widely throughout the body tissues, accumulating primarily in adipose tissue. Half-life is 18-159 days.
- Plasma concentrations can be detected 10 weeks after administration, and fatty tissue concentrations persist for up to 20 months.

USUAL DOSE AND SCHEDULE
Adrenocortical Cancer, Functional and Nonfunctional

- Adults: initially, 1-6 g/day orally (low dose), given in three to four divided doses, then increased to 8-10 g/day orally (usual dose) as tolerated

SIDE EFFECTS

- Adrenocortical insufficiency
- Nausea
- Vomiting
- Diarrhea
- CNS depression
- Vertigo
- Lethargy
- Dizziness
- Confusion
- Hemorrhagic cystitis (rare)

STORAGE

- Store at room temperature between 59° and 86° F (15°-30° C) away from light and moisture

DRUG INTERACTIONS

- Mitotane decreases the effects of phenytoin, warfarin and phenobarbital.
- Mitotane should be used cautiously with other drugs that may cause central nervous system (CNS) depression including alcohol, opiate agonists, tricyclic antidepressants, phenothiazines, anxiolytics, sedatives and hypnotics, and sedating histamine 1 blockers.
- Spironolactone decreases the pharmacological effect of mitotane.
- Vaccines may have increased adverse effects.

PREGNANCY

Category C

SPECIAL CONSIDERATIONS

- Supplemental glucocorticoid and mineralocorticoid therapy may be necessary because mitotane inhibits normal steroid synthesis.
- Nausea and vomiting can be dose-limiting toxicities.
- Neurological assessments should be performed on patients who take mitotane for more than 2 years; prolonged therapy can cause severe neurological problems, including brain damage and functional impairment.

PATIENT EDUCATION

- Administration of antidiarrheal medicine may be necessary.
- If diarrhea occurs, ensure adequate hydration with fluids.

- Lethargy may occur; avoid activities that require mental alertness.
- Report nausea, vomiting, and diarrhea to prescriber because dose adjustment may be necessary.
- Report all neurological symptoms to prescriber.

BILIOGRAPHY

Clinical Pharmacology. (2006). *Mitotane*. Retrieved May 25, 2006, from http://cpip.gsm.com (subscription required).
Medicine Net. (2005). *Mitotane—oral*. Retrieved May 30, 2006, from http://www.medicinenet.com/mitotaneoral/article.htm.
Wilkes, G., & Barton-Burke, M. (2005). *2005 Oncology nursing drug handbook* (pp. 226-227). Sudbury, MA: Jones & Bartlett.

Mitoxantrone (Novantrone)

Barbara Holmes Gobel and Deborah Mast

DRUG CLASS

- Anthracenediones

ROUTE OF ADMINISTRATION

- Intravenous (IV)

Off-Label

- Intrapleural
- Intra-arterial
- Intraperitoneal

HOW TO ADMINISTER

- IV push over at least 3 minutes into a free-flowing infusion of compatible solution
- IV bolus over 5-30 minutes

PRETREATMENT GUIDELINES

- Liver function tests; dose reduction may be needed.
  ○ Total bilirubin between 1.5-3 mg/dL, administer 50% of the normal dose
- Total bilirubin >3 mg/dL, administer 25% of the normal dose

- Complete blood cell count (CBC) with differential and platelets and chemistry profile
- Baseline left ventricular ejection fraction. Hold for <50%.

USE

- Prostate cancer (treatment of severe pain)
- Acute myelogenous leukemia

Off-Label Uses

- Breast cancer
- Ovarian cancer
- Pleural effusion
- Bone marrow ablation
- Hepatocellular cancer
- Non-Hodgkin lymphoma
- Acute lymphocytic leukemia
- Chronic myelogenous leukemia
- Stem cell transplant preparation
- Multiple sclerosis

PHARMACOKINETICS

- Initial alpha half-life is 2-15 minutes.
- Initial beta half-life is 17 minutes to 3 hours.
- Terminal half-life is 23-215 hours; median is 75 hours.

USUAL DOSE AND SCHEDULE
Prostate Cancer

- Adults, for the treatment of severe pain related to advanced hormone-refractory prostate cancer in combination with corticosteroids: 12-14 mg/m^2 every 21 days in combination with corticosteroids

Acute Myelogenous Leukemia

- Adults, for induction therapy: 12 mg/m^2/day on days 1-3 in combination with cytarabine
- Adults, second induction course for incomplete response: 12 mg/m^2/day for 2 days in combination with cytarabine
- Adults, consolidation therapy: 12 mg/m^2/day for 2 days in combination with cytarabine for 5 days

SIDE EFFECTS
Vesicant Potential

- Nausea

- Alopecia
- Diarrhea
- Vomiting
- Chest pain
- Conjunctivitis
- Tumor lysis syndrome
- Bluish-colored sclera and urine
- Mucositis, stomatitis, esophagitis
- Myelosuppression (can be dose-limiting toxicity)
- Congestive heart failure from decreased left ventricular ejection fraction (LVEF)

NADIR

- 9-10 days after drug administration, recovery 21 days

STORAGE
Unreconstituted Powder

- Store unopened vials between 59°-77° F (15°-25° C).

Reconstituted Powder or Solution

- Once vial stopper is penetrated, the undiluted concentrate may be stored at 59°-77° F (15°-25° C) for 7 days or under refrigeration for 14 days; do not freeze.

MIXING INSTRUCTIONS

- Dilute to at least 50 mL with normal saline solution (NS) or 5% dextrose in water (D5W).
- Product is a dark blue solution.

COMPATIBILITY WITH OTHER DRUGS/INTRAVENOUS FLUIDS

- Ondansetron
- D5W
- Sodium chloride 0.9%

DRUG INTERACTIONS

- Ciprofloxacin: oral absorption is decreased.
- Anticoagulants, nonsteroidal anti-inflammatory drugs (NSAIDs), and platelet inhibitors can add to the risk of bleeding.
- Trastuzumab: concurrent use can increase incidence of ventricular dysfunction.

PREGNANCY

Category D

SPECIAL CONSIDERATIONS

- Cardiotoxicity risk increased with cumulative doses of >160 mg/m²; in patients with previous anthracycline treatment and radiation to chest in cardiac area, risk increases at lower cumulative doses of mitoxantrone.
- Patients with baseline LVEF <50% should not receive mitoxantrone unless benefit of treatment outweighs risk.

PATIENT EDUCATION

- Mitoxantrone is a dark blue solution; urine, fingernails, and sclera may turn a blue-green color.
- Report signs of infection to prescriber.
- Report signs of bleeding to prescriber.
- Instruct patient to report swollen feet or ankles, shortness of breath, chest pain, or wheezing to prescriber.

BIBLIOGRAPHY

Clinical Pharmacology. (2006). *Mitoxantrone*. Retrieved May 25, 2006, from http://cpip.gsm.com/ (subscription required).

Medicine Net. (2005). *Mitoxantrone—injection*. Retrieved May 25, 2006, from http://www.medicinenet.com/ mitoxantrone-injection/article.htm.

U.S. Food and Drug Administration. (2002). *Mitoxantrone*. Retrieved May 30, 2006, from www.accessdata.fda.gov/ scripts/cder/onctools/labels.cfm?GN= mitoxantrone.

Wilkes, G., & Barton-Burke, M. (2005). *2005 Oncology nursing drug handbook* (pp. 227-230). Sudbury, MA: Jones & Bartlett.

Oxiliplatin (Eloxatin)

Barbara Holmes Gobel and Deborah Mast

DRUG CLASS

- Alkylating agent

ROUTE OF ADMINISTRATION

- Intravenous (IV)

HOW TO ADMINISTER

- Administer IV over 2 hours.
- Avoid extravasation; tissue irritation and necrosis have been reported.

PRETREATMENT GUIDELINES

- Renal function; consider holding dose for creatinine clearance <20 mL/min
- Neurological function (toxicity from previous dose may warrant dose reduction or increasing infusion time from 2 to 6 hours)
- Gastrointestinal function (toxicity from previous dose may warrant dose reduction)
- Complete blood cell count (CBC) (hematological toxicity from previous dose may warrant dose reduction)
- Absolute neutrophil count >1,500/mm²
- Platelet count >75,000/mm²

USE

- Colorectal cancer

Off-Label Uses

- Breast cancer
- Mesothelioma
- Ovarian cancer
- Testicular cancer
- Pancreatic cancer
- Head and neck cancer
- Non-Hodgkin lymphoma

PHARMOCOKINETICS

- Rapid and extensive biotransformation to active and inactive metabolites in the plasma
- Terminal half-life is 391 hours.

USUAL DOSE AND SCHEDULE
Colorectal Cancer

- Adults (FOLFOX4):
  - Day 1: Give oxiliplatin 85 mg/m² IV infusion in combination with leucovorin 200 mg/m² IV infusion, both given over 2 hours at same time in separate bags with use of a Y-line, followed by 5-fluorouracil (5-FU) 400 mg/m² IV bolus over 2-4 minutes, followed by 5-FU 600 mg/m² IV infusion over 22 hours.
  - Day 2: Give leucovorin 200 mg/m² IV over 2 hours followed by 5-FU 400 mg/m² IV bolus over 2-4 minutes, followed by 5-FU 600 mg/m² IV infusion over 22 hours.

SIDE EFFECTS
Vesicant Potential
Neurotoxicity—Acute and Chronic

- Cold-induced dysesthesias
- Pharyngolaryngeal dysesthesia—cold-induced
- Nausea
- Fatigue
- Alopecia
- Diarrhea
- Bleeding
- Vomiting
- Stomatitis
- Hematuria
- Constipation
- Hypersensitivity reactions with first dose
- Cumulative hypersensitivity after 10-12 cycles (anaphylaxis and severe hypersensitivity)

STORAGE
Unreconstituted Powder

- Store unopened vials of the concentrated solution at 59°-86° F (15°-30° C).
- Do not freeze.
- Protect from light.

Reconstituted Powder or Solution

- Shelf life is 6 hours at room temperature, 68°-77° F (20°-25° C).

- May be stored up to 24 hours under refrigeration, 36°-46° F (2°-8° C)

MIXING INSTRUCTIONS
Reconstitution and Dilution of Lyophilized Powder

- Reconstitute with sterile water for injection, USP, or 5% dextrose in water (D5W).NEVER mix with sodium chloride or chloride-containing solutions.
- Lyophilized powder is first reconstituted by adding 10 mL (for the 50-mg vial) or 20 mL (for the 100-mg vial) of sterile water for injection, USP, or D5W.
- Dilute the reconstituted solution in 250-500 mL of 5% dextrose injection, USP before administration.

Dilution of the Aqueous Solution

- The concentration of aqueous solution is 5 mg/mL.
- The aqueous solution MUST be diluted with additional 250-500 mL of 5% dextrose injection, USP.

Product Stability

- Must be used within 6 hours if left at room temperature, 68°-77° F (20°-25° C).
- May be stored up to 24 hours under refrigeration, 36°-46° F (2°-8° C)

COMPATIBILITY WITH OTHER DRUGS/INTRAVENOUS FLUIDS

- Incompatible with normal saline solution
- Leucovorin, compatible at Y-site
- D5W

DRUG INTERACTIONS

- Concomitant use with anticoagulants, nonsteroidal anti-inflammatory drugs (NSAIDs), platelet inhibitors, and salicylates may increase the risk of bleeding.
- Caution with other nephrotoxic drugs which could increase oxiliplatin nephrotoxicity

PREGNANCY
Category D

- May cause fetal harm when administered to a pregnant woman
- It is not known whether oxiliplatin is excreted in breast milk; breast-feeding should be discontinued or treatment delayed.

SPECIAL CONSIDERATIONS

- If nausea, vomiting, or other acute symptoms occur, infusing oxiliplatin over a period of up to 6 hours may reduce peak serum levels and lessen toxicities.
- Should not be used in patients allergic to platinum compounds, such as carboplatin or cisplatin
- Dose reductions may be needed for patients with peripheral neuropathy, gastrointestinal toxicity, or hematological toxicities.
- Premedication with antiemetics should occur.

PATIENT EDUCATION

- Cold-induced dysesthesias and pharyngolaryngeal dysesthesia can be greatly reduced by avoiding cold objects, cold drinks and foods, and breathing cold air for 3 to 7 days after administration.
- Instruct patient to report signs of infection to prescriber.
- Instruct patient to report diarrhea to prescriber.
- Cumulative peripheral neuropathy

BIBLIOGRAPHY

Clinical Pharmacology. (2006). *Oxiliplatin*. Retrieved May 30, 2006, from http://cpip.gsm.com (subscription required).

Medicine Net. (2005). *Oxiliplatin—injection*. Retrieved May 30, 2006, from http://www.medicinenet.com/oxaliplatin-injection/article.htm.

Polovich, M., White, J. M., & Kelleher, L. O. (2005). *Chemotherapy and biotherapy guidelines and recommendations for practice* (2nd ed., pp. 22, 169.). Pittsburgh, PA: Oncology Nursing Service.

UpToDate Online. (2006). *Oxiliplatin*. Retrieved June 15, 2006, from http://www.uptodateonline.com/utd/content/topic.do?topicKey=drug_l_z/58721&type=A&selectedTitle=2~21 (subscription required).

U.S. Food and Drug Administration. (1999). *Oxiliplatin*. Retrieved May 30, 2006, from http://www.accessdata.fda.gov/scripts/cder/onctools/labels.cfm?GN=oxaliplatin.

Wilkes, G., & Barton-Burke, M. (2005). *2005 Oncology nursing drug handbook* (pp. 234-238). Sudbury, MA: Jones & Bartlett.

Paclitaxel (Taxol)

Linda U. Krebs

DRUG CLASS

- Plant alkaloid, taxane, mitotic inhibitor

ROUTE OF ADMINISTRATION

- Intravenous (IV) route by intermittent or continuous infusion

HOW TO ADMINISTER

- IV infusion over 3-24 hours depending on cancer type
- Use in-line filtration (0.22-micron filter) during administration.

PRETREATMENT GUIDELINES

- Premedicate with dexamethasone, diphenhydramine (or equivalent), and histamine 2 (H_2) antagonists to prevent severe hypersensitivity reactions (severe hypersensitivity reactions occur in approximately 2%-4% of patients).
- Monitor complete blood cell count (CBC), liver and renal function, intake and output (I&O), and vital signs (VS).

USE

- Advanced ovarian cancer
- Non–small cell lung cancer
- Breast cancer
- Acquired immunodeficiency syndrome (AIDS)–related Kaposi's syndrome (KS)

PHARMACOKINETICS

- Metabolized by liver, eliminated by bile
- Small amounts secreted unchanged in the urine

Cancer Management

- Biphasic half-life: initial very rapid, followed by slower decline in plasma levels
- Not removed by hemodialysis

USUAL DOSE AND SCHEDULE
Single Agent

- 100-175 mg/m² IV over 3 hours every 3 weeks
- 80 mg/m² IV over 1 hour weekly

Combination Therapy

- Doses as noted under single agent followed by cisplatin or carboplatin

Continuous Infusion

- 135-175 mg/m² over 24 hours every 3 weeks

Other

- Lower dose; weekly dosage regimens are common with 80 mg/m²

SIDE EFFECTS

- Alopecia
- Anemia
- Neutropenia
- Leukopenia
- Thrombocytopenia
- Infections
- Bleeding
- Peripheral neuropathy (especially in the elderly)
- Myalgia/arthralgia
- Nausea/vomiting
- Diarrhea
- Mucositis
- Asthenia
- Onycholysis
- Bradycardia—particularly during administration
- Hypotension—particularly during administration
- Hypertension (HTN)—particularly during administration
- Severe conduction abnormalities
- Injection site reactions: irritant, potential vesicant

NADIR

- Neutrophils: 11days; platelets: 8-9 days

STORAGE
Unreconstituted Powder

- Refrigerate unopened vials.

Reconstituted Powder or Solution

- Stable for 27 hours; store at 25° C (77° F); protect from light.

MIXING INSTRUCTIONS

- Mix with 0.9% sodium chloride (NaCl) injection, 5% dextrose injection, 5% dextrose/0.9% NaCL, or 5% dextrose in Ringer's injection to final concentration of 0.3-1.2 mg/mL.
- Use non–di(2-ethylhexyl) phthalate (DEHP) plasticized solution containers and administration sets.

Product Stability

- Stable for 27 hours; store at 25° C (77° F); protect from light.

COMPATIBILITY WITH OTHER DRUGS/INTRAVENOUS FLUIDS

- Compatible with 0.9% NaCl injection, 5% dextrose injection, 5% dextrose/0.9% NaCl, or 5% dextrose in Ringer's injection
- Incompatible with amphotericin B, hydroxyzine, liposomal doxorubicin, methylprednisolone, mitoxantrone

DRUG INTERACTIONS

- Increases doxorubicin levels
- Caution with CYP450, 2C8, and 3A4 substrates or inhibitors
- More profound myelosuppression when given following cisplatin
- Paclitaxel metabolism is inhibited if given with cyclosporine, diazepam, doxorubicin, felodipine, ketoconazole, midazolam, retinoic acid, or troleandomycin.
- Paclitaxel metabolism is increased if given with: carbamazepine or phenobarbital.
- May increase live virus vaccine side effects and decrease body's vaccine antibody response

PREGNANCY
Category D

- Do not use if pregnant or while nursing.

SPECIAL CONSIDERATIONS

- Anaphylaxis and severe hypersensitivity reactions occur in 2%-4%. Premedicate with H₂ antagonist, corticosteroids, and diphenhydramine (or equivalent). If reaction occurs, stop infusion and administer supportive care. Infusion may be resumed at a decreased infusion rate once reaction has subsided.

Dose Modifications

- Modify dose for hepatic impairment, myelosuppression, and significant neuropathies.
- Toxicity enhanced with elevated liver enzymes
- Contains dehydrated alcohol

Contraindications

- Do not administer to those with hypersensitivity or drugs developed with Cremophor EL (polyoxyethylated castor oil).

PATIENT EDUCATION

- Instruct patient to immediately report any wheezing, shortness of breath, difficulty breathing, chest pain, or other signs/symptoms of anaphylaxis or hypersensitivity reaction.
- Instruct patient to report any signs of bleeding, bruising, infection, fever, shortness of breath, fatigue, or numbness or tingling in fingers and toes.
- Advise patient about possibility of joint pain for 2-3 days after initiation of therapy, which usually resolves within several days.
- Instruct patient to avoid receiving vaccinations and to refrain from being in crowds or around those with known infections.
- Instruct patient to avoid pregnancy and to use effective contraceptive measures.

BIBLIOGRAPHY

Elsevier. (2006). *The Elsevier guide to oncology drugs and regimens* (pp. 285-288). Huntington, NY: Elsevier Oncology.

Hodgson, B. B., & Kizior, R. J. (2006). *Mosby's 2006 drug consult for nurses* (pp. 338-341). St. Louis: Mosby.

Hughes, T. E. (2005). Paclitaxel (Taxol). In J. Abraham, C. J. Allegra, & J. Gulley (Eds.). *Bethesda handbook of clinical oncology* (2nd ed., pp. 650-651). Philadelphia: Lippincott Williams & Wilkins.

Kelleher, L. O. (2005). Principles of chemotherapy. In M. Polovich, J.M. White, & L.O. Kelleher (Eds.). *Chemotherapy and biotherapy guidelines and recommendations for practice* (2nd ed.) (pp. 18-35). Pittsburgh, PA: Oncology Nursing Society.

MedlinePlus. (2003). *Paclitaxel*. Retrieved on January 21, 2007, from http://www.nlm.nih.gov/medlineplus/druginfo/uspdi/202682.html.

PDR oncology pocket guide (2nd ed., pp. 68-69). (2005). Montvale, NJ: Thompson PDR.

RxList. (2005). *Taxol*. Retrieved on January 21, 2007, from http://www.rxlist.com/cgi/generic/paclitaxel.htm.

Spratto, G. R., & Woods, A. L. (2005). *2005 PDR nurses drug handbook* (pp. 918-921). Clifton Park, NY: Thomson Delmar Learning.

Wilkes, G. M., & Barton-Burke, M. (2006). *2006 Oncology nursing drug handbook* (pp. 243-250). Sudbury, MA: Jones & Bartlett.

Paclitaxel Protein-Bound Particles (Abraxane)

Linda U. Krebs

DRUG CLASS

- Taxane, plant alkaloid, antimicrotubule agent

ROUTE OF ADMINISTRATION

- Intravenous (IV) route by infusion

HOW TO ADMINISTER

- IV infusion over 30 minutes

PRETREATMENT GUIDELINES

- Premedication to prevent hypersensitivity reactions is not required.
- Monitor complete blood cell count (CBC) and liver and renal function.
- Do not administer if baseline neutrophils count is <1,500 cells/mm^3.

USE

- Metastatic and recurrent breast cancer (relapse within 6 months of adjuvant therapy)

PHARMACOKINETICS

- Small amounts secreted unchanged in the urine; approximately 20% excreted in feces
- Metabolized by the liver
- Biphasic half-life: initial very rapid, followed by slower decline in plasma levels
- Terminal half-life approximately 27 hours

USUAL DOSE AND SCHEDULE
Single Agent

- 260 mg/m^2 IV over 30 minutes every 3 weeks

SIDE EFFECTS

- Alopecia
- Anemia
- Neutropenia
- Leukopenia
- Thrombocytopenia
- Infections
- Bleeding
- Fatigue
- Peripheral neuropathy (especially in the elderly)
- Myalgias/arthralgias
- Asthenia
- Nausea/vomiting
- Diarrhea
- Mucositis
- Visual disturbances (keratitis, blurred vision at higher than recommended doses)
- Cough/dyspnea
- Pneumonia
- Lower extremity edema
- Injection site reactions
- Hypersensitivity reactions—day of administration
- Bradycardia—during administration
- Hypotension—during administration
- Severe conduction abnormalities
- Severe cardiovascular events

NADIR

- Neutropenia, which occurs frequently, is dose dependent and dose limiting.

STORAGE
Unreconstituted Powder

- Store in original carton and protected from light at 20° to 25° C (68° to 77° F) until stamped package date.

Reconstituted Powder or Solution

- May be stored for up to 8 hours at 2° to 8° C (36° to 46° F) (preferable to use immediately after reconstitution)

MIXING INSTRUCTIONS

- Mix with 20 mL of 0.9% sodium chloride injection, slowly injecting fluid onto the sidewall of the vial (injecting fluid onto lyophilized cake will cause foaming). Let sit 5 minutes and then gently swirl or invert vial over 2 minutes to ensure that cake has dissolved.
- Prevent foaming (if foaming or clumping occurs, allow vial to stand for 15 minutes until foam subsides).
- Reconstituted fluid will be milky but without particles.
- Do not filter.

Product Stability

- Should be used immediately but may be stored for up to 8 hours at 2° to 8° C (36° to 46° F)

COMPATIBILITY WITH OTHER DRUGS/INTRAVENOUS FLUIDS

- Compatible with 0.9% sodium chloride injection

DRUG INTERACTIONS

- Caution with CYP450, 2C8, and 3A4 substrates or inhibitors
- May increase live virus vaccine side effects and decrease body's vaccine antibody response

PREGNANCY

Category D
- Do not use if pregnant or while nursing.
- Teratogenic

SPECIAL CONSIDERATIONS

- Before treatment with paclitaxel protein-bound particles, the patient should have received prior therapy with an anthracycline, unless contraindicated.
- Do not substitute paclitaxel protein-bound particles for other formulations of paclitaxel.
- Do not administer if baseline neutrophils count is <1,500 cells/mm^3.

Dose Modifications

- Modify dose for severe neutropenia (<500/mm^3 lasting >1 week):
  - 220 mg/m^2 IV every 3 weeks
  - If neutropenia recurs, further reduce dose to 180 mg/m^2 IV every 3 weeks.
- Hold dose for grade 3 sensory neuropathy until symptoms decrease to grade 1 or 2; modify all further doses.
- Use cautiously with the elderly and in those with cardiovascular disease, elevated serum bilirubin levels, or hepatic impairment.
- Drug levels may be increased with concomitant intake of pomegranates and grapefruit.
- Serum creatinine elevation occurs in approximately 11% (does not require dose modification).

PATIENT EDUCATION

- Advise patient to immediately report any irritation/inflammation at injection site.
- Instruct patient to report any signs of bleeding, bruising, infection, fever, shortness of breath, fatigue, mouth sores, or numbness or tingling in fingers and toes. Advise patient about possibility of joint pain for 2-3 days after initiation of therapy, which usually resolves with several days.
- Advise patient to avoid intake of pomegranates and grapefruit; use herbs (e.g., licorice, valerian, echinacea) with caution.
- Instruct patient to avoid receiving vaccinations and to refrain from being in crowds or around those with known infections.
- Instruct patient to minimize sun exposure, use sun protective clothing, and use sunscreen of sun protection factor (SPF) 15 or higher.
- Instruct patient to drink at least 2-3 L of fluid/day (unless otherwise instructed).
- Instruct patient to avoid pregnancy and use effective contraceptive measures.

BIBLIOGRAPHY

AstraZeneca. (2006). *Abraxane*. Retrieved on February 3, 2007, from http://abraxane.com/professional/index.html.

Chemocare. (2005). *Paclitaxel protein-bound*. Retrieved on February 2, 2007, from http://www.chemocare.com/bio/paclitaxel_proteinbound.asp.

Elsevier. (2006). *The Elsevier guide to oncology drugs and regimens* (pp. 288-290). Huntington, NY: Elsevier Oncology.

National Cancer Institute. (2006). *Paclitaxel albumin-stabilized nanoparticle formulation*. Retrieved on February 2, 2007, from http://www.cancer.gov/cancertopics/druginfo/fda-nanoparticle-paclitaxel.

RxList. (2005). *Abraxane*. Retrieved on February 2, 2007, from http://www.rxlist.com/drugs/drug-92630-Abraxane+IV.aspx?drugid=92630&drugname=Abraxane+IV.

U.S. Food and Drug Administration. (2005). *Abraxane*. Retrieved on February 2, 2007, from http://www.fda.gov/cder/foi/label/2005/021660lbl.pdf.

Wilkes, G. M., & Barton-Burke, M. (2006). *2006 oncology nursing drug handbook* (p. 1151). Sudbury, MA: Jones & Bartlett.

Pemetrexed (Alimta)

Linda U. Krebs

DRUG CLASS

- Multitargeted antifolate (antimetabolite)

ROUTE OF ADMINISTRATION

- Intravenous (IV) route by IV piggyback

HOW TO ADMINISTER

- Administer over 10 minutes.
- Wait 30 minutes to begin cisplatin (for common combination regimen).

PRETREATMENT GUIDELINES

- Evaluate complete blood cell count (CBC), renal function.
- Premedicate with corticosteroids by using dexamethasone 4 mg twice daily given the day before, the day of, and the day after treatment to reduce risk of rash.
- Vitamin supplementation:
  - Low-dose folic acid or multivitamin with folic acid daily (350-1,000 mcg; most common dose 400 mcg); begin 1 week before starting therapy with a minimum of five daily doses before therapy; continue for 21 days after completion of therapy.
  - Vitamin B$_{12}$—1,000 mcg intramuscular (IM) injection during week before starting therapy and then every 9 weeks thereafter

USE

- Malignant pleural mesothelioma
- Non–small cell lung cancer (NSCLC)

PHARMACOKINETICS

- Not metabolized; 70%-90% remains unchanged
- Eliminated mainly through urine
- Half-life is 3.5 hours; prolonged terminal half-life is 20 hours.
- Peak plasma level in 30 minutes

USUAL DOSE AND SCHEDULE
Single Agent
- 500 to 600 mg/m^2 given on day 1 every 3 weeks

Combination Therapy
- 500 mg/m^2 on day 1 every 3 weeks with cisplatin

SIDE EFFECTS
- Anorexia
- Constipation
- Chest pain
- Depression
- Dysphagia
- Dyspnea
- Fatigue
- Fever
- Hypertension
- Infection
- Myelosuppression
- Nausea/vomiting
- Pharyngitis
- Rash/desquamation
- Stomatitis

NADIR
- Neutrophils: 8-9.6 days; recovery 4.2-7.5 days later

STORAGE
Unreconstituted Powder
- Store at room temperature.

MIXING INSTRUCTIONS
- Reconstitute vials with 20 mL of preservative-free 0.9% sodium chloride (NaCl).
- Swirl vial until powder is dissolved.
- Further dilute in 100 mL of preservative-free 0.9% NaCl.

Product Stability
- Reconstituted powder or solution: store up to 24 hours either refrigerated or at 25° C (77° F).

COMPATIBILITY WITH OTHER DRUGS/INTRAVENOUS FLUIDS
- Compatible with preservative-free 0.9% NaCl
- Incompatible with any diluents containing calcium (Ringer's solution or Ringer's lactate)

DRUG INTERACTIONS
- In mild to moderate renal insufficiency, avoid nonsteroidal anti-inflammatory drugs (NSAIDs) with short elimination half-lives 2 days before and 2 days after administration. NSAIDs with longer half-lives: stop 5 days before to 2 days after treatment.
- Delayed clearance with nephrotoxic or tubularly secreted drugs (e.g., probenecid)

PREGNANCY
Category D
- Do not use if nursing; fetotoxic and teratogenetic in mice; no studies in pregnant women

SPECIAL CONSIDERATIONS
Dose Modification
- Withhold dose if creatinine clearance (CrCl) <45 mL/min.
- If concurrently using NSAIDs, use with caution if CrCl <60 mL/min.
- Modify dose for hematological toxicity (modification based on toxicity grade).
- Discontinue for grade 3 or 4 neurotoxicity.
- Other medical conditions, including kidney disease and third space fluids, such as ascites and effusions, may affect drug elimination and enhance toxicities. It is preferable to eliminate effusions before beginning treatment.
- It is essential that vitamin B$_{12}$ and folate are administered daily throughout treatment.
- Evaluate carefully for skin rash or desquamation.

PATIENT EDUCATION
- Instruct patient to take vitamin B12 and folate as ordered.
- Instruct patient to conscientiously follow oral hygiene measures.
- Instruct patient to report any signs of bleeding, bruising, infection, fever, shortness of breath, fatigue, or numbness or tingling in fingers and toes.
- Instruct patient to avoid receiving immunizations without prior provider approval.
- Instruct patient to refrain from being in crowds or around those with known infections.
- Instruct patient to avoid pregnancy and to use effective contraceptive measures.

BIBLIOGRAPHY
Elsevier. (2006). *The Elsevier guide to oncology drugs and regimens* (pp. 294-296). Huntington, NY: Elsevier Oncology.

Hodgson, B. B., & Kizior, R. J. (2006). *Mosby's 2006 drug consult for nurses* (pp. 333-335). St. Louis: Mosby.

Hughes, T. E. (2005). Pemetrexed (Alimta). In J. Abraham, C. J. Allegra, & J. Gulley (Eds.). *Bethesda handbook of clinical oncology* (2nd ed., pp. 652-653). Philadelphia: Lippincott Williams & Wilkins.

Kelleher, L. O. (2005). Principles of chemotherapy. In M. Polovich, J. M. White, & L. O. Kelleher (Eds.). *Chemotherapy and biotherapy guidelines and recommendations for practice* (2nd ed., pp. 18-35). Pittsburgh, PA: Oncology Nursing Society.

MedlinePlus Drug Information. (2004). *Pemetrexed*. Retrieved January 21, 2007, from http://www.nlm.nih.gov/medlineplus/druginfo/uspdi/500515.html.

PDR oncology pocket guide (2nd ed., pp. 16-17). (2005). Montvale, NJ: Thompson PDR.

RxList. (2005). *Alimta*. Retrieved January 21, 2007, from http://www.rxlist.com/cgi/generic3/alimta.htm.

Wilkes, G. M., & Barton-Burke, M. (2006). *2006 oncology nursing drug handbook* (pp. 259-263). Sudbury, MA: Jones & Bartlett.

Pentostatin (Nipent)

Linda U. Krebs

DRUG CLASS
- Antimetabolite, adenosine deaminase inhibitor

ROUTE OF ADMINISTRATION
- Intravenous (IV) route

HOW TO ADMINISTER
- Administer as an IV bolus over 3-5 minutes or diluted over 20-30 minutes.

PRETREATMENT GUIDELINES

- Hydrate with 500-1000 mL of IV fluid before and after each dose.
- Monitor complete blood cell count (CBC).
- Monitor serum creatinine; consider withholding drug if creatinine clearance (CrCl) <60 mL/min. Reduce dose by 50% for creatinine clearance between 50-60 mL/min, hold if <50 mL/min.

USE

- Interferon alfa refractory hairy cell leukemia
- Cutaneous T-cell lymphoma

PHARMACOKINETICS

- Half-life is 2.6-15 hours.
- Drug is eliminated essentially unchanged in urine.

USUAL DOSE AND SCHEDULE
Single Agent

- Give 4 mg/m^2 IV every other week over 3-5 minute or over 20-30 minutes diluted in a larger volume.

SIDE EFFECTS

- Rash
- Nausea
- Vomiting
- Leukopenia
- Anemia
- Thrombocytopenia
- Fever
- Infection
- Fatigue
- Mental confusion
- Numbness or tingling in fingers and toes
- Stomatitis
- Insomnia
- Hypotension
- Allergic reaction
- Myalgias

NADIR

- May cause neutropenia and thrombocytopenia with nadir at 7 days and recovery between days 10 and 14

STORAGE
Unreconstituted Powder

- Refrigerate at 2°-8° C (35°-46° F).

Reconstituted Powder or Solution

- Store reconstituted vials, including those further diluted, at room temperature under normal light.

MIXING INSTRUCTIONS

- Mix with 5 mL of sterile water for injection to a final solution of 2 mg/mL.
- Solution can be diluted further with 25-50 mL of 5% dextrose injection or normal saline solution.
- Do not use if solution is discolored or contains particles.

Product Stability

- Reconstituted solution should be used within 8 hours.

COMPATIBILITY WITH OTHER DRUGS/INTRAVENOUS FLUIDS

- Compatible with sterile water for injection, 5% dextrose for injection, and normal saline solution

DRUG INTERACTIONS

- Fatal pulmonary toxicity has occurred when administered with fludarabine.
- Pulmonary edema and hypotension have occurred when administered with carmustine or high doses of cyclophosphamide.

PREGNANCY

Category D
- Do not use if pregnant or nursing.

SPECIAL CONSIDERATIONS

- Do not use pentostatin in combination with fludarabine.
- Withhold dose if patient has a severe rash.
- Myelosuppression may require prophylactic antibiotics.

Dose Modification

- Modify dose for myelosuppression and renal impairment.
- Use cautiously in those with renal or hepatic impairment or infection.

- Use with caution if taking allopurinol, vidarabine, or vitamins.

Response to Therapy

- Evaluate at 6 months; if no response, discontinue therapy.
- If only partial response at 12 months, discontinue therapy.

PATIENT EDUCATION

- Have patient report any bruising, bleeding, signs of infection, fever, or fatigue.
- Have patient report any shortness of breath or difficulty breathing.
- Instruct patient to avoid pregnancy and use effective contraceptive measures.

BIBLIOGRAPHY

Antimetabolite antineoplastics. (2005). In Springhouse. *Nursing rapid-fire drug facts* (pp. 38-40). Philadelphia: Lippincott Williams & Wilkins.

Chemocare. (2005). *Pentostatin*. Retrieved January 31, 2007, from http://www.chemocare.com/bio/pentostatin.asp.

Elsevier. (2006). *The Elsevier guide to oncology drugs and regimens* (pp. 297-299). Huntington, NY: Elsevier Oncology.

Hughes, T. E. (2005). Pentostatin (Nipent). In J. Abraham, C. J. Allegra, & J. Gulley (Eds.). *Bethesda handbook of clinical oncology* (2nd ed., pp. 653). Philadelphia: Lippincott Williams & Wilkins.

Kelleher, L. O. (2005). Principles of chemotherapy. In M. Polovich, J. M. White, & L. O. Kelleher (Eds.). *Chemotherapy and biotherapy guidelines and recommendations for practice* (2nd ed., pp. 18-35). Pittsburgh, PA: Oncology Nursing Society.

MedlinePlus Drug Information. (2003). *Pentostatin*. Retrieved on January 21, 2007, from http://www.nlm.nih.gov/medlineplus/druginfo/medmaster/a692004.html.

RxList. (2005). *Nipent*. Retrieved on January 21, 2007, from http://www.rxlist.com/drugs/drug-161-Nipent+IV.aspx?drugid=161&drugname=Nipent+IV.

SuperGen Inc. (1999). *Nipent, pentostatin*. San Ramon, CA: SuperGen Inc.

Procarbazine (Matulane)

Linda U. Krebs

DRUG CLASS

- Miscellaneous agent (mechanism of action unclear, probably alkylating agent)

ROUTE OF ADMINISTRATION

- Orally

HOW TO ADMINISTER

- Administer orally in single or divided doses (50-mg capsules).
- Give with food or fluids if patient has difficulty swallowing or has severe gastrointestinal side effects.

PRETREATMENT GUIDELINES

- Evaluate kidney and liver function, uric acid (monitor uric acid, aminotransferases, liver function tests [LFTs] weekly during treatment).
- Evaluate complete blood cell count (CBC) with differential, reticulocytes.

USE

- Stage III/IV Hodgkin lymphoma

PHARMACOKINETICS

- Metabolized in the liver and kidneys to cytotoxic products
- Approximately 70% eliminated through the urine as metabolites within 24 hours
- Half life: 10 minutes
- Crosses blood brain barrier and distributes into the CSF

USUAL DOSE AND SCHEDULE
Single Agent

- Adults:
  - 2-4 mg/kg orally daily for 7days; then 4-6 mg/kg orally daily until maximal response obtained
  - Maintenance dose: 1-2 mg/kg orally daily
- Children:
  - 50 mg/m^2 orally daily for 7 days and then 100 mg/m^2 until maximal response obtained

- Maintenance dose: 50 mg/m^2 orally daily

Combination Therapy

- 100 mg/m^2 orally daily for 14 days

SIDE EFFECTS

- Alopecia
- Anemia
- Anorexia
- Confusion
- Constipation
- Diarrhea
- Hyperpigmentation
- Fever
- Hallucinations
- Insomnia
- Lethargy
- Leukopenia
- Myalgia/arthralgia
- Nausea/vomiting
- Nightmares
- Paresthesias
- Pruritus
- Stomatitis
- Thrombocytopenia
- Xerostomia

NADIR

- Nadir occurs 14-21 days after initiation of therapy and recovers by day 28.

STORAGE

- Store away from heat, moisture, and direct light.

DRUG INTERACTIONS

- Avoid sympathothomimetics, tricyclic antidepressants, tyramine-containing drugs/foods, alcohol (may cause disulfiram-type [Antabuse] reaction), tobacco.
- Extreme caution with barbiturates, antihistamines, narcotics, hypotensives, phenothiazines
- Decreases plasma levels of digoxin
- Increases hypoglycemic effect of insulin and oral hypoglycemic agents
- Increases methotrexate toxicity

PREGNANCY
Category D

- Do not use while pregnant or nursing.

SPECIAL CONSIDERATIONS
Dosing

- Adult dosing based on body weight (in kilograms) (if the patient is particularly obese, use lean body weight). Pediatric dosing is based on body surface area (square meters).
- Toxicity may be seen as renal or hepatic impairment.
- Discontinue if central nervous system (CNS) symptoms occur (paresthesias, neuropathies, confusion).
- Discontinue for diarrhea, stomatitis, hemorrhage, hypersensitivity.
- Discontinue for severe myelosuppression (monitor every 3-4 days).
- Multiple drug and food interactions

PATIENT EDUCATION

- Instruct patient to avoid alcoholic beverages and tyramine-rich foods (e.g., yeasts, yogurt, caffeine, chocolate, aged cheese, liver, beer, non-alcoholic beer, wine, smoked or pickled fish).
- Instruct patient to avoid sympathomimetic drugs and tricyclic antidepressants.
- Teach patient to consume adequate fluids and prevent dehydration.
- Teach patient to avoid exposure to the sun because of the potential for photosensitivity (sun sensitivity).
- Instruct patient to report any signs of bleeding, bruising, infection, fever, shortness of breath, fatigue, rash, or prolonged constipation.
- Instruct patient to avoid pregnancy and to use effective contraceptive measures.

BIBLIOGRAPHY

Elsevier. (2006). *The Elsevier guide to oncology drugs and regimens* (pp. 305-308). Huntington, NY: Elsevier Oncology.

Hodgson, B. B., & Kizior, R. J. (2006). *Mosby's 2006 drug consult for nurses* (pp. 425-426). St. Louis: Mosby.

Cancer Management

Hughes, T. E. (2005). *Procarbazine* (Matulane). In J. Abraham, C. J. Allegra, & J. Gulley (Eds.). *Bethesda handbook of clinical oncology* (2nd ed., pp. 655). Philadelphia: Lippincott Williams & Wilkins.

Kelleher, L. O. (2005). Principles of chemotherapy. In M. Polovich, J. M. White, & L. O. Kelleher (Eds.). *Chemotherapy and biotherapy guidelines and recommendations for practice* (2nd ed., pp. 18-35). Pittsburgh, PA: Oncology Nursing Society.

MedlinePlus. (2002). *Procarbazine*. Retrieved on January 21, 2007, from http://www.nlm.nih.gov/medlineplus/druginfo/uspdi/202484.html.

PDR oncology pocket guide (2nd ed.) (pp. 48-49). (2005). Montvale, NJ: Thompson PDR.

RxList. (2005). *Procarbazine*. Retrieved on January 21, 2007, from http://www.rxlist.com/cgi/generic3/procarb.htm.

Spratto, G. R., & Woods, A. L. (2005). *2005 PDR nurses drug handbook* (pp. 1019-1121). Clifton Park, NY: Thomson Delmar Learning.

Wilkes, G. M., & Barton-Burke, M. (2006). *2006 Oncology nursing drug handbook* (pp. 268-271). Sudbury, MA: Jones & Bartlett.

Raltitrexed (Tomudex)— Investigational

Linda U. Krebs

DRUG NOT AVAILABLE IN UNITED STATES

DRUG CLASS

- Antimetabolite folate antagonist

ROUTE OF ADMINISTRATION

- Intravenous (IV) route by IV infusion

HOW TO ADMINISTER

- IV infusion over 15 minutes

PRETREATMENT GUIDELINES

- Evaluate creatinine clearance (CrCl); dose reduced for renal impairment, do not administer if CrCl <25 mL/min.
- Do not give if patient has diarrhea.

- Do not give if there is any history of hypersensitivity.
- Evaluate complete blood cell count (CBC) with differential, hepatic and renal function.
- Assess baseline weight and nutritional status.
- Evaluate presence of diarrhea, mucosal integrity.

USE

- Colorectal cancer

PHARMACOKINETICS

- Peak plasma levels during or immediately after administration
- Drug metabolized into polyglutamates
- Half-life of polyglutamates approximately 8-100 hours
- Excreted unchanged in urine and feces

USUAL DOSE AND SCHEDULE
Single Agent

- 3 mg/m^2 IV over 15 minutes every 3 weeks
- Renal dosing
  - For CrCl 55-65 mL/min, 75% of normal dose, every 4 weeks
  - For CrCl 25-54 mL/min, give % equivalent to mL/min, i.e. for CrCl of 30 mL/min, give 30% of normal dose, every 4 weeks
  - Hold dose for CrCl <25 mL/min

SIDE EFFECTS

- Allergic reactions (with first dose—rare)
- Alopecia (rare)
- Anemia
- Anorexia
- Neutropenia
- Thrombocytopenia
- Diarrhea
- Fatigue
- Fever
- Nausea/vomiting
- Pain
- Rash
- Stomatitis

NADIR

- Neutrophils: usually occurs around day 8, but may be delayed as late as day 21. Recovery usually begins on day 10.

STORAGE
Unreconstituted Powder

- Until date stamped on package; store at 2°-8° C (35°-46° F).

Reconstituted Powder or Solution

- Refrigerate; stable for 24 hours.

MIXING INSTRUCTIONS

- Mix with 4 mL of sterile water for injection; withdraw and further dilute with 50-250 mL of 0.9% normal saline solution (NS) or 5% dextrose in water (D5W).

Product Stability

- Once mixed, the solution is stable for 24 hours if refrigerated.

COMPATIBILITY WITH OTHER DRUGS/INTRAVENOUS FLUIDS

Compatible with 0.9% NS and D5W; do not mix with other drugs.

DRUG INTERACTIONS

- Folate and folic acid decrease cytotoxicity.
- Competes for renal tubular excretion with methotrexate, penicillin, and indomethacin
- May displace warfarin from serum proteins resulting in an increased INR

PREGNANCY
Category D

- Do not use if pregnant or while nursing.
- Drug is embryolethal and teratogenic.

SPECIAL CONSIDERATIONS
Dose Modifications

- Reduce dose for myelosuppression, gastrointestinal (GI) toxicities, and renal dysfunction as identified in individual protocols.
- Hold dose for uncontrolled diarrhea.
- Use carefully in those who have been heavily pretreated with prior cancer therapies.
- Use with caution in those taking highly protein-bound (warfarin)

and renally excreted (nonsteroidal anti-inflammatory drugs [NSAIDs]) drugs.

PATIENT EDUCATION

- Instruct patient to report any signs of bleeding, bruising, infection, fever, shortness of breath, fatigue, or diarrhea.
- Advise patient about possibility of experiencing joint pain for 2-3 days after initiation of therapy, which usually resolves within several days.
- Instruct patient to refrain from being in crowds or around those with known infections.
- Instruct patient to avoid pregnancy and to use effective contraceptive measures.
- Instruct patient not to take folate of any type, including folate-containing vitamins.
- Instruct to immediately report any signs/symptoms of diarrhea and to take antidiarrheals as prescribed.
- Teach appropriate oral and skin care.

BIBLIOGRAPHY

Canadian Pharmacist Association. (2006). *Compendium of pharmaceuticals and specialties 2006.* Publisher: Canadian Pharmaceutical Association.

Kelleher, L. O. (2005). Principles of chemotherapy. In M. Polovich, J. M. White, & L. O. Kelleher (Eds.). *Chemotherapy and biotherapy guidelines and recommendations for practice* (2nd ed., pp. 18-35). Pittsburgh, PA: Oncology Nursing Society.

MedlinePlus. (2000). *Raltitrexed.* Retrieved on January 21, 2007, from http://www.nlm.nih.gov/medlineplus/druginfo/uspdi/500167.html.

Norum, J., Balteskard, L., Edna, T. H., et al. (2002). Raltitrexed (Tomudex) or Nordic-FLv regimen in metastatic colorectal cancer: a randomized phase II study focusing on quality of life, patients' preferences and health economics. *Journal of Chemotherapy, 14,* 301-308.

Wilkes, G. M., & Barton-Burke, M. (2006). *2006 Oncology nursing drug handbook* (pp. 275-278). Sudbury, MA: Jones & Bartlett.

Streptozocin (Zanosar)

Linda U. Krebs

DRUG CLASS

- Alkylating agent (nitrosourea)

ROUTE OF ADMINISTRATION

- Intravenous (IV) route

HOW TO ADMINISTER

- Administer over 1-2 hours (too-rapid infusion increases risk of renal toxicity)

PRETREATMENT GUIDELINES

- Use with caution in renal impairment.
- Premedicate with antiemetics.
- Monitor complete blood cell count (CBC), liver function tests (LFTs), renal function, uric acid, and glucose before treatment and weekly throughout therapy.

USE

- Metastatic islet cell carcinoma of the pancreas

PHARMACOKINETICS

- Unchanged drug and metabolites excreted in the urine

Initial Half-Life

- Unchanged drug: 35 minutes
- Metabolites: up to 40 hours

USUAL DOSE AND SCHEDULE
Single Agent

- 500 mg/m^2 IV daily for 5 days every 6 weeks
- 1 g/m^2 IV weekly for two doses then may escalate to achieve a response if no significant toxicity (maximum single dose not to exceed 1,500 mg/m^2)

SIDE EFFECTS

- Diarrhea
- Elevated liver enzymes
- Hypoalbuminemia
- Glucose tolerance abnormality; rare insulin shock with hypoglycemia
- Hypophosphatemia
- Myelosuppression
- Nausea
- Vomiting
- Azotemia
- Anuria

NADIR

- Neutrophils: 10 days; recovery in 14 to 17 days

STORAGE
Unreconstituted Powder

- Store unopened vials under refrigeration and protected from light (preferably stored in carton).

Reconstituted Powder or Solution

- Stable for 12 hours; store in refrigerator (contains no preservatives; do not store longer than 12 hours).

MIXING INSTRUCTIONS

- Reconstitute with 9.5 mL of dextrose injection or 0.9% sodium chloride for injection. Solution will be pale gold and will contain 100 mg/mL streptozocin and 22 mg/mL citric acid.
- May be diluted further with either dextrose injection or 0.9% sodium chloride

PRODUCT STABILITY

Once mixed, the solution is stable no longer than 12 hours.

COMPATIBILITY WITH OTHER DRUGS/INTRAVENOUS FLUIDS

- Dextrose injection or 0.9% sodium chloride injection

DRUG INTERACTIONS

- Additive toxicity with other cytotoxic drugs
- Avoid other nephrotoxic drugs.
- May prolong doxorubicin half-life (consider reducing doxorubicin dose)
- Concomitant phenytoin decreases cytotoxic effects of streptozocin.

Cancer Management

PREGNANCY
Category D
- Do not use if pregnant or nursing; mutagenic and teratogenic.

SPECIAL CONSIDERATIONS
Irritant
- Injection site reactions common; extravasation may cause tissue lesions and necrosis.

Dose-Related Renal Toxicity
- Renal complications are dose related and cumulative; monitor renal function before and after each course of therapy.
- Obtain uric acid, blood urea nitrogen (BUN), serum creatinine, electrolytes, and creatinine clearance before and at least weekly during and for 4 weeks after therapy; may need to reduce dose.
- Mild proteinuria is usually an early sign of impending renal dysfunction.
- Adequate hydration is essential (usually 2 to 3 L/day)
- Do not treat with other nephrotoxic drugs.

Elderly
- Use with caution; may impair mental and physical functioning.

Measurement of Therapeutic Response
- Functional tumors: a biochemical response can be determined by serial monitoring of fasting insulin levels.
- Functional and nonfunctional tumors: evaluate for measurable reductions in tumor size.

PATIENT EDUCATION
- Instruct patient to consume 2 to 3 L of fluid/day.
- Teach patient to watch for signs and symptoms of kidney dysfunction (decreased urine output, changes in urine color).
- Instruct patient to report any signs of bleeding, bruising, infection, fever, shortness of breath, or fatigue.
- Instruct patient to refrain from being in crowds or around those with known infections.
- Instruct patient to avoid pregnancy and use effective contraceptive measures.

BIBLIOGRAPHY
Elsevier. (2006). *The Elsevier guide to oncology drugs and regimens* (pp. 322-324). Huntington, NY: Elsevier Oncology.

Hughes, T. E. (2005). Streptozotocin (Zanosar). In J. Abraham, C. J. Allegra, & J. Gulley (Eds.). *Bethesda handbook of clinical oncology* (2nd ed., pp. 656-657). Philadelphia: Lippincott Williams & Wilkins.

Kelleher, L. O. (2005). Principles of chemotherapy. In M. Polovich, J. M. White, & L. O. Kelleher (Eds.). *Chemotherapy and biotherapy guidelines and recommendations for practice* (2nd ed., pp. 18-35). Pittsburgh, PA: Oncology Nursing Society.

MedlinePlus. (2003). *Streptozocin*. Retrieved on January 21, 2007, from http://www.nlm.nih.gov/medlineplus/druginfo/medmaster/a684053.html.

PDR oncology pocket guide (2nd ed., p. 81). (2005). Montvale, NJ: Thompson PDR.

RxList. (2005). *Zanosar*. Retrieved on January 21, 2007, from http://www.rxlist.com/cgi/generic/zanosar.htm.

Spratto, G. R., & Woods, A. L. (2005). *2005 edition PDR nurses drug handbook* (pp. 1145-1146). Clifton Park, NY: Thomson Delmar Learning.

Wilkes, G. M., & Barton-Burke, M. (2006). *2006 Oncology nursing drug handbook* (pp. 283-288). Sudbury, MA: Jones & Bartlett.

Temozolomide (Temodar)

Linda U. Krebs

DRUG CLASS
- Alkylating agent/imidazotetrazine derivative

ROUTE OF ADMINISTRATION
- Oral

HOW TO ADMINISTER
- Administer whole capsule on an empty stomach with a glass of water.
- May be taken at bedtime
- If patient is unable to swallow, capsule may be opened and mixed with applesauce or apple juice (do not allow contents to touch skin).
- Obtain complete blood cell count (CBC) at day 22 and weekly thereafter; do not start treatment until hematological parameters are acceptable (as noted in pretreatment guidelines).

PRETREATMENT GUIDELINES
- Monitor absolute neutrophil count (ANC); must be $>1.5 \times 10^9$/L before treatment.
- Monitor platelet count, must be $>100 \times 10^9$/L before dosing.
- Dose is adjusted on the basis of the nadir of the previous cycle and immediate pretreatment platelet and granulocyte counts.
- Administer appropriate antiemetics.

USE
- Newly diagnosed glioblastoma
- Refractory anaplastic astrocytoma

PHARMACOKINETICS
- Peak plasma levels occur at 1 hour.
- Prodrug, metabolized to active form under physiologic conditions in all tissues to which the drug distributes
- Half-life: 1.8 hours
- Metabolized by hydrolysis; excreted primarily through the urine
- Crosses the blood-brain barrier

USUAL DOSE AND SCHEDULE
Single Agent (Glioblastoma)
- 75 mg/m² orally once daily for 42 days (usually given concomitantly with focal radiotherapy of 60 Gy divided into 30 fractions).
- Begin six cycles of maintenance therapy 4 weeks after end of primary treatment at 150 mg/m² orally once daily for 5 days followed by 23 days without treatment. Dose may be escalated at subsequent cycles.

Single Agent (Anaplastic Astrocytoma)

- Initial dose of 150 mg/m² orally once daily for 5 consecutive days every 28 days
- If no adverse events occur and hematological parameters are acceptable at nadir and at dosing, dose may be increased to 200 mg/m² orally daily for 5 consecutive days for 28-day treatment cycle (review package insert).

SIDE EFFECTS

- Asthenia
- Anxiety
- Constipation
- Convulsions
- Diarrhea
- Dizziness
- Drowsiness
- Fatigue
- Fever
- Headache
- Hemiparesis
- Incoordination
- Insomnia
- Myelosuppression
- Nausea/vomiting
- Peripheral edema
- Thrombocytopenia
- Urinary incontinence

NADIR

- Neutrophils: by day 28; platelets: by day 26. Recovery occurs in about 14 days.

STORAGE

- Store at 25° C (77° F).

DRUG INTERACTIONS

- Valproic acid decreases the clearance of temozolomide, clinical significance unknown.
- May increase live virus vaccine side effects and decrease body's vaccine antibody response.

PREGNANCY

Category D
- Do not use if pregnant or nursing.
- May cause fetal harm during pregnancy

SPECIAL CONSIDERATIONS

- Caution in elderly or those with renal/hepatic impairment
- Women and elderly may have increased myelosuppression.
- Contraindicated if hypersensitive to dacarbazine (DTIC)
- All foods will decrease drug absorption.
- Contents of pill (active drug) are cytotoxic; do not allow contents to come in contact with skin.

PATIENT EDUCATION

- Instruct patient to not open capsules but to swallow whole with water.
- Instruct patient to take on an empty stomach because food reduces both amount and rate of absorption; may be taken at bedtime.
- Instruct that, if unable to swallow, may open pill and mix with either apple juice or applesauce; teach not to touch contents of opened capsule (contents cytotoxic).
- Instruct patient to report any signs of bleeding, bruising, infection, fever, shortness of breath, or fatigue.
- Instruct patient to avoid driving or other hazardous activities until temozolomide's effects on vision, concentration, and alertness have been assessed.
- Instruct patient to avoid receiving vaccinations and to refrain from being in crowds or around those with known infections.
- Instruct patient to avoid pregnancy and to use effective contraceptive measures.

BIBLIOGRAPHY

Elsevier. (2006). *The Elsevier guide to oncology drugs and regimens* (pp. 329-330). Huntington, NY: Elsevier Oncology.

Hodgson, B. B., & Kizior, R. J. (2006). *Mosby's 2006 drug consult for nurses* (pp. 426-428). St. Louis: Mosby.

Hughes, T. E. (2005). Temozolomide (Temodar). In J. Abraham, C. J. Allegra, & J. Gulley (Eds.). *Bethesda handbook of clinical oncology* (2nd ed., p. 658). Philadelphia: Lippincott Williams & Wilkins.

Kelleher, L. O. (2005). Principles of chemotherapy. In M. Polovich, J. M. White, & L. O. Kelleher (Eds.). *Chemotherapy and biotherapy guidelines and recommendations for practice* (2nd ed., pp. 18-35). Pittsburgh, PA: Oncology Nursing Society.

MedlinePlus. (2005). *Temozolomide.* Retrieved on January 21, 2007, from http://www.nlm.nih.gov/medlineplus/druginfo/uspdi/500076.html.

PDR oncology pocket guide (2nd ed., pp. 70-71). (2005). Montvale, NJ: Thompson PDR.

RxList. (2006). *Temodar.* Retrieved on January 21, 2007, from http://www.rxlist.com/cgi/generic2/temoz.htm.

Spratto, G. R., & Woods, A. L. (2005). *2005 PDR nurses drug handbook* (pp. 1175-1176). Clifton Park, NY: Thomson Delmar Learning.

Wilkes, G. M., & Barton-Burke, M. (2006). *2006 Oncology nursing drug handbook* (pp. 288-292). Sudbury, MA: Jones & Bartlett.

Teniposide (Vumon, VM-26)

Linda U. Krebs

DRUG CLASS

- Plant alkaloid (derivative of the mandrake plant, epipodophyllotoxin)

ROUTE OF ADMINISTRATION

- Intravenous (IV) route by IV infusion

HOW TO ADMINISTER

- IV over 30-60 minutes; rapid infusion may result in hypotension.
- Monitor the patient for at least 60 minutes after the infusion.

PRETREATMENT GUIDELINES

- Monitor complete blood cell count (CBC) with differential, renal function, and liver function.
- Consider premedication with corticosteroids or antihistamines if plan is to retreat after a hypersensitivity reaction.

USE

- Refractory childhood acute lymphocytic leukemia (ALL)

PHARMACOKINETICS

- Half-life: 5 hours
- Significantly bound to plasma proteins
- Metabolized renally, excreted primarily through the urine

USUAL DOSE AND SCHEDULE
Combination Therapy

- 165 mg/m² IV over 30-60 minutes twice weekly for eight to nine doses
- 250 mg/m² IV over 30-60 minutes weekly for four to eight doses

SIDE EFFECTS

- Alopecia
- Anaphylaxis
- Anemia
- Diarrhea
- Hypersensitivity
- Hypotension (if infused too rapidly)
- Mucositis
- Myelosuppression
- Nausea/vomiting
- Peripheral neurotoxicity
- Rash
- Renal dysfunction
- Thrombophlebitis

NADIR

- Neutrophils: days 10-12. Recovery by day 21

STORAGE
Unreconstituted

- Store until expiration date at 2°-8° C (35°-46° F) and protect from light.

Reconstituted Powder or Solution

- Give within 4 hours to decrease possibility of precipitation; do not refrigerate.

MIXING INSTRUCTIONS

- Dilute with 5% dextrose injection or 0.9% sodium chloride injection to a concentration of 0.1 mg to 1.0 mg/mL.
- Only use non-DEHP plasticized solution containers and administration sets, lipid administration sets or low-DEHP-containing nitroglycerin sets, glass containers or polyolefin plastic bags.
- Gloves essential for reconstitution

Product Stability

- Stable for 24 hours at room temperature; precipitation may occur.

COMPATIBILITY WITH OTHER DRUGS/INTRAVENOUS FLUIDS

- Compatible with 0.9% sodium chloride injection and 5% dextrose injection

DRUG INTERACTIONS

- High doses of teniposide plus pretreatment with antiemetics may result in acute central nervous system (CNS) depression and hypotension.
- Decreased methotrexate clearance leading to increased methotrexate-related toxicities
- Increased side effects when given with sodium salicylate, sulfamethizole, or tolbutamide
- Increased peripheral neuropathy may occur when given with vincristine.
- Heparin solution can cause precipitation.
- May increase live virus vaccine side effects and decrease body's vaccine antibody response

PREGNANCY

Category D
- Do not use if pregnant or nursing.

SPECIAL CONSIDERATIONS

- Observe patient for at least 60 minutes after administration.
- Drug is cytotoxic; avoid contact with skin.
- Extravasation may result in potential tissue necrosis or thrombophlebitis.
- Anaphylaxis is possible in hypersensitivity reactions.
- Dose should be modified for patient with both leukemia and Down syndrome because increased sensitivity to the drug has been observed.
- Do not administer to those with hypersensitivity to etoposide or drugs developed with Cremophor EL (polyoxyethylated castor oil).

PATIENT EDUCATION

- Instruct patient to report any signs of bleeding, bruising, infection, fever, shortness of breath, or fatigue.
- Instruct patient to avoid receiving vaccinations and to refrain from being in crowds or around those with known infections.
- Instruct patient to take antiemetics as ordered because nausea and vomiting are common.
- Prepare patient for alopecia, inform that hair will regrow after therapy, but new hair may have a different texture or color.
- Instruct patient to avoid pregnancy and to use effective contraceptive measures.

BIBLIOGRAPHY

Elsevier. (2006). *The Elsevier guide to oncology drugs and regimens* (pp. 331-333). Huntington, NY: Elsevier Oncology.

Hodgson, B. B., & Kizior, R. J. (2006). *Mosby's 2006 drug consult for nurses* (pp. 428-430). St. Louis: Mosby.

Hughes, T. E. (2005). Teniposide (Vumon). In J. Abraham, C. J. Allegra, & J. Gulley (Eds.). *Bethesda handbook of clinical oncology* (2nd ed., p. 659). Philadelphia: Lippincott Williams & Wilkins.

Kelleher, L. O. (2005). Principles of chemotherapy. In M. Polovich, J. M. White, & L. O. Kelleher (Eds.). *Chemotherapy and biotherapy guide-lines and recommendations for practice* (2nd ed., pp. 18-35). Pittsburgh, PA: Oncology Nursing Society.

MedlinePlus. (2003). *Teniposide*. Retrieved January 21, 2007, from http://www.nlm.nih.gov/medlineplus/druginfo/medmaster/a692045.html.

RX list. (2004). *Vumon*. Retrieved January 21, 2007, from http://www.rxlist.com/cgi/generic2/teniposide.htm.

Spratto, G. R., & Woods, A. L. (2005). *2005 PDR nurses drug handbook* (pp. 1178-1179). Clifton Park, NY: Thomson Delmar Learning.

Wilkes, G. M., & Barton-Burke, M. (2006). *2006 Oncology nursing drug handbook* (pp. 292-294). Sudbury, MA: Jones & Bartlett.

Thioguanine (Tabloid, 6-Thioguanine, 6-TG)

Linda U. Krebs

DRUG CLASS

- Thiopurine antimetabolite

ROUTE OF ADMINISTRATION

- Administer by mouth

HOW TO ADMINISTER

- Orally in a single daily dose

PRETREATMENT GUIDELINES

- Consider prophylaxis for possible tumor lysis syndrome.
- Monitor uric acid; pretreat with hydration and allopurinol.
- Monitor liver function tests (LFTs) before starting therapy and then monthly.

USE

- Induction, consolidation, and maintenance therapy for acute nonlympholytic leukemias

PHARMACOKINETICS

- Half-life approximately 80 minutes
- Metabolized by the liver and excreted through the urine

USUAL DOSE AND SCHEDULE
Single Agent (Adults and Children)

- 2 mg/kg orally daily in a single dose
- If no clinical improvement at above dose by 4 weeks, can increase dose to 3 mg/kg orally as a single daily dose

Combination Therapy

- Varies with different regimens

SIDE EFFECTS

- Anorexia
- Headache
- Hepatotoxicity
- Hyperuricemia
- Myalgias/arthralgias
- Myelosuppression
- Nausea/vomiting
- Stomatitis
- Intestinal necrosis and perforation (with multiple-drug chemotherapy that includes thioguanine)
- Liver toxicity associated with vascular endothelial damage (when given over a long period; not recommended)

NADIR

- Neutrophils: between day 7 and day 28

STORAGE

- Scored tablets, store at 15°-25° C (59°-77° F) in a dry place.

DRUG INTERACTIONS

- May be cross-resistant with mercaptopurine
- Caution with TPMT (thiopurine methyltransferase) inhibitors such as aminosalicylate derivatives (e.g., olsalazine, mesalazine, sulfasalazine) because the combination can increase the risk of myelosuppression; may need dose reduction with other drugs whose primary toxicity is myelosuppression
- Esophageal varices reported when given with busulfan.
- Veno-occlusive liver disease reported with combination chemotherapy.

PREGNANCY

Category D
- Do not use while pregnant or nursing.
- Potentially mutagenic and teratogenic

SPECIAL CONSIDERATIONS

- Avoid long-term therapy (increased risk of liver toxicity).
- Evaluate for TPMT (inherited deficiency of the enzyme thiopurine methyltransferase). If present, rapid bone marrow suppression may develop with therapy; may require significant dose reductions.

PATIENT EDUCATION

- Instruct patient to conclude all dental work before beginning therapy.
- Teach patient good oral hygiene measures.
- Instruct patient to take on an empty stomach.
- Teach patient to drink plenty of fluids and to urinate frequently.
- Instruct patient to report any signs of bleeding, bruising, infection, fever, shortness of breath, fatigue, or yellowing of skin.
- Instruct patient to avoid pregnancy and to use effective contraceptive measures.

BIBLIOGRAPHY

Antimetabolite antineoplastics. (2005). In *Nursing rapid-fire drug facts* (pp. 38-40). Philadelphia: Lippincott Williams & Wilkins.

Elsevier. (2006). *The Elsevier guide to oncology drugs and regimens* (pp. 337-339). Huntington, NY: Elsevier Oncology.

Hughes, T. E. (2005). Thioguanine (Tabloid). In J. Abraham, C. J. Allegra, & J. Gulley (Eds.). *Bethesda handbook of clinical oncology* (2nd ed., p. 660). Philadelphia: Lippincott Williams & Wilkins.

Kelleher, L. O. (2005). Principles of chemotherapy. In M. Polovich, J. M. White, & L. O. Kelleher (Eds.). *Chemotherapy and biotherapy guidelines and recommendations for practice* (2nd ed., pp. 18-35). Pittsburgh, PA: Oncology Nursing Society.

MedlinePlus. (2003). *Thioguanine*. Retrieved January 21, 2007, from http://www.nlm.nih.gov/medlineplus/druginfo/medmaster/a682099.html.

PDR oncology pocket guide (2nd ed., pp. 67-68). (2005). Montvale, NJ: Thompson PDR.

RxList. (2004). *Thioguanine*. Retrieved January 21, 2007, from http://www.rxlist.com/cgi/generic2/thioguanine.htm.

Spratto, G. R., & Woods, A. L. (2005). *2005 edition PDR nurses drug handbook* (pp. 1203-1205). Clifton Park, NY: Thomson Delmar Learning.

Wilkes, G. M., & Barton-Burke, M. (2006). 2006 *Oncology nursing drug handbook*, (pp. 295-296). Sudbury, MA: Jones & Bartlett.

Cancer Management

Thiotepa (Thioplex, Triethylene-thiophosphoramide)

Linda U. Krebs

DRUG CLASS

- Alkylating agent

ROUTES OF ADMINISTRATION

- Intravenous (IV)
- Intravesical instillation
- Intracavitary instillation
- Intrathecal

HOW TO ADMINISTER

- IV: administer by rapid infusion over 1-2 minutes or infused over 10-60 minutes.
- Intravesical: instill into bladder; allow to remain for approximately 2 hours; may reposition the patient every 15 minutes.
- Intracavitary: instill through tubing used to remove effusion.

PRETREATMENT GUIDELINES

- IV administration:
  - Monitor complete blood cell count (CBC) with differential, uric acid; be sure of adequate hydration; may need to pretreat with allopurinol.
  - Monitor CBC at least weekly during therapy and for 3 weeks after therapy.
- Intravesical instillation:
  - Patient should be dehydrated for 8-10 hours before instillation in bladder.
  - Standard volume is 60 mL; may decrease to 30 mL if patient complains of discomfort.

USE

- Superficial papillary carcinoma of the bladder
- Ovarian cancer
- Breast cancer
- Lymphoma
- Bronchogenic carcinoma
- Peritoneal, pleural, or pericardial infusions as a result of metastatic tumors

PHARMACOKINETICS

- Extensive hepatic metabolism
- Half-life approximately 2.3 hours
- Approximately 85% excreted in the urine, mostly as metabolites

USUAL DOSE AND SCHEDULE
Single Agent

- 1. IV:
  - 0.3-0.4 mg/kg IV for one dose; repeat at 1- to 4-week intervals
  - 0.2 mg/kg for 4-5 days every 2-4 weeks
- Intravesical: 60 mg mixed in 30-60 mL of sodium chloride for injection (if discomfort at 60 mL can reduce to 30 mL) every 6 weeks
- Intracavitary: 0.6-0.8 mg/kg for every 1 to 4 weeks
- Intrathecal 10-15mg/kg diluted in 1-5 ml normal saline or Elliot's B solution

SIDE EFFECTS

- Alopecia
- Amenorrhea
- Anaphylaxis
- Cystitis (may be hemorrhagic)
- Decreased spermatogenesis
- Dizziness
- Fatigue
- Fever
- Headache
- Hematuria (after intravesical administration)
- Hypersensitivity reactions
- Myelosuppression
- Pain at injection site
- Rash
- Stomatitis
- Urticaria
- Weakness

NADIR

- Neutrophils: days 10-14. Bone marrow effects may last as long as 30 days.

STORAGE
Unreconstituted Powder

- Store in refrigerator; protect from light at all times.

Reconstituted Powder or Solution

- If reconstituted with sterile water for injection, store in refrigerator and use within 8 hours.
- Reconstituted solutions that have been further diluted with sodium chloride solutions should be used immediately.

MIXING INSTRUCTIONS

- Reconstitute with 1.5 mL of sterile water for injection resulting in a drug concentration of approximately 10 mg/mL.
- Resulting solution is hypotonic and may be further mixed or should be given with 0.9% sodium chloride, 5% dextrose, dextrose with 0.9% sodium chloride or Ringer's solution.
- Filter solutions through a 0.22-micron filter before administration; discard solutions that are opaque or have a precipitate. Final concentration of 1mg/ml in 0.9% NaCl is considered isotonic for IV push.

Product Stability

- Use within 8 hours.

COMPATIBILITY WITH OTHER DRUGS/INTRAVENOUS FLUIDS

- Compatible with multiple drugs (check package insert)
- Incompatible with cisplatin and filgrastim

DRUG INTERACTIONS

- Increased toxicity when given with other chemotherapeutic agents
- Decreased effectiveness of antigout medications
- Prolonged muscle relaxation and respiratory depression when combined with pancuronium (skeletal muscle relaxant)
- Increased risk of apnea in patients treated with succinylcholine
- May increase live virus vaccine side effects and decrease body's vaccine antibody response

PREGNANCY

Category D
- Do not use if pregnant or nursing.
- Can cause fetal damage or death.

SPECIAL CONSIDERATIONS

- Carcinogenic and mutagenic
- Use with caution in renal and hepatic dysfunction.
- Dose individualized on the basis of the clinical response and the level of associated side effects
- Interrupt therapy for rapidly decreasing platelet or white blood cell count (WBC) or if platelets fall below 150,000/mm³ or WBC count falls below 3,000/mm³.

PATIENT EDUCATION

- Instruct patient to conclude all dental work before beginning therapy.
- Teach patient good oral hygiene.
- For intravesicular instillation into the bladder, teach patient to take nothing by mouth for 6 hours after instillation; report bloody urine or painful urination.
- Instruct patient to report any signs of bleeding, bruising, infection, fever, shortness of breath, or fatigue.
- Instruct patient to avoid receiving vaccinations and to refrain from being in crowds or around those with known infections.
- Instruct patient to avoid pregnancy and to use effective contraceptive measures.

BIBLIOGRAPHY

Elsevier. (2006). *The Elsevier guide to oncology drugs and regimens* (pp. 339-341). Huntington, NY: Elsevier Oncology.

Hodgson, B. B., & Kizior, R.J. (2006). *Mosby's 2006 drug consult for nurses* (pp. 292-294). St. Louis: Mosby.

Hughes, T. E. (2005). Thiotepa (Thioplex). In J. Abraham, C. J. Allegra, & J. Gulley (Eds.). *Bethesda handbook of clinical oncology* (2nd ed., pp. 660-661). Philadelphia: Lippincott Williams & Wilkins.

Kelleher, L. O. (2005). Principles of chemotherapy. In M. Polovich, J. M. White, & L. O. Kelleher (Eds.). *Chemotherapy and biotherapy guidelines and recommendations for practice* (2nd ed., pp. 18-35). Pittsburgh, PA: Oncology Nursing Society.

MedlinePlus. (2003). *Thiotepa*. Retrieved on January 21, 2007, from http://www.nlm.nih.gov/medlineplus/druginfo/medmaster/a682821.html.

RxList. (2004). *Thiotepa*. Retrieved on January 21, 2007, from http://www.rxlist.com/cgi/generic2/thiotep.htm.

Spratto, G. R., & Woods, A. L. (2005). *2005 PDR nurses drug handbook* (pp. 1205-1206). Clifton Park, NY: Thomson Delmar Learning.

Thiotepa. In *Nursing rapid-fire drug facts* (pp. 559-560). (2005). Philadelphia: Lippincott Williams & Wilkins.

Wilkes, G. M., & Barton-Burke, M. (2006). *2006 Oncology nursing drug handbook* (pp. 297-299). Sudbury, MA: Jones & Bartlett.

Topotecan Hydrochloride (Hycamptin)

Linda U. Krebs

DRUG CLASS

- Topoisomerase I inhibitor

ROUTE OF ADMINISTRATION

- Intravenous (IV) route by IV infusion

HOW TO ADMINISTER

- Administer by IV infusion over 30 minutes, 2 hours, or 24 hours.

PRETREATMENT GUIDELINES

- Do not treat unless neutrophil count is >1,000 cells/mm³, platelet count is >100,000 cells/mm³, and hemoglobin level is >9 mg/dL (may require transfusion).
- Monitor renal function; reduce dose for renal impairment.
  - For creatinine clearance: 20-39 mL/min, administer 50% of normal dose
  - Hold for CrCl <20 mL/min
- Monitor serum bilirubin, aspartate aminotransferase (AST), and alanine aminotransferase (ALT).
- Premedicate with antiemetics as indicated.

USE

- Ovarian cancer
- Small cell lung cancer (SCLC)
- Esophageal cancer

PHARMACOKINETICS

- Half-life 2-3 hours
- Approximately 48% excreted through the urine

USUAL DOSE AND SCHEDULE
Single Agent

- 1.5 mg/m² IV over 30 minutes daily for 5 consecutive days (days 1-5) of a 21-day cycle (four cycles recommended)
- 1.3-1.6 mg/m² IV infusion over 30 minutes, 2 hours, or 24 hours

SIDE EFFECTS

- Alopecia
- Injection site reactions: erythema, ecchymosis
- Myelosuppression
- Nausea
- Vomiting
- Stomatitis
- Anorexia
- Diarrhea
- Constipation
- Abdominal pain
- Fatigue
- Asthenia
- Headache
- Increased serum bilirubin, AST, and ALT

NADIR

- Neutrophils: days 11-12; not cumulative. Recovery at 3 weeks.
- Platelets: day 15
- Red blood cells (RBCs): day 15

STORAGE
Unreconstituted Powder

- Stable until date on package; store in original package between 20°-25° C (68°-77° F).

Reconstituted Powder or Solution

- Use immediately (some references suggest that the product is stable for 24 hours).

Cancer Management

MIXING INSTRUCTIONS

- Reconstitute each single-dose vial with 4 mL of sterile water for injection and then further dilute in 0.9% sodium chloride or 5% dextrose for IV infusion.

Product Stability

- Lyophilized form contains no preservatives and should be used immediately.

COMPATIBILITY WITH OTHER DRUGS/INTRAVENOUS FLUIDS

- Compatible with 0.9% sodium chloride and 5% dextrose
- Incompatible with carboplatin, cisplatin, cyclophosphamide, dexamethasone, doxorubicin, etoposide, 5-fluorouracil, gemcitabine, granisetron, mitomycin C, ondansetron, paclitaxel, vincristine

DRUG INTERACTIONS

- Causes worsening of neutropenia if given with granulocyte colony-stimulating factor (G-CSF); do not administer growth factor for at least 24 hours after last dose of topotecan.
- Giving with cisplatin or other bone marrow depressant drugs may increase the severity of myelosuppression.
- May increase live virus vaccine side effects and decrease body's vaccine antibody response

PREGNANCY

Category D
- Do not use if pregnant or nursing.

SPECIAL CONSIDERATIONS

- Essential to monitor renal and hepatic function, especially in the elderly

Dose Modifications

- Reduce dose for moderate renal impairment (creatinine clearance [CrCl] 20-39 mL/min).

- Modify dose for myelosuppression; for severe myelosuppression consider G-CSF.

PATIENT EDUCATION

- Teach patient to be aware of the potential for diarrhea late in therapy.
- Teach patient to be aware of signs and symptoms of dehydration/electrolyte depletion.
- Instruct patient to report any signs of bleeding, bruising, infection, fever, shortness of breath, fatigue, nausea, vomiting, or diarrhea.
- Instruct patient to avoid receiving vaccinations and to refrain from being in crowds or around those with known infections.
- Help patient prepare for alopecia; inform that hair will regrow after therapy and that new hair may have a different texture or color.
- Instruct patient to avoid pregnancy and to use effective contraceptive measures.

BIBLIOGRAPHY

Elsevier. (2006). *The Elsevier guide to oncology drugs and regimens* (pp. 342-343). Huntington, NY: Elsevier Oncology.

Hodgson, B. B., & Kizior, R. J. (2006). *Mosby's 2006 drug consult for nurses* (pp. 430-432). St. Louis: Mosby.

Hughes, T. E. (2005). Topotecan (Hycamtin). In J. Abraham, C. J. Allegra, & J. Gulley (Eds.). *Bethesda handbook of clinical oncology* (2nd ed., pp. 661). Philadelphia: Lippincott Williams & Wilkins.

Kelleher, L. O. (2005). Principles of chemotherapy. In M. Polovich, J. M. White, & L. O. Kelleher (Eds.). *Chemotherapy and biotherapy guidelines and recommendations for practice* (2nd ed., pp. 18-35). Pittsburgh, PA: Oncology Nursing Society.

MedlinePlus. (2003). *Topotecan hydrochloride*. Retrieved January 21, 2007, from http://www.nlm.nih.gov/medlineplus/druginfo/medmaster/a697006.html.

PDR oncology pocket guide (2nd ed., pp. 42). (2005). Montvale, NJ: Thompson.

RxList. (2005). *Topotecan IV*. Retrieved January 21, 2007, from http://www.rxlist.com/drugs/drug-13492-Topotecan+IV.aspx?drugid=13492&drugname=Topotecan+IV.

Spratto, G. R., & Woods, A. L. (2005). *2005 PDR nurses drug handbook* (pp. 1233-1234). Clifton Park, NY: Thomson Delmar Learning.

Topotecan. In *Nursing rapid-fire drug facts* (pp. 596-597). (2005). Philadelphia: Lippincott Williams & Wilkins.

Wilkes, G. M., & Barton-Burke, M. (2006). *2006 Oncology nursing drug handbook* (pp. 300-302). Sudbury, MA: Jones & Bartlett.

Tretinoin (Vesanoid®)

Linda U. Krebs

DRUG CLASS

- Retinoid

ROUTE OF ADMINISTRATION

- Administer by mouth (for cancer treatment)
- Topical preparations (for treatment of acne and wrinkles)

HOW TO ADMINISTER

- Administer orally in 2 divided doses (discontinue 30 days after remission is achieved or at 90 days if no remission, whichever comes first)

PRETREATMENT GUIDELINES

- Be sure patient is not pregnant prior to beginning therapy; repeat pregnancy test routinely throughout therapy
- Monitor CBC, differential, coagulation profile, liver function (discontinue if LFTs > 5 times the upper limit of normal), triglyceride and cholesterol levels.

USE

- APL

PHARMACOKINETICS

- Peak plasma levels are achieved in 1-2 hours
- 95% bound to plasma protein.
- Half-life of Tretinoin is 0.5-2 hours

- Metabolized by the liver and primarily excreted through the urine.

USUAL DOSE AND SCHEDULE
Single Agent

- Adults and Children: 45 mg/m²/day in 2 evenly divided doses

SIDE EFFECTS

- Malaise
- Shivering
- Hemorrhage
- Infection
- Peripheral edema
- Bone and flank pain
- Chest discomfort
- Edema
- DIC
- Weight change
- Dyspnea
- Pleural effusion
- Respiratory insufficiency
- Pneumonia
- Hypercholesterolemia (reversible)
- Hypertriglyceridemia (reversible)

STORAGE

- 10 mg. capsule, store at 15°-30°C, protect from light

DRUG INTERACTIONS

- Possible interactions with drugs that affect the CYP450 system (inducers: e.g., phenobarbital and inhibitors: e.g., cyclosporine) which may alter pharmacokinetic properties.
- Certain herbs such as bergamot and St. John's wort may increase risk of photosensitivity.

PREGNANCY

Category D; do not use if pregnant or nursing

- High risk of teratogenetic effects; may cause abortion or fetal abnormalities
- Use 2 methods of birth control during and for 1 month following completion of therapy.

SPECIAL CONSIDERATIONS

- Risk of retinoic-acid-APL syndrome (unexplained fever, acute respiratory distress, weight gain, radiographic pulmonary infiltrates, pleural and/or pericardial effusions leading to multi-organ failure) in about 25% of patients (treat with high-dose steroids at first sign of syndrome, usually 10 mg dexamethasone IV every 12 hours for 3 days or until symptoms resolve)
- Should not be given to those with a sensitivity to parabens.
- Monitor closely for respiratory compromise.
- Monitor closely for leukocytosis (occurs in approximately 40% with resultant increased risk of life-threatening complications; full dose chemotherapy may be added for those with a WBC count >5x10⁹/L).
- Observe for early signs of pseudotumor cerebri (nausea, vomiting, papilledema, visual disturbances and headache), particularly in children.
- Absorption is increased when taken with food.

PATIENT EDUCATION

- Instruct patient to take tretinoin with food to enhance absorption.
- Instruct patient to immediately report the signs and symptoms of retinoic acid-APL syndrome (unexplained fever, dyspnea, weight gain).
- Instruct patient to use 2 reliable forms of contraception during treatment and for 1 month following therapy.
- Teach patient to avoid sun exposure and use sun protection methods and products.
- Instruct patient to not skip any doses and to notify provider if a dose is missed for any reason.
- Instruct patient to refrain from donating blood while taking tretinoin.

BIBLIOGRAPHY

The Elsevier guide to oncology drugs and regimens (pp. 352-354). (2006). Huntington, NY: Elsevier Oncology.

Food and Drug Administration. (2004). *Tretinoin*. Retrieved on January 21, 2007 from http://www.fda.gov/cder/foi/label/2004/20438s004lbl.pdf.

Hughes, T.E. (2005). Tretinoin (Vesanoid). In J. Abraham, C.J. Allegra, & J. Gulley (Eds.). *Bethesda handbook of clinical oncology*, (2nd. ed., pp. 663). Philadelphia, PA: Lippincott, Williams & Wilkins.

MedlinePlus Drug Information. (2004). *Tretinoin*. Retrieved on January 21, 2007 from http://www.nlm.nih.gov/medlineplus/druginfo/uspdi/203663.html.

PDR *oncology pocket guide* (2nd. ed., pp. 77). (2005). Montvale, NJ: Thompson PDR.

Spratto, G.R. & Woods, A.L. (2005). *2005 edition PDR nurses drug handbook*, (pp. 1247-1250). Clifton Park, NY: Thomson Delmar Learning.

Wilkes, G.M., & Barton-Burke, M. (2006). 2006 *oncology nursing drug handbook*, (pp. 530-533). Sudbury, MA: Jones and Bartlett Publishers.

Trimetrexate (Neutrexin)

Linda U. Krebs

DRUG CLASS

- Antimetabolite (folate antagonist)

ROUTE OF ADMINISTRATION

- Administer intravenously (IV) by IV infusion.

HOW TO ADMINISTER

- Before administration, the reconstituted solution should be further diluted with 5% dextrose.
- Administer by IV infusion over 60-90 minutes; do not mix with leucovorin or a chloride ion (immediate precipitation).
- Dose must be followed by leucovorin as directed (either IV or orally; if IV, flush line with at least 10 mL of 5% dextrose between drugs).

PRETREATMENT GUIDELINES

- Monitor complete blood cell count (CBC) with differential.
- Monitor hepatic and renal function.
- Assess pulmonary status.

USE

- *Pneumocystis carinii* pneumonia (PCP)
- Advanced recurrent or metastatic colorectal cancer (investigational)

PHARMACOKINETICS

- Metabolized by the liver; 10%-20% excreted by kidneys within 24 hours
- Metabolized by P450 enzyme system
- Half-life 9-18 hours

USUAL DOSE AND SCHEDULE
Single Agent

- For PCP: administer 45 mg/m^2 IV over 60 to 90 minutes daily for 21 days.
- Must be given concurrently with oral or intravenous leucovorin at prescribed doses (usually 20 mg/m^2 IV every 6 hours or 20 mg/m^2 orally four times daily) to reduce occurrence of life-threatening toxicities. Leucovorin is continued for 72 hours after the last does of trimetrexate.

Combination Therapy

- Investigational for colorectal cancer: 110 mg/m^2 IV over 60 minutes weekly on days 1, 8, 15, 22, 29, and 36 (6 weeks) followed by a 2-week rest (given with capecitabine or 5-fluorouracil [5-FU]).
- Must be given with oral leucovorin at a dose of 15 mg every 6 hours for four doses starting 24 hours after each trimetrexate dose to avoid life-threatening toxicities (other dosing regimens may be ordered; round oral leucovorin dose up to the next 25-mg increment).

SIDE EFFECTS

- Hypersensitivity or allergic-type infusion reactions
- Headache
- Paresthesias
- Nausea/vomiting
- Stomatitis
- Diarrhea
- Rash
- Thrombocytopenia
- Leukopenia
- Alopecia
- Dyspnea
- Elevated liver function test (LFT) results
- Mental confusion
- Anorexia
- Fatigue

NADIR

- White blood cells (WBC): day 8 with recovery by day 16.
- Platelets: day 14

STORAGE
Unreconstituted Powder

- Store at room temperature; protect from light.

Reconstituted Powder or Solution

- Solution is stable for 6 hours at room temperature (some references state stability up to 24 hours) or 24 hours if refrigerated.

MIXING INSTRUCTIONS

- Reconstitute with 2 mL of 5% dextrose in water (D5W) or sterile water for injection to a concentration of 12.5 mg/mL (do not use other solutions because precipitation may occur).
- Reconstituted, the fluid should appear clear, pale yellowish-green.
- Filter with a 22-micron filter and then further dilute with 5% D5W to a final concentration of 0.25 to 2.0 mg/mL.

PRODUCT STABILITY

- Once reconstituted, trimetrexate is stable at room temperature for 6 hours or under refrigeration for 24 hours.
- When the solution is diluted further for patient administration, the solution is stable for 24 hours at room temperature or under refrigeration.

COMPATIBILITY WITH OTHER DRUGS/INTRAVENOUS FLUIDS

- Incompatible with leucovorin and chloride solutions (immediate precipitation)

DRUG INTERACTIONS

- Trimetrexate is metabolized by P450 enzyme system; drugs that induce or inhibit this system may cause interactions affecting trimetrexate plasma concentrations. Avoid drugs such as cimetidine, erythromycin, zidovudine, fluconazole, rifampin, and ketoconazole. If concomitant administration cannot be avoided, monitor patient closely.

PREGNANCY
Category D

- Do not use if pregnant or nursing; drug is embryotoxic and fetotoxic.

SPECIAL CONSIDERATIONS

- Leucovorin must be given to decrease toxicities of trimetrexate. Leucovorin may be given either before or after trimetrexate dose (per treatment protocol). If given IV, be sure line is well flushed to prevent interaction between drugs. Do not use a chloride-containing solution because precipitation will occur.

Dose Modifications

- Hold therapy if serum creatinine increases to >2.5 mg/dL or aminotransferases or alkaline phosphatase increase to >5 times the upper limit of normal.
- Dose of trimetrexate and leucovorin should be modified on the basis of hematological toxicity (neutrophils and platelets).

PATIENT EDUCATION

- Teach patient importance of taking oral leucovorin as prescribed. Stress not missing a dose and taking each dose on time. Instruct to report any missed dose immediately.
- Instruct patient to conscientiously follow oral hygiene measures.
- Instruct patient to report any signs of bleeding, bruising, infection, fever, mouth sores, skin rash, shortness of breath, fatigue,

seizures, or rapid/pounding/ irregular heartbeat.

- Teach patient that headache is common, that acetaminophen may be taken for relief, and that a continued headache should be reported.
- Instruct patient to avoid pregnancy and to use effective contraceptive measures.

BIBLIOGRAPHY

Kelleher, L. O. (2005). Principles of chemotherapy. In M. Polovich, J. M. White, & L. O. Kelleher (Eds.). *Chemotherapy and biotherapy guidelines and recommendations for practice* (2nd ed., pp. 18-35). Pittsburgh, PA: Oncology Nursing Society.

Medimmune Oncology. (2000). *Neutrexin*. Retrieved January 21, 2007, from http://www.fda.gov/cder/foi/label/ 2002/20326s11s13lbl.pdf.

MedlinePlus. (2003). *Trimetrexate glucuronate*. Retrieved January 21, 2007, from http://www.nlm.nih.gov/medl ineplus/druginfo/medmaster/a694019. html.

RxList. (2006). *Neutrexin*. Retrieved January 21, 2007, from http://www. rxlist.com/cgi/generic2/trimetrexate. htm.

Stewart, J. A. (1988). Safety and tolerance of trimetrexate: results of a phase II multicenter study in patients with metastatic cancer refractory to conventional therapy or for which no conventional therapy exists. *Seminars in Oncology, 15*, 10-16.

WebMD. (2007). *Trimetrexate IV*. Retrieved January 21, 2007, from http://www. webmd.com/drugs/drug-8950- Trimetrexate.aspx?drugid=8950&dru gname=Trimetrexate.

Wilkes, G. M., & Barton-Burke, M. (2006). *2006 Oncology nursing drug handbook* (pp. 304-307). Sudbury, MA: Jones & Bartlett.

UFT (Ftorafur [Tegafur], Uracil)

Linda U. Krebs

DRUG NOT AVAILABLE IN UNITED STATES

DRUG CLASS

- Combination of antimetabolite and alkylating agents, dihydropyrimidine dehydrogenase inhibitory fluoropyrimidines (fluorouracil prodrug)

ROUTE OF ADMINISTRATION

- Administer by mouth.

HOW TO ADMINISTER

- Administer in a single or three evenly divided doses (8 hours apart) on an empty stomach.

PRETREATMENT GUIDELINES

- Monitor complete blood cell count (CBC) with differential, calcium, potassium, magnesium, liver function, and coagulation profile.
- Premedicate with antiemetics.
- Assess oral mucosa.

USE

- Metastatic colorectal cancer

PHARMACOKINETICS

- Metabolized in the liver to 5-fluorouracil (5-FU)
- Excreted as respiratory carbon dioxide with a small amount excreted by kidneys

USUAL DOSE AND SCHEDULE
Single Agent

- 300-350 mg/m^2/day in three divided doses for 28 days

Combination Therapy

- 200 mg/m^2/day for 28 days per cycle; may be combined with 5 or 50 mg of leucovorin given concomitantly throughout each cycle

- 300 mg/m^2/day orally in three divided doses for 28 days with 1-week rest period combined with leucovorin 75-90 mg/day in three divided doses throughout each cycle

SIDE EFFECTS

- Skin pigmentation changes
- Asthenia
- Paresthesias
- Headache
- Nausea/vomiting
- Diarrhea
- Stomatitis
- Fatigue
- Rash
- Myelosuppression

NADIR

- Severe myelosuppression not common

STORAGE

- Capsules: store at temperatures not exceeding 25° C (77° F).

DRUG INTERACTIONS

- Unknown

PREGNANCY

Category D
  - Do not use if pregnant or nursing.

SPECIAL CONSIDERATIONS

- Single daily dose increases diarrhea.
- Does not cause hand-foot syndrome
- Use with caution in patients with a history of heart disease.

PATIENT EDUCATION

- Instruct patient to report any bruising, bleeding, mouth ulcers, fever, or signs of infection.
- Instruct patient to take on an empty stomach with a full glass of water (at least 1 hour before or 2 hours after a meal).
- Instruct patient in good oral hygiene and self-examination practices.
- Teach patient to report diarrhea and to take prescribed antidiarrheals as ordered.

- Teach patient that hair may thin but will begin to regrow after completion of therapy.
- Teach patient that nails may become brittle and ridged and eyes may become sore, itchy, and tear excessively.
- Instruct patient to avoid pregnancy and to use effective contraceptive measures.

BIBLIOGRAPHY

Cancerbackup. (2006). *Tegafur-uracil (Uftoral)*. Retrieved January 21, 2007, from http://www.cancerbackup.org.uk/ Treatments/Chemotherapy/Individual drugs/Tegafur-uracil.

Kelleher, L. O. (2005). Principles of chemotherapy. In M. Polovich, J. M. White, & L. O. Kelleher (Eds.). *Chemotherapy and biotherapy guidelines and recommendations for practice* (2nd ed., pp. 18-35). Pittsburgh, PA: Oncology Nursing Society.

Netdoctor.co.uk. (2006). *Uftoral*. Retrieved January 21, 2007, from http://www.netdoctor.co.uk/medicines/ 100004526.html.

Shirao, K., Hoff, P. M., Ohtsu, A., et. al. (2004). Comparison of the efficacy, toxicity and pharmacokinetics of a Uracil/ Tegafur (UFT) plus oral leucovorin (LV) between Japanese and American patients with advanced colorectal cancer: Joint United States and Japanese study of UFT/LV. *Journal of Clinical Oncology, 22*, 3466-3474.

Wilkes, G. M., & Barton-Burke, M. (2006). *2006 Oncology nursing drug handbook* (pp. 307-310). Sudbury, MA: Jones & Bartlett.

Vinblastine Sulfate (Velban)

Linda U. Krebs

DRUG CLASS

- Plant alkaloid (periwinkle plant)

ROUTE OF ADMINISTRATION

- Administer by the intravenous (IV) route; fatal if given intrathecally.

HOW TO ADMINISTER

- Administer IV no more frequently than every 7 days.
- Inject into tubing of free-flowing IV over at least 1 minute.
- May be given as a continuous infusion over 96 hours

PRETREATMENT GUIDELINES

- Monitor complete blood cell count (CBC); administer only if white blood cell count (WBC) is 4,000 cells/mm^3.
- Modify the dose by 50% if bilirubin between 1.5-3 mg/dL, decrease normal dose by 75% if total bilirubin between 3.1-5 mg/dL, and hold drug for total bilirubin >5 mg/dL.
- Monitor uric acid and renal function.

USE

- Hodgkin disease
- Non-Hodgkin lymphoma
- Mycosis fungoides
- Testicular cancer
- Kaposi's sarcoma
- Choriocarcinoma
- Bladder cancer
- Breast cancer
- Cervical cancer
- Head and neck cancer
- Kidney cancer
- Ovarian cancer
- Lung cancer
- Melanoma

PHARMACOKINETICS

- Triphasic half-life lasting between 3.7-24.8 hours
- Almost completely metabolized by the liver; metabolites excreted in the bile
- 99% bound to plasma proteins

USUAL DOSE AND SCHEDULE
Single Agent or Combination Therapy

Adults

- 6-10 mg/ m^2 IV every 2 to 4 weeks
- If given weekly or at more frequent intervals, dose is incrementally increased from a starting dose of 3.7 mg/m^2 IV to a maximum dose of 18.5 mg/m^2 IV.
- For maintenance dosing, give one dose level down from final weekly (or more frequent) dosing.

Children

- If given weekly or at more frequent intervals, dose is incrementally increased from a starting dose of 2.5 mg/m^2 IV to a maximum dose of 12.5 mg/m^2 IV.
- For maintenance dosing, give one dose level down from final weekly (or more frequent) dosing.

Continuous Infusion

- 1.7 to 2.0 mg/m^2/day weekly or over a period of 96 hours by IV infusion

SIDE EFFECTS
Vesicant

- Leukopenia
- Anemia
- Thrombocytopenia
- Alopecia
- Constipation
- Anorexia
- Nausea
- Vomiting
- Abdominal pain
- Diarrhea
- Hypertension
- Acute shortness of breath
- Bronchospasm
- Aspermia
- SIADH

NADIR

- Nadir occurs in 4-10 days and lasts for 7-14 days.

STORAGE
Unreconstituted Powder

- Store vials in refrigerator at 2°-8° C (36°-46° F).

Reconstituted Powder or Solution

- May be stored in refrigerator up to 30 days if bacteriostatic sodium chloride is used for reconstitution (discard all other solutions)

MIXING INSTRUCTIONS

- Supplied as 1 mg/mL vials and 10 mg powder for injection vials
- Reconstitute 10 mg powder for injection vials with 10 mL of bacteriostatic sodium chloride or sodium chloride injection (unpreserved) to a solution

of 1 mg/mL. Solution should be clear and colorless.

Product Stability

- Once mixed with preserved normal saline solution, the drug may be stored for up to 30 days in the refrigerator.

COMPATIBILITY WITH OTHER DRUGS/INTRAVENOUS FLUIDS

- Compatible with preserved and unpreserved sodium chloride, allopurinol, cisplatin, cyclophosphamide, doxorubicin, etoposide, 5-fluorouracil, gemcitabine, granisetron, heparin, leucovorin, methotrexate, ondansetron, paclitaxel, and vinorelbine.
- Incompatible with any solutions that raise or lower the pH from between 3.5 and 5.5 and with cefepime and furosemide.

DRUG INTERACTIONS

- Causes reduced levels of phenytoin and is associated with increased seizure activity; adjust dose of phenytoin by monitoring serial blood levels.
- Increased toxicity when given concurrently with CYP3A4 inhibitors such as azole antifungals, erythromycin, or verapamil. CYP3A4 inducers may decrease the levels/effects of vinblastine (including phenobarbital, phenytoin, carbamazepine).
- Vinblastine may decrease effects of antigout medications.
- If given with other bone marrow suppressants, may increase risk of myelosuppression
- Synergistic if given with bleomycin
- May potentiate virus replication, increase vaccine side effects, and decrease the patient's antibody response to the live virus vaccine

PREGNANCY

Category D

- Do not use if pregnant or nursing.

- May be carcinogenic, mutagenic, or teratogenic

SPECIAL CONSIDERATIONS

- Avoid in those with malignant infiltration of bone marrow.
- Avoid in those with cachexia or ulcerated skin, especially the elderly.
- Vesicant; manage extravasation immediately by institutional protocol (usually hyaluronidase and heat).
- Lethal if given intrathecally.
- Hepatic insufficiency increases risk of treatment-related toxicities.
- There is an increased risk of acute shortness of breath and bronchospasm when used with mitomycin C; may occur within minutes to weeks of concomitant medications.
- May cause severe eye irritation; wash the eye immediately with water.

PATIENT EDUCATION

- Teach patient to immediately report pain, burning, swelling, or irritation that occurs at the injection site during administration.
- Instruct patient to report signs of bruising, bleeding, infection, fever, shortness of breath, fatigue, nausea, vomiting, mouth ulcers or soreness, any numbness or tingling in hands or feet, or difficulty walking.
- Instruct patient on potential for jaw and tumor area pain.
- Teach patient to prevent constipation through diet and increased fluids.
- Teach patient to avoid contact with crowds and those with known infections.
- Teach patient to avoid vaccinations.
- Instruct patient on good oral hygiene.
- Teach patient that alopecia is reversible; new hair will regrow and may have a different texture and color.

- Instruct patient to avoid pregnancy and to use effective contraceptive measures.

BIBIOLOGRAPHY

Elsevier. (2006). *The Elsevier guide to oncology drugs and regimens* (pp. 359-361). Huntington, NY: Elsevier Oncology.

Hodgson, B. B., & Kizior, R. J. (2006). *Mosby's 2006 drug consult for nurses*, (pp. 341-344). St. Louis: Mosby.

Hughes, T. E. (2005). Vinblastine (Velban). In J. Abraham, C. J. Allegra, & J. Gulley (Eds.). *Bethesda handbook of clinical oncology* (2nd ed., pp. 665). Philadelphia: Lippincott Williams & Wilkins.

Kelleher, L. O. (2005). Principles of chemotherapy. In M. Polovich, J. M. White, & L. O. Kelleher (Eds.). *Chemotherapy and biotherapy guidelines and recommendations for practice* (2nd ed., pp. 18-35). Pittsburgh, PA: Oncology Nursing Society.

MedlinePlus. (2000). *Vinblastine.* Retrieved January 21, 2007, from http://www.nlm.nih.gov/medlineplus/druginfo/uspdi/202593.html.

PDR oncology pocket guide (2nd ed., pp. 78-79). (2005). Montvale, NJ: Thompson PDR.

RxList. (2004). *Vinblastine sulfate.* Retrieved January 21, 2007, from http://www.rxlist.com/cgi/generic3/vinblastine.htm.

Spratto, G. R., & Woods, A. L. (2005). *2005 PDR nurses drug handbook* (pp. 1301-1303). Clifton Park, NY: Thomson Delmar Learning.

Vinblastine. In *Nursing rapid-fire drug facts* (p. 566). (2005). Philadelphia: Lippincott Williams & Wilkins.

Wilkes, G. M., & Barton-Burke, M. (2006). *2006 Oncology nursing drug handbook* (pp. 313-316). Sudbury, MA: Jones & Bartlett.

Vincristine Sulfate (Oncovin)

Linda U. Krebs

DRUG CLASS

- Plant alkaloid (periwinkle plant)

ROUTE OF ADMINISTRATION

- For intravenous (IV) use only. Fatal if administered intrathecally.
- By IV push or infusion through a properly placed catheter or central line

Cancer Management

HOW TO ADMINISTER

- Administer dose over 1 minute either into the tubing of a running IV infusion or directly into a vein through a catheter or central line.
- To prevent potential for intrathecal administration, may administer IV piggyback.
- If extravasation occurs, immediately stop the infusion and follow institutional procedure for vincristine extravasation (usually hyaluronidase and heat).

PRETREATMENT GUIDELINES

- Monitor complete blood cell count (CBC), liver and renal function, and serum uric acid level.
- Carefully calculate dosage of vincristine; overdose may result in serious toxicity or fatality.
  ○ Decrease the dose by 50% if total bilirubin between 1.5-3 mg/dL
  ○ Decrease normal dose by 75% if total bilirubin between 3.1-5 mg/dL
  ○ Hold drug for total bilirubin >5 mg/dL
- Should not be used in those receiving radiation therapy given to areas that include the liver

USE

- Acute leukemia
- Hodgkin disease
- Non-Hodgkin lymphoma
- Rhabdomyosarcoma
- Neuroblastoma
- Wilms' tumor

PHARMACOKINETICS

- Metabolized in the liver; primarily eliminated in feces (80%; with 20% in urine)
- Does not cross the blood-brain barrier
- Half-life of 24 hours

USUAL DOSE AND SCHEDULE
Single Agent or Combination Therapy

- Adults, elderly: 0.4-1.4 mg/m² once a week. Doses are often capped at 2 mg.

- Children: 1-2 mg/m² once a week (in children who weigh less than 10 kg or who have a body surface area less than 1 m², the dose is 0.05 mg/kg with a maximum dose of 2 mg).

Continuous Infusion

- 0.5 mg/day to 0.5 mg/m²/day for 4 days

SIDE EFFECTS
Vesicant

- Alopecia
- Abdominal cramps
- Weight loss
- Nausea
- Vomiting
- Diarrhea
- Constipation
- Paralytic ileus
- Hypertension
- Hypotension
- Polyuria
- Dysuria
- Urinary retention
- Paresthesias
- Jaw pain
- Neuritic pain, peripheral neuropathy
- Motor difficulties
- Rash
- Fever
- Weakness

NADIR

- Neutrophils: by day 10, with recovery in 21 days

STORAGE

- Refrigerate unopened vials.
- The solution normally appears clear and colorless. Discard if discolored or has a precipitate.
- Stable for at least 30 days at room temperature

MIXING INSTRUCTIONS

- Premixed liquid, 1 mg/mL; may be administered undiluted.

PRODUCT STABILITY

- Stable for 24 hours

COMPATIBILITY WITH OTHER DRUGS/INTRAVENOUS FLUIDS

- Incompatible with cefepime, furosemide, and idarubicin

DRUG INTERACTIONS

- Causes reduced levels of phenytoin and is associated with increased seizure activity; adjust dose of phenytoin by monitoring serial blood levels.
- There is an increased risk of acute shortness of breath and bronchospasm when used with mitomycin C; may occur within minutes to weeks of concomitant medications.
- Asparaginase and other neurotoxic medications may increase the risk of neurotoxicity.
- Vincristine may decrease effects of antigout medications.
- Actions of methotrexate and anticoagulants are increased if used concomitantly.
- Increased toxicity when given concurrently with CYP3A4 inhibitors such as azole antifungals, erythromycin, or verapamil. CYP3A4 inducers may decrease the levels/effects of vinblastine (including phenobarbital, phenytoin, carbamazepine).
- When combined with doxorubicin, the risk of myelosuppression is increased.
- May potentiate virus replication, increase vaccine side effects, and decrease the patient's antibody response to the live-virus vaccine.

PREGNANCY
Category D

- Do not use if pregnant or nursing.

SPECIAL CONSIDERATIONS

- Vesicant: if extravasation occurs, use appropriate institutional protocol.
- Concurrent administration of mitomycin C increases the risk of acute shortness of breath and bronchospasm.
- Foot or wrist drop, difficulty walking, slapping gait, ataxia, and

muscle wasting may occur, especially with prolonged administration or higher doses; assess Achilles tendon reflex for evidence of peripheral neuropathy.

- Handle with extreme care during preparation and administration; may be carcinogenic, mutagenic, or teratogenic.
- Use cautiously in those with hepatic impairment, neurotoxicity, or preexisting neuromuscular disease.
- Assess for daily bowel activity and consistency of stools.
- Lethal if given intrathecally
- Contraindicated in those receiving radiation therapy to liver
- Elderly more likely to have neurotoxic side effects.

PATIENT EDUCATION

- Teach patient to prevent constipation through use of stimulant laxatives, diet, and, increased fluids.
- Have patient report signs of bruising, bleeding, infection, fever, shortness of breath, fatigue, nausea, vomiting, any numbness or tingling in hands or feet, or difficulty walking.
- Instruct patient to avoid vaccinations.
- Instruct patient to avoid alcohol intake.
- Teach patient to immediately report pain, burning, swelling, or irritation at the injection site during administration.
- Teach patient to avoid contact with crowds and those with known infections.
- Teach patient that alopecia is reversible; new hair will regrow and may have a different texture and color.
- Instruct patient to avoid pregnancy and to use effective contraceptive measures.

BIBLIOGRAPHY

Elsevier. (2006). *The Elsevier guide to oncology drugs and regimens* (pp. 362-364). Huntington, NY: Elsevier Oncology.

Hodgson, B. B., & Kizior, R. J. (2006). *Mosby's 2006 drug consult for nurses*, (pp. 344-346). St. Louis: Mosby.

Hughes, T. E. (2005). Vincristine (Oncovin and others). In J. Abraham, C. J. Allegra, & J. Gulley (Eds.). *Bethesda handbook of clinical oncology* (2nd ed., pp. 665-666). Philadelphia: Lippincott Williams & Wilkins.

Kelleher, L. O. (2005). Principles of chemotherapy. In M. Polovich, J. M. White, & L. O. Kelleher (Eds.). *Chemotherapy and biotherapy guidelines and recommendations for practice* (2nd ed., pp. 18-35). Pittsburgh, PA: Oncology Nursing Society.

MedlinePlus. (2003). *Vincristine*. Retrieved January 21, 2007, from http://www.nlm. nih.gov/medlineplus/ druginfo/medm aster/a682822.html.

PDR oncology pocket guide (2nd ed., pp. 79-80). (2005). Montvale, NJ: Thompson PDR.

RxList. (2004). *Vincristine sulfate*. Retrieved January 21, 2007, from http://www.rxlist.com/cgi/generic3/vi ncristine.htm.

Spratto, G. R., & Woods, A. L. (2005). *2005 PDR nurses drug handbook* (pp. 1303-1305). Clifton Park, NY: Thomson Delmar Learning.

Vincristine. In *Nursing rapid-fire drug facts* (pp. 584). (2005). Philadelphia: Lippincott Williams & Wilkins.

Wilkes, G. M., & Barton-Burke, M. (2006). 2006 *Oncology nursing drug handbook* (pp. 316-318). Sudbury, MA: Jones & Bartlett.

Vinorelbine Tartrate (Navelbine)

Linda U. Krebs

DRUG CLASS

- Semisynthetic vinca alkaloid (derived from vinblastine), antimitotic agent

ROUTE OF ADMINISTRATION

- Intravenous (IV) route for IV infusion only; fatal if given intrathecally

HOW TO ADMINISTER

- Use extreme caution to prevent extravasation.
- Administer IV over 6-10 minutes into the side port of a freely flowing IV; flush well with 75 to 125 mL of one of the compatible solutions.

PRETREATMENT GUIDELINES

- Evaluate complete blood cell count (CBC) with differential, liver function.
  - Decrease dose by 50% if total bilirubin between 1.5-3 mg/dL
  - Decrease normal dose by 75% if total bilirubin between 3.1-5 mg/dL
  - Hold drug for total bilirubin >5 mg/dL
- Contraindicated if granulocytes <1,000 cells/mm^3
  - If ANC = 1500 cells/mm^3 give 100% of dose
  - If ANC = 1000-1499 cells/mm^3, give 50% of normal dose
- Do not administer growth factors within 24 hours before or after administration.

USE

- Non–small cell lung cancer (NSCLC)
- Investigational for many tumor types

PHARMACOKINETICS

- Vinorelbine is metabolized in the liver and excreted through urine and feces. It has a half-life of 28-43 hours.

USUAL DOSE AND SCHEDULE
Single Agent

- 30 mg/m^2 IV weekly

Combination Therapy (Usually with Cisplatin)

- 25 mg/m^2 IV weekly
- 30 mg/m^2 IV days 1 and 29; then every 6 weeks

SIDE EFFECTS
Vesicant

- Alopecia
- Anemia
- Asthenia
- Chest pain
- Diarrhea
- Dyspnea
- Fatigue
- Granulocytopenia
- Injection site reaction/pain
- Intestinal obstruction, necrosis, or perforation
- Leukopenia

- Mucositis
- Nausea/vomiting
- Paralytic ileus
- Peripheral neuropathy
- Phlebitis
- Severe constipation
- Thrombocytopenia

NADIR

- Neutrophils: between days 7-10

STORAGE

Unopened Vials/Unreconstituted Powder

- Refrigerate and protect from light.
- Stable at room temperature for up to 72 hours.

Reconstituted Powder or Solution

- Diluted solutions stable up to 24 hours at 5°-30° C (41°-86° F).

MIXING INSTRUCTIONS

- Dilute with 5% dextrose injection or 0.9% sodium chloride injection to a concentration of 1.5-3.0 mg/mL.
- Further dilute for infusion to final concentration of 0.5-2.0 mg/mL.

Product Stability

- Stable for up to 24 hours at room temperature and in standard room lighting if stored in polyvinyl chloride bags or polypropylene syringes.

COMPATIBILITY WITH OTHER DRUGS/INTRAVENOUS FLUIDS

- Compatible with 5% dextrose, 0.45% or 0.9% sodium chloride, Ringer's solution, or Ringer's lactate
- Incompatible with amphotericin B, 5-fluorouracil, furosemide, ampicillin, methylprednisolone, sodium bicarbonate; multiple other drugs (review package insert)

DRUG INTERACTIONS

- May increase myelosuppression when given with other myelosuppressive drugs.
- May produce an acute pulmonary reaction if given with mitomycin C.
- May increase live virus vaccine side effects and decrease body's vaccine antibody response.
- May increase risk of neuropathies if given with or used sequentially with paclitaxel.
- Increased toxicities if given with azole antifungals.

PREGNANCY

Category D
- Do not use while pregnant or nursing.
- Drug is embryotoxic and teratogenic.

SPECIAL CONSIDERATIONS

- Vesicant; manage extravasation per institutional guidelines.
- Bronchospasms and acute shortness of breath may occur in those with underlying pulmonary disease/dysfunction or if receiving concurrent mitomycin C.
- Patient may have profound myelosuppression.

Dose Modification

- Dose should be decreased or held if granulocyte count <1,500 cell/mm³; if three consecutive doses need to be held due to granulocytopenia, vinorelbine should not be restarted.
- Modify dose for hyperbilirubinemia if treatment related.
- Modify dose for neurotoxicity.
- Lethal if given intrathecally

PATIENT EDUCATION

- Have patient notify nurse if any pain, stinging, burning, redness, or swelling occurs during drug administration.
- Instruct patient to practice good oral hygiene.
- Instruct patient to report any signs of bleeding, bruising, infection, fever, shortness of breath, fatigue, or numbness or tingling in fingers and toes.
- Advise patient about possibility of experiencing joint pain for 2-3 days after initiation of therapy, which usually resolves within several days.
- Instruct patient to avoid receiving live vaccines or vaccinations and to refrain from being in crowds or around those with known infections.
- Instruct patient to avoid pregnancy and to use effective contraceptive measures.

BIBLIOGRAPHY

Elsevier. (2006). *The Elsevier guide to oncology drugs and regimens* (pp. 364-366). Huntington, NY: Elsevier Oncology.

Hodgson, B. B., & Kizior, R. J. (2006). *Mosby's 2006 drug consult for nurses* (pp. 346-349). St. Louis: Mosby.

Hughes, T. E. (2005). Vinorelbine (Navelbine). In J. Abraham, C. J. Allegra, & J. Gulley (Eds.). *Bethesda handbook of clinical oncology* (2nd ed., pp. 666-667). Philadelphia: Lippincott Williams & Wilkins.

Kelleher, L. O. (2005). Principles of chemotherapy. In M. Polovich, J. M. White, & L. O. Kelleher (Eds.). *Chemotherapy and biotherapy guidelines and recommendations for practice* (2nd ed., pp. 18-35). Pittsburgh, PA: Oncology Nursing Society.

MedlinePlus. (2003). *Vinorelbine*. Retrieved January 21, 2007, from http://www.nlm.nih.gov/medlineplus/druginfo/uspdi/203542.html.

PDR oncology pocket guide (2nd ed., pp. 54-55). (2005). Montvale, NJ: Thompson PDR.

RxList. (2005). *Navelbine*. Retrieved January 21, 2007, from http://www.rxlist.com/cgi/generic2/vinor.htm.

Spratto, G. R., & Woods, A. L. (2005). *2005 PDR nurses drug handbook* (pp. 1305-1307). Clifton Park, NY: Thomson Delmar Learning.

Vinorelbine. In *Nursing rapid-fire drug facts*. (pp. 597). (2005). Philadelphia: Lippincott Williams & Wilkins.

Wilkes, G. M., & Barton-Burke, M. (2006). *2006 Oncology nursing drug handbook* (pp. 321-324). Sudbury, MA: Jones & Bartlett.

Targeted Therapy

Sandra E. Remer

INTRODUCTION

This chapter is intended to assist oncology nurses to understand a very complex and newer treatment modality: targeted therapies. This newer view of cancer care encompasses the molecular and genetic biology of cancer, thus creating a need for the oncology nurse to understand cancer treatment from basic cell functioning. Nurses must now relearn not only the processes involved in the growth and development of normal and malignant cells but also the processes involved in the signaling pathways. The signaling pathways control all the cellular processes. Relearning these processes will in turn provide the oncology nurse with the information needed to develop more appropriate patient care and effective education for both patients and their families.

One important issue to keep in mind is that none of the signaling pathways works independently of the other pathways. All cells in the human body contain many different receptors on the cell's surface, as well as the surrounding microenvironment, which contains many different ligands (i.e., proteins, enzymes) that are set into motion by various steps produced to regulate the normal processes of growth, differentiation, apoptosis, cell adhesion, and angiogenesis. The receptors remain dormant until a specific ligand binds with the receptor, thus initiating a cascade of intracellular signaling pathways, such as the binding of transforming growth factor (TGF)-alpha with the epidermal growth factor receptor (EGFR). A list of terminology specific to the signaling pathways can be found in the box on page 288. The new targeted therapies enhance current treatments, providing the possibility of survival from a disease that has such widespread impact. A list of approved targeted therapies may be found in the table on page 289.

Historical View

For decades, cancers have been treated with various types of treatment modalities. Surgery, the removal of the tumor or abnormal growth, has been the mainstay for most cancer treatment and has been recorded as far back as 3,000 BCE (Niederhuber, 2000). Surgery not only reduces tumor burden as part of the treatment plan but may also be used as prophylaxis, to determine the histologic diagnosis, in determination of disease stage, to relieve pain, and to eliminate or minimize the symptoms of the disease itself.

Chemotherapy is a drug designed to "kill" cancer cells by interfering with deoxyribonucleic acid (DNA) during some point in the cell cycle. Chemotherapy therefore inhibits tumor cell growth and development or proliferation. Chemotherapy has been in use since the 1950s as either a single agent or in combination with other chemotherapy drugs or other treatment modalities. It is a systemic therapy reaching all areas of the body, affecting healthy cells as well as tumor cells.

Radiation therapy is the use of high-energy radiation sources to destroy cancer cells. Radiation goals are to completely destroy the tumor or to shrink the tumor for symptom control.

All these modalities have their own limitations to improving cancer care. Surgery may not remove all the cancer cells. Microscopic disease may still remain, even with the most all-inclusive resections under highly technical navigational systems. Because neither chemotherapy nor radiation therapy differentiates between healthy and cancerous tissues, they cause a variety of nonspecific toxicities sustained by the healthy normal tissues. Poor tolerance of chemotherapy or radiation therapy may result in subtherapeutic dosing or delays in therapy administration schedules or may even necessitate the discontinuation of therapy completely. Furthermore, toxicities to healthy tissues may prevent dose escalation (Herbst & Shin, 2002). In addition, some cancer cells simply may not respond to treatments because of the cellular ability to repair damage or resist drug therapy by expelling chemotherapeutic agents from the tumor cells (Wood & Muehlbauer, 2003). Despite the advances in surgical technology, the refinements in conventional chemotherapy and radiation and development of newer chemotherapeutic agents, many cancers still remain a challenge. Therefore, the new initiative to attack cancer involves treatment that targets specific cellular processes.

MECHANISM OF ACTION

Normally, cells grow and divide as the body needs them. Old cells die and new ones take their place. However, in cancer, genetic changes take place in which the normal cell death process is lost. Cells are then allowed to grow out of control and not die (apoptosis) when they are supposed to. At the same time, the cancer cells have developed the ability to create a new vascular system within their environments that provides nutrition which promote continual growth of the tumor. Thus, molecular targeted therapies have been developed.

Molecular targeted therapies are a new class of drugs whose goal is directed at blocking any of the signaling processes responsible for the growth and spread of cancer cells.

Targeted therapies work differently from chemotherapy in that they interfere with the specific molecules involved in the process of carcinogenesis, tumor growth, and metastasis. The specific molecule being targeted may be the "switch" that regulates growth and development of the tumor cell or the "switch" that allows the cancer cell to enter the process of apoptosis (Wood & Muehlbauer, 2003).

Additionally, targeted therapies have been directed at several of the other cellular changes specific to cancer cells, such as migration of cancer cells or the development

Targeted Therapy Terminology

Angiogenesis: the process by which new blood vessels form by sprouting from existing blood vessels

Apoptosis: programmed cell death. The normal process by which damaged cells are eliminated. Apoptosis is a tightly controlled process of normal cell function.

Cell-signaling cascades: groups of factors that are linked and pass on messages from the cell surface to the inside of the cell

Comedone: a blackhead, discolored dried sebum plugging an excretory duct of the skin

Cross-talk: the activation of cell signaling pathway without growth factor binding; activation of a receptor by another activated receptor in the absence of ligand binding

Cytokine: a small protein or biological factor that is released by cells and has a specific effect on cell-cell interactions, communication, and behavior of other cells

Cytoplasm: the intracellular portion of a cell where biochemical reactions take place

Degradation: the breaking down of a substance

Dimerization: the reaction of the receptor by the ligand when two monomers (identical molecules) are paired having little structural change

Domain: the functional region or component of a protein

Downstream regulation: changes that take place below the site of a signaling inhibition

Endothelial cells: the cells that line the vascular system. They act as a barrier between the bloodstream and target cells that hormones must pass through to reach their receptors and exert their biological action.

Epidermal growth factor (EGF): one of a family of ligands (growth factors) that bind to receptors, resulting in stimulation of cell growth

Epidermal growth factor receptor (EGFR): a family member composed of four similarly structured transmembrane receptor–tyrosine kinases; activation of these tyrosine kinases is usually dependent on ligand binding to the external portion of the receptor; ErB1 is also referred to as HER-1 (human EGF receptor), and is commonly referred to as EGFR. Other members of this reception family are ErB2 (HER-2/*neu*), ErB3 (HER-3), and ErB4 (HER-4). These receptors are large proteins residing in the cell membrane.

Epidermal growth factor receptor–tyrosine kinase (EGFR-TK): the intracellular (cytoplasm) portion of the EGFR protein; the EGFR-TK domain is essential for signaling transduction.

Expression: proteins of messenger ribonucleic acids that result from transcription and translation of specific genes

Extracellular matrix (ECM): the material that surrounds cells. Important regulatory molecules in the extracellular matrix promote, inhibit, or guide growth of cells.

Genetic alteration: changes in the instruction makeup of a cell that can cause a disruption in its signaling process so that the cell no longer grows and divides normally or dies when it should

Growth factor: a substance made by the body that functions to regulate cell division and cell survival. It is produced by normal cells during embryonic development, tissue growth, and wound healing.

Heterodimerization: the pairing of two different (hetero) receptors

Homodimerization: the pairing of two of the same (homo) receptors

Integrins: cell surface proteins that bind to extracellular matrix components

Keratin: a protein that helps keep the skin hydrated by preventing water evaporation. It can also absorb water, further aiding hydration.

Keratinocytes: cells of the hair, nails, and skin

Kinase: an enzyme that catalyzes transfer of a phosphate molecule from adenosine triphosphate (ATP) to an acceptor molecule resulting in a cascade of kinase-mediated activation reactions

Ligand: a molecule such as growth factor that binds to another molecule and activate receptors on the surface of a cell

Ligand binding: the process by which the ligand attaches itself to a specific receptor on the cell surface and activates the receptor, initiating the signaling pathway

Lymphocytic perifolliculitis: a lymphocytic (white blood cell) inflammation surrounding hair follicle

Malignant: cancerous, a cell/mass that divides and grows without control and order

Matrix metalloproteinases (MMP): a family of proteins that dissolve (degrade) the extracellular matrix ahead of sprouting of vessels

Monomer: a single receptor in an inactivated state, a molecule of protein

Oncogene: mutated or overexpressed version of a normal gene that can release the cell from normal restraints on growth and promote or allow continuous growth and division, converting a cell into a tumor cell

Papulopustular eruption: a small circumscribed superficial elevation of the skin containing pus, elevation of the skin with an inflamed base or a pimple

Paronychial: an acute of chronic infection of the folds of skin surrounding the nail

Pericytes: cells associated with the wall of small blood vessels; neither smooth muscle cells nor endothelial cells

Phosphorylation: the creation or generation of free phosphorus that results from an ATP molecule binging to the tyrosine receptor site on the intracellular portion of the receptor

Proteases: enzymes that aid in the breakdown of proteins in the body

Receptor: a structure on the outside or inside of a cell (cell membrane protein) that selectively binds to a specific drug, hormone, or chemical mediators to alter cell function

Signaling pathway: a series of interdependent proteins responsible for transmitting growth signals to the nucleus of the cell

Targeted therapy: an anticancer agent used to block a specific cellular cycle or pathway. The goal of targeted therapy is to prevent replication or invasion while preserving normal cells as a result of reduced toxicity

Transcription: the process by which DNA passes genetic information to ribonucleic acid (RNA). Transcription is the first step in producing proteins. The transfer of the genetic information on a gene from a molecule of DNA to a molecule of messenger RNA.

Transmembrane: refers to across the cell membrane or through the cell membrane

Tumorigenesis: the change of a normal cell into tumor cells

Tumor suppressor gene: a normal gene that signals the cell to slow down growth and division

Tyrosine kinase: an enzyme that catalyzes the transfer of a phosphate molecule from adenosine triphosphate (ATP) to a tyrosine residue in proteins

Tyrosine kinase receptor: the intracellular portion of the EGFR. Activation of the TK receptor stimulates several events (proliferation, invasion, angiogenesis, metastasis, and inhibition of apoptosis)

Upstream regulation: changes that take place above the site of a signaling inhibition

Vascular endothelial growth factor (VEGF): a growth factor essential to angiogenesis; binds to receptors on endothelial cells

Data from *CancerWeb Project on-line dictionary.* (1997-2007). Center for Cancer Education, University of Newcastle-upon-Tyne: http://cancerweb.ncl.ac.uk/cgi-bin/; National Cancer Institute Web site: http://cancer.gov/cancertopics; Esper, P., & Knoop, T. (2005). *Current topics in colorectal cancer—targeting VEGF for oncology nurses.* Institute for Medical Education & Research: www.imeronline.com, Project ID:04 2605 ES16; McCorkle, M., Gailoto, M., Oestreicher, P., Barkley, D. (2005). *Targeted therapies in non-small cell cancer* (pp. 1-32). Pittsburgh, PA: Oncology Education Service; Wujcik, D., & Thomas, M. (2005). *Current topics in colorectal cancer—targeting EGFR for oncology nurses.* Institute for Medical Education & Research: www.imeronline.com, Project ID: 2735 ES 16.

Summary of Targeted Therapies Currently Food and Drug Administration Approved or in Clinical Development

EGFR Inhibitors	PDGFR Inhibitors	VEGFR Inhibitors	PKC Inhibitors	EGFR-TK Inhibitors	VEGFR-TK Inhibitors
Gefitinib (Iressa oral) ZD1839	Imatinib mesylate (Gleevec) (oral)	Valatanib	Tamoxifen	Gefitinib Oral ZD1839	SU5416 (semaxanib)
Erlotinib (Tarceva) oral	PTK787/ZK-222584 (oral)	Sorafenib (nexavar) (oral)	Enzastaurin (LY317615)	Erlotinib (Tarceva) oral	PTK787/ZK-222584 (oral)
Lapatinib (GW572016) AEE778 ZD6474 (Zactima) EKB569	SU011248 Sunitinib (oral) Sutent Raf kinase inhibitor Sorafenib oral(Nexavar) (BAY 43-9006)	Sunitinib Sutent (oral) SU011248 AEE788 AZD2171 ZD6474 (Zactima) CEP-7055		CI-1033 (canertinib) PKI-166 GW572016 (lapatinib)	
Cetuximab (Erbitux) Panitumumab					

Many drugs affect multiple targets. *EGF*, Epidermal growth factor; *EGFR*, EGF receptor; *PDGFR*, platelet-derived growth factor receptor; *PKC*, protein kinase C; *VEGF*, vascular endothelial growth factor; *VEGFR*, VEGF receptor.

Cetuximab (Erbitux):Anti-EGFR monoclonal antibody, ImClone Systems, Inc. New York, NY; Zactima (ZD6474), AstraZeneca Pharmaceuticals; BAY 43-9006, Sorafenib Oral-Nexavar, Bayer Pharmaceuticals Corporation, West Haven, CT, and Onyx Pharmaceuticals, Emeryville, CA; Iressa and AZD2171, AstraZeneca Pharmaceuticals, Wilmington, DE; CEP-7055, Sanofi-Aventis, Bridgewater, NJ; Tarceva, OSI Pharmaceuticals; Tarrytown, NY/Genentech, South San Francisco, CA; Gleevec,- Novartis Pharmaceuticals Corp; East Hanover, NJ; PTK787/ZK, 222584, Novartis Pharmaceutical Corp and Schering AG Corp.; Enzastaurin (LY317615), Eli Lilly and Company, Indianapolis; GW572016 (Lapatinib), GlaxoSmithKline, Middlesex, United Kingdom; EBK569, Wyeth, Madison, NJ; CI-1033 (canertinib), Pfizer, New York, NY; panitumumab (ABX-EGF) fully human monoclonal antibody, Amgen, Inc., Thousand Oaks, CA.

Data from Janmaat & Giaccone, 2003; Marques & McCreery, 2003; Perez-Soler & Saltz, 2005;Reardon & Wen, 2006; Segaert & Van Cutsem, 2005; Vlahovic & Crawford, 2003).

of new blood vessels. Because targeted therapies focus on specific molecules or cellular changes, they may be more effective and less harmful to normal cells than other modalities currently available. The benefit of target therapy is a reduction in treatment-related side effects and improvement in quality of life. Targeted therapies are used alone or in combination with other chemotherapeutic agents.

The combination of a molecular targeted therapy and radiation therapy is another promising therapeutic option. Overactivity of the EGFR pathway is associated with radiation resistance. Therefore, combination therapy may increase the effectiveness of radiation (Baumann & Krause, 2004). Because each type of cancer involves a different set of genes and proteins involved in growth and spread, targeted therapies used to control each type of cancer are different. Once tumors can be more accurately classified by molecular and genetic mutations, treatments may then be modified to the individual tumor. The most effective treatment may very well combine the previous modalities of surgery, radiation, and chemotherapy with the newer molecular targeted therapies. The concept of targeted therapies has rapidly expanded just within the last 3 to 5 years and targeted therapies have now become one of the most exciting treatment modalities entering the field of oncology.

ANTIANGIOGENESIS

Angiogenesis is a naturally occurring process in the human body throughout growth and development and

Angiogenesis Inhibitors

PROTEINS
Angiostatin
Endostatin
Interferons
Platelet factor 4
Prolactin 16-kd fragment
Thrombospondin
TIMP-1 (tissue inhibitor of metalloproteinase-1)
TIMP-2 (tissue inhibitor of metalloproteinase-2)
TIMP-3 (tissue inhibitor of metalloproteinase-3)

Data from National Cancer Institute Web site: http://cancer:gove/cancertopics/understandingcancer; Rosen, L.S. (2005). VEGF-targeted therapy: therapeutic potential and recent advances. *The Oncologist, 10*, 382-391. Available at www.TheOncologist.com.

specific times during adult life. For the period of embryo development, vasculogenesis is the process that creates the primary network of vascular endothelial cells that become the major vessels (Ferrara, 2004; National Cancer Institute, 2006). Angiogenesis continues throughout fetal development, transforming the new blood vessels and capillaries into a completed circulatory system. From this point and throughout the adult human life the vascular system is generally associated with maintenance controlled by angiogenesis inhibitors. (See the box above for a list of angiogenesis inhibitors.) In the adult, new vessel formation is infrequent and generally associated with the repair of tissue during wound healing and cardiovascular injury (Wood, Sandler, & Muehlbauer, 2005). In women, angiogenesis is also active a few days each month with the formation of new blood vessels in the lining of the uterus during the menstrual cycle.

Angiogenesis is responsible for the maintenance of the vascular system that controls the delivery of oxygen and nutrients with a corresponding elimination of metabolic waste and carbon dioxide. Oxygen and nutrients are necessary for growth, maintenance, and survival of tissues supplied by the vasculature system. (See the figure below.)

Angiogenesis is defined as the process by which new blood vessels form by sprouting from existing blood vessels (Wujcik & Thomas, 2005). *Tumor angiogenesis* is the development of blood vessels that are structurally and functionally abnormal. Both normal physiological and tumor angiogenesis are regulated by a variety of growth factors in their microenvironments. See the boxes on page 289 and right for a designation of inhibitors and activators of angiogenesis. These agents are needed to support the cellular microenvironment of the vascular system.

The microenvironment surrounding the cell is very specific for each type of tissue throughout the human body. Proteins located within the microenvironment perform important activities for the cell. Proteins are needed for the extracellular matrix to physically support the cell structure. Proteins can alter the behavior of the cell's matricellular proteins, growth factors, and proteases through interaction with membrane receptors (growth factor receptors, proteases) and adhesion proteins (such as integrins).

Other biological functions including extracellular matrix breakdown, proliferation, apoptosis, angiogenesis, and motility are influenced by the reactions created when signals from within the microenvironment influence the ligand binding on the cell surface, creating a signaling cascade inside the cell to the nucleus where the gene transcription is altered and cell functions change (Rempel & Mikkelsen, 2006).

EGFR and vascular endothelial growth factor (VEGF) signaling pathways are two components that play a major role in the process of angiogenesis and the growth and spread of cancer cells. (See the figure on page 291.)

VEGF (a cytokine), as it is commonly called, is also known as VEGF-A. It stimulates vascular endothelial cell growth, survival, and proliferation. It plays a significant role in the development of new blood vessels (angiogenesis). VEGF is a member of a family of six structurally related proteins (see table on page 291) that regulate the growth and differentiation of multiple components of the vascular

Activators of Angiogenesis

PROTEINS
Acidic fibroblast growth factor
Angiogenin
Basic fibroblast growth factor (bFGF)
Epidermal growth factor (EGF)
Granulocyte colony-stimulating factor
Hepatocyte growth factor
Interleukin-8
Placental growth factor (PGF)
Platelet-derived endothelial growth factor (PDEGF)
Scatter factor
Transforming growth factor-alpha
Tumor necrosis factor-alpha
Vascular endothelial growth factor (VEGF)

SMALL MOLECULES
Adenosine
1-Butyryl glycerol
Nicotinamide
Postaglandins E1 and E2

Data from National Cancer Institute Web site: http://cancer.gov/cancer-topics/understandingcancer; Retrieved 02/10/2007 Ferrara, N. (2004). Vascular endothelial growth factor as a target for anticancer therapy. *The Oncologist, 9*(suppl 1), 2-10: www.TheOncologist.com; Rosen, L. S. (2005). VEGF-targeted therapy: therapeutic potential and recent advances. *The Oncologist,. 10*, pp 382-391: www.TheOncologist.com.

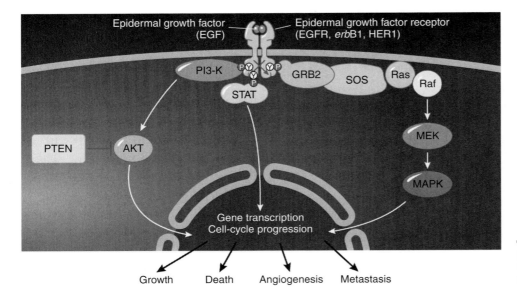

Pathophysiology of Tumor Angiogenesis

The growth of a tumor is dependent on its vascular supply. Absorption of oxygen and nutrients is possible only within 1 to 2 mm of the tumor borders (co-opting or appropriating vessels from the surrounding tissue); therefore, further growth requires a process through which new vessels develop toward the tumor (Ferrara, 2004; Rosen, 2005).

Endothelial cells, the primary building blocks of vessels, are the cells that line the walls of blood vessels. The endothelial cell has the extraordinary ability to divide and migrate; however, most of the time the endothelial cell remains dormant. The formation of new vessels involves the recruitment of circulating endothelial cells.

Many factors activate angiogenesis, with hypoxia being an important stimulator of tumor angiogenesis (Carmeliet, 2003; Wood & Muehlbauer, 2003).

When a tumor can no longer obtain an adequate supply of oxygen and nutrients, its cellular environment secretes increased amounts of VEGF through up-regulation into the surrounding tissue while at the same time down-regulating proteins that inhibit angiogenesis within the tumor and its

microenvironment. This activation is referred to as the angiogenic switch. VEGF then binds to the appropriate receptor on the endothelial cell surface, activating the tyrosine kinase (TK) portion located inside the cell, which in turn initiates the signaling pathway. The signaling pathway then transmits a series of molecules (proteins) to the nucleus, where gene transcription is altered causing the stimulation of new endothelial cell growth. The extracellular matrix is degraded (broken down) so that the endothelial cells are able to invade the matrix (migrate through the capillary basement membrane) and begin to divide and proliferate. As the endothelial cells divide, they form a string of the endothelial cells, which then forms a hollow tube, creating a new network of blood vessels, making tissue growth and repair possible.

These new structures are tortuous, leaky, less organized, and less stable than normal blood vessels (Jain, 2001). These leaky, less stable vessels enhance the permeability of the vasculature and then increase migration and proliferation of the endothelial cells, thus providing the pathway for metastasis. In his article on normalizing tumor vasculature, Jain has also suggested that blocking of VEGF and its receptor leads to apoptosis (programmed cell death) of the endothelial cells and a decrease in vessel diameter, density, and permeability, which decreases interstitial fluid pressure and in some tumors increases oxygen tension, thus improving the microenvironment of the tumor. This in turn would allow not only for improved delivery of nutrients but also of increased delivery of therapeutic agents (Jain, 2001).

Other triggers of VEGF expression include the following (Esper & Knoop, 2005; Ferarra, 2004; Ferarra, Gerber, & LeCouter, 2003; Hicklin & Ellis, 2005; Wood & Muehlbauer, 2003):

- EGFR (HER-1) activation associated with solid tumors such as breast, lung, colorectal, prostate, renal cell, and ovarian
- Human epidermal receptor (HER-2) overexpression associated with VEGF production in colon, pancreatic, gastric, breast, renal cell, non–small cell lung cancer, and glioblastoma multiforme
- Insulin-like growth factor 1 receptor, which is also associated with increased VEGF production in

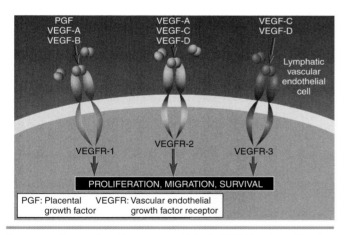

Targeting Tumor Vasculature. Copyright © 2007 Oncology Nursing Society. Reprinted with permission.

Vascular Endothelial Growth Factor Family Receptors and Functions

VEGF Family	Receptors	Functions
VEGF (VEGF-A)	VEGFR-1, VEGFR-2, neuropilin-1	Angiogenesis, vascular maintenance
VEGF-B	VEGFR-1	Not established
VEGF-C	VGFR-2, VGFR-3	Lymphangiogenesis
VEGF-D	VGFR-2, VGFR-3	Lymphangiogenesis
VEGF-E (viral factor)	VGFR-2	Angiogenesis
PLGF (placental growth factor)	VGFR-1, neuropilin-1	Angiogenesis and inflammation

VEGF, Vascular endothelial growth factor.
Data from Carmeliet, 2003; Ferrara, Gerber, & LeCouter, 2003; Hicklin & Ellis, 2005.

system, especially blood and lymph vessels. It is also known as for its permeability activity.

breast, endometrial, pancreatic, and colorectal cancers

Oncogenes and tumor suppressor genes are associated with increased production of VEGF, as described in the table VEGF on tumors on page 291. A few of these include C-Src, which regulates VEGF expression and promotes neovascularization in existing tumors; BCR-ABL oncogenes have been identified as having a key role in the pathogenesis of leukemia, which are considered angiogenesis-dependent malignancies; the Ras oncogene is associated with increased VEGF production in pancreatic, colon, and non–small cell lung cancer; and the p53 tumor suppressor gene is also found in solid tumors such as colorectal, breast, and endometrial cancer and astrocytomas. The gene functions as the regulator of the cell cycle on DNA damage-inducing apoptosis when the damage is beyond repair (Esper & Knoop, 2005; Ferarra, 2004; Ferrara, Gerber, & LeCouter, 2003; Hicklin & Ellis, 2005; Wood & Muehlbauer, 2003).

Two other mechanisms for the activation of VEGF expression are the link between the prostaglandin cyclooxygenase 2 in several solid tumors including gastric, colon, prostate, breast, and pancreas and the platelet-derived growth factor in the regulation of host-derived VEGF for sustaining angiogenesis (Esper & Knoop, 2005; Ferrara, 2004; Ferrara, Gerber, & LeCouter, 2003; Hicklin & Ellis, 2005; Wood & Muehlbauer, 2005).

EPIDERMAL GROWTH FACTOR

One of the first molecules to be identified was the epidermal growth factor receptor (EGFR) and its ligands, epidermal growth factor (EGF) and TGF-alpha by Nobel Laureate Dr. Stanley Cohen in the 1960s (Mendelsohn, 2001; Wujcik & Thomas, 2005).

The autocrine mechanism, involving autostimulation of EGF receptors on the surface of cancer cells by TGF-alpha,

which cancer cells produce, was described in a landmark paper by Drs. Michael Sporn and George Todar in 1980. In 1981, Chinkers and Cohen published an article depicting that the EGFRs and the *src* oncogene product have the novel enzymatic activity of a TK (Mendelsohn, 2001; Mendelsohn & Baselga, 2000).

Since that time, other members of the EGFR (HER receptor family, naturally occurring cell-membrane bound protein receptors) have been identified. EGFR is known as HER-1 (*erb*B1). The other family members are HER-2 (*erb*B2), discovered in 1985, HER-3 (*erb*B3), and HER-4 (*erb*B4). (See the EGFR family figure below.)

In addition, kinases (serine, threonine, and tyrosine), also discovered in the 1980s, play a significant role in a variety of cellular processes such as growth and differentiation. EGFR (HER-1) and HER-2 are the two most highly studied and well understood of the family. These proteins are found on the surface or inside of most normal cells and are overexpressed in many cancers. See the table on EGFR overexpression in tumors on page 293.

The EGF/HER molecule is a membrane-bound protein that structurally is divided into three distinctive regions. Region 1 is the extracellular ligand-binding region located on the outside of the cell, region 2 is the transmembrane lipophilic section that spans the cell membrane and holds the receptor to the cell, and region 3 is the intracellular (cytoplasmic) region, which has TK activity and regulatory function, as seen in the figure on page 293. Each region plays an important role in cell function, growth, and interaction for the development and metastasis of malignant tumors.

In normal cells, EGFR signaling is very tightly controlled; however, oncogenic activation of this pathway occurs as a result of EGFR mutation, overexpression, structural rearrangements of genes, or release of its normal autoinhibitory and regulatory constraints (Ritter & Arteaga, 2003).

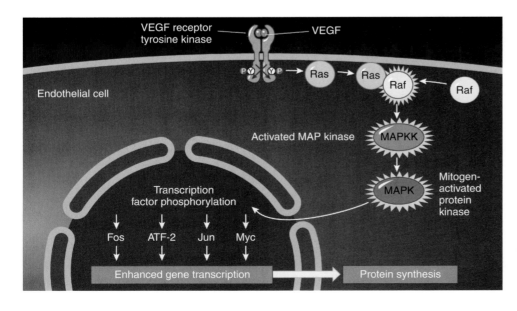

HER Family of Receptors. Copyright © 2006 Oncology Nursing Society. Reprinted with permission.

EPIDERMAL GROWTH FACTOR—TYROSINE KINASE

The EGFR is a 170-kd cell membrane protein structurally composed of an extracellular ligand-binding domain, a transmembrane domain, and an intracellular TK domain.

EGFR is a TK of the *erb*B family that is commonly altered in epithelial tumors. EGFR-TK, as seen in the table on page 294, is overexpressed or abnormally activated in most common solid tumors, including non–small cell lung, breast, prostate, colon, pancreatic, gastric, head and neck, and ovarian cancer and gliomas.

The primary ligands that bind to the extracellular domain are EGF and TGF-alpha, both playing significant roles in epidermal cell biology. TK activity is central in signal transduction, acting as a relay for an intricate network of interdependent signaling molecules that ultimately affects gene transcription within the nucleus (Marques & McCreery, 2003; Pao & Miller, 2005; Pizzo, 2004; Vlahovic & Crawford, 2003).

Epidermal Growth Factor Receptor Overexpression in Solid Tumors

Tumor Type EGFR (%)	Frequency of Overexpression in Solid Tumors
Hereditary small cell lung cancer	80%-100%
Non–small cell lung cancer	40%-80%
Prostate	40%-70%
Glioma	40%-63%
Gastric	25%-77%
Breast	14%-91%
Colorectal	25%-77%
Pancreatic	30%-50%
Ovarian	35%-70%
Renal cell carcinoma	50%-90%
Bladder	31%-48%

EGFR, Epidermal growth factor receptor.
Data from Ciardiello & Tortora, 2002; Herbst & Shin, 2002; Salomon et al., 1995.

EGFR-TK activity in the normal cell is strictly controlled, allowing only limited cell growth for the processes of maintenance and repair. In tumor activity, EGFR-TK activation contributes to tumor development and progression, by means of proliferation, differentiation, invasion, metastases, and inhabitation of apoptosis (Marques & McCreery, 2003; Pao & Miller, 2005; Pizzo, 2004; Vlahovic & Crawford, 2003). It also influences tumor angiogenesis by upstream regulation of VEGF and interleukin-8. Additionally, cross-talk with other signaling molecules, such as G protein–coupled receptors and integrins, increases the range of impact EGFR-TK (Prenzel et al., 2001).

Approximately 90 TKs have been identified, 58 of which are the transmembrane receptor type and 32 the cytoplasmic nonreceptor type (Blume-Jensen & Hunter, 2001; Vlahovic & Crawford, 2003). The nonreceptor type of TK is found in the cytoplasm of the cell lacking the transmembrane domain segment and functions downstream of the receptor tyrosine kinases. Bcr-Abl fusion protein and c-Scrc are examples of nonreceptor TKs. Bcr-Abl is the fusion protein created by the chromosomal translocation that generates the Philadelphia chromosome found in some forms of leukemia, and c-Scrc is a TK implicated in control of cell division, production of autocrine growth factors, cell survival response, and cell motility. c-Scrc was the first oncogene to be discovered and the first TK (Courtneidge, 2002).

Activation of the receptor occurs when a ligand, either the EGF or the TGF-alpha, binds to the extracellular domain on the cell surface, resulting in dimerization with either another EGFR protein or another ErbB receptor; ErbB-2 is the preferred partner (Janmaat & Giaccone, 2003). This dimerization triggers autophosphorylation of TK at the intracellular domain segment, activating appropriate downstream signaling molecules. EGFR-activated pathways include Akt and signal transducer and activator of

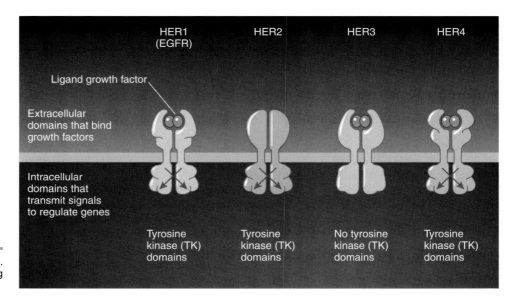

Epidermal Growth Factor Receptor–Tyrosine Kinase Overexpression in Human Solid Tumors

Tumor	% of Overexpression
Non–small cell lung cancer	40-80
Prostate	40
Head and neck (squamous cell cancer)	80-100
Colorectal	25-77
Breast	14-91
Ovarian	35-70
Pancreatic	30-50
Gastric	33
Glioblastoma	>60

Data from Hanahan & Weinberg, 2000; Marques & McCreery, 2003; Reardon & Wen, 2006; Souliers et al., 2004.

of transcription cascades important for cell survival and the mitogen-activated protein pathway, which induces proliferation. EGFR can also be activated by stimuli that do not directly bind to the receptor (nonreceptor) such as hormones, lymphokines, and stress factors (Pao & Miller, 2005).

High expression levels or mutations, as well as other potential mechanisms, can provoke abnormal EGFR-TK activity such as ligand overexpression, heterodimerization with other ErbB members, especially HER-2, and transactivation by heterologous signaling networks. This combined with the ability of EGFR-TK to affect tumor growth, including cell proliferation, angiogenesis, invasion, metastases, and survival, provides a rationale for inhibition of EGFR-TK as an anticancer therapy (Janmaat & Giaccone, 2003; Mendelsohn, 2001; Mendelsohn & Baselga, 2000).

The number of biological agents being developed for treating cancer is growing. Agents targeting the EGFR/HER-1 are receiving primary consideration because the EGFR/HER-1 and TK molecules are overexpressed in 30% to 100% of all solid tumor types. Some of the tumor cells producing an overexpression of EGFR also produce a high level of their corresponding ligands, creating an autocrine activation loop that is thought to promote independent tumor growth (Perez-Soler & Saltz, 2005). In addition, overexpression of EGFR activity is often correlated with chemoresistance and poor survival in patients with these tumors (Herbst & Shin, 2002; Perez-Soler & Saltz, 2005; Segaert & VanCutsem, 2005).

TOXICITIES

This new class of drug has a more promising safety profile with fewer of the nonspecific toxicities than standard chemotherapy and generally does not exert an effect on the hematopoietic system. The change in the type and degree of toxicity makes targeted therapy an effective agent for use as a primary treatment or in combination therapy with other treatment modalities. Some of the common side effects of this new class of drug are rash, nail and hair changes, xerosis, diarrhea, ophthalmological toxicity, interstitial lung disease, infusion reactions, and drug interactions. See the individual drug monographs for specific toxicities.

Rash

Papulopustular eruptions are one of the most common side effects of the EGFR inhibitors, although little is known about the etiology and pathophysiology of the rash. The rash (folliculitis) develops primarily on the face, neck, shoulders, and upper torso. The rash is characterized by interfollicular and intrafollicular papulopustules, usually occurring within the first 2 weeks of treatment. The rash affects approximately two thirds of patients being treated with EGFR inhibitor agents. The rash is generally mild to moderate, although there have been some reports of severe rashes. The rash is generally considered dose dependent and usually resolves after the discontinuation of treatment or with treatment interruptions (often within 1-2 weeks). However, the rash may spontaneously clear up despite therapy continuation.

Currently the EGFR rash is classified according to Common Toxicity Criteria from the National Cancer Institute. This criterion categorizes rashes according to whether patients are symptomatic from the rash, how much of the body is affected by the rash, and whether there is a need for some type of management intervention. How much of the body affected is considered either localized (<50% of the body) or spread (>50% of the body). One of the main problems with this type of classification system is that the dermatological reactions are not commonly seen with the use of standard chemotherapy. Therefore, the grading scale does not accurately depict the true nature of the EGFR inhibitor rash.

Because the EGFR rash has a pustular appearance, it is often compared with acne vulgaris. The EGFR-related rash has been called acneiforme-like skin reaction, acneiforme follicular rash, maculopapular skin rash, and monomorphic pustular lesion (Dick & Crawford, 2005; Perez-Soler & Saltz, 2005; Marques & McCreery, 2003; Perez-Solar et al., 2005; Segaert & Van Cutsem, 2005; Shah et al., 2005). The distinguishing feature separating the EGFR rash from acne vulgaris is the lack of comedones (blackheads or whiteheads); therefore, these descriptive names should not be used.

Pathophysiology of Rash. The actual etiology of this type of rash is not yet completely understood. It is well known, however, that EGFR/HER-1 is expressed in epidermal and follicular keratinocytes, sebaceous epithelium, and various other epithelial and connective tissue cells. These are the known areas for reactions. The largest study of the EGFR rash to date was presented by Busam and colleagues in 2001. The rash was characterized by lymphocytic perifolliculitis or suppurative superficial folliculitis, without an infectious etiology and the rash happened as a result of the follicular rupture. Histologic inspection of the rash revealed that sebaceous (oil) glands were not affected and there was no presence of microcomedones or comedones.

Sterile neutrophils were noted within the follicle along with a strong inflammatory element. As more targeted therapies are developed and used, more accurate descriptions and classification of these rashes will lead to a better understanding of the rash's etiology, thus providing a comprehensive pathway to specific treatment. Management of this rash is crucial to the quality of life for patients. Should the rash not be properly managed, quality of life may cause premature discontinuation of treatment.

Management of Rash. In 2004, the HER-1/EGFR Inhibitor Rash Management Forum made many recommendations for caring for the patient with an EGFR rash. The forum also put together recommendations for the investigation of additional treatments for the rash. It is critical to continuously review the literature to effectively manage the symptoms patients are discussing with their health care providers.

Currently EGFR rashes are treated symptomatically. In addition to the rash itself, patients may also have erythema, dry skin, itching, and a burning sensation (Lacouture et al., 2006). Complications such as herpes zoster and secondary infections may also occur. Patients should be referred to a dermatologist for the following:

- Atypical rash
- Symptoms of infection
- Necrosis
- Blistering
- Petechia

Patients should also be instructed that the rash is not an allergic rash and to notify their physicians as soon as a rash develops.

Because the EGFR rash is unlike acne, the use of a makeup to hide the rash will not make it worse. A dermatologist-approved brand of makeup may be used; however, most water-based foundations are acceptable. (See the box, right for product recommendations.) Makeup should be removed with a gentle hypoallergenic cleanser such as those listed below.

To prevent further dryness of the skin, products containing alcohol or benzoyl peroxide should be avoided because these will dry the skin, making it worse. Patients should be encouraged to use emollients to alleviate skin dryness, applying them after showering. Tepid water will increase absorption of the emollients. Mild nonperfumed skin cleansers such as Basis soap, Ivory, Dove, or Neutrogena should be used during showering. Patients should avoid direct sunlight. Use of a sun block and hats and protective clothing is recommended when outdoors. Sun blocks should be reapplied frequently.

Painful rashes may be treated with standard analgesics. Patients should be encouraged to discuss the pain with their physicians. For itching, medications such as diphenhydramine or hydroxyzine hydrochloride may be used. However, their effectiveness is considered minimal. Typical low-potency corticosteroids may also be considered.

Product Recommendations for Epidermal Growth Factor Receptor Skin Rash

MILD SOAPS AND CLEANSERS
- Basis
- Neutrogena
- Cetaphil
- Dove
- Ivory Skin Cleansing Liquid-Gel
- Aveeno Shower Gel

MAKEUP
- Dermablend makeup
- Hypoallergenic brands of makeup (i.e., Almay, Clinique)

SUNSCREEN
- AntiHelios Sunscreen

EMOLLIENTS FOR DRY SKIN
- Eucerin Cream
- Eucerin Dry Skin Therapy
- Cetaphil cream
- Aquaphor healing ointment
- Bag Balm
- Udderly Smooth Udder Cream
- Zim's Crack Cream products
- Neutrogena Norwegian Formula Cream (hand/body)
- Vaseline Intensive Care Advanced Healing Lotion

PRURITUS
- Gold Bond powder
- Aveeno baths
- Sween cream
- Benadryl (diphenhydramine) lotion or oral tablets (25 mg) every 6 hours

CRACKS AND FISSURES
- Band-Aid Brand Liquid Bandage applied into cracks/fissures to relieve pain and promote healing
- Bag Balm for soothing fissures on palms of hands and sole of feet
- Zim's Crack Cream products
- Aquaphor healing ointment
- Products available at most local drug stores or pharmacies

Data from Culkin. (2006); Dick, A. E., & Crawford, G. H. (2005). Managing cutaneous side effects of epidermal growth factor receptor (HER1/EGFR) inhibitors. *Community Oncology, 2*, 492-496; Halpern & Agero (2006); Peréz-Soler, R., Delord, J. P., Halpern, A., Kelly, K., Krueger, J., Sureda, B. M., et al. (2005). HER1/EGFR inhibitor-associated rash: future directions for management and investigation outcomes from the HER1/EFGR inhibitor rash management forum. *The Oncologist, 10*, 345-356.

Recommendations have been made for the prophylactic use of intranasal mupirocin daily to prevent secondary infections (Culkin, 2006; Dick & Crawford, 2005; Perez-Soler et al., 2005). If a secondary infection develops, the use of antibiotics is based on the bacterial strain, and cultures should be obtained. A short course of oral antibiotics such as tetracycline or doxycycline is indicated. These antibiotics are used for their anti-inflammatory property and coverage of *Staphylococcus aureus*, one of the most common skin infections. Signs of an *S. aureus* infection are yellowish-brown crust overlying the inflammatory lesions with significant fluid oozing from the lesion. Topical clindamycin, pimecrolimus (Elidel), or tacrolimus (Protopic) may also be applied.

See Section Seven for patient education material for common skin conditions caused by targeted treatment.

Nail Changes

Nail changes refer to paronychia, which is an inflammation of the lateral nail folds. This usually occurs in a delayed fashion between 4 weeks to 6 months with a medium onset of 2 months after the start of therapy. Incidence is between 6% and 50% of patients being treated with EGFR inhibitors. Patients present with painful, erythematous, and edematous lateral nail folds, ingrown nails, and proliferation of granulation tissue. Fungal cultures are routinely negative; however, bacterial cultures may show the presence of *S. aureus*. Treatment with antibiotic therapy will be necessary to prevent further complications. Paronychial inflammation may interfere with activities of daily living. Patients should be advised to avoid tight-fitting shoes, pushing back the cuticles around the nail beds, clipping nails too short, and biting nails. When nail lesions are severe, application of silver nitrate, antiseptic soaks, and cushioning may also be recommended.

Hair Alterations

Alterations in the hair of patients treated with EGFR inhibitors are less common than the rash and are generally not seen until 2 to 3 months after the start of therapy. The common complaint is that of brittle, finer, and curly hair, with frontal alopecia gradually developing. Progressive growth of facial hair and eyelashes may be particularly noticeable in some female patients. Trichomegaly of eyelashes may be seen and will need to be trimmed with scissors if too long. Unwanted facial hair may be cosmetically treated with wax depilation or electrolysis.

Xerosis

Dry skin is very common side effect of EGFR inhibitors. The mechanism for xerosis is similar to dry skin associated with the use of retinoids. Dry skin on the fingertips may result in painful fissures. Treatment with emollients containing 5% to 10% urea or 10% salicylic acid is recommended. Patients should be advised to avoid alcohol-containing lotions and gels and hot baths and showers, which tend to cause drying. Measures should be taken to avoid the development of folliculitis. Acral erythema has also been seen 2 to 4 weeks after treatment with EGFR inhibitors, appears to be dose dependent, then disappears after therapy is stopped. Acral erythema presents as painful symmetrical erythematous and edematous areas on the palms and soles, similar to the "hand-foot syndrome" with the use of some chemotherapy agents. There may be paresthesias which can be aggravated by warmth. Although the palms and soles are the most common sites, other areas of the body may be affected. The use of mild soaps and shower gel and skin care products that promote and maintain hydration is indicated; see box on page 295 for recommendations.

CONCLUSION

Nursing knowledge of mechanism of action, potential side effects, and symptom management for targeted therapy will impact patient outcomes. Thorough nursing care involves adequate teaching about targeted therapy, prompt recognition of side effects, and evidence-based treatment recommendations. Informed nurses will promote quality of life for patients undergoing treatment with targeted therapy.

BIBLIOGRAPHY

Agero, A.L., Dusza, S.W., Benvenuto-Andrade, C., et al. (2006). Dermatologic side effects associated with the epidermal growth factor receptor inhibitors. *Journal of American Academy of Dermatology, 55* (4), 657-670.

Areteaga, C.L. (2001). The epidermal growth factor receptor: From mutant oncogene in nonhuman cancers to therapeutic target in human neoplasia. *Journal of Clinical Oncology, 19*, 32s-40s.

Baumann, M., & Krause, M. (2004). Targeting the epidermal growth factor receptor in radiotherapy: Radiobiological mechanisms, preclinical and clinical results. *Radiotherapy Oncology, 72*, 257-266.

Blume-Jensen, P. & Hunter, T. (2001). Oncogenic kinase signaling. *Nature, 411* (6835), 355-365.

Busam, K.J., Capodieci, P., Motzer, R. et al. (2001). Cutaneous side effects in cancer patients treated with antiepidermal growth factor receptor antibody C225. *British Journal of Dermatology, 144*, 1169-1176.

Carmeliet, P. (2003). Angiogenesis in health and disease. *Natural Medicine, 9*, 653-660.

Chinkers, M. & Cohen, S. (1981). Purified EGF receptor-kinase interacts specifically antibioties to Rous sarcoma virus transforming protein. *Nature, 290* (5806), 516-519.

Ciardiello, F., & Tortora, G. (2002). Anti-epidermal growth factor receptor drugs in cancer therapy. *Expert Opinion on Investigational Drugs, 11*, 755-768.

Cohen, S. (1962). Isolation of a mouse submaxillary gland protein accelerating incisor eruption and eyelid opening in the new born animal. *Journal of Biological Chemistry, 237*, 1555-1562.

Courtneidge, S.A. (2002). Role of Src in signal transduction pathways. *Biochemical Society Transactions, 30* (part 2), 11-17.

Culkin, A. (2006). Nursing management: questions and answers. In *Current topics In lung cancer: Targeting EGFR*. Institute for Medical Education & Research, North Miami, Florida, p. 4. Accessed on 10/1/2007 at http://www.imeronline.com/109_lung_cancer/lung_cancer_4.html.

Dick, A. E., & Crawford, G. H. (2005). Managing cutaneous side effects of epidermal growth factor receptor (HER1/EGFR) inhibitors. *Community Oncology, 2*, 492-496.

Esper, P., & Knoop, T. (2005). *Current topics in colorectal cancer—targeting VEGF for oncology nurses*, Institute for Medical Education and Research, Project ID:04 2605 ES16. Retrieved from www.imeronline.com, Retrieved January 31, 2007.

Ferrara, N. (2004). Vascular endothelial growth factor as a target for anticancer therapy. *The Oncologist, 9*(suppl 1), 2-10.

Ferrara, N., Gerber, H.-P., & LeCouter, J. (2003). The biology of VEGF and its receptors. *Nature Medicine, 9*, 669-676.

Frankel, C. (2004). *Anti-VEGF therapy: clinical perspective, nursing implications, and patient management strategies clinical implications of targeting VEGF in solid tumors*. Meniscus Educational Institute. Presented at the Oncology Nursing Society, April 30, 2004. Anaheim, CA. Genentech Bio-Oncology.

Hanahan, D., and Weinberg, R.A. (2000). The hallmarks of cancer. *Cell, 100*, 57-70.

Herbst, R. S., & Shin, D. M. (2002). Monoclonal antibodies to target epidermal growth factor receptor-positive tumors: a new paradigm for cancer therapy. *Cancer, 94*, 1593-1611.

Heymach, J. V., Desai, J., Manola, J. et al. (2004). Phase II study of the antiangiogenic agent SU5416 in patients with advanced soft tissue sarcomas. *Clinical Cancer Research, 10*, 5732-5740

Hicklin D. J., & Ellis, L. M. (2005). Role of the vascular endothelial growth factor pathway in tumor growth and angiogenesis. *Journal of Clinical Oncology, 23*, 1011-1027.

Jain, R. K. (2001). Normalizing tumor vasculature with anti-angiogenic therapy: a new paradigm for combination therapy. *Nature Medicine, 7*, 987-989.

Janmaat, M. L., & Giaccone, G. (2003). Small-molecule epidermal growth factor receptor tyrosine kinase inhibitors. *The Oncologist, 8*, 576-586.

Knopp, T. (2005). *Nursing management of patients receiving angiogenesis inhibitors.* Current topics in colorectal cancer: targeting VEGF, IMER Institute for Medical Education & Research. Retrieved from www.imeronline.com on January 31, 2007.

Lacouture, M. E., Basti, S., Patel, J., et al. (2006). The SERIES clinic: an interdisciplinary approach to the management of toxicities of EGFR inhibitors. *The Journal of Supportive Oncology, 4*, 236-238.

Marques, C., & McCreery, H. (2003). *Inhibition of EGFR-TK in solid tumors: implications for practice* (pp. 1-26). AstraZeneca Pharmaceuticals: Birmingham, AL.

McCorkle, M., Gailoto, M., Oestreicher, P.M. et al. (2005). *Targeted therapies in non-small cell cancer* (pp. 1-32). Pittsburgh, PA: Oncology Education Service.

Mendelsohn, J. (2001). The epidermal growth factor receptor as a target for cancer therapy. *Endocrine-Related Cancer, 8*, 3-9.

Mendelsohn, J., & Baselga, J. (2000). The EGF receptor family as targets for cancer therapy. *Oncogene, 19*, 6550-6565.

National Cancer Institute. (2006). *Angiogenesis.* Retrieved April 7, 2007, from www.nci.nih.gov/cancertopics/understanding-cancer/angiogenesis.

Niederhuber, J. E. (2000). Surgical therapy. In M. D. Abeloff, J. O. Armitage, A. S., Lichter, et al. (Eds.). *Clinical oncology* (2nd ed., pp. 471-481). New York: Churchill Livingstone.

Pao, W., & Miller, V. A. (2005). Epidermal growth factor receptor mutations, small-molecule kinase inhibitors, and non-small-cell lung cancer: current knowledge and future directions. *Journal of Clinical Oncology, 23*, 2556-2568.

Peréz-Soler, R., Delord, J. P., Halpern, A., et al. (2005). HER1/EGFR inhibitor-associated rash: future directions for management and investigation outcomes from the HER1/EFGR inhibitor rash management forum. *The Oncologist, 10*, 345-356.

Peréz-Soler, R. & Saltz, L. (2005). Cutaneous adverse effects with HER1/EGFR-targeted agents: is there a silver lining? *Journal of Clinical Oncology, 23*, 5235-5246.

Pizzo, B. (2004). New directions in oncology nursing care: focus on gefitinib in patients with lung cancer. *Clinical Journal of Oncology Nursing, 8*, 385-392.

Prenzel, A., Fischer, O.M., Streit, S., et al. (2001) The epidermal growth factor receptor family as a central element for cellular signal transduction and diversification. Endocrin-Related *Cancer, 8*, 11-31.

Purdom, M. (2004). Management of acneiform rashes related to gefitinib therapy. *Clinical Journal of Oncology Nursing, 8*, 316-317.

Readon, D.A., and Wen, P. Y. (2006). Therapeutic Advances in the Treatment of Glioblastoma: Rational and Potential Role of Targeted Agents. *The Oncologist, 11*, 152-164.

Rempel, S., & Mikkelsen, T. (2006). Tumor invasiveness and anti-invasion strategies. In H. B. Newton, (Ed.), *Handbook of brain tumor chemotherapy* (pp. 193-218). San Francisco: Elsevier and Academic Press.

Research VEGF. Retrieved February 9, 2007, from www.researchvegf.com.

Ritter, C. A., & Arteaga, C. L. (2003). The epidermal growth factor receptor-tyrosine kinase: a promising therapeutic target in solid tumors. *Seminars in Oncology, 30*(suppl 1), 3-11.

Robert, C., Soria, J.-C., Spatz, A., et al. (2005). Cutaneous side-effects of kinase inhibitors and blocking antibodies. *Lancet Oncology, 6*, 491-500.

Rosen, L. S. (2005). VEGF-targeted therapy: therapeutic potential and recent advances. *The Oncologist, 10*, 382-391.

Salomon, D. S., Brandt, R., Ciardiello, F., et al. (1995). Epidermal growth factor-related peptides and their receptors in human malignancies. *Critical Reviews in Oncology/ Hematology, 19*, 183-232.

Segaert, S., & Van Cutsem, E. (2005). Clinical signs, pathophysiology, and management of skin toxicity during therapy with epidermal growth factor receptor inhibitors. *Annals of Oncology, 16*, 1425-1433.

Shah, N. T., Kris, M.G., Pao, W., et al. (2005). Practical management of patients with non-small cell lung cancer treated with gefitinib. *Journal of Clinical Oncology, 23*, 165-174.

Shu, K. Y., Kindler, H. L., Medenica, M., et al. (2006) Doxycycline for the treatment of paronychia induced by the epidermal growth factor receptor inhibitor cetuximab. *British Journal of Dermatology, 154*, 191-192.

Smith, B. D., Levis, M., Beran, M., et al. (2004). Single-agent CEP-701, a novel FLT3 inhibitor, shows biologic and clinical activity in patients with relapsed or refractory acute myeloid leukemia. *Blood, 103*, 3669-3676.

Soulieres, D., Senzer, N.N., Vokes, E.E., et al. 2004 Multicenter phase II study of erlotinib, an oral epidermal growth factor receptor tyrosine kinase inhibitor, in patients with recurrent or metastatic squamous cell cancer of the head and neck. *Journal of Clinical Oncology, 22*, 77-85.

Sporn, M. B., & Todaro, G.J. (1980). Autocrine secretion and malignant transformation of cells. *New England Journal of Medicine, 303* (15), 878-880.

S.T.E.P.S Program. (2006). Retrieved December 28, 2006, from http://www.thalomide.com/thalomid_history.aspx.

Vlahovic, G., & Crawford, J. (2003). Activation of tyrosine kinases in cancer. *The Oncologist, 8*, 531-538.

Wujcik, D., & Thomas, M. (2005) *Current topics in colorectal cancer—targeting EGFR for oncology nurses.* Presented at the Oncology Nursing Society 30th Annual Congress, April 28, 2005.

Wood, L. S., & Muehlbauer, P. M. (2003). Molecular and targeted therapies in cancer care. In *Concept to chairside* (pp. 3-25). Oncology Education Service.. Pittsburgh, PA.

Wood, L. S., Sandler, A. B., & Muehlbauer, P. (2005). *Targeting VEGF and EGFR pathways: translating science into clinical practice.* Presented at the Institution for Medical Education & Research. Educational Dinner Symposium Retrieved from www.imeronline.com on January 31, 2007.

Targeted Therapy Agents

Bevacizumab (Avastin)

Sandra E. Remer

DRUG CLASS

- Antiangiogenesis agent

ROUTE OF ADMINISTRATION

- Intravenous (IV) route by IV infusion
- DO NOT ADMINISTER AS AN IV PUSH OR BOLUS.

HOW TO ADMINISTER

- The initial infusion should be given over 90 minutes after the chemotherapy.
- If the first infusion is well tolerated, the second infusion may be given over 60 minutes.
- If the 60-minute infusion is well tolerated, subsequent infusions may be given over 30 minutes.

PRETREATMENT GUIDELINES

- No dose adjustments for hepatic or renal impairments

USE

- To be used in combination with a chemotherapeutic agent:
  - Colorectal cancer
  - Lung cancer

Off-Label Uses

- Renal cell cancer
- Malignant glioma
- Metastatic breast cancer

PHARMACOKINETICS

- Estimated half-life is approximately 20 days (range 11-50 days).
- Predicted time to reach steady state is 100 days. Drug excreted through kidneys.
- Clearance varies by body weight, sex, and tumor burden.
- No studies have been conducted to examine pharmacokinetics of bevacizumab in patients with renal or hepatic impairment.

USUAL DOSE AND SCHEDULE

- First-line treatment for metastatic colorectal cancer: adults: 5 mg/kg IV every 14 days until disease progression. There are no recommended dose reductions.
- Treatment of advanced and metastatic non–small cell lung cancer: adults: 15 mg/kg IV given on day 1 every 3 weeks in combination with paclitaxel 200 mg/m^2 and carboplatin AUC = 6 (each given on day 1)
- Treatment of metastatic renal cell cancer: adults: 10 mg/kg IV given every 2 weeks
- Treatment for malignant glioma in a phase II clinical trial is a 6-week cycle of 5 mg/kg every other week × 2, in combination with CPT-11 125 mg/m^2 every week × 4 followed by a 2-week rest period
- Efficacy as a single agent in colorectal cancer has not been established.

MAXIMUM DOSE LIMITS
Adults and Elderly

- The maximum tolerated dose has not been established.
- In clinical trials, the highest dose was 20 mg/kg IV.

Adolescents, Children, and Infants

- Safe and effective use of bevacizumab in infants and children has not been established.

SIDE EFFECTS
Serious/Life Threatening

- Gastrointestinal perforation*
- Wound healing*
- Hemorrhage*
- Arterial thromboembolic event

---

*Boxed warnings

- Hypertension
- Proteinuria (nephrotic syndrome)
- Congestive heart failure
- Infusion-related reaction

Common

- Asthenia
- Alopecia
- Pain
- Abdominal pain
- Headache
- Hypertension
- Dizziness
- Diarrhea
- Nausea
- Vomiting
- Anorexia
- Stomatitis
- Constipation
- Upper respiratory infection
- Epistaxis
- Dyspnea
- Exfoliative dermatitis
- Skin discoloration
- Proteinuria

NADIR

- No neutropenia observed
- Anemia and thrombocytopenia observed

STORAGE

- Store vial under refrigeration at 2°-8° C (36°-46° F).
- Protect from light.
- Store in the original carton until time of use.
- DO NOT FREEZE OR SHAKE.

MIXING INSTRUCTIONS

- Visually inspect vial for particulate matter and discoloration before mixing.
- Withdraw the appropriate amount of bevacizumab from vial(s).
- Dilute in a total volume of 100 mL of 0.9% sodium chloride injection.
- Do not mix or administer with dextrose solutions.
- Discard any unused portion left in vial because product contains no preservative.

PRODUCT STABILITY

- Diluted bevacizumab solution may be stored 2°-8° C (36°-46° F) for up to 8 hours.

COMPATIBILITY WITH OTHER DRUGS/INTRAVENOUS FLUIDS

- No incompatibilities between drug and polyvinylchloride or polyolefin bags have been observed.

DRUG INTERACTIONS

- No formal drug interaction studies with antineoplastic agents have been done.

PREGNANCY

Category C

- Angiogenesis is critical to fetal development and the inhibition of angiogenesis after the administration of drug is likely to result in adverse effects on pregnancy. Before beginning therapy, patients should be counseled regarding the potential risk to the developing fetus. Adequate contraception should be used.
- It is not known whether drug is secreted in human milk. Because human immunoglobulin G1 is secreted into human milk, the potential for absorption and harm to the infant after ingestion is unknown. Women should be advised to discontinue nursing during treatment and for a prolonged period of time after use, taking into account the estimated half-life of 20 days with a range between 11 and 50 days.

SPECIAL CONSIDERATIONS

- Use with caution in patients with known hypersensitivity to drug or any component of drug product.
- Therapy should NOT be initiated for at least 28 days after major surgery. The surgical incision should be fully healed before initiation of therapy.

- Because of the potential for impaired wound healing, suspend use before elective surgery. Although the appropriate interval between the last dose and elective surgery is unknown, the estimated half-life of 20 days should be taken into consideration when planning surgery.

PATIENT EDUCATION

- Teach patients about the role of angiogenesis in cancer development.
- Advise patients of side effects related to infusion reaction.
- Advise patients of life-threatening side effects, such as gastrointestinal perforation, severe bleeding, wound healing complications, congestive heart failure, pulmonary embolus and blood clots.
- Advise patients to check with health care professional before stopping or starting any medications.
- Advise patients to inform health care professional of recent surgery, the consideration of surgery, or if wound has not healed.

BIBLIOGRAPHY

Frankel, C. (2004). *Anti-VEGF therapy: Clinical perspective, nursing implications, and patient management strategies. clinical implications of targeting VEGF in solid tumors.* Meniscus Educational Institute. Continuing Education presentation. Oncology Nursing Society Congress, Anaheim, CA. Sponsored by Genentech Bio-Oncology, April 30, 2004.

Genentech, Inc. (2006). *Avastin (bevacizumab) package insert.* Retrieved September 24, 2007, from http://www.gen.com/gen/products/information/pdf/avastin-prescribing.pdf.

Knopp, T. (2005). *Nursing management of patients receiving angiogenesis inhibitors: current topics in colorectal cancer: targeting VEGF.* Retrieved February 1, 2007 from www.imeronline.com.

U.S. BL 125085 *Supplement Amendment: AVASTIN.* Genentech, Inc. 17 of 28/1048: 125085s45lbl.doc.

Cetuximab (Erbitux)

Sandra E. Remer

DRUG CLASS

- Endothelial growth factor receptor (EGFR) inhibitor

ROUTE OF ADMINISTRATION

- Intravenous (IV)

HOW TO ADMINISTER

- DO NOT ADMINISTER AS AN IV PIGGYBACK OR BOLUS.
- MUST be administered with the use of a low-protein-binding 0.22 micron in-line filter
- Can be administered by infusion pump or syringe pump
  - Piggyback into the patient's infusion line.
  - After infusion, a 1-hour observation period is recommended.
  - Maximum infusion rate should not exceed 5 mL/min.

PRETREATMENT GUIDELINES

- Use with caution in patients with known hypersensitivity to drug, murine proteins, or any component of product.
- Premedication with an H_1 antagonist (e.g., diphenhydramine 50 mg IV) is recommended.
- Monitor serum calcium, magnesium, and potassium levels before and during treatment.

USE

- Metastatic colorectal carcinoma
- Head and neck carcinoma

Off-Label Uses

- Pancreatic carcinoma

PHARMACOKINETICS

- In clinical trials, drug had a mean half-life of 118 hours (ranging from 75-188 hours).
- In studies there were no proven effects on pharmacokinetics for

Cancer Management

race, age, sex, or hepatic and renal function.

- Cetuximab has not been studied in pediatric populations.

USUAL DOSE AND SCHEDULE

- Adults: initial infusion dose of 400 mg/m² over 2 hours in combination with irinotecan or as monotherapy. Then, administer subsequent weekly infusions at 250 mg/m² IV over 60 minutes.
- Treatment is continued until progression of disease.

SIDE EFFECTS
Boxed Warnings

- Infusion reactions
- Cardiopulmonary arrest
- Pulmonary toxicity

Severe

- Infusion reactions may occur. Caution must be exercised with every infusion because a severe reaction may occur during any infusion.
- Severe reaction includes rapid onset of airway obstruction; bronchospasm, stridor, hoarseness, urticaria, or hypotension.
- Interstitial lung disease has been reported. Onset of symptoms has occurred between the fourth and eleventh doses in all reported cases.
- Dermatological toxicity— acneiform rash, dry skin, or exfoliative dermatitis occurred in 88% of patients as well as paronychial inflammation— associated swelling of the lateral nail folds of the toes and fingers.

Common

- Asthenia/malaise
- Diarrhea
- Nausea/vomiting
- Abdominal pain
- Anorexia
- Constipation
- Headache
- Dehydration with electrolyte imbalance
- Dyspnea
- Dyspepsia
- Fatigue

- Stomatitis
- Weakness
- Weight loss

NADIR

- Little to no neutropenia or thrombocytopenia has been reported with monotherapy.
- Leukopenia reported in 25% of patients receiving combination of drug with irinotecan.
- Anemia reported in patients with advanced colorectal cancer.

STORAGE

- Store vials under refrigeration at 2° to 8° C (36° to 46° F).
- DO NOT FREEZE.
- Preparations are chemically and physically stable for up to 12 hours at 2° to 8° C (36° to 46° F) and up to 8 hours at controlled room temperatures 20° to 25° C (68° to 77° F).
- Discard any unused portion of the solutions after either 8 hours at controlled room temperatures or 12 hours at 2° to 8° C (36° to 46° F).
- Discard any unused portion of the vial.

MIXING INSTRUCTIONS

- Supplied as a 50-mL, single-dose vial containing 100 mg of cetuximab at a concentration of 2 mg/mL in phosphate-buffered saline solution.
- The solution should be clear and colorless and may contain a small amount of easily visible white amorphous particles.
- DO NOT SHAKE OR DILUTE.

DRUG INTERACTIONS

- No drug interactions of clinical significance have been reported.
- There is no evidence of any interaction between cetuximab and irinotecan.

PREGNANCY
Category C

- There are no adequate or well-controlled studies in pregnant women. Drug should only be given to a pregnant woman or any woman not using adequate

contraception if the potential benefit justifies the potential risk to the fetus.

- All patients should be counseled before initiation of therapy regarding the potential risk to the developing fetus.
- If the patient becomes pregnant while receiving this drug, she should be apprised of the potential hazard to the fetus or the potential risk for loss of the pregnancy.

SPECIAL CONSIDERATIONS

- No dosage adjustments are necessary for hepatic or renal impairment.
- Maximum dosage limits have not been established; however, doses higher than 500 mg/m² have not been tested.

PATIENT EDUCATION

- Recommend that patients wear sunscreen and hats and limit sun exposure because sunlight can exacerbate any skin reactions that may occur.
- Women of childbearing age should be advised to avoid pregnancy and use contraception during treatment.
- Women should not breast-feed during treatment or for 60 days after the last dose.
- Tell your doctor or health care professional if you have any lung disease, especially lung fibrosis, any unusual reaction to drug, mouse proteins, other medications, foods, dyes, or preservatives.
- It is important not to miss a dose. Notify your doctor or health care professional if you are unable to keep an appointment.
- Tell your doctor or health care professional if you frequently drink beverages that contain caffeine or alcohol or if you smoke or use recreational drugs because these may affect the way your medicine works.
- Tell your doctor or health care professional before you start or stop any of your medicines.

- Tell your doctor or health care professional as soon as possible if you have any of the following:
  - ○ Difficulty breathing or shortness of breath anytime during your treatment
  - ○ Extreme tiredness or weakness
  - ○ Eye inflammation
  - ○ Mouth sores
  - ○ Pain, tingling, or numbness of the hands or feet
  - ○ Reactions during the infusion or the drug (especially difficulty breathing, wheezing, shortness of breath, hives, faintness, or dizziness)
  - ○ Skin rash, redness, or severe dry skin.

BIBLIOGRAPHY

Cetuximab (Erbitux). (2006). Henry Ford Hospital Clinical Pharmacology customized monograph. Retrieved January 31, 2007, from http://www.fda.gov/cder/consumer.info/druginfo/erbitux.htm.

Erbitux (cetuximab). (2006) Retrieved January 31, 2007, from http://www.bms.com.

ERLOTINIB (TARCEVA)

Sandra E. Remer

DRUG CLASS

Epidermal growth factor (HER1/EGFR) tyrosine kinase inhibitor

ROUTE OF ADMINISTRATION

- Oral white-film coated tablet (25 mg, 100 mg and 150 mg)

HOW TO ADMINISTER

- Orally
- Do not chew or crush tablet

PRETREATMENT GUIDELINES

- Liver function tests including AST, ALT and bilirubin must be monitored

USE
FDA Approved

- Non-small cell lung cancer
- Pancreatic cancer

Non-FDA Approved

- Glioblastoma multiforme
- Recurrent metastatic squamous cell of the head and neck
- Ovarian cancer
- Mesothelioma
- Breast cancer
- Bladder cancer
- Colorectal cancer
- Prostate cancer

PHARMACOKINETICS

- Cleared primarily by the liver. The half-life is approximately 36 hours.
- Bioavailability following a 150 mg dose is about 60% and peak plasma levels occur after 4 hours.
- Food increases bioavailability to almost 100%.

USUAL DOSE AND SCHEDULE
NSCLC

- Daily dose of 150 mg at least one hour before or 2 hours after food.
- Treatment should continue until progression or unacceptable toxicity

Pancreatic Cancer

- Daily dose of 100 mg at least one hour before or 2 hours after food.
- Treatment should continue until progression or unacceptable toxicity.

SIDE EFFECTS
Warning

- Pulmonary toxicity
- Myocardial infarction/ischemia
- Cerebrovascular accident
- Microangiopathic hemolytic anemia with thrombocytopenia

Common

- Rash and diarrhea

Additional side effects

- Anorexia
- Fatigue
- Dyspnea
- Cough
- Nausea/vomiting
- Abdominal pain

NADIR

In clinical studies, erlotinib did not show some of the side effects of traditional chemotherapy, such as lowering of white cell count.

STORAGE

Store at 25° C (77° F); excursions permitted to 15°–30° C (59°–86° F)

MIXING INSTRUCTIONS

- Oral medication, therefore no mixing instructions are necessary.
- Keep erlotinib out of the reach of children.

DRUG INTERACTIONS

- Caution should be used when taking erlotinib in co-treatment with ketoconazole and other strong CYP3A4 enzyme inhibitors such as atazanavir, clarithromycin, indinavir, itraconazole, nefazodone, nelfinavir, ritonavir, saquinavir, telithromycin, troleandomycin (TOA), and voriconazole. These medications may increase the effect of erlotinib.
- Pre-treatment with CYP3A4 inducers such as rifampicin, rifabutin, rifapentine, Phenytoin, carbamazepine, Phenobarbital and St. John's Wort decrease the effectiveness of erlotinib. Use of alternate drugs is recommended otherwise dosing of erlotinib should be adjusted per dose modification schedule.

PREGNANCY
Category D

- There are no adequate and well controlled studies in pregnant women.
- Women of childbearing potential should be advised to avoid pregnancy while on therapy.
- Adequate contraceptive methods should be used during therapy, and for at least 2 months after completing therapy.
- Treatment should only be continued in pregnant women if the potential benefit to the mother outweighs the risk to the fetus.
- If used during pregnancy, the patient should be apprised of the potential hazard to the fetus or

Cancer Management

potential risk for the loss of the pregnancy.

SPECIAL CONSIDERATIONS

- Used with caution in patient with hepatic impairment.
- It is not known whether erlotinib is excreted in human milk. Because many drugs are excreted in human milk and because of the effects on infants have not been studied, women should be advised against breast-feeding while receiving therapy.

PATIENT EDUCATION

- Take every day as prescribed
- Take at the same time every day at least one hour before or 2 hours after food. Taking with food may increase risk of side effects.
- If you miss a day, take your normal dose the next day. DO NOT take a double dose. Tell your doctor if you miss a dose.
- Avoid grapefruit or grapefruit juice. It may affect the way the drug works.
- Tell your doctor or nurse if you are taking any other medications including vitamins and herbals. Tell your doctor is you are taking a blood thinner such as Coumadin, as it may increase your risk of bleeding.
- Follow all instructions on how to take the drug.
- Do not stop taking the drug unless your doctor tells you.
- Call your doctor if you experience any of the following symptoms:
  - Severe or persistent diarrhea
  - Nausea, loss of appetite or vomiting
  - Onset or worsening of any unexplained shortness of breath or cough
  - Eye irritation

BIBLIOGRAPHY

McKorkle, M. (2005). Oncology Education Service, Inc. *Targeted Therapies in Non-Small Cell Lung Cancer. A Continuing Educational Monograph for Oncology Nurses.*
New Product Bulletin-Tarceva™ (erlotinib). (2004). American Pharmacy Association Washington, DC.
Tarceva (erlotinib) Tablets. Retrieved January 31, 2007, from http://www.tarceva.com.
Tarceva package insert. Retrieved January 30, 2007, from http://www.gen.com/gen/products/information/pdf/tarceva-prescribing.pdf.
Tarceva Monograph (2006). Henry Ford Clinical Pharmacy. Retrieved January 30, 2007, from http://hfhs.org.

Gefitinib (Iressa)

Sandra E. Remer

DRUG NOT AVAILABLE IN THE UNITED STATES EXCEPT FOR CLINICAL TRIAL USE

DRUG CLASS

Epidermal growth factor receptor inhibitor-tyrosine kinase

ROUTE OF ADMINISTRATION

- Oral; round, brown, film-coated 250-mg tablet

HOW TO ADMINISTER

- Orally
- Distribution of gefitinib will be limited under a risk management plan called the "Iressa Access Program."

PRETREATMENT GUIDELINES

- Liver function tests, including aspartate aminotransferase, alanine aminotransferase, and bilirubin must be monitored.
- Monitor prothrombin time, international normalized ratio if patient is taking warfarin.

USE

- Locally advanced or metastatic non–small cell lung cancer

Off-Label Use

- Head and neck cancer (squamous cell)

PHARMACOKINETICS

- Half-life is approximately 48 hours.
- Slowly absorbed with peak plasma levels at 3-7 hours after dosing
- Primarily cleared through the liver via CYP3A4 enzyme
- Gefitinib and its metabolites are not significantly excreted via the kidneys.

USUAL DOSE AND SCHEDULE

- Adults: 250-mg tablet daily with or without food
- Maximum dosage limits: adults/elderly 500 mg/day
- Adolescents and children: safe and effective use not established

SIDE EFFECTS
Serious

- Pulmonary toxicity (interstitial lung disease), including pneumonia, pneumonitis, and alveolitis

Common

- Diarrhea
- Rash
- Xerosis
- Nausea/vomiting
- Pruritus
- Anorexia
- Asthenia/weakness
- Weight loss

Infrequent

- Peripheral edema
- Amblyopia
- Dyspnea
- Conjunctivitis
- Vesicular rash
- Bullous rash
- Oral ulceration
- Stomatitis
- Elevation of hepatic enzymes

NADIR

In clinical studies, gefitinib did not show some of the side effects of traditional chemotherapy, such as lowering of white blood cell count.

STORAGE

Store at room temperature of 20-25°C (68-77 F).

MIXING INSTRUCTIONS

- Oral medication; therefore no mixing instructions are necessary.
- For patients who have difficulty swallowing, tablets may be dispersed in a half a glass of noncarbonated drinking water. NO other liquids should be used. Drop

the tablet into the water without crushing it. Stir until tablet is dispersed (approximately 10 minutes) and drink liquid immediately. Rinse glass immediately.
- The liquid may also be administered via a nasogastric (NG) tube.

DRUG INTERACTIONS
- Metabolized by cytochrome P450 (CYP3A4) and CYP2D6. Caution should be used when administering CYP3A4 or CYP2D6 drugs with gefitinib.
  - ○ **Inducers of CYP3A4** include: barbiturates, bosentan, carbamazepine, dexamethasone, nevirapine, oxcarbazepine, phenytoin or fosphenytoin (possible ethotoin), rifampin, rifabutin, rifapentine, and St. John's wort.
  - ○ **Inhibitors of CYP3A4** are: amiodarone, antiretroviral protease inhibitors, clarithromycin, dalfopristin, quinupristin, delavirdine, efavirenz, erythromycin, fluvoxamine, fluoxetine, grapefruit juice, imatinib, STI-571, mifepristone, RU-486, nefazodone, and selected azole antifungals.
  - ○ **CYP2D6 agents include:** amoxapine, atomoxetine, certain beta-blockers (e.g., carvedilol, metoprolol, propranolol, and timolol), clozapine, codeine, darifenacin, dextromethorphan, donepezil, encainide, flecainide, fluoxetine, haloperidol, hydrocodone, maprotiline, methadone, methamphetamine, mexiletine, morphine, paroxetine, perphenazine, propafenone, risperidone, thioridazine, tramadol, trazodone, tricyclic antidepressants, or venlafaxine.

PREGNANCY
Category D
- May cause fetal harm when administered to pregnant women.
- There are no adequate, well-controlled studies in pregnant women. Women of childbearing potential should be advised to avoid pregnancy while receiving therapy.
- Adequate contraceptive methods should be used during therapy and for at least 2 months after completing therapy.
- Treatment should only be continued in pregnant women if the potential benefit to the mother outweighs the risk to the fetus.
- If used during pregnancy, the patient should be apprised of the potential hazard to the fetus or potential risk for the loss of the pregnancy.

Nursing Mothers
- It is not known whether gefitinib is excreted in human milk. Because many drugs are excreted in human milk and because of the potential for serious adverse reactions in nursing infants, women should be advised against breastfeeding while receiving therapy.

SPECIAL CONSIDERATIONS
- Gefitinib should be used with caution in patients with hepatic disease.

PATIENT EDUCATION
- Take every day as prescribed.
- Do not crush or chew tablets.
- Do NOT take with grapefruit or grapefruit juice.
- Notify health care professional at the first sign of side effects, such as diarrhea or rash.
- Notify health care professional of all medications, including prescription, over-the-counter, vitamins, and herbal preparations.
- Tell your health care professional if you are taking a blood thinner such as warfarin (Coumadin), because it may increase your risk of bleeding.
- Store all medication at room temperature way from humid or warm places such as bathrooms or kitchen sinks.
- May be taken with or without food.
- Gloves are not needed to handle gefitinib; no hazardous waste precautions are necessary for stool, emesis, or urine.
- Follow all instructions on how to take gefitinib.
- Notify health care professional of any new onset of eye pain or signs or symptoms of infection (chills, cough, or burning/pain with urination).

BIBLIOGRAPHY
Henry Ford Clinical Pharmacy. (2006). *Gefitinib (Iressa) monograph.* Retrieved January 31, 2007 from http://cpip. gsm.com.
Iressa (gefitinib). (2007). Retrieved January 31, 2007 from www.astrazeneca-us.com.
McKorkle, M. (2005). *Targeted therapies in non-small cell lung cancer: A continuing educational monograph for oncology nurses.* Pittsburgh, PA: Oncology Education Service, Inc.
Oncology Nursing Society. (2003). *Gefitinib/Iressa.* Retrieved January 31, 2007 from http://www.ons.org/patientEd/Treatment/PatientMeds/gefitinib.shtml.

Imatinib Mesylate (Gleevec)

Sandra E. Remer

DRUG CLASS
- Protein tyrosine kinase inhibitor

ROUTE OF ADMINISTRATION
- Oral

HOW TO ADMINISTER
- Oral tablet (100 and 400 mg brownish-orange tablet)
- Imatinib is taken by mouth once or twice a day with a meal and large glass of water. Tablets may be cut in half if instructed by physician for dose prescribed.
- Tablets may be dispersed in a glass of water, orange juice, or apple juice if patient is unable to swallow tablets.
- DO NOT TAKE WITH GRAPEFRUIT, GRAPEFRUIT JUICE, OR CAFFEINE-CONTAINING PRODUCTS (and avoid grapefruit, grapefruit juice, or caffeine-containing products for 1 hour before and after taking the drug).

Cancer Management

- Swallow tablet whole. DO NOT CHEW THEM. Sit up for 1 hour after taking this medication.
- If daily dose is 800 mg or greater, the 400-mg tablet should be used to limit patient exposure to iron.

PRETREATMENT GUIDELINES

- Complete blood cell counts and liver function tests

USE

- Chronic myelogenous leukemia (CML)
- Gastrointestinal stromal tumors (GIST)
- Acute lymphocytic leukemia (ALL)
- Hypereosinophilic syndrome/chronic eosinophilic leukemia
- Philadelphia chromosome–positive ALL (PH+ ALL)
- Aggressive systemic mastocytosis (ASM)
- Myelodysplastic syndrome (MD)

Off-Label Uses

- Desmoid tumors

Clinical Trials

- Recurrent glioblastoma
- Advanced melanoma
- Recurrent non–small cell lung cancer (NSCLC)
- Metastatic colorectal cancer
- Metastatic breast cancer
- Extensive small cell lung cancer
- Prostate cancer
- Pancreatic, chordoma, and gastric adenocarcinoma

PHARMACOKINETICS

- Imatinib is given orally and is well absorbed. It is metabolized by the liver by cytochrome P450 (CYP) 3A4 isoenzyme.
- The mean half-lives of imatinib and its active metabolite are 18 and 40 hours, respectively.
- Drugs that induce imatinib metabolism may decrease the clinical activity of imatinib, whereas drugs which inhibit imatinib metabolism may lead to toxic side effects. (See Drug Interactions.)

USUAL DOSE AND SCHEDULE

- Patients receiving P450 inducers such as rifampin or phenytoin should have their doses increased by at least 50% and clinical responses should be closely monitored.

Adults

- Ph+ CML (chronic phase initial/failure): 400 mg orally once daily
- Ph+ CML in accelerated phase or blast crisis: 600 mg orally daily
- Ph+ ALL (resistant or relapsed): 300-1,000 mg/day orally
- Kit (CD117) + unresectable or metastatic GIST: 400-600 mg orally once daily
- Hypereosinophilic syndrome and other eosinophilic disorders: 100-400 mg/day orally
- Desmoid tumors: 400 mg orally twice daily

Pediatric

- Ph+ chronic-phase CML (recurred after hematopoietic stem cell transplant or resistant to interferon alfa) >3 years: 260 mg/m^2/day orally as single dose or divided dose (AM/PM)
- Ph+ newly diagnosed CML is 340 mg/m^2/day orally (not to exceed 600 mg)

MAXIMUM DOSE LIMITS

- Adults: 800 mg/day orally
- Elderly: 800 mg/day orally
- Adolescents: 340 mg/m^2 day orally
- Children ≥3 years: 340 mg/m^2 day orally
- Children <3 years: Safe and effective use not established.

SIDE EFFECTS

- Nausea/vomiting
- Fluid retention and edema
- Diarrhea
- Muscle cramps
- Fatigue
- Skin rash
- Abdominal pain and indigestion

NADIR

- Bone marrow suppression often occurs during imatinib therapy

and is dependent on the stage of the underlying disease.

- Complete blood cell counts should be performed at least weekly for the first month, then biweekly the second month, and periodically after as clinically indicated.
- Dosage adjustments for neutropenia and thrombocytopenia are recommended (see package insert).

STORAGE

- Store at room temperature 15°-30° C (59°-86° F).
- Protect from moisture.
- Do not store on a windowsill or in the bathroom.
- Ask your nurse of pharmacist how to dispose of any medication you do not use.
- Keep out of the reach of children.

MIXING INSTRUCTIONS

- No mixing instructions, product is tablet for oral use only.
- Do not chew tablet.
- Tablets may be dispersed in a large glass of water, orange juice, or apple juice for patients unable to swallow tablets.

DRUG INTERACTIONS

- Avoid aspirin, acetaminophen, or aspirin- or acetaminophen-containing products; birth control pills (oral contraceptives); blood thinners (warfarin); herbal products (e.g., St. Johns Wort); erythromycin; phenytoin (e.g., Dilantin); heart medicines (e.g., calcium channel blockers); antifungal medicines; and antidepressants.
- Drug interaction list is long; please check with a pharmacist or package insert for complete list.

PREGNANCY

Category D

- There is evidence of human fetal risk, but the benefits from use in pregnant women may be acceptable despite its potential risk.
- Imatinib mesylate may interfere with the normal menstrual

cycle in women and may stop sperm production in men. Women and men considering taking imatinib therapy must use a reliable method of birth control.

- Women who are pregnant or would like to become pregnant should discuss this with their health care provider before taking this drug.

SPECIAL CONSIDERATIONS

- Imatinib is often associated with edema and serious fluid retention; give with caution in the elderly patient or those with impaired renal or cardiac function.
- Patients with hepatic disease should be monitored closely.
- Imatinib is a potent inhibitor of cytochrome P450 (enzyme metabolism) and all drugs both prescription and nonprescription, including herbals and vitamins, should be closely monitored by physician or health care professional.
- No medications should be started or stopped without the approval of the health care provider.
- Studies have not been done on children under the age of 3 years old.

PATIENT EDUCATION

- Notify your doctor or nurse if you have any of the following:
  - Bleeding problems
  - Dental problems
  - Infection (especially cold sores, shingles, painful or difficulty urinating because these products mask a fever)
  - Heart disease (e.g., heart failure)
  - Jaundice (yellowing of the skin or eyes)
  - Kidney disease
  - Liver disease
  - An unusual or allergic reaction to imatinib, other medications, food, dyes, or preservatives.
  - Pregnant or trying to become pregnant or breast-feeding
  - Sores or white patches in your mouth

- Puffiness around the eyes or ankles
- Pinpoint red spots on your skin
- Weight gain of 5 pounds over your baseline weight
- Avoid taking aspirin, nonsteroidal anti-inflammatory drugs (such as acetaminophen, ibuprofen, and naproxen) unless prescribed by your doctor. These products mask a fever.
- Do not have any vaccinations without approval of your doctor. Avoid anyone who has recently received a polio vaccine.
- Notify your doctor if you need to have surgery or any other procedures.
- Be careful when you are brushing or flossing your teeth or using a toothpick while on imatinib therapy to avoid infections and bleeding.

BIBLIOGRAPHY

Henry Ford Hospital Clinical Pharmacy. (2006). *Imatinib mesylate (Gleevec)*. Retrieved January 31, 2007, from http://cpip.gsm.com/apps/products.

Imatinib mesylate (Gleevec). Retrieved January 31, 2007, from http://www.ons.org/patientED/Treatment/PatientMeds/imatinib.shtml.

Imatinib mesylate (Gleevec). Retrieved January 31, 2007, from http://www.gleevec.com/info/ page/home. Novartis Oncology.

Novartis. (2007). *Imatinib mesylate (Gleevec): full prescribing information*. Retrieved January 31, 2007, from http:// www.novartis.com.

Lapatinib (Tykerb)

Joyce Marrs

DRUG CLASS

- Tyrosine kinase inhibitor. Acts on the epidermal growth factor receptors HER-1 and HER-2.

ROUTE OF ADMINISTRATION

- Oral

HOW TO ADMINISTER

- Taken by mouth daily 1 hour before or 1 hour after a meal.

PRETREATMENT GUIDELINES

- Review current medication list for drugs that are metabolized by the CYP3A4 or CYP2C8 pathway.
- Measure baseline left ventricular ejection fraction.
- Measure baseline liver function tests and electrolytes.
- May want to consider baseline electrocardiogram because of potential for QT interval prolongation.
- Women of childbearing potential should be screened for pregnancy.

USE

- Used in combination with capecitabine for advanced or metastatic HER-2/*neu*-positive breast cancer that has been previously treated with a taxane, an anthracycline, and trastuzumab

PHARMACOKINETICS

- Drug half-life is 24 hours.
- Steady state achieved in 6 to 7 days when administered daily.
- When taken with food, drug concentration is increased.

USUAL DOSE AND SCHEDULE

- Full dosage is 1,250 mg per day.
- Consider holding drug for toxicities >grade 2. Once toxicity has resolved to grade 1 or less, resume at 1,250 mg per day. If problem recurs, decrease dose to 1,000 mg per day.

SIDE EFFECTS
Warnings and Precautions

- Decreased left ventricular ejection fraction (LVEF) may occur.
- Diarrhea may be severe and require interventions such as electrolyte replacement and intravenous fluids.
- QT interval prolongation
- Severe liver impairment may necessitate dose reduction.

More Common

- Diarrhea
- Nausea

Cancer Management

- Vomiting
- Rash
- Hand-foot syndrome
- Fatigue

Less Common

- Stomatitis
- Dyspepsia
- Dry skin
- Inflammation of the mucosa
- Dyspnea
- Back pain
- Insomnia
- Pain in extremities

STORAGE

- Product should be stored at 25° C (77° F). A range between 15°-30° C (59°-86° F) is permitted.

DRUG INTERACTIONS

- Lapatinib interacts with CYP3A4 inhibitors such as:
  - Ketoconazole
  - Itraconazole
  - Clarithromycin
  - Atazanavir
  - Indinavir
  - Nefazodone
  - Nelfinavir
  - Ritonavir
  - Saquinavir
  - Telithromycin
  - Voriconazole
  - Grapefruit and grapefruit juice
- Lapatinib interacts with CYP3A4 inducers such as:
  - Dexamethasone
  - Phenytoin
  - Rifampin
  - Carbamazepine
  - Rifabutin
  - Rifapentine
  - Phenobarbital
  - St. John's Wort

PREGNANCY

Category D

SPECIAL CONSIDERATIONS

- Lapatinib should be stopped if LVEF is decreased. After a minimum of 2 weeks, drug may be reinitiated at a reduced dose if patient is asymptomatic and the LVEF has recovered.
- Drug dose may need to be adjusted when liver impairment is present.

PATIENT EDUCATION

- Take medication 1 hour before or after a meal.
- Avoid eating grapefruit or drinking grapefruit juice while on lapatinib.
- Instruct patient to take the whole dose once a day at about the same time.
- If a daily dose is forgotten, the missed dose should not be made up.
- Patients should report palpitations, dyspnea, or fatigue.

BIBLIOGRAPHY

Tykerb. (n.d.). *Full prescribing information*. Retrieved April 2, 2007, from http://ws.gsk.com/products/assets/us_tykerb.pdf.

Lenalidomide (Revlimid)

Sandra E. Remer

DRUG CLASS

- Antiangiogenesis agent (thalidomide analog)

ROUTE OF ADMINISTRATION

- Oral capsule

HOW TO ADMINISTER

- Oral capsule only available under a special restrictive distribution program called "RevAssist."
- May only be prescribed by licensed health care providers who are registered in the RevAssit program and understand the potential risk of teratogenicity.
- May only be dispensed by a licensed pharmacy that is registered in the RevAssist program and may only be given to patients who are registered in the RevAssist program and who agree to adhere to the program.

PRETREATMENT GUIDELINES

- Monitor renal function, complete blood cell count with platelets.
- Women must use an effective contraception for at least 4 weeks before beginning therapy and during treatment. Contraception must be continued during dose interruptions and for 4 weeks after the discontinuation of drug therapy. Two reliable forms of contraception must be used simultaneously unless the woman has been postmenopausal for 24 consecutive months or has had a hysterectomy.
- Before lenalidomide is prescribed, women of childbearing potential should have two negative pregnancy tests, the first done within 10-14 days and the second test within 24 hours before prescribing, with results verified by the prescriber.
- Pregnancy tests should occur weekly during the first 4 weeks of use, and then testing should be repeated every 4 weeks in women with regular menstrual cycles. If menstrual cycles are irregular, pregnancy testing should occur every 2 weeks.
- It is not known whether lenalidomide is present in the semen of male patients receiving the drug. Therefore, men must always use a latex condom during sexual contact with women of childbearing potential even if they have undergone successful vasectomies.

USE

- Multiple myeloma
- Myelodysplastic syndrome (MDS)

PHARMACOKINETICS

- Rapidly absorbed after oral administration with maximum plasma concentrations between 0.625 and 1.5 hours
- Coadministration with food does NOT alter the extent of the absorption.
- Metabolic profile in humans has not been studied.

- Eliminated through urinary excretion. Half-life of elimination is 3 hours.

USUAL DOSE AND SCHEDULE
- The recommended starting dose is 10 mg daily taken with water.
- Dosing is continued or modified on the basis of clinical and laboratory findings.

SIDE EFFECTS
- **WARNING: POTENTIAL FOR HUMAN BIRTH DEFECTS:** Lenalidomide is an analog of thalidomide. Thalidomide is a known human teratogen that causes severe life-threatening human birth defects. If lenalidomide is taken during pregnancy, it may cause birth defects or death to an unborn baby. Women should be advised to avoid pregnancy while taking lenalidomide.

Severe
- Hematological toxicity (neutropenia and thrombocytopenia)
- Deep vein thrombosis and pulmonary emboli (significantly increased risk)

Common
- Diarrhea
- Constipation
- Itching
- Rash
- Dry skin
- Tiredness
- Dyspnea
- Nausea
- Anorexia
- Cough
- Dizziness and headache
- Fatigue
- Insomnia
- Muscle cramps
- Arthralgia
- Peripheral edema
- Pharyngitis
- Night sweats
- Back pain
- Nasopharyngitis

NADIR
- During the major study for indication, 48% of patients had grade 3 or 4 neutropenia; the median onset was 42 days and median time to recover was 17 days.
- Grade 3 or 4 thrombocytopenia median onset was 28 days and mean recovery was 22 days.

STORAGE
- At 25° C (77° F); excursions permitted to 15°-30° C (59°-86° F). (See *United States Pharmacopeia* controlled room temperature.)

MIXING INSTRUCTIONS
- Oral medication. Do NOT break, chew, or open capsule.
- Dose is continued or modified on the basis of clinical and laboratory findings.

DRUG INTERACTIONS
- Anticoagulants, nonsteroidal anti-inflammatory drugs, platelet inhibitors, salicylates, thrombolytic agents, vaccines
- Drug is not metabolized by nor inhibits or induces the P450 pathway.

PREGNANCY
Category X
- Lenalidomide is an analog of thalidomide. Thalidomide is a known human teratogen that causes severe life-threatening human birth defects. If lenalidomide is taken during pregnancy, it may cause birth defects or death to an unborn baby. Women should be advised to avoid pregnancy while taking lenalidomide.

SPECIAL CONSIDERATIONS
Women
- Lenalidomide should be used in females of childbearing potential only when all of the following conditions are met:
  - Appears to understand the risks associated with the drug and is thought to be able to reliably carry out instructions

- Is capable of complying with the contraceptive measures, pregnancy testing, patient registration, and patient survey as described in the RevAssist program
- Has received both oral and written warnings of the potential risks of taking lenalidomide during pregnancy and of exposing a fetus to the drug
- Has received both oral and written warnings of the risk of possible contraception failure and of the need to use two reliable form of contraception simultaneously, unless continuous abstinence form heterosexual contact is the chosen method. Sexually mature females who have not undergone a hysterectomy or who have not been postmenopausal for at least 24 consecutive months are considered to be females of childbearing potential.
- Acknowledges, in writing, her understanding of these warnings and of the need to use two reliable methods of contraception for 4 weeks before beginning lenalidomide therapy, during lenalidomide therapy, and during the dose interruptions and for 4 weeks after discontinuation of lenalidomide therapy
- Has had two negative pregnancy tests with a sensitivity of at least 50 mIU/mL within 10-14 days and 24 hours before beginning therapy
- If the patient is between 12 and 18 years of age, parents or legal guardian are to read the educational materials and agree to try and ensure compliance with the above.

Men
- Lenalidomide should be used in sexually active males when the all of the following conditions are met:
  - Appears to understand the risks associated with the drug and is thought to be able to reliably carry out instructions

Cancer Management

- ○ Is capable of complying with the contraceptive measures that are appropriate for men, patient registration, and patient survey as described in the RevAssist program
- ○ Has received both oral and written warnings of the potential risks of taking lenalidomide and of exposing a fetus to the drug
- ○ Has received both oral and written warnings of the risk of possible contraception failure and that it is unknown whether lenalidomide is present in semen. Has been instructed that he must always use a latex condom during any sexual contact with females of childbearing potential even if he has undergone a successful vasectomy
- ○ Acknowledges, in writing, his understanding of these warnings and of the need to use a latex condom during sexual contact with women of childbearing potential even if he has undergone a successful vasectomy. Women of childbearing potential are considered to be sexually mature females who have not undergone a hysterectomy or who have not been postmenopausal for at least 24 consecutive months (i.e., who have had menses at anytime in the preceding 24 consecutive months).
- ○ If the patient is 12 to 18 years of age, parents or legal guardian are to read the educational materials and agree to try and ensure compliance with the above.

PATIENT EDUCATION

- Patients on lenalidomide therapy should have their complete blood cell counts monitored weekly for the first 8 weeks of therapy and at least monthly thereafter. Patients may require dose interruption or reduction. Patients may require

use of blood product support or growth factors.
- Patients should be instructed to inform their health care providers or seek emergency medical care if they have the following signs or symptoms:
  - ○ Shortness of breath
  - ○ Chest pain
  - ○ Arm or leg swelling
- Swallow capsules whole with water once a day. Do not break, chew, or open the capsule.
- Do not give blood while taking drug.
- Do not share this medication with anyone even if they have the same symptoms you have.
- If you miss a dose, take it as soon as you remember that day. Do NOT take two doses at the same time.
- Keep lenalidomide out of the reach of children.

BIBLIOGRAPHY

Henry Ford Clinical Pharmacy. (2006). *Revlimid (lenalidomide)* [monograph]. Retrieved January 31, 2007, from http://cpip.g.com/apps/products. *Revlimid (lenalidomide)* [package insert]. (2006). Retrieved January, 31, 2007, from www.Celgene.com.

Panitumumab (Vectibix)

Joyce Marrs

DRUG CLASS

- Epidermal growth factor receptor (EGFR) inhibitor

ROUTE OF ADMINISTRATION

- Intravenous (IV) infusion

HOW TO ADMINISTER

- As an IV infusion over 1 hour
- For doses higher than 1,000 mg, infuse over 90 minutes.
- Administer with use of a low-protein-binding in-line 0.22-micron filter.

- Do not administer as an IV bolus or push.

PRETREATMENT GUIDELINES

- Premedication for hypersensitivity reaction was not uniform in clinical trial.
- Have equipment and medications available for possible infusion reaction.

USE

- Metastatic colorectal cancer positive for EGFR expression that has progressed while on or after treatment with fluoropyrimidine-, oxiliplatin-, and irinotecan-based chemotherapy regimens

PHARMACOKINETICS

- Average half-life is 7.5 days.

USUAL DOSE AND SCHEDULE

- Administer at a dose of 6 mg/kg every 14 days.

MAXIMUM DOSE LIMITS

- No data identified in clinical trial for overdosage. Highest dose administered was 9 mg/kg every 3 weeks.

SIDE EFFECTS
Most Frequent

- Acneform eruptions, dry skin, skin fissure, generalized exfoliative dermatitis, paronychia, pruritus, rash
- Hypomagnesemia
- Abdominal pain, constipation, diarrhea, nausea, vomiting
- Fatigue
- Ocular toxicity

Serious

- Dermatological toxicity may lead to infection, sepsis, and death.
- Hypomagnesemia
- Infusion reactions
- Pulmonary fibrosis
- Ocular toxicity

Precautions

- Dermatological toxicity may be exacerbated by sun exposure.
- Administration of panitumumab in conjunction with irinotecan, 5-fluorouracil, and leucovorin is not

recommended. Diarrhea incidence and severity will increase when given in combination with this regimen.

- Monitor for symptoms of hypomagnesemia and hypocalcemia.

Black Box Warnings

- Severe dermatological toxicities may require that dose be reduced or held.
- Severe infusion reactions occurred in approximately 1% of patients. Stop infusion at first sign of infusion reaction.

STORAGE

- Refrigerate at 2°-8° C (36°-46° F) until time to use.
- Do not freeze.
- Protect from sunlight.

MIXING INSTRUCTIONS

- Inspect vial for discoloration. There may be small translucent to white particles in vial that will be removed with in-line filter. DO NOT SHAKE THE VIAL.
- Dilute dose in a total of 100 mL of normal saline solution for dose under 1,000 mg. A total volume of 150 mL is used for doses greater than 1,000 mg.
- Final concentration should be <10 mg/mL.
- Do not shake vial or diluted solution. Mix by gentle inversion.

PRODUCT STABILITY

- Use within 6 hours of mixing when stored at room temperature.
- Solution good for 24 hours when stored at 2°-8° C (36°-46° F).
- Do not freeze.

DRUG INTERACTIONS

- Drug interaction studies have not been conducted.
- Flush line with normal saline solution before and after infusion.
- Do not mix with other drugs or IV solutions.

PREGNANCY

Category C
- Drug crosses the placental barrier.

- Women of childbearing potential should be advised to use birth control while receiving panitumumab and for 6 months after completion of therapy.

SPECIAL CONSIDERATIONS

- Monitor electrolyte levels throughout treatment and for 8 weeks after completion of therapy for hypomagnesemia and hypocalcemia.

PATIENT EDUCATION

- Instruct patients to wear sunscreen and hats to limit exposure to sun. Sunlight may worsen skin reactions.
- Instruct patient to notify health care provider if diarrhea occurs.
- Instruct patient to report cough or difficulty breathing.

BIBLIOGRAPHY

Vectibix (panitumumab) [package insert]. (2006). Thousand Oaks, CA: Amgen.

Sorafenib Tosylate (Nexavar)

Laura S. Wood

DRUG CLASS

- Angiogenesis inhibitor
- Targeted therapy—multiple receptor tyrosine kinase inhibitor. Inhibits KIT, vascular endothelial growth factors (VEGFR1, VEGFR2, BEGFR3), and platelet-derived growth factors (PDGFR-alpha and PDGFR-beta).

ROUTE OF ADMINISTRATION

- Oral

PRETREATMENT GUIDELINES

- None

USE

- Advanced renal cell carcinoma

PHARMACOKINETICS

- Peak plasma concentrations approximately 3 hours after oral

administration. Steady-state concentrations achieved within 7 days. Mean elimination half-life is approximately 25-48 hours. Bioavailability is similar when sorafenib is taken in a fasted state or with a moderate-fat meal. With a high-fat meal, bioavailability reduced by 29%. It is recommended that sorafenib be administered without food (1 hour before meals or 2 hours after eating).

USUAL DOSE AND SCHEDULE

- 400 mg (2 × 200 mg tablets) twice daily continuously without food (1 hour before or 2 hours after eating)

Dose Modifications

- Dose reduction to 400 mg once daily with additional dose reductions to 400 mg every other day if needed. Mean maximum concentration and area under the curve are higher with daily administration rather than twice daily.

Maximum Dosage Limits

- The highest dose studied clinically is 800 mg twice daily. No recommendations for dose escalation are currently available.

Pediatric Use

- The safety and efficacy of sorafenib in pediatric patients has not been studied in clinical trials.

SIDE EFFECTS
Serious/Life Threatening

- Increased risk of bleeding may occur. If any bleeding event necessitates medical intervention, permanent discontinuation of sorafenib should be considered.
- The incidence of treatment-emergent cardiac ischemia/ infarction events was higher in the sorafenib group (2.9%) compared with the placebo group (0.4%).

Common Side Effects

- Diarrhea
- Fatigue

- Hypertension
- Rash/desquamation
- Hand-foot syndrome
- Pruritus
- Alopecia
- Nausea

NADIR

- Mild leukopenia, neutropenia, thrombocytopenia, and anemia.
- Myelosuppression nadirs have not been identified because of the continuous administration schedule and mild suppression not requiring dose interruption.

STORAGE

- Dry place at room temperature

DRUG INTERACTIONS

- Grapefruit
- Sorafenib metabolism unlikely to be altered by CYP3A4 inhibitors (ketoconazole)
- Sorafenib does not appear to inhibit CYP2C9 substrates (warfarin).
- CYP3A4 inducers (dexamethasone, rifampin, St. John's wort, phenytoin, phenobarbital) are expected to increase metabolism and decrease sorafenib concentrations.

PREGNANCY

Category D
- Women of childbearing potential should avoid getting pregnant or breast-feeding while on treatment.

SPECIAL CONSIDERATIONS

- Infrequent bleeding events or elevations in prothrombin time (PT)/international normalized ratio (INR) have been reported in some patients taking warfarin while on sorafenib therapy. Patients taking concomitant warfarin should be monitored regularly for changes in PT, INR, or clinical bleeding episodes.

PATIENT EDUCATION

- Teach patients about the process of angiogenesis and its role in cancer.
- Advise patients about neutropenia, thrombocytopenia, and risk of bleeding.
- Teach patients about hand-foot syndrome and skin care.
- Instruct patient taking warfarin about possible increased risk of bleeding and the need for more frequent PT/INR monitoring.
- Emphasize the importance of timely notification of health care professionals for the development of hand-foot syndrome or bleeding.

BIBLIOGRAPHY

Kidney Cancer Association. *Therapies for advanced kidney cancer.* Retrieved September 23, 2007 from www.kidney cancer.org/index.cfm?page10-40.
Sorafenib tosylate [package insert]. (2007). Leverkusen, Germany: Bayer HealthCare AG. Retrieved September 23, 2007, from www.nexavar.com.
Wood, L.S. (2006). Managing the side effects of sorafenib and sunitinib. *Community Oncology* 3: 558-562.
Wood, L.S, Manchen, B. (2007). Sorafenib: A promising new targeted therapy for renal cell carcinoma. *Clinical Journal of Oncology Nursing 11(5)*, 649-656.

Sunitinib Malate (Sutent)

Laura S. Wood

DRUG CLASS

- Angiogenesis inhibitor
- Targeted therapy: multiple receptor tyrosine kinase inhibitor. Inhibits KIT, vascular endothelial growth factors (VEGFR1, VEGFR2, BEGFR3), and platelet-derived growth factors (PDGFR-alpha and PDGFR-beta).

ROUTE OF ADMINISTRATION

- Oral

PRETREATMENT GUIDELINES

- None

USE

- Advanced renal cell carcinoma and gastrointestinal stromal tumor for patients with disease progression on imatinib or intolerance to imatinib

PHARMACOKINETICS

- Maximum plasma concentration 6-12 hours after oral administration. Food has no effect on bioavailability. Steady-state concentrations achieved within 10-14 days. Terminal half-life of sunitinib and its primary metabolite are approximately 40-60 hours and 80-110 hours, respectively.
- Formulation: 50 mg, 25 mg, and 12.5 mg capsules

USUAL DOSE AND SCHEDULE

- 50 mg once daily, on a schedule of 4 weeks on treatment followed by 2 weeks off. May be taken with or without food
- Dose modifications: dose increase or reduction of 12.5 mg increments (37.5 mg and 25 mg) on the basis of side effects, tolerability, and concomitant medications

Maximum Dosage Limits

- Dose escalation to a maximum of 87.5 mg daily should be considered if sunitinib must be coadministered with CYP3A4 inducer.

Pediatric Use

- The safety and efficacy of sunitinib in pediatric patients has not been studied in clinical trials.

SIDE EFFECTS
Serious/Life Threatening

- Left ventricular dysfunction/congestive heart failure (CHF)
- Gastrointestinal or tumor bleeding
- Gastrointestinal perforation

Common Side Effects

- Fatigue
- Hypertension
- Diarrhea
- Nausea
- Mucositis/stomatitis
- Dyspepsia
- Vomiting

- Constipation
- Abdominal pain
- Rash
- Skin discoloration
- Dry skin, hair depigmentation
- Hand-foot syndrome
- Taste alterations
- Anorexia
- Arthralgias
- Headache
- Neutropenia
- Thrombocytopenia
- Epistaxis

NADIR

- Timing of neutropenia and thrombocytopenia is variable.

STORAGE

- Store at room temperature.

DRUG INTERACTIONS

- Grapefruit
- Strong CYP450 inhibitors (ketoconazole) may increase sunitinib plasma concentrations.
- CYP3A4 inducers (dexamethasone, phenobarbital, phenytoin, St. John's wort) may decrease sunitinib plasma concentrations.

PREGNANCY

Category D
- Women of childbearing potential should avoid becoming pregnant or breast-feeding while on treatment.

SPECIAL CONSIDERATIONS

- Monitor complete blood cell count (CBC) with differential and chemistry panel at the beginning of each cycle, and CBC with differential at the end of 28-day dosing.
- Patients should be carefully monitored for clinical signs and symptoms of CHF. Baseline and periodic evaluation of left ventricular ejection fraction should be considered.
- Limited data on effect of sunitinib on wound healing. Careful consideration should be taken when planning surgery whenever possible.

PATIENT EDUCATION

- Teach patients about the process of angiogenesis and its role in cancer.
- Advise patients about neutropenia, thrombocytopenia, and risk of bleeding.
- Teach patients about hand-foot syndrome and skin care.
- Emphasize the importance of timely notification of health care professionals for fever, bleeding, or the development of hand-foot syndrome.

BIBLIOGRAPHY

Kidney Cancer Association. (2007). *We have kidney cancer: a practical guide for patients and families.* Retrieved September 23, 2007 from Kidney Cancer Association: www.kidneycancer.org

MacIntyre J. 2007. Pharmacologic application of sunitinib malate in the management of gastrointestinal stromal tumors. *Clinical Journal of Oncology Nursing 11,* 237-241.

Pfizer. (2007). *Sutent.* Retrieved September 23, 2007, from Pfizer: www.sutent.com.

Pfizer Labs, Division of Pfizer Pharmaceuticals. (2007). *Sunitinib (Sutent)* [package insert]. Pfizer Labs, Division of Pfizer Pharmaceuticals: New York, NY.

Wood, L.S. (2006). Managing the side effects of sorafenib and sunitinib. *Community Oncology 3,* 558-562.

Thalidomide (Thalomid)

Sandra E. Remer

DRUG CLASS

- Antiangiogenesis agent

ROUTE OF ADMINISTRATION

- Oral

HOW TO ADMINISTER

- Only in compliance with all of the terms outlined in the System for Thalidomide Educational and Prescribing Safety (STEP) program. Thalomide may only be prescribed by physicians registered with the STEPS program.
- May only be dispensed by pharmacists registered with the STEPS program
- All patients must complete an informed consent and participate in a mandatory confidential monitoring registry.

PRETREATMENT GUIDELINES
Women

- Women of childbearing age **MUST** have pregnancy test with in 24 hours of starting therapy.
- Female patients must use the mandatory two methods of contraception, one highly effective and one additional method.
- Highly effective: intrauterine contraceptive device, hormonal (birth control pills, injections, or implants), tubal ligation, or partner's vasectomy
- Other method: latex condom, diaphragm, or cervical cap

Men

- Because thalidomide is present in the semen of patients receiving it, males must always use a latex condom during sexual contact with women of childbearing potential even if he has undergone a successful vasectomy.

USE

- Erythema nodosum leprosum (ENL)
- Myelodysplastic syndrome (MDS)

Off-Label Uses

- Primary malignant brain tumors (orphan drug status)
- Graft-versus-host disease (GVHD) (orphan drug status)
- GVHD prophylaxis (orphan drug status)
- Kaposi's sarcoma (orphan drug status)
- Multiple myeloma (orphan drug status)
- Renal cell cancer
- Acquired immunodeficiency syndrome (AIDS)–associated wasting syndrome and cancer cachexia (orphan drug status)

Studies

- Also studied in breast cancer and prostate cancer
- Also used in other noncancer disease processes. Currently Celgene (Summit, NJ) is pursuing an additional indication, now in review.

PHARMACOKINETICS

- Thalidomide is given orally and is slowly absorbed from the gastrointestinal tract.
- The half-life range is 5-7 hours. Less than 1% of the dose is excreted in the urine as unchanged drug and is indictable in urine after 48 hours.
- Renal or hepatic dosing has not been determined.

USUAL DOSE AND SCHEDULE

- Usual dose is 200 mg daily at bedtime.
- Thalidomide has been given up to 1200 mg/day divided into three to four daily doses with the larger part of the dose given in the evening to minimize the sedation effects.

Disease-Specific Doses

- Malignant glioma: 200-400 mg orally at bedtime, increasing as directed
- GVHD: 800-1600 mg/day orally at bedtime
- GVHD prophylaxis: 800-1600 mg/day at bedtime
- Kaposi's sarcoma: 200 mg/day increasing every 2 weeks as tolerated to maximum 1,000 mg/day
- Multiple myeloma: 200 mg/day orally with dose increased by 200 mg/day every 2 weeks to tolerance or a maximum of 800 mg/day
- MDS: 100 mg/day orally increased to 400 mg/day
- Renal cell cancer: 200 mg/day orally increased to 800-1,200 mg/day
- AIDS-associated wasting syndrome and cancer cachexia: 100 mg/day with a range from 50-200 mg/day

SIDE EFFECTS

- **WARNING: SEVERE LIFE-THREATENING HUMAN BIRTH DEFECTS:** Thalomide must never be taken by a pregnant woman or one who could become pregnant while taking this drug.

Severe

- Peripheral neuropathy
- Neutropenia
- Hypertension
- Bradycardia
- Stevens-Johnson syndrome
- Toxic epidermal necrolysis
- Seizures and thrombotic events

Common

- Drowsiness
- Somnolence
- Dizziness
- Orthostatic hypotension
- Bradycardia
- Rash
- Diarrhea
- Fever
- Chills
- Headache
- Increased appetite
- Weight gain
- Dry mouth
- Confusion
- Amnesia
- Mood changes
- Photosensitivity
- Increase in human immunodeficiency virus (HIV) viral load

NADIR

- The incidence of neutropenia is <1%; however, there is an increased incidence of neutropenia in HIV-positive patients of 2%-20%.
- Anemia and lymphadenopathy is more commonly reported in immunosuppressed patients.
- Neutropenic fever has also been reported.

STORAGE

- Room temperature (15°-30° C [59°-86° F]) and protect from light.
- Keep this drug out of the reach of children.

DRUG INTERACTIONS

- Thalidomide may enhance the sedative effects of barbiturates, ethanol, chlorpromazine, and reserpine as well as other drugs, including amitriptyline, amoxapine, anxiolytics, sedatives and hypnotics, butorphanol, clomipramine, clozapine, doxepin, droperidol, entacapone, haloperidol, sedating H_1 blockers, imipramine, maprotiline, mirtazapine, molindone, nalbuphine, nefazodone, nortriptyline, olanzapine, opiate agonists, pentazocine, phenothiazines, pimozide, pramipexole, quetiapine, risperidone, ropinirole, skeletal muscle relaxants, tolcapone, tramadol, and trazodone.
- Use with caution in combination with drugs known to be associated with peripheral neuropathy.
- Drugs that interfere with hormonal contraception: concomitant use of HIV-protease inhibitors, griseofulvin, modafinil, penicillins, rifampin, phenytoin, carbamazepine, or certain herbal supplements such as St. John's wort with hormonal contraceptive agents may reduce the effectiveness of the contraceptive for up to 1 month after the discontinuation of these drugs.

PREGNANCY

Category X

- Contraindicated; positive evidence of serious fetal abnormalities in humans. Thalidomide may cause severe birth defects or death to an unborn baby.

SPECIAL CONSIDERATIONS

- Thalidomide is the most heavily regulated drug in the United States and may only be obtained through approved physicians and pharmacies registered in the System for Thalidomide Education and Prescribing Safety (STEPS) Program.

○ The patient understands that severe birth defects can occur with the use of thalidomide.

○ The patient has been warned by his or her physician that an unborn baby will most certainly have severe birth defects and can even die if a woman is pregnant or becomes pregnant while taking thalidomide.

○ Thalomide will be prescribed to the patient and MUST not be shared with anyone, even someone who has similar symptoms.

○ Thalidomide must never be given to women who are able to have children.

○ The patient cannot donate blood while taking thalidomide.

○ The patient has read the thalidomide patient brochure or viewed the videotape "Important information for Men and Women taking Thalomid (thalidomide)" and understands the contents, including other possible health problems from thalidomide side effects.

○ The patient's physician has answered any questions the patient has asked.

○ The patient must participate in a telephone survey and patient registry while taking thalidomide.

PATIENT EDUCATION

- Keep thalidomide out of the reach of children.
- NEVER share this medication with anyone.
- Return any unused thalidomide to the pharmacy where your prescription was filled. Your pharmacy will accept all unused thalidomide as part of controlled distribution program.
- Tell your physician or other health care professional about ALL the medication you are taking, including nonprescription drugs.
- Report side effects to your physician or health care professional as soon as possible: irregular menstrual bleeding or a missed menstrual period, new or increased tingling or numbness in hands or feet, muscle cramps, rash, seizures, unusual swelling or pain in arms or legs.

- Thalidomide causes drowsiness; be careful driving or operating machinery while taking thalidomide.
- Thalidomide may cause dizziness; sit upright for a few minutes before standing to avoid falling.
- All patients will receive counseling about potential birth defects and MUST follow the conditions of the STEPS Program.

BIBLIOGRAPHY

Henry Ford Clinical Pharmacy. (2006). *Thalidomide*. Retrieved January 31, 2007, from http://cpip.gsm.com/apps/products.

Oncology Nursing Society. (2003) *Thalomid (thalidomide)*. Retrieved January 31, 2007, from http://www.ons.org/patientEd/Treatments/PatientMeds/thalidomide.shtml.Supp:Nov/Dec 2003.

STEPS program. (2006). Retrieved January 31, 2007, from http://www.thalomide.com/thalomid_history.aspx.

Thalidomide. (2007). Retrieved January 31, 2007, from http://rxonline.epocrates.com. February 12, 2006.

Thalomid (thalidomide) [package insert]. Retrieved January 31, 2007, from www.Celegen.com.2005.

Cancer Management

Hormonal Therapy

Kristi Orbaugh

INTRODUCTION

As early as the 19th century, investigators began to recognize the importance of hormonal suppression in the treatment of breast cancer. In 1896, George Beatson observed an association between surgical removal of the ovaries and reduction in some of the breast tumors (Beatson, 1896). Since that time, investigators have attempted to suppress estrogen through many different avenues. Because hormonal therapies are very specific in their ability to block specific receptors and various feedback loops, these therapies were the first form of targeted therapy. Although hormone therapy was first used in the treatment of breast cancer, it was quickly added to the treatment regimens of prostate, endometrial, and ovarian cancers. Tumor growth that is stimulated by testosterone or estrogen can be suppressed by blocking these hormones from communicating with the cancer cells.

ADRENOCORTICOIDS

Adrenocorticoids are mainly responsible for the control of glucose metabolism, gluconeogenesis, and immune systems regulation. The major forms of adrenocorticoids are cortisol and corticosterone. Adrenocorticoids are manufactured in the adrenal cortex and regulated through the action of adrenocorticotropic hormone (ACTH). ACTH is produced in the anterior pituitary. The regulation of ACTH depends on a precise sensitive balance between serum levels and stimulation from the nervous system. The feedback effects are mediated from the nervous system. The most commonly used corticosteroids in clinical practices are cortisone acetate, hydrocortisone, prednisolone, methylprednisolone, and dexamethasone. Studies of tissue culture demonstrated that lymphoid cells are most sensitive to glucocorticoids and resulted in a great decrease in deoxyribonucleic acid, ribonucleic acid, and protein synthesis (Cohen, 1989). Adrenocorticoids or glucocorticoids inhibit lymphocyte proliferation by encouraging apoptosis (Cohen, 1989). These agents are used commonly in acute lymphoblastic leukemia, chronic lymphocytic leukemia, Hodgkin disease, non-Hodgkin lymphoma, and multiple myeloma. In addition, the drugs may be used as adjuvant treatment with routine antiemetics, pain medicine, and to reduce edema from central nervous system metastasis.

The most common side effects from this class of drugs are hypersensitivity, appearance of Cushing's syndrome, osteoporosis, diabetes mellitus, and profound immune system suppression. Additional side effects include euphoria, peptic ulcer disease, and steroid psychosis.

ANDROGENS

The generic term for the major sex steroid in males is androgens. The testes produce testosterone, which is the primary male hormone. The main functions of the androgens are male development, spermatogenesis, inhibition of fat deposition, and muscle mass and brain development. The most well-known adrenal androgen is testosterone. Other androgens include the following:

- *Dehydroepiandrosterone* is a steroid produced from cholesterol in the adrenal cortex. This is the primary precursor of natural testrogens.
- *Androstenedione* is produced by the testes, adrenal cortex, and ovaries. Androstenediones are metabolically converted to androgens, including testosterone. In females this androgenic steroid is the parent structure of estrone. This steroid had been banned by many sporting organizations for athletic or body building supplements.
- *Androstanediol* is a steroid metabolite that acts as the main regulator of gonadotropin secretion.
- *Androsterone* is a chemical byproduct created during the breakdown of androgens or progesterone. It also exerts minor masculinizing effects. This is found in equal amounts in the urine and plasma in both male and females.
- *Dehydrotesterone* is a metabolite of testosterone. It is an extremely potent androgen and binds strongly to androgen receptors.

ANTIESTROGENS

It has been apparent to observant clinicians for more than a century that estrogen played an important role in the pathophysiological mechanisms of breast cancer. It became known in the early 1900s that approximately one third of premenopausal women with advanced breast cancer would respond to an oophorectomy (Boyd, 1990; Jordan & Kennedy, 1997). In the same way, some postmenopausal women responded to adrenalectomies and hypophysectomy (Pearson, Ray, & Harold, 1956). With the discovery of the estrogen receptor (Jensen & Jacobson, 1962; Toft & Gorski, 1966) the mechanisms of actions for estrogen on the various target tissues became more apparent. The two most common drug classes used for their antiestrogen-like effects include selective estrogen receptor modulators (SERMs) and estrogen-receptor down-regulators (ERD).

Selective Estrogen Receptor Modulators

SERMs work by occupying the estrogen receptors inside cells. This blocks the action of estrogen in breast and other estrogen-sensitive tissues. SERMs do not block all estrogen receptors. As the name suggests, they selectively inhibit certain estrogen receptors, such as those in breast tissue, while allowing stimulation of estrogen receptors in other organs. The most prescribed SERM is tamoxifen (Nolvadex). Toremifene (Fareston) is not prescribed frequently in the United States.

Estrogen-Receptor Down-Regulators

ERDs work by blocking or breaking down the estrogen receptors. Fewer cancer cells receive the signal telling them to grow and divide because fewer estrogen receptors are available. ERDs destroy the estrogen receptors. But unlike SERMs, they do not act like weak estrogens elsewhere in the body. ERDs cause fewer hot flashes and other menopausal symptoms than the SERMs because the ERDs do not seem to affect the estrogen receptors in the brain, which can affect the body's thermostat.

AROMATASE INHIBITORS

Two major routes exist for estrogen production. The routes are ovarian production and peripheral aromatization. In premenopausal women, both routes are active. In postmenopausal women, only the peripheral aromatization is active. Since the early 1970s, the aromatase enzyme has been a target for drug inhibition (Rieber & Theriault, 2005). Aminoglutethimide was the first drug used to block the aromatase enzyme in women with metastatic breast cancer (Smith, 2003). In most postmenopausal women androstenedione is released from the adrenal glands. This adrenal steroid goes through several metabolic steps before coming into contact with the aromatase enzyme. Eventually it is converted to estrogen. This is called aromatization. This enzymatic conversion occurs at peripheral sites such as breast tissue, liver, muscles, and fat cells. The conversion is catalyzed by the aromatase enzyme complex. By blocking or inhibiting the aromatase enzyme the conversion to estrogen is not possible. Two major classes of aromatase inhibitors are currently used. They include nonsteroidal aromatase inhibitors and steroidal aromatase inhibitors.

Nonsteroidal aromatase inhibitors are also called competitive aromatase inhibitors. These drugs bind reversibly to the receptor site on the enzymes and prevent the formation of estrogen for as long the aromatase inhibitors occupy the receptor site.

Steroidal aromatase inhibitors, also called noncompetitive aromatase inhibitors, are derivatives of androstenedione. This class of aromatase inhibitors retains their androgenic properties. Because these agents bind irreversibly to the aromatase enzyme, they are also called suicide inhibitors. New enzymes must be synthesized to overcome this inhibitor even after the drug has been cleared from the body. Although studies have not shown this to be true, hypothetically these agents should improve efficacy compared with the reversible inhibitors.

LUTEINIZING HORMONE RELEASING HORMONE AGONISTS

Ovarian ablation has been recognized as an effective means of treating breast cancer for well over a century

(Boyd, 1990) in the same way orchiectomy has been used to treat prostate cancer. Historically, surgical removal or irradiation of the ovaries or testes has been used to ablate hormonal stimulation, which can cause proliferation to sensitive tissues. These methods have been used with some success with ranges from 21% or 37% (Sarma & Schottenfeld, 2002). The development of luteinizing hormone releasing hormone (LHRH) agonists has allowed ovarian or testicular ablation to be achieved through chemical means. The use of a LHRH agonist minimizes morbidity, thereby providing a preferable alternative to the other more decisively invasive procedures. The LHRH agonist mimics the naturally occurring substance in the body and produces the same physiological effects. By mimicking the normal LHRH, the agonists fill the receptor in the pituitary. An agonist will occupy the receptors for a longer period of time than the endogenous LHRH. LHRH agonist suppresses ovarian production of estrogen by binding to the LHRH pituitary receptors. This results in down-regulation of the receptors. With continued administration, estrogen and progesterone production are greatly reduced. Estrogen initially surges because of the primary stimulating effects on the receptors. After approximately 2 to 4 weeks of treatment, the negative feedback mechanism will be activated and the desired inhibition of luteinizing hormone (LH) and follicle-stimulating hormone (FSH) will be achieved. Estrogen and progesterone levels will then begin to fall. This exact process happens the same way in males, resulting in decreased LH and FSH stimulation on the testicles and ultimately a decrease in testosterone production.

LUTEINIZING HORMONE RELEASING HORMONE ANTAGONISTS

The LHRH antagonists are a class of peptide analogs representing important oncologic and gynecologic applications. The antagonists act on the same receptor site as LHRH. This causes immediate inhibition of the release of gonadotropins and sex steroids. The "flare response" is prevented because the antagonists induce immediate suppression. Just as with LHRH agonists, the ovaries are no longer stimulated to produce estrogen and the testes are not stimulated to release testosterone.

PROGESTINS

In normal day-to-day physiological functioning, progesterone is involved in the differentiation of a broad spectrum of tissues. The specific effect of progesterone appears to depend on the type of tissue (Dunn, Wickerham, & Ford, 2005). For example, progesterone is required for the maintenance of pregnancy and it produces changes in the uterus and breast during the menstrual cycle. Progestins exert their action on the hypothalamic-pituitary axis. This results in the inhibition of gonadotropin-releasing hormone and indirectly affects tissue growth. In addition, progestins appear to have a direct effect on cellular proliferation. This can result in either growth or inhibition of cellular condition. The cellular effects are mediated through the progesterone receptor located in the cell nucleus.

Before the development of third-generation aromatase inhibitors, progestins were used as second-line hormonal therapy for estrogen receptor or progesterone-receptor positive breast cancer in postmenopausal women. With the development the new aromatase inhibitors, progestins are now generally considered third or fourth line in the treatment of breast cancer.

CONCLUSION

The past century has brought many changes and advances to the oncology field. One type of treatment that remains consistent is hormonal manipulation and hormone blockade. Tumors that are stimulated to grow from hormones attaching to specific receptor sites frequently respond to treatment that attempts to interrupt the communication between the hormone and the specific receptor. Hormonal treatment has been used successfully since the 19th century and will continue to be used and perfected in the future.

REFERENCES

Beatson, G. T. (1896). On the treatment of inoperable cases of carcinoma of the mamma: suggestions for a new method of treatment, with illustrative cases. *Lancet, 2,* 104-107.

Boyd, S. (1990). On oophorectomy in cancer of the breast. *British Medical Journal, 2,* 1161-1167.

Cohen, J. J. (1989). Lymphocyte cell death induced by glucocorticoids. In R. P. Scheimer, H. N. Claman, & A. L. Dronsky (Eds). *Anti-inflammatory steroid action: Basic and clinical aspects.* (pp. 110-121). San Diego: Academic Press.

Dunn, B. K., Wickerham, D. L., & Ford, L. G. (2005). Prevention of hormone-related cancers: breast cancer. *Journal of Clinical Oncology, 23,* 357-367.

Jenson, E. V., & Jacobson, H. I. (1962). Basic guideline on the mechanism of estrogen action. *Recent Progress in Hormone Research, 8,* 387-414.

Jordan, D. T., & Kennedy, B. J. (1977). Tamoxifen therapy in advanced breast cancer. *Annals of Internal Medicine, 87,* 687-690.

Pearson, O. H., Ray, B. S., & Harold, C. C. (1956). Hypophysectomy in the treatment of advanced cancer. *Journal of the American Medical Association, 161,* 17-21.

Rieber, A. G., & Theriault, R. L. (2005). Aromatase inhibitors in postmenopausal breast cancer patients. *Journal of the National Comprehensive Cancer Network, 3,* 309-314.

Sarma, A. V., & Schottenfeld, D. (2002). Prostate cancer incidence, mortality and survival trends in the United States 1981-2001. *Seminars in Urologic Oncology, 20,* 3-9.

Smith, I. E. (2003). Drug therapy: aromatase inhibitors in breast cancer. *New England Journal of Medicine, 348,* 2431-2442.

Toft, D., & Gorski, J. (1966). A receptor molecule for estrogens: isolation from the rat uterus and preliminary characterization. *Proceedings of the National Academy of Science, USA, 55,* 1574-1581.

Abarelix (Plenaxis)

DRUG CLASS
- Luteinizing hormone releasing hormone antagonist

ROUTE OF ADMINISTRATION
- Intramuscular (IM) injection

PRETREATMENT GUIDELINES
- Baseline tumor marker (if appropriate)
- Baseline testosterone level
- Baseline liver function test
- Baseline electrocardiogram

USE
- Advanced prostate cancer

PHARMACOKINETICS
- Competitively blocks gonadotropin-releasing hormone receptors in the pituitary
- Suppresses luteinizing hormone and follicle-stimulating hormone secretion
- Reduces secretion of testosterone by the testes
- Excreted in the urine
- No initial increase in testosterone.

USUAL DOSE AND SCHEDULE
- 100 mg IM on days 1, 15, and 29
- Every 4 weeks thereafter

SIDE EFFECTS
- Immediate-onset systemic allergic reaction resulting in hypotension and syncope have occurred.
- Possible prolongation of QT interval
- Edema
- Gynecomastia
- Impotence
- Fatigue
- Urinary hesitation
- Histamine release
- Urinary frequency
- Hot flashes
- Weight gain

DRUG INTERACTIONS
- Antiarrhythmic medication
- Amiodarone, procainamide, quinidine, sotalol

PREGNANCY
Category X

SPECIAL CONSIDERATION
- After getting the injection, the patient must stay in the office for at least 30 minutes.

PATIENT EDUCATION
- Report history of osteoporosis.
- Report any history of heart disease.
- Report history of allergies.

BIBLIOGRAPHY
Sarma, A. V., & Schottenfeld, D. (2002). Prostate cancer incidence, mortality, and survival trends in the United States 1981-2001. *Seminars in Urologic Oncology, 20,* 3-9.

Schellhammer, P. F. (2000). Therapy of advanced cancer of the prostate. *Report to the 95th Annual Meeting of the American Urological Association,* April 29–May 4, 2000, Atlanta, GA.

Aminoglutethimide (Cytadren)

DRUG CLASS
- Adrenal suppressant

ROUTE OF ADMINISTRATION
- Oral

PRETREATMENT GUIDELINES
- Baseline liver function tests
- Baseline complete blood cell count
- Baseline thyroid function
- Baseline vital signs

USE
- Prostate cancer
- Breast cancer

PHARMACOKINETICS
- "Chemical adrenalectomy"
- Interferes with the conversion of enzymes, thereby effectively inhibiting the synthesis of corticosteroids, estrogens, and androgens
- Adrenals are suppressed and the growth of malignances that need estrogen or testosterone to thrive is also suppressed.

USUAL DOSE AND SCHEDULE
- 750-2000 mg orally daily in divided doses
- Give with 40 mg of hydrocortisone daily

SIDE EFFECTS
- Drowsiness
- Fatigue
- Skin rash (usually noticed during the first week of treatment, resolves over time)
- Mild nausea
- Clumsiness
- Ataxia
- Dizziness
- Malaise
- Fever

DRUG INTERACTIONS
- May diminish the effects of warfarin, theophylline, digitoxin, dexamethasone, and medroxyprogesterone
- Drug side effects potentiated by alcohol.
- Must use hydrocortisone as a glucocortoid replacement.
- Aminoglutethimide enhances dexamethasone metabolism.

PREGNANCY

Category D

SPECIAL CONSIDERATIONS

- Adjuvant corticosteroids should be administered.
- Most side effects will decrease in severity and incidence after the first 2 to 6 weeks of therapy.
- Adrenal hypofunction may develop with stressful situations such as acute illness, surgery, or trauma. Additional steroids may be required to ensure normal response to stress.
- Approximately 50% of patients will require mineralocorticoid replacement with fludrocortisone.
- Frequently monitor blood pressure.

PATIENT EDUCATION

- Emphasize importance of not stopping the hydrocortisone abruptly.
- Warn patient of possible transient drowsiness.
- Avoid hazardous activities that require alertness until sedative effects subside.
- Stand up slowly to avoid dizziness.
- Take this medication with 8 ounces of water.
- Do not take on an empty stomach.
- If a skin rash develops when starting therapy and the rash persists more than 5 days, therapy should be temporarily discontinued.
- May restart therapy after rash resolves.
- Elderly may be more sensitive to central nervous system adverse events.
- Avoid breast-feeding.

BIBLIOGRAPHY

Honig, S. F. (1996). Treatment of metastic disease: hormonal therapy and chemotherapy. In J. R. Harris, M. E. Lippman, & M. Morrow (Eds.). *Disease of the breast.* (pp. 669-734). Philadelphia: Lippincott-Raven.

Stege, R., Grande M., Carlstrom K., et al. (2000). Prognostic significance of tissue prostate-specific antigen in endocrine-treated prostate carcinoma. *Clinical Cancer Research, 6,* 160-165.

Anastrozole (Arimidex)

DRUG CLASS

- Nonsteroidal aromatase inhibitor, competitive aromatase inhibitor

ROUTE OF ADMINISTRATION

- Oral

PRETREATMENT GUIDELINES

- Consider baseline bone density study.
- Baseline complete blood cell count
- Baseline comprehensive metabolic panel

USE

- First-line treatment in postmenopausal women with advanced or locally advanced breast cancer that is hormone receptor positive or unknown receptor status.
- Advanced breast cancer in postmenopausal women with progression of disease after tamoxifen therapy.
- Adjuvant treatment of postmenopausal early breast cancer that is hormone receptor positive.

PHARMACOKINETICS

- Binds reversibly to the aromatase enzyme
- Resulting in inhibition, the conversion of androgens to estrogens
- Decreased biosynthesis of estrogen in all tissue
- Has no effect on adrenal corticosteroids or aldosterone formation
- Well absorbed from the gastrointestinal tract
- Food does not affect absorption.
- Metabolized by the liver
- Metabolites are excreted in the urine.

USUAL DOSE AND SCHEDULE

- 1 mg every day

SIDE EFFECTS

- Hot flashes
- Arthralgias
- Myalgias
- Decreased bone density
- Vomiting
- Nausea
- Fatigue
- Edema
- Anorexia
- Mild leukopenia
- Headache
- Decreased libido

DRUG INTERACTIONS

- Tamoxifen

PREGNANCY

Category D

SPECIAL CONSIDERATIONS

- Consider calcium and vitamin D supplements.
- Dosage adjustment is not necessary for renal or hepatic dysfunction.
- Coadministration of corticosteroids not necessary

PATIENT EDUCATION

- Encourage weight-bearing exercise.
- Use reliable birth control.
- Report any unusual side effects such as shortness of breath or pain.
- Do not abruptly stop drug without consulting health care provider.

BIBLIOGRAPHY

Rieber, A., & Theriault, R. (2005). Aromatase inhibitors in postmenopausal breast cancer patients. *Journal of the National Comprehensive Cancer Network, 3,* 309-314.

Smith, I. E. (2003). Drug therapy: aromatase inhibitors in breast cancer. *New England Journal of Medicine, 348,* 2431-2442.

Bicalutamide (Casodex)

DRUG CLASS
- Antineoplastic agent, antiandrogen

ROUTE OF ADMINISTRATION
- Oral

PRETREATMENT GUIDELINES
- Baseline complete blood cell count
- Baseline comprehensive metabolic profile
- Baseline prostate-specific antigen

USE
- Prostate cancer

PHARMACOKINETICS
- Competitively inhibit the action of androgens by binding to androgen receptors in the target tissues.
- Well absorbed after oral administration
- Route or amount absorbed not affected by food intake.
- Metabolized in the liver
- Both the parent drug and metabolites are eliminated in the urine and feces.

USUAL DOSE AND SCHEDULE
- 50 mg once every day in combination with a luteinizing hormone releasing hormone analog

PATIENT EDUCATION
- Do not abruptly stop taking this medication.
- Should be taken at the same time each day.
- If hot flashes occur, cool, light clothing, cool cloths applied to the head, and cool environment are recommended.

BIBLIOGRAPHY
Boccardo, F., Rubagotti A., Barichello M., et al. (1999). Bicalutamide monotherapy versus flutamide plus goserelin in prostrate cancer patients: results of an Italian Prostate Cancer Project Study. *Journal of Clinical Oncology, 17,* 2027-2038.

Trachienberg, J., Gittelman, M., Steidle, C., et al. (2000). Abarelix—depot (A-D) versus leuprolide acetate (L) plus bicalutamide (casodex©), for prostate cancer: results of a multi-institutional, randomized phase III study in 255 patients. In *Proceedings and Abstracts of the American Society of Clinical Oncology,* Abstract 1307.

Buserelin (Suprefact)

DRUG CLASS
- Luteinizing hormone releasing hormone antagonist
- Available for use in the United Kingdom and Canada only. **Not available in the United States.**

ROUTE OF ADMINISTRATION
- Nasal solution
- Injection

PRETREATMENT GUIDELINES
- Baseline prostate-specific antigen or other tumor marker, if appropriate
- Baseline weight

USE
- Advanced prostate cancer

PHARMACOKINETICS
- Blocks the luteinizing hormone receptor in the pituitary gland.
- Greatly reduces or eliminates production of luteinizing hormone
- Because the testes are not being stimulated by luteinizing hormone, testosterone levels fall.

USUAL DOSE AND SCHEDULE
- Nasal dosage: 200 mcg (two sprays) into each nostril every 8 hours
- Injection dosage: 500 mcg (0.5 mg) subcutaneously every 8 hours
- May at some point lower dosage to 200 mcg (0.2 mg) once every day.

SIDE EFFECTS
- Nasal irritation
- Tumor flare
- Hot flashes
- Gynecomastia
- Injection site irritation
- Edema
- Decreased libido
- Impotence
- Weight gain
- Nausea
- Vomiting
- Fatigue

DRUG INTERACTIONS
- None reported

PREGNANCY
Category X

SPECIAL CONSIDERATIONS
- May cause sterility. Consider sperm banking, if appropriate.
- Assess for allergies
- Not commercially available in the United States

PATIENT EDUCATION
- Report nasal irritation.
- Report injection site reaction.
- Discuss possibility of sterility.
- If a dose is missed, do not double dose.
- Report increase in bone pain.

BIBLIOGRAPHY
Sarma, A. V., & Schottenfeld, D. (2002). Prostate cancer incidence, mortality, and survival trends in the United States 1981-2001. *Seminars in Urologic Oncology, 20,* 3-9.

Exemestane (Aromasin)

DRUG CLASS
- Steroidal aromatase inhibitor

ROUTE OF ADMINISTRATION
- Oral

PRETREATMENT GUIDELINES
- Baseline complete blood cell count
- Baseline comprehensive metabolic panel

Cancer Management

- Baseline liver function tests
- Baseline bone density study

USE

- Treatment of advanced breast cancer in postmenopausal women, after disease progression after tamoxifen treatment
- Adjuvant treatment of postmenopausal women with estrogen receptor–positive early breast cancer who have had 2-3 years of tamoxifen. Then stay on exemestane for a completion of a 5-year regimen.

PHARMACOKINETICS

- Orally active and selective type 1 aromatase inhibitor
- A derivative of androstenedione
- Binds to the steroid-binding site of aromatase
- Converted by the normal catalytic mechanism of the enzyme
- The binding of the substrate results in inactivation of the aromatase.
- Enzymatic activity is blocked and no estrogen can be produced until a new enzyme is synthesized.
- Metabolites are excreted from the kidneys and from the liver.
- Clinical relevance of the irreversible binding properties is not yet clear.

USUAL DOSE AND SCHEDULE

- 25 mg every day

SIDE EFFECTS

- Depression
- Headache
- Fatigue
- Peripheral edema
- Sweating
- Nausea and vomiting
- Flu-like syndrome
- Arthralgia
- Insomnia
- Weight changes
- Hypertension
- Skeletal pain
- Dizziness
- Hot flashes

DRUG INTERACTIONS

- Metabolized by the P4503A4 (CYP3A9) isoenzyme system. Use with caution with known inducers of the enzyme system. Serum levels may be decreased.

PREGNANCY

Category D

SPECIAL CONSIDERATIONS

- Consider calcium and vitamin D supplementation.
- Follow up appropriate laboratory values.

PATIENT EDUCATION

- Encourage weight-bearing exercise.
- Use reliable birth control.
- Report any persistent or intolerable side effects.
- Instruct patient not to stop medication abruptly.

BIBLIOGRAPHY

Rieber, A., & Theriault, R. (2005). Aromatase inhibitors in postmenopausal breast cancer patients. *Journal of the National Comprehensive Cancer Network, 3*, 309-314.

Smith, I. E. (2003). Drug therapy: aromatase inhibitors in breast cancer. *New England Journal of Medicine, 348*, 2431-2442.

Flutamide (Eulexin)

DRUG CLASS

- Nonsteroidal antiandrogen

ROUTE OF ADMINISTRATION

- Oral

PRETREATMENT GUIDELINES

- Baseline comprehensive metabolic panel
- Baseline liver function tests
- Baseline prostate-specific antigen

USE

- Treatment of metastatic prostate cancer given in combination with luteinizing hormone releasing hormone analogs

PHARMACOKINETICS

- Inhibits uptake of androgen or inhibits receptor and nuclear binding of androgen in target tissues
- Absorption is rapid and complete after oral administration.
- Animal studies indicate that the drug concentrates in the prostate.
- Rapid metabolism with more than 97% of the drug metabolized within the first hour of administration.
- More than 95% of the drug is excreted in the urine.
- 96% is bound to plasma proteins.

USUAL DOSE AND SCHEDULE

- 250 mg by mouth every 8 hours

SIDE EFFECTS

- Loss of libido
- Hot flashes
- Galactorrhea
- Nausea and vomiting
- Rash
- Drowsiness
- Gynecomastia
- Impotence
- Elevated liver functions

DRUG INTERACTIONS

- None reported

PREGNANCY

Category D

SPECIAL CONSIDERATIONS

- Almost always given with luteinizing hormone releasing hormone analog
- Monitor prostate-specific antigen for changes.

PATIENT EDUCATION

- Report bothersome hot flashes to health care provider for symptom management.
- Flutamide should not be stopped abruptly without instruction from health care provider.

BIBLIOGRAPY

Eisenberger, M. A., Blumenstein, B.A., Crawford, E.D., et al. (1998). Bilateral orchiectomy with or without flutamide for metastic prostate cancer. *New England Journal of Medicine, 339*, 1036-1042.

Fulvestrant (Faslodex)

DRUG CLASS
- Estrogen receptor antagonist

ROUTE OF ADMINISTRATION
- Intramuscular (IM)

PRETREATMENT GUIDELINES
- Baseline complete blood cell count
- Baseline tumor marker (if appropriate)

USE
- Hormone receptor–positive metastatic breast cancer in postmenopausal women, with disease progression after antiestrogen therapy

PHARMACOKINETICS
- Estrogen receptor antagonist that binds to the estrogen receptor
- No agonist effect as with other antiestrogens
- Estrogen receptor is degraded so that it is lost from the cell.
- Once it binds to the site, it causes the receptor to break down, preventing cellular response to estrogen.

USUAL DOSE AND SCHEDULE
- 250 mg IM every 4 weeks

SIDE EFFECTS
- Nausea
- Vomiting
- Edema
- Headache
- Constipation
- Abdominal pain
- Rash
- Thromboembolic phenomenon
- Hot flashes
- Cold-like symptoms
- Vaginal bleeding
- Bone pain
- Diarrhea
- Injection site reaction

PREGNANCY
Category D

SPECIAL CONSIDERATIONS
- Use with extreme caution in patients with moderate to severe hepatic impairment.
- Document thromboembolic events.
- Follow up appropriate laboratory values.

PATIENT EDUCATION
- Use reliable birth control method.
- Report swelling, redness, or pain in the extremities.
- Report history of deep venous thrombosis.
- Report acute shortness of breath.
- Report any persistent or intolerable side effects.

BIBLIOGRAPHY
Pietras, R. J., Marquis, D. C., Chen, H. W., et al. (2003). Improved antitumor therapy with Faslodex for dual targeting of HER-2 and estrogen receptor signaling pathways in human breast cancers with oversuppression of HER-2 neu gene. *Breast Cancer Research, 82,* S12-S13.

Goserelin Acetate (Zoladex, Zoladex LA)

DRUG CLASS
- Luteinizing hormone-releasing hormone agonist (LHRH). Synthetic analog of LHRH

ROUTE OF ADMINISTRATION
- Subcutaneous (SQ) implant

PRETREATMENT GUIDELINES
- Baseline tumor markers if appropriate
- Baseline comprehensive metabolic panel
- Baseline lipid profile

USE
- Palliative treatment of advanced prostate carcinoma as an alternative to orchiectomy
- With flutamide before and during radiation therapy for early-stage prostate cancer.
- Endometriosis
- Palliative treatment of advanced breast cancer
- Endometrial thinning before ablation for dysfunctional uterine bleeding.

PHARMACOKINETICS
- Potent inhibitor of gonadotropin secretion from the pituitary gland
- Initial increase in serum levels of luteinizing hormone and follicle-stimulating hormone
- Followed by long-term suppression of pituitary gonadotropins

USUAL DOSE AND SCHEDULE
- SQ implant, 3.6 mg every 28 days
- SQ implant, 10.8 mg every 12 weeks

SIDE EFFECTS
- Sexual dysfunction
- Gynecomastia
- Renal insufficiency
- Urinary frequency
- Depression
- Pain at injection site
- Nausea and vomiting
- Hot flashes
- Tumor flare
- Elevated cholesterol levels
- Lethargy

DRUG INTERACTIONS
- None reported

PREGNANCY
Category X

SPECIAL CONSIDERATIONS
- Watch for tumor flare response.
- Patients with impending urethral obstruction or spinal cord compression should have appropriate treatment before the start of goserelin.
- Use with caution in patients with abnormal renal function.

PATIENT EDUCATION
- Report weakness or numbness in lower extremities.

Cancer Management

- Report injection site reactions.
- Report weight gain of 2 pounds or more in 1 day.
- Report urinary retention.
- May have increased bone pain at the start of treatment.
- Importance of compliance to 28-day cycle
- Identify appropriate resources for counseling and for support with alteration in sexual activity.

BIBLIOGRAPHY

Boccardo, F., Rubagotti, A., Barichello, M., et al. (1999). Bicalutamide monotherapy versus flutamide plus goserelin in prostate cancer patients: results of an Italian Prostate Cancer Project Study. *Journal of Clinical Oncology, 17,* 2027-2038.

Letrozole (Femara)

DRUG CLASS

- Aromatase inhibitor (nonsteroidal)

ROUTE OF ADMINISTRATION

- Oral

PRETREATMENT GUIDELINES

- Baseline bone density scan
- Baseline comprehensive metabolic profile
- Baseline complete blood cell count
- Baseline tumor marker if appropriate

USE

- Advanced breast cancer in postmenopausal women
- Adjuvant breast cancer in postmenopausal women with hormone receptor positivity
- First-line treatment of advanced or metastatic breast with hormone-positive or hormone unknown disease
- Treatment of advanced breast cancer with disease progression after antiestrogen therapy
- Extended adjuvant treatment of early breast cancer in postmenopausal women after 5 years of tamoxifen therapy

PHARMACOKINETICS

- A nonsteroidal competitive inhibitor of aromatase
- Results in inhibition of conversion of androgens to estrogens
- Decreased biosynthesis of estrogen in all tissues
- Does not cause increase in serum follicle-stimulating hormone levels
- Does not affect synthesis of adrenocorticosteroids, aldosterone, or thyroid hormones
- Inactive liver metabolites are excreted in urine.
- Highly selective potent agent that significantly suppresses serum estradiol levels within 14 days

USUAL DOSE AND SCHEDULE

- 2.5 mg orally every day
- Reduction of dose recommended in patients with cirrhosis and severe hepatic dysfunction.

SIDE EFFECTS

- Hot flashes
- Arthralgia
- Night sweats
- Weight increases
- Nausea
- Fatigue
- Edema
- Myalgia
- Bone fractures
- Vaginal bleeding

DRUG INTERACTIONS

- Tamoxifen

PREGNANCY

Category D

SPECIAL CONSIDERATIONS

- Use caution with patients with severe hepatic impairment.
- Use caution with renal impairment.
- Monitor bone density.
- Consider added calcium and vitamin D.

PATIENT EDUCATION

- Use reliable birth control.
- Do not stop drug without notifying the medical provider.
- Encourage patient to do weight-bearing exercises.

BIBLIOGRAPHY

Lipton, A., Ali, S. M., Leitzel, K., et al. (2003). Serum HER-2/neu and response to the aromatase inhibitor letrozole versus tamoxifen. *Journal of Clinical Oncology, 21,* 1967-1972.

Leuprolide Acetate (Lupron)

DRUG CLASS

- Luteinizing hormone releasing hormone agonist (LHRH); synthetic analog

ROUTES OF ADMINISTRATION

- Intramuscular (IM)
- Subcutaneous (SQ)

PRETREATMENT GUIDELINES

- Baseline complete blood cell count
- Baseline comprehensive metabolic panel
- Baseline weight
- Baseline symptoms
- Baseline tumor marker if applicable

USE

- Prostate cancer
- Breast cancer
- Ovarian cancer
- Endometrial cancer
- Benign endometriosis
- Infertility
- Benign prostate hypertrophy

PHARMACOKENETICS

- Direct effect on ovaries and testes
- Peptide analog of luteinizing releasing hormones
- LHRH analogs affect follicle-stimulating hormone and luteinizing hormone secretion, thereby affecting the pituitary-ovarian axis and ultimately decreasing the release of estrogen to postmenopausal levels.
- In the male population, testosterone levels are greatly diminished.

- This analog is approximately 100 times more potent than the natural hormone.

USUAL DOSE AND SCHEDULE

- 1 mg/day SQ or depot IM 7.5 mg every month, 22.5 mg every 3 months, or 30 mg every 4 months

SIDE EFFECTS

- Hot flashes
- Impotence
- Decrease in libido
- Edema
- Breast pain
- Tumor flare response
- Sweating
- Depression
- Gynecomastia
- Increase in cholesterol levels
- General loss of strength

DRUG INTERACTIONS

- None reported

PREGNANCY

Category X

SPECIAL CONSIDERATIONS

- With depot form do not use needles less than 22 gauge.
- Follow manufacturer's guidelines when reconstituting.
- Always reconstitute with the diluent provided.

PATIENT EDUCATION

- Record weight at baseline.
- Report weight gains of greater than or equal to 2 pounds/day.
- Report weakness, numbness, respiratory difficulty, or impaired urination.
- Identify appropriate resources for counseling and for support of alteration in sexual activity.
- May have increase in bone pain at the start of therapy
- Report induration or erythema at injection site.

BIBLIOGRAPHY

D'Amico, A., Schultz, D., Loffredo, M., et al. (2000). Biochemical outcome following external beam radiation therapy with or without androgen suppression therapy for clinically localized prostate cancer. *Journal of the American Medical Association, 284,* 1280-1283.
Trachienberg, J., Gittelman, M., Steidle, C., et al. (2000). Abarelix—depot (A-D) versus leuprolide acetate (L) plus bicalutamide [casodex (C)], for prostate cancer: results of a multi-institutional, randomized phase III study in 255 patients. *Proceedings and Abstracts of the American Society of Clinical Oncology,* Abstract 1307.

Megestrol (Megace, Megase ES)

DRUG CLASS

- Progesterone; synthetic progestin

ROUTE OF ADMINISTRATION

- Oral (tablet or liquid suspension)

PRETREATMENT GUIDELINES

- Baseline complete blood cell count
- Baseline comprehensive metabolic profile
- Baseline weight
- Note any thromboembolic events or hypercoagulability syndrome.

USE

- Breast cancer
- Endometrial cancer
- Anorexia
- Cachexia

PHARMACOKINETICS

- Precise mechanism of action is unknown.
- Suppresses gonadotropins, having an antiluteinizing effect
- May down-regulate estrogen or progesterone receptors

USUAL DOSE AND SCHEDULE

- Breast cancer: 40 mg four times a day
- Endometrial cancer: 40-320 mg/day in divided doses
- Appetite stimulant: 800 mg/day
- Adjust to 400 mg/day after 1 month for appetite stimulation

SIDE EFFECTS

- Weight gain
- Edema
- Breakthrough menstrual bleeding
- Vaginal itching
- Vaginal irritation
- Vaginal discharge
- Hypertension
- Thromboembolism.

DRUG INTERACTIONS

- Aminoglutethimide

PREGNANCY

Category X (as appetite stimulant)
Category D (for carcinoma)

SPECIAL CONSIDERATIONS

- Use extreme caution in patients with a history of thromboembolic disease.
- Long-term use may increase risk of respiratory infection.
- May cause secondary adrenal suppression
- Note sensitivity to tartrazines.
- Use with caution with patients with diabetes mellitus.

PATIENT EDUCATION

- Report unusual shortness of breath.
- Report pain or leg swelling.
- May take with food if gastrointestinal upset.
- Report vaginal bleeding.
- Report edema.
- Practice reliable birth control.

BIBLIOGRAPHY

Dawson, N. A. (1995). Dramatic prostate specific antigen decrease in response to discontinuation of megestrol acetate in advanced prostate cancer: expansion of the antiandrogen withdrawal syndrome, *Journal of Urology, 153,* 1946-1947.

Cancer Management

Nilutamide (Nilandron)

DRUG CLASS

- Antiandrogen

ROUTE OF ADMINISTRATION

- Oral

PRETREATMENT GUIDELINES

- Baseline liver function tests
- Baseline comprehensive metabolic profile
- Baseline chest x-ray film
- Baseline prostate-specific antigen (PSA)

USE

- Used in combination with surgical castration for the treatment of metastatic prostate cancer
- Used in combination with luteinizing hormone releasing hormone analog

PHARMACOKINETICS

- Binds to the androgen receptor, which prevents normal androgenic response
- Absorbed completely and rapidly from the gastrointestinal tract
- Metabolites excreted through the urine

USUAL DOSE AND SCHEDULE

- 300 mg by mouth every day for 30 days
- Followed by 150 mg by mouth once daily thereafter

SIDE EFFECTS

- Hot flashes
- Gynecomastia
- Breast pain
- Impaired adaptation of night vision
- Elevated liver functions
- Decreased libido
- Galactorrhea
- Impotence
- Photophobia
- Interstitial pneumonitis

DRUG INTERACTIONS

- Demonstrated inhibition of the liver cytochrome P450 and therefore may decrease the metabolism of compounds requiring these systems
- Could delay the elimination of drugs with a low therapeutic margin such as theophylline, phenytoin, and vitamin K antagonists

PREGNANCY

Category C

SPECIAL CONSIDERATIONS

- Use with caution in patients with severe hepatic impairment.
- Use with caution in patients with severe respiratory insufficiency.
- Hypersensitivity to nilutamides
- Consider baseline pulmonary function tests.
- Monitor vital signs, PSA, and electrocardiogram.

PATIENT EDUCATION

- Review dosage and dosing frequency guidelines.
- May take with or without food.
- Wear tinted glasses to prevent delay in adaptation to darkness.
- Use extreme caution when driving through tunnels or at night.
- Report any chest pain, shortness of breath, or cough immediately.
- Do not abruptly stop this medication without notifying the health care provider.
- Take medication at the same time every day.

BIBLIOGRAPHY

D'Amico, A., Schultz, D., Loffredo, M., et al. (2000). Biochemical outcome following external beam radiation therapy with or without androgen suppression therapy for clinically localized prostate cancer. *Journal of the American Medical Association, 284,* 1280-1283.

Tamoxifen (Nolvadex, Soltamox)

DRUG CLASS

- Antiestrogen/selective estrogen receptor modulator

ROUTE OF ADMINISTRATION

- Oral

PRETREATMENT GUIDELINES:

- Baseline complete blood cell count (CBC)
- Baseline comprehensive metabolic panel

PHARMACOKINETICS

- Nonsteroidal antiestrogen with weak estrogen agonist effects
- Competes with estrogen for estrogen-binding sites in target tissue (breast tissue).
- Blocks uptake of estradiol

USE

- Adjuvant treatment in axillary node–negative breast cancer after surgical resection
- Adjuvant therapy in axillary node–positive breast cancer in postmenopausal women after surgical resection
- Metastatic breast cancer in women and men
- Endometrial cancer
- Chemoprevention in high-risk women

USUAL DOSE AND SCHEDULE

- 20 mg daily, by mouth

SIDE EFFECTS

- Hot flashes
- Nausea
- Vomiting
- Vaginal bleeding/discharge
- Menstrual irregularities
- Vaginal dryness
- Fluid retention
- Peripheral edema
- Tumor flare pain

- Myelosuppression (rare)
- Transient thrombocytopenia
- Triglyceride elevation
- Headache
- Dizziness
- Hair thinning
- Rash
- Pruritus
- Deep vein thrombosis
- Pulmonary embolism
- Superficial phlebitis
- Endometrial hyperplasia

PREGNANCY

Category D

DRUG INTERACTIONS

- Warfarin
- Bromocriptine
- Drugs activated by P450 system
- Drugs metabolized by liver P450 enzymes
- Aminoglutethimides
- Cytotoxic drugs
- Letrozole
- Medroxyprogesterone
- Rifamycins

SPECIAL CONSIDERATIONS

- Use with caution with patients with abnormal liver function.
- Use with caution with patients who have a personal or family history of thromboembolic disease or hypercoagulable states.
- Monitor blood counts and chemistry panel.

PATIENT EDUCATION

- Notify physician of menstrual irregularities, abnormal pelvic pain, abnormal vaginal bleeding.
- Report unusual leg pain.
- Stress the importance of regular routine gynecological examinations.

BIBLIOGRAPHY

Fisher, B., Dignam, J., Bryant, J., et al. (2001). Five versus more than five years of tamoxifen for lymph node negative breast cancer: updated findings from the National Surgical Adjuvant Breast and Bowl Project B-14 randomized trial. *Journal of the National Cancer Institute*, *93*, 684-690.

Toremifene Citrate (Fareston)

DRUG CLASS

- Antiestrogen (selective estrogen receptor modulator [SERM])

ROUTE OF ADMINSTRATION

- Oral

PRETREATMENT GUIDELINES:

- Baseline prothrombin time (PT)/international normalized ratio (INR)
- Baseline complete blood cell count (CBC)
- Baseline comprehensive metabolic panel
- Baseline eye examination

USE

- Metastatic breast cancer in postmenopausal women with estrogen receptor positivity or unknown estrogen status

PHARMACOKINETICS

- Synthetic analog of tamoxifen
- Nonsteroidal antiestrogen
- Binds directly to estrogen receptors
- Blocks downstream intracellular signal transduction pathways
- Inhibition of cell growth and induction of apoptosis
- Extensively metabolized by the liver by the P450 enzyme system
- Well absorbed by the gastrointestinal tract
- Absorption not affected by food
- Extensively metabolized in the liver

USUAL DOSE AND SCHEDULE

- 60 mg every day

SIDE EFFECTS

- Hot flashes
- Sweating
- Menstrual irregularity
- Milk production in breast
- Transient tumor flare
- Nausea and vomiting
- Anorexia

- Alopecia
- Hypercalcemia
- Peripheral edema
- Rash
- Mild leukopenia
- Mild thrombocytopenia
- Cataract formation
- Depression
- Dry eyes

DRUG INTERACTIONS

- Carbamazepine
- Clonazepam
- Erythromycin
- Phenytoin
- Cyclosporine
- Ketoconazole
- Macrolide antibiotics
- Phenobarbital
- Warfarin

PREGNANCY

Category D

SPECIAL CONSIDERATIONS

- Watch for hypercalcemia.
- Use with caution with patients with brain metastasis or vertebral metastasis.
- Note any history of thromboembolic disorders.

PATIENT EDUCATION

- Report vaginal bleeding.
- Get baseline, then biannual eye examination.
- Report swelling, pain, or redness in extremities.
- Report family history of thrombolic events.
- Use reliable birth control. Toremifene may induce ovulation.

BIBLIOGRAPHY

Honig, S. F. (1996). Treatment of metastic disease: hormonal therapy and chemotherapy. In J. R. Harris, M. E. Lippman, & M. Morrow (Eds.). *Disease of the breast* (pp. 669-734). Philadelphia: Lippincott-Raven.

Cancer Management

Complementary and Alternative Medicine (CAM)   *Dorothy Lynn Crider*

DEFINITIONS

Complementary and alternative medicine (CAM) includes conventional medical treatment and alternative therapies (natural modalities). Often the health care professional is not aware that the patient is using additional therapies.

Integrative medicine is a practice where the health care practitioner and patient work together to combine conventional medical treatments and alternative therapies. This provides a collaborative and holistic approach to health care.

Alternative medicine is generally considered a method where the patient rejects the conventional medical treatment and chooses "natural healing modalities" instead.

Some 28% to 91% of cancer patients are reported to use some form of CAM. Among cancer patients using CAM, 40% to 70% are not reporting their use of CAM to their health care practitioners. Users of CAM are most likely to be female, highly educated, of higher socioeconomic class and to use more than one CAM at a time.

WHAT ARE NATURAL HEALING METHODS?

Most of the natural methods are based on the idea that the body can heal itself and the therapies are aimed at assisting the body to do so. Many natural methods also embrace the concept of treating the whole person by addressing physical, emotional, mental, and spiritual needs. Natural modalities also place value on promoting health, preventing illness, and working with the body to restore health when disease occurs.

People turn to natural healing modalities for a variety of reasons including the following:
- Rising health care costs
- Untoward side effects of medications/procedures
- Failure of conventional treatment
- Decreased personal attention from conventional medical practitioners
- A desire for more control over health
- Feelings of depersonalization with increased technology in conventional medicine
- A belief that combining natural healing and medicine would net better results
- Conventional health care providers are suggesting CAM

WHAT ARE THE NATURAL SYSTEMS/THERAPIES THAT PEOPLE ARE TRYING?

It is well documented that more and more people include some type of natural healing in their own self-care. The research varies depending on which modalities are being tested, but we see that billions of dollars are spent by Americans every year on "natural healing" supplements and treatments. There is a wide range of natural healing practices and modalities that patients engage in. Examples include prayer, yoga, qigong, breath work, guided imagery, chiropractic, diet, herbs, meditation, energy-based healing, acupuncture, massage, dance, art, sound healing, magnetics, radionics, aromatherapy, thought field therapy, naturopathy, and vibrational healing. Some patients may also try whole health system approaches from other cultures such as traditional Chinese medicine, ayurveda, or Tibetan medicine. These approaches are very integrated and may require life style commitments such as diet and routines for exercise and sleep.

WHAT IS THE NURSE'S ROLE IN WORKING WITH PATIENTS WHO CHOOSE COMPLEMENTARY AND ALTERNATIVE MEDICINE?

- With the availability of the Internet, the variety of modalities being used is somewhat daunting. Because there is much we still do not know about the combining of conventional and alternative healing, nurses have an important role to play in gathering information and helping promote safe health care. It may help to focus assessments in terms of products, practices, and therapies: Establish a collaborative tone with patients.
- Assess which, if any, alternative therapies patients are using with each patient contact.
- Assess any side effects or changes in the patient's condition at each appointment.
- Assist the patient to search for reliable information regarding the combining of therapies.

RESEARCH

Acceptable Western research methods do not work well with alternative therapies. Western medicine has traditionally used the double-blind study with a control group and strives to remove researcher bias or influence. We tend to focus on one symptom and one treatment. We also expect that one treatment will be good for most patients with the diagnosis. CAM by its very nature focuses on the entire individual and all the symptoms/systems and relies on collaboration with the patient (expects influence to occur), and placebos are not easy to develop because of the interactive nature of CAM treatments. CAM supports the idea that what works for one patient may not work for the next and that each individual requires a personal plan.

The challenge really lies in developing new acceptable methods for research. The good news is that research is becoming available through reliable sources from the National Institutes of Health as well as universities and medical centers.

COSTS

The cost of products, practices, and therapies varies greatly. Some can be easily learned by watching a DVD from the local library, whereas others may cost thousands of dollars and involve lengthy stays at healing centers. Cost can also be affected by quality of the product or locale (what part of the country you live in). Many natural products are also now marketed through multilevel marketing companies. Encourage patients to investigate the quality of the company and length of time the product has been in use.

BENEFITS AND RISKS

Some practice methods have a high level of safety and benefit, such as qigong, meditation, and guided imagery. Other methods rely on the skill of the practitioner, such as massage, chiropractic, and acupuncture. For oral supplementation, we could see positive or negative synergistic effects when combined with medications.

CAM requires patients to have good self-body awareness skills and health care professionals to have good assessment skills. Then patients and professionals must collaborate to discover what really benefits and what could be damaging. We may all need to learn new ways of assessing, such as kinesiology. The key to increasing benefit and decreasing risk will be open, clear, communication, and keen observations of patient's responses.

BIBLIOGRAPHY

Bauer, B. (2007). *Mayo clinic guide to alternative medicine* (pp. 7-21). New York, New York: Time Inc.

Chong, O. (2006). An integrative approach to addressing clinical issues in complementary and alternative medicine in an outpatient oncology center. *Clinical Journal of Oncology Nursing, 10,* 83-88.

Duke Center for Integrative Medicine, Liebowitz, R., & Smith, L. (2006). *The Duke encyclopedia of new medicine, conventional and alternative medicine for all ages* (pp. 18-25). London, UK: Rodale.

Smith, A. (2005). Opening the dialogue: herbal supplementation and chemotherapy. *Clinical Journal of Oncology Nursing, 9,* 447-450.

Cancer Management

Complementary and Alternative Medicine Therapies

Acupuncture/ Acupressure

Dorothy Lynn Crider

DEFINITION

- Acupuncture is based on the belief that the body has energy that runs through pathways, called meridians, in the body. This energy supports the organs and basic physical, emotional, and spiritual health. Blood tends to follow the energy, or qi (pronounced "chee").
- Too much or too little qi results in the potential for disease to develop.
- The acupuncturist affects the flow of energy by influencing some of the 400 points on the meridians, called acupoints.
- The acupuncturist may use needles, pellets, cupping, or herbs to affect the flow of energy.
- The goal is to bring the energy back into balance.
- Acupressure uses the same acupoints, but the therapist uses finger pressure to stimulate or sedate the points.
- Acupuncture is one aspect of traditional Chinese medicine (TCM). TCM includes acupuncture, herbology, diet, massage, and qigong (exercise that integrates movement, breath, and meditation).

WHO PERFORMS THIS SERVICE?

- The National Certification Commission for Acupuncture and Oriental Medicine awards three types of certificates: Diplomate in Acupuncture, Diplomate in Herbology, and Diplomate in Oriental Medicine (includes both acupuncture and herbology).
- Clients should ask about the practitioner's credentials.
- There is some difference in practice standards from state to state.

COST

- The initial or first visit fee is often higher because of the extensive assessment. Cost varies from $65-$150 per session.
- Treatment time varies; however, the initial visit is typically 1 hour with subsequent visits lasting 30 minutes to 1 hour.
- Frequency of visits varies by condition and could be several times a week to once a month.
- Needles are left in for 15 to 30 minutes. The practitioner generally leaves the room after placing the needles and will reassess the client during the session.

BENEFITS

- Promote overall health, prevent pain, treat disease
- Provide analgesia
- Relieve pain
- Reduce nausea
- Reduce itching
- Reduce anxiety
- Improve sleep
- Improve depression
- Reduce swelling
- Facilitate relaxation and release at time of death
- Increase relaxation

RISKS

- Contraindications are specific to the medical condition. Practitioner evaluates at each visit.

RESOURCE

- National Certification Commission for Acupuncture and Oriental Medicine: www.NCCAOM.org

BIBLIOGRAPHY

Bauer, B. (2007). *Mayo clinic guide to alternative medicine* (pp. 76-77). New York: Time Inc.
Beinfield, H., & Korngold, E. (1991). *Between heaven and earth, a guide to Chinese medicine* (pp. 240-249). New York: Ballantine Books.
Duke Center for Integrative Medicine,

Liebowitz, R., & Smith, L. (2006). *The Duke encyclopedia of new medicine, conventional and alternative medicine for all ages* (pp 446-450, 464, & 465). London, UK: Rodale Books.

Aromatherapy

Dorothy Lynn Crider

DEFINITION

- For thousands of years, essential oils have been used to promote physical, psychological, and spiritual well-being.
- Each essential oil is made up of several different chemicals that determine its therapeutic effects.
- These natural chemicals are easily recognized and used by the body. Methods of use for essential oils include inhalation, diffusion, massage, embrocation (a lotion that relieves muscle or joint pain), compresses, application to reflex/ acupuncture points, and baths.
- The more commonly used oils by cancer patients include frankincense, niaouli, peppermint, lavender, cypress, lemongrass, tea tree oil, and marjoram.

WHO PERFORMS THIS SERVICE

- Aromatherapist, massage therapist, reflexologist, acupressure practitioner
- Some certification programs exist, so clients should ask about the therapist's training.

COST

- $60-$100 per hour. This cost may also include making a specific blend for the client to use at home; however, this service may be an additional cost depending on oil prices.

BENEFITS

- Simultaneous treatment of emotional and physical concerns

- Each single essential oil can have several indications for treatment depending on the chemical makeup.
- Examples of indications are antitumoral, antibacterial, antifungal, antidepressive, analgesic, antispasmodic, antiinflammatory, lymphatic decongestant, expectorant, antiemetic, bronchodialating, and antianxiety.

RISKS

- Check resources for safety precautions for each oil before use:
  - Oils should be diluted with a carrier oil such as grapeseed or apricot.
  - Check the Food and Drug Administration's GRAS (generally regarded as safe) list.
  - Check for skin sensitivity and oils that can increase skin sensitivity to sun exposure.
  - Check for oils that can be hepatotoxic and nephrotoxic with prolonged use.
  - Check for estrogenic effects that would make oil contraindicated in estrogen-sensitive tumors.
  - Some essential oils may compete for receptor sites with chemotherapy, so keep the oil dose low (1-2 drops/1ounce of carrier oil) or no oils for 9-10 days after chemotherapy.

RESOURCES

- International Federation of Aromatherapists: http://www.ifaroma.org/
- Young Living Essential Oils: www.youngliving.com
- Duke Center for Integrative Medicine: www.dcim.org

BIBLIOGRAPHY

Balz, R. (1990). *The healing power of essential oils* (pp. 13, 35, 36, 56-59, 96, 107, 111, 118). Twin Lakes, WI: Lotus Light Publications.
Duke Center for Integrative Medicine, Liebowitz, R., & Smith, L. (2006). *Duke encyclopedia of new medicine, conventional & alternative medicine for all ages* (pp. 548-549). London, UK: Rodale.
Enteen, S. (2007). Aromatherapy for clients with special needs. *Massage Today, 7*, 5.
Schnaubelt, K. (1998). *Advanced aromatherapy, the science of essential oil therapy* (pp. 31-50). Rochester, VT: Healing Arts Press.

Art Therapy

Dorothy Lynn Crider

DEFINITION

- Art therapy uses different art mediums to help clients explore and express feelings with a therapist. This modality provides a safe way for unconscious feelings and thoughts to come into awareness. The therapist assists the client toward expression and self-understanding. This is particularly helpful with clients who have a difficult time recognizing and expressing their feelings.
- No artistic skills are required by the client.
- A wide variety of artistic modalities may be used, such as print, paint, clay, crayon, collage, and sand.
- Can be performed one-on-one with a therapist or in a group setting

WHO PERFORMS THE SERVICE

- Art therapists have formal education and training. Ask about their training/degrees.

COST

- Depend on whether the client chooses individual or group session and varies with geographical location. Individual sessions usually last 50 minutes. Group sessions can last from 1-3 hours.

BENEFITS

- Increased self-awareness
- Release of emotions
- Identification of issues for further therapy
- Stress reduction
- Relief of trauma
- Increased coping skills

RISKS

- Safely conducted with the therapist

RESOURCES

- American Art Therapy Association: http://www.arttherapy.org

BIBLIOGRAPHY

American Art Therapy Association. *Art therapy*. Retrieved February 11, 2007, from http://www.arttherapy.org.
Duke Center for Integrative Medicine, Liebowitz, R., & Smith, L. (2006). *Duke encyclopedia of new medicine, conventional & alternative medicine for all ages* (pp. 491-493). London, UK: Rodale.

Guided Imagery

Dorothy Lynn Crider

DEFINITION

- The purposeful use of the mind to affect changes in the body, mind, and emotions
- Cultures for thousands of years have used imaging to promote health and heal disease.
- Guided imagery is one of the most widely used of the complementary healing modalities.
- Research demonstrates that mental images can result in changes in physiological, biochemical, and immunological responses of the body.
- The same areas of the brain used for imagination control vital functions such as heart rate, respiratory rate, and digestion. Images can serve as a bridge between the mind and body.

WHO PERFORMS THE SERVICE

- Guided imagery can be facilitated by a trained health care professional or can be self-guided. Many different types of health care practitioners use guided imagery (physicians, nurses, social workers, psychologists, chaplains).
- CDs, DVDs, and books are also available for self-use.

COST

- Depends on the type of health care professional seen

- DVDs, CDs, and books can be purchased or found at the library.

BENEFITS

- Enhanced performance and energy
- Pain relief
- Improve immune system functioning
- Ease symptoms or side effects from drugs
- Improve recovery time after medical procedures
- Decreased anxiety
- Improvement in sleep
- Reduced stress response
- Improvement in digestion
- Lowered blood pressure
- Improvement in emotional control

RISKS

- Persons with a history of psychotic episodes are advised to work with a health care professional.
- Otherwise considered a very safe modality

RESOURCES

- University of California, San Diego Medical Center, Moores Cancer Center, Complementary and Alternative Therapies for Cancer Patients: http://cancer.ucsd.edu/outreach/ publiceducation/CAMS/guidedima gery.asp
- Well Baskets: http://www.wellbaskets.com
- Belleruth Naparstek's Guided Imagery Center, Health Journeys: http://www.healthjourneys.com/

BIBLIOGRAPHY

Bauer, B. (2007). *Mayo clinic guide to alternative medicine* (p. 61). New York: Time Inc.
Duke Center for Integrative Medicine, Liebowitz, R., & Smith, L. (2006). *The Duke encyclopedia of new medicine, conventional and alternative medicine for all ages* (pp. 520-522). London, UK: Rodale.

Healing Touch

Dorothy Lynn Crider

DEFINITION

- The goal of healing touch is to affect the energy field within and around the body to promote physical, emotional, and spiritual health. Healing touch uses a number of different energy healing techniques to restore the client's energy to its highest potential.
- Energy healing has been a part of many cultures for thousands of years.
- The client and practitioner are viewed as working together.
- The practitioner may lightly touch the client or work with hands close to but off the body. The client remains fully clothed, in either a sitting or lying down position.

WHO PERFORMS THIS SERVICE

- Ask the practitioner about completed courses or certifications.
- The American Holistic Nurse's Association and Healing Touch International have certification programs.

COST

- Some hospitals, clinics, and churches offer the service free or on a sliding scale.
- Some practitioners are also in private practice, and costs vary from $45-$85 per hour.
- Sessions may last from 30 minutes to 1 hour.

BENEFITS

- Overall relaxation
- Improved sense of well-being
- Decreased pain
- Faster wound healing
- Decreased anxiety
- Decreased blood pressure, heart rate, and respiratory rate
- Increased sense of attentive caring

RISKS

- None; however, check that healing touch fits with the client's belief system.

RESOURCES

- Healing Touch International: http://www.healingtouchinternati onal.org/

BIBLIOGRAPHY

Bauer, B. (2007). *Mayo clinic guide to alternative medicine* (p. 78). New York: Time Inc.
Duke Center for Integrative Medicine, Liebowitz, R., & Smith, L. (2006). *Duke encyclopedia of new medicine, conventional & alternative medicine for all ages* (pp. 562 & 563). London, UK: Rodale.
Hover-Kramer, D. (1996). *A resource for health care professionals* (pp. 6, 11-13, 27, 30-37). Albany, NY: Delmar.

Herbal, Vitamin, and Oral Supplementation

Dorothy Lynn Crider

DEFINITIONS

- Oral supplementation includes vitamins, herbs, minerals, enzymes, amino acids, juices, probiotics, hormones, transfer factors, fatty acids, organ tissues, glandular extracts, and other compounds extracted from plants or animal products.
- Many persons believe that, as a result of overuse of farm lands, overuse of chemicals and petrochemical pollution, our food sources no longer supply us with enough of the proper nutrients. Also eating of prepared and preserved foods with decreased vitality has led to increased health problems. Hence, many people choose to supplement their diets.
- The scope of oral supplementation available today is overwhelming. This text reviews some of the more commonly used supplements. The reader is

encouraged to explore the resources for more specific information.

VITAMINS
Definition

- Vitamins are substances derived from foods that the body requires but does not produce (except for vitamin D, which the skin produces, and niacin, which is produced by the liver in small amounts).
- Four of the 13 vitamins (A, D, E, and K) are fat soluble, which means that if they are taken in excess they can become toxic.
- Nine of the vitamins are water soluble. Water-soluble vitamins are not stored in the body, except for folate and vitamin B_{12}, which can be stored in the liver.

Risks

- When taken in excess can lead to toxicity and stress the liver or kidneys

MINERALS
Definition

- Minerals are found as naturally occurring in our food.
- Some minerals are needed in larger amounts daily and some are useful in very small amounts (trace minerals).
- Minerals are produced in several forms: inorganic salts, colloidal, ionic, and nano (smallest).

Benefits

- Minerals play a role in our health as:
  ○ Components of skeleton and teeth
  ○ Important structural elements of cells
  ○ Regulation of fluid balance
  ○ Regulation of nerve impulses
  ○ Cellular respiration

Risks

- Can become toxic in excessive doses

ENZYMES
Definition

- Enzymes are substances that speed up the rate of biological reactions and are not used by the body (biological catalysts).
- Sprouted seeds, nuts, and raw juices also make enzymes more available to the body.

Benefits

- Enzyme supplementation may be used to promote and improve digestion (protease, amylase, and lipase).
- Other enzyme supplements might be used to "digest" nonessential tissues, such as tumors or growths (Venus flytrap plant, silkworm).

Risks

- More research is needed with the category used to "digest nonessential tissues."

HERBS
Definition

- Herbs are healing plants that were the basis for most ancient medical systems before modern drug development.
- Many people continue to use herbs today feeling that "natural plant" medicines are more likely to be recognized and used by the body than synthetically compounded drugs.
- Herbal therapy can use the bark, flower, root, seed, or leaves of a plant.
- Herbs may be used in their dry form, made into tinctures, teas, compresses, ointments, creams, or even used in baths.

Benefits

- Because herbs have multiple chemical constituents, one herb may have several therapeutic indications.

Risks

- Includes untoward side effects and lack of regulation of the industry, which can result in contamination or inconsistent dosing
- The chemical constituents of herbs when combined with conventional drugs may result in synergistic or antagonistic effects.
- Some herbs may compete with chemotherapy for receptor sites.

PROBIOTICS
Definition

- Probiotics are products that contain live microorganisms, which can affect the microflora of the gut and promote health
- Probiotics can be found in fermented milk products such as yogurt or in supplemental forms such as capsules or tablets.

Risks

- Potential for diarrhea in sensitive individuals

JUICE THERAPY
Definition

- Consuming freshly prepared raw vegetables, fruits, grasses, or nuts is considered juice therapy.

Benefits

- Benefits are thought to include the ability to extract vitamins, minerals, and enzymes more completely from the food.
- This method also allows people to take in larger amounts of vegetables.
- Some juice diets aim to cleanse, detoxify, and alkalize the body.
- Some cancer patients use juicing to try to increase nutrition.

Risks

- Potential for diarrhea and rapid detoxification responses in some individuals

FLOWER ESSENCES
Definition

- Flower essences contain the energy of the flower and are taken to promote balance so the body can heal itself.
- The remedies are intended to correct emotional and personality patterns. Dr. Bach's Rescue Remedy is a blend often used at times of great shock or trauma.

RESOURCES

- Skidmore-Roth, L. (2006). *Mosby's handbook of herbs & natural*

Cancer Management

supplements (3rd ed.). St. Louis: Elsevier Mosby.

- American Cancer Society. *How to know what is safe: choosing and using dietary supplements: what you need to know first:* http://www.cancer.org/docroot/ETO/content/ETO_5_3x_How_to_Know_What_Is_Safe_Choosing_and_Using_Dietary_Supplen ts.asp.

BIBLIOGRAPHY

Bauer, B. (2007). *Mayo clinic guide to alternative medicine* (pp. 23-57). New York:Time Inc.

Decker, G. (2006). The ten cardinal rules of herb use. *Clinical Journal of Oncology Nursing, 10,* 279.

Duke Center for Integrative Medicine, Liebowitz, R., & Smith, L. (2006). *The Duke encyclopedia of new medicine, conventional and alternative medicine for all ages* (pp. 530 - 545, 550 - 559). London, UK: Rodale.

Hoffman, D. (1993). *An elders' herbal* (pp. 179-181). Rochester, VT: Healing Arts Press.

Montbriand, M. (2004). Herbs or natural products that decrease cancer growth. *Oncology Nursing Forum, 31,* 1-27.

Montbriand, M. (2004). Herbs or natural products that increase cancer growth or recurrence. *Oncology Nursing Forum, 31,* 1-23.

Montbriand, M. (2004). Herbs or natural products that protect against cancer growth. *Oncology Nursing Forum, 31,* 1-30.

Montbriand, M. (2005). Herbs or natural products that may cause cancer or harm. *Oncology Nursing Forum, 32,* 1-15.

Humor

Michele L. Musella

DEFINITION

- Humor therapy is the use of techniques that encourage laughter.
- The ability to laugh fosters a positive and hopeful outlook and renders one less likely to become depressed. Humor enables patients to put their problems in perspective.
- Laughter or humor therapies are used primarily to temporarily reduce pain and suffering.

- Humor therapy can lead to relaxation either by passive participation such as seeing or reading something humorous or by active engagement such as finding humor in life's everyday situations.

WHO PERFORMS THIS SERVICE

- Humor therapists receiving therapeutic recreational training through the American Therapeutic Recreation Association

COST

- There is no fee associated with this therapy.

BENEFITS

- There is no scientific evidence that humor is effective in treating cancer, but there are findings that it does produce positive effects:
  - Research shows that humor therapy integrates and balances activity on both sides of the brain, producing neurochemical changes that create immune-enhancing effects.
  - Humor increases the number and activity of natural killer cells that target some types of cancer and tumor cells.
  - Humor supports the immune system while activating immunoglobulin A, which fights upper respiratory infections, and interferon gamma, which turns on the immune system.
  - Humor decreases stress hormones, particularly epinephrine.
- Laughter reduces hypertension, produces muscle relaxation, provides cardiac conditioning, and acts as an aerobic workout.
- Studies have shown that humor therapy administered before pain medication has fostered a decreased pain level compared with patients who did not receive this therapy.
- It is felt that humor therapy enhances conventional medical therapies and is an accepted tool used to combat disease and help patients cope with illness.

- One of the greatest benefits is that it is free and usually has few negative side effects (except an occasional pain in the side from laughing).

RISKS

- Humor therapy is generally considered safe unless it is used to avoid situations that are important to the patient and their family. Laughter may lead to increased pain at the surgical site if the patient is immediately postoperative.This is a temporary side effect.

RESOURCES

- American Therapeutic Recreation Association: www.atra-tr.org

BIBLIOGRAPHY

American Cancer Society. *Complementary and alternative methods: humor therapy.* Retrieved February 6, 2007, from *http://www.cancer.org/docroot/ETO/content/ETO_5_3X_Humor_Therapy.asp?sitearea=ETO.*

Klein, A. (1998). *The courage to laugh: humor, hope and healing in the face of death and dying.* Los Angeles, CA: Tarcher/Putnam.

MacDonald, C. (2004). A chuckle a day keeps the doctor away: therapeutic humor and laughter. *Journal of Psychosocial Nursing and Mental Health Services, 42,* 18-25.

Massage

Michele L. Musella

DEFINITION

- Massage is a range of therapeutic approaches with use of the practitioner's hands, elbows, forearms, and instruments, for the purpose of muscle and soft tissue kneading, rubbing, or manipulation.The object is to improve health and well-being.
- There are many types of massage including Swedish, shiatsu, trigger point, neuromuscular, therapeutic, myotherapy, and hot stone massage.

WHO PERFORMS THIS SERVICE

- Certified massage therapists who may be licensed by a state or national certification board provide this service.
- Therapists may be certified in specific types of massage.

COST

- The average session lasts usually from 30 minutes to 1 hour. Fees range from $60 to $100 per hour.

BENEFITS

- Practitioners have seen that massage reduces depression, pain, and stress and relieves anxiety. Massage can both stimulate and relax the mind and body.
- It leads to increased circulation, which aids cellular replenishment, and it serves as a detoxifier.
- Massage improves muscle tone and mobility and eases aching limbs. Myotherapy is used to alleviate muscle pain; some studies show that caregivers have learned how to provide this therapy for homebound oncology patients.
- Massage has been reported to promote digestion, nutrient assimilation, and elimination.
- Other benefits include endorphin production and lactic acid detoxification, which lead to reduced pain, anxiety, and stress in oncology patients. Massage fosters a feeling of relaxation and overall well-being.
- The American Cancer Society has recognized the benefits of massage therapy as an important complementary therapy and recommends it for cancer patients because it provides both physical and psychological benefits. When stone temperatures are monitored, hot stone massage has been shown to provide a great deal of comfort to oncology patients.

RISKS

- Improper pressure in treatments performed by an unskilled provider may lead to pain.
- Some believe that tissue manipulation may cause cancer cells to migrate throughout the body. It is recommended that massage near tumors be avoided until more research has been done to validate or refute this theory.
- Massage should be avoided if the skin is broken, if the patient has open wounds or a rash, or if the patient has blood clots or broken bones, or osteoporosis.
- All patients with cancer should consult their providers before receiving treatments that involve joint or tissue manipulation.

RESOURCES

- American Massage Therapy Association: www.amtamassage.org
- New York State Society of Medical Massage Therapists: www.nysmassage.org
- National Certification Board for Therapeutic Massage and Body Work: www.ncbtmb.com

BIBLIOGRAPHY

Ernst, E. (Ed.). (2001). *The desktop guide to complementary and alternative medicine*. St. Louis: Mosby.

Evans, M.B. (2003). *Yoga, tai chi, massage, therapies and healing remedies*. London: Anness.

Springhouse. (2002). *Professional guide to complementary and alternative therapies*. Philadelphia: Springhouse/ Lippincott Williams & Wilkins.

Meditation

Michele L. Musella

DEFINITION

- It is believed that the body's chi (energy) follows the mind's intent.
- When the mind is in focus and harmony, the body remains healthy. Disease occurs when the mind is confused.
- Meditation includes practices that involve training one's attention to encourage oneness between the mind and body.
- There are many forms of meditation, but the most common include concentration and mindfulness meditation.

- ○ *Concentrative meditation* focuses on an image, sound, mantra, or breath in an effort to quiet the mind, allowing clarity and awareness to emerge. Therapists believe there is a strong connection between one's state of mind and breathing patterns. When using concentrative meditation, the patient is taught to study each breath, remaining focused until the breathing pattern is slow, deep, and regular. Once this is achieved, the mind becomes calm and peaceful.
- ○ *Mindfulness meditation* is the act of calming the mind as the subject passively opens his or her attention to sensations as they are presented. In this type of meditation, the patient focuses on events as they happen. Rather than manipulating the thoughts, the patient is taught to encourage the mind to remain uninvolved in an effort to foster a calm, clear, and nonreactive mindset.
- ○ *Five yin color meditation*, is another type of traditional Chinese medicine meditation that combines concentrative meditation, visualization, and traditional Chinese theory. Each of the five major organs (lungs, heart, spleen, liver, and kidneys) represents an emotion and is represented by a color. This form of meditation requires the patient to be seated and to be in a concentrative meditative state. The patient focuses on one organ at a time visualizing the color in the most powerful way possible, expelling dull color and negative energy and breathing in positively charged vibrant color. Once all five colors are coursing through the body the patient is said to be fully grounded. Chi and the mind intent have reached a state of equilibrium.

WHO PERFORMS THIS SERVICE

- Certified yoga and meditation practitioners

Cancer Management

COST

- Cost varies among practitioners. Private sessions are around $50 for 1 half hour.

BENEFITS

- The best benefits are derived when twice-daily sessions lasting 10-20 minutes are done regularly.
- Physical benefits include the following:
  - Reduction in blood pressure
  - Lower cholesterol levels
  - Deep rest
  - Decreased metabolic rate
  - Reduced workload on the heart
  - Improved aeration of the lungs
  - Easier breathing
  - Increased harmony of brain wave activity
- Psychological benefits reported are increased emotional stability, feelings of vitality and rejuvenation. Decreases in irritability, depression, and anxiety have also been seen. The National Institutes of Health National Center for Complementary and Alternative Medicine reports favorable results on pain reduction, lower blood cortisol levels, and improved mood and immune function with the regular practice of meditation.

RISKS

- Meditation should be avoided with clients who are paranoid, overwhelmed by anxiety, or those in danger of developing delusions as a result of altered states of consciousness.

RESOURCES

- American Institute of Health Care Professionals, Inc. for certification as a meditation instructor: http://www.aihcp.org/meditation.htm.
- National Center for Complementary and Alternative Medicine: Meditation for health purposes: http://nccam.nih.gov/health/meditation/.

BIBLIOGRAPHY

Ernst, E. (Ed.) (2001). *The desktop guide to complementary and alternative medicine*. St. Louis: Mosby.

Evans, M. B. (2003). *Yoga, tai chi, massage therapies, and healing remedies*. London: Anness.

Springhouse. (2002). *Professional guide to complementary and alternative therapies*. Philadelphia: Springhouse/Lippincott Williams & Wilkins.

Music Therapy

Michele L. Musella

DEFINITION

- Music therapy can involve singing, playing an instrument, drumming, or listening to live or recorded music.
- It is used to engage the patient both musically or socially to encourage emotional expression and relieve symptoms.

WHO PERFORMS THIS SERVICE

- Trained music therapists

COST

- If accessed through an acute-care setting, there is no cost. If used privately, cost involves fees for equipment.

BENEFITS

- When used in conjunction with medical treatment, music therapy can help reduce anxiety, pain, and chemotherapy side effects such as nausea and vomiting.
- It has been shown to lower blood pressure and heart rates and slow respiratory rates.
- Medical experts believe music therapy aids healing and improves movement and the patient's quality of life.

RISKS

- Music therapy is generally safe and produces positive effects. Musical intervention by those lacking training may cause increased stress and discomfort. Musical selections may bring back bad memories, so it is important to consult the patient when making choices.

RESOURCES

- American Music Therapy Association, Inc.: www.musictherapy.org

BIBLIOGRAPHY

Gold, C., Heldal, T. O., Dahle, T., et al. (2005). Music therapy for schizophrenia or schizophrenia-like illnesses. *Cochrane Database of Systematic Reviews, 18*, CD004025.

Davis, K. The Healing Power of Music. Retrieved March 30, 2000, from *www.discoveryhealth.com*

Johnston, K., Rohaly-Davis, J. (1996.) An introduction to music therapy: helping the oncology patient in ICU. *Critical Care Nursing Quarterly* 18(4), 54-60.

Polarity Therapy

Michele L. Musella

DEFINITION

- Polarity therapy is a holistic type of hands-on electromagnetic therapy used to realign and unite the mind, body, and spirit. The American Polarity Therapy Association (APTA) is promoting this therapy as the premier wellness treatment of our time.
- The term polarity refers to universal pulsation and the attraction and repulsion of energy.
- Polarity practitioners subtly manipulate the joints by using massage, hydrotherapy, reflexology, and the holding of pressure points. This is done to unblock stagnant energy between the body's negative and positive poles by using the body's six chakras in conjunction with the five elements of traditional Chinese medicine: ether, air, water, earth, and fire.
- It is believed that polarity helps develop balance and promotes creativity, flexibility, and spontaneity and fosters the ability to meet life's challenges.

- Polarity therapy has four areas of concentration:
  - Special polarity exercises
  - A health-enhancing nutritional plan
  - Touch
  - The creation of a positive attitude

WHO PERFORMS THIS SERVICE

- Certified polarity therapists complete at least 500 hours of training from an accredited program.

COST

- The cost for this service ranges from $60-$100 for a 1-hour treatment. This fee varies among practitioners because the length of a session may vary.

BENEFITS

- Polarity balances the flow of energy in the body.
- The therapy is used to detoxify the body and reduce stress and anxiety while promoting relaxation.
- Polarity programs encourage the client to adopt a healthy lifestyle and have been shown to be very effective for oncology patients.

RISKS

- When done by a trained therapist, this treatment is safe. Injury may result from improperly applied techniques.
- Oncology patients should consult with their providers before engaging in muscle or joint manipulation activities.

RESOURCES

- American Polarity Therapy Association: www.polaritytherapy.org

BIBLIOGRAPHY

American Polarity Therapy Association. (2003). *American Polarity Therapy Association standards for practice and education* (4th ed.). Retrieved April 28, 2007, from http://polaritytherapy.myst rategicmarketer.com/assets/images/prod uctpics/aptastandards_2003.pdf.

Decker, G. (1999). Manual healing methods. In *An introduction to complementary & alternative therapies* (pp. 135-137). Pittsburgh, PA: Oncology Nursing Press.

Seidman, M. (1991). *A guide to polarity therapy: the gentle art of hands-on healing*. Boulder, CO: Elan Press.

Stone, R. (1986). *Polarity therapy, The completed collected works*. CRCS. Pubns

Reflexology

Michele L. Musella

DEFINITION

- Reflexology is a holistic therapy that encourages self-healing of the body, thereby restoring a balance in energy flow.
- It is also known as zone therapy and it is the application of pressure with the thumbs or fingers to specific points on the hands and feet that correspond to different organs and parts of the body.
- It is thought that reflexology stimulates the nerve endings, which encourages the release of endorphins to decrease pain and increases lymphatic flow. Reflexology is believed to stimulate internal organs and increase circulation.
- This treatment is not intended as a diagnostic tool or a treatment of disease processes to replace conventional medical therapies.

WHO PERFORMS THIS SERVICE

- Reflexologists who have completed appropriate training perform this service. Verify that the practitioner has the appropriate background and training.

COST

- The initial cost ranges from $80 to $100 for a 1- to 2-hour session. Further sessions will last between 30 minutes to 1 hour.

BENEFITS

- Reflexology links the body systems with areas mapped onto the feet and hands.
- When reflexology is performed, symptoms from various disorders can be relieved.
- Reflexology does provide relaxation and caring touch, which provide symptom relief. The patient may experience the following:
  - Reduced stress
  - Feelings of deep relaxation
  - Improved circulation
  - A state of overall balance
  - A sense of revitalization
- Initial treatments may leave the patients experiencing a type of healing catharsis seen in temporary symptoms of headache, sinus congestion, and nausea. The patient may also experience sensations of tiredness or tingling related to the release of toxins and the clearing of blocked energy.
- Research shows that the following conditions improve by the use of reflexology:
  - Anxiety
  - Premenstrual syndrome
  - Headaches/migraines
  - Cancer pain
  - Foot edema
  - Multiple sclerosis—specifically motor and sensory symptoms

RISKS

- Reflexology should not be administered to a patient with:
  - Pregnancy
  - New foot injury
  - Surgery with an unhealed wound
  - Fever
  - Gallstones
  - Kidney stones
  - Gout
  - Osteoarthritis
  - Presence of a pacemaker
  - Active infections
  - Mental illness
  - Unstable blood pressure
- Other risks would occur if the practitioner were to diagnose illness, or if the patient chose to use this therapy exclusively rather than as a complementary therapy.

Cancer
Management

RESOURCES

- Reflexology Association of America: http://www.reflexology-usa.org

BIBLIOGRAPHY

Association of Reflexologists. (n.d.) *Reflexology*. Retrieved July 4, 2005, from http://www.aor.org.uk info@aor.org.uk

Decker, G. (1999). Manual healing methods. In *An introduction to complementary & alternative therapies* (pp. 135-137). Pittsburgh, PA: Oncology Nursing Press.

Vonner, V. (2005). Get quick pain relief anytime, anywhere. In *Reflexology across America,* [spring newsletter]. Retrieved July 4, 2005, from http://www.reflexology-usa.org/.

Reiki

Michele L. Musella

DEFINITION

- Reiki is the Japanese term for "universal life energy." The premise of this therapy is that healing energy is channeled through the practitioner to the patient to activate the patient's natural healing powers.
- Practitioners believe that energy paths of the body are blocked, resulting in distress or disease.
- The belief is that reiki can achieve the following:
  - Realign the body's chakra system
  - Strengthen the flow of energy
  - Decrease pain
  - Ease tension
  - Assist those who are suffering
  - Enhance the natural self-healing abilities of the body

- Reiki is not used to diagnose medical conditions, but it is thought to correct the underlying issues that have created the physical or emotional condition leading to the disease.
- Reiki treatments can be done by the laying on of hands, which can be done by a level 1 reiki practitioner or from a distance by advanced practitioners.
- This therapy is used to treat both psychological and emotional distress as well as acute and chronic physical ailments.
- Practitioners use reiki to correct imbalances, eliminate blocked energy, and enhance the body's natural ability to heal itself. Initial treatments have been found effective in helping in every type of illness.
- It can be used effectively as a complement to all forms of medical intervention to reduce side effects and enhance the patient's quality of life.

WHO PERFORMS THIS SERVICE

- Trained certified reiki practitioners provide this service. Level 1 reiki is done in person; level 2 may be done as a distance healing treatment.

COST

- Sessions range in price from $45-$80 but this varies with practitioner and length of the session. Best results have been seen when a patient has three sessions within a short time frame. They take a break and then repeat the process.

BENEFITS

- Studies show that reiki aids meditation, releases stress, eases depression, reduces fear, and decreases pain.
- After reiki therapy, oncology patients have reported a reduction in symptoms of nausea and vomiting associated with chemotherapy.
- Other studies validate pain reduction for these patients after reiki sessions.

RISKS

- Reiki is considered a safe, noninvasive treatment.
- Reiki may have initial effects of causing emotional release in the form of laughter, crying, or loquaciousness; gastric upset, mild cases of nausea or diarrhea; headaches; or overall tingling sensations. These are temporary conditions and may be a result of body detoxification and part of the healing process.

RESOURCES

- American Reiki Institute, Tacoma, Washington: www.americanreikiinstitute.com

BIBLIOGRAPHY

Burack, M. (1995). *Reiki—healing yourself and others*. Encinitas, CA: Reiki Healing Institute.

Stuart, C. (Ed). (2005). *The illustrated guide to massage and aromatherapy* (pp. 398-477). London: Hermes House.

Stein, D. (1996). *Essential reiki: a complete guide to an ancient healing art*. Freedom, CA: Crossing Press.

Principles of Symptom Management

Alopecia

Wendy Vogel

DEFINITION

- The absence or loss of hair
- Can result from genetic factors, aging, local or systemic disease or can be therapy induced
- Minimal hair loss is considered less than 25%, moderate hair loss is 25%-50%, and severe hair loss is more than 50%.
- At least 50% of hair must be lost for it to be noticeable.
- In oncology settings, toxic alopecia generally occurs because of chemotherapeutic agents or radiation therapy.
- Toxic alopecia is usually temporary and can include body hair as well as hair of the head.
- The average daily hair loss is approximately 100 hairs.
- Because hair follicles are mitotically active structures, they are at risk for damage from radiation and chemotherapy.
- Scalp hair is the most sensitive to damage, followed by the male beard, eyebrows, axilla, pubis, and fine hair.
- The degree of alopecia depends on the treatment given, the dose, the schedule, and the route of administration.
- Bolus-dosing schedules of chemotherapy will cause more alopecia than cumulative doses given over extended periods.
- Radiation doses at 2500-3000 cGy fractionated over 2 or 3 weeks will cause hair loss. A single dose as small as 500 cGy may cause hair loss.
- Radiation doses of more than 4500 cGy may cause permanent alopecia.
- More than 6000 cGy may cause sebaceous and sweat glands to stop functioning.

PATHOPHYSIOLOGY AND CONTRIBUTING FACTORS

- When cells in the hair bulb absorb the chemotherapeutic agent or damage to the cells from radiation occurs, cellular division and protein synthesis can be suppressed or halted.
- Cells can enter the telogen phase early, enabling the hair to be shed.
- Hair loss will usually occur within 2-3 weeks after the first exposure to the toxin.
- Continued loss can occur over the next 3-4 weeks, although this varies according to chemotherapeutic agent.
- Generally, hair loss will begin on the crown and the sides of the head above the ear.
- Regrowth will occur within 3-5 months. New hair growth may be of different texture, color, or consistency.
- Regrowth may occur before the end of therapy because of the tricyclic nature of hair growth phases.

SIGNS AND SYMPTOMS

- Loss of hair usually begins 2-3 weeks after exposure. The scalp may become sensitive before loss.

ASSESSMENT TOOLS

- Thorough history
  - Comorbid diseases
  - Nutrition
  - Drug history
  - Psychiatric history
- Physical examination
  - Inspection for a pattern of hair loss
  - Density of remaining hair
  - Color (dull or bright)
  - Condition of scalp
  - Length and texture of hair
- A hair pull test involves gentle traction on about 50 hairs. If two or three or more hairs are dislodged, then an accelerated hair loss is likely.
- Common Terminology Criteria for Adverse Events (version 3.0)
  - Grade 1 indicates thinning or patchy hair.
  - Grade 2 is complete hair loss.
- Eastern Cooperative Oncology Group grading scale
- World Health Organization toxicity grading criteria

LABORATORY AND DIAGNOSTIC TESTS

- None

DIFFERENTIAL DIAGNOSES

- Malnutrition
- Hypothyroidism
- Noncytoxic drugs such as allopurinol, amphetamines, anticoagulants, antithyroid drugs, heavy metals, hypocholesterolemic drugs, levodopa, oral contraceptives, propranolol, and retinoids
- Chronic stress
- Postpartum state
- Lupus erythematosus
- Alopecia of different etiologies such as congenital, alopecia areata, androgenetic alopecia, trauma, tinea capitis, folliculitis decalvans, and alopecia neoplastica

INTERVENTIONS

- Prevention has been a subject of debate since the 1960s.
- Various preventive methods have been used, including scalp tourniquets and scalp hypothermia. Discomfort and the risk of creating a "drug-free area" that could be a site for recurrence have discouraged these practices.

Pharmacologic Interventions

- None used as standard of care
- Several agents for prevention and treatment of alopecia have been studied with varying results:
  - Tocopherol
  - ImuVert
  - Minoxidil

Nonpharmacologic Interventions

- Alopecia can cause the skin to be sensitive or tender. Warmth, lotions, massage, or other symptomatic treatments may be used, although there are no guidelines in the medical literature to advise these.
- Patients should be reassured that hair regrowth will occur.
- Psychosocial adjustment should be continually assessed throughout the treatment period until regrowth.

PATIENT TEACHING

- Instruct as to when hair loss will occur.
- Advise the patient to obtain a wig or head covering if desired before hair loss, while a good color and style match can be made.
- Sunscreen and the use of hats should be encouraged.
- Care should be taken to avoid cuts or nicks to the scalp if the head is shaved.
- Refer to patient teaching sheet in Section Seven

FOLLOW-UP

- Hair should begin to regrow within 3-5 months after therapy ends. The rate of growth will depend on the individual's growth rate. If hair has not begun to regrow within 6 months, alopecia may be permanent.

RESOURCES

- American Academy of Dermatology: www.aad.org/default.htm
- Cancer Care.org: www.cancercare.org
- Cancer Symptoms.org: www.cancersymptoms.org
- Oncolink: www.oncolink.com

BIBLIOGRAPHY

Camp-Sorrell, D. (2005). Chemotherapy toxicities and management. In C. Yarbro, M. Frogge, & M. Goodman (Eds.). *Cancer nursing principles and practice* (6th ed., pp. 412-457). Sudbury, MA: Jones & Bartlett.

Common terminology criteria for adverse events, version 3.0. (2003). Retrieved January 5, 2006, from http://ctep.cancer.gov/forms/CTCAEv3.pdf.

Ferri, F. (2005). *Ferri's clinical advisor*. St. Louis: Mosby.

Groenwald, S., Frogge, M., Goodman, M., et al. (1997). *Cancer nursing principles and practice.* Sudbury, MA: Jones & Bartlett.

Reeves, D. (1999). Alopecia. In C. Yarbro, M. Frogge, & M. Goodman (Eds.). *Cancer symptom management* (2nd ed., pp. 275-284). Sudbury, MA: Jones & Bartlett.

Viale, P. (2006). Chemotherapy and cutaneous toxicities: Implications for oncology nurses. *Seminars in Oncology Nursing, 22,* 144-151.

Wiedemeyer, K., Schill, W., & Loser, C. (2004). Disease of hair follicles leading to hair loss. Part I: nonscarring alopecias. *SKINmed 3,* 209-214.

Alterations in Sexuality

Wendy H. Vogel

DEFINITION

- Human sexuality is more than just sexual function. It is defined as a combination of feelings and behaviors that are unique for each person and includes sexual response, intimacy, emotions, fertility, and hormonal function.
- Sexual function is a specific aspect of sexuality that includes gender and involves the mind and body.
- Sexuality is an important part of normal life for most people and important to their quality of life.
- Sexual dysfunction can occur in 20%-100% of cancer patients, depending on the cancer site.
- Long-term sexual dysfunction has been documented in at least 50% of breast, prostate, colorectal, or gynecological cancer patients.
- Although sexual dysfunction is common, fewer than 20% of men or women seek medical help.

Pathophysiology and Contributing Factors

- Cancer or cancer treatments may damage one of the physiological systems, such as hormonal, vascular, neurological, or psychological systems, needed for healthy sexual responses.
- The most common sexual problem diagnosed after cancer treatment is loss of desire for sex in both men and women, erectile dysfunction in men, and dyspareunia in women.
- Less likely to resolve over time, unlike other cancer treatment side effects

- Pelvic surgery, radiation, chemotherapy, or hormonal agents may affect sexuality:
  - Chemotherapy
    - Dependent on the agent used
    - Affects the granulose cells and the oocyte
    - Alkylating agents, antimetabolites, and antitumor antibiotics can cause amenorrhea, oligospermia, azoospermia, decreased libido, ovarian dysfunction, and erectile dysfunction. Combinations of these drugs may prolong infertility.
    - Alkylating agents may cause primary ovarian failure resulting in amenorrhea, decreased estradiol, and elevated gonadotropin levels.
    - Women who are age 40 years or older have a higher risk of permanent menopause than younger women.
    - 80% of women less than age 25 years recover normal menses after chemotherapy.
    - When used without an alkylating agent, doxorubicin, bleomycin, vinblastine, or dacarbazine cause gonadal dysfunction in up to 50% of patients.
    - Alkylating agents cause the most damage in men to sexuality and fertility.
    - There is limited literature available about the effects of biotherapy on sexuality, but most changes in sexual function can be related to the biological agent's side effects such as fatigue, dry mucous membranes, and flu-like syndrome.
  - Radiation therapy
    - In men, prostate, bladder or rectal surgery, radiation to the pelvis (including brachytherapy), or hormonal therapy may contribute to impotence.

- Testicular damage is dose dependent and the specific drug and age of the patient has less importance.
- Drugs associated with impotence:
  - Antihypertensives such as sympatholytics, alpha-adrenergic blockers, beta-adrenergic blockers, vasodilators, diuretics
  - Psychotropic agents such as major tranquilizers, antidepressants, antianxiety agents
  - Controlled substances such as alcohol, cocaine, narcotics, nicotine
  - Hormonal agents
  - Anticholinergics
  - Histamine H_2-receptor blockers
  - Clofibrate
  - Digoxin
  - Finasteride
- Rule of thumb: If fertility is to be recovered in men, the sperm counts will return to normal within 3 years after therapy completion.

SIGNS AND SYMPTOMS

- Women:
  - Decreased libido
  - Dyspareunia
  - Difficulty reaching orgasm
  - Altered body image
  - Amenorrhea
  - Menopausal symptoms
  - Infertility
  - Abnormal hormone levels
- Men:
  - Decreased libido
  - Erectile dysfunction
  - Difficulty maintaining erection
  - Premature ejaculation
  - Difficulty reaching orgasm
  - Altered body image
  - Infertility

ASSESSMENT TOOLS

- Should be part of the initial new patient history and routine follow-up
  - Cancer diagnosis
  - Age of patient
  - Sex
  - Preillness sexual functioning and relationships

- Ethnic background and cultural norms
- Body image
- Concomitant physical and psychological illnesses
- Medications
- Gynecological history, including any history of sexually transmitted diseases
- Obstetrical history
- Men should be questioned regarding alcohol intake, drug abuse, tobacco use, and whether he has morning erections.
- A quiet, private, nonthreatening environment should be provided and confidentiality ensured.
- The PLISSIT model addresses both assessment and rehabilitation:
  - **P**ermission
  - **L**imited **I**nformation
  - **S**pecific **S**uggestions
  - **I**ntensive **T**herapy
- The ALARM model for the assessment of sexual functioning:
  - **A**ctivity
  - **L**ibido
  - **A**rousal
  - **R**esolution
  - **M**edical history relevant to sexuality
- Physical assessment should include:
  - Women: Pelvic and adnexal examination and also rectal examination
  - Men: Genital examination, rectal examination. The bulbocavernosus reflex and the pudendal-evoked response should also be assessed.

LABORATORY AND DIAGNOSTIC TESTS

- Women:
  - Luteinizing hormone, follicle-stimulating hormone, serum estradiol
  - Serum testosterone level
  - Erythrocyte sedimentation rate, white blood cells
  - Wet mount; cervical, vaginal cultures
  - Urinalysis
  - Pelvic/abdominal ultrasonography

- Men:
  - Serum follicle-stimulating hormone and morning testosterone levels; fasting glucose; thyroid profile
  - Rigiscan to differentiate between psychogenic and organic erectile dysfunction
  - Postage stamp test: securely place a length of postage stamps around the circumference of the shaft of the penis before the man goes to bed at night. If the stamps have separated, it may indicate the man had an erection during the night.
  - Serum prolactin if pituitary adenoma is suspected

DIFFERENTIAL DIAGNOSES

- Menopausal changes
- Dyspareunia
- Atrophic tissue
- Impaired lubrication
- Psychogenic versus organic
- Inadequate foreplay
- Vaginismus
- Endometriosis
- Chronic pelvic pain
- Surgical adhesions
- Infection
- Tubal prolapse
- Uterine prolapse
- Rectocele, cystocele, enterocele
- Postcoital cystitis
- Previous sexual abuse
- Interstitial cystitis
- Erectile dysfunction
- Psychiatric condition such as depression or obsessive-compulsive disorder

INTERVENTIONS

- Giving permission to patients to discuss sexual concerns legitimizes concerns.
- Dispel myths.
- Specific suggestions may be given when patients require more information than addressed in the general, limited information process.
- Intensive therapy may be required for some patients:
  - With troubled relationships
  - History of past abuse

- Need for surgical intervention
- A proactive approach is needed rather than waiting until the patient asks for information.
- Discussions should occur before treatment decision making. Patients should be well informed about the potential and expected side effects of each treatment option.
- Fertility preservation should be considered in those who are of childbearing years.
  - Sperm banking
  - Egg storage
- Sexual rehabilitation should include both behavior changes and partner involvement, addressing such problems as
  - Men: erectile dysfunction, decreased libido, difficulty reaching orgasm, and pain with ejaculation
  - Women: loss of libido, dyspareunia, vaginal stenosis, and difficulty reaching orgasm
- Written information for the patient and partner to review in private is also helpful.
- If the health care provider is unable to provide the required information or treatment, then an appropriate referral should be made.
- Erectile dysfunction:
  - Sildenafil 50 mg or vardenafil 10 mg orally 1 hour before sexual activity. Avoid concomitant nitrate use.
  - Intracavernosal injections of vasodilators such as papaverine, alprostadil, or prostaglandin E_1 pellet. This approach may be associated with penile scarring over time.
  - Vacuum device. If other approaches fail, penile prosthesis may be considered, but these do not address issues of libido or orgasm.
  - Oral medications such as pentoxifylline and yohimbine have been used with limited success.
  - Testosterone therapy in elderly, hypogonadal males may be considered.

- Psychogenic erectile dysfunction will spontaneously resolve in 15%-30% of cases.
  - Referral for intensive therapy if psychotherapy, sex therapy, or surgical treatment is required.
- Dyspareunia:
  - Discontinue exacerbating activity and irritants.
  - Advise the use of nonirritating lubricants.
  - Consider position changes during coitus, perhaps with the woman in the superior position.
  - Muscle exercises, relaxation techniques, and stress reduction techniques may be helpful.
  - For pain, topical lidocaine could be considered. Mild oral analgesics may also be considered.
  - Antidepressants could be helpful if depression is a concern, but consideration should be given to sexual side effects of many antidepressants.
  - Encourage regular sexual activity.
  - For vaginal atrophy resulting from hormonal changes, water-based lubricants, vaginal moisturizers, or a low-dose estrogen (vaginal ring or suppository) may be considered.
  - To prevent vaginal stenosis in women who have had pelvic radiation therapy, vaginal dilation should be taught.
  - Hormone replacement therapy may be considered after a benefit-risk discussion with the patient.
  - Vaginal reconstruction could be considered after complete or partial vaginectomy.
  - Topical lidocaine, corticosteroids, or anti-infective agents as appropriate.
- Control physical symptoms before sexual relations:
  - Nausea and vomiting
    - Antiemetics 1 hour and light meal or crackers before sexual activity

- Partner should avoid perfumes, colognes, or scented candles.
  - Pain
    - Medication 1 hour before sexual activity
    - Relaxation techniques, massage, warm bath before sexual activity
    - Support painful areas with cushions/pillows.
  - Fatigue
    - 30-60 minute nap before sexual activity
    - Avoid large meal before sexual activity.
  - Dyspnea
    - Sexual positioning that requires minimal effort on part of the patient

PATIENT TEACHING

- Refer to Section Seven for patient teaching tool regarding sexuality.
- Times in the disease trajectory patients need information about sexuality:
  - Diagnosis
  - During treatment
  - During recovery and resumption of sexual activity
- Rebuilding sexuality is a continuing process.
- Patient education materials should include the following:
  - Safe sexual practices
  - Avoidance of sexual relations during times of serious immunosuppression
  - Contraception during treatment and for a period of time after treatment
  - Exploration of other means of sexual expression besides intercourse
  - Information to dispel myths
  - Hints for coping with specific problems
  - Education sheets may facilitate communications (See Section Seven).

FOLLOW-UP

- Referral for psychotherapy, surgery, urology, endocrinology, or gynecology as appropriate
- Follow-up assessment of intervention success periodically

RESOURCES

- American Cancer Society: www.cancer.org
- Chemocare.org: www.chemocare.org
- Female sexual dysfunction: www. femalesexualdysfunctiononline. com
- Fertile Hope: www.fertilehope.org
- National Cancer Institute: www.cancer.gov
- The North American Menopausal Society (NAMS): www.menopause.org
- Oncology Nursing Society's CancerSymptoms.org: www.cancersymptoms.org
- SusanLoveMD.org: www.susanlovemd.org

BIBLIOGRAPHY

Bokhour, B., Clark, J., Inui, T., et al. (2001). Sexuality after treatment for early prostate cancer: exploring the meanings of "erectile dysfunction." *Journal of General Internal Medicine, 16,* 649-655.

Bostwick, D. G., Crawford, E. D., Higano, C. S., et al. (Eds.). (2005). *American Cancer Society's complete guide to prostate cancer.* Atlanta: American Cancer Society.

Bruner, D., & Iwamoto, R. (1999). Altered sexual health. In C. Yarbro, M. Frogge, & M. Goodman (Eds.), *Cancer symptom management* (2nd ed., pp. 549-566). Sudbury, MA: Jones & Bartlett.

Fenstermacher, K., & Hudson, B. (2000). *Practice guidelines for family nurse practitioners* (2nd ed.). Philadelphia: W. B. Saunders.

Ferri, F. (2005). *Ferri's clinical advisor, 2005.* Philadelphia: Elsevier Mosby.

Fincannon, J. L., & Bruss, K. V. (2003). *Couples confronting cancer.* Atlanta: American Cancer Society.

Katz, A. (2005). The sounds of silence: Sexuality information for cancer patients. *Journal of Clinical Oncology, 23,* 238-241.

Krebs, L. (2005). Sexual and reproductive dysfunction. In C. Yarbro, M. Frogge, & M. Goodman (Eds.). *Cancer symptom management* (6th ed., pp. 841-869). Sudbury, MA: Jones & Bartlett.

Mick, J., Hughes, M., & Cohen, M. (2004). Using the BETTER model to assess sexuality. *Clinical Journal of Oncology Nursing, 8,* 84-86.

Penson, R., Gallagher, J., Gioiella, M., et al. (2000). Sexuality and cancer. *The Oncologist, 5,* 336-344.

Polovich, M., White, J., & Kelleher, L. (2005). *Chemotherapy and biotherapy guidelines and recommendations for practice* (2nd ed.). Pittsburgh, PA: Oncology Nursing Society.

Schover, L. (2005). Sexuality and fertility after cancer. *American Society of Hematology, Educational Program,* 523-527.

Schwartz, S., & Plawcki, H. (2002). Consequences of chemotherapy on the sexuality of patients with lung cancer. *Clinical Journal of Oncology Nursing, 6,* 212-216.

Anorexia

*Laura M. Benson
and Kristin A. Cawley*

DEFINITION

- The loss of desire to eat
- Weight loss greater than 10% within a 6-month period
- Occurs in as many as 40% of cancer patients at diagnosis and up to 70% in patients in advanced stages
- Highest incidences occur in patients with gastrointestinal cancers.
- Often associated with cachexia (lean tissue wasting)
- Weight loss is a major cause of morbidity and mortality in patients with advanced cancer.
- Associated with a lower quality of life, poor response to chemotherapy, reduced performance status, and shorter survival times

PATHOPHYSIOLOGY AND CONTRIBUTING FACTORS

- End result of altered central and peripheral neurohormonal signals that govern appetite
- Involuntary systemic effect of underlying disease
- Predisposed by disease progression
- Direct result of supportive treatment modalities, including surgery, radiation, and chemotherapy
- Secondary effect of:
  - Taste alterations
  - Pain
  - Nausea
  - Lowered immune competence
- Humoral and inflammatory responses:
  - Production of inflammatory cytokines

- Local effects of tumor:
  - Dysphagia
  - Gastric obstruction
- Psychological factors, including depression
- Metabolic disturbances

SIGNS AND SYMPTOMS

- Lack of appetite
- Weight loss
- Muscle wasting
- Early satiety
- Fatigue
- Nausea
- Vomiting
- Weakness
- Sleep disturbances

ASSESSMENT TOOLS

- Patient history and physical examination
- Patient Generated Subjective Global Assessment
- Rotterdam Symptom Checklist
- Psychosocial Adjustment to Illness Scale
- Hospital Anxiety and Depression Scale

LABORATORY AND DIAGNOSTIC TESTS

- Complete blood cell count
- Creatinine
- Albumin, prealbumin, transferrin, and retinol-binding protein

DIFFERENTIAL DIAGNOSES

- Malnutrition
- Dehydration
- Fatigue
- Depression
- Hypercalcemia

INTERVENTIONS

- Treat underlying etiologies

Pharmacologic Interventions

- Progestational agents:
  - Megestrol acetate (Megace)
  - Medroxyprogesterone
- Corticosteroids
  - Dexamethasone
- Cannabinoids
  - Dronabinol
- Cytoheptadine
- Dietary supplements
- Treat hypercalcemia if present

Symptom Management

Nonpharmacologic Interventions

- Increased food intake
- Screening at diagnosis and regular intervals
  - Weight change
  - Dietary intake
  - Physical examination findings
  - Laboratory findings
- Management of underlying etiologies
  - Nausea
  - Constipation
  - Mucositis
- Nutritional counseling
- Parenteral nutrition
- Minimizing factors that decrease food intake

PATIENT TEACHING

Refer to patient teaching sheet in Section Seven.

- Eat small frequent meals.
- Decrease energy expenditure.
- Minimize factors that decrease food intake.
- Avoid offensive odors.
- Eat energy-dense foods.
- Limit fat intake.
- Avoid extremes in taste and smell of food.
- Enhance presentation of food.

FOLLOW-UP

- Nutrition/dietician consultation as needed
- Assess new onset of or continuing weight loss

RESOURCES

- Oncology Nursing Society: Cancer Symptoms: www.cancersymptoms.org
- Oncology Nursing Society: www.ons.org

BIBLIOGRAPHY

Brown, J. K. (2002). A systematic review of the evidence on symptom management of cancer-related anorexia and cachexia. *Oncology Nursing Forum, 29,* 517-532.

Cope, D. (2002). Management of anorexia, cachexia, and weight loss in patients with advanced cancer. *Clinical Journal of Oncology Nursing, 6,* 241-242.

Davis, M. P., Dreicer, R., Walsh, D., et al. (2004). Appetite and cancer-associated anorexia: A review. *Journal of Clinical Oncology, 22,* 1510-1517.

Esper, P., & Heidrich, D. (2005). Symptom clusters in advanced illness. *Seminars in Oncology Nursing, 21,* 20-28.

Laviano, A., Meguid, M., & Rossi-Fanelli, F. (2003). Cancer anorexia: Clinical implications, pathogenesis, and therapeutic strategies. *The Lancet Oncology, 4,* 686-694.

Molassiotis, A. (2003). Anorexia and weight loss in long-term survivors. *Journal of Clinical Nursing, 12,* 925-927.

Von Meyenfeldt, M. (2005). Cancer-associated malnutrition: An introduction. *European Journal of Oncology Nursing, 9,* S35-S38.

Yavuzen, T., Davis, M. P., Walsh, D., et al. (2005). Systematic review of the treatment of cancer-associated anorexia and weight loss. *Journal of Clinical Oncology, 23,* 8500-8511.

Anxiety

Denice Economou

DEFINITION

- Subjective feeling of distress, apprehension, tension, insecurity, or uneasiness, usually without a known stimulus or cause
- Most often rated as mild, moderate, or severe

PATHOPHYSIOLOGY AND CONTRIBUTING FACTORS

- Thought to result from an inappropriate activation of the sympathetic nervous system
- Increased levels of norepinephrine with decreased levels of serotonin and gamma-aminobutyric acid
- Hormonal input such as hypothalamus, pituitary, and adrenal glands interfere with normal processes, leading to feelings of panic or a sense of dread.
- Cardiovascular abnormalities contribute to anxiety as a result of altered regulation of the autonomic nervous system.
- Medication induced: see list under "Assessment Tools"
- Withdrawal from alcohol or nicotine
- Disease stage—anxiety increases as disease advances or physical status declines
- Difficulty with treatment regimens or lifestyle changes and financial concerns
- Dealing with family issues or conflicts and facing death
- Family and staff anxiety can contribute to the patient's level of anxiety and vice versa.

SIGNS AND SYMPTOMS

- Restlessness, panic, tachycardia, difficulty concentrating, palpitations, sweating, dizziness, urinary frequency, abdominal discomfort, sleep disturbances
- Chest pain, irritability, headache, apprehension, and anorexia
- Any repetitive behaviors to prevent discomfort (pacing, rubbing hands)
- Vital signs: elevated heart rate, blood pressure, or respiratory rate and temperature
- Skin examination may reveal endocrine-associated changes that contribute to anxiety—dry skin in thyroid disorder, Addison's disease symptoms—facial puffiness, and increased skin pigmentation. Skin turgor may predict poor appetite, dehydration, or hypernatremia.

ASSESSMENT TOOLS

- Depression and anxiety screening. Tools to help evaluate subjective feelings of anxiety and level patient is experiencing. Can rate anxiety on a visual analog scale or verbal rating scale like pain ratings, 0-10
- Ask questions such as: "Do you feel nervous?" "Do you worry about your diagnosis or treatment?" Goal is to understand what may be contributing to the anxiety.
- History should include any history of psychosocial disorders, adjustment disorders, or panic attacks.
- Any history of generalized anxiety disorders or phobias or history of agitated depression

- What are the presenting symptoms, including precipitating factors, onset, and duration?
- What makes the symptoms better or worse?
- How does the patient cope with anxiety? What methods does the patient use to manage anxiety?
- Medication history, including over-the-counter medications. Medications associated with anxiety include stimulants, thyroid replacement medications, corticosteroids, bronchodilators and decongestants, epinephrine, antihypertensives, antihistamines, anticholinergics, anesthetics, and analgesics.
- Uncontrolled pain, hypoxia, sepsis, adverse drug effects, and withdrawal can lead to anxiety.
- Cardiac examination to identify irregular heart rate or abnormal heart sounds
- Pulmonary examination to rule out hypoxia related to pneumonia, pleural effusions, or embolus
- Neurological examination to identify cranial nerve palsies and neuropathies

LABORATORY AND DIAGNOSTIC TESTS

- Complete blood cell count to identify infections
- Thyroid-stimulating hormone to detect thyroid abnormalities
- Oxygen saturation for respiratory conditions
- Electrocardiogram to evaluate cardiac functioning
- Chest x-ray film to rule out pneumonia, pleural effusion, or embolus

DIFFERENTIAL DIAGNOSES

- Phobic disorders
- Panic attack
- Obsessive-compulsive disorder
- Posttraumatic stress disorder

INTERVENTIONS

- Treating anxiety is related to the patient's subjective level of distress.
- Moderate to severe anxiety can interfere significantly with the patient's ability to comply with treatments.

Pharmacologic Interventions

- Benzodiazepines: diazepam, alprazolam, temazepam
- Azapirones: buspirone
- Antidepressants: amitriptyline, imipramine, nortriptyline, doxepin, fluoxetine, sertraline, paroxetine, venlafaxine
- Other medications used for anxiety include propranolol and haloperidol.
- Atypical neuroleptics: olanzapine, risperidone

Nonpharmacologic Interventions

- Initiate a discussion of concerns that may be contributing to the feeling of anxiety, such as pain, fear, dependence issues. Use open-ended questions and clarification remarks.
- Help patient identify what has helped him or her get through times like this before. Talk about how we can help you use those strategies now.
- Encourage the patient to identify people who can support him or her through this anxiety.
- Recognize that as patients move through anxiety from mild to severe the cause may be lost as the anxiety takes over. Preventive strategies can be useful to minimize anxiety or stabilize the escalation.
- Increase opportunities for control
- Evaluate dietary intake to reduce caffeine products and alcohol to promote sleep.
- Relieve pain.

PATIENT TEACHING

- Provide patient and family education to support reduction of fear and anticipatory reactions. Give instructions on medications and side effect management. Goal of education is to reduce stress and anxiety.
- Increase patient and family participation in activities.
- Encourage hope.

- Use a family member or friend as the support person to stay present to help the patient.
- Provide accurate information to help restructure unrealistic fearful beliefs.
- Teach anxiety-reducing interventions such as relaxation, visualization, deep breathing, massage, touch, and physical exercise.
- Stress management may also include music and art therapy, yoga.

FOLLOW-UP

- Refer patients to supportive psychiatric care when necessary.
- Multidisciplinary management can be the most effective way to achieve relief of anxiety. Social workers and chaplains should be part of the team to help support and manage patients experiencing anxiety.

RESOURCES

- MentalHelp.Net: www.mentalhelp.net

BIBLIOGRAPHY

Breitbart, W., Chochinov, H. M., & Passik, S. (2004). Psychiatric symptoms in palliative medicine. In D. Doyle, G. Hanks, N. Cherny, et al. (Eds.). *Oxford textbook of palliative medicine* (3rd ed., pp. 746-771). New York: Oxford University Press.

Dahlin, C. (2006). Anxiety. In D. Camp-Sorrell, & R. A. Hawkins (Eds.). *Clinical manual for the oncology advanced practice nurse* (pp. 1105-1111). Pittsburgh: Oncology Nursing Society.

End-of-Life Nursing Education Consortium. (2006). *Oncology-module 3: Symptom management*. Duarte, CA: American Association of Colleges of Nursing.

Pasacreta, J., Minarik, P. A., & Nield-Anderson, L. (2006). Anxiety and depression. In B. Ferrell & N. Coyle (Eds.). *Textbook of palliative nursing*. (2nd ed., pp. 375-399). New York: Oxford University Press.

Arthralgias and Myalgias

Carol S. Blecher

DEFINITION

- Arthralgias: pains in the joints
- Myalgias: diffuse generalized muscle pains
- Both may be accompanied by a general feeling of malaise.

PATHOPHYSIOLOGY AND CONTRIBUTING FACTORS

- Generally the pathophysiology is unclear.
- Proposed theories include the following:
  - Response to a noxious stimulus or trauma that damaged muscle tissue releases bradykinin and stimulates the muscle nociceptors
  - Related to the taxanes and vinca alkaloids. May have a relationship to microtubule stabilization or inflammatory reaction to the drug.
- Risk factors include the following:
  - History of peripheral neuropathy
  - History of diabetes
  - Alcohol use
  - Drugs such as paclitaxel (especially in combination with cisplatin), docetaxel, vincristine, vinblastine, vinorelbine, rituximab, etoposide, bacille Calmette-Guérin (BCG), filgrastim, sargramostim, interferon, interleukin-2, dacarbazine, altretamine, topotecan, gemcitabine, procarbazine, fludarabine, letrozole (aromatase inhibitors as a class), azacytidine, cladribine, L-asparaginase
  - Age
  - Prior neurotoxic chemotherapy
  - History of arthritis
  - History of neuromuscular disease

SIGNS AND SYMPTOMS
Myalgias

- Generalized or localized muscle aches
- Edema
- Induration
- Fever
- Warm, flushed skin
- Tachycardia
- Shortness of breath
- Headache
- Thirst

Arthralgias

- Painful joints
- Swelling and redness of joints
- Fever and chills
- Fatigue
- Depression

ASSESSMENT TOOLS

- Assessment of the patient with arthralgias or myalgias should include the following:
  - History, including diagnosis and cancer treatment, current medications, presenting symptoms, precipitating factors, location, and duration
  - Vital signs
    - Elevated temperature
    - Tachycardia
    - Tachypnea
  - Musculoskeletal system
    - Edema
    - Spasm
    - Erythema
    - Warmth and tenderness
    - Strength and range of motion
  - Complete pain assessment
    - Character of the pain
    - Location
    - Quality
    - Onset
    - Factors that cause pain to worsen
    - Factors that alleviate pain
      - Current medication
      - Severity of the pain— current pain score, worst pain score, best pain score, and pain goal
      - Effects of pain on activities of daily living (ADLs) and quality of life (QOL)
  - National Cancer Institute Common Toxicity Criteria and

Common Terminology Criteria for Adverse Events
- Grade 1: mild pain not interfering with function
- Grade 2: moderate pain, pain or analgesics interfering with function but not interfering with ADLs
- Grade 3: severe pain, pain or analgesics severely interfering with ADLs
- Grade 4: disabling

LABORATORY AND DIAGNOSTIC TESTS

- Complete blood cell count (CBC) with differential to evaluate neutropenia and rule out infection
- Chemistries to rule out hypo- or hyperkalemia, hypomagnesemia, hypocalcemia, hypo- or hypernatremia, hypophosphatemia
- Creatinine kinase levels to rule out muscle inflammation or damage
- Urinalysis focusing on red blood cells
- Thyroid-stimulating hormone (TSH)
- Blood cultures if neutropenia is suspected
- Electromyelogram (EMG) to differentiate myelopathy from neuropathy
- Muscle biopsy to identify specific myopathies

DIFFERENTIAL DIAGNOSES

- Cancer or metastatic disease
- Hematoma
- Ruptured tendon
- Thrombophlebitis
- Pyomyositis
  - Bacterial infection of the skeletal muscles that results in a pus-filled abscess
  - Most often caused by *Staphylococcus aureus*
- Fasciitis
- Sarcoidosis
- Ischemia or infarct
- Alcoholic myopathy
- Exertional muscle damage
- Fibromyalgia
- Inflammation
- Infections such as toxoplasmosis, trichinosis, influenza, herpes

- Electrolyte imbalance such as hypo- or hyperkalemia, hypomagnesemia, hypocalcemia, hypo- or hypernatremia, hypophosphatemia
- Hypothyroidism
- Drugs: steroid withdrawal, paclitaxel (especially in combination with cisplatin), docetaxel, vincristine, vinblastine, vinorelbine, rituximab, etoposide, bacille Calmette-Guérin, filgrastim, sargramostim, interferon, interleukin-2, dacarbazine, altretamine, topotecan, gemcitabine, procarbazine, fludarabine, letrozole (aromatase inhibitors as a class), azacytidine, cladribine, L-asparaginase
- Amyloidosis
- Osteomalacia
  - The adult equivalent of the disease rickets
  - Mineralization of newly formed bone matrix is defective
- Guillain-Barré syndrome
- Polymyalgia rheumatica
- Fabry's disease
  - An X-linked recessive inherited lysosomal storage disease
- Parkinson's disease

INTERVENTIONS

- Treatment of the underlying disease
- Frequent rests interspersed with activity
- Maintain adequate nutrition

Pharmacologic Interventions

- Add medications as needed using the World Health Organization ladder as a reference
  - Acetaminophen (Tylenol) 650 mg orally every 4 hours as needed not to exceed 4 grams per day
  - Ibuprofen (Motrin, Advil, Nuprin) 200-400 mg every 6 hours
  - Indomethacin (Indocin) 25 to 50 mg orally twice or three times a day not to exceed 200 mg per day
  - Prednisone 10 mg orally twice a day for 5 days after chemotherapy

Nonpharmacologic Interventions

- Use a heating pad or hot water bottle on the painful area.
- Use an ice pack on the painful area.
- Take warm baths.
- Complementary therapies such as massage, relaxation techniques, whirlpool, magnets

PATIENT TEACHING

- See Section Seven for patient teaching materials for muscle aches and joint pain.

FOLLOW-UP

- Pain service referral
- Physical therapy
- Occupational therapy

Call your health care provider if:

- You have new and increasingly severe back pain.
- You have a new symptom of numbness and tingling down your legs.
- You have weakness or decreased sensation in the lower extremities.
- You have a loss of bowel function or bladder control.

RESOURCES

- iVillage Total Health: Pain & Arthritis: http://pain.health.ivillage.com/index.cfm

BIBLIOGRAPHY

Arthralgias and myalgias. (2007). Retrieved September 29, 2007, from http://www.lungcanceronline.org/effects/arthralg ias.html.

Chemotherapy and pain, myalgias, arthralgias. (2005). Retrieved February 7, 2007, from www.Chemocare.com/managing.

Common terminology criteria for adverse events, version 3. (2006). Retrieved February 7, 2007, from http://ctep.cancer.gov/forms/CTCAEv3.pdf.

Martin, V. R. (2004). Arthralgias and myalgias. In C. H. Yarbro, M. H. Frogge, & M. Goodman (Eds.). *Cancer symptom management* (pp. 27-28). Sudbury, MA: Jones & Bartlett.

MedlinePlus Medical Encyclopedia. (n.d.). *Joint pain.* (08/22/06.) Retrieved February 7, 2007, from http://www.nlm.nih.gov/medlineplus/ency/article/003261.htm.

MedlinePlus Medical Encyclopedia. (05/17/07.) *Muscle aches.* Retrieved September 29, 2007, from http://www.nlm.nih.gov/medlineplus/ency/article/003178.htm.

Myalgias and arthralgias: long term consequences of the aromitase inhibitors. (2005). Retrieved December 30, 2006, from http://www.medscape.com/viewarticle/516882_4.

Rumsey, K. A. (2000). Myalgia. In D. Camp-Sorrell & R. A. Hawkins (Eds.). *Clinical manual for the oncology advanced practice nurse* (pp. 775 - 781). Pittsburgh: Oncology Nursing Press.

Confusion

Carol S. Blecher

DEFINITION

- Confusion, or cognitive failure, is a symptom or a description of a person's mental state.
- It is a number of different subjective symptoms and objective behaviors.
- May be operationally defined as behaviors that fall into the following four categories:
  - Disorientation to time, place, or person
  - Inappropriate communication
  - Inappropriate behavior
  - Illusions, misinterpretation of real stimuli, or hallucinations, which are subjective sensory perceptions without real stimuli
- End-of-life confusion can be used to refer to cognitive failure caused by metastatic cancer and multiorgan system failure.

PATHOPHYSIOLOGY AND CONTRIBUTING FACTORS

- Pathogenesis is not well understood.
- May include:
  - Reduced cerebral oxygen metabolism
  - Damaged neuronal enzyme synthesis
  - Neurotransmitter imbalance
  - Neuronal loss
  - Metabolic abnormality

Symptom Management

SIGNS AND SYMPTOMS

- Hypoactive behavior such as mental slowness, a generalized slowing down, or somnolence
- Hyperactive behavior such as restlessness, pacing, searching, or picking
- Delusions
- Paranoia
- Poor memory or forgetfulness
- Inability to concentrate
- Changes in personality
- Changes in habits or ability to care for self

ASSESSMENT TOOLS

- Brief cognitive assessment/mini mental status examination including:
  - Orientation to time and place
  - Memory test through the repetition of three unrelated objects
  - Attention and calculation with serial numbers testing
  - Language testing through the identification of two items, repetition of a sentence
  - Following a multistep command, writing a sentence, and then copying a sentence
- Common terminology criteria (CTC) for adverse events
  - Grade 1: transient confusion, disorientation, or attention deficit
  - Grade 2: confusion, disorientation, or attention deficit interfering with function but not interfering with activities of daily living (ADLs)
  - Grade 3: confusion or delirium interfering with ADLs
  - Grade 4: harmful to others or self, hospitalization indicated
  - Grade 5: death
- Physical examination to rule out neurologic problems
- Cardiovascular examination to rule out cardiac abnormalities
- Pulmonary examination to rule out adventitious breath sounds

LABORATORY AND DIAGNOSTIC TESTS

- Chemistry panel to evaluate for metabolic abnormalities
  - Hypernatremia
  - Hyponatremia
  - Hypercalcemia
  - Hypomagnesemia
  - Hyperglycemia
  - Hypoglycemia
- Complete blood cell count (CBC) to evaluate for
  - Hyperleukocytosis
  - Anemia
- Serum therapeutic drug levels of
  - Digoxin
  - Lithium
  - Alcohol
  - Phenytoin
  - Gabapentin
- Ammonia level
- Magnetic resonance imaging (MRI) of the head to rule out brain metastases or hemorrhage
- Pulse oximetry or arterial blood gas analysis (ABG) to rule out hypoxia
- Lumbar puncture (LP) to assess for carcinomatous meningitis
- Electroencephalogram (EEG)

DIFFERENTIAL DIAGNOSES

- Electrolyte abnormalities
- Dehydration
- Renal failure
- Cirrhosis
- Sepsis
- Hypothermia
- Hyperthermia
- Meningitis
- Airway obstruction
- Syndrome of inappropriate antidiuretic hormone (SIADH) secretion
- Tumor lysis syndrome
- Drug-induced confusion related to:
  - Cardiac drugs such as procainamide, propranolol, quinidine, lidocaine, clonidine, methyldopa, reserpine, digitalis
  - Gastrointestinal drugs such as atropine, belladonna, phenothiazine, scopolamine, cimetidine, ranitidine, metoclopramide
  - Musculoskeletal drugs such as corticosteroids, indomethacin, salicylate, diazepam
  - Neurologic/psychiatric drugs such as barbiturates, phenytoin, levodopa, amantadine, chloral hydrate, glutethimide,

benzodiazepines, lithium salts, antidepressants
  - Respiratory/allergic drugs such as chlorpheniramine, cyproheptadine, diphenhydramine, theophylline
  - Analgesics such as narcotics
  - Antidiabetic drugs such as insulin, oral hypoglycemics
  - Antineoplastic agents such as methotrexate, mitomycin, procarbazine, ifosfamide, interferon, L-asparaginase, cytarabine

INTERVENTIONS
Pharmacologic Interventions

- Haloperidol (Haldol)
  - Mild confusion: 0.5 to 1.0 mg orally, intramuscularly (IM), or intravenously (IV) twice a day
  - Agitated confusion: 1-2 mg every 30-60 minutes. When agitation is controlled, assess the 24-hour dose and adjust to a twice-daily dose.
  - Terminal confusion: treat as per protocol for mild confusion.
- Lorazepam (Ativan) for use in confusion associated with alcohol withdrawal and hepatic encephalopathy. Dose is 0.5-2.0 mg every 1-4 hours orally, IM, or IV.
- Phenothiazine (Thorazine) for use in severe symptoms when sedation is required. Usual dose is 12.5-50 mg every 12 hours orally, IM, or IV.
- Diazepam (Valium) may be used but with caution because the active metabolites may cause prolonged sedation. Dose is 2-10 mg orally or IV two to four times a day.
- Midazolam (Versed) used only when all other methods fail to control symptoms. Short half-life, so titration is easy. Dose is 1-4 mg continuous IV or subcutaneous infusion.

Nonpharmacologic Interventions

- Correct or manage causative factors.
- Orient frequently with calendars, clocks, and reorientation to place.

- Ensure safety:
  - Keep bed in low position and if patient is hospitalized, keep call bell within reach.
  - Assist with toileting, ambulation, and positioning.
  - Check often for thirst, dry mouth, indigestion, hunger, pain, and hypothermia or hyperthermia.
  - Have people stay with the patient and avoid restraints.
  - Encourage the patient to use hearing aids and glasses if necessary.
  - Patient is not to drive.
  - Reassure patient frequently.

PATIENT TEACHING

- If the patient only has grade 1 or 2 confusion, aim patient teaching toward offering reassurance, frequent orientation, and encouraging the safety mechanisms listed above while correcting or managing the causative factors.
- If the patient has grade 3 or 4 confusion, direct education efforts toward the significant others, offering reassurance and teaching them how to assist the patient according to the nonpharmacologic interventions listed above.

FOLLOW-UP

- Short term:
  - Monitor the effectiveness of the drug regimen over the first 24-48 hours.
  - Correct the underlying cause of confusion and monitor for clearing of confusion.
  - Continue safety measures to reduce risk for falls or self-injury.
  - In terminal-stage confusion, balance sedation with wakefulness to facilitate patient/significant other communication.
- Long term:
  - Follow at-risk patients closely.
  - Refer to psychiatrist or psychologist.
  - Refer for home care.
  - Refer to hospice if appropriate.

RESOURCES

- Common terminology criteria for adverse events: http://ctep.cancer.gov/forms/CTC AEv3.pdf
- MedlinePlus Medical Encyclopedia. Confusion: www.nlm.nih.gov/medlineplus/ency/article/003205.htm
- National Comprehensive Cancer Network palliative care guidelines: nccn.org/patients/patient_gls/.../ NCCN Palliative Care Guidelines.pdf

BIBLIOGRAPHY

Boyle, D. M. (2000). Confusion/delirium. In D. Camp-Sorrell & R. A. Hawkins (Eds.). *Clinical manual for the oncology advanced practice nurse* (pp. 721-728). Pittsburgh, PA: Oncology Nursing Press.

Chernecky, C. C. (1998). *Advanced and critical care oncology nursing: managing primary complications* (pp. 60, 193, 111, 288, 306, 362, 629, 647). Philadelphia: W. B. Saunders.

Cohen, M. Z., & Armstrong T. (2004). Cognitive dysfunction. In C. H. Yarbro, M. H. Frogge, & M. Goodman (Eds.). *Cancer symptom management* (pp. 635-650). Sudbury, MA: Jones & Bartlett.

Keubler, K. K., English, N., & Heidrich, D. E. (2001). Delirium, confusion, agitation, and restlessness. In B. R. Ferrell, & N. Coyle (Eds.). *Textbook of palliative nursing* (pp. 290-308). New York: Oxford University Press.

Smith, H. (2002). Delirium/acute confusion. In K. K. Kuebler, & P. Esper (Eds.). *Palliative practices A-Z* (pp. 81-83). Pittsburgh, PA: Oncology Nursing Society.

Constipation

Carolyn Grande

DEFINITION

- Passage of hard, dry stools with difficulty or discomfort
- Decrease in frequency of defecation
- Obstipation
  - A more severe form of constipation
  - Absence of bowel movement despite large volumes of stool in the bowel.
- Constipation occurs in approximately 50% of cancer patients and as much as 75% of terminally ill patients.
- Constipation is more common in women and the elderly.

PATHOPHYSIOLOGY AND CONTRIBUTING FACTORS

- Bowel function is determined by the state of intestinal motility and management of fluid in terms of absorption and secretion.
- Primary causes—related to extrinsic/lifestyle factors include the following:
  - Age
  - Low-fiber diet
  - Dehydration
  - Decreased activity
  - Weakness/poor muscle tone
  - Extreme fatigue
- Secondary causes are related to medical conditions or disease processes that may cause hypomotility or obstruction.
- Iatrogenic causes result from pharmacological agents or medical interventions:
  - Drug classes
    - Opioids
    - Anticonvulsants
    - Anesthetics
    - Anticholinergics
    - Tricyclic antidepressants
    - Diuretics
    - Iron supplements
    - Serotonin antagonists
    - Vinca alkaloids
- Surgical anastomosis may lead to narrowing of the colon lumen from scar tissue.

SIGNS AND SYMPTOMS

- Abdominal fullness
- Bloating
- Nausea
- Vomiting
- Excessive gas
- Cramping
- Change in bowel patterns, size and consistency of stools

ASSESSMENT TOOLS

- Comprehensive history including:
  - Extent of cancer and past/current treatment
  - Dietary habits including fluid intake

Symptom Management

○ Alcohol use
○ Medication list of prescribed and over-the-counter drugs with doses and frequency
○ Previous laxative or enema use and its effect
- Baseline frequency pattern of bowel elimination
- Description of last bowel movement including:
  ○ When
  ○ Amount
  ○ Consistency and color of stool
  ○ Presence of blood
  ○ Distinct odor change
- Comprehensive physical examination including:
  ○ Abdominal examination: auscultate for bowel sounds, percuss all four quadrants, palpate for masses or hepatomegaly
  ○ Examine anus for fissures, external hemorrhoids, inflammation
  ○ Rectal or stoma examination for masses, fecal impaction, or stricture
  ○ Examine stool for occult blood
- Accurate assessment tools are lacking in making the diagnosis of constipation. Given the subjective nature of constipation, the Rome criteria were developed to assist in diagnosing this symptom. Criteria to establish a diagnosis of constipation required that a patient experienced the following in the past 3 months:
  ○ Straining with defecation
  ○ Hard stools
  ○ Incomplete evacuation
  ○ Anorectal blockage
  ○ Disimpaction
  ○ Fewer than three bowel movements in a week
  ○ The patient should not have
    ▪ loose stools
    ▪ symptoms of irritable bowel syndrome
- The U.S. Department of Health and Human Services, the National Institutes of Health, and the National Cancer Institute have outlined a grading system for adverse events to assist in categorizing the severity of

the event. The grading system spans from 1 through 5 on the basis of patient assessment. Grading for constipation is as follows:
  ○ Grade 1: occasional or intermittent symptoms; occasional use of stool softeners, laxatives, dietary modification or enema
  ○ Grade 2: persistent symptoms with regular use of laxatives or enemas indicated
  ○ Grade 3: symptoms interfering with activities of daily living, obstipation with manual evacuation indicated
  ○ Grade 4: life-threatening consequences (e.g., obstruction, toxic megacolon)
  ○ Grade 5: death

LABORATORY AND DIAGNOSTIC TESTS

- Complete blood cell count, electrolyte panel including calcium and potassium, renal and liver function tests, thyroid function tests
- Supine and upright x-ray films to differentiate between mechanical obstruction and ileus
- Computed tomography (CT) of abdomen and pelvis if an extraluminal site is suspected
- Barium enema
- Sigmoidoscopy/colonoscopy

DIFFERENTIAL DIAGNOSIS

- Cancer
  ○ Mass obstruction
- Spinal cord tumor compression at T8-L3
- Metabolic
  ○ Hypercalcemia
  ○ Hypokalemia
  ○ Uremia
  ○ Hypothyroidism
- Diseases/conditions
  ○ Anorectal abscess
  ○ Anal fissure
  ○ Cirrhosis
  ○ Depression
  ○ Diabetes
  ○ Diverticulosis
  ○ Hepatic porphyria
  ○ Intestinal obstruction

○ Irritable bowel syndrome
○ Mesenteric artery ischemia
- Other
  ○ Dehydration
  ○ Nutritional compromise
  ○ Extreme fatigue/weakness
  ○ Poor muscle tone

INTERVENTIONS
Pharmacologic Interventions

- Laxatives and cathartics are divided into categories on the basis of the mechanism of action:
- Bulk formers: onset of effect 12 hours–3 days
  ○ Psyllium (Metamucil)
  ○ Methylcellulose (Cologel, Citrucel)
- Bowel stimulants: onset of effect 6-10 hours, rectally 15-60 minutes
  ○ Phenolphthalein (in Ex-lax, Feen-a-mint, Correctol)
  ○ Bisacodyl (Dulcolax), 5 mg tablet one to three times a day. Suppository 10 mg as needed
  ○ Senna (Senokot), 187 mg tablet, maximum eight per day
  ○ Cascara sagrada, 5 mL or 1 tablet as needed at bedtime
  ○ Casanthranol, 30 mg usually in combination with docusate
- Osmotic laxatives
  ○ MiraLax: onset of effect 2 to 4 days; 1 tablespoon (17 grams) in 4-8 ounces of water, juice, soda, coffee, or tea daily
  ○ Lactulose: onset of effect 24-48 hours
    ▪ Cephulac, 30-45 mL three or four times/day or hourly to induce rapid effect
    ▪ Chronulac, 15-30 mL/day, maximum 60 mL/day
    ▪ Sorbitol, 3-150 mL/day
  ○ Polyethylene glycol electrolyte solution: onset of effect within 1 hour
    ▪ GoLYTELY, 8 ounces orally every 15 minutes as tolerated over 3-4 hours until 1 liter taken or diarrhea results
  ○ Glycerin suppositories: onset of effect within 30 minutes of use. Take one or two per day as needed or 5-15 mL as enema
- Lubricants: onset of effect within 8 hours

○ Mineral oil, 15-40 mL/day, once or in divided doses; as retention enema 60-150 mL/day
- Detergent laxatives: onset of effect 24-72 hours
  ○ Docusate, 50-500 mg/day 1 or divided doses
    - Docusate sodium (Colace)
    - Docusate calcium (Surfak)
- Saline laxatives
  ○ Magnesium salts:
    - Magnesium citrate, $1/2$ to 1 full bottle orally as needed, onset of effect 30 minutes–6 hours dose dependent
    - Magnesium hydroxide (milk of magnesia), 30-60 mL/day orally in single or divided doses, onset of effect 4-8 hours
  ○ Sodium salts:
    - Sodium phosphate (Fleet Phospho-soda), 20-30 mL as a single dose, onset of effect 3-6 hours
    - Fleet enema, onset of effect 3-5 minutes
- Use of these agents can be initiated with a four-step approach. Advancement to the next step is indicated if the prior step at maximal doses was ineffective. Allow at least 48 hours to evaluate effectiveness of intervention:
  ○ Step 1: bulk laxatives or milk of magnesia
  ○ Step 2: docusate sodium, senna, or milk of magnesia
  ○ Step 3: sorbitol or lactulose
  ○ Step 4: magnesium citrate or GoLYTELY
- Drug and dosage should be determined by patient condition, response, and tolerance of side effects. For patients receiving opioids for chronic pain or who have vinca alkaloid–containing chemotherapy regimens, prophylaxis for constipation with a stool softener and a stimulant laxative should be used.

Nonpharmacologic Interventions
- Increase daily intake of dietary fiber, gradually titrate 3-4 g/day to total of 10-20 g/day. For patients with structural blockage this method should be avoided because it may increase the obstruction. Sources of fiber include the following:
  ○ Wheat bran
  ○ Whole grain breads
  ○ Peanuts
  ○ Peanut butter
  ○ Peas
  ○ Unpeeled pears
  ○ Dried apricots
  ○ Beans
- Increase fluid intake to six to eight 8-ounce glasses of water/day. Avoid coffee, tea, and grapefruit juices because they can have a diuretic effect.
- Establish a toileting routine after breakfast, when contractions within the intestines are strongest.
- Increase exercise to improve gastrointestinal motility.

PATIENT TEACHING
- Prevention of constipation is the goal.
  ○ Recommend that patients consistently carry a water bottle to sip on throughout the day.
  ○ Develop a routine for toileting, the same time each day.
  ○ Establish an exercise routine of at least 30 minutes/day.
  ○ Incorporate at least 10 grams of dietary fiber/day into meal plan.
  ○ Initiate bowel regimen per doctor/nurse concurrently with chronic opioid use for pain management.
  ○ Initiate prophylactic bowel regimen per doctor/nurse in chemotherapy regimens containing vincristine or vinblastine.

FOLLOW UP
- Contact the nurse or physician for persistent constipation or if pain ensues.

RESOURCES
- National Cancer Institute. Common terminology criteria for adverse events: http://ctep.cancer.gov.

BIBLIOGRAPHY
Gerber, L., Hicks, J., & Shah, J. (2001). Rehabilitation of the cancer patient. In V.T. DeVita, S. Hellman, & S.A. Rosenberg (Eds.), *Cancer principles and practice in oncology* (p. 3099). Philadelphia: Lippincott Williams & Wilkins.

Gross, J. (1994). Functional alterations: Bowel. In J. Gross & B. L. Johnson (Eds.). *Handbook of oncology nursing* (pp. 517-528). Sudbury, MA: Jones & Bartlett.

Lagman, R. L. (2006). Constipation—not a mundane symptom. *The Journal of Supportive Oncology, 4,* 223-224.

Sykes, N. P. (2006). The pathogenesis of constipation. *The Journal of Supportive Oncology, 4,* 213-218.

Thomas, J. (2006). Strategies to manage constipation. *The Journal of Supportive Oncology, 4,* 220-223.

Tuchmann, L. (1997). Constipation. In R.A. Gates & R.M. Fink, (Eds.). *Oncology nursing secrets: questions and answers about caring for patients with cancer* (pp. 216-225). Philadelphia: Hanley & Belfus.

Cough

Ruth Canty Gholz

DEFINITION

- A pulmonary protective reflex
- An explosive expiration for clearing the tracheobronchial tree
- Categorized as acute or chronic
- May become excessive and nonproductive, possibly harming the airway mucosa
- Present in 38% of advanced cancer patients, in 60% of those with lung cancer, and in 80% having cough before death

PATHOPHYSIOLOGY AND CONTRIBUTING FACTORS

- Common causes include asthma, gastroesophageal reflux disease, and upper airway cough syndrome (formerly called postnasal drip syndrome).
- Results from aspiration, inhalation of matter, pathogens, inflammation, and inflammatory mediators
- May be voluntary or involuntary

Symptom Management

- Starts with inspiratory gasp to the closing of the glottis, a Valsalva maneuver, ending with an expiratory release
- Vagal afferent nerves initiate the cough reflex. They are plentiful in the airway mucosa and airway wall.
- "Cough center" in the medulla generates an efferent signal.
- During cough, intrathoracic pressures rise and expiratory pressures may near 500 miles per hour.
- Excessive cough interferes with breathing and sleep and may cause headache, pain, nausea, vomiting, syncope, and urinary incontinence.

SIGNS AND SYMPTOMS

- Patients present with cough interfering with quality of life.
- Cough is persistent.
- Frequent throat clearing
- May be accompanied by wheezing or dyspnea
- Becomes worse with exposure to fragrance, cold dry air, or pollutants
- May be productive or nonproductive of sputum
- May have air flow obstruction

ASSESSMENT TOOLS

- Patient history
- Medication review
- Character and timing of cough
- Precipitating factors
- Smoking history or exposure to environmental or occupational irritants
- Physical assessment
  - Oropharynx examination: assess for mucus or erythema
  - Pulmonary examination: assess respiratory muscles, lung sounds
  - Cardiovascular examination: jugular venous distention, wet lung sounds

LABORATORY AND DIAGNOSTIC TESTS

- Sputum cytology, sputum culture, arterial blood gases
- Chest x-ray film

- Computed tomography (CT) of chest, bronchoscopy, pulmonary function tests, if indicated

DIFFERENTIAL DIAGNOSIS

- Asthma/chronic obstructive pulmonary disease (COPD))/pulmonary fibrosis/interstitial lung disease
- Infection/aspiration/superior vena cava syndrome
- Obstruction/pericardial or pleural effusion/endobronchial tumor
- Lymphangitis/paraneoplastic syndrome
- Gastroesophageal syndromes
- Esophagorespiratory fistulas

INTERVENTIONS

- Must treat the underlying disease process as well as the cough

Pharmacologic Interventions

- Centrally acting antitussives: codeine, hydrocodone, dextromethorphan
- Peripherally acting antitussives: benzonatate levodropropizine, moguisteine
- Antihistamine/decongestant combination
- Guaifenesin
- Over-the-counter lozenges
- Nasal spray, ipratropium bromide
- Inhaled bronchodilators or inhaled corticosteroids
- Antibiotic if infection present
- Palliative chemotherapy/radiation
- If no improvement: inhaled cromolyn sodium or lidocaine, nebulized morphine, paroxetine, benzodiazepines

Nonpharmacologic Interventions

- Warm humidified air
- Deep breathing exercises
- Sleeping or resting laying on side
- Splinting with pillow to reduce strain

PATIENT TEACHING

- Take medications as prescribed.
- Reduce exposure to irritants.
- Stop smoking, smoke-free environment

- Coughing and deep breathing exercises including splinting with cough
- Sleep in semiupright position
- Add warm humidified air to room.
- Keep journal to document the course of the cough.

FOLLOW-UP

- Report change in sputum production, change in color, odor, or blood tinged.
- Report fevers or chills.
- Report sudden onset of chest pain or shortness of breath.

RESOURCES

- AstraZeneca, United States: www.lungcancerinfo.net
- Lungcancer.org: www.lungcancer.org
- Oncology Nursing Society: www.ons.org

BIBLIOGRAPHY

Berry, P. (2002). Cough. In K. Kuebler, P. Berry, & D. Heidrich (Eds.). *End of life care: Clinical practice guidelines* (pp. 235-241). Philadelphia: W. B. Saunders.

Bolser, D. (2006). Cough suppressant and pharmacologic protrusive therapy. *Chest, 1*, 238S-249S.

Braunwald, E., Fauci, A., Kasper, D., et al. (Eds.) (2001). *Harrison's principles of internal medicine* (15th ed., pp. 203-205). New York: McGraw-Hill.

Canning, B. J. (2006.) Anatomy and neurophysiology of the cough reflex. *Chest, 1*, 33S-47S.

Estfan, B., & Legrand, S. (2004). Management of cough in advanced cancer. *Journal of Supportive Oncology, 6*, 523-527.

Irwin, R. (2006). Complications of cough. *Chest, 1*, 54S-58S.

Kvale, P. (2006). Chronic cough due to lung tumors. *Chest, 1*, 147S-153S.

McCool, F., & Rosen, M. (2006). Nonpharmacologic airway clearance therapies. *Chest, 1*, 250S-259S.

McDermott, M. (2000). Cough. In D. Camp-Sorrell & R. A. Hawkins (Eds.). *Clinical manual for the oncology advanced practice nurse* (pp. 127-130). Pittsburgh: Oncology Nursing Press.

Pratter, M., Brightling, C., Boulet, L., et al. (2006). An empiric integrative approach to the management of cough: ACCP evidence-based clinical practice guidelines. *Chest, 1*, 222S-230S.

Silvestri, R., & Weinberger, S. (2006). *Evaluation of chronic cough in adults.*

Retrieved May 24, 2006, from www.uptodate.com

Weisberger, S., & Silvestri, R. (2006). *Treatment of chronic cough in adults.* Retrieved May 12, 2006, from www.uptodate.com.

Depressed Mood

Denice Economou

DEFINITION

- Major depressive disorder is diagnosed according to the Diagnostic and Statistical Manual of Mental Disorders (DSM-IV).
- Patients report a depressed mood or state they have experienced a loss of interest or pleasure in almost all of their activities for at least 2 weeks.
- Four of the following additional conditions must exist:
  - Decreased energy
  - Feelings of guilt or lack of worth
  - Difficulty concentrating or making decisions
  - Recurrent thoughts of death or suicidal thoughts or plans
  - Changes in appetite
  - Changes in sleep patterns
- Many of the physical symptoms that relate to appetite, concentration, and lack of energy can be the result of a cancer patient's treatment regimen. For this reason the diagnosis of depression in oncology patients is often missed or undertreated.

PATHOPHYSIOLOGY AND CONTRIBUTING FACTORS

- Both biological and psychosocial factors influence mood disturbances in patients.
- Genetic factors may make some patients more susceptible to the development of depression.
- Physiological stressors including medications, endocrine or nutritional disturbances, or infections can induce biochemical changes that precipitate depression.

- Developmental events or multiple losses may sensitize a patient, causing the patient to lose the ability to cope with the illness.
- These factors contribute to changes in neurotransmission, affecting mood, motivation, and psychomotor function. Norepinephrine and serotonin are neurotransmitters most often associated with depression. Medications used to manage depression are related to regulation of these transmitters.
- Medication classes associated with depressive side effects include analgesics, anticonvulsants, antihypertensives, anti-inflammatory agents, antimicrobials, antineoplastics, cytotoxics, hormones, immunosuppressive agents, sedatives, steroids, stimulants, tranquilizers, and benzodiazepines.
- Cancer diagnosis causes fear of pain, dependence, and altered body image, distress.
- Psychological factors contribute to the feelings of depression (i.e., coping ability, emotional maturity, disruption of life's plans).
- Social factors associated with depressed mood include financial stability, emotional support from family or friends, occupational successes or failures.
- Mood state of depression includes feelings of gloom, despair, numbness, emptiness, lack of worth.

SIGNS AND SYMPTOMS

- Mood seems depressed for at least 2 weeks.
- Unable to find pleasure in activities that used to be enjoyable
- Feelings of worthlessness
- Difficulty concentrating
- Difficulty sleeping or sleeping too much
- Fatigue
- Verbalizes thoughts of dying or committing suicide

ASSESSMENT TOOLS

- One of the most accurate screening measurements is a single question: "Are you depressed most of the day nearly every day?" A positive response necessitates further evaluation. A study found in 197 advanced cancer patients that this question showed 100% sensitivity and 100% specificity for depression.
- The Beck's Depression Inventory (BDI) is a 21-item questionnaire that takes about 2-5 minutes to complete and has an average specificity of 90%.
- Hospital Anxiety and Depression Scale
- Distress Thermometer Scale
- Assessment should include the following:
  - Report of depression
  - Signs and symptoms (4 or more from list in Definition)
  - History of depression or substance abuse (drugs or alcohol)
  - Medications associated with depression
  - Patients with head and neck, gastrointestinal, or lung cancer are at higher risk for suicide.
  - Unrelieved pain
- Social worker assessment can be beneficial to assist with evaluation and management of appropriate problems.
- Predictors for patients at risk are patients with a history of poor coping or psychological adjustment skills. Patients with a history of clinically significant anxiety or depression or major psychiatric syndromes should be monitored closely throughout treatment.
- Social support: Patients who are able to maintain close connections with family and friends cope more effectively with their illness and outlook for the future.
- Cultural considerations: What is the language used to describe feelings of depression? Latino and Mediterranean cultures may complain of nerves or headaches. Asian or Chinese cultures may use

Symptom Management

words related to weakness, tiredness, or imbalance. Middle Eastern cultures may refer to problems of the heart or feeling heartbroken.

LABORATORY AND DIAGNOSTIC TESTS

- There are no laboratory or diagnostic tests to screen for depressed mood. Refer to assessment tools above.

DIFFERENTIAL DIAGNOSES

- Fatigue
- Hypothyroidism
- Bipolar disorder

INTERVENTIONS
Pharmacologic Interventions

- Antidepressant medications:
  - Especially when used in conjunction with behavioral interventions and follow-up
  - Tricyclic antidepressants (TCAs), selective serotonin reuptake inhibitors (SSRIs), atypical antidepressants, psychostimulants, and an older class of medications, monoamine oxidase inhibitors (MAOIs).
  - When prescribing, consider the short- and long-term side effects, possible interactions with other medications and other illnesses, and prior response to antidepressants.
  - Monitor patients who are on psychotropic medications for dosing accuracy, especially when therapies change or invasive procedures such as surgery, chemotherapy, or disease progression occur.

Nonpharmacologic Interventions

- If a patient verbalizes thoughts or plans for committing suicide, immediate evaluation is necessary. If a patient verbalizes thoughts of jumping out a window, shooting himself or herself, or self-harm in other ways, the nurse must assess whether the patient has access to

complete these threats and must remove the patient from harm.
- Statements such as "I should just kill myself" or "I have no reason to go on living" require further evaluation.

PATIENT TEACHING

- Patients with depressed mood are at higher risk for noncompliance with their treatments. Monitor and encourage adherence.
- Reinforce hope and educate the family and caregivers on patient's needs as appropriate.
- Common side effects of antidepressants can include sedation, anticholinergic effects, orthostatic hypotension, and weight gain.
- If suicidal thoughts have been identified, caregivers must be aware of these feelings and preventive actions should be taken in the home to remove items that may be used to complete these threats (e.g., guns, knives, ropes are removed from the home).
- Discuss plans with the patient so that suicide is not thought of as an automatic solution to problems. Interventions should be provided to relieve extreme symptoms and improve quality of life.
- Feelings of hopelessness and worthlessness need to be discussed and the patient's ability to mobilize personal support systems needs to be established.
- Caregiver support is essential.

FOLLOW-UP

- If a patient screens positively for depression, notify the physician for a referral to a psychiatric professional for further assessment.
- If a patient reports a desire to commit suicide, discuss with patient the plan and notify the physician immediately. Take necessary steps to protect the patient from self-harm and arrange for immediate psychiatric follow-up.

- Ask specific questions regarding mood. Be aware of statements made that refer to feelings of hopelessness, burden to their family, financial concerns, or unrelieved symptoms.
- Assess distress levels related to fatigue, pain, mood, or family and financial concerns.
- Continue to provide hope and support.

BIBLIOGRAPHY

American Cancer Society/National Comprehensive Cancer Network. (2005). Distress—treatment guidelines for patients. *Version II/July 2005*, 9404-9401.

Albright, A. V., & Valente, S. (2006). Depression and Suicide. In R. M. Carroll-Johnson, L. M. Gorman, & N. J. Bush (Eds.), *Psychosocial nursing care along the cancer continuum* (pp. 241-274). Pittsburgh: Oncology Nursing Press.

Badger, T. A., Braden, C. J., & Mishel, M. H. (2001). Depression burden, self-help interventions, and side effect experience in women receiving treatment for breast cancer. *Oncology Nursing Forum, 28*, 567-574.

Barsevick, A. M., & Kehs Much, J. (2004). Depression. In H. C. Yarbro, H. M. Frogge, & M. Goodman (Eds.). *Cancer symptom management* (3rd ed., pp. 668-692). Boston: Jones & Bartlett.

Chochinov, J. H. (1997). Are you depressed? Screening for depression in the terminally ill. *American Journal of Psychiatry, 154*, 674-676.

Massie, M. J., & Popkin, M. K. (1998). Depressive disorders. In J. Holland (Ed.). *Psycho-oncology* (pp. 518-540). New York: Oxford University Press.

Pasacreta, J. V., Minarik, P. A., & Nield-Anderson, L. (2006). Anxiety and depression. In B. R. Ferrell & N. Coyle (Eds.), *Textbook of palliative nursing* (pp. 375-399). New York: Oxford University Press.

Diarrhea

Carolyn Grande

DEFINITION

- The increase in frequency, volume, and consistency of stool
- The passage of ≥200 grams of stool/day

- Can be acute or chronic and is experienced by 10% of advanced cancer patients and 43% of bone marrow transplant patients
- Diarrhea classifications:
  - *Osmotic diarrhea* is related to mechanical disturbances resulting from ingestion of hyperosmolar substances such as sorbitol or enteral feeding solutions (J-tubes, G-tubes). The diarrhea is watery and voluminous, resolving when the causative agent is withdrawn.
  - *Secretory diarrhea* is related to biochemical disturbances causing a mechanical response. The origins of these disturbances are enterotoxin-producing pathogens such as *Clostridium difficile* and *Escherichia coli* or endocrine tumors. The diarrhea is watery and voluminous.
  - *Exudative diarrhea* is often the toxicity of radiation therapy to the bowel mucosa. This diarrhea is characterized by high frequency of more than six stools per day with variable volume, although less than 1,000 mL/day. Stools are characterized by mucus and blood.
  - *Malabsorptive diarrhea* is related to both mechanical and biochemical disturbances. These disturbances can result from enzyme deficiencies. Stools are voluminous, foul smelling, and steatorrhea type.
  - *Dysmotility-associated diarrhea* is related to a mechanical disturbance or peristaltic dysfunction that results in rapid transit time of stool through the small and large intestine. Stools are small, semisolid/liquid consistency with variable volume and frequency.
  - *Chemotherapy-induced diarrhea* results from mechanical and biochemical disturbances resulting from effects of chemotherapy on the bowel mucosa. Stools are watery or semisolid.

PATHOPHYSIOLOGY AND CONTRIBUTING FACTORS

- Gastrointestinal motility involves processes that promote the absorption of nutrients. Movement through the gastrointestinal tract requires coordination of intraluminal pressures and smooth muscle contractions controlled by the enteric nervous system and peptide hormonal release. Diarrhea is due to an imbalance in the physiologic mechanisms of the gastrointestinal tract. It is the result of impaired absorption and excessive secretion.
- Decreased absorption of fluid and electrolyte can result from:
  - Presence of osmotically active substances in the lumen
  - Increased intestinal motility
- Increased secretion of fluid and electrolytes can result from:
  - Endogenous secretions
  - Exogenous toxins
- In radiation that involves the abdomen or pelvis and in chemotherapy-induced diarrhea, acute damage to the epithelial crypt cells results in necrosis, inflammation, and ulceration of the intestinal mucosa. Atrophy and fibrosis of the lining can occur over time, resulting in decreased absorption of water and electrolytes, producing diarrhea.
- Risk factors for diarrhea:
  - Chemotherapy
    - Diarrhea from previous chemotherapy cycles
    - Types of chemotherapeutic agents include fluropyrimidines, topoisomerase I inhibitors (irinotecan, topotecan), antitumor antibiotic (actinomycin D), toxoid (paclitaxel)
  - Other factors, such as the presence of primary tumor
  - Radiation therapy (RT)
    - Diarrhea is dependent on
      - □ Total RT dose
      - □ Size of the RT field
      - □ Site being irradiated
      - □ Dose per fraction

SIGNS AND SYMPTOMS

- Increased number of stools/day
- Nocturnal stool
- Incontinence
- Cramping
- Patient may have other symptoms:
  - Nausea/vomiting
  - Hypotension
  - Dizziness
  - Decreased skin turgor
  - Dry mouth
  - Perianal irritation

ASSESSMENT TOOLS

- Comprehensive history:
  - Cancer diagnosis and past/current treatment
  - Sites of metastasis
  - Complete medication list:
    - Laxatives
    - Opioids or recent opioid withdrawal
    - Recent antibiotic therapy
    - Regular/as-needed prescription medications
    - Over-the-counter medications
    - Herbal and vitamin supplements
    - Chemotherapy/biotherapy agents
- Hallmark assessment tool is patient report. Refer to patient assessment sheet in Section Seven
  - Description of baseline bowel movements and current bowel movement history:
    - When
    - Amount
    - Consistency and color of stool
    - Incontinence
    - Presence of blood
    - Distinct odor change
- Assess for signs and symptoms of dehydration:
  - Orthostatic hypotension
  - Dry mouth
  - Excessive thirst
  - Dizziness
  - Feelings of weakness
  - Decreased urination
  - Weight loss

Symptom Management

- Comprehensive physical examination
  - Abdomen
    - Palpate for tenderness, distention
    - Percuss—dullness may indicate obstruction, fecal impaction
    - Auscultate for bowel sounds
- The U.S. Department of Health and Human Services, the National Institutes of Health, and the National Cancer Institute have outlined a grading system for adverse events to assist in categorizing the severity of the event. The grading system spans from 1 through 5 on the basis of patient assessment. Grading for diarrhea is as follows:
  - Grade 1: increase of fewer than four stools per day over baseline; mild increase in ostomy output compared with baseline
  - Grade 2: increase of four to six stools per day over baseline; intravenous (IV) fluids indicated for less than 24 hours; moderate increase in ostomy output compared with baseline; not interfering with activities of daily living (ADLs)
  - Grade 3: increase of seven or more stools per day over baseline; incontinence; IV fluids for equal to or greater than 24 hours or longer; hospitalization; severe increase in ostomy output compared with baseline; interfering with ADLs
  - Grade 4: life-threatening consequences (e.g., hemodynamic collapse)
  - Grade 5: death
- Diarrhea includes diarrhea of the small bowel or colonic origin or ostomy diarrhea.
- Refer to chemotherapy-induced diarrhea in Section Seven.

LABORATORY AND DIAGNOSTIC TESTS

- Complete blood cell count
- Check stool for occult blood.
- Metabolic panel to assess electrolyte levels, blood urea nitrogen (BUN)/creatinine, albumin
- Stool cultures for enteric pathogens, *clostridium difficile* (*C. difficile*), and ova and parasites
- Flat plate of the abdomen or obstruction series (as indicated by history and physical examination)

DIFFERENTIAL DIAGNOSES

- Carcinoid syndrome
- Chemotherapy-induced diarrhea
- Radiation therapy–induced diarrhea
- *C. difficile* infection
- Enzyme deficiency
- Crohn's disease
- Acute viral, bacterial, or protozoal infections
- Intestinal obstruction
  - Tumor
  - Stool
  - Scar tissue
- Irritable bowel disease
- Ischemic bowel disease
- Lactose intolerance
- Pseudomembranous enterocolitis
- Rotavirus gastroenteritis
- Thyrotoxicosis
- Ulcerative colitis
- Laxative overuse
- Opioid withdrawal

INTERVENTIONS
Pharmacologic Interventions

Antidiarrheal agents are divided into categories on the basis of mechanism of action:
- Opioids
  - Lomotil: 2.5 mg diphenoxylate with 0.025 mg atropine sulfate/tablet. May load with two tablets then one to two tablets four times a day, not to exceed eight tablets/day
  - Codeine: 15-60 mg orally every 4 to 6 hours as needed
  - Opium tincture: 10% opium liquid (10 mg morphine/mL with 19% alcohol). 0.3-1 mL orally every 2-6 hours until controlled. Not to exceed 6 mL/24 hours.
  - Paregoric: 0.4 mg morphine/mL orally one to four times/day or 4 mL every 4 hours
- Nonopioids
  - Imodium (loperamide): 2-mg capsules or liquid 1 mg/mL or 1 mg/5 mL; may load 4 mg orally then 2 mg after each loose stool. Not to exceed 16 mg/day
- Absorbents
  - Bismuth subsalicylate (Pepto-Bismol): chewable tablets 262 mg or suspensions 262 mg/15 mL or 524 mg/15 mL. Dosing 524 mg every 30 minutes, not to exceed 5 grams/day
  - Kaopectate (5.85 gm kaolin and 130 mg pectin/30 mL): 2-6 grams every 4 hours as needed
- Somatostatin analog
  - Octreotide acetate: 50-200 mcg subcutaneously three times/day

Nonpharmacologic Interventions

- Diet modifications, including:
  - Foods that build stool consistency, low in fiber, pectin containing
  - Eat foods high in potassium.
  - Eat foods at room temperature to minimize peristalsis.
  - Maintain a lactose-free diet if indicated.
  - Increase fluid intake to at least 3 L/day.

PATIENT TEACHING

- Encourage foods that are low in fiber and that contain pectin:
  - Beets
  - Applesauce (without spice)
  - Peeled apple
  - White rice
  - Banana*
  - Baked potato without skin
  - White bread
  - Plain pasta
  - Avocados*
  - Asparagus tips*
- Encourage foods high in potassium:
  - Peach and apricot nectar

---

*Also high in potassium.

- Boiled or mashed potatoes without skin
- Lactose-free milk
- Fish
- Bananas
- Avoid high-fiber, high-fat, greasy, or spicy foods or caffeine-containing foods:
  - Whole grain breads or cereals
  - Raw vegetables
  - Nuts
  - Seeds
  - Popcorn
  - Relishes or pickles
  - High-fat spreads or dressings
  - Chocolate
  - Coffee/tea
- Increase fluids to at least 3 L/day
  - Bouillon
  - Fruitades
  - Gatorade, Propel, or other sports drinks
  - Pedialyte or Pedialyte ice pops
  - Ice pops
  - Gelatin
- Avoid alcohol and carbonated beverages
- Maintain a lactose-free diet when indicated
  - Avoid milk and dairy products
  - May use lactose-free dairy products or soy milk products
- Maintain skin integrity
  - Cleanse rectal area after each bowel movement with soft wipes; pat rather than rub perianal area when cleansing
  - Apply topical skin barrier ointments such as Desitin and A&D ointment
  - Sitz baths as needed
- Take anti-diarrheal medication as prescribed

FOLLOW-UP

- Have patient or caregiver record number and consistency of stools.
- Call physician or nurse if diarrhea persists in frequency and volume >24 hours after following outlined plan of care.

RESOURCE

- National Cancer Institute. Common terminology criteria for adverse events: http://ctep.cancer.gov

BIBLIOGRAPHY

Anthony, L. (2003). New strategies for the prevention and reduction of cancer treatment-induced diarrhea. *Seminars in Oncology Nursing, 19,* 17-21.

Benson, A. B., III, Ajani, J. A., & Catalano, R. B., et al. (2004). Recommended guidelines for the treatment of cancer treatment-induced diarrhea. *Journal of Clinical Oncology, 22,* 2918-2926.

Friedman, L. S., & Isselbacher, K. J. (1994). Diarrhea and constipation. In K. J. Isselbacher, E. Braunwald, & J. D. Wilson, et al. (Eds.). *Harrison's principles of internal medicine* (13th ed., pp. 213-219). New York: McGraw-Hill.

Gwede, C. K. (2003). Overview of radiation- and chemoradiation-induced diarrhea. *Seminars in Oncology Nursing, 19*(4 suppl 3), 6-10.

Hogan, C. M. (1998). The nurse's role in diarrhea management. *Oncology Nursing Forum, 25,* 879-886.

Rutledge, D. N., & Engelking, C. (1998). Cancer-related diarrhea: selected findings of a national survey of oncology nurse experiences. *Oncology Nursing Forum, 25,* 861-873.

Viale, P. H., Fung, A., & Zitella, L. (2005). Advanced colorectal cancer: current treatment and nursing management with economic considerations. *Clinical Journal of Oncology Nursing, 9,* 541-552.

Viele, C. (2003). Overview of chemotherapy-induced diarrhea. *Seminars in Oncology Nursing, 19,* 2-5.

Dizziness and Vertigo

Ruth Canty Gholz

DEFINITION

- Described in terms of sensations
- Lightheadedness, fainting, spinning, confusion, blurred vision, tingling
- Nonspecific
- Clustered with vertigo, dizziness, disequilibrium, and presyncope (prodromal symptom for fainting or near fainting)
- Unsteadiness
- Must fit patient into category of dizziness, vertigo, or presyncope

PATHOPHYSIOLOGY AND CONTRIBUTING FACTORS

- Vertigo (a symptom of dizziness) is caused from a disturbance in the vestibular system: sensory, visual, or somatosensory. The vestibular system includes apparatus in inner ear, vestibular nerve and nucleus in the medulla, and connections from the cerebellum.
- May be specific or nonspecific
- Never continuous
- Made worse by movement of the head and or cervical spine
- Disruption between vestibular apparatus and the brain
- Pyschologic disorder

SIGNS AND SYMPTOMS

- Lightheadedness
- Feeling of spinning (similar to coming off a roller coaster or when spun multiple times)
- Imbalance, tipping to one side
- Nausea and vomiting with the spinning
- Visual changes
- Auditory changes
- May be episodic or regular, in short or long duration
- Out of body feeling
- May have additional paresthesias of face or limbs

ASSESSMENT TOOLS

- Patient history
- Identify what dizziness means to patient, full sensations, duration, aggravating and alleviating factors
- Neurological examination
- Orthostatic assessment
- Ear examination
- Medication review
- Assessment for nystagmus, hearing loss, ataxic gait, nausea, vomiting, visual changes, numbness, incoordination
- Social history
- Psychological assessment

LABORATORY AND DIAGNOSTIC TESTS

- Complete blood count (CBC), blood glucose level, and thyroid-stimulating hormone level (TSH)
- Range of motion with emphasis on cervical spine
- Cervical spine x-ray film
- Vestibular function tests
- Stimulate to hyperventilate

Symptom Management

DIFFERENTIAL DIAGNOSES

- Meniere's disease
- Diseases of the central nervous system (CNS)
- Cerebrovascular disease
- Orthostasis
- Neurological deficit
- Dehydration
- Hyperventilation
- Parkinson's disease
- Medication side effect
- Labyrinthitis
- Malignancy
- Cervical spine disorders

INTERVENTIONS
Pharmacologic Interventions

- Antihistamines: meclizine
- Anticholinergics: scopolamine
- Benzodiazepines
- Antiemetics as needed

Nonpharmacologic Interventions

- Hydration
- Repositioning
- Vestibular rehabilitation
- Bed rest if needed
- Treat the cause
- Physical and occupational therapy
- Sodium-restricted diet

PATIENT TEACHING

- Avoid sudden changes in position.
- Chief concern is safety.
- Sit or lie down if feeling dizzy.
- Increase fluids; drink 3 liters per day.
- Ensure good lighting.
- Use cane as needed for support.
- Do not drive or use machinery if dizzy.
- Do not use alcohol, tobacco, or caffeine.
- Use energy conservation techniques.

FOLLOW-UP

- Seek immediate medical assistance if change in level of consciousness, respiratory difficulty, or sudden loss of vision or hearing.
- Patient to alert health care provider if sudden, severe ear pain or for a temperature greater than 100.5° F.
- Report ear infections, sinus congestion, or respiratory complaints.
- Ensure that the patient's environment remains safe.

RESOURCES

- Mayo Clinic (Mayo Foundation for Medical Education and Research): www.mayoclinic.com
- WebMD: www.webmd.com
- Chemo Care (Cleveland Clinic): www.chemocare.com
- People Living With Cancer (American Society of Clinical Oncology): www.plwc.org

BIBLIOGRAPHY

Branch, W., & Barton, J. (2006). *Approach to the patient with dizziness*. Retrieved May, 26, 2006, from www.uptodate.com.

Braunwald, E., Fauci, A., Kasper, D., et al. (Eds.). (2001). *Harrison's principles of internal medicine* (15th ed., pp. 111-118). New York: McGraw-Hill.

Maher, K. (2006). Dizziness/vertigo. In D. Camp-Sorrell & R. A. Hawkins (Eds.). *Clinical manual for the oncology advanced practice nurse* (2nd ed., pp. 884-895). Pittsburgh: Oncology Nursing Society.

Dysphagia

Laura M. Benson and Kristin A. Cawley

DEFINITION

- Difficulty swallowing
- Occurs in 96% of patients treated for head and neck cancers
- Common symptom in head and neck cancer
- Described by patients as food getting "stuck" and choking
- Classifications:
  - *Oropharyngeal dysphagia*—difficulty initiating the swallowing process and propelling food through esophagus
  - *Esophageal dysphagia*—ability to swallow food, yet having sensation in which food is not able to pass from esophagus into the stomach (often associated with pain)
- Chemotherapy and radiation often reduce symptoms of dysphagia, thus prolonging life.
- May compromise quality of life and cause life-threatening complications

PATHOPHYSIOLOGY AND CONTRIBUTING FACTORS

- Narrowing (stricture) of the lower part of the esophagus
- Inflammatory changes in the esophagus
- Results from any condition that weakens or damages the muscles and nerves involved in swallowing:
  - Obstructive lesions
  - Tumors
  - Inflammatory masses
  - Trauma/surgical resection
  - Zenker's diverticulum
  - Esophageal webs
  - Extrinsic structural lesions
  - Anterior mediastinal masses
  - Esophageal spasms
  - Mucositis
  - Xerostomia
  - Postirradiation sequelae
  - Laryngeal penetration
  - Age-related factors

SIGNS AND SYMPTOMS

- Difficulty swallowing
- Pain with swallowing
- Weight loss
- Dehydration
- Taste alterations
- Atrophy of neck muscles
- Aspiration
- Infection

ASSESSMENT TOOLS

- History and physical examination
- Character and quality of pain
- Precipitating factors

LABORATORY AND DIAGNOSTIC TESTS

- Complete blood cell count (CBC)
- Comprehensive metabolic panel (creatinine)
- Albumin, prealbumin, transferrin, and retinol-binding protein
- Barium study (esophagram)/ barium swallow

- Fiberoptic endoscopic examination of swallowing (FEES)
- Nasopharyngoscopy
- Endoscopy
- Manometry—measures pressure within the esophagus
- Chest x-ray film

DIFFERENTIAL DIAGNOSES

- Xerostomia
- Anorexia
- Malnutrition
- Dehydration
- Pain
- Cough
- Mucositis
- Gastroesophageal reflux
- Tissue fibrosis
- Aspiration pneumonia
- Anxiety
- Infection
- Depression
- Isolation
  - May avoid social gatherings where food is involved

INTERVENTIONS

- Treat underlying etiologies

Pharmacologic Interventions

- Histamine-2 receptor antagonists (blockers)
- Proton pump inhibitors
- Prokinetic agents
- Antacids
- Hydration
- Pain management

Nonpharmacologic Interventions

- Laborious exercises:
  - Chin tuck for improved airway closure
  - Head rotation to modify pharyngeal pressure
- Parenteral nutrition
- Esophageal dilation
- Pharyngeal electrical stimulation

PATIENT TEACHING

- Eat sitting upright at a 90-degree angle.
- Avoid lying down after meals.
- Keep head of bed elevated while sleeping.
- Avoid solid, abrasive foods. Incorporate pureed, liquid diet.
- Medication compliance

FOLLOW-UP

- Nutritional counseling
- Speech pathologist consultation
- Surgery consultation
- Call health care provider if experiencing the following:
  - Difficulty or pain when you swallow
  - Pain not relieved with pain medication
  - Continuing weight loss

RESOURCES

- Dysphagia Resource Center: www.dysphagia.com
- Oncology Nursing Society: www.ons.org

BIBLIOGRAPHY

Dysphagia: hard to swallow. (2004). *The Mayo Clinic Health Letter, 22,* 1-3.

Levy, L. (2005). An alternative approach to treating dysphagia. *Radiation Therapist: The Journal of Radiation Oncology Sciences, 14,* 55-58.

Mercadante, S., Casuccio, A., & Fulfaro, F. (2000). The course of symptom frequency and intensity in advanced cancer patients followed at home. *Journal of Pain & Symptom Management, 20,* 104-112.

Rosenthal, D. I., Lewin, J. S., & Eisbruch, A. (2006). Prevention and treatment of dysphagia and aspiration after chemoradiation for head and neck cancer. *Journal of Clinical Oncology, 24,* 2636-2643.

Skeat, J. (2005). Outcome measurement in dysphagia: Not so hard to swallow. *Dysphagia, 20,* 113-122.

Dyspnea

Ruth Canty Gholz

DEFINITION

- An uncomfortable sensation or awareness of breathing
- A subjective experience of breathing discomfort that consists of qualitative distinct sensations that vary in intensity. Derived from interactions among multiple physiological, psychological, social, and environmental factors and may induce secondary physiological and behavioral responses
- Shortness of breath

- Subjective sensation of breathlessness
- Inability to get air
- Feeling of suffocation
- Severity may be related to the perception of dyspnea.
- Heavy or hard breathing
- Described as air hunger
- Occurs in up to 75% of persons with advanced cancer
- Most common symptom in lung cancer

PATHOPHYSIOLOGY

- Not completely understood
- Multifactorial
- Respiratory center controls breathing, yet dyspnea results from cortical stimulation.
- Cortex overrides the respiratory center, stimulating chemoreceptors in the lung and respiratory muscles and mechanoreceptors.
- Respiratory effort increases.
- Increased use of respiratory muscles
- Amplification of ventilatory requirements
- May be divided into respiratory system dyspnea or cardiovascular dyspnea
- Acute or chronic, occurs with exertion or at rest
- Contributing factors:
  - Hypoxia
  - Hypercapnia
  - Interstitial lung disease
  - Pleural or cardiac effusion
  - Malignancy: direct tumor effects, indirect tumor effects, or treatment-related causes
  - Chronic obstructive pulmonary disease (COPD)
  - Neuromuscular weakness
  - Bronchoconstriction or spasm
  - Air flow obstruction
  - Myocardial dysfunction
  - Anemia
  - Pain
  - Deconditioning
  - Thyroid disorders
  - Cardiovascular disease
  - Aspiration
  - Pneumonia
  - Anxiety
  - Radiation pneumonitis

Symptom Management

SIGNS AND SYMPTOMS

- Air hunger
- Feeling of suffocation
- Cyanosis, pallor
- Anxiety
- Tachypnea
- Tachycardia
- Use of accessory muscles when breathing

ASSESSMENT TOOLS

- Visual analog scale for dyspnea
- Borg 10-point scale with descriptors
- Subjective descriptors/self-report
- Functional assessment tools: shuttle walking test, reading aloud of numbers
- Medical, social, smoking, exposure history
- Physical examination with review of systems
- Respiratory rate and quality, use of accessory muscles
- Cardiopulmonary examination
- Onset, aggravating or alleviating factors

LABORATORY AND DIAGNOSTIC TESTS

- Pulse oximetry
- Complete blood count and chemistries
- Pulmonary function tests
- Maximal inspiratory pressure (MIP)
- Arterial blood gas measurement
- Computed tomographic (CT) scans
- Chest x-ray films
- Echocardiograms

DIFFERENTIAL DIAGNOSES

- Lung cancer
- COPD
- Pulmonary embolism
- Myocardial infarction
- Congestive heart failure
- Cardiomyopathy
- Anxiety/panic attack
- Pain
- Asthma
- Obesity

INTERVENTIONS
Pharmacologic Interventions

- Treat underlying cause.
- Opioids
- Anxiolytics
- Glucocorticoids for spasm or inflammation
- Bronchodilators
- Diuretics
- No strong evidence to support nebulized opioids for dyspnea

Nonpharmacologic Interventions

- Oxygen for hypoxia
- Cool air blowing on the face
- Cognitive/behavioral interventions
- Breathing exercises

PATIENT TEACHING

- Take medications as directed.
- Keep a dyspnea diary.
- Report changes in sputum production.
- Receive extra oxygen; cool air from a fan may be as effective.
- Monitor temperature and report if greater than 100.5° F.
- Pursed lip breathing
- Relaxation techniques
- Diaphragmatic breathing
- Inspiratory muscle training
- Positioning for comfort; keep head tilted
- Exercise
- Nutrition
- Energy conservation and pacing
- Get rid of smoking and pet dander in the home.

RESOURCES

- Oncology Nursing Society: www.ons.org
- Chemo Care (Cleveland Clinic): www.chemocare.com
- Oncology Nursing Society: www.cancersymptoms.org
- People Living With Cancer (American Society of Clinical Oncology): www.plwc.org

BIBLIOGRAPHY

Inzeo, D., & Tyson, L. (2003). Nursing assessment and management of dyspnea in patients with lung cancer. *Clinical Journal of Oncology Nursing, 7*, 332-333.

Jantarakupt, P., & Porock, D. (2005). Dyspnea management in lung cancer: Applying the evidence for chronic obstructive pulmonary disease. *Oncology Nursing Forum, 32*, 785-795.

Joyce, M., & Beck, S. (2006) *Measuring oncology nursing-sensitive outcomes: evidence-based summary: dyspnea.* Retrieved May 12, 2006, from http://www.ons.org/outcomes/clinical/pdf/DyspneaEvidenceSummary.pdf.

Meek, P., Schwartzstein, R., Adams, R., et al. (1999). American Thoracic Society: dyspnea: mechanisms, assessment and management: consensus statement. *American Journal of Respiratory Critical Care Medicine, 159*, 321-341.

National Cancer Institute. (2006) *Dyspnea and coughing in patients with advanced cancer.* Retrieved May 12, 2006, from http://www.cancer.gov/cancertopics/pdq/supportivecare/cardiopulmonary/HealthProfessional.

Schwartzstein, R. (2006) *Approach to the patient with dyspnea.* Retrieved May 12, 2006, from.do?topicKey=copd/12483&type=A&selectedTitle=1~111.

Thomas, J., & Von Gunten, C. (2003). Management of dyspnea, *Journal of Supportive Oncology, 1*, 23-24.

Wickman, R. (2002). Dyspnea: recognizing and managing an invisible problem. *Oncology Nursing Forum, 29*, 925-923.

Esophagitis

Kristin A. Cawley
and Laura M. Benson

DEFINITION

- Inflammation of the lining of the esophagus, the tube that carries food from the throat to the stomach
- If left untreated, this condition can become very uncomfortable, causing problems with swallowing, ulcers, and scarring of the esophagus. In rare instances, a condition known as "Barrett's esophagus" may develop, which is a risk factor for cancer of the esophagus.

PATHOPHYSIOLOGY AND CONTRIBUTING FACTORS

- Breakdown of rapidly dividing epithelial cells caused by chemotherapy and radiation treatment, primarily in the gastrointestinal (GI) tract
- History of esophagitis or mucositis
- Poor oral hygiene, prior dental disease

- Treatment regimen
- History of alcohol consumption and smoking

SIGNS AND SYMPTOMS

- Difficult or painful swallowing
- Heartburn or acid reflux
- Mouth sores
- Bleeding
- Infection
- A feeling of something of being stuck in the throat
- Nausea
- Vomiting

ASSESSMENT TOOLS

- History, physical, and oral examinations
- Nutritional status
- Symptomatic functional assessment based on ability to swallow
- Pain, using 0-10 or categorical (none-mild-moderate-severe)

LABORATORY AND DIAGNOSTIC TESTS

- Complete blood cell count (CBC)
- Blood, urine, sputum culture
  - Upper endoscopy
  - Biopsy of esophageal tissue sample
  - Upper GI series (or barium swallow)

DIFFERENTIAL DIAGNOSES

- Gastroesophageal reflux disease (GERD)
- Esophageal stricture
- Dysphagia
- Pain

INTERVENTIONS

- *Treat the underlying condition.*
- Endoscopy to remove any lodged pill fragments
- Surgery to remove the damaged part of the esophagus

Pharmacologic Interventions

- Antacids
- Antibiotics, antifungals, or antivirals to treat an infection
- Pain medications that can be gargled or swallowed
- Corticosteroid medication to reduce inflammation

- Intravenous nutrition to allow the esophagus to heal and to reduce the likelihood of malnourishment or dehydration

Nonpharmacologic Interventions

- Nutritional
- Salt and soda rinses

PATIENT TEACHING

- Dental evaluation before treatment is initiated
- Dental cleaning
  - Brush with soft toothbrush.
  - Continue despite thrombocytopenia or neutropenia unless uncontrolled bleeding develops
  - Fluoride toothpaste
- Flossing
  - Patients who floss regularly should continue to do so unless there is uncontrolled bleeding, platelets <20,000, or absolute neutrophil count (ANC) <1.
- Rinsing
  - Normal saline solution (NS), sodium bicarbonate ($NaHCO_3$), $NS/NaHCO_3$, water
  - Nonalcoholic unsweetened mouthwash
  - Rinse every 4-6 hours, increasing to every 2 hours as needed for comfort (swish/gargle 15-30 seconds).
- Dental appliances
  - Should be left out as much as possible once mucous membranes become irritated
- Report any pain that is unrelieved with pain medication.
- Dietary modifications
- Report any fever of 100.5° F or greater.

FOLLOW-UP

- Assess for increased risk of esophagitis with continuing treatments.
- Assess for pain unrelieved with pain medication.
- Reinforce importance of communication to physician and nurse.

RESOURCES

- National Cancer Institute. Oral complications of chemotherapy and head/neck radiation (PDQ): http://www.cancer.gov/cancertopi cs/pdq/supportivecare/oralcompli cations/healthprofessional

BIBLIOGRAPHY

Carr, E. (2005). Head and neck malignancies. In C. H. Yarbro, M. H. Frogge, & M. Goodman (Eds.). *Cancer nursing: Principles and practice* (6th ed., pp. 1294-1324). Sudbury, MA: Jones & Bartlett.

Clarkson, J. E., Worthington, H. V., & Eden, O. B. (2005). Interventions for preventing oral mucositis for patients with cancer receiving treatment (review). *Cochrane Database System Review,* 2007, Oct 17(4): CD 000978.

McGuire, D. B. (2003). Barriers and strategies in implementation of oral care standards for cancer patients. *Supportive Care in Cancer, 11,* 435-441.

Mendenhal, W. M., Hinerman, R. W., Amdur, R.J., et al. (2004). Larynx. In C. A. Perez, L. W. Brady, E. C. Halperin, et al. (Eds.). *Principles and practice of radiation oncology* (4th ed., pp. 1094-1116). Philadelphia: Lippincott Williams & Wilkins.

Sonis, S. T., Elting, L. S., Keefe, D., et al. (2004). Perspectives on cancer therapy-induced mucosal injury: Pathogenesis, measurement, epidemiology, and consequences for patients. *Cancer, 100* (Suppl), 1995-2025.

Fatigue

Susan Newton

DEFINITION

- Cancer-related fatigue is a subjective feeling of weariness or tiredness that is different from any other fatigue that a person has experienced.
- A persistent subjective sense of tiredness related to cancer or cancer treatment that interferes with usual functioning
- Typically is not relieved by sleep or rest
- A serious detrimental effect on the cancer patient's quality of life
- Affects as many as 80%-100% of cancer patients

Symptom Management

- 78% of patients reported fatigue during cancer and its treatment.

PATHOPHYSIOLOGY AND CONTRIBUTING FACTORS

- Exact pathophysiological mechanism unknown
- Many contributing factors:
  - Underlying disease
  - Treatment-related toxicity:
    - Chemotherapy
    - Radiation therapy
    - Surgery
    - Biotherapy
  - Cytokines
  - Performance status
  - Anemia
  - Infection
  - Malnutrition
  - Metabolic disturbances
  - Sleep disorders
  - Depression

SIGNS AND SYMPTOMS

- Reported as the most distressing symptom associated with cancer and its treatment.
- Rated as more distressing than pain, nausea, and vomiting, which can frequently be treated with medications
- Patient reports whole-body tiredness; inability to perform basic tasks.
- Other reported physical symptoms:
  - Shortness of breath
  - Heart palpitations
  - Depressed mood
  - General lack of energy
- Often presents with other symptoms:
  - Pain
  - Insomnia
  - Depression or anxiety
- Five factors associated with fatigue:
  - Anemia
  - Pain
  - Emotional distress
  - Sleep disturbances
  - Hypothyroidism

ASSESSMENT TOOLS

- Key assessment finding is the patient's self-report.

- Fatigue is whatever the patient says it is.
- Clinicians, family members, or anyone else cannot judge fatigue level.
- Other assessment information:
  - Physical examination
  - Related laboratory data
  - Caregiver information
- Methods and tools measuring fatigue. These include:
  - FACT-G (general)
  - FACT-F (fatigue)
  - FACT-An (anemia)
  - Brief Fatigue Inventory (BFI)
  - Linear Analog Scale Assessment (LASA)
  - Visual Analog Scale (VAS)
  - Piper Fatigue Scale
  - Multidimensional Fatigue Symptom Inventory (MFSI)
  - MFI-20

LABORATORY AND DIAGNOSTIC TESTS

- Laboratory tests to assess for the *cause of fatigue:*
  - Complete blood cell count (CBC) to check for anemia
  - Iron testing, including transferrin, total iron-binding capacity, ferritin, and iron levels
  - Folic acid and vitamin B_{12}
  - Thyroid function, including thyroxine (T_4) total, tri-iodothyronine (T_3) uptake, thyroid-stimulating hormone (TSH)
- There are no diagnostic tests to screen for fatigue.

DIFFERENTIAL DIAGNOSES

- Anemia
- Depression
- Infection
- Sleep disturbances
- Malnutrition
- Hypothyroidism
- Dehydration
- Medications that cause fatigue

INTERVENTIONS
Pharmacologic Interventions

- Erythropoietin, if fatigue is related to anemia
  - Epoetin alfa (Procrit)
  - Darbepoetin alfa (Aranesp)

- Both drugs have demonstrated the ability to decrease transfusions and increase hemoglobin levels in cancer patients receiving them.
- There are also data to support that patients who receive erythropoietin have an increase in energy level, activity level, and overall quality of life.
- Antidepressants, if depression is suspected.
  - The prevalence and incidence of depression in patients with cancer varies widely, depending on the diagnostic criteria and the instruments used; however, a significant number of patients with cancer have depression.
  - Patients who are at greatest risk of depression are those with advanced disease, those who have uncontrolled physical symptoms, and those who have had previous psychiatric disorders.
  - The drug class most frequently used in the treatment of depression is the group of selective serotonin reuptake inhibitors (SSRIs), including:
    - Citalopram (Celexa)
    - Escitalopram (Lexapro)
    - Paroxetine (Paxil)
    - Fluoxetine (Prozac, Sarafem)
    - Sertraline (Zoloft)
  - Each of these drugs has varying side effects.
  - Oncology professionals should seek the expertise of mental health providers if they have questions regarding the prescribing of antidepressants or for referral to cognitive/psychological counseling.
- Psychostimulants are being tested in patients with advanced cancers and in patients with chronic diseases that cause fatigue. No randomized, placebo-controlled studies have been conducted to evaluate the effect of psychostimulants in patients with cancer; however, much of the research that has been conducted has been testing the effect of methylphenidate (Ritalin)

on fatigue levels in this patient population. A study evaluated patient-controlled methylphenidate for the management of fatigue in 31 patients with advanced cancer. Results showed an improvement in fatigue levels, a number of other symptoms, and overall quality of life. Further studies should be conducted to verify and confirm these results.

- Corticosteroids such as methylprednisolone (prednisone) have been shown to reduce the significance of fatigue in some patient populations, such as those with chronic fatigue syndrome. However, because of the side effects associated with long-term use of these drugs (alterations in bone metabolism, adrenal suppression), they are not good options for the cancer population.

Nonpharmacologic Interventions

- Exercise, such as walking on a regular basis
- Delegating tasks
- Energy conservation principles
- Frequent rest periods that do not interfere with nighttime sleep
- Stress reduction techniques

PATIENT TEACHING

- Instruct patient regarding factors that contribute to fatigue:
  ○ Cancer itself
  ○ Cancer treatments
  ○ Anemia
  ○ Nutritional problems
  ○ Sleep problems
- Teach patient to recognize the signs of fatigue:
  ○ Feeling weary or exhausted. It may be physical, emotional, or mental exhaustion.
  ○ Body may feel heavy, especially arms and legs.
  ○ Less desire to do normal activities such as eating or shopping
  ○ Difficulty concentrating or thinking clearly
- Instruct patient regarding ways to manage fatigue:
  ○ Take time to rest, but be aware that too much rest can decrease energy levels

○ Stay as active as possible, take part in activities that the patient enjoys, at least three times a week
○ Eat nutritious foods and drink plenty of liquids.
○ Conserve energy when possible
○ Watch for signs of stress

FOLLOW-UP

Fatigue is the number one side effect experienced by patients with cancer. Because of this, patients will need education before beginning therapy for their cancer and continuing evaluation and support to help them through the effects of this symptom.

RESOURCES

- Oncology Nursing Society: www.ons.org
- CancerCare, Inc.: www.cancercare.org
- Abramson Cancer Center of the University of Pennsylvania: www.oncolink.com
- Oncology Nursing Society: www.cancersymptoms.org
- Johnson & Johnson Consumer Products Company: www.strengthforcaring.com
- Cancer Symptoms: http://www.cancersymptoms.org/fatigue/managing.shtml
- http://www.cancersymptoms.org/fatigue/suggested.shtml
- http://www.cancersymptoms.org/fatigue/caregivers.shtml

BIBLIOGRAPHY

Breitbart, W. (1995). Identifying patients at risk for, and treatment of major psychiatric complications of cancer. *Supportive Care in Cancer, 3*, 45-60.

Bruera, E., Driver, L., Barnes, E. A., et al. (2003). Patient-controlled methylphenidate for the management of fatigue in patients with advanced cancer: a preliminary report. *Journal of Clinical Oncology, 21*, 4439-43.

Cella, D., Lai, J., Chang, C., et al. (2002). Fatigue in cancer patients compared with fatigue in the general United States population. *Cancer, 94*, 528-538.

Cope, D. G. (2003). Oncology patient evidence-based notes (OPEN): Cancer-related fatigue. *Oncology Nursing Forum, 7*, 601-602.

Demetri, G. D., Kris, M., Wade, J., et al. (1998). Quality-of-life benefit in chemotherapy patients treated with epoetin alfa is independent of disease response or tumor type: results from a prospective community oncology study. Procrit Study Group. *Journal of Clinical Oncology, 16*, 3412-425.

Iop, A., Manfredi, A. M., & Bonura, S. (2004). Fatigue in cancer patients receiving chemotherapy: An analysis of published studies, *Annals of Oncology, 15*, 712-20.

Littlewood, T. J., Bajetta, E., Nortier, J. W. R., et al. (2001). Effects of epoetin alfa on hematologic parameters and quality-of-life in cancer patients receiving nonplatinum chemotherapy: Results of a randomized, double blind, placebo-controlled trial. *Journal of Clinical Oncology, 19*, 2865-2874.

Morrow, G. R., Abhay, R. S., Roscoe, J. A., et al. (2005). Management of cancer-related fatigue. *Cancer Investigation, 23*, 229-239.

Nail, L. M. (2002). Fatigue in patients with cancer. *Oncology Nursing Forum, 29*, 537-544.

National Comprehensive Cancer Network, v.2.2007. (2007). *The complete library of NCCN clinical practice guidelines in oncology (June, 2007)* (CD-ROM). Rockledge, PA: Author.

National Comprehensive Cancer Network. (2005). *Practice guidelines in oncology: Cancer-related fatigue, version 2.2005*. Retrieved December 30, 2005, from http://www.NCCN.org.

Ream, E., & Richardson, A. (2005). From theory to practice: Designing interventions to reduce fatigue in patients with cancer. *Oncology Nursing Forum, 26*, 1295-1305.

Schwartzberg, L. S., Yee, L. K., Senecal, F. M., et al. (2004). A randomized comparison of every two-week darbepoetin alfa and weekly epoetin alfa for the treatment of chemotherapy-induced anemia in patients with breast, lung, or gynecologic cancer. *The Oncologist, 9*, 696-707.

Sharp, K. (2005). Depression: The essentials. *Clinical Journal of Oncology Nursing, 9*, 519-525.

Theobald, D. E. (2004). Cancer pain, fatigue, distress, and insomnia in cancer patients. *Clinical Cornerstone, 6*(Suppl), 15-21.

Vogelzang, N., Breitbart, W., Cella, D., et al. (the Fatigue Coalition). (1997). Patient, caregiver, and oncologist perceptions of cancer-related fatigue: Results of a tri-part survey. *Seminars in Hematology, 34*, 4-12.

Waltzman, R., Croot, C., Justice, G. R., et al. (2005). Randomized comparison of epoetin alfa (40,000 U weekly) and darbepoetin alfa (200 μg every two weeks) in anemic patients with cancer receiving chemotherapy. *The Oncologist, 10*, 642-650.

Symptom Management

Winningham, M. L., & Barton-Burke, M. (2000). *Fatigue in cancer: A multidimensional approach*. Sudbury, MA: Jones & Bartlett.

Fever

Ruth Canty Gholz

DEFINITION

- Elevation of core body temperature
- Mean oral temperature is 98.6° F (plus or minus 0.7) or 37° C (plus or minus 0.4)
- A single temperature of 101° F or 38.3° C is significant.
- An emergency in a person with neutropenia or immunosuppression

PATHOPHYSIOLOGY AND CONTRIBUTING FACTORS

- Hypothalamus regulates and controls body temperature in the thermoregulatory center.
- Balances heat production with heat dissipation
- When the balance is disrupted (elevation of the hypothalamic set point), vasoconstriction and heat production occur.
- Fever can be induced from disease or pyrogens.
- Exogenous pyrogens occur from outside of the person. Primarily infectious agents, toxins, tumors
- Pyrogenic cytokines cause fever when activated. Includes interleukins, interferons, and tumor necrosis factor
- Fever has three phases: chill, fever, and flush.
- Elderly are more susceptible to temperature change and may have apyrexia and lower fever than others.
- Persons with cancer may have fever from infection, drugs, tumor, thrombosis, graft-versus-host disease, or a blood transfusion.

SIGNS AND SYMPTOMS

- Vasoconstriction of hands and feet
- Shivering, followed by need for warmth
- Chills, rigors
- Flush
- Dry skin
- Diaphoresis

ASSESSMENT TOOLS

- Determine whether patient is at high or low risk of febrile neutropenia if on chemotherapy.
- High-risk assessment of fever:
  - Inpatient
  - Comorbidity
  - Neutropenia
  - Elevated serum creatinine level
  - Liver function tests
- Low-risk assessment of fever:
  - Outpatient
  - No comorbidity
  - Short duration of neutropenia
  - Good performance status
- Risk assessment tools:
  - Multinational Association for Supportive Care in Cancer (MASCC) Risk Score
  - Talcott Risk Assessment
  - History and physical examination
- Areas to examine:
  - Skin assessment for areas of pressure, sores, or wounds
  - Vascular access devices as source of infection
  - Lungs and sinuses
  - Mouth, pharynx, esophagus, rectum, bowel
  - Vagina, anus
  - Examination of lymph nodes
- Assess for nausea, vomiting, diarrhea
- Review of medical history
- Medications
- Review potential exposures
- Time from last chemotherapy and drugs received
- Neurological assessment because confusion can occur with high fevers
- Vital signs: assess signs of sepsis; check temperature frequently
- In persons with cancer, consider infection as cause of fever unless proven otherwise

LABORATORY AND DIAGNOSTIC TESTS

- Complete blood cell count (CBC) with differential, sedimentation rate
- Renal panel
- Chest x-ray film
- Cultures: urine, sputum, blood, stool, vascular access device

DIFFERENTIAL DIAGNOSES

- Tumor/paraneoplastic fever
- Transfusion associated
- Drug-associated fever
- Infection: neutropenic fever—bacterial, viral, fungal
- Fever of unknown origin (FUO)

INTERVENTIONS

- Determined by cause of fever
- Treat the cause of fever

Pharmacologic Interventions

- Antipyretics to reduce temperature, myalgias, chills
- Empirical broad-spectrum antibiotic
- Anaerobic therapy as needed
- Specific therapy for documented infection sites or pathogens
- Prophylaxis to prevent future episodes of fever

Nonpharmacologic Interventions

- Hydration
- Nutritional support
- Comfort care, oral care, keep mucous membranes moist, sponge bathing with cool or cold cloths, changing bed linen and clothes, use of a fan for cooling

PATIENT TEACHING

- Prevention: good hand washing and hygiene
- Report fevers (above 38.5° C or 100.5° F) or chills to health care provider as soon as possible.
- Take complete course of antibiotics or other medications as ordered.
- Check temperature at least two times daily at home throughout duration of chemotherapy.

- For future chemotherapy, may need to use a colony-stimulating factor.
- Contact health care provider if any unusual symptoms or signs of infection or bleeding.
- When a neutropenic person will not experience the usual signs of infection (i.e., redness, swelling, pus), fever may be the first sign of infection.
- Do not take any rectal medications or treatments.
- Avoid contact with anyone who is ill.
- No dental work unless approved by health care provider

FOLLOW-UP

- Daily follow up when hospitalized
- Outpatient daily follow-up for the first 72 hours at home or in the clinic and as needed for signs and symptoms of persistent or recurrent fever

RESOURCES

- Chemo Care (Cleveland Clinic): www.chemocare.com
- National Comprehensive Cancer Network: www.NCCN.org
- Oncology Nursing Society: www.ons.org
- National Cancer Institute: www.cancer.gov
- American Cancer Society: www.cancer.org

BIBLIOGRAPHY

Braunwald E., Fauci A., Kasper D., et al. (Eds.) (2001). *Harrison's principles of internal medicine* (15th ed., pp. 90-94). New York: McGraw-Hill.
Dalal, S., & Zhukovsky, D., (2006). Pathophysiology and management of fever. *Journal of Supportive Oncology, 4*, 9-16.
Ezzone, S. (2006). Fever. In D. Camp-Sorrell & R.A. Hawkins (Eds.), *Clinical manual for the oncology advanced practice nurse* (pp. 979-988). Pittsburgh: Oncology Nursing Society.
Klastersky, J. (2004). Management of fever in neutropenic patients with different risks of complications. *Clinical Infectious Diseases, 39*(Suppl 1), S37: 532-537.
Mackowiak, P. (2006). Pathophysiology and management of fever—we know less than we should. *Journal of Supportive Oncology, 4*, 21-22.
National Comprehensive Cancer Network. (2006). *Fever and neutropenia: clinical practice guidelines in oncology, v. 1.* Retrieved April 1, 2007, from http://www.nccn.org/professionals/physician_gls/PDF/fever.pdf.
Porat, R., & Dinarello, C. (2006). *Pathophysiology and treatment of fever in adults.* Retrieved July 31, 2006, from www.uptodate.com.

Flu-Like Syndrome

Ruth Canty Gholz

DEFINITION

- Cluster of constitutional symptoms similar to the flu, may occur in different combinations
- Not the flu
- Characterized by fever, chills, rigors, myalgias/arthralgias, malaise, headache, cough, and nasal congestion
- Occurs after specific oncologic therapies
- Symptoms resolve within a specific time frame and lessen with each exposure to the anticancer agent

PATHOPHYSIOLOGY AND CONTRIBUTING FACTORS

- Occurs as a result of pyrogens causing an increase in the thermoregulatory set point
- Pyrogens may be exogenous (virus, bacteria, neoplastic cells, or drugs) or endogenous (cytokines)
- Chill is a muscle contraction in response to the rise in temperature.
- Occurs with the following agents:
  ○ Interferons
  ○ Interleukins
  ○ Granulocyte colony-stimulating factor (G-CSF)
  ○ Granulocyte-macrophage colony-stimulating factor (GM-CSF)
  ○ Monoclonal antibodies
  ○ Tumor necrosis factor
  ○ Bacille Calmette-Guérin (BCG)
  ○ Bleomycin
  ○ Cladribine
  ○ Cytarabine
  ○ Dacarbazine
  ○ Fluorouracil
  ○ L-Asparaginase
  ○ Monoclonal antibodies
  ○ Paclitaxel
  ○ Pamidronate disodium
  ○ Procarbazine
  ○ Trimetrexate
  ○ Zoledronic acid

SIGNS AND SYMPTOMS

- Chills or rigors that occur 3-6 hours after therapy
- Fever occurs average of 30-90 minutes after a chill
- Myalgia or arthralgia
- Headache
- Malaise
- Fatigue
- Nausea or vomiting
- Anorexia
- Diarrhea

ASSESSMENT TOOLS

- Physical examination with review of systems: cardiopulmonary, abdomen, lymph nodes, musculoskeletal, and skin
- Assess vital signs: blood pressure, temperature, pulse, and respirations
- Neurological assessment

LABORATORY AND DIAGNOSTIC TESTS

- Complete blood cell count (CBC) to determine whether related to neutropenia
- If neutropenic need to pan culture and rule out infection
- Chest x-ray film if neutropenic

DIFFERENTIAL DIAGNOSIS

- Infection
- Toxic shock syndrome
- Flu
- Cold
- Drug-induced symptoms

Symptom Management

INTERVENTIONS
Pharmacologic Interventions

- Antipyretics (acetaminophen, nonsteroidal anti-inflammatory drugs [NSAIDs])
- Antihistamines
- Opiate to relieve rigors (meperidine, morphine, hydromorphone)
- Monitor temperature patterns; if no response to antipyretics, may be infectious process.
- Analgesics for headache, myalgias, arthralgias
- Premedicate before administration of causative agent to potentially block flu-like syndrome.

Nonpharmacologic Interventions

- Provide warm blankets, heating pads, warm bath.
- Provide quiet dark room for headache.
- Increase fluids.
- Relaxation techniques
- Emotional support and reassurance
- Provide for rest.

PATIENT TEACHING

- Teach patient that this is a possible side effect of therapy.
- Use of antipyretic for fever
- Warm blankets and water to relieve chills
- NSAID or acetaminophen for myalgias or arthralgias
- Instruct patient that this side effect is short lived and reduces with future drug administration.

FOLLOW-UP

- Report fevers or chills not controlled with above interventions.
- Obtain care if vomiting, seizures, mental status change or uncontrolled fever
- Patients have emergency numbers for contact

RESOURCES

- Oncology Nursing Society: www.ons.org/patientEd
- People Living With Cancer: http://www.plwc.org/

BIBLIOGRAPHY

Lawary, N. (2005). Flu-like symptoms. In Hickey, M., Newton, S. (Eds.). *Telephone triage for oncology nurses* (pp. 122-135). Pittsburgh, PA: Oncology Nursing Society.

Polovich, M., White, J., & Kelleher, L. (Eds.) (2005). *Chemotherapy and biotherapy guidelines and recommendations for practice* (pp.156-158). Pittsburgh: Oncology Nursing Society.

Shelton, R. (2001). Flu-like syndrome. In P. Reiger (Ed.). *Biotherapy: a comprehensive review* (pp. 519-543). Boston: Jones & Bartlett.

Stempkowski, L. (2000). Flu-like syndrome. In D. Camp-Sorrell, & R.A. Hawkins (Eds.). *Clinical manual for the oncology advanced practice nurse* (pp. 825-830). Pittsburgh, PA: Oncology Nursing Society.

Wilkes, G., & Barton-Burke, M. (2005). *Oncology nursing drug handbook*. Boston: Jones & Bartlett.

Hand-Foot Syndrome (HFS)

Laura S. Wood

DEFINITION

- Dermatologic reaction associated with certain anti-cancer therapies
- Presentation varies depending on agent, dose, and patient characteristics
- Involvement of hands and feet are most common, but can involve other skin surfaces
- Also known as:
  - Palmar-plantar erythrodysesthesia (PPE)
  - Acral erythema
  - Hyperkeratosis
  - Hand-foot reaction

PATHOPHYSIOLOGY AND CONTRIBUTING FACTORS

- Cutaneous eruption of the integument of the hands and feet
- Drugs with sustained serum levels such as liposomal doxorubicin and capecitabine are most likely to cause HFS
- Results from prolonged drug exposure via superficial capillaries

- Dependent of both peak drug concentration and total cumulative dose
- May occur earlier and more severely with bolus or short-term dose-intensive therapy
- May result from friction and pressure (weight-bearing) on hands and feet or other areas
- Patients with diabetes or peripheral vascular disorders are at increased risk
- Cytochrome P450 subsystem inhibitors must be considered as potential contributing factors

SIGNS AND SYMPTOMS

- Often characterized by initial paresthesias (tingling sensations, numbness, or sensitivity to warmth) followed by erythema
- May occur concurrently with dry skin
- May include hyperkeratosis and callus formation
- May include blisters, bullae, or fissures
- Acral erythema is painful symmetrical erythematous and edematous areas
- Dry or moist desquamation may occur
- May include swelling or edema
- Can become painful, interfere with function and activities of daily living
- Can have a negative impact on quality of life

ASSESSMENT TOOLS

- Patient history
- Medication review during each interaction
- Physical exam of hands and feet should be done prior to initiation of therapy, and at every clinic visit
- Common Toxicity Criteria (CTC version 3.0)
  - Grade 1 (mild)
  - Grade 2 (moderate)
  - Grade 3 (severe)
  - Grade 4 (life threatening)

LABORATORY AND DIAGNOSTIC TESTS

- No specific laboratory tests
- Physical exam and patient-reported symptoms facilitate accurate diagnosis
- Patients with diabetes, peripheral vascular disease, and peripheral neuropathy should have more frequent examination of hands and feet

DIFFERENTIAL DIAGNOSES

- Cellulitis
- Rash
- Contact dermatitis
- Allergic reaction

INTERVENTIONS

Pharmacologic Interventions

- Dexamethasone for severe HFS not responsive to other interventions
- Pyridoxine for pruritus associated with HFS
- Treatment interruption and/or dose reduction for severe HFS

Nonpharmacologic Interventions

- Prevention is not possible. Patient education regarding frequent self-assessment and compliance with skin care regimen is critical to minimizing risk of severe or treatment-limiting HFS
- Initiation of skin care regimen with first dose of therapy
  - Avoidance of deodorant or fragrant-based soaps and lotions
  - Frequent application of moisturizing lotion (Bag balm, Udder Butter, Eucerin cream)
  - Avoidance of activities resulting in excessive friction or pressure involving hands or feet
  - Minimize duration of exposure to heat (i.e. bathing or dishwashing)
  - Well fitting, cushioned, comfortable shoes
  - Gel insole liners
- Early notification for development of symptoms associated with HFS
- Exfoliating agents for hyperkeratotic areas
- Use of sunscreen for any potential periods of sun exposure

PATIENT TEACHING

- Emphasize compliance with skin care regimen
- Emphasize early notification for development of symptoms associated with HFS
- If the skin blisters, soak the area with cool water for 10 minutes, then apply petroleum jelly to the wet skin to trap the moisture.

FOLLOW-UP

- If patient reports any changes to the palms of their hands or soles of their feet, a physical assessment and diagnosis/treatment plan must be made.

RESOURCES

- www.chemocare.com
- www.cancersymptoms.org
- http://ctep.cancer.gov/forms/CTCAEv3.pdf

BIBLIOGRAPHY

Bardia, A., Loprinzi, C.L., Goetz, M.P. (2006). Hand-foot syndrome after dose-dense adjuvant chemotherapy for breast cancer: A case series. *Journal of Clinical Oncology, 24*(13), 18-19.

Conrad, K.J. (2001). Cutaneous reactions. In Yasko, J. M., (Ed). *Nursing Management of Symptoms Associated with Chemotherapy,* 5th ed., (pp. 191-204). Meniscus HealthCare Communications.

Laack, E., Mende, T., Knuffmann, C., et al. (2001). Hand-foot syndrome associated with short infusions of combination chemotherapy with gemcitabine and vinorelbine. *Annals of Oncology, 12*(12), 1761-1763.

Nagore, E., Insa, A., & Sanmartin, O. (2000). Antineoplastic therapy-induced palmar plantar erythrodysesthesia ('Hand Foot') syndrome: Incidence, recognition, and management. *American Journal of Clinical Dermatology,* 1(4), 225-234.

Pike, K. (2001). Clinical challenges: Hand-foot syndrome. *Oncology Nursing Forum, 28*(10), 1519-1520.

Robert, C., Soria, J.C., Spatz, A., et al (2005). Cutaneous side effects of kinase inhibitors and blocking antibodies. *The Lancet Oncology,* 6, 491-500.

Wilkes, G. M. & Doyle, D., (2005). Palmar-plantar erythrodysesthesia. *Clinical Journal of Oncology Nursing, 9*(1), 103-106.

Headache

Carol S. Blecher

DEFINITION

- Headaches are defined as pain that is referred to the surface of the head from deep structures.

PATHOPHYSIOLOGY AND CONTRIBUTING FACTORS

- Can be caused by some other physical disorder, or they can be an independent disorder.
- When there is damage to the venous sinuses or to the membranes that cover the brain, intense pain may occur, although the brain itself is almost completely insensitive to pain.
- Three major types:
  - *Tension (or stress):* caused by the tightening of muscles in the head and neck
  - *Migraine:* caused by dilation of the blood vessels in the brain
  - *Cluster:* a form of chronic, recurrent headache. Characterized by a sudden onset with no specific cause, although it appears to be related to a sudden release of histamine or serotonin
- Contributing factors vary with the type of headache: most frequent causes of headaches in cancer patients are related to:
  - Primary brain tumors or brain metastases
  - An increase in intracranial pressure either from mass effect or edema
  - Radiation therapy which initially increases edema and causes headaches.
  - Intrathecal chemotherapy causing headaches, and the procedure of administering chemotherapy by omaya reservoir or lumbar puncture.
  - Chemotherapy and biotherapy agents including
    - Erythropoietin
    - Granulocyte colony-stimulating factor (G-CSF)

- Granulocyte-macrophage colony-stimulating factor (GM-CSF)
- Oprelvekin (Neumega)
- Immunoglobulin (IgG)
- Interferon
- Interleukin
- Levamisole
- All-trans retinoic acid (ATRA)
- Monoclonal antibodies in general
- Tumor necrosis factor
- Dacarbazine
- Gemcitabine
- Paclitaxel

SIGNS AND SYMPTOMS

- Patients with brain tumors may have headaches that are worse in the morning.
- Initially these headaches ease during the day but ultimately become persistent.
- Pain is usually described as dull, but if it occurs while the patient is sleeping, it wakes the patient up.
- The pain may be associated with morning nausea and vomiting, papilledema, and seizures.

ASSESSMENT TOOLS

- History, including diagnosis and cancer treatment, current medications, presenting symptoms, precipitating factors, location, and duration. Assess for any associated symptoms.
- Neurological examination, evaluating for confusion, a decrease in attention span, memory loss, drowsiness, or ataxia
- Vital signs: changes in vital signs may be indicative of an increase in intracranial pressure (ICP). Blood pressure should be monitored for a widened pulse pressure as well as hypertension. Heart rate monitoring for bradycardia.
- Examine the head for signs of trauma, skull tenderness (subdural hematoma), poor dentition or grinding of the teeth, bogginess of the sinuses, papilledema, otitis media, and mastoiditis.
- Examine the neck for nuchal rigidity, tenderness of the

shoulders or neck, and decreased range of motion.
- National Cancer Institute (NCI) common toxicity criteria (CTC) and common terminology criteria for adverse events:
  - Grade 1: mild pain not interfering with function
  - Grade 2: moderate pain, pain or analgesics interfering with function, but not interfering with activities of daily living (ADLs)
  - Grade 3: severe pain, pain, or analgesics severely interfering with ADLs
  - Grade 4: disabling

LABORATORY AND DIAGNOSTIC TESTS

- Complete blood cell count (CBC) to rule out infection or anemia
- Chemistries to rule out renal failure and other underlying systemic diseases
- Prothrombin time (PT)/partial thromboplastin time (PTT) to identify a risk for intercranial bleeding
- Arterial blood gas analysis (ABGs) to asses for hypoxia
- Drug screening for cocaine and amphetamines
- Computed tomography (CT) scan of the head to identify a tumor, metastases, or edema
- Magnetic resonance imaging (MRI) of the head to identify a tumor, metastases, or edema
- Lumbar puncture to assess infection (meningitis or encephalitis) or meningeal carcinomatosis

DIFFERENTIAL DIAGNOSES

- Migraine
- Subarachnoid hemorrhage
- Meningitis
- Subdural hematoma
- Stroke
- Arteriovenous malformation
- Dental abscess
- Sinusitis
- Acute glaucoma
- Hypertension
- Systemic lupus erythematosus
- Trigeminal neuralgia
- Meningeal carcinoma

- Brain metastases
- Primary brain tumor
- Drug-related headaches from chemotherapy and biotherapy agents including:
  - Erythropoietin
  - G-CSF
  - GM-CSF
  - Oprelvekin (Neumega)
  - IgG
  - Interferon
  - Interleukin
  - Levamisole
  - All-trans retinoic acid
  - Monoclonal antibodies in general
  - Tumor necrosis factor
  - Dacarbazine
  - Gemcitabine
  - Paclitaxel
- Drug-related headaches from analgesics including:
  - Butabarbital (Fiorinal/Esgic/Bellergal)
  - Narcotics
  - Tranquilizers/muscle relaxers
  - Caffeine
  - Ergot preparations
  - Acetaminophen (Tylenol).
- Drug-related headaches from other agents including:
  - Amphotericin B
  - Azathioprine
  - Aztreonam
  - Cyclosporine
  - Foscarnet
  - Ganciclovir
  - Pamidronate
  - Rifampicin

INTERVENTIONS
Treatment of the Underlying Disease

- Primary brain tumor surgery, radiation therapy, chemotherapy
- Metastatic brain tumor radiation therapy
- Edema of the brain treated with dexamethasone

Pharmacologic Interventions

- Aspirin
- Acetaminophen (Tylenol)
- Naproxen (Naprosyn, Anaprox, Aleve)
- Ibuprofen (Motrin, Advil, Nuprin)
- Indomethacin (Indocin)

- Ketorolac (Toradol)
- Ergotamine tartrate/caffeine (Cafergot, Wigraine, Ergomar)
- Sumatriptan (Imitrex)
- Aspirin/butalbital/caffeine
- Beta-blockers (propranolol [Inderal], nadolol [Corgard], metoprolol [Lopressor])
- Calcium channel blockers (verapamil [Calan])
- Tricyclic antidepressants (amitriptyline [Elavil, Endep], and nortriptyline [Pamelor])

Nonpharmacologic Interventions

- Complementary therapies such as biofeedback, acupuncture, massage, relaxation, transcutaneous electrical nerve stimulation (TENS)
- Dietary modifications: avoid dairy products, caffeinated drinks, chocolate, salted or preserved meats, and food containing monosodium glutamate (MSG).
- Herbal and nutrient therapies suggested for relief of headaches include skullcap, rosemary, thyme, chamomile, feverfew, valerian, white willow, vitamin B complex, vitamin E, calcium, and magnesium.

PATIENT TEACHING

- Treatment for headache is determined on the basis of the following:
  - Age, health status, and medical history
  - Severity of symptoms
  - Individual tolerance of specific medications, procedures, or therapies
  - Expectations for the course of the condition
  - Personal opinions/preferences
- Treatment may include the following:
  - Drug therapy (medication)
  - Biofeedback training
  - Stress reduction
  - Dietary evaluation to eliminate food that might contribute to headaches
  - Regular exercise, such as swimming or vigorous walking
  - Use of cold packs

FOLLOW-UP

- Call health care provider if:
  - This is the first time the person has had a headache
  - The headache occurs rapidly or is persistent
  - It is associated with fever, stiff neck, or uncontrollable vomiting
  - The headache is associated with confusion, seizures, or loss of consciousness
  - There is numbness, weakness, or vision loss with the headache
  - The headache interferes with the ability to function normally
  - You take medication for the headache more than 2 days per week
- Also consider:
  - Pain service referral
  - Headache center referral
  - Physical therapy
  - Occupational therapy

RESOURCES

- American Council for Headache Education: www.achenet.org
- National Headache Foundation: www.headaches.org

BIBLIOGRAPHY

Common terminology criteria for adverse events, version 3. (2006). Retrieved 02/08/07 from http://www.fda.gov/cder/cancer/toxicityframe.htm.

Hickman, J. L. (1998). Managing primary complications. In C. C. Chernecky (Ed.). *Advanced and critical care oncology nursing* (pp. 371-383). Philadelphia: W. B. Saunders.

MedlinePlus Medical Encyclopedia. (05/16/06.). *Headache.* Retrieved 02/08/07 from http://www.nlm.nih.gov/medlineplus/ency/article/003024.htm.

Shelton, B. K. (2004). Flulike syndrome. In C. H. Yarbro, M. H. Frogge, & M. Goodman (Eds.). *Cancer symptom management* (pp. 61-76). Sudbury, MA: Jones & Bartlett.

Sherman, D.W. (2001). Patients with acquired immune deficiency syndrome. In B. R. Ferrell, & N. Coyle (Eds.). *Textbook of palliative nursing* (pp. 467-499), New York: Oxford University Press.

Strohl, R. A. (2000). Headache. In D. Camp-Sorrell & R. A. Hawkins (Eds.). *Clinical manual for the oncology advanced practice nurse* (pp. 775-781). Pittsburgh: Oncology Nursing Press.

Hiccups

Denice Economou

DEFINITION

- Sudden, involuntary diaphragmatic spasm causing a sudden inhalation and interrupted by a spasmodic closure of the glottis
- Three types:
  - *Benign*—lasting as long as 48 hours
  - *Persistent or chronic*—lasting longer than 48 hours but less than 1 month
  - *Intractable*—lasting longer than 1 month

PATHOPHYSIOLOGY AND CONTRIBUTING FACTORS

- Reflex arc in the cervical spine (C3-C5) travels afferent pathways over fibers of the phrenic and vagus nerves and thoracic segments T6-T12
- Response to vagus and phrenic nerve irritation
- Conditions causing hiccups are organized under four conditions:
  - Structural
  - Metabolic
  - Inflammatory
  - Infectious
- Hiccups can contribute to fatigue and exhaustion, especially when sleep and eating are interrupted.
- Unrelieved hiccups can also lead to feeling of depression, anxiety, and frustration over the long term.
- Common causes in terminal illness include stroke, brain tumors, sepsis, and nerve irritation such as gastric distention, gastritis, gastroesophageal reflux disease (GERD), pancreatitis, *Helicobacter pylori* infection, hepatitis, and myocardial infarction.
- Excessive drinking or smoking
- Medications that may contribute to hiccups:
  - Steroids
  - Chemotherapy
  - Nicotine
  - Opioids
  - Muscle relaxants

Symptom Management

SIGNS AND SYMPTOMS

- Brief, irritable spasms of the diaphragm

ASSESSMENT TOOLS

- Obtain a history of presenting symptoms.
- Precipitating factors: triggers such as eating, drinking, or positioning.
- Medical history regarding abdominal, thoracic, or neurological surgery; social history of alcohol use
- Level of distress hiccups are causing
- Interference with activities of daily living (ADLs) including eating and sleeping
- Observe patient for other causes of hiccups.
- Oral examination to identify any swelling or obstruction that may be contributing to hiccups
- Evaluate for infection or septic process.
- Pneumonia or pericarditis or abdominal distention or ascites
- Peritumor edema in the abdominal area

LABORATORY AND DIAGNOSTIC TESTS

- Complete blood cell count (CBC) and electrolytes to rule out infection or renal failure
- Chest x-ray film to rule out pulmonary processes

DIFFERENTIAL DIAGNOSES

- Diaphragmatic or phrenic nerve irritation
- Gastric dilation
- Hiatal hernia
- Pancreatitis
- Alcohol abuse
- Central nervous system (CNS) dysfunction
- Psychogenic cause

INTERVENTIONS
Pharmacologic Interventions

- Chlorpromazine (Thorazine)
- Attempt to decrease gastric distention with medications such as simethicone and metoclopramide. Nasogastric (NG) tube or fasting may be necessary to help relieve this symptom.
- Additional medications include muscle relaxants, anticonvulsants, or dopamine agonists.

Nonpharmacologic Interventions

- Respiratory measures may help. Consider having the patient hold the breath. Rebreathing in a paper bag, causing sneeze or cough with spices.
- Drink large gulps of water, swallowing sugar, or sucking on a lemon wedge may interfere with hiccups.
- Psychological interventions include distraction techniques and breathing exercises.
- Intractable hiccups may require anesthetic block of the phrenic and cervical nerves or acupuncture.
- Peppermint water helps to relax lower esophagus.

PATIENT TEACHING

- Provide education and information regarding different classes of medications used for relief along with nonpharmacologic approaches.

FOLLOW-UP

- Gastrointestinal (GI) consultation if the cause is GI related
- Anesthesia consult if nerve block is necessary
- Provide support to the patient and continual assessment of interventions until patient's hiccups are relieved.

RESOURCES

- Mayo Clinic http:www.mayoclinic.com/health/ hiccups/DS00975

BIBLIOGRAPHY

Camp-Sorrell, D. (2006). Hiccups. In D. Camp-Sorrell & R. A. Hawkins (Eds.). *Clinical manual for the oncology advanced practice nurse* (pp. 13-17). Pittsburgh: Oncology Nursing Society.

Dahlin, C., & Goldsmith, T. (2006). Dysphagia, xerostomia, and hiccups. In B. R. Ferrell & N. Coyle (Eds.). *Textbook of palliative nursing* (2nd ed., pp. 195-218). New York: Oxford University Press.

Smith, H. S., & Busracamwongs, A. (2003). Management of hiccups in the palliative care population. *AJHPC, 20,* 149-154.

Lymphedema

Wendy H. Vogel

DEFINITION

- Swelling from abnormal production of lymph fluid or because of an obstruction in the lymph circulation
- Occurs in approximately 20% of patients after a radical mastectomy and in 6%-7% after modified radical mastectomy
- Lower-extremity lymphedema after pelvic or inguinal lymphadenectomy occurs in about 20% of patients.

PATHOPHYSIOLOGY AND CONTRIBUTING FACTORS

- Primary lymphedema is rare, most often occurring as a birth defect.
- Secondary lymphedema usually develops as the result of an obstruction of the lymphatic system by a tumor or trauma such as infection, surgery, or radiation therapy.
  - May occur acutely or chronically, years after treatment
  - Acute lymphedema subsides within a few weeks after surgery when collateral circulation has developed
  - The most common sites of lymph obstruction are the axillary, pelvic, or inguinal nodes.
- After surgery, if lymph fluid does not get rerouted or collateral circulation does not develop, then the lymph system may not be able to accommodate the demand for drainage and fluid accumulates in the interstitial spaces, and the result is edema.
- If edema persists, the high protein concentration causes fibrosis of the subcutaneous tissue, which causes irreversible damage to the lymph system.
- More common in women who have undergone axillary dissection and radiation therapy with more than 46 Gy

- Risk factors:
  - Lymph node dissection (the greater the number of lymph nodes removed, the greater the risk of lymphedema)
  - Radiation therapy
  - Infection
  - Obesity
  - Age
  - Breast cancer, ovarian cancer, lymphoma, and prostate cancer

SIGNS AND SYMPTOMS

- Swollen limb
- Swollen axilla or groin area
- Edema may extend to the face, neck, or genitals.
- Signs of infection or inflammation may be present.

ASSESSMENT TOOLS

- Obtain a thorough history:
  - Possible sources, signs and symptoms of infection
  - Any unusual or heavy lifting or activity
  - Repetitive-type movements
  - Time frame with regard to surgery or trauma
  - Activity level
  - Nutrition
  - Comorbid conditions
- Psychosocial:
  - Assess impact on body image, sexuality, social activities, job.
  - Assess for anger, social avoidance, sexual dysfunction, poor adjustment.
- Assess for pain.
- Physical examination:
  - Measure the affected limb, using anatomic landmarks for follow-up assessment accuracy.
  - Assess for signs and symptoms of infection.
  - Pulses and range of motion
  - Strength of the affected limb
  - Affected areas for presence of suspicious masses or tumor recurrence
  - Grade the severity:
    - Mild—2-3 cm difference from one limb to another, feelings of heaviness, throbbing or soreness
    - Moderate—3-5 cm difference, visibly noticeable,

skin may be stretched and shiny, pitting edema may be present, tissue is soft
    - Severe—greater than 5 cm difference, skin stretched and discolored to purple or brown, tough, brawny, with peau d'orange appearance, tissue may be firm, nonpitting

LABORATORY AND DIAGNOSTIC TESTS

- Rule out venous swelling such as venous obstruction or thrombus with color flow Doppler ultrasonogram or venogram.
- Computed tomography (CT) or magnetic resonance imaging (MRI) of the axilla or groin to rule out tumor recurrence
- Lymphoscintigraphy as indicated
- Blood urea nitrogen (BUN), creatinine, liver function tests, albumin, urinalysis, liver function tests to rule out possible systemic causes

DIFFERENTIAL DIAGNOSIS

- Thrombus
- Infection
- Cirrhosis
- Nephrosis
- Congestive heart failure
- Myxedema
- Hypoalbuminemia
- Chronic venous stasis
- Obstruction from pelvic or abdominal malignancy

INTERVENTIONS

- Gold standard: complete decongestive physiotherapy (CDP):
  - Phase I: therapist administers manual lymphatic massage, compression bandaging, exercises, and skin care.
  - Phase II: patient self-care activities including use of compression garments, night wrappings, and continued exercises
- Elevation of edematous extremity
- Refer to physical therapy or surgery as indicated.
- Pain management

- Refer to support group as appropriate.
- Diuretics, if used, should be used only temporarily. Effects are generally minimal.
- Prevention is key:
  - Encourage exercise, particularly strengthening exercises and aerobic activity.
  - No heavy, dependent lifting of more than 15 pounds.
  - Prevent infection or prompt treatment if infection occurs.
  - Encourage good hygiene and precautions against trauma.
  - Encourage well-balanced, low-sodium, high-fiber diet.
  - Maintain ideal body weight.

PATIENT TEACHING

- Avoid trauma to affected extremity.
- Use good hygiene to avoid introduction of bacteria to potential open areas of affected extremity
- Avoid heavy, dependent lifting or vigorous repetitive motions against resistance.
- Avoid venipuncture, chemotherapy or blood product administration, injection or assessment of blood pressure in affected extremity unless needs of moment outweigh potential consequences.
- Be aware of and report signs and symptoms of infection.
- Avoid having limb in dependent position for long periods of time, as with air travel.
- Refer to patient teaching sheet in Section Seven.

FOLLOW-UP

- Periodically assess for intervention success.
- Referrals as appropriate; especially for CDP if necessary

RESOURCES

- American Cancer Society: www.cancer.org
- Breast cancer.org www.breastcancer.org
- Chemocare.org: www.chemocare.org
- Circle of Hope Lymphedema Foundation: www.lymphedemacircleofhope.org

Symptom Management

- National Cancer Institute: www.cancer.gov
- Oncology Nursing Society, CancerSymptoms.org: www.cancersymptoms.org
- SusanLoveMD.org: www.susanlovemd.org
- The National Lymphedema Network: www.lymphnet.org

BIBLIOGRAPHY

Chapman, D., & Moore, S. (2005). Breast cancer. In C. Yarbro, M. Frogge, & M. Goodman (Eds.). *Cancer nursing principles and practice*, (6th ed, pp. 1022-1088). Sudbury, MA: Jones & Bartlett.

Ferri, F. (2005). *Ferri's clinical advisor, 2005*. New York: Elsevier Mosby.

Golshan, M., & Smith, B. (2006). Prevention and management of arm lymphedema in the patient with breast cancer. *Journal of Supportive Oncology, 4*, 381-386.

Herd-Smith, A., Russo, A., Muraca, M., et al. (2001). Prognostic factors for lymphedema after primary treatment of breast carcinoma. *Cancer, 92*, 1783-1787.

Kalinowski, B. (1999). Lymphedema. In C. Yarbro, M. Frogge, & M. Goodman (Eds.). *Cancer symptom management* (2nd ed., pp. 457-486). Sudbury, MA: Jones & Bartlett.

Ridner, S. (2002). Breast cancer lymphedema: Pathophysiology and risk reduction guidelines. *Oncology Nursing Forum, 29*, 1285-1293.

Ridner, S. (2006). Breast cancer treatment-related lymphedema—a continuing problem. *Journal of Supportive Oncology, 4*, 389-390.

Menopausal Symptoms

Wendy H. Vogel

DEFINITION

- Menopause is a hormonal change that occurs when estrogen and progesterone levels begin to drop.
- Usually occurs between ages 45 and 55 years; however, can also be surgically or chemically induced.
- The average age of menopause in the United States is 51 years.
- There are increasing numbers of women who have menopausal symptoms after treatment for cancer.
- Early menopause can have long-lasting effects on a woman's quality of life.

PATHOPHYSIOLOGY AND CONTRIBUTING FACTORS

- Physiological menopause is due to exhaustion of the ovarian follicles that contain the germ cells that produce the steroid hormones estrogen and progesterone.
- Premature ovarian failure is cessation of ovarian function before age 40 years.
- Ovarian failure may be induced by radiation, chemotherapy, surgery, or infection.
- When a decreased level of hormone is detected by the hypothalamus, the pituitary gland will secrete follicle-stimulating hormone (FSH) and luteinizing hormone (LH). The ovaries are unable to respond to the FSH and LH; therefore, estrogen deficiency occurs, ovulation does not occur, and thus the woman is amenorrheic.
- Vasomotor instability (a hot flash) is caused by dysfunction of the thermoregulatory center in the hypothalamus.
  - There is a sharp rise in epinephrine, which stimulates heart function, rise in blood pressure, and an intense feeling of warmth throughout the upper body with flushing and perspiration that may last as little as a few seconds or as long as 20 minutes.
  - Estrogen influences the firing rate of the thermosensitive neurons in the preoptic area of the hypothalamus and affects how responsive vascular smooth muscle is to vasoactive substances such as epinephrine and norepinephrine.
  - Cancer survivors, especially those who have had breast cancer, may experience more vasomotor symptoms and at an earlier age.
- A few years after estrogen deprivation, women will begin to experience genitourinary symptoms, primarily as a result of decreased arterial blood flow to vagina and vulva.
  - Atrophy of the vaginal wall
  - Vaginal dryness, infections, bleeding, and burning sensations
  - Dyspareunia
  - Urinary symptoms may occur as a result of urogenital atrophy.
  - Decreased libido may occur because loss of ovarian function will also decrease serum androgen levels.
- Psychological changes:
  - Estrogen increases the degradation rate of monoamine oxidase, the enzyme that catabolizes serotonin.
  - Serotonin deficiency is believed to contribute to depression.
  - Decreased bone density occurs because of the imbalance of bone resorption and formation. Early estrogen deprivation can lead to osteoporosis and potential fractures.
  - Increased risk for heart disease because risk is reactive to the age at which estrogen deprivation occurs.

SIGNS AND SYMPTOMS

- The symptoms of menopause can be mild or severe.
- Change in or cessation of menses
- Vasomotor symptoms such as hot flashes and night sweats
- Vaginal atrophy, thinning of vaginal wall, dryness, dyspareunia, postcoital bleeding
- Urinary symptoms such as urgency, stress incontinence, frequent urinary tract infections
- Emotional lability, mood changes, irritability
- Cognitive changes such as forgetfulness or decreased ability to concentrate or make decisions; depression
- Weight gain in hips and thighs
- Sleep disturbances
- Decreased skin elasticity

ASSESSMENT TOOLS

- Pelvic examination; observing for vaginal atrophy and associated difficulties

LABORATORY AND DIAGNOSTIC TESTS

- FSH
- LH
- Serum estradiol
- Mean estrone
- Urinalysis of presence of urinary tract symptoms
- Bone density testing
- Lipid panel

DIFFERENTIAL DIAGNOSES

- Ovarian abnormalities
- Polycystic ovarian syndrome
- Pregnancy hypothalamic dysfunction
- Hypothyroidism
- Pituitary tumors
- Adrenal abnormalities
- Ovarian neoplasm
- Tuberculosis
- Bone loss
- Lipid profile elevations

INTERVENTIONS
Pharmacologic Interventions

- Hormone replacement therapy (HRT) is a controversial subject in postmenopausal women because of various health risks, including breast cancer.
  - Hormonal replacement options have different doses of estrogen and combinations of estrogen and progesterone or testosterone, varying levels of systemic absorption dependent on the route of administration.
  - HRT is contraindicated in patients with stroke or thromboembolic event, recent myocardial infarction, acute liver or pancreatic disease, and undiagnosed vaginal bleeding.
  - For menopausal symptoms, HRT may be considered but should be given for the shortest amount of time possible (ideally less than 5 years).
  - HRT should be chosen to match the specific menopausal complaints and to provide maximum safety.
  - HRT options include oral estrogens, vaginal estrogens, and transdermal estrogens. Each option has various

combinations. A full discussion of benefits and risk of HRT should ensue between the patient and the health care provider.
  - In the oncology patient, careful consideration should be given to hormone-related cancer, and the risks of cancer stimulation should be evaluated.
  - The lowest dose possible of estrogen should be chosen. Oral doses and vaginal doses as low 0.3 mg may provide relief from hot flashes and vaginal discomfort, although lower doses may have a somewhat delayed response. Consider adding a progestin if a patient remains symptomatic.
  - Local estrogen products may be used for vaginal and urinary complaints and have less systemic absorption.
  - Minimizing progestin exposure decreases the rate of endometrial hyperplasia. Progestins may be given less frequently, for example, quarterly or biyearly, for women on lower-dose estrogens.
  - Topical estrogens may be useful for vaginal and urinary symptoms, but potential risks should be reviewed with the patient.
  - Zoledronic acid is in clinical trials for the prevention of bone loss in postmenopausal women with breast cancer who are on an aromatase inhibitor.
- Nonhormonal pharmacological options for vasomotor symptoms include the following:
  - Clonidine, oral or transdermal
  - Venlafaxine, fluoxetine, or paroxetine
  - Bellergal or Bellergal-S
  - Propranolol
  - Lofexidine
  - Vitamin E 400 international units twice a day; also vitamins B and C
  - Ginseng
  - Megace acetate and medroxyprogesterone have been used; however, the safety in patients with a hormonally

sensitive tumor is not fully known. Progestins can stimulate proliferation of the endometrium when given alone. Potential risks of treatment and the benefits must be considered carefully and discussed with the patient.
  - Phytoestrogens and black cohosh have been used, but the safety of these is not known, and the results in many studies show effects similar to placebo.
  - Gabapentin is being evaluated in clinical trials for the treatment of hot flashes, but side effects may limit its use.

Nonpharmacologic Interventions

- Hot flashes
  - Acupuncture
  - Paced respirations
  - Trained relaxation techniques
  - Avoidance of hot flash triggers such as alcohol, hot drinks, or spicy foods
- Dietary issues (low-fat diet), smoking cessation, low to moderate alcohol intake, maintenance of healthy weight, and sedentary lifestyle
- Weight reduction and moderate exercise of 30 minutes or more on most days of the week should be recommended.
- Vaginal lubricants, such as Replens (Auspharm, Australia), may be helpful for vaginal dryness (refer to Alterations in Sexuality, page 340).
- Insomnia may be treated both pharmacologically and nonpharmacologically (refer to Sleep Disturbances, page 389).
- Osteoporosis prevention and treatment
  - Bisphosphonates may be prescribed for those with osteopenia or osteoporosis.
  - Raloxifene, a selective receptor modulator, is also approved for the prevention and treatment of osteoporosis. Should not be given with an aromatase inhibitor or tamoxifen. Raloxifene may increase hot flashes.

○ Patients should be advised to take calcium and vitamin D, perform weight-bearing exercise, and avoid smoking and excess alcohol intake.

PATIENT TEACHING

- Patients should understand the fertility risks and the potential for early menopause before undergoing cancer treatment.
- If HRT is considered, the risks and benefits must be fully explored with the patient.
- Prevention and screening for osteoporosis

FOLLOW-UP

- As needed to assess symptom management
- Sleep hygiene or bladder training as appropriate

RESOURCES

- American Cancer Society: www.cancer.org
- Breastcancer.org: www.breastcancer.org
- Chemocare.org: www.chemocare.org
- National Cancer Institute: www.cancer.gov
- Oncology Nursing Society's CancerSymptoms.org: www.cancersymptoms.org
- SusanLoveMD.org: www.susanlovemd.org

BIBLIOGRAPHY

Batur, P., Blixen, C., Moore, H., et al. (2006). Menopausal hormone therapy in patients with breast cancer. *Maturitas, 53*, 123-132.

Epocrates, Inc. (2006). *Epocrates Rx Pro clinical data base*, version 7.50. Retrieved 10/5/07 from http://www.epocrates.com/index.html.

Fenstermacher, K., & Hudson, B. (2000). *Practice guidelines for family nurse practitioners* (2nd ed.). Philadelphia: W. B. Saunders.

Ferri, F. (2005). *Ferri's clinical advisor, 2005.* Philadelphia: Elsevier Mosby.

Gainford, M., Simmons, C., Nguyen, H., et al. (2005). A practical guide to the management of menopausal symptoms in breast cancer patients. *Supportive Care in Cancer, 13*, 573-578.

Goodman, M. (1999). Menopausal symptoms. In C. Yarbro, M. Frogge, & M. Goodman (Eds). *Cancer symptom*

management (2nd ed., pp. 95-111). Sudbury, MA: Jones & Bartlett.

Hackley, B., & Rousseau, M. (2004). Managing menopausal symptoms after the Women's Health Initiative. *Journal of Midwifery & Women's Health, 49*, 87-95.

Hickey, M., Saunders, C., & Stuckey, B. (2005). Management of menopausal symptoms in patients with breast cancer: an evidence-based approach. *Lancet Oncology, 6*, 687-695.

Kendall, A., Dowsett, M., Folkerd, E., et al. (2006). Caution: Vaginal estradiol appears to be contraindicated in post-menopausal women on adjuvant aromatase inhibitors. *Annals of Oncology, 17*, 584-587.

Mom, C., Buijs, C., Willemse, P., et al. (2006). Hot flashes in breast cancer patients. *Critical Reviews in Oncology and Hematology, 57*, 63-77.

Thewes, B., Meiser, B., Taylor, A., et al. (2006). Fertility- and menopause-related information needs of younger women with a diagnosis of early breast cancer. *Journal of Clinical Oncology, 23*, 5155-5165.

Mucositis

*Kristin A. Cawley
and Laura M. Benson*

DEFINITION

- Commonly associated with chemotherapy, radiation therapy, and bone marrow transplantation
- Can occur anywhere along the digestive tract from the mouth to the anus.
- Occurs in 20%-40% of patients treated with chemotherapy alone and up to 50% of patients receiving combination radiation and chemotherapy.
- Nearly 100% of patients receiving chemotherapy and radiation therapy for the treatment of head and neck cancer and as many as 90% of patients undergoing bone marrow transplantation experience mucositis.
- The most debilitating symptom reported by cancer patients

PATHOPHYSIOLOGY AND CONTRIBUTING FACTORS

- Breakdown of rapidly dividing epithelial cells caused by chemotherapy and radiation

treatment, primarily in the gastrointestinal tract
- Previous history of mucositis
- Poor oral hygiene, prior dental disease
- Treatment regimen
- Ill fitting-dentures
- History of alcohol consumption and smoking

SIGNS AND SYMPTOMS

- Dry, cracked lips
- Pain and difficulty swallowing
- Ulcers or sores in the mouth, on gums and tongue; the sores may be reddish and may have white centers.
- Swelling
- Irritation
- Mucosal bleeding
- Sensitivity to hot and cold foods
- Xerostomia
- Infection
- Weight loss
- Dehydration

ASSESSMENT TOOLS

- Beck's Oral Examination Guide
- Eiler's Oral Assessment Guide
- Schubert et al.'s Oral Mucositis Index
- Sonis' Oral Mucositis Assessment Scale
- Common Toxicity Criteria Common Terminology Criteria for Adverse Events v3.0 (CTCAE)
- History and physical examination, clinical examination based on inspection of oral cavity
- Risk for mucositis
- Current oral hygiene and dental care
- Nutritional status
- Symptomatic functional assessment based on ability to swallow
- Pain, using 0-10 or categorical (none-mild-moderate-severe)

LABORATORY AND DIAGNOSTIC TESTS

- Complete blood cell count (CBC)
- Blood, urine, sputum culture

DIFFERENTIAL DIAGNOSES

- Pain
- Malnutrition
- Infection
- Dysphagia

- Anorexia
- Xerostomia
- Dehydration

INTERVENTIONS
- Treat underlying etiology.

Pharmacologic Interventions
- Palifermin (Kepivance)
- Bioadherent gel (Gelclair)
- Viscous lidocaine
- Opioid narcotics

Nonpharmacologic Interventions
- Nutritional
- Cryotherapy
- Salt and soda rinses

PATIENT TEACHING
- Dental evaluation before initiation of treatment
- Cleaning:
  - Brush with a soft toothbrush.
  - Continue despite thrombocytopenia or neutropenia unless develop uncontrolled bleeding.
  - Fluoride toothpaste
- Flossing
  - Patients who floss regularly should continue unless there is uncontrolled bleeding, platelets <20,000, or absolute neutrophil count (ANC) <1.
- Rinsing:
  - Normal saline solution (NS), sodium bicarbonate ($NaHCO_3$), $NS/NaHCO_3$, water
  - Nonalcoholic unsweetened mouthwash
  - Rinse every 4-6 hours, increasing to every 2 hours as needed for comfort (swish/gargle 15-30 seconds).
- Dental appliances should be left out as much as possible once mucous membranes become irritated.
- Report any fever of 100.5° F or greater.
- Report any pain unrelieved with pain medication.
- Dietary modifications

FOLLOW-UP
- Assess for increased risk of mucositis with continuing treatments.
- Assess for pain unrelieved with pain medication.
- Reinforce importance of communication to physician and nurse.

RESOURCES
- Joanna Briggs Institute. Prevention and treatment of oral mucositis in cancer patients: http://www.joannabriggs.edu.au/best_practice/bp5.php
- Manage mucositis professional Web site: www.managemucositis.com
- National Cancer Institute. Oral complications of chemotherapy and head/neck radiation (PDQ): http://www.cancer.gov/cancertopics/pdq/supportivecare/oralcomplications/healthprofessional
- National Institute of Dental and Craniofacial Research. Oral Complications of Cancer Treatment: What the Oncology Team Can Do: http://www.nidcr.nih.gov/NR/rdonlyres/285A30FC-F618-47D8-A840-756BB494A019/4580/WhatTheOncologyTeamCanDo.pdf
- Oncology Nursing Society. Measuring Oncology Nursing-Sensitive Patient Outcomes: Evidence-Based Summary Review (Mucositis): http://onsopcontent.ons.org/toolkits/evidence/Clinical/pdf/MucositisSummary.pdf

BIBLIOGRAPHY

Clarkson, J. E., Worthington, H. V., & Eden, O. B. (2005). Interventions for preventing oral mucositis for patients with cancer receiving treatment [review]. *The Cochrane Collaboration*, Issue 1.

Eilers, J. E. (2004). Nursing interventions and supportive care for the prevention and treatment of oral mucositis associated with cancer treatment. *Oncology Nursing Forum, 31*, 13-23.

Epstein, J. B., & Schubert, M. M. (2003) Oropharyngeal mucositis in cancer therapy: review of pathogenesis, diagnosis, and management. *Oncology, 17*, 1767-1779.

Keefe, D. M., Schubert, M. M., Elting, L. S., et al. (2007). Updated clinical practice guidelines for the prevention and treatment of mucositis. *Cancer, 109*, 820-831.

McGuire, D. B. (2003). Barriers and strategies in implementation of oral care standards for cancer patients. *Support Care Cancer, 11*, 435-441.

Plevova, P. (1999). Prevention and treatment of chemotherapy- and radiotherapy-induced oral mucositis: a review. *Oral Oncology, 35*, 453-470.

Rubenstein, E. B., Peterson, D. E., Schubert, M., et al. (2004). Clinical practice guidelines for the prevention and treatment of cancer therapy-induced oral and gastrointestinal mucositis. *Cancer, 100*(9 Suppl), 2026-2046.

Silverman, S. (2007). Diagnosis and management of oral mucositis. *Journal of Supportive Oncology, 5*(2 suppl 1), 13-21.

Sonis, S. T., Elting, L. S., Keefe, D., et al. (2004). Perspectives on cancer therapy-induced mucosal injury: pathogenesis, measurement, epidemiology, and consequences for patients. *Cancer, 100*(9 Suppl), 1995-2025.

Stricker, C. T., & Sullivan, J. (2003). Evidence-based oncology oral care clinical practice guidelines: development, implementation, and evaluation. *Clinical Journal of Oncology Nursing, 7*, 222-227.

Sutherland, S. E., & Browman, G. P. (2001). Prophylaxis of oral mucositis in irradiated head and neck cancer patients: a proposed classification scheme of interventions and meta-analysis of randomized controlled trials. *International Journal of Radiation Oncology, Biology, Physics, 49*, 917-930.

Worthington, H. V., Clarkson, J. E., & Eden, O. B. (2004). Interventions for treating oral mucositis for patients with cancer receiving treatment. *The Cochrane Database of Systematic Reviews*, Issue 2.

Nausea and Vomiting

Carolyn Grande

DEFINITION
Nausea

- A sensation of profound revulsion to food or of impending vomiting. A feeling of being sick at the stomach
- Can be classified as anticipatory, acute, delayed, or breakthrough
- Severity can lead to poor compliance with treatment regimen and decreased quality of life.

Vomiting

- Forceful expulsion of gastric contents from stomach through the mouth

Symptom Management

- Eject matter from stomach through the mouth
- Patterns of nausea/vomiting
  - *Anticipatory:* a conditioned response that occurs before chemotherapy
  - *Acute:* onset occurs within a few minutes to several hours after drug administration and usually resolves within 24 hours
  - *Delayed:* onset develops more than 24 hours after chemotherapy. Achieves maximum intensity 48 to 72 hours after chemotherapy and can last up to 7 days
  - *Breakthrough:* occurs if preventive regimen fails

PATHOPHYSIOLOGY AND CONTRIBUTING FACTORS

- Activation of afferent impulses to the vomiting center (medulla) in the brain from the chemotherapy trigger zone (CTZ), peripheral mechanisms in the gastrointestinal (GI) tract; vestibular mechanisms; cortical mechanisms or alterations of taste and smell
- Efferent impulses sent from the medulla (vomiting center) set a series of events in motion, leading to vomiting. Several neuroreceptors are involved in emesis, most notably serotonin (5-hydroxytryptamine [5-HT3]) and neurokinin-1 (NK-1). Anticipatory nausea and vomiting involves a psychological mechanism because the experience is not related to the administration of chemotherapy or radiation therapy.
- The exact mechanism of radiation-induced vomiting is not clear; however, it is believed that a peripheral mechanism in the GI tract or central mechanisms in the CTZ may contribute.
- Many contributing factors:
  - Underlying tumor
  - Treatment-related toxicity:
    - Surgery
    - Chemotherapy
    - Radiation therapy
    - Bone marrow transplantation

- Patient-specific factors:
  - Sex—women more susceptible
  - Age—younger patients more susceptible
  - Alcohol history—higher consumption correlates with lower incidence
  - Performance status—lower performance status correlates with higher incidence
  - History of morning sickness or motion sickness more susceptible
  - Level of chemotherapy emetogenicity: low, moderate, or high
  - Tumor burden: more susceptible as tumor burden increases
  - Combined-modality therapy: more susceptible than monotherapy
  - Dehydration increases incidence.
  - Comorbid conditions: anxiety, GI malignancies, intestinal obstruction, impaired liver or renal function, hypercalcemia, hepatitis, pancreatitis, peritonitis, cerebellar metastasis

SIGNS AND SYMPTOMS

- Ill feeling of the stomach
- Hypersalivation
- Diaphoresis
- Tachycardia
- Tachypnea

ASSESSMENT TOOLS

- Hallmark assessment tool is patient report.
- Other assessment information:
  - Physical examination including vital signs and weight
  - Laboratory data
  - Caregiver report
- U.S. Department of Health and Human Services, National Institutes of Health and National Cancer Institute Grading System for Nausea:
  - Grade 1: loss of appetite without alteration in eating habits
  - Grade 2: oral intake decreased without significant weight loss, dehydration, or malnutrition; intravenous (IV) fluids indicated for less than 24 hours

  - Grade 3: inadequate oral caloric or fluid intake; IV fluids, tube feedings, or total parenteral nutrition (TPN) indicated for 24 hours or longer
  - Grade 4: life-threatening consequences
  - Grade 5: death
- U.S. Department of Health and Human Services, National Institutes of Health and National Cancer Institute Grading System for Vomiting:
  - Grade 1: one episode in 24 hours
  - Grade 2: two to five episodes in 24 hours; IV fluids indicated for less than 24 hours
  - Grade 3: six episodes in 24 hours; IV fluids or TPN indicated for 24 hours or longer
  - Grade 4: life-threatening consequences
  - Grade 5: death

LABORATORY AND DIAGNOSTIC TESTS

- Laboratory tests to assess for primary cause or secondary complications from persistent nausea and vomiting. Diagnostic tests performed to rule out differential diagnosis. There are no diagnostic tests for nausea/vomiting.
- Complete blood cell count (CBC), electrolyte panel including sodium, potassium, chloride; carbon dioxide; blood urea nitrogen (BUN) and creatinine, liver function tests
- Flat plate of the abdomen
- Obstruction series

DIFFERENTIAL DIAGNOSES

- Chemotherapy induced
- Radiation therapy induced
- Underlying disease
- Intestinal obstruction
- Cholecystitis
- Cirrhosis
- Diverticulitis
- Gastritis
- Hepatitis
- Migraine headache
- Pancreatitis
- Medications that cause nausea

INTERVENTIONS

- Prevention of nausea and vomiting is the goal.

Pharmacologic Interventions

- Anticipatory nausea or vomiting: alprazolam (Xanax) 0.5-2 mg orally, three times a day, starting the night before treatment, or lorazepam (Ativan) 0.5-2 mg orally the night before treatment and the morning of treatment
- Acute and delayed nausea or vomiting: highly emetogenic chemotherapy
  - Before chemotherapy:
    - NK1 receptor antagonist—aprepitant (Emend) 125 mg orally, day 1, 80 mg orally daily on days 2 and 3, *and*
    - Corticosteroid—dexamethasone (Decadron) 12 mg orally or IV on day 1, 8 mg orally or IV on days 2 and 3, *and*
    - 5-HT3 receptor antagonist (select one)
      - Dolasetron (Anzemet) 100 mg orally or IV on day 1, *or*
      - Granisetron (Kytril) 2 mg orally, 1 mg orally twice a day, or 1 mg IV on day 1, *or*
      - Ondansetron (Zofran) 16-24 mg orally or 8-12 mg IV on day 1, *or*
      - Palonosetron (Aloxi) 0.25 mg IV on day 1, *and*
      - Benzodiazepine-lorazepam 0.5-2 mg orally, IV, or sublingually (SL) every 4-6 hours on days 1-4 (may or may not be given because of sedating effects)
- Acute and delayed nausea/vomiting: moderately emetogenic chemotherapy
  - Before chemotherapy:
    - Aprepitant 125 mg orally, day 1, 80 mg orally daily on days 2 and 3, *and*
    - Dexamethasone 12 mg orally or IV on day 1, 8 mg orally or IV days 2 and 3, *and one of the following 5-HT3 receptor antagonists*

- Dolasetron 100 mg orally or IV on day 1, *or*
- Granisetron 2 mg orally, 1 mg orally BID or 1 mg IV on day 1, *or*
- Ondansetron 16-24 mg orally or 8-12 mg IV on day 1, *or*
- Palonosetron 0.25 mg IV on day 1, *and*
- Lorazepam 0.5-2 mg orally, IV, SL every 4-6 hours on days 1-4 (may or may not be given because of sedating effects)
  - On treatment days 2-4:
    - Aprepitant 80 mg orally on days 2 and 3 only if used on day 1, *and*
    - Dexamethasone 8 mg orally or IV daily or 4 mg orally or IV twice daily with or without lorazepam 0.5-2 mg orally, IV, or SL every 4-6 hours (may or may not be given because of sedating effects), *or*
    - Dexamethasone 8 mg orally or IV daily or 4 mg orally or IV twice daily (preferred), *or select one of the following 5-HT3 receptor antagonists:*
      - Dolasetron 100 mg orally or IV *or*
      - Granisetron 1-2 mg orally daily, 1 mg orally twice daily or 1 mg IV, *or*
      - Ondansetron 8 mg orally twice daily, 16 mg orally daily, or 8 mg IV *or*
      - Substituted benzamide-metoclopramide (Reglan) 0.5 mg/kg orally or IV every 6 hours or 20 mg orally four times a day with or without diphenhydramine (Benadryl) 25-50 mg orally or IV every 4-6 hours as needed
- Acute and delayed nausea/vomiting: low emetogenic chemotherapy
  - No antiemetic agent, *or*
  - Dexamethasone 12 mg orally or IV on day of treatment, *or*
  - Phenothiazine-prochlorperazine (Compazine) 10 mg orally

---

or IV every 4-6 hours or 15-mg spansule every 8-12 hours, *or*
  - Metoclopramide 20-40 mg orally every 4-6 hours or 1-2 mg/kg every 3-4 hours with or without diphenhydramine 25-50 mg orally or IV every 4-6 hours as needed, *or*
  - Lorazepam 0.5-2 mg orally, IV, or SL every 4-6 hours (may or may not be given because of sedating effects)
- Breakthrough nausea or vomiting:
  - General rule is to consider administering an additional agent from a different class not previously given.
  - Corticosteroid: dexamethasone 12 mg orally or IV daily, *or select one of the following 5-HT3 receptor antagonists:*
    - 5-HT3 receptor antagonist: dolasetron 100 mg orally or IV, *or*
    - Granisetron 1-2 mg orally daily, 1 mg orally twice daily, or 1 mg IV, *or*
    - Ondansetron 8 mg orally or IV daily, *or*
    - Phenothiazine-prochlorperazine 25 mg suppository every 12 hours, 10 mg orally or IV every 4-6 hours, or 15-mg spansule every 8-12 hours, *or*
    - Substituted benzamide: metoclopramide 20-40 mg orally every 4-6 hours or 1-2 mg/kg every 3-4 hours with or without diphenhydramine 25-50 mg orally or IV every 4-6 hours as needed, *or*
    - Butyrophenones: haloperidol (Haldol) 1-2 mg orally every 4-6 hours or 1-3 mg IV every 4-6 hours, *or*
    - Benzodiazepine: lorazepam 0.5-2 mg orally every 4-6 hours, *or*
    - Cannabinoid: dronabinol (Marinol) 5-10 mg orally every 3-6 hours, *or*

- Antipsychotic: olanzapine (Zyprexa) 2.5-5 mg orally twice daily as needed

Nonpharmacologic Interventions

- Behavioral management
- Acupuncture/acupressure
- Guided imagery/progressive muscle relaxation
- Music therapy

PATIENT TEACHING

- Take antinausea medication on a timed schedule before nausea begins.
- Eat small, frequent meals. Nausea is more likely to occur on an empty stomach.
- Avoid spicy, greasy, or fatty foods and overly sweet foods.
- Cold foods, salty foods, dry crackers, and dry toast may be more tolerable.
- Consider diversionary activities (i.e., music therapy, relaxation techniques).
- Avoid unpleasant odors.

FOLLOW-UP

- If vomiting is severe, restrict diet to clear liquids and call your doctor or nurse.
- If emesis is red or brown (coffee-ground appearance), recall foods eaten and call your doctor or nurse.

RESOURCES

- National Comprehensive Cancer Network. NCCN clinical practice guidelines in oncology-antiemesis: http://www.NCCN.org
- Tipton, J., McDaniel, R., Barbour, L., et al. (2006). *What interventions are effective in preventing and treating chemotherapy-induced nausea and vomiting (CINV)?* [Brochure: PEP card]. Pittsburgh: Oncology Nursing Society.

BIBLIOGRAPHY

American Society of Health System Pharmacists Commission on Therapeutics. (1999). ASHP therapeutic guidelines on the pharmacologic management of nausea and vomiting in adult and pediatric patients receiving chemotherapy or radiation therapy or undergoing surgery. *American Journal of Health-System Pharmacy, 56*, 729-764.

Berger, A. M., & Clark-Snow, R. A. (2001). Adverse effects of treatment. In V. T. DeVita Jr., S. Hellman, & S.A. Rosenberg (Eds.). *Cancer principles and practice in oncology* (pp. 2869-2879). Philadelphia: Lippincott Williams & Wilkins.

Collins, K. B., & Thomas, D. J. (2004). Acupuncture and acupressure for the management of nausea and vomiting. *Journal of the American Academy of Nurse Practitioners, 16*, 76-80.

Dirckx, J. H. (Ed.) (1997). *Stedman's concise medical dictionary for the health professions* (3rd ed., pp. 582 and 953). Baltimore: Williams & Wilkins.

King, C. R. (1997). Nonpharmacologic management of chemotherapy-induced nausea and vomiting. *Oncology Nursing Forum, 24*(7 Suppl.), 41-48.

Kowalak, J. P., & Hughes, A. S. (Eds.) (2002). *Handbook of signs & symptoms* (2nd ed., pp. 404-406, 605-608). Philadelphia: Lippincott Williams & Wilkins.

Luebbert, K., Dahme, B., & Hasenbring, M. (2001). The effectiveness of relaxation training in reducing treatment-related symptoms and improving emotional adjustment in acute non-surgical cancer treatment: A meta-analytical review. *Psycho-Oncology, 10*, 490-502.

O'Bryant, C. L., Gonzales, J.A., & Bestul, D. (2004). *Guide to the prevention and management of nausea and vomiting in the oncology setting.* New York: McMahon.

Pain

Denice Economou

DEFINITION

- Pain is an unpleasant sensory and emotional experience associated with actual or potential tissue damage.
- One third of patients actively receiving treatment for their cancer and two thirds of patients with end-stage cancer have pain.
- Pain is whatever the person says it is, experienced whenever the person says it is.

PATHOPHYSIOLOGY AND CONTRIBUTING FACTORS

- The basic causes of cancer pain are related to pain caused by the tumor, pain caused by the treatment for the cancer, and iatrogenic causes of pain unrelated to the cancer or its treatment.
- Somatosensory primary afferent fibers carry sensory information to the spinal cord; grouped on the basis of transduction properties of the individual nerve fibers.
- Noxious stimuli activate nociceptors Ad and C fibers in the peripheral nerve.
- Nociceptors are polymodal and respond to mechanical, thermal, and chemical stimuli, which leads to the action potentials, which are conducted by the axon to the dorsal horn of the spinal cord and brainstem.
- Transmission of acute pain involves the activation of sensory receptors on peripheral C-fibers (nociceptors).
- Once tissue damage and inflammation occur, prostaglandins, bradykinin, histamine, adenosine triphosphate (ATP), and acetylcholine act on excitatory receptors on the sensory ending and play a major role in sensitization and activation.
- Impaired nerve fibers either at the site of nerve injury or in the cell body of impaired fibers in the dorsal root ganglia have ectopic discharges that are characterized as neuropathic pain.
- Multiple factors come together to determine the patient's perception of pain and his or her ability to get relief from the pain. Gender, culture, and social and societal input affects a patient's pain response.
- Major barriers to pain management continue to be related to the patient's belief in myths associated with the management of pain and include fear of tolerance, addiction, and dependence.
  - *Tolerance:* the physiological response of receptors being continually exposed to the opioids in circulation and the need to increase the dose of medication in an effort to

achieve the same level of pain relief. In cancer patients, tolerance is not an issue because studies have shown the primary reason for oncology patients to need an increase in dose is related to a change in the source of their pain (e.g., metastasis, bone fractures, impingement of nerves from growing tumors). Oncology patients on stable doses of opioids over time can reduce the dose of their medications and achieve the same level of pain relief.

○ *Addiction:* a neurobehavioral syndrome with genetic and environmental influences that result in psychological dependence on the use of substances for their psychic effects. Characterized by compulsive use despite harm. This describes the state of addiction and identifies the contributing factors that play a role in a person's propensity to become addicted to the opioids. Using opioids to relieve pain cannot in and of itself lead to a person becoming addicted to the medications.

○ *Physiological dependence:* the symptoms of withdrawal are experienced when opioids are discontinued immediately without tapering of the medication. The experience of dependence does not signify addiction. The receptors are used to being bathed in this medication; therefore, abrupt withdrawal leads to acute symptoms.

SIGNS AND SYMPTOMS

- There is no true objective test to establish a patient's experience of pain.
- Verbal report of pain is the **single most accurate tool** in identifying pain.
- Subjective signs may include the following:
  ○ Facial grimacing
  ○ Furrowed brow

○ Contracted muscles
○ Moaning
○ Guarding or decreased movement
○ Agitation or restlessness
- Cognitive responses: withdrawn behaviors, inability to concentrate, or irritability
- Associated symptoms may include lack of appetite, depressed mood, and sleep disorders.

ASSESSMENT TOOLS

- Visual analog scale (VAS) may be used with anchor words or numbers (0-10).
- Verbal scale
- Faces (Wong-Baker or Revised Faces Scale [RFS])
- Pain assessment is the most important intervention for the successful management of pain.
  ○ *Pain history:* past experience with pain or pain medications. Include the family or caregiver when assessing pain (e.g., the patient may be stoic and may underreport the pain or family may overrate their loved one's pain). What do they call the pain (e.g., discomfort, hurt)? Is this pain acute, meaning less than 1 to 3 months, or chronic, meaning pain that exists for longer than 1 to 3 months?
  ○ *Location:* where the patient reports pain. May have more than one site of pain. If the patient complains of pain all over, assess the emotional state of the patient for depression, anxiety, fear, or hopelessness.
  ○ *Intensity:* how does the patient rate the level of pain? The most common tool is the numerical rating scale that asks the patient to rate the pain on a 0-10 scale. The VAS is a 10-cm line where the patient marks on the line how intense the pain is and the line is measured. Zero is on the left end and convert the mark to a number from 0-10. Children over 3 years old and adults who

have difficulty using the 0-10 scale may use the faces scale.
  ○ *Description:* what words does the patient use to describe the pain: sharp, shooting, dull, aching? These are indicators to the potential source of pain.
- General sources of pain include the following:
  ○ *Myofascial:* pain in soft tissue or muscle. Usually can point to specific area of pain. Responds to heat/cold, massage, transcutaneous electrical nerve stimulation (TENS), nonopioids such as acetaminophen or nonsteroidal anti-inflammatory drugs (NSAIDs)
  ○ *Visceral:* pain related to the stretching of viscera surrounding organs. Characteristically vague in distribution and quality. Deep, dull, aching, squeezing can be associated with nausea, vomiting, and diaphoresis. Called referred pain when area that hurts is related to nerve distribution and not specific site. Feels like the pain travels. Opioids and adding additional nonopioids and nonpharmacologic approaches may be beneficial.
  ○ *Bone pain:* described as dull and achy. Associated with known bone metastasis or possible fracture resulting from cancer in that area. Pain is present with weight bearing or movement. Radiation therapy, steroids, opioids, calcitonin, bisphosphonates, NSAIDs are used to treat.
  ○ *Neuropathic:* injury to some element of the nervous system.
- Dysesthesia: burning, tingling, numbing, shooting.
- Hyperalgesia: increased response to normally painful stimulus. Allodynia: stimulus that is not normally painful (light touch). Treatments include antidepressants, antiseizure medications such as

gabapentin, Lyrica, membrane stabilizers.
- Aggravating and relieving factors: what makes the pain better or worse?
- Effect on physical or social functioning: does the pain affect the patient's ability to complete activities of daily living (ADLs) or to withdraw from normal activities?
- Medication history: what opioids has the patient tolerated in the past? This aids in treatment planning. If the patient has had pain relief with an opioid previously, will likely happen again.
- Physical examination:
  - Examine the site of pain and any patterns of referred pain.
  - Perform a neurologic examination as appropriate to the site of pain.
    - Head and neck pain: cranial nerve and funduscopic evaluation
    - Back and neck pain: examine patient for motor and sensory function in limbs, gross motor weakness or sensory deficit. Report deficits to physician immediately.
    - Bowel and bladder control: assess the patient's control of urinary and rectal sphincter control. Report deficits to physician immediately.
- Diagnostic evaluation: evaluate disease status as appropriate to cancer diagnosis and treatment, including tumor markers and radiological examinations (e.g., computed tomographic [CT] scan, bone scan, and magnetic resonance imaging [MRI] scan).
- Reassess pain frequently. Patient comfort is the primary indicator of successful pain management.

LABORATORY AND DIAGNOSTIC TESTS
- No blood test can identify the existence of pain. Laboratory testing would be important for documentation of possible disease

recurrence or metastasis (carcinoembryonic antigen [CEA] or cancer antigen [CA] 125 levels).
- Diagnostic testing will be related to location of pain and or known disease locations. These could include CT scans, positron emission tomographic (PET) scans, radiology examinations.

DIFFERENTIAL DIAGNOSES
- Rule out history of nonmalignant chronic pain
- Arthritis
- Neuralgia
- Chronic abdominal pain
- Fibromyalgia
- Headaches
- Low back pain
- Peripheral neuropathy related to diabetes
- Acquired immunodeficiency syndrome (AIDS)
- Phantom limb pain
- Reflex sympathetic dystrophy
- Sickle cell disease

INTERVENTIONS
- The World Health Organization offers a three-step analgesic ladder to help guide medication management of patients with newly diagnosed pain. Based on the level of pain a patient describes, the appropriate medication class combination can be initiated (on the basis of pain rating scale [VAS]).
  - 0-3 = mild pain, nonopioid/adjuvants
  - 4-7 = moderate pain, opioid/nonopioid/adjuvants
  - 8-10 = severe pain, opioid/ nonopioid/adjuvants/etc.

  NOTE: If patient's pain is rated as severe (8-10 on a 0-10 scale), the route of choice should be subcutaneous or intravenous to allow for rapid effect from the medication in a shorter amount of time.

Pharmacologic Interventions
- Compounded medications: acetaminophen with codeine (Tylenol #3), hydrocodone with acetaminophen (Vicodin),

---

> ## Types of Pharmacologic Interventions
>
> **OPIOIDS**
> Morphine, hydromorphone, oxycodone, hydrocodone, methadone, fentanyl (transdermal and transmucosal)
>
> **NONOPIOIDS**
> Aspirin, acetaminophen, nonsteroidal anti-inflammatory drugs (NSAIDs)
>
> **ADJUVANTS**
> Steroids, antidepressants, anticonvulsants, bisphosphonates, benzodiazepines

hydrocodone with acetaminophen (Norco), oxycodone with acetaminophen (Percocet), and hydrocodone with ibuprofen (Vicoprofen) offer combined opioid/nonopioid medications.
- Compounded opioids are dose limited because of milligrams of acetaminophen and NSAIDs. Recommend no more than 4,000 mg total dose of acetaminophen or NSAIDs in 24 hours.
- Pain medication must be titrated for effectiveness. Increasing or decreasing the dose for comfort is essential to achieve effective management of a patient's pain.
- If patients are not receiving effective management of their pain and are experiencing multiple side effects related to their medication, opioid rotation may be necessary. Another opioid may provide more effective pain management with fewer side effects.
- If a patient becomes overly sedated from the medication and is experiencing respiratory distress, reversal of the opioid dose may be necessary. Dilute naloxone in 10 mL of normal saline solution and titrate until alertness and respirations are improved.
- Anesthesia consultation for management with appropriate pain blocks
- Radiopharmaceuticals for bone pain when appropriate

- Spinal infusion of medications for pain relief (epidural/intrathecal)

Nonpharmacologic Interventions

- Radiation therapy for pain related to bone metastases
- Heat or cold compresses for musculoskeletal pain (myofascial)
- Surgical interventions
- Physical activity to maintain mobility and prevent secondary pain sources
- Cutaneous stimulation (TENS), massage, pressure, or vibration for pain associated with muscle tension or muscle spasm
- Relaxation or visualization techniques for distraction
- Acupuncture
- Community resources such as pastoral care and psychosocial care

PATIENT TEACHING

- Help the patient understand how to rate the pain and document the tool and words they use to describe their pain.
- The right dose is the one that relieves a patient's pain with minimal side effects.
- Anticonstipation medications should be started as soon as pain medication is started.
- Anticonstipation medications must include both a laxative and softener combination for relief of opioid-related constipation.

FOLLOW-UP

- Reassess patient's pain ratings daily or per shift if inpatient and no pain is reported.
- Reassess patient's comfort level 30 minutes after an intravenous or subcutaneous injection and 1 hour after oral medications. If pain is not improved, the physician or advanced practice nurse must be notified to increase or change management plan as necessary.
- Documentation is the most important follow-up intervention. Communicating patient's medication regimen and response can prevent patients from suffering needlessly.

RESOURCES

- Pain Medicine and Palliative Care at Beth Israel NY: www.stoppain.org
- Pain Resource Center at City of Hope: http://prc.coh.org
- People Living with Cancer: www.PLWC.org

BIBLIOGRAPHY

Agency for Health Care Policy & Research. (1994). *Clinical practice guidelines: Management of cancer pain.* Rockville, MD: AHCPR publication #94-0592.

American Pain Society. (2003). *Principles of analgesic use in the treatment of acute pain and cancer pain* (5th ed.). Glenview, IL: American Pain Society.

Fink, R., & Gates, R. (2006). Pain assessment. In Ferrell, B., & Coyle, N. (Eds.). *Oxford textbook of palliative nursing care* (pp. 97-125). New York: Oxford University Press.

Flor, H., Fyrich, T., & Turk, D. C. (1992). Efficacy of multidisciplinary pain treatment centers: A meta-analytic review. *Pain, 49,* 221-230.

McCaffery, M., & Pasero, C. (1999). *Pain clinical manual* (2nd ed.). St. Louis: Mosby.

Miaskowski, C., Zimmer, E. F., Barrett, K. M., et al. (1997). Differences in patients; and family caregivers' perceptions of the pain experience influence patient and caregiver outcomes. *Pain, 72,* 217-226.

Potter, J., & Higginson, I. J. (2004). Pain experienced by lung cancer patients: A review of prevalence, causes and pathophysiology. *Lung Cancer, 43,* 247-257.

Redinbaugh, E. M., Baum, A., DeMoss, C., et al. (2002). Factors associated with the accuracy of family caregiver estimates of patient pain. *Journal of Pain and Symptom Management, 23,* 31-38.

Schaible, H. G., & Richter, F. (2004). Pathophysiology of pain. *Langenbeck's Archives of Surgery, 389,* 237-243.

Simpson, K. H., & Budd, K. (Eds.) (2000). *Cancer pain management? A comprehensive approach.* New York: Oxford University Press.

Wong, D. L., Hockenberry, M., Wilson, D., et al. (2001). *Wong's essentials of pediatric nursing* (6th ed., p. 1301). St Louis: Mosby.

Peripheral Neuropathy

Carol S. Blecher

DEFINITION

- A disorder of the motor, sensory, and autonomic neurons that lead from the skin, joints, and muscles of the face, arms, legs, and torso to the central nervous system.
- Causes a lack of communication between the brain and the periphery
- Characterized by symptoms of pain and numbness

PATHOPHYSIOLOGY AND CONTRIBUTING FACTORS

- Direct damage to the neurons
- Chemotherapy-induced peripheral neuropathy is caused by damage to the nerve fibers through demyelinization of the large fiber sensory nerves (cisplatinum), microtubule inhibition resulting in axonal degeneration (vinca alkaloids), or axonal degeneration and demyelination (taxanes).
- Tumor pressing on the nerves
- Many contributing factors, including:
  - Alcohol abuse
  - Diabetes mellitus
  - Nutritional imbalance
  - Human immunodeficiency virus (HIV) infection/ acquired immunodeficiency syndrome (AIDS)
  - Hypothyroidism
  - Arthrosclerosis/ischemic disease
  - Vitamin B_{12} deficiency
  - Concurrent neuropathic medication (isoniazid, gentamicin, ciprofloxacin hydrochloride, phenytoin)
  - Treatment-related toxicity
    - Radiation
    - Phantom limb pain
    - Postherpetic neuralgia

Symptom Management

SIGNS AND SYMPTOMS

- Pain, which may be described as burning, sharp, stabbing, or an electric type of pain
- Numbness or tingling and loss of feeling
- A perception of wearing a sock or glove when there is none present
- Muscle weakness and loss of dexterity/coordination
- Extreme sensitivity to touch

ASSESSMENT TOOLS

- Sensory, motor, autonomic, and cranial nerve functions
- History, including risk factors for the development of neuropathy such as diabetes or alcoholism
- Any concomitant medications that cause neuropathy
- Symptom assessment should include onset, intensity, location, quality, intermittent or constant, alleviating and aggravating factors, accompanying symptoms, impact on ability to perform activities of daily living (ADLs) and quality of life.
- Physical examination should include monitoring for orthostatic hypotension, cranial nerve examination, assessment of motor function, reflexes, and sensory function
- Common terminology criteria (CTC) for adverse events:
  ○ Neuropathy, motor
    - Grade 1—asymptomatic; weakness on examination/ testing only
    - Grade 2—symptomatic weakness interfering with function, but not interfering with ADLs
    - Grade 3—weakness interfering with ADLs, bracing or assistance needed to walk (e.g., cane or walker indicated)
    - Grade 4—life threatening, disabling (e. g., paralysis)
    - Grade 5—death
  ○ Neuropathy, sensory
    - Grade 1—asymptomatic: loss of deep tendon reflexes or paresthesias (including tingling), but not interfering with function
    - Grade 2—sensory alteration or paresthesia (including tingling), interfering with functioning, but not interfering with ADLs
    - Grade 3—sensory alteration or paresthesia interfering with ADLs
    - Grade 4—disabling
    - Grade 5—death
- Toxicity grading scales
  ○ World Health Organization (WHO) toxicity criteria
  ○ Eastern Cooperative Oncology Group (ECOG)
  ○ National Cancer Institute of Canada (NCIC) Common Toxicity Criteria:
    - Sensory neuropathy
    - Motor neuropathy
  ○ Ajani Motor Neuropathy: tool for assessing chemotherapy-induced neuropathy in patients with cancer:
    - Sensory neuropathy
    - Motor neuropathy
  ○ Total neuropathy scale
    - Sensory symptoms
    - Motor symptoms
    - Pin sensibility
    - Vibration sensibility
    - Reflex
    - Autonomic symptoms
    - Vibration sensation
    - Sural amplitude: The sural nerve is the nerve leading from the tibial nerve that enervates the gastrocnemius and lateral portion of the leg. The conduction amplitude may be decreased in chemotherapy-induced peripheral neuropathies.
    - Peroneal amplitude: The peroneal nerve is the nerve leading from the sciatic nerve to the biceps and gastrocnemius muscles. The conduction amplitude may be decreased in chemotherapy-induced peripheral neuropathies.
  ○ National Cancer Institute (NCI) common terminology criteria for adverse events:
    - Neuropathy cranial
    - Neuropathy motor
    - Neuropathy sensory
  ○ Functional Assessment of Cancer Therapy/Gynecologic Oncology Group— Neurotoxicity (FACT/GOG-Ntx)
  ○ Functional Assessment of Cancer Therapy—Taxane
  ○ Peripheral Neuropathy Scale

LABORATORY AND DIAGNOSTIC TESTS

- Nerve conduction studies to identify the severity and location of the peripheral neuropathy
- Electromyelogram (EMG) to evaluate axonal neuropathy and muscle atrophy related to the neuropathy
- Audiometry to assess hearing
- Nerve biopsy: a procedure in which a small portion of the nerve is removed to assess for abnormalities
- Blood screening for:
  ○ Diabetes
  ○ Vitamin deficiency
  ○ Lupus erythematosus
  ○ Lyme disease
  ○ Hepatitis

DIFFERENTIAL DIAGNOSES

- Motor neuron disease
- Disorders of the neuromuscular junction
- Myopathy
- Myelopathy
- Syringomyelia
- Dorsal column disorders
  ○ Tabes dorsalis
- Hysterical disorders

INTERVENTIONS
Pharmacologic Interventions

- Vitamin B_{12} supplements
- Over-the-counter pain relievers:
  ○ Acetaminophen
  ○ Nonsteroidal anti-inflammatory drugs (NSAIDs)
- Anticonvulsants
  ○ Phenytoin
  ○ Carbamazepine
  ○ Gabapentin

- Pregabalin (Lyrica)
- Lidocaine patches
- Tricyclic antidepressants
  - Amitriptyline (Elavil)
  - Nortriptyline (Pamelor)
  - Desipramine (Norpramin)
  - Imipramine (Tofranil)
- Opioid analgesics

Nonpharmacologic Interventions

- Treatment of the underlying disease
- Physical therapy
- Massage
- Exercise
- Occupational therapy
- Transcutaneous electrical nerve stimulation (TENS)
- Biofeedback
- Acupuncture
- Hypnosis
- Relaxation techniques
- Support groups
- Safety measures
  - Orthotics
  - Ergonomic chairs
  - Braces
  - Splints
  - Positioning
  - Adequate lighting
  - Rails or other appliances to promote safety
  - Removal of obstacles such as loose rugs
  - Bed frames to keep sheets off tender body parts

PATIENT TEACHING

- Help patients to describe their symptoms. Is it:
  - Pain
  - Numbness or tingling and loss of feeling
  - Feeling like you are wearing a sock or glove
  - Muscle weakness and loss of dexterity/coordination
  - Burning pain
  - Sharp stabbing or electric type of pain
  - Extreme sensitivity to touch
- Prevention
  - Avoid alcohol.
  - Increase intake of B vitamins.
  - Avoid repetitive activities that may place stress on a nerve such as golf, tennis, playing a

musical instrument, typing at a computer keyboard.

- Management
  - Controlling diabetes
  - Correction of vitamin deficiency
  - Relieving nerve pressure by eliminating the source of the pressure if possible or through surgical repair of the problem
  - Medications: pain relief medication following the World Health Organization (WHO) ladder, antiseizure medication, lidocaine patches, tricyclic antidepressants
  - Therapies: TENS, biofeedback, acupuncture, hypnosis, relaxation techniques
- Safety
  - Orthotics
  - Ergonomic chairs
  - Braces
  - Splints
  - Positioning
  - Adequate lighting
  - Rails or other appliances to promote safety
  - Removal of obstacles such as loose rugs
  - Bed frames to keep sheets off tender body parts
- Coping skills
  - Setting priorities
  - Getting out of the house
  - Seeking and accepting support
- Mayo Clinic Patient Education Tool
- Follow-up
  - Physician
  - Physical therapy
  - Occupational therapy
  - Laboratory data for underlying disease state
  - Have the patient call the health care team immediately for tingling/weakness in hands or feet or for pain that is new.

RESOURCES

- After Shingles (Visiting Nurse Associations of America): www.aftershingles.com
- The Neuropathy Association: www.neuropathy.org
- Neuropathy Trust: www.neuropathy-trust.org

- National Institute of Neurological Disorders and Stroke: Peripheral Neuropathy Information: www.ninds.nih.gov/disorders/peripheralneuropathy/peripheralneuropathy.htm
- Pain Medicine and Palliative Care at Beth Israel NY: www.stoppain.org
- American Society of Clinical Oncology: People Living With Cancer: www.PLWC.org
- Nervous System Disturbances: http://www.plwc.org/nervoussystem
- Common Terminology Criteria for Adverse Events, Version 3, pp. 51 and 56: http://ctep.cancer.gov/forms/CTAEv3.pdf
- Mayo Clinic Patient Education Tool: http://www.mayoclinic.com/print/peripheralneuropathy/DS00131/DSECTION=all&MET

BIBLIOGRAPHY

Peripheral neuropathy. (2005). Retrieved August 27, 2006, from http://www.mayoclinic. com/print/peripheralneuropathy/DS00131/DSECTION=all&MET.

Peripheral neuropathy. (2006). Retrieved August 27, 2006, from http://www.cancersymptoms.org.

Measuring oncology nursing sensitive patient outcomes: evidence based summary. (2006). Retrieved August 27, 2006, from http://www.ons.org.

Medline Plus Medical Encyclopedia. (2004). *Peripheral neuropathy.* Retrieved August 27, 2006, from http://ww.nlm.nih.gov/medlineplus/ency/article/000593.htm.

Poncelet, M. D., & Noelle, A. (1998). An algorithm for the evaluation of peripheral neuropathy [electronic version]. *American Family Physician, 57,* 755-764.

Wilkes, G. M. (2004). Peripheral neuropathy. In C. H. Yarbro, M. H. Frogge, & M. Goodman (Eds.). *Cancer symptom management* (pp. 333-358). Sudbury, MA: Jones & Bartlett.

Symptom Management

Pleural Effusion

Laura S. Wood

DEFINITION

- Accumulation of excess fluid in the pleural space
- Associated with lung or breast cancer, lymphoma, occasionally with gastrointestinal, genitourinary, and carcinoma of unknown primary
- Classified as transudative (from a systemic problem) or exudative (from a local, pulmonary dysfunction).

PATHOPHYSIOLOGY AND CONTRIBUTING FACTORS

- Excess fluid is formed in or decreased fluid is removed from the pleural space resulting from imbalance between the osmotic and hydrostatic pressure controlling the secretion and reabsorption of pleural fluid.
- May be nonmalignant or malignant
- May result from direct tumor involvement or indirect sequelae of disease progression
- Superior vena cava syndrome (SVC)
- Pericardial constriction
- Obstruction of lymphatics by tumor
- Obstruction of pulmonary vessels by tumor
- Shedding of malignant cells into the pleural space

SIGNS AND SYMPTOMS

- Depend on the amount and rate of fluid accumulation
- Malignant pleural effusions usually develop slowly.
- Presenting symptoms:
  - Resting or exertional dyspnea
  - Cough
  - Chest discomfort
  - Weight loss
  - Anorexia
  - Malaise

ASSESSMENT TOOLS

- Patient history (both medical and oncologic)

- Physical examination
  - Vital signs
  - Lung auscultation and percussion
  - Assessment of peripheral capillary refill
- Common toxicity criteria (CTC version 3.0):
  - Grade 1 (mild)
  - Grade 2 (moderate)
  - Grade 3 (severe)
  - Grade 4 (life threatening)

LABORATORY AND DIAGNOSTIC TESTS

- Resting and ambulatory pulse oximetry
- Chest x-ray film
- Chest computed tomographic (CT) scan
- Ventilation-perfusion scan (VQ scan) to rule out pulmonary emboli
- Arterial blood gases
- Cytological analysis of pleural fluid obtained from thoracentesis procedure

DIFFERENTIAL DIAGNOSES

- Congestive heart failure
- Nephrotic syndrome
- Cirrhosis
- Infection
- Malignancy
- Hemothorax
- Pulmonary embolism
- Pancreatitis

INTERVENTIONS
Pharmacologic Interventions

- Diuretics if clinically appropriate

Nonpharmacologic Interventions

- Oxygen therapy if clinically appropriate
- Thoracentesis procedure
- Chest tube placement for drainage
- Pleurx catheter
- Talc or chemical pleurodesis procedure for large or recurrent pleural effusions
- External beam radiation therapy
- Pleuroperitoneal shunt

PATIENT TEACHING

- Assessment and diagnosis of pleural effusion

- Information about procedures
- Treatment plan
- Follow-up plan for early diagnosis and intervention for recurrent pleural effusions

FOLLOW-UP

- Patient and family will need support and education to help them through the effects of this symptom. It should be clear when the patient or family needs to contact the physician, such as if dyspnea occurs as a result of the effusion.

RESOURCES

- Chemo Care (The Cleveland Clinic Foundation): www.chemocare.com
- Oncology Nursing Society: www.cancersymptoms.org
- Common Terminology Criteria for Adverse Events, Version 3, page 49: http://ctep.cancer.gov/forms/CTCAEv3.pdf

BIBLIOGRAPHY

Brubacher, S., & Gobel, B. H. (2003). Use of the Pleurx pleural catheter for the management of malignant pleural effusions. *Clinical Journal of Oncology Nursing, 7*, 35-38.

Cope, D. G. (2005). Malignant effusion and edema. In Yarbro, Frogge, Goodman, et al. *Cancer nursing: principles and practice* (6th ed., pp. 825-840). Sudbury, MA: Jones & Bartlett.

Erasmus, J. J., Goodman, P. C., & Patz, E. F. (2000). Management of malignant pleural effusions and pneumothorax. *Radiologic Clinics of North America 38*, 375-383.

Huether, S. F., & McCance, K. L. (2004). *Understanding pathophysiology* (3rd ed.). St. Louis: Mosby.

Shuey, K., & Payne, Y. (2005). Malignant pleural effusion. *Clinical Journal of Oncology Nursing, 9*, 529-532.

Spiegler, P. A., Hurewitz, A. N., & Groth, M. L. (2003). Rapid pleurodesis for malignant pleural effusions. *Chest, 123*, 1895-1898.

Pruritus

Denice Economou

DEFINITION

- Pruritus refers to the pathological condition that is a stimulus for the sensory discomfort, and itching is a symptom related to localized and systemic diseases.
- Itching can affect patients on many different levels.
- Itching is subjective and affects patients' quality of life in all domains.
- Words used to describe itching include stinging, pins and needles, tickle, crawling sensation, and pain.

PATHOPHYSIOLOGY AND CONTRIBUTING FACTORS

- Pruritus begins in the free nerve endings in the epidermis and dermis and is transmitted through C fibers to the dorsal horn of the spinal cord and to the cerebral cortex by the spinothalamic tract.
- A spinal reflex response, scratching, is as innate as a deep tendon reflex.
- Itching most commonly occurs in skin and is exacerbated by skin inflammation, dry or hot weather conditions, sunburn, skin vasodilation, and psychological stressors.
- Chemical causes include caustic substances and perfumes and cleaning products.
- Repeated scratching itself can promote itching.

SIGNS AND SYMPTOMS

- Occurs when the nerves in the skin react to the release of chemicals such as histamine. The signals from these nerves are processed in the brain and perceived as itching.
- What makes it better or worse? Applying heat may make it worse, whereas ice or cool cloths may have some relief. Hodgkin disease and myeloid metaplasia are two diseases where heat or hot showers worsen the itch. This may be the symptom that leads the patient to the physician for diagnosis.

ASSESSMENT TOOLS

- Assessment is aimed at identifying the cause.
- Assessment should include psychosocial and physical symptoms.
- Understanding the intensity of the discomfort or distress can be identified using the 0-10 rating system.
- Check the area for signs of secondary infection.
- Check family history for allergies, exposure to known infectious agents/insect bites, or other family members who may also be experiencing itching symptoms.
- Evaluate medication profile for potential causes including chemotherapy/biological medications.
- Physical examination:
  - Follow a systematic approach as in pain assessment.
  - Location of itch: general or specific site or pattern. This information may tell you whether this is related to fungal infection in skin creases, for instance, or suggest scabies mite infestation. Also assess whether the pattern of itch is following a dermatomal distribution, which may relate to a past herpes zoster infection.
  - Is there a rash related to the itch? A rash is usually not related to a systemic cause. Evaluate if "rash" is really skin irritation related to physical scratching of the site. Focal rash may be indicative of a contact sensitivity or infection.
  - Quality of the itch: is the itch relieved even briefly by scratching? Is it described as tickling sensation (usually associated with contact dermatitis) or burning/painful sensation (usually associated with herpes zoster)?
  - Chemotherapy drugs associated with itching or rash: asparaginase, cisplatin, carboplatin, cytarabine, etoposide, interferon alfa-2a and interferon alfa-2b, doxorubicin, melphalan, and daunorubicin. Gemcitabine is associated with perianal pruritus.
  - Thorough history of any new products being used, any recent travel, exposure to outdoor plants (poison oak or poison ivy), or pets in the home. Any new medications or use of over-the-counter herbals or vitamins.

LABORATORY AND DIAGNOSTIC TESTS

- Complete blood count (CBC), including a differential leukocyte count.
- Liver function tests (alkaline phosphatase, serum bilirubin)
- Renal function tests (blood urea nitrogen, creatinine)
- Thyroid panel (free thyroxine [FT_4], thyroid-stimulating hormone [TSH])
- Serum iron and ferritin
- Stool examination for occult blood, ova, and parasites
- Human immunodeficiency virus (HIV) testing
- Skin biopsy may be necessary (assess whether related to chemotherapy—biopsy may not be necessary).

DIFFERENTIAL DIAGNOSES

- Dry skin
- Hives
- Rash
- Eczema
- Psoriasis
- Chickenpox
- Insect bite
- Medications
- Hormonal changes
- Infestations of the skin with a parasite, such as scabies or head lice
- Allergic reactions
- Shingles

- Blood disorders, such as anemia, polycythemia, and multiple myeloma
- Kidney failure
- Liver disease, including hepatitis C and cirrhosis
- Thyroid disease
- Diabetes
- Acquired immunodeficiency syndrome (AIDS)

INTERVENTIONS

Managing pruritus requires multiple approaches to reduce the symptoms. Depending on the severity and cause, use of topical, systemic, and behavioral interventions may be necessary.

- Preventive treatment when possible. Prevent dry skin or skin breakdown.
- Topical treatments related to source of pruritus:
  - Xerosis (dry skin): hydrate the skin by soaking in a warm bath and then patting dry and applying an occlusive moisturizer to trap in the moisture.
  - Lotions should be alcohol and fragrance free (Aquaphor, Vanicream, Moisturel, and Eucerin or Cetaphil). If cost is an issue, cooking shortening such as Crisco can be used.
- Soothing oatmeal baths and the use of cold packs can be helpful.

Pharmacologic Interventions

- Systemic interventions to improve pruritus include:
  - Opioid antagonists (Narcan) for systemic or intraspinal opioid-associated itching
  - Systemic corticosteroids when itch is generalized and related to inflammatory conditions can be helpful, but long-term use is contraindicated and may increase preexisting pruritus.
  - Antihistamines are useful in itching associated with histamine-mediated causes such as hives. Unfortunately, the side effect of sedation may make its use less attractive. Using this approach at bedtime is most helpful.

- Local anesthetics such as mexiletine have been used in patients with intractable itching with relief.
- Antidepressants have been used with some relief when itching is related to neuropathic pain. (Doxepin may be most effective because it is most "antihistaminic.") Histamine 1 (H1) antagonist, antiserotonergic at 5-hydroxytryptamine (5-HT) 2 and 5-HT3 receptor, sites is associated with reducing itching.
- Topical lotions containing calamine and Benadryl as an antihistamine or menthol-containing ointments may also have a local anesthetic or cooling response that relieves the itch. Capsaicin cream applied four to five times per day can also be helpful. It reduces substance P, decreasing both pain and itching sensations.
- Antidepressant-compounded creams may decrease pain and itching by local inhibition of H1 and H2 receptors and antiserotonergic effects (doxepin, Zonalon).
- Topically applied corticosteroids can reduce the sensation of itch, but long-term use can cause secondary problems such as skin infections, acne, and thinning of the skin.
- Use the higher percent ointment or cream initially and decrease as itching improves. The choice of ointment depends on area to be covered and percent potency needed. Ranging from high to low potency includes Diprolene 0.05% and Topicort 0.25%, mid range Kenalog 0.1% and Valisone 0.1%. Low-potency preparations include hydrocortisone ointment 1%.
- Applying topical steroids to skin that has been hydrated will improve local absorption.
- Typical causes of itching include fungal infections such as *Candida albicans*, which is especially present in skin folds. Topical

antifungal medications such as nystatin, ketoconazole, and the newest group allylamine/benzalamine drugs can cure the infection and relieve the itch.
- Fungal infections not responding to topical antifungals may require systemic treatments.
- Tar products can be used to reduce inflammation and itching. These products can reduce the need for topical steroids in patients with chronic pruritus, but the smell and staining associated with these products make them less preferred than other products.

Nonpharmacologic Interventions

- Acupuncture can be helpful in reducing pruritus.
- Distraction and relaxation techniques may also reduce the sensation of itching.

PATIENT TEACHING

- Moisturize skin with lubricants frequently, especially after bathing.
- Avoid known irritants such as pet hair, cleaning products, and so forth.
- Wear loose-fitting cotton clothing.
- Drink plenty of fluids.
- Keep a humid and cool environment.
- Keep fingernails cut short to limit damage from scratching and wear soft mittens and socks at bedtime.
- Skin cleansing is important if skin breakdown has occurred related to scratching or open lesions. Skin cleansers must have a neutral pH. Dove, Oil of Olay, and Aveeno are some products that can be used.

RESOURCE

- Oncology Nursing Society: www.cancersymptoms.org

BIBLIOGRAPHY

Moses, S. (2003). Pruritus. *American Family Physician*, 68, 1135-1146.
Polovich, M., White, J. M., & Kelleher, L. O. (2005). Side effects of cancer therapy. In *Chemotherapy and biotherapy guidelines and recommendations for practice* (2nd ed., pp. 207-208). Pittsburgh: Oncology Nursing Press.
Rhiner, M., & Slatkin, N. E. (2005). Pruritus, fever, and sweats. In N. Coyle & B. Ferrell (Eds.). *The Oxford textbook*

of palliative nursing (2nd ed., pp. 345-354). New York: Oxford University Press.

Roebuck, H. L. (2006). For pruritus, combination therapy works best. The Nurse Practitioner, 31, 12-13.

Yarbro, C. H., & Seiz, A. M. (2003). Pruritus. In C. H Yarbro, M. H. Frogge, & M. Goodman (Eds). Cancer symptom management (3rd ed., pp. 97-110). Boston: Jones & Bartlett.

Seizures

Carol S. Blecher

DEFINITION

- Seizures may be defined as a change in neurological function caused by an overactivation of the cerebral neurons.

PATHOPHYSIOLOGY AND CONTRIBUTING FACTORS

- Seizures are a symptom of irritation of the central nervous system (CNS) that results in an abnormal discharge of neurons.
- Cerebral function is disturbed by electrical discharges that are synchronous, abnormal, and excessive.
- This abnormal discharge of neurons can cause an alteration of consciousness or any other cerebral cortical function.
- Classification is either focal or generalized, but all seizures are characterized by sudden involuntary contraction of groups of muscles.
- Causes:
  - Neuronal loss or scarring from surgery or head trauma
  - Primary brain cancer or metastatic brain tumors
  - Acquired immunodeficiency syndrome (AIDS) or a history of seizures
  - Metabolic disturbances such as syndrome of inappropriate antidiuretic hormone secretion (SIADH), hypoglycemia, hyponatremia, hypercalcemia, hypocalcemia, hypomagnesemia, renal or hepatic failure, alcohol or drug withdrawal

- Chemotherapeutic agents including busulfan, carmustine, cisplatin, cyclosporine, high-dose 5-fluorouracil (5-FU), ifosfamide, intrathecal methotrexate
- Types
  - Primary generalized seizures
    - Absence
    - Atypical absence
    - Myoclonic
    - Atonic
    - Tonic
    - Clonic
    - Tonic-clonic
  - Partial seizures: preceded by an aura.
    - Simple partial: characterized by focal activity with no loss of consciousness
    - Complex partial: characterized by loss of consciousness
    - Secondarily generalized
- Absence (petit mal): brief, characterized by no obvious motor symptoms
- Unclassified epileptic seizures characterized by abrupt onset, unconsciousness, involuntary motor activity, involuntary sensory activity, and incontinence. There is also a postictal state after the seizure that is characterized by somnolence or headache.

SIGNS AND SYMPTOMS

- Change in level of consciousness
- Aura before the event: an unusual feeling, smell, or sensation
- Change in muscle tone and movement
- Activity is involuntary and uncontrolled
- A postictal state after the seizure characterized by somnolence or headache
- No memory regarding the event

ASSESSMENT

- History, including diagnosis and cancer treatment, current medications, presenting symptoms, changes in activities of daily living (ADL), social history, family history, and history of recent infections

- Signs and symptoms, including clinical symptoms regarding the episode. May have to obtain this information from the individual who observed the event because the patient may have no memory of the seizure
- Neurological examination evaluating for automatism (repetitive movements), hyperreflexia, positive Babinski sign, localized neurological deficits
- Vital signs: orthostatic changes
- Skin examination for signs of intravenous (IV) drug abuse or trauma, including lacerations, bruises, and oral trauma
- National Cancer Institute (NCI) common toxicity criteria:
  - Grade 0: none
  - Grade 1: none
  - Grade 2: seizure is self-limited and consciousness is preserved
  - Grade 3: seizure in which consciousness is altered
  - Grade 4: Seizures of any type that are prolonged, repetitive, or difficult to control (e.g., status epilepticus, intractable epilepsy)
- Common terminology criteria for adverse events:
  - Grade 1: none
  - Grade 2: one brief generalized seizure, seizures well controlled by anticonvulsants, or infrequent focal motor seizures not interfering with ADLs
  - Grade 3: seizure in which consciousness is altered, poorly controlled seizure disorder with breakthrough generalized seizures despite medical intervention
  - Grade 4: seizures of any kind that are prolonged, repetitive, or difficult to control (e.g., status epilepticus, intractable epilepsy)
  - Grade 5: death

LABORATORY AND DIAGNOSTIC TESTS

- Complete blood cell count (CBC) to rule out thrombocytopenia, which can cause intracerebral bleeding

- Chemistries to assess for SIADH, hypoglycemia, hyponatremia, hypercalcemia, hypocalcemia, hypomagnesemia, renal or hepatic failure
- Pregnancy test for women of childbearing age; because anticonvulsives are pregnancy category D, they can cause harmful effects to the fetus.
- Drug screening for cocaine, crack cocaine, and heroin because these medications or their withdrawal can cause seizures
- Drug levels of current anticonvulsive medications
- Alcohol blood level
- Computed tomographic (CT) scan of the head to identify tumor, metastases, or head trauma
- Electroencephalogram (EEG) will differentiate seizure activity from psychogenic symptoms and motor activity caused by neuromuscular conditions.
- Lumbar puncture to assess infection (meningitis, abscess, toxoplasmosis) or meningeal carcinomatosis

DIFFERENTIAL DIAGNOSES
- Cerebrovascular event
- Tumor: primary brain tumor or metastatic disease
- Trauma
- Infectious meningitis, abscess, toxoplasmosis
- Migraine headache
- Alcohol withdrawal
- Drug toxicity: busulfan, carmustine, cisplatin, cyclosporine, high-dose 5-FU, ifosfamide, intrathecal methotrexate, cocaine, crack cocaine, and heroin
- Psychiatric disorders

INTERVENTIONS
Nonpharmacologic Interventions
- During an active seizure:
  - Secure airway
  - Obtain IV access
  - Protect from injury
  - Oxygen supplementation
  - Obtain blood work: blood sugar for hypoglycemia

- If patient has a history of seizures and is on antiseizure medications, monitor serum levels of anticonvulsants.
- If the seizure is caused by underlying metabolic disturbances, these should be corrected and any medications contributing to the conditions should be discontinued.
- If appropriate, transfer patient to the nearest emergency department.

Pharmacologic Interventions
- Lorazepam (Ativan)
- Diazepam (Valium)
- Midazolam (Versed)
- Valproic acid (Depakote)
- Carbamazepine (Tegretol)
- Phenytoin (Dilantin)
- Ethosuximide (Zarontin)
- Clonazepam (Klonopin)
- Phenobarbital
- Lamotrigine (Lamictal)
- Gabapentin (Neurontin)

PATIENT TEACHING
- Instructions should include the following:
  - Seizure precautions
  - Do not drive or operate dangerous machinery.
  - Report blurred vision, ataxia, or drowsiness caused by your anticonvulsive medications to your health care provider immediately.
  - Avoid alcohol while taking anticonvulsants.
  - Call your health care provider if:
    - This is a first-time seizure.
    - A seizure lasts more than 2 to 5 minutes.
    - The person does not awaken or have normal behavior after a seizure.
    - Another seizure starts soon after a seizure ends.
    - The person had a seizure in water.
    - The person is pregnant, injured, or has diabetes.
    - The person does not have a medical ID bracelet (instructions explaining what to do).

- There is anything different about this seizure compared with the person's usual seizures.
- Epilepsy Foundation of America
- MedlinePlus Patient Education Tools
- Ohio State University Patient Education Tool

FOLLOW-UP
- Monitor the patient's clinical state, seizure frequency, and serum anticonvulsant levels.
- CBC, chemistries, liver enzymes to assess for myelosuppression and monitor renal and hepatic function
- Patients who have a 2-year seizure-free period and no risk factors may be taken off the antiseizure medications. Patients with risk factors should be maintained on medication for 5 years.
- If the patient's disease is terminal, the seizure activity should be controlled with lorazepam or a barbiturate.
- Referrals should be made to a neurologist, a radiation oncologist, and an epilepsy center.

RESOURCES
- Common Terminology Criteria for Adverse Events: http://ctep.cancer.gov/forms/CTCAEv3.pdf
- Epilepsy Foundation of America: www.efa.org

BIBLIOGRAPHY
Kernich, C. A. (1998). Seizures. In Chernecky, C. C. (Ed.). *Advanced and critical care oncology nursing. Managing primary complications* (pp. 536-548). Philadelphia: W. B. Saunders.

MedlinePlus Medical Encyclopedia. *Convulsions.* Retrieved January 16, 2007, from http:// www.nlm.nih.gov/ medlineplus/ency/ article/000021.htm.

MedlinePlus Medical Encyclopedia. *Febrile seizure.* Retrieved July 27, 2007, from http://www.nlm. nih.gov/medlineplus/ency/article/000 980.htm.

MedlinePlus Medical Encyclopedia. *Generalized tonic-clonic seizure.* Retrieved February 8, 2007 from http://www.nlm.nih.gov/medlineplus/ency/article/000695. htm.

MedlinePlus Medical Encyclopedia. *Partial complex seizure.* Retrieved September 28, 2007, from http://www. nlm.nih.gov/medline plus/ency/article/ 000699.htm.

MedlinePlus Medical Encyclopedia. *Petit mal seizure.* Retrieved February 8, 2007, from http://www.nlm.nih.gov/medline-plus/ency/article/ 000696.htm.

Minchin, A.C. (2000). Seizures. In D. Camp-Sorrell & R. A. Hawkins (Eds.). *Clinical manual for the oncology advanced practice nurse* (pp. 775-781). Pittsburgh: Oncology Nursing Press.

Ohio State University patient education tool: epilepsy and seizures. Retrieved September 29, 2007, from http:// medicalcenter.osu.edu/patientcare/ healthinformation/dise asesandcondi-tions/nervous/seizures/.

Paice, J. A. (2001). Neurological distur-bances. In Ferrell, B. R., & Coyle, N. (Eds.). *Textbook of palliative nursing* (pp. 262-268). New York: Oxford University Press.

Wilkes, G. M. (2004). Increased intercranial pressure. In C. H. Yarbro, M. H. Frogge, & M. Goodman (Eds.). *Cancer symptom management* (pp. 374-385). Sudbury, MA: Jones & Bartlett.

Zielke, K. A. (2002). Seizures. In Kuebler, K. K., & Esper, P. (Eds.), *Palliative practices A-Z* (pp. 211-213). Pittsburgh: Oncology Nursing Society.

Sleep Disturbances

Wendy H. Vogel

DEFINITION

- Sleep disturbances include insomnia or hypersomnia.
  - *Insomnia* is the inability to sleep when needed and may include difficulty falling asleep, maintaining sleep, or early morning awakenings with difficulty resuming sleep.
  - *Hypersomnia* is the inability to maintain wakefulness when needed.
- Sleep disturbances are a common problem in oncology patients and can be transient, chronic, and recur-ring and can affect quality of life.

PATHOPHYSIOLOGY AND CONTRIBUTING FACTORS

- Sleep disturbances are common in oncology patients.
- The most common cause of insomnia is uncontrolled pain.

- Insomnia or hypersomnia can also occur because of use of certain medications, withdrawal from certain medications, anxiety, depression, hypoxia, urinary frequency, pruritus, endocrine disorders, hot flashes, restless legs, sleeping during the day, caffeine intake, change in environment, or psychological stress.
- Insomnia could also be an independent disorder with no known etiology, called primary insomnia.
- Cancer patients often complain of daytime sleepiness and night time insomnia.
- Sleep deprivation is linked to changes in mentation, such as a decline in cognitive function and behavioral changes.
- Studies have shown a decrease in certain immune functions associated with insomnia.
- There are two stages of sleep, non–rapid eye movement (NREM) sleep and rapid eye movement (REM) or dreaming sleep. Circadian factors control the wake and sleep patterns over a 24-hour period. NREM sleep, REM sleep, and circadian rhythms may be disrupted in oncology patients.
- The normal amount of sleep needed to maintain healthy functioning varies from 6-10 hours per night.
- Types:
  - Transient: less than 2 weeks
  - Short-term: between 2 and 4 weeks
  - Chronic: more than 4 weeks
- Incidence:
  - The incidence of sleep disturbances range from 25%-95% in oncology patients.
  - About 50% of these sleep disturbances are insomnias (in the general population, insomnia occurs in 30%-35% of people).
  - Sleep disturbances are more likely during the initial diagnosis, during cancer treatments, and at the end-of-life period.

- Up to 44% of patients continue to report insomnia several years after diagnosis and treatment.

SIGNS AND SYMPTOMS

- Inability to fall asleep/sleeping too much
- Awakenings in the night, early morning awakening and inability to return to sleep, difficulty staying asleep

ASSESSMENT TOOLS

- Assess the type of sleep disturbance that is present, onset, and duration.
- Knowing the patient's normal sleep habits will enable the health care provider to establish a baseline normal.
- Amount and timing of daily physical exercise
- Bed partner/family member's perceptions of sleep disturbance
- Bedtime/wake times
- Diet, caffeine, and alcohol intake
- Environmental conditions (lighting, noise, ventilation, bedding, temperature, positioning)
- Medication review
- Patient's belief about cause of sleep disturbance
- Presence of daytime napping
- Presleep routines (food and fluid intake, hygiene, stimulation)
- Total hours slept during a 24-hour period
- Assess for risk factors:
  - Active chemotherapy treatment
  - Chronic medical illness
  - Depression/anxiety
  - Distress of symptoms such as pain, nausea, diarrhea, etc.
  - Fatigue
  - Female sex
  - Lower educational level
  - Lower socioeconomic status
  - Menstruation
  - Older age
  - Perimenopause
  - Personal or family history of insomnia
  - Recent life stressors
  - Specific cancer types such as breast, colorectal, prostate, ovarian, lung, hematological, and malignant melanoma

Symptom Management

- ○ Unpleasant environment
- ○ Use of alcohol
- Assess for medications known to cause insomnia:
  - ○ Amphetamines
  - ○ Anticonvulsants
  - ○ Biologicals such as interferons, interleukins, and tumor necrosis factor
  - ○ Bronchodilators
  - ○ Caffeine
  - ○ Chemotherapy
  - ○ Corticosteroids
  - ○ Decongestants
  - ○ Dieting agents
  - ○ Hormonal agents
  - ○ Illicit drugs
  - ○ Long-term use of analgesic medications
  - ○ Monoamine oxidase inhibitors (MAOIs)
  - ○ Selective serotonin reuptake inhibitors (SSRIs)
  - ○ Theophyllines
- Physical examination:
  - ○ Neurological assessment
  - ○ Oropharyngeal examination, observing for anatomical obstruction

LABORATORY AND DIAGNOSTIC TESTS

- No standard quantitative criteria exist to diagnose insomnia.
- A sleep study (polysomnogram) may be useful in a primary sleep disorder such as narcolepsy or parasomnias. (Not indicated for evaluation of transient or chronic insomnia or insomnia associated with psychiatric disorders.)
- It is useful to determine cause factors for sleep disturbances, such as obstructive sleep apnea and periodic leg movements.
- A sleep journal may be helpful in obtaining the specific information noted in the assessment above.
- Underlying physical and emotional causes should be ruled out and treated as necessary. This could include obtaining a urinalysis and a complete blood cell count.

DIFFERENTIAL DIAGNOSES

- It is important to differentiate between a primary cause of sleep

disturbance such as narcolepsy or parasomnia from secondary causes of sleep disturbance.
- Cancer-related fatigue

INTERVENTIONS

- Rule out any physical or emotional causes of sleep disturbances. Management of these causes (such as uncontrolled pain or depression) may correct the sleep disturbance.

Pharmacologic Interventions

- For insomnia, benzodiazepines or sedative-hypnotics
- Medications should be closely monitored.
- Tolerance to short-acting benzodiazepines could occur in as little as 2 weeks, and these should be used intermittently and for as short a period as possible (ideally no more than 3-4 weeks).
- Tapering and then discontinuing the medication once a therapeutic point is reached should be considered.
- Pharmacotherapy is not recommended for chronic insomnia, except for a short-term period and only as an adjunct to other treatment, such as cognitive behavioral treatment (see table on page 391).
- Alternative treatments for insomnia:
  - ○ Melatonin
  - ○ Valerian root extract
- Treatment for hypersomnia:
  - ○ Psychostimulants such as methylphenidate or a cholinesterase inhibitor such as donepezil.
  - ○ Modafmil, a nonamphetamine stimulant may be considered. Use in small doses and give early in the day, and this may help in preventing daytime napping, thus improving insomnia as well.

Nonpharmacologic Interventions

- Review medications; adjust timing so that patient does not have to awaken to take medications. Ensure that medications such as

diuretics are taken no later than 3 PM.
- Instruct in good sleep hygiene (refer to Sleep Hygiene in Section Seven).
- Cognitive control techniques such as counting, refocusing, meditation, or guided imagery may assist in controlling racing thoughts or worries.
- Thought stopping is repeating the word "the" or "stop" every 3 seconds.
- Relaxation training including progressive muscle relaxation, biofeedback, yoga, or hypnosis.

PATIENT TEACHING

- Educate the patient on sleep hygiene (specific behaviors that promote good sleep). Refer to Section Seven for patient education sheet on sleep hygiene.
  - ○ Stay in the bed only during hours intended for sleep.
  - ○ Establish a routine wake and bedtime.
  - ○ Avoid stimulants such as caffeine.
  - ○ Refrain from exercising at least 6 hours before bedtime.
  - ○ Decrease or eliminate nighttime use of tobacco products.
  - ○ Determine the best sleep environment.
  - ○ Do not nap during the day, or limit naps to 20 minutes, avoiding all naps after 3 PM.
  - ○ Create a bedtime routine
  - ○ If not asleep within 15-20 minutes, get out of bed and do a nonstimulating activity until sleepy, then return to bed.
  - ○ Avoid heavy foods at bedtime.
  - ○ Keep a sleep log.
  - ○ Remove bedroom clock.

FOLLOW-UP

- As indicated to assess pharmacological success and as need for cognitive-behavioral training.

RESOURCES

- American Cancer Society: www.cancer.org

Pharmacologic Treatment for Short-Term Insomnia

Class	Drugs	Benefits	Complications
Benzodiazepines	Clonazepam Lorazepam Oxazepam	Class of choice for short-term treatment Useful in insomnia caused by anxiety or restless legs Useful in insomnia that is refractory to other treatments	Long-acting agents may have daytime drowsiness, dizziness, cognitive impairment. Short-acting agents may have tolerance and dependence issues, rebound insomnia, daytime anxiety.
Nonbenzodiazepines	Zaleplon Zolpidem Zopiclone	More receptor selectivity Fewer residual side effects the next day Do not lead to tolerance, less potential for abuse Quick onset of action	May cause amnesias, paresthesias, arthralgias, flu-like symptoms
Tricyclic antidepressants with sedative effects	Amitriptyline Doxepin Nortriptyline	Useful in depressed patients, or insomnia from neuropathic pain. High sedative effects	May cause dry mouth, somnolence, dizziness, constipation, palpitations
Second-generation antidepressants with sedative effects	Trazodone (low dose) Nefazodone Mirtazapine	Useful in depressed patients Mirtazapine can stimulate appetite and decrease nausea	May cause dry mouth, somnolence, dizziness, constipation
Antihistamines	Diphenhydramine Hydroxyzine	Useful for sedation, reducing nausea and vomiting	May cause daytime sedation and delirium, especially in elderly May cause constipation, urinary retention, and confusion

- American Insomnia Association: http://www.americaninsomniaass ociation.org/aboutaia.htm
- National Cancer Institute: www.cancer.gov
- Abramson Cancer Center of the University of Pennsylvania: Oncolink: www.oncolink.com

BIBLIOGRAPHY

Graci, G. (2005). Pathogenesis and management of cancer-related insomnia. *Supportive Oncology, 3*, 349-359.

Kua, H., Chiu, M., Liao, W., et al. (2006). Quality of sleep and related factors during chemotherapy in patients with stage I/II breast cancer. *Journal of the Formosan Medical Association, 105*, 64-69.

O'Donnell, J. (2004). Insomnia in cancer patients. *Clinical Cornerstone, 6*(suppl1D), S6-14.

Savard, J., Simard, S., Ivers, H., et al. (2005). Randomized study on the efficacy of cognitive-behavioral therapy for insomnia secondary to breast cancer, part I: immunologic effects. *Journal of Clinical Oncology, 23*, 6097-6106.

Savard, J., Simard, S., Ivers, H., et al. (2005). Randomized study on the efficacy of cognitive-behavioral therapy for insomnia secondary to breast cancer, part I: sleep and psychological effects. *Journal of Clinical Oncology, 23*, 6083-6096.

Yellen, S., & Dyonzak, J. (1999). Sleep disturbances. In C. Yarbro, M. Frogge, & M. Goodman (Eds.). *Cancer symptom management* (2nd ed., pp 161-180). Sudbury, MA: Jones & Bartlett.

Xerostomia

Kristin A. Cawley and Laura M. Benson

DEFINITION

- Abnormal dryness of the mouth from a lack of salivary secretion
- Ranges from mild, moderate, to severe
- Associated with cancer of the head and neck; complication associated with radiation therapy
- The most common complaint reported by cancer patients in quality of life (QOL) studies (95%), causing severe distress (89%)
- Often chronic, affecting quality of life

PATHOPHYSIOLOGY AND CONTRIBUTING FACTORS

- Radiation therapy to the head and neck damages blood vessels supplying salivary glands.
- Major and minor salivary glands become atrophic and fibrotic.
- Saliva consistency changes from thin and watery to thick, ropy, tenacious secretions.
- Damage depends on the total dose and volume of tissue irradiated.
- Surgical excision of head and neck tumors involving salivary glands
- Chemotherapy agents, such as adriamycin
- Pharmacological causes: anticholinergics, antidepressants, antihistamines, antihypertensives, diuretics, opiates, phenothiazines, sedatives
- Gastroesophageal reflux

SIGNS AND SYMPTOMS

- Dry mouth
- Dysphagia
- Gingival bleeding
- Ulcerations in the oral cavity
- Tenacious secretions
- Weight loss
- Increased frequency in expectorations
- Pain, mild to burning
- Taste alterations
- Impaired speech
- Infection
- Malnutrition
- Dehydration

ASSESSMENT TOOLS

- Common Toxicity Criteria Common Terminology Criteria for Adverse Events v3.0 (CTCAE)

- History and physical, clinical examination based on inspection of oral cavity
- Current oral hygiene and dental care
- Nutritional status
- Symptomatic functional assessment based on ability to swallow
- Pain, using 0-10 or categorical (none-mild-moderate-severe)

LABORATORY AND DIAGNOSTIC TESTS

- Complete blood cell count (CBC)
- Blood, urine, sputum culture
- Sialometry—the measurement of the rate of saliva production

DIFFERENTIAL DIAGNOSES

- Sjögren's syndrome
- Pain
- Malnutrition
- Infection
- Dysphagia
- Anorexia
- Mucositis
- Dehydration

INTERVENTIONS

- Treat underlying etiology.

Pharmacologic Interventions

- Artificial saliva
- Nonalcoholic mouthwashes
- Pilocarpine (Salagen)
- Amifostine (Ethyol)
- Viscous lidocaine
- Opioid narcotics

Nonpharmacologic Interventions

- Oral mouth care regimen
- Monitor nutritional status.
- Sugar-free candy and sugar-free gum
- Increase fluid intake during and between meals, such as water and nonacidic juices.
- Avoid eating dry foods.
- Avoid irritants such as tobacco, alcohol, carbonated beverages, caffeine, and spicy or acidic foods.

PATIENT TEACHING

- Have a comprehensive dental evaluation before treatment is initiated.
- Report any pain, tenderness, or burning sensations in the oral cavity.
- Practice oral care daily using fluoride treatments during radiation therapy; wait 30 minutes after to rinse, eat, or drink.
- Brush teeth three to four times daily.
- Floss daily with unwaxed dental floss.
- Rinse with nonalcoholic mouthwashes (Biotene).
- On completion of therapy, patients require dental follow-up every 3 to 4 months to monitor for oral complications because they can deteriorate rapidly in irradiated patients with head and neck cancer.
- Report any fever of 100.5° F or greater.
- Report any pain unrelieved with pain medication.
- Dietary modifications

FOLLOW-UP

- Assess patients' current oral intake and ability to maintain adequate hydration and nutrition.
- Assess for pain unrelieved with pain medication.
- Reinforce importance of communication to physician and nurse.

RESOURCES

- National Cancer Institute. Oral complications of chemotherapy and head/neck radiation (PDQ): http://www.cancer.gov/cancertopics/pdq/supportivecare/oralcomplications/healthprofessional
- National Institute of Dental and Craniofacial Research. Oral Complications of Cancer Treatment: What the Oncology Team Can Do: http://www.nidcr.nih.gov/NR/rdonlyres/285A30FC-F618-47D8-A84056BB494A019/4580/WhatTheOncologyTeamCanDo.pdf
- Oncology Nursing Society. Measuring Oncology Nursing-Sensitive Patient Outcomes: Evidence-Based Summary Review (Mucositis):http://onsopcontent.ons.org/toolkits/evidence/Clinical/pdf/MucositisSummary.pdf

BIBLIOGRAPHY

Bruce, S. D. (2004). Radiation-induced xerostomia: how dry is your patient? *Clinical Journal of Oncology Nursing*, 8, 61-67.

Dirix, P., Nuyts, S., & Van den Bogaert, W. (2006). Radiation-induced xerostomia in patients with head and neck cancer: a literature review. *Cancer, 107*, 2525-2534.

Epstein, J., Roberson, M., Emerson, S., et al. (2001). Quality of life and oral function in patients treated with radiation therapy for head and neck cancer. *Head and Neck, 23*, 389-398.

Jemal, A., Murray, T., Samuels, A., et al. (2003). Cancer statistics, 2003. *CA: A Cancer Journal for Clinicians, 53*, 5-26.

McGuire, D. B. (2003). Barriers and strategies in implementation of oral care standards for cancer patients. *Support Care Cancer, 11*, 435-441.

Mautner, B. D., Maher, K., & Zampint, K. (2003). *Late side effects in radiation therapy*. Presented at the Oncology Nursing Society 28th Annual Congress, Denver, CO.

Plevova, P. (1999). Prevention and treatment of chemotherapy- and radiotherapy- induced oral mucositis: a review. *Oral Oncology, 35*, 453-470.

Sonis, S.T., Elting, L. S., Keefe, D., et al. (2004). Perspectives on cancer therapy-induced mucosal injury: pathogenesis, measurement, epidemiology, and consequences for patients. *Cancer, 100* (9 Suppl), 1995-2025.

Stricker, C. T., & Sullivan, J. (2003). Evidence-based oncology oral care clinical practice guidelines: development, implementation, and evaluation. *Clinical Journal of Oncology Nursing, 7*, 222-227.

Sutherland, S. E., & Browman, G. P. (2001). Prophylaxis of oral mucositis in irradiated head and neck cancer patients: a proposed classification scheme of interventions and meta-analysis of randomized controlled trials. *International Journal of Radiation Oncology, Biology, Physics, 49*, 917-930.

Oncologic Emergencies

Structural Emergencies

Barbara J. Murphy

Bowel Obstruction

DEFINITION

- The interference or cessation of the normal passage of intestinal contents through the gastrointestinal tract
- The obstruction may be partial or complete
- May involve either the small or large bowel
- Paralytic ileus is a failure of normal motility in the absence of any mechanical obstruction.
- Obstipation refers to acute abdominal pain with the ability to pass flatus but not bowel movements.

EPIDEMIOLOGY

- The risk for the development of bowel obstruction is high in any patient with a history cancer and is considered a common occurrence in abdominal and pelvic disease. However, minimal data are available regarding incidence. (Note: constipation is a frequent occurrence in palliative care with a conservative estimate of 50% of all patients admitted to hospice care.)
- Nonmalignant obstructions: adhesions from previous surgeries, hernia, inflammatory bowel disease, fecal impaction, and bowel ischemia
- Malignant obstructions: a possible primary neoplasm in any part of the bowel, abdomen, or pelvis or as metastasis from multiple sites
- Posttreatment for malignancy can also cause obstruction: fibrosis from radiation, neurotoxic complications from chemotherapy

RISK FACTORS

- History of abdominal or pelvic malignancies
- Previous abdominal surgery (potential for adhesions)
- Inflammatory bowel disease
- Herniations in the abdominal wall
- Opioid use
- Immobility
- Chemotherapy drugs—in particular vinca alkaloids and thalidomide and its derivatives
- Low fiber and fluid intake

PATHOPHYSIOLOGY

- Mechanical bowel obstruction, whether it is located in the large or small bowel, is the result of a physical block to the onward passage of intestinal contents.
- Functional bowel obstruction is caused by a loss of propulsive peristalsis (e.g., paralytic ileus, occurring after surgery).

SIGNS AND SYMPTOMS

- Presenting symptoms will vary depending on the site of the obstruction. The bowel secretes approximately 6-8 L daily.
- Anorexia, nausea, vomiting, abdominal distention, abdominal fullness, early satiety, dyspepsia, diminished or absent bowel sounds, abdominal or pelvic cramping, pain, constipation or conversely liquid stool
- Dyspnea may accompany abdominal distention.

DIAGNOSTIC TESTS

- Abdominal x-ray films, computed tomographic (CT) or positron emission tomographic (PET) scans
- Complete blood cell count (CBC): elevated white blood cell count (WBC) suggests strangulation; elevated hematocrit may point to dehydration.
- Electrolyte studies: acid-base disturbances are common in small bowel obstruction.

TREATMENT
Pharmacologic Management

- Octreotide inhibits the release of several gastrointestinal hormones and reduces gastrointestinal secretions.
- Role of corticosteroids in treating bowel obstruction is still controversial but may be useful as adjuvant antiemetic.
- Laval and colleagues studied 80 cases of malignant obstruction by using a series of staged interventions:
  - Stage I included treatment for 5 days with a corticosteroid, antiemetic, anticholinergic, and analgesic.
  - Stage II provided a somatostatin analog if vomiting persisted.
  - Obstruction relief with symptom control was obtained by medical treatment in 29 cases and symptom control occurred alone in an additional 32 cases. This suggests that a staged protocol for the treatment of inoperable malignant bowel obstruction is highly effective in relieving symptoms.

Nonpharmacologic Management

- Immediate treatment is bowel rest and intravenous fluid replacement.
- Nasogastric tubes are useful to decompress and drain. A venting gastrostomy may be a palliative option.
- Surgical intervention has been traditional with the creation of an ostomy or a resection (removal of a portion of bowel). Recently, colorectal stents, implanted with use of endoscopy and fluoroscopy, are an option for palliative treatment.

BIBLIOGRAPHY

Laval, G., Arvieux, C., Stefani, L., et al. (2006). Protocol for the treatment of malignant

Oncologic Emergencies

inoperable bowel obstruction: A prospective study of 80 cases at Grenoble University Hospital Center. *Journal of Pain and Symptom Management, 31,* 502-512.

Ptok, H., Meyer, F., Marusch, F., et al. (2006). Palliative stent implantation in the treatment of malignant colorectal obstruction. *Surgical Endoscopy, 20,* 909-914.

Von Gunten, C., & Muir, J. C. (2002). Medical management of bowel obstruction. *Journal of Palliative Medicine, 5,* 739-740.

Cystitis

DEFINITION

- A painful bladder disorder caused by inflammation of the bladder epithelium (hemorrhagic, inflammatory, or infectious)
- Occurs when an inflammatory lesion or process compromises the ability to store urine in lower urinary tract
- Associated with cancer symptoms, treatment side effects, or disease sequelae
- Hemorrhagic cystitis: often the sudden onset of hematuria combined with bladder pain and irritative bladder symptoms

EPIDEMIOLOGY

- In the individual with cancer, cystitis is most frequently related to:
  - Carcinoma of the bladder: 75%-85% present with hematuria (gross or microscopic)
  - Irritable bladder symptoms (IBS) about 20% of cases
  - Drug-induced cystitis: (intravesical chemotherapy 49%)
    - Unchanged drug is excreted in the urine.
    - Damages tissues
  - Radiation induced after external beam therapy and pelvic irradiation

PATHOPHYSIOLOGY

- Problems are generally with the urothelium or with neuromuscular function.
- The mucosal lining of the bladder is made of multiple layers of epithelial cells.
- Distinction needs to be made among causes of symptoms:
  - Tumor invasion
  - Infection
  - Chemotherapy induced
  - Radiation therapy induced
- Symptoms may be similar, but tumor invasion is usually more insidious and gross hematuria is present.
- In chemotherapy induced cystitis, metabolites of cytotoxic drugs are excreted into renal system and reside in the bladder for extended periods of time.
  - Some symptoms are expected consequences of immune stimulation and inflammatory reaction (bacillus Calmette-Guérin [BCG]).
- Radiation cystitis caused by external beam or interstitial therapy to the pelvis:
  - External beam can damage urethra, impair blood flow, and induce fibrosis, stricture, or atrophy.

SIGNS AND SYMPTOMS

- Urinary frequency
- Mild burning to excruciating pain in bladder, lower abdomen, perineum, vagina
- Low back pain
- Urinary urgency
- May or may not have presence of white blood cells (WBCs) or red blood cells (RBCs)

CANCERS ASSOCIATED WITH DISORDER

- Bladder cancer or invasion of bladder by tumors within the pelvis
- Ovary, cervix, uterus, rectum, prostate, or colon cancers
- Any tumor type treated with systemic cytotoxic drugs
  - Cyclophosphamide (Cytoxan)
  - Ifosfamide (Ifex)
  - Busulfan (Busulfex)
- Intravesical treatment with BCG

DIAGNOSTIC TESTS

- Detailed urinalysis
  - Dipstick
  - pH
  - Microscopic analysis
- Urine culture (midstream or sterile specimen)
- Urine cytological examination
- Intravenous pyelogram (IVP)
- Cystoscopy
- Renal and bladder ultrasonography

TREATMENT

- Type of treatment will be determined by cause and severity of cystitis.
- Preventive strategies, particularly in the immunocompromised, are key.
- Severity of bladder symptoms/disturbances can be evaluated by a Common Toxicity criteria scale.

Pharmacologic Management

- Antibiotics
- Systemic administration of thiols can prevent or ameliorate the bladder damage—most widely used is mercaptoethane sulfonate (mesna).
- Symptomatic management of BCG-induced cystitis includes analgesics; urinary specific/opioids, antispasmodics.

Nonpharmacologic Management

- Hydration
- Warm moist heat to lower back
- Soaking in bath water

PATIENT TEACHING

- Hydration (at least 1,500 mL daily)
- Encourage emptying bladder contents frequently.
- Create a voiding diary.
- Pelvic floor exercises (Kegel exercises)
- Minimize foods/fluids known to promote acidic, concentrated urine.
- Avoid caffeine/alcohol/carbonated beverages.
- Avoid catheterization.

BIBLIOGRAPHY

Fitzgerald, M. (2004). *Urinary tract infection: Providing the best care.* Retrieved November 1, 2006, from http://www.medscape.com/viewprogram/1920.

Gray, M., & Campbell, F. G. (2001). Urinary tract disorders. In B. Ferrell, & N. Coyle (Eds.). *Palliative nursing* (pp. 175-191). New York: Oxford.

Gupta, K., & Stamm, W. (2005). *Urinary tract infections.* Retrieved November 1, 2006, from http://www.medscape.com/viewarticle/505095.

Neoplastic Cardiac Tamponade

DEFINITION

- Compression of the heart caused by accumulation of excessive fluid within the pericardial sac

EPIDEMIOLOGY

- Many go undetected until there is a significant decrease in cardiac output.
- Approximately 20% of patients are shown to have metastatic disease to the pericardium on autopsy.

PATHOPHYSIOLOGY

- Pericardium is a two-layered sac that encloses the heart and the great vessels that come off the heart.
- The pericardial space is created between the two layers that protect the heart (parietal and visceral) with normally a very small amount of fluid (50 mL) that serves as a lubricant.
- Collection of pericardial fluid accumulates (pericardial effusion), increasing pressure and compressing the heart. To maintain cardiac output, body attempts to compensate by increasing heart rate and peripheral vasoconstriction.
- Develops slowly or rapid onset. A slow onset can stretch to accommodate almost 4 L of fluid.
- Five grades of toxicity associated with pericardial effusion

  - Grade 4 is cardiac tamponade and requires aggressive life support or end-of-life care if aggressive measures are not appropriate.

SIGNS AND SYMPTOMS

- Initially difficult to detect until the fluid accumulation is significant (slowly developing effusions allow the pericardium to stretch)
- Hoarseness, cough or hiccups, difficulty swallowing (compression of trachea, esophagus, and nerves)
- Muffled heart sounds
- Pericardial friction rub may be heard.
- Increased jugular venous distention (JVD)
- Kussmal's sign (deep gasping respirations, frequently associated with diabetic coma)
- Systolic blood pressure decreases and diastolic pressure will rise (narrowing of pulse pressure).
- Paradoxical pulse (decline in systolic blood pressure on inspiration)
- Other signs of decreased cardiac output include tachycardia, anxiety, restlessness, peripheral cyanosis, oliguria, and shock.

CANCERS ASSOCIATED WITH DISORDER

- Tumors most often associated with pericardial metastasis are lung cancer, breast cancer, leukemia, Hodgkin disease, and melanoma.
- Primary tumors are rare and are usually mesotheliomas and sarcomas.
- Lung and breast cancers can spread by direct extension or lymphatic metastasis.
- Lymphomas and leukemias typically spread by hematogenous routes.
- Radiation therapy of 4,000 rad or greater to the mediastinum can lead to immediate or long-term complications.

DIAGNOSTIC TESTS

- Routine chest x-ray films initially reveal subtle changes and enlarged pericardial silhouette.

- Electrocardiogram (ECG) findings may be nonspecific—sinus tachycardia.
- Echocardiography—96% accuracy
- Computed tomography (CT) and magnetic resonance imaging (MRI) are noninvasive and reveal pleural effusion, masses, or pericardial thickening.
- Percutaneous pericardiocentesis
  - Used only with large effusions or cardiac tamponade.
  - Fluid is aspirated and assessed for transudate versus exudate
  - Cytologic studies have confirmed that 80% to 90% have malignant cells.

TREATMENT

- Primary goal to remove the fluid and relieve/prevent impending cardiac collapse
- Degree of intervention based on underlying status of the patient, comorbid conditions, and previous treatment

Pharmacologic Management

- Mild tamponade may respond to diuretics and steroids (usually temporary).
- Chemotherapy: primarily effective in chemotherapy-sensitive tumor types
- Pericardial sclerosis: instillation of agents that cause irritation and subsequent fibrosis (50% success rate)

Nonpharmacologic Management

- Surgical interventions:
  - Pericardial "window": permits drainage of fluid into pleural space; 90% response rate
  - Pericardioperitoneal shunt
- Radiation:
  - Used successfully in radiosensitive tumors
  - Cardiac tolerance a consideration factor (3,500-4,000 rad)

PATIENT TEACHING

- Early identification of signs and symptoms

Oncologic Emergencies

- Maximize safety concerns in activities of daily living (ADLs) and ambulation
- Interventions to minimize severity of symptoms:
  - Elevate head of bed
  - Oxygen
  - Energy expenditure
  - Pain and dyspnea management
- Measures to enhance adaptation and rehabilitation

BIBLIOGRAPHY

Carlson, R. (2002). *Oncologic emergencies: Cardiovascular emergencies*. Retrieved January 16, 2007 from http://www. medscape.com/viewarticle/534544.

Ewer, M. S., Benjamin, R. S., & Yeh, E. T. H. (2003). Cardiac complications. In D. W. Kufe, R. E. Pollock, R. R. Weichselbaum, et al, (Eds). *Cancer medicine* (pp. 2525-2541). Hamilton, ON: BC Decker.

Goldman, D. (2004). Effusions. In C. Yarbro, M. Frogge, & M. Goodman, (Eds.). *Cancer symptom management* (pp. 359-373). Sudbury, MA: Jones & Bartlett.

Radiation Pneumonitis

DEFINITION

- A constellation of clinical, radiographic, and histologic findings reflecting acute toxicity causing inflammation of lung tissue exposed to radiation therapy
- Incidence and severity are related to:
  - Volume of lung radiated
  - Dose, rate, and quality of radiation
  - Concomitant chemotherapy (Bleomycin, Paclitaxel)
  - History of previous radiation

EPIDEMIOLOGY

- Symptomatic injury may occur in up to 20%, ranging from mild cough and dyspnea on exertion to respiratory failure.
- Usually occurs 2 weeks to 6 months after exposure

- High-risk groups include:
  - Low pretreatment performance status
  - Comorbid lung disease
  - Smoking history
  - Low pulmonary function tests
  - Tends to be more severe in the elderly

PATHOPHYSIOLOGY

- Radiation causes direct injury to the endothelial and epithelial cells, which results in alveolitis.
- Accumulation of inflammatory and immune cells takes place in the alveolar walls and spaces.
- Accumulation is believed to play a role in the subsequent development of pulmonary fibrosis or chronic inflammation and distorts the normal structures.
- Fibrosis is the repair process that follows: thickens alveolar walls.
- Evolves over months to years after initial damage

SIGNS AND SYMPTOMS

- Cough (dry) is initially experienced related to irritation of main bronchus and decreased mucus production
- 1-3 months post: symptoms include dyspnea, productive cough, fever, and night sweats
- More severe symptoms include acute respiratory distress with significant cough, dyspnea, fever, and tachycardia.

CANCERS ASSOCIATED WITH DISORDER

- Any tumor type that requires direct radiation or combination chemotherapy and radiation to the chest and lung fields

DIAGNOSTIC TESTS

- Chest x-ray films may show diffuse haziness progressing to infiltrates within the irradiated area.
- Pulmonary function tests (PFTs)
- Arterial blood gases
- Complete blood cell count (CBC) with differential: elevated white blood cell count and increased sedimentation rate

TREATMENT

- Prevention is the primary goal, including appropriate preassessment of underlying pulmonary impairment.
- Chemoprotective agents, such as amifostine, are thought to be helpful with administration before radiation therapy.

Pharmacologic Management

- Corticosteroid therapy
- Antibiotics may be needed for a secondary infection.
- Bronchodilators and sedatives may be effective in supportive relief.

Nonpharmacologic Management

- Oxygen therapy
- Monitor activities to minimize energy.
- Monitor adequate relief of symptoms.

PATIENT TEACHING

- Patient and family can identify critical symptoms or changes in status and be able to report accordingly:
  - Increased pain
  - Increased difficulty breathing
  - Skin changes
  - Use of accessory muscles
- Understands measures to minimize energy expenditure:
  - Frequent rest periods
  - Use of ready-made meals
  - Items used frequently within easy reach
- Understands and uses supportive therapies (i.e., morphine, oxygen, sedation)

BIBLIOGRAPHY

Houlihan, N. (2004). Symptom management of lung cancer. In N. Houlihan (Ed.). *Lung cancer*. (pp. 103-124). Pittsburgh: Oncology Nursing Society.

McManamen, L. (2003). Interstitial densities following radiotherapy. *Clinical Journal of Oncology Nursing, 7*, 209-211.

Spinal Cord Compression

DEFINITION

- A direct injury/compression to the spinal cord that leads to sensory and motor deficits
- Results from a tumor that advances and/or metastasizes to press on, encircle, or displace the spinal cord

PATHOPHYSIOLOGY

- Tumor may invade the spinal cord or cause collapse of the vertebrae by lytic destruction of vertebral bodies or pedicles.
- Pathology produces edema, inflammation, and mechanical compression, which causes direct neural injury and vascular damage and oxygenation impairment.
- Not life threatening, but represents a medical emergency
- Classifications are based on:
  - Location (extradural, intradural)
  - Level of cord involvement (cervical, thoracic, lumbar, sacral, cauda equina)

RISK FACTORS

- Bone is the third most common site of metastasis
- Occurs in 5%-30% of oncology patient population
- Second most frequent neurological complication of cancer
- Primary tumors are a possibility (5%).
- Solid tumors (lung, breast, prostate, and kidney) provide highest risk.
- Hematological malignancies; lymphomas and multiple myeloma

SIGNS AND SYMPTOMS

- Depends on level of cord involvement
- Back pain: pain may be progressive and occur up to 6 months before diagnosis.
- Leg (one or both) weakness, with or without sensory loss
- Muscle atrophy in lower extremities
- Loss of bowel and bladder function

DIAGNOSTIC TESTS

- Complete blood cell count (CBC) with differential, sedimentation rate: helps to determine spinal cord compression versus infection
- Chemistry profile including calcium and liver function tests
- Imaging studies: plain x-ray films, magnetic resonance imaging (MRI), computed tomographic (CT) scan, and positron emission tomographic (PET) scan. Plain films frequently associated with vertebral blastic or lytic lesions. However, contrast-enhanced MRI provides the best definition of spinal lesions.
- *Lumbar punctures are contraindicated because removal of cerebrospinal fluid may worsen the spinal cord compression.*

TREATMENT

- Prompt diagnosis and treatment is crucial.
- Treatment is primarily palliation of symptoms and prevention of permanent disabilities.

Pharmacologic Management

- Corticosteroids
  - Reduces edema
  - Dose and duration based on patient response
- Pain management
- Chemotherapy
  - Indicated in chemotherapy-sensitive tumors: lymphoma or Hodgkin disease
  - Adjuvant therapy in combination with irradiation or surgery

Nonpharmacologic Management

- Radiation therapy
  - Produces symptom reduction
  - Initiated immediately after diagnosis
  - Usual course 2-4 weeks
- Surgery:
  - Surgical decompression is treatment of choice for patients not radiosensitive.
  - Indicated if there is evidence of spinal instability or rapidly progressing loss of function

PATIENT TEACHING

- Early recognition of signs and symptoms
- Mobility/safety
- Skin integrity
- Pain management
- Coping strategies with potential limitations

BIBLIOGRAPHY

Heary, R. F. (2003). *Metastatic spinal tumors*. Retrieved January 16, 2007 from http://www.medscape.com/view article/421498.

Osowski, M. (2002). *Spinal cord compression: An obstructive oncologic emergency*. Retrieved January 16, 2007 from http://www.medscape.com/viewarticle/442735.

Wilkes, G. (2004). Spinal cord compression. In C. Yarbro, M. Frogge, & M. Goodman (Eds.). *Cancer symptom management* (pp. 359-373). Sudbury, MA: Jones & Bartlett.

Superior Vena Cava Syndrome

DEFINITION

Superior vena cava (SVC) syndrome is a complex of symptoms and physical findings associated with compression of or obstruction to the superior vena cava.

- Tumor or thrombus
- Result is compromised venous drainage of the head, neck, and upper extremities

EPIDEMIOLOGY

- 75%-85% of cases of SVC syndrome have a malignant etiology.
- Lung cancer up to 80%: most frequently small cell lung cancer

Oncologic Emergencies

RISK FACTORS

- Lung cancer
- Lymphoma involving the mediastinum
- Central venous catheters and pacemakers
- Previous radiation therapy to the mediastinum

PATHOPHYSIOLOGY

- The SVC is a thin-walled, low-pressure major blood vessel.
- Primary function is to carry venous drainage from head, upper extremities to the heart.
- SVC is surrounded by rigid structures in the mediastinum and multiple lymph node chains.
- Easily compressed by direct tumor invasion, enlarged lymph nodes, or a thrombus within the vessel
- Results in:
  - Increase in venous pressure
  - Decrease in cardiac output

SIGNS AND SYMPTOMS

- Progression of physical findings can be insidious or acute. Slower progression allows some collateral circulation to develop.
- Facial swelling
- Swelling of neck, arms, hands
  - Men may have a problem with buttoning shirt collar (Stoke's sign)
- Neck and thoracic vein distention
- Dyspnea (most common)
- Nonproductive cough
- Cyanosis of upper torso
- Late signs include the following:
  - Severe headache
  - Irritability
  - Visual disturbances
  - Change on level of consciousness
  - Stridor
  - Horner's syndrome (ptosis, meiosis, and anhidrosis)

DIAGNOSTIC TESTS

- X-ray films (approximately 15% will have a normal chest film)
  - Superior mediastinal widening in approximately 66%
  - 25% may have pleural effusions.
  - Hilar mass: 12%
- Computed tomographic (CT) scan/magnetic resonance imaging (MRI): better reveal whether the obstruction is thrombus related
- Laboratory data:
  - Arterial blood gases (ABGs)
  - Coagulation studies

TREATMENT

- Early identification of clients at risk is essential.
- Goal is to provide rapid palliation/relief of symptoms and attempt to cure underlying condition.

Pharmacologic Management

- Corticosteroids may reduce inflammatory component and improve venous blood flow.
- Chemotherapy for chemotherapy-sensitive tumors
- Fibrinolytic/anticoagulation therapy in appropriate situations
- Diuretics

Nonpharmacologic Management

- Radiation therapy
  - Indicated as urgent in cases of acute respiratory distress
  - A variety of radiation fractionation protocols are effective.
- Removal of central venous catheter combined with anticoagulation
- Interventional
  - Percutaneous implantation of endovascular stents: associated with high success rate and low morbidity
- Supportive management includes:
  - Oxygen therapy to relieve dyspnea
  - Anxiety reduction

PATIENT TEACHING

- Early recognition and reporting of signs and symptoms
- Maximize environmental safety:
  - Side rails, low bed, items in easy reach
  - Eliminate throw rugs, use of walker
- Interventions to reduce symptoms of respiratory distress:
  - Elevate head of bed
  - Oxygen use
  - Anxiety management
    - Use of morphine, antianxiety medications
- Interventions to reduce symptoms of circulatory compromise:
  - Remove rings and restrictive clothing
  - Avoid venipunctures/blood pressure measurement on upper extremities
  - Monitor skin integrity
  - Elevate upper arms to promote venous return

BIBLIOGRAPHY

Carlson, R. (2002). *Oncologic emergencies: Cardiovascular emergencies.* Retrieved January 16, 2007 from http://www.medscape.com/viewarticle/ 534544.

Flounders, J. A. (2003). Oncology emergency modules: Superior vena cava syndrome. *Oncology Nursing Forum, 30,* E84-E90. Retrieved January 16, 2007 from http:/www.ons.org/Publications/ journals/ONF/Volume30/Issue4/3004513.asp.

Urinary Tract Infection

DEFINITION

- Lower urinary tract infection (UTI): bladder epithelium undergoes inflammatory changes when colonized with infectious agents.
- Bacteriuria is present.

EPIDEMIOLOGY

- One of the most common conditions treated by physicians
- Highest in elderly, also the age group most likely to have cancer
  - 20% in women over 65 years old
  - 10% in men over 65 years old
- Most common bacteria: *Escherichia coli, Enterobacter,* and *Staphylococcus* species

RISK FACTORS

- Men have increased "protective" factors:
  - Longer urethral length
  - Scrotum provides a physical barrier
- Common causes of male dysuria:
  - Foreskin in early life
  - Prostate in mid and later life
- Inefficient bladder emptying
- Estrogen deficiency in postmenopausal women
- Women's use of spermicide, vaginally or with condoms
- Children and elders with constipation

PATHOPHYSIOLOGY

- The urinary tract, adjacent to the bacteria-rich lower gastrointestinal tract, produces and stores urine
- The periurethral area is typically colonized with gut and other flora, some capable of causing UTI.
- Urination flushes bacteria from the urethral orifice. Periurethral pathogens on occasion enter the urethra and ascend, reaching the bladder and resulting in UTI.
- Can involve mucosal tissue (cystitis) or soft tissue (pyelonephritis, prostatitis)
- In urethritis, the inflammation and infection is limited to the urethra only, or urethra and vagina in women—usually a sexually transmitted pathogen.
- Acute pyelonephritis is an infection of the renal parenchyma and renal pelvis caused by an ascending cystitis.

SIGNS AND SYMPTOMS

- Asymptomatic bacteriuria:
  - Urine culture reveals a significant growth of a pathogen, but the patient has no symptoms of UTI.
- Symptomatic UTI:
  - Bladder irritability
  - Dysuria
  - Urgency
  - Frequency
  - Fever
  - Strong to foul odor

DIAGNOSTIC TESTS

- Urine dipstick
  - Leukocyte esterase (LE): enzyme present in white blood cells (WBC) indicates presence of neutrophils. Results not valid in neutropenic patient.
  - Protein
  - pH
- Urine culture
- Microscopic analysis

DIFFERENTIAL DIAGNOSIS

Differentiation between UTI and bacteriuria:
- Pyuria alone = inflammation
- Bacteriuria without pyuria = colonization
- Pyuria + bacteriuria + nitrites = infection

TREATMENT
Pharmacologic Management
- Antimicrobial therapy

Nonpharmacologic Management
- Hydration
- Use of alternative therapy not yet supported by conclusive research
- Long-term adherence to blueberry/cranberry products and expected benefit may be overestimated

PATIENT TEACHING
- Identification and reporting of signs and symptoms
- Adequate fluid intake
- Proper toileting techniques
- Avoid bladder irritants that may induce acidic urine.
- Avoid catheterizations.

BIBLIOGRAPHY
Fitzgerald, M. (2004). *Urinary tract infection: Providing the best care.* Retrieved November 1, 2006, from http://www.medscape.com/viewprogram/1920.
Gupta, K., & Stamm, W. (2005). *Urinary tract infections.* Retrieved November 1, 2006, from http://www.medscape.com/viewarticle/505095.

Urinary Tract Obstruction

DEFINITION
- A drop in urine outflow may indicate failure of the kidneys to filter blood and produce urine (oliguria or anuria).
- Urinary stasis or blockage of urine transport from upper to lower urinary tracts indicates an obstruction.
- Obstruction of the urinary tract may occur at multiple levels and involves a blockage of the flow of urine, causing it to back up and damage one or both kidneys.
  - Ureter
  - Bladder
  - Urethra
- Involvement can be by direct extension, encasement, or invasion. Obstruction can also occur from metastatic deposits involving these same sites.

EPIDEMIOLOGY
- Many cases go undetected until there is a significant decrease in urinary output.
- Bladder outlet obstruction most common in men: benign prostatitic hypertrophy (BPH)
- Cervical cancers cause most ureteral obstructions in women.
- Retroperitoneal fibrosis resulting from radiation therapy

RISK FACTORS
- Urinary tract stones
  - Ureteral stones
  - Bladder stones
- Urinary tract tumors
- Retroperitoneal fibrosis
- BPH (enlarged prostate)
- Tumors of nearby organs
- Colon cancer
- Cervical cancer
- Uterine cancer

PATHOPHYSIOLOGY
- Urine is transported from the renal papilla to the bladder

Oncologic Emergencies

through the upper urinary tract to the lower urinary tract (bladder, urethra).

- Active transport depends on smooth muscle contractibility.
- Any blockage will cause an accumulation of urine and subsequent distention.
- Pressure builds directly on the tissue and causes structural damage.
- Tubular filtrate pressure may increase within the nephron because drainage anywhere within the urinary collecting system is impaired.
- Acute or chronic renal failure results.
- Renal failure with uremia and elevated serum potassium levels will compromise cardiac function.

SIGNS AND SYMPTOMS

- Symptoms vary depending on whether the obstruction is acute or chronic, unilateral or bilateral, complete or partial, and caused by:
  - Flank pain
    - Bilateral or unilateral
    - Colicky or severe
  - Urinary tract infection
  - Fever
  - Difficulty or pain while urinating
  - Nausea or vomiting
  - Hypertension
  - Renal failure
  - Edema

- Decreased urine output
- Hematuria (microscopic or gross)

DIAGNOSTIC TESTS

- X-ray studies:
  - Kidney, ureter, and bladder (KUB) x-ray
  - Intravenous pyelogram (IVP)
  - Abdominal ultrasonography
  - Renal ultrasonography
  - Abdominal computed tomographic (CT) scan
- Laboratory studies:
  - Complete blood cell count (CBC)
  - Blood urea nitrogen (BUN) and creatinine
  - Urinalysis

TREATMENT
Pharmacologic Management

- Pain management
- Urine alkalinization: prevention of stone formation
- Steroids
- Antibiotics to manage any infection present
- Chemotherapy

Nonpharmacologic Management

- Radiation therapy: useful in management of invasive disease
- Extracorporeal shock wave lithotripsy (SWL), a noninvasive means of stone management
- Surgical:
  - Although temporary relief from the obstruction can be achieved

without surgery, the cause of the obstruction must be removed and the urinary system repaired.
  - Stents in the ureter or in the renal pelvis may provide short-term relief of symptoms. Nephrostomy tubes, which drain urine from the kidneys through the back, may be used to bypass the obstruction.
- Foley catheter, to manage urethral obstruction, may also be helpful.

PATIENT TEACHING

- Recognize and report early signs of urinary problems.
- Hypertension management, frequent monitoring of blood pressure
- Hydration
- Minimize foods/fluids known to promote acidic, concentrated urine.
- Pain management
- Appropriate management of any drainage tubes

BIBLIOGRAPHY

Gray, M., & Campbell, F. G. (2001). Urinary tract disorders. In B. Ferrell & N. Coyle (Eds.). *Palliative nursing* (pp. 175-191). New York: Oxford.

Stoller, M., & Stackhouse, B. (2006). *Advances in the management of urinary stone disease.* Retrieved November 1, 2006, from http://www.medscape.com/viewprogram/4949.

Metabolic Emergencies

Adrenal Failure

Jean Rosiak

DEFINITION

- Condition in which the adrenal gland is unable to produce adequate amounts of cortical hormones in

response to physiological demands
  - Glucocorticoids are required for normal function of all cells in the body and are secreted from the adrenal cortex in large quantities during times of physiological stress to maintain homeostasis.

- Potentially lethal complication that can lead to deterioration of cardiovascular status and death if untreated

EPIDEMIOLOGY

- Bilateral adrenal metastasis: 8.6%-27% overall incidence at autopsy; only 4% become symptomatic
  - Breast cancer 58%

- ○ Malignant melanoma 50%
- ○ Lung cancer 42%
- ○ Non-Hodgkin lymphoma 25%
- Radiation dose >5,000 cGy to pituitary: 18%-35% incidence of adrenal insufficiency (AI) after 5-15 years

PATHOPHYSIOLOGY

- Adrenal failure results from destruction or dysfunction of the hypothalamic-pituitary-adrenal axis.
- Primary AI/adrenal failure:
  - ○ Caused by processes that damage the adrenal glands or by drugs that block cortisol synthesis
- Secondary AI/adrenal failure
  - ○ Results from processes that reduce the secretion of corticotropin-releasing hormone (CRH) by the hypothalamus or adrenocorticotropin hormone (ACTH) by the pituitary gland as a result of pituitary or hypothalamic conditions
  - ○ Most common cause of secondary adrenal insufficiency is abrupt discontinuation of long-term administration of glucocorticoids.
- Causes of AI/adrenal failure:
  - ○ Consequence of sudden withdrawal of exogenous corticosteroids
  - ○ Bilateral adrenal hemorrhage or venous thrombosis
  - ○ Adrenal tumor or metastatic involvement
  - ○ Pituitary hemorrhage or tumor
  - ○ Autoimmune disorders
  - ○ Medications inhibiting cytochrome P-450 isoenzymes necessary for adrenal steroidogenesis:
    - ■ Ketoconazole
    - ■ Aminoglutethimide
    - ■ Megestrol acetate (used to increase appetite in cachectic patients)
  - ○ Infections:
    - ■ Tuberculosis
    - ■ Acquired immunodeficiency syndrome (AIDS)
    - ■ Meningococcemia
    - ■ Histoplasmosis

SIGNS AND SYMPTOMS

- More than 80%-90% of both adrenal glands must be nonfunctioning before clinical signs result
  - ○ May not be symptomatic unless severe stress is induced
- Slow onset:
  - ○ Chronic fatigue
  - ○ Joint pain/muscle cramps
  - ○ Anorexia/unintentional weight loss
  - ○ Abdominal pain
  - ○ Nausea
  - ○ Diarrhea
- Acute symptoms
  - ○ Fever
  - ○ Tachycardia
  - ○ Loss of vasomotor tone
  - ○ Hypotension, acute shock
  - ○ Cardiovascular collapse
  - ○ Death
- Primary AI (associated with lack of aldosterone and cortisol)
  - ○ Salt craving
  - ○ Dehydration resulting from renal salt wasting
  - ○ Postural hypotension
  - ○ Electrolyte abnormalities: hyperkalemia, hyponatremia
  - ○ Hyperpigmentation of skin and buccal mucosa (ACTH related)
- Secondary AI
  - ○ Pallor
  - ○ Amenorrhea/diminished libido
  - ○ Scanty axillary and pubic hair
  - ○ Headache and visual symptoms

CANCERS ASSOCIATED WITH DISORDER

- Breast cancer
- Malignant melanoma
- Lung cancer
- Non-Hodgkin lymphoma
- Medication-induced adrenal insufficiency
  - ○ Prostate cancer treated with ketoconazole
  - ○ Prostate or breast cancer treated with aminoglutethimide
  - ○ Cachexia treated with megestrol acetate

DIAGNOSTIC TESTS

- Early morning serum cortisol and ACTH levels
  - ○ Serum cortisol level peaks in the early morning hours.

- Cortisol level >18 mcg/dL = normal adrenal function
- Cortisol level <3 mcg/dL = adrenal insufficiency
  - ○ Cortisol level may be falsely low in patients with albumin level <2.5 g/dL.
  - ○ ACTH level elevated in primary AI
  - ○ ACTH level low or normal (when cortisol level decreased) in secondary AI
- ACTH stimulation test: evaluate for adrenal insufficiency (on the basis of inability of adrenal gland to respond acutely to injection of ACTH by secreting cortisol)
  - ○ Draw baseline cortisol level.
  - ○ Administer cosyntropin 0.25 mg (250 mcg) intravenously (IV).
  - ○ Draw cortisol levels at 30 and 60 minutes after dose.
    - ■ Failure to increase serum cortisol at least 5 mcg/dL above baseline and at least to a level of 15 mcg/dL at either 30 or 60 minutes is diagnostic of adrenal insufficiency.
    - ■ Serum cortisol level of >18 mcg/dL at either time point is a normal response.
- Serum potassium
  - ○ Elevated in primary AI
  - ○ Normal in secondary AI
- Serum sodium: decreased
- Serum glucose level: decreased

DIFFERENTIAL DIAGNOSIS

- Primary adrenal failure (Addison's disease)
  - ○ Autoimmune adrenalitis
  - ○ Infection: tuberculosis, AIDS-related infections
- Secondary adrenal failure
  - ○ Pituitary adenomas

TREATMENT

- Prompt replacement of corticosteroids
  - ○ Glucocorticoid: main form of therapy for all forms of adrenal failure
    - ■ Hydrocortisone 10-12.5 mg/m^2/day: usually

given as 20 mg orally every morning and 10 mg orally every evening

- □ May require lower dose, particularly in secondary AI
- □ Smallest dose that improves symptoms is recommended.
  - ■ Short half-life mimics normal cortisol circadian rhythm.
- ○ Stress-dose steroids before any surgical procedure
  - ■ Hydrocortisone 5 mg/hr IV during surgery
  - ■ For first 24 hours after surgery, a total of 150-200 mg is administered.
  - ■ Taper by 50% per day if the postoperative period is without complications.
- ○ Stress-dose steroids: sepsis, fever >38° C, dental procedures, invasive procedures (gastroscopy, colonoscopy, cystoscopy, bronchoscopy)
  - ■ Maximal recommended dose is 50 mg every 8 hours.
- ○ Mineralocorticoid: needed in addition to glucocorticoids in patients with primary AI
  - ■ Required for patients with concomitant aldosterone deficiency resulting in persistent hyperkalemia
  - ■ Fludrocortisone 0.05-0.2 mg daily, usually in a single dose
  - ■ Dose is adjusted according to symptoms

PATIENT TEACHING

- Patient and caregiver awareness regarding the condition and appropriate treatment is important.
- Wear a medical alert bracelet or necklace stating the need for glucocorticoids in event of an emergency.
- Go to the emergency department if experiencing multiple episodes of vomiting or diarrhea.

FOLLOW-UP

- Consider endocrinology consultation.

- Hydrocortisone may be needed during periods of stress.
- Monitor symptoms for signs of crisis.

BIBLIOGRAPHY

Choi, C. H., Tiu, S. C., Shek, C. C., et al. (2002). Use of low-dose corticotropin stimulation test for the diagnosis of secondary adrenocortical insufficiency. *Hong Kong Medical Journal, 8*, 427-434.

Dirix, L. Y., & van Oosterom, A. T. (2002). Metabolic complications: Adrenocortical insufficiency. In R. L. Souhami, I. Tannock, P. Hohenberger, et al. (Eds.). *Oxford textbook of oncology* (2nd ed., pp. 923-925). Oxford: Oxford University Press.

Dorin, R. I., Qualls, C. R., & Crapo, L. M. (2003). Diagnosis of adrenal insufficiency. *Annals of Internal Medicine, 139*, 194-204.

Gonzalez, H., Nardi, O., & Annane, D. (2006). Relative adrenal failure in the ICU: An identifiable problem requiring treatment. *Critical Care Clinics, 22*, 105-118.

McCullough, D. M. (2003). Adrenal gland disorders. In T. M. Buttaro, J. Trybulski, P. P. Bailey, et al. (Eds.). *Primary care: A collaborative practice* (2nd ed., pp. 990-993). St. Louis: Mosby.

Nieman, L. K. (2003). Dynamic evaluation of adrenal hypofunction. *Journal of Endocrinological Investigation, 26*, 74-82.

O'Connor, T., & Trump, D. L. (2004). Endocrine complications. In M. D. Abeloff, J. O. Armitage, J. E. Niederhuber, et al. (Eds.), *Clinical oncology* (3rd ed., pp. 1287-1294). St. Louis: W. B. Saunders.

Salvatori, R. (2005). Adrenal insufficiency. *Journal of the American Medical Association, 294*, 2481-2488.

Stempkowski, L. M. (2000). Adrenal metastasis. In D. Camp-Sorrell & R. A. Hawkins (Eds.). *Clinical manual for the oncology advanced practice nurse* (pp. 529-533). Pittsburgh, PA: Oncology Nursing Press.

Strohl, R. A. (1999). Radiation therapy. In C. Miaskowski & P. Buchsel (Eds.). *Oncology nursing: Assessment and clinical care* (p. 75). St. Louis: Mosby.

Torrey, S. P. (2005). Recognition and management of adrenal emergencies. *Emergency Medicine Clinics of North America, 23*, 687-702.

Hypercalcemia

Jean Rosiak

DEFINITION

- Serum calcium >11 mg/dL or ionized calcium is >1.35 mmol/L.
- Rate of calcium mobilization from bone exceeds renal threshold for calcium excretion.
- Prognostic factor for survival of less than 1 year (median survival 3 months)

EPIDEMIOLOGY

- 10%-20% overall incidence in adult patients with advanced cancer (0.5%-1% in children)
- Adult T-cell lymphoma/ leukemia: 50%
- Multiple myeloma: 20%-40%
- Breast cancer: 17%-40%
- Squamous cell lung cancer: 35%

PATHOPHYSIOLOGY

- Calcium is essential in maintaining cell membrane permeability (transmission of nerve impulses, cardiac contractility), bone formation, normal clotting mechanisms, regulating numerous cellular processes affecting multiple organ systems.
- 99% of calcium is stored in bone.
- Bone is a constantly changing tissue; continual process of bone remodeling: bone formation and resorption.
  - ○ Osteoblasts: responsible for bone formation by secreting a specialized extracellular matrix that subsequently mineralizes
  - ○ Osteoclasts: responsible for bone resorption/breakdown by releasing a proteolytic enzyme that dissolves bone matrix, releasing calcium into the extracellular space
- Hypercalcemia results when more calcium is resorbed from bone than deposited in bone, and renal excretion of excessive calcium is impaired.

- Local osteolytic hypercalcemia (20%-30%)
  - Tumor cells infiltrating bone (bone metastasis) secrete local cytokines that directly stimulate osteoclasts and inhibit osteoblasts.
  - Results in release of calcium into the extracellular fluid/systemic circulation
- Humoral hypercalcemia of malignancy (80%)
  - Systemic cytokines secreted by tumor cells
    - Promotes release of calcium and phosphate from bone
    - Increases calcium reabsorption in the kidney
    - Parathyroid hormone–related protein (PTHrP): principal mediator of cancer-related hypercalcemia in patients with solid tumors

SIGNS AND SYMPTOMS
- Can be vague and attributable to other conditions
- Gastrointestinal:
  - Anorexia, nausea, vomiting
  - Constipation, ileus, abdominal pain
- Musculoskeletal:
  - Fatigue, muscle weakness
  - Bone pain
  - Pathological fractures
- Renal:
  - Polyuria, polydipsia, nocturia
  - Oliguric renal failure, azotemia
- Neurological:
  - Restlessness, apathy
  - Mental status changes/disorientation
  - Lethargy: can progress to stupor and coma
- Cardiovascular:
  - Hypertension
  - Electrocardiographic (ECG) changes
- Death can result if hypercalcemia is untreated.

CANCERS ASSOCIATED WITH DISORDER
- Multiple myeloma (usually the result of local factors in bone secreted by tumor)

- Solid tumors (usually the result of systemic factors associated with tumor)
  - Breast, lung, renal, prostate, and head and neck cancer

DIAGNOSTIC TESTS
- Serum calcium
  - Normal calcium level: 8.5-10.5 mg/dL
  - Mild hypercalcemia: <12 mg/dL
  - Moderate hypercalcemia: 12-14 mg/dL
  - Severe hypercalcemia: >14-16 mg/dL
  - Life-threatening hypercalcemia: >16 mg/dL
- Ionized serum calcium: >1.35 mmol/L
- Serum albumin
  - Decreased albumin level may give false-normal calcium value.
  - Corrected calcium level = total serum calcium (mg/dL) + (4.0 − serum albumin [g/dL]) × 0.8
- Parathyroid hormone level (measured with immunoradiometric assay)
  - Elevated in primary hyperparathyroidism
  - Usually low in malignancy
- PTHrP
  - Level greater than 1 pmol/L is specific indicator of malignancy.

DIFFERENTIAL DIAGNOSIS
- Primary or secondary hyperparathyroidism
- Renal failure
- Paget's disease of bone
- Medications (thiazides, lithium, large doses of vitamins A or D)

TREATMENT
Pharmacologic Management
- Only effective long-term management is to treat the underlying disease.
- Continuing management requires pharmacologic measures to inhibit bone resorption and promote renal calcium excretion.
- Immediate goal is to restore fluid and electrolyte balance.
- Hydration: 1-2 L of isotonic (0.9%) saline solution over 2 hours (may

administer 100-250 mL/hr for 24-48 hours)
  - Hydration results in approximately 2 mg/dL decrease in serum calcium level.
  - Clinical improvement usually seen within 24 hours; effect is temporary.
- Diuresis: furosemide 20-40 mg intravenously (IV) every 12 hours
  - Enhances calcium excretion
  - Thiazide diuretics contraindicated because they inhibit urinary excretion of calcium
- Bisphosphonates: one of the most effective therapies for hypercalcemia
  - Inhibit normal and pathological bone resorption by effects on osteoclasts
  - May inhibit adhesion of tumor cells to bone matrix
  - Administered IV because of poor oral absorption
  - Pamidronate (Aredia) 90 mg IV over 2-24 hours (60-mg dose can be used in patients with lower calcium levels)
    - Response rate: 90% within 3-4 days
    - Duration of response: 7-30 days
  - Zoledronate (Zometa) 4 mg IV over 15 minutes every 3-4 weeks
    - Response rate: more than 90% within 4-10 days
    - Duration of response: 4-6 weeks
- Gallium nitrate 200 mg/m^2/day as a 5-day continuous infusion (100 mg/m^2/day may be considered in patients with mild hypercalcemia and minimal symptoms)
  - Inhibits bone resorption and stimulates bone formation
  - Inhibits tubular calcium reabsorption and parathyroid hormone (PTH) secretion
  - Response rate: 72%-82%
  - Duration of response: 6-8 days
  - More effective than bisphosphonates in treating hypercalcemia in patients with

tumors of epidermoid histology (high-level PTHrP expression)

- Mithramycin (Plicamycin) 25 mcg/kg IV over 3-6 hours
  - Blocks ribonucleic acid (RNA) synthesis in osteoclasts
  - Response rate: 30%-50% within 12 hours, with maximum effect at 48 hours
  - Duration of response: several days, requiring repeated doses every 3-7 days
- Calcitonin 4-8 International Units/kg intramuscularly or subcutaneously every 6-8 hours
  - Inhibits osteoclast-mediated bone resorption
  - Promotes urinary calcium and sodium excretion
  - Decreases serum calcium within 2-6 hours
  - Duration of response: 24-72 hours
  - Resistance to effects develop within a few days of instituting therapy.
- Corticosteroids: prednisone 40-60 mg/day orally or hydrocortisone 100-150 mg IV every 12 hours
  - Decrease calcium resorption from the gastrointestinal tract
  - Inhibits bone resorption and increases urinary calcium excretion
  - Not a first-line treatment: complications of long-term steroid use limit its usefulness
  - May take 1-2 weeks for calcium-lowering effect
- Dialysis

PATIENT TEACHING

- Educate the patient and caregiver regarding sign and symptoms of hypercalcemia.
- Importance of maintaining hydration: 1-3 L of fluid per day unless contraindicated
- Importance of maintaining activity: immobility can worsen hypercalcemia.

FOLLOW-UP

- Monitor serum calcium or ionized calcium level.
- Monitor renal function/hydration status.
- Be alert for signs and symptoms of recurrent hypercalcemia.

BIBLIOGRAPHY

Body, J. J. (2004). Hypercalcemia of malignancy. *Seminars in Nephrology, 24,* 48-54.

Davidson, T. G. (2001). Conventional treatment of hypercalcemia of malignancy. *American Journal of Health-System Pharmacy, 58,* S8-S15.

Fojo, A. T. (2005). Metabolic emergencies: Hypercalcemia and cancer. In V. DeVita, S. Hellman, & S. A. Rosenberg, (Eds.). *Cancer principles and practice* (pp. 2297-2299). Philadelphia: Lippincott Williams & Wilkins.

Hutton, E. (2005). Evaluation and management of hypercalcemia. *Journal of the American Academy of Physician Assistants, 18,* 30-35.

Leyland-Jones, B. (2004). Treating cancer-related hypercalcemia with gallium nitrate. *Journal of Supportive Oncology, 2,* 509-516.

Li, E. C., & Davis, L. E. (2003). Zoledronic acid: A new parenteral bisphosphonate. *Clinical Therapeutics, 25,* 2669-2708.

Miaskowski, C. (1997). Hypercalcemia. In *Oncology nursing: An essential guide for patient care.* (pp. 230). Philadelphia: W. B. Saunders.

Miaskowski, C. (1999). Oncologic emergencies: Hypercalcemia. In C. Miaskowski & P. Buchsel, (Eds.), *Oncology nursing: Assessment and clinical care* (pp. 223-227). St. Louis: Mosby.

National Cancer Institute. (2005). *Hypercalcemia (PDQ).* Retrieved June 14, 2006, from http://www.cancer.gov/cancertopics/pdq/supportivecare/hypercalcemia/healthprofessional/allpages.

Richerson, M. T. (2004). Electrolyte imbalances: Hypercalcemia. In C. H. Yarbro, M. H. Frogge, & M. Goodman (Eds.), *Cancer symptom management* (3rd ed., pp. 440-446). Sudbury, MA: Jones & Bartlett.

Shuey, K. M. (2004). Hypercalcemia of malignancy: Part I. *Clinical Journal of Oncology Nursing, 8,* 209-210.

Shuey, K. M., & Brant, J. M. (2004). Hypercalcemia of malignancy: Part II. *Clinical Journal of Oncology Nursing, 8,* 321-323.

Smith, W. J. (2000). Hypocalcemia/hypercalcemia. In D. Camp-Sorrell & R. A. Hawkins (Eds.). *Clinical manual for the oncology advanced practice nurse* (pp. 849-858). Pittsburgh: Oncology Nursing Press.

Wickham, R. S. (2000). Hypercalcemia. In C. H. Yarbro, M. H. Frogge, M. Goodman, et al. (Eds.). *Cancer nursing: principles and practice* (5th ed., pp. 776-791). Sudbury, MA: Jones & Bartlett.

Williams, J. (2003). Oncology complications and paraneoplastic syndromes: Hypercalcemia. In T. M. Buttaro, J. Trybulski, P. P. Bailey, et al. (Eds.). *Primary care: A collaborative practice* (2nd ed., pp. 1209-1210). St. Louis: Mosby.

Hyperuricemia

Jean Rosiak

DEFINITION

- Elevation in serum uric acid level resulting from rapid release and breakdown of intracellular nucleic acids from malignant cells caused by cell lysis
  - Cell lysis may occur spontaneously in rapidly growing tumors but most often is due to cytotoxic therapy.
  - Breakdown of tumor cells yields large amounts of uric acid.
- Most common manifestation of tumor lysis syndrome

EPIDEMIOLOGY

- 21.4%: acute lymphoblastic leukemia (ALL)
- 19.6%: non-Hodgkin lymphoma (NHL)
- 14.7%: acute myelogenous leukemia (AML)

CANCERS ASSOCIATED WITH DISORDER

- Large tumor burden/high proliferative rate
  - ALL/AML/NHL
  - Bulky adenopathy
  - Hepatosplenomegaly
- Tumors highly responsive to cytotoxic therapy

PATHOPHYSIOLOGY

- Uric acid level elevation may be present before initiation of cytotoxic therapy.
  - Caused by spontaneous tumor cell breakdown

- Usually caused by chemotherapy or other cytotoxic treatment
  - Massive breakdown of tumor cells releases nucleic acids from cells
  - Rapid breakdown of nucleic acids → hypoxanthine → xanthine → uric acid
- Facilitated by the enzyme xanthine oxidase
- Elevated uric acid level usually develops within 1-2 days of initiation of cytotoxic treatment.
  - Can lead to acute renal failure
  - Renal capacity for uric acid clearance exceeded
  - Precipitation of uric acid crystals in renal tubules
  - Renal obstruction

SIGNS AND SYMPTOMS

- Cloudy sedimented urine, oliguria, anuria, acute renal failure
- Nausea, vomiting, diarrhea, anorexia
- Hypertension
- Lethargy
- Flank pain

DIAGNOSTIC TESTS

- Serum uric acid level: elevated
- Monitor renal function: creatinine, blood urea nitrogen (BUN), intake and output

DIFFERENTIAL DIAGNOSIS

- Tumor lysis syndrome
- Tumor infiltration of the kidney/tumor-associated obstructive uropathy
- Drug-associated nephrotoxicity
- Intrinsic kidney disease
- Acute sepsis
- Hereditary gout

TREATMENT

- Hydration
  - Aggressive hydration with a slightly hypotonic saline or isotonic solution
    - 3000 mL/m²/day (200 mL/kg/day if weight <10 kg)
- Diuresis (if no acute obstructive uropathy or hypovolemia)
  - Keep urine output >100 mL/m²/hour (3 mL/kg/hour if weight <10 kg).

- Furosemide 0.5-1.0 mg/kg
- Mannitol 0.5 mg/kg
- Dopamine 5 mcg/kg/min can be given to improve renal perfusion.
- Urine alkalinization: controversial
  - Improves solubility of uric acid (maximum solubility at pH of 7.5) and hypoxanthine, but not xanthine
  - Xanthine may precipitate in the kidneys at pH >6.5, leading to xanthine nephropathy.
- Allopurinol (see figure below)
  - Inhibits xanthine oxidase, the enzyme responsible for uric acid formation (hypoxanthine → xanthine → uric acid)
  - Increases urinary concentration and excretion of precursors of uric acid: hypoxanthine and xanthine
  - No effect on existing uric acid load
    - May not significantly affect uric acid level for several days

- Begin 12-24 hours before start of chemotherapy
- Adverse effects
  - Inhibition of xanthine oxidase can lead to increased plasma levels of hypoxanthine and xanthine, which may precipitate in renal tubules and lead to obstruction and acute renal failure
  - Reduces the degradation of 6-mercaptopurine (6-MP)
  - Dose reduction of 6-MP to 25%-33% dose required
- Oral allopurinol: recommended dosage is 300-800 mg daily (200-400 mg/m²/day) as single or divided doses
- Allopurinol (Aloprim): intravenous (IV)
  - Daily IV dose equivalent to recommended oral dosage
  - Adults—200-400 mg/m²/day, maximum daily dose 600 mg
  - Pediatric—200 mg/m²/day

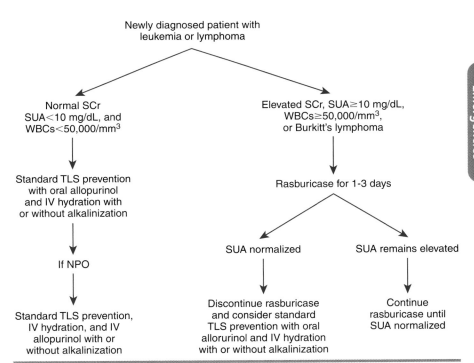

Decision algorithm for the use of rasburicase and IV allopurinol in a patient newly diagnosed with leukemia or lymphoma. SCr, Serum creatinine; SUA, serum uric acid; WBCs, white blood cells; TLS, tumor lysis syndrome; NPO, = nothing by mouth. (From Holdsworth, M. T., & Nguyen, P. (2003). Role of I.V. allopurinol and rasburicase in tumor lysis syndrome. *American Journal of Health-System Pharmacy, 60,* p. 2221. Copyright 2003 by the American Society of Health-System Pharmacists, Inc. Reprinted with permission.

Oncologic Emergencies

- Administer as single infusion or in equally divided doses at 6-, 8-, or 12-hour intervals
- Mean time to response—5 days for adults, 1 day for children
- Cost significantly higher than oral formulation: reserve for critically ill patients, convert to oral form as soon as possible
- Rasburicase (Elitek (see figure on page 407)
  - Promotes the conversion of uric acid to allantoin: 5-10 times greater solubility than uric acid, allowing rapid urinary excretion
  - Reduces serum uric acid level within 2-4 hours of administration
  - Indicated for initial management of elevated uric acid levels
  - Considerably more expensive than standard therapy (oral Allopurinol and hydration)
    - Oral allopurinol—<$0.25 for 300-mg tablet
    - IV allopurinol—$432/day for 300 mg/m^2/day (1.65 m^2)
    - Rasburicase—$2,532/day for 0.2 mg/kg/day (1.65 m^2)
    - Recommended dosage: 0.15-0.2 mg/kg IV once daily over 30 minutes for 1-5 days
    - Begin 4-24 hours before start of chemotherapy
  - Adverse effects
    - Hemolytic anemia or methemoglobinemia in patients with glucose-6-phosphate dehydrogenase deficiency (G6PD)
    - Possible loss of efficacy from production of antirasburicase antibodies (5%-15% incidence)
    - Interference with uric acid measurements: sample must remain refrigerated and be tested within 4 hours of collection

- Hemodialysis
  - Indicated for uric acid level >10 mg/dL unresponsive to other measures

PATIENT TEACHING

- Avoid dietary sources of purines.
- Avoid alcohol and salicylates.

FOLLOW-UP

- Monitor uric acid levels for indication or resolution of hyperuricemia.
- Monitor renal function.

BIBLIOGRAPHY

Annemans, L., Moeremans, K., Lamotte, M., et al. (2003). Incidence, medical resource utilization and costs of hyperuricemia and tumour lysis syndrome in patients with acute leukaemia and non-Hodgkin's lymphoma in four European countries. *Leukemia & Lymphoma, 44*, 77-83.

Bessmertny, O., Robitaille, L. M., & Cairo, M. S. (2005). Rasburicase: A new approach for preventing and/or treating tumor lysis syndrome. *Current Pharmaceutical Design, 11*, 4177-4185.

Brant, J. M. (2002). Rasburicase: An innovative new treatment for hyperuricemia associated with tumor lysis syndrome. *Clinical Journal of Oncology Nursing, 6*, 12-16.

Bynum, D. T. (2003). Gout. In T. M. Buttaro, J. Trybulski, P. P. Bailey, et al. (Eds.). *Primary care: A collaborative practice* (2nd ed., pp. 852-856). St. Louis: Mosby.

Cairo, M. S. (2002). Prevention and treatment of hyperuricemia in hematological malignancies. *Clinical Lymphoma, 3*, S26-S31.

Cairo, M. S., & Bishop, M. (2004). Tumour lysis syndrome: New therapeutic strategies and classification. *British Journal of Haematology, 127*, 3-11.

DelToro, G., Morris, E., & Cairo, M. S. (2005). Tumor lysis syndrome: Pathophysiology, definition, and alternative treatment approaches. *Clinical Advances in Hematology & Oncology, 3*, 54-61.

Fojo, A. T. (2005). Oncologic emergencies. In V. DeVita, S. Hellman, & S. Rosenberg (Eds.). *Cancer principles and practice* (pp. 2292-2295). Philadelphia: Lippincott Williams & Wilkins.

Holdsworth, M. T., & Nguyen, P. (2003). Role of I.V. allopurinol and rasburicase in tumor lysis syndrome. *American Journal of Health System Pharmacists, 60*, 2213-2222.

Locatelli, F., & Rossi, F. (2005). Incidence and pathogenesis of tumor lysis syndrome. *Contributions to Nephrology, 147*, 61-68.

Nabi Biopharmaceuticals. (2003). *Aloprim (allopurinol sodium) for injection [full prescribing information]*. Retrieved June 14, 2006, from http://www.nabi.com/products/resource.php?id=8&sec=products.

Sanofi-Aventis (2005). *Elitek (rasburicase) [prescribing information]*. Retrieved June 14, 2006, from http://www.sanofiaventis.us:80/live/us/en/layout.jsp?scat=8D52920D-5655-4CCB-A499-EE05C6172519.

Williams, J. (2003). Tumor lysis syndrome/hyperuricemia. In T. M. Buttaro, J. Trybulski, P. P. Bailey, et al. (Eds.). *Primary care: A collaborative practice* (2nd ed., pp. 1210-1211). St. Louis: Mosby.

Yarpuzlu, A. A. (2003). A review of clinical and laboratory findings and treatment of tumor lysis syndrome. *Clinica Chimica Acta, 333*, 13-18.

Hypoglycemia

Jean Rosiak

DEFINITION

- Potentially life-threatening decrease in serum glucose levels
- May result from a paraneoplastic syndrome in which tumor cells secrete insulin-like substances (i.e., insulin-like growth factor-2) that bind with insulin receptors, resulting in decrease in blood glucose level associated with low insulin level
- Glucose level <40 mg/dL requires immediate treatment and is considered an endocrine emergency.

EPIDEMIOLOGY

- Mortality rate among cancer patients who have hypoglycemia is 18%.
- 17% of patients without diabetes who have hypoglycemia have a cancer diagnosis.
- Of the non-insulin-producing tumors, those producing insulin-like growth factors:
  - Mesenchymal tumors: 50%
    - Fibrosarcoma
    - Mesothelioma

- ■ Neurofibroma
- ■ Leiomyosarcoma
- ■ Rhabdomyosarcoma
- ○ Hepatocellular carcinoma: 25%
- ○ Adrenocortical carcinoma: 5%-10%
- ○ Gastrointestinal carcinoma: 5%-10%
- ○ Lymphoma: 5%-10%

PATHOPHYSIOLOGY

- Normally insulin is produced by the pancreas, circulates with a very short half-life, and interacts with insulin receptors primarily on liver, fat, and muscle cells to affect glucose, fat, and protein metabolism
- Paraneoplastic syndrome may occur in which tumor cells secrete insulin-like growth factor-2 (IGF-2)
  - ○ IGF-2 interacts with insulin receptors and IGF receptors, leading to stimulation of glucose uptake by muscle and fat, and potentially also by tumor cells, while hepatic glucose output is suppressed.
  - ○ IGF-2 may be a "survival" signal for oncogene-induced abnormal cancer cell growth.
    - ■ Increased glucose consumption/use by the tumor
    - ■ Inhibition of apoptosis
- Hepatocellular carcinoma or extensive liver metastasis may deplete glycogen stores and impair gluconeogenesis.

SIGNS AND SYMPTOMS

- May be asymptomatic unless fasting
  - ○ Occurs most often at night or on waking
- Diaphoresis/cold sweats
- Pallor
- Dizziness
- Headache
- Heart pounding
- Blurred vision
- Trembling/nervousness
- Personality changes, irritability
- Confusion: may progress to stupor/coma
- Convulsions

CANCERS ASSOCIATED WITH DISORDER

- Pancreatic beta-cell cancer
- Non-islet cell tumors
- Mesenchymal tumors
- Hepatoma/hepatocellular carcinoma
- Fibrous pleural tumor

DIAGNOSTIC TESTS

- Blood glucose level
  - ○ Hypoglycemia: National Cancer Institute: Common Terminology Criteria for Adverse Events:
    - ■ Grade 1: <lower limit of normal (LLN): 55 mg/dL
    - ■ Grade 2: <55-40 mg/dL
    - ■ Grade 3: <40-30 mg/dL
    - ■ Grade 4: <30 mg/dL
    - ■ Grade 5: death
  - ○ <40 mg/dL establishes severe hypoglycemia
- Serum insulin level
  - ○ Increased with insulinoma (insulin-producing tumor of the pancreas)
  - ○ Increased with exogenous insulin administration
  - ○ Decreased with tumor-associated hypoglycemia
- Serum C peptide level
  - ○ Increased with insulinoma
  - ○ Decreased with tumor-associated hypoglycemia
  - ○ Decreased if hypoglycemia from exogenous insulin administration

DIFFERENTIAL DIAGNOSIS

- Drug-induced hypoglycemia
  - ○ Surreptitious or therapeutic insulin administration
  - ○ Oral hypoglycemic agents
- Infection/sepsis
- Insufficient food intake/starvation
- Chronic liver disease
- Adrenal or pituitary failure

TREATMENT

- Only effective treatment is removal or treatment of underlying malignancy
  - ○ Removal of the tumor often leads to complete resolution of hypoglycemia.

- Severe hypoglycemia or coma requires immediate treatment.
- Rapid intravenous (IV) infusion of 50 mL of 50% dextrose solution
- Glucose <40 mg/dL or if symptomatic and glucose <60 mg/dL
  - ○ Continuous IV infusion of 20% glucose at 50-150 mL/hr
    - ■ Adjust rate to maintain glucose level higher than 60 mg/dL
    - ■ Measure glucose level every 3-4 hours until stabilized
  - ○ Glucagon 1 mg intramuscularly (IM) or 0.06-0.3 mg/hr IV
    - ■ Promotes glycogenolysis and gluconeogenesis
- Octreotide can decrease insulin hypersecretion in insulinomas but not helpful in tumor-associated hypoglycemia due to IGF-2
- Glucocorticoids may be temporarily beneficial.

PATIENT TEACHING

- Education of patient and caregiver regarding signs/symptoms of hypoglycemia
- Education regarding management of hypoglycemia
  - ○ Two to three glucose tablets or liquids or foods containing sugar (i.e., regular soda, fruit juice) followed by a protein source
  - ○ If unconscious, do not give anything by mouth.
- Eat regular meals divided over the day and at night.

FOLLOW-UP

- Regular monitoring of glucose level
- Continuous treatment may eventually be required.

BIBLIOGRAPHY

Baird-Powell, S. (2000). Diabetes mellitus, types 1 and 2. In D. Camp-Sorrell & R. A. Hawkins (Eds.), *Clinical manual for the oncology advanced practice nurse* (pp. 837-848). Pittsburgh, PA: Oncology Nursing Press.

Cancer Therapy Evaluation Program (2003). *Common terminology criteria for adverse events* (version 3.0). Washington, DC: National Institutes of Health/U.S. Department of Health and

Human Services. Retrieved June 14, 2006, from http://ctep.cancer.gov/reporting/ctc.html.

Carlson, H. E. (2004). Metabolic complications: Hypoglycemia. In D. A. Casciato (Ed.). *Manual of clinical oncology* (5th ed., pp. 561-562). Philadelphia: Lippincott Williams & Wilkins.

Dirix, L. Y., & vanOosterom, A. T. (2002). Metabolic complications: Hypoglycemia in malignancy. In R. L. Souhami, I. Tannock, P. Hohenberger, et al. (Eds.). *Oxford textbook of oncology* (2nd ed., pp. 918-920). Oxford: Oxford University Press.

LeRoith, D. (2004). Non-islet cell hypoglycemia. *Annals of Endocrinology, 65,* 99-103.

Mendoza, A., Kim, Y. N., & Chernoff, A. (2005). Hypoglycemia in hospitalized patients without diabetes. *Endocrine Practice, 11,* 91-96.

Syndrome of Inappropriate Antidiuretic Hormone

Jean Rosiak

DEFINITION

- Syndrome of inappropriate antidiuretic hormone secretion (SIADH) is a paraneoplastic syndrome in which excessive amounts of antidiuretic hormone (ADH) are produced by tumor cells, causing excessive water retention and dilutional decrease in sodium level.
  - Malignant cells are capable of synthesizing, storing and releasing ADH independent of normal physiological controls.
- Hyponatremia, commonly defined as serum sodium level <135 mEq/L, resulting from ectopic production of antidiuretic hormone by a tumor or central secretion
  - Mild: 125-135 mEq/L
  - Moderate: 115-125 mE/L
  - Severe: <115 mEq/L (medical emergency)

- Water intoxication results and can become a life-threatening oncologic emergency.

EPIDEMIOLOGY

- Occurs in 1%-2% of adults with cancer
- Small cell lung cancer (SCLC): accounts for 80% of all SIADH cases
  - 10%-30% of patients with SCLC have hyponatremia
  - 9%-14% are symptomatic
- Non–small cell lung cancer = 1% incidence
- Head and neck cancer = 3% incidence

CANCERS ASSOCIATED WITH DISORDER

- Small cell lung cancer
  - Does not negatively correlate with stage of disease, response to treatment, or survival
- Tumors with squamous cell or neuroendocrine histologic features
- Primary and metastatic lesions to brain and lung

PATHOPHYSIOLOGY

- Water balance is normally regulated through a negative feedback loop.
  - ADH produced by the hypothalamus is stored in the posterior pituitary
    - Released in response to increased osmolality or decreased plasma volume
    - Inhibited by decreased osmolality and increased plasma volume.
  - ADH acts by increasing water reabsorption from the renal collecting tubules.
- SIADH is characterized by unregulated tumor production of ADH, resulting in excessive water retention by the renal tubules and excessive urinary loss of sodium.
  - Reduced serum sodium level (dilutional)
  - Increased free water is distributed intracellularly, not interstitially; therefore edema is rare.

- Cerebral edema leads to disruption of neural function and may lead to death.

SIGNS AND SYMPTOMS

- Severity of symptoms is related to degree of hyponatremia and rapidity of onset.
- Early manifestations:
  - Thirst
  - Anorexia
  - Mild nausea and vomiting
  - Weight gain without edema
  - Muscle cramps
  - Headache
  - Weakness
  - Mild lethargy/irritability
- More symptomatic as sodium falls below 120 mg/dL (resulting from cerebral edema):
  - Hyporeflexia
  - Confusion/combativeness
  - Oliguria
- Severe hyponatremia: <110-115 mg/dL:
  - Seizures
  - Coma
  - Death may result if hyponatremia is severe or rapid in onset.

DIAGNOSTIC TESTS

- Serum sodium: <130 mEq/L
- Serum osmolality: <280 mOsm/kg
- Urine sodium: >20 mEq/L
- Urine osmolality: >300 mOsm/kg (urine osmolality > serum osmolality)
- Blood urea nitrogen (BUN): normal or decreased (often <10 mg/dL)
- Creatinine: normal or decreased
- Serum ADH: elevated

DIFFERENTIAL DIAGNOSIS

- Central nervous system (CNS) infection or trauma
- Pulmonary infections: tuberculosis, abscess, pneumonia
- Drug effect: cyclophosphamide, vincristine, vinblastine, cisplatin, ifosphamide, tricyclic antidepressants, narcotics, barbiturates
- Renal failure

TREATMENT

- Identify and treat the underlying malignancy: only potential cure for SIADH
- Severe hyponatremia <115 mEq/L is an oncologic emergency.
  - 3% saline solution by slow infusion at rate sufficient to increase serum sodium level by 0.5-1.0 mEq/L/hr
    - 300-500 mL intravenously (IV) over 4-6 hours
    - 1-2 mL/kg IV over 2-3 hours
  - Furosemide 40-80 mg IV (1 mg/kg) every 6-8 hours simultaneously with hypertonic saline solution infusion
    - Induce loss of free water
  - Monitor sodium and electrolytes every 1-3 hours
  - Discontinue when sodium concentration >120 mEq/L and neurological symptoms subside.
  - Untreated SIADH or too rapid correction may result in severe neurological impairment or death.
    - Osmotic demyelination syndrome can occur within 2-6 days of too-rapid correction.
    - Damage to endothelial cells in the brain resulting from brain cell dehydration
    - Breakdown of the blood-brain barrier
    - Characterized by seizures, paralysis, coma, and possibly death
  - If seizures result with too-rapid correction of sodium, dexamethasone 10-20 mg and mannitol 50 g IV should be given immediately.
- Moderately severe hyponatremia:
  - Fluid restriction
    - Sodium <125 mEq/L: limit fluid intake to 500 mL/24 hours
    - Sodium >125 mEq/L: limit fluid intake to 800-1000 mL/24 hours
    - Correction occurs in 3-5 days
    - May be required for long-term management

- Demeclocycline (Declomycin) 600-1200 mg/day in divided doses (150-300 mg orally four times daily)
  - Impairs effect of ADH on renal tubule
  - Facilitates free water excretion
  - Effective within 5-7 days of start of treatment
  - Fluid restriction not required when used
  - Side effects include hematological changes, nephrotoxicity, and photosensitivity.
- Mild hypovolemic hyponatremia may be treated with isotonic (0.9%) saline solution IV or, if tolerated, oral salt tablets (may result in little or no net change in sodium level)
  - Recommend rate of correction no more than 12 mEq/L per day over 2-3 days.

PATIENT TEACHING

- Instruction regarding syndrome and rationale for/importance of treatment:
  - Untreated SIADH will lead to coma and death.
- Monitor weight and report increase.
- Instruction regarding importance of fluid restriction and measures to control thirst:
  - Plan timing/schedule of allowed fluid intake.
  - Frequent oral hygiene, avoid mouthwash containing alcohol, frequent saline solution mouth rinses, use of artificial saliva or sugarless gum, avoid smoking
- Stress management and pain control
  - Pain and stress increase ADH production.

FOLLOW-UP

- Maintain high index of suspicion in patients with lung cancer or history of SIADH.
- Monitor weight and intake and output.
  - Be alert for increase of intake over output.

- Monitor serum and urine sodium and osmolality levels.
- Monitor for use of medications that may contribute to SIADH:
  - Tricyclic antidepressants, nicotine, narcotics, and barbiturates can increase ADH secretion.

BIBLIOGRAPHY

Carlson, H. E. (2004). Metabolic complications: Hyponatremia—syndrome of inappropriate antidiuretic hormone (SIADH). In D. A. Casciato (Ed.). *Manual of clinical oncology* (5th ed., pp. 554-558). Philadelphia: Lippincott Williams & Wilkins.

Fojo, A. T. (2005). Metabolic emergencies: Cancer and hyponatremia. In V. DeVita, S. Hellman, & S. A. Rosenberg (Eds.). *Cancer principles and practice* (pp. 2295-2296). Philadelphia: Lippincott Williams & Wilkins.

Haapoja, I. S. (2000). Syndrome of inappropriate antidiuretic hormone. In C. H. Yarbro, M. H. Frogge, M. Goodman, et al. (Eds.). *Cancer nursing: Principles and practice* (5th ed., pp. 913-919). Sudbury, MA: Jones & Bartlett.

Heideman, R. L., & Heideman, N. H. (2004) Hyponatremia. In M. D. Abeloff, J. O. Armitage, J. E. Niederhuber, et al. (Eds.). *Clinical oncology* (3rd ed., pp. 973-982). St. Louis: W. B. Saunders.

Langfeldt, L. A., & Cooley, M. E. (2003). Syndrome of inappropriate antidiuretic hormone secretion in malignancy: Review and implications for nursing management. *Clinical Journal of Oncology Nursing, 7,* 425-430.

Lindaman, C. (1992). SIADH: Is your patient at risk? *Nursing92 (June) 22,* 60-63.

Miaskowski, C. (1997). Syndrome of inappropriate antidiuretic hormone secretion. In *Oncology nursing: An essential guide for patient care* (pp. 241). Philadelphia: W. B. Saunders.

Miaskowski, C. (1999). Oncologic emergencies: Syndrome of inappropriate antidiuretic hormone secretion. In C. Miaskowski & P. Buchsel (Eds.). *Oncology nursing: assessment and clinical care* (pp. 236-243). St. Louis: Mosby.

Richerson, M. T. (2004). Electrolyte imbalances: Syndrome of inappropriate antidiuretic hormone secretion. In C. H. Yarbro, M. H. Frogge, & M. Goodman (Eds.). *Cancer symptom management* (3rd ed., pp. 446-449). Sudbury, MA: Jones & Bartlett.

Williams, J. (2003). Oncology complications and paraneoplastic syndromes: Syndrome of inappropriate antidiuretic hormone. In T. M. Buttaro, J. Trybulski,

P. P. Bailey, et al. (Eds.). *Primary care: A collaborative practice* (2nd ed., pp. 1211-1212). St. Louis: Mosby.

Tumor Lysis Syndrome

Jeanene "Gigi" Robison

DEFINITION

- A group of metabolic disorders that can occur after cytotoxic therapy is initiated
- Can lead to life-threatening hemodynamic and renal complications

EPIDEMIOLOGY

- Risk increases when associated with:
  - Tumors with rapid response to effective therapy, usually chemotherapy given for a hematological malignancy
  - Tumors larger than 8-10 cm (e.g., abdominal mass, mediastinal mass)
  - Tumors with a high proliferation rate
  - Extensive lymph node involvement
  - Multiple metastasis
  - Bulky tumors associated with lymphadenopathy or hepatosplenomegaly
  - Elevated white blood cell count (WBC)
  - Elevated pretreatment lactate dehydrogenase (LDH) level
  - Preexisting renal impairment or metabolic disturbances
  - Dehydration
- The most frequent cause of tumor lysis syndrome (TLS) is the administration of cytotoxic therapy.
- Any form of cancer therapy that causes rapid cell lysis and necrosis of a tumor mass can induce this syndrome.
- Rarely, pretreatment TLS has occurred in persons with Burkitt's lymphoma and acute myelogenous leukemia (AML), which is most likely caused by rapid tumor lysis.
- In several studies, the incidence of clinically significant TLS varies from 3% to 6%, despite preventive measures in many patients.
- The incidence of silent laboratory evidence of TLS is seen in 42% to 70% of those with high risk for development of TLS.
- Advanced age may predispose a person to impaired renal function, which may result in a reduced capacity to dispose of tumor lysis byproducts.
  - This factor may contribute to the increased occurrence of TLS in older persons.
- No increased incidence is associated with sex or ethnicity.

CANCERS ASSOCIATED WITH DISORDER

- Lymphoma
  - Most common complication of Burkitt's lymphoma
  - Frequent cases occur in lymphoblastic lymphoma
- Acute leukemias
  - More common in acute lymphocytic leukemia (ALL) than AML and in those with high WBC.
- Highest risk for development:
  - Burkitt's lymphoma
  - Lymphoblastic non-Hodgkin lymphoma
  - Acute leukemias, especially T-cell ALL, and including AML
- Moderate risk for development:
  - Low-grade non-Hodgkin lymphoma
  - Multiple myeloma
  - Chronic leukemia, especially CML in blast crisis
  - Myelodysplastic syndrome (MDS)
  - Breast cancer
  - Small cell lung carcinoma
  - Germ cell tumors, such as seminoma or ovarian cancer
  - Ewing's sarcoma
- Lowest risk for development:
  - Low-grade lymphoma treated with interferon
  - Medulloblastoma
  - Merkel cell carcinoma
  - Gastrointestinal adenocarcinoma

PATHOPHYSIOLOGY

- A metabolic imbalance that can occur after cytotoxic therapy is initiated
- The result of rapid tumor cell destruction and, concurrently, the rapid release of intracellular components, primarily potassium, phosphorus, and uric acid, into the bloodstream
- Metabolic abnormalities associated with TLS:
  - Hyperkalemia
  - Hyperuricemia
  - Hyperphosphatemia
  - Hypocalcemia
- The inability of the kidneys to clear these intracellular byproducts from the blood stream can lead to life-threatening hemodynamic and renal complications
  - Cardiac arrhythmias
  - Renal failure
  - Acute respiratory distress syndrome (ARDS)

SIGNS AND SYMPTOMS

- Most likely to occur within 24 to 48 hours of starting chemotherapy treatment
- May last up to 7 days after therapy is completed
- Early signs:
  - Weakness
  - Muscle cramps
  - Nausea and vomiting
  - Diarrhea
  - Lethargy
  - Paresthesias
- Late signs:
  - Paralysis
  - Bradycardia
  - Hypotension
  - Oliguria
  - Edema
  - Cardiac irritability
  - Laryngospasm
  - Flank pain
  - Hematuria
  - Crystalluria
  - Tetany
  - Renal failure

- ○ Seizures
- ○ Cardiac arrest

DIAGNOSTIC TESTS

- Before initiation of chemotherapy, measure:
  - ○ Electrolytes (potassium, phosphorus, calcium), renal function (blood urea nitrogen [BUN], creatinine), LDH, uric acid, and magnesium levels
  - ○ Electrocardiogram (ECG) in clients identified with hyperkalemia
- Continuing evaluations:
  - ○ Monitor electrolytes, renal function, uric acid, magnesium levels, and urine pH every 6 to 8 hours

DIFFERENTIAL DIAGNOSIS

- Acute nephrocalcinosis
- Acute renal failure

TREATMENT

- Identification of those persons at increased risk for development of TLS
- Initiate preventive measures.

Pharmacologic Management

- Prevention:
  - ○ Intravenous (IV) hydration administered in amounts of 4-5 L per day, or 3 L/m^2/24 hours, to induce a urine output of at least 3 L/day.
  - ○ Amount of hydration may vary, depending on the patient's age and comorbidities.
  - ○ Normal saline solution or dextrose 5% in water (D5W) is used as hydration fluids before, during, and after treatment.
  - ○ Excessive hydration is contraindicated in those persons with poor cardiac status—may lead to fluid overload.
  - ○ Reduction of uric acid in serum with the use of allopurinol, which may be given orally or by IV (Aloprim).
    - ■ Blocks the enzyme xanthine oxidase to decrease the production of uric acid.

- ■ Deposits of uric acid in the kidney are decreased.
  - ○ Rasburicase (Elitek) for pediatric patients to treat high uric acid levels in children with TLS.
  - ○ Alkalinization of urine by addition of sodium bicarbonate to IV fluids.
    - ■ Goal is to maintain a urine pH between 7.0 and 7.5 and decrease the solubility of uric acid.
    - ■ Use of sodium bicarbonate is controversial; calcium and phosphate can precipitate in the renal tubules if the urine becomes too alkaline.
    - ■ Alkaline urine is determined by a pH >7.5.
    - ■ Sodium bicarbonate infusion is stopped when serum bicarbonate level is 30 mEq/L, urine pH is greater than 7.5, serum uric acid levels have normalized, or serum phosphorus is elevated.
    - ■ An alternative method to alkalinize the urine is the IV administration of acetazolamide at 250-500 mg/day (5 mg/kg/day).
  - ○ Avoid nephrotoxic medicines.
  - ○ Avoid endogenous sources of potassium and phosphorus.
- Management:
  - ○ Manage hyperkalemia.
    - ■ Treat mild hyperkalemia (e.g., potassium less than 6.5 mEq/L) with exchange resins, such as sodium polystyrene sulfonate (Kayexalate), orally or by retention enema. In addition to the potassium level, sodium polystyrene sulfonate will assist in lowering phosphorus levels.
    - ■ Treat severe hyperkalemia (e.g., potassium greater than 6.5 mEq/L or ECG changes) with calcium gluconate, if ECG changes are apparent; hypertonic glucose (e.g., dextrose 50%) IV along with

insulin; sodium bicarbonate; or loop diuretics.
  - ○ Manage hypocalcemia
    - ■ Calcium level not corrected unless symptomtomatic or a positive Chvostek or Trousseau sign present.
    - ■ Calcium gluconate is administered. If potassium level is over 6.5 mEq/L, calcium gluconate is given as a cardioprotectant.
  - ○ Manage hyperuricemia
    - ■ Allopurinol administered at 600-900 mg/day with a maximum dose of 500 mg/m^2/day either orally or IV.
    - ■ Uricase available in Europe; limited availability in the United States.
      - □ Converts uric acid to metabolites that are water soluble.
      - □ Dose: 50-100 units/kg/day given intramuscularly (IM) or IV.
  - ○ Manage hyperphosphatemia.
    - ■ Give phosphate binding, aluminum-containing antacids.
  - ○ Forced diuresis
    - ■ If adequate urine output not achieved by hydration alone, loop diuretics may be administered to maintain urinary output.
    - ■ Mannitol is given if hydration and loop diuretics do not induce adequate urine output.

Nonpharmacologic Management

- Monitor laboratory tests, especially electrolytes (potassium, phosphorus, calcium), magnesium, uric acid, BUN, creatinine, and LDH. Usually blood for testing is drawn every 6 to 8 hours during the first 48 to 72 hours after treatment is initiated.
- Acute TLS with renal failure:
  - ○ Hemodialysis when potassium is greater than 6 mEq/L, uric acid is greater than 10 mEq/L, or phosphorus level is greater than 10 mEq/L.

Oncologic
Emergencies

○ Hemodialysis preferred over peritoneal dialysis because of increased clearance rates with hemodialysis.

○ Continuous hemodialysis may be more beneficial than intermittent hemodialysis.

PATIENT TEACHING

- Goal is to prevent or reverse renal failure and maintain normal electrolyte levels.
- Define TLS and describe the process of cell breakdown and release of byproducts into the bloodstream and the consequences of this.
- Describe the signs and symptoms of TLS.
- Explain the purpose of frequent laboratory draws and the need to closely monitor these results. Provide patient with a copy of laboratory results.
- Explain the nursing care and treatments for TLS.
- Encourage patient to increase fluid intake before and after chemotherapy (8-10 glasses/day).
- Patient is to report any decreased urine output, increase in weight, an alteration in mental status function, nausea, vomiting, diarrhea, or anorexia.

FOLLOW-UP

- Continue to monitor for signs and symptoms of TLS.
- Monitor laboratory findings as to the continuation or resolution of TLS.

BIBLIOGRAPHY

Annemans, L., Moeremans, K., Lamotte, M., et al. (2003). Incidence, medical resource utilization and costs of hyperuricemia and tumour lysis syndrome in patients with acute leukaemia and non-Hodkin's lymphoma in four European countries. *Leukemia Lymphoma, 44*, 77-83.

Brant, J. (2002). Rasburicase: An innovative new treatment for hyperuricemia associated with tumor lysis syndrome. *Clinical Journal of Oncology Nursing, 6*, 12-16.

Cairo, M., & Bishop, M. (2004). Tumour lysis syndrome: New therapeutic strategies and classification. *British Journal of Haematology, 127*, 3-11.

Chielens, D. (1999). Chronic myelogenous leukemia. In C. Miakowski & P. Buchsel, (Eds.). *Oncology nursing: Assessment and clinical care* (pp. 1239-1261). St. Louis: Mosby.

Gobel, B. (2005). Metabolic emergencies. In J. Itano & K. Taoka, (Eds.). *ONS core curriculum in oncology nursing* (4th ed., pp. 383-421). St. Louis: Elsevier Saunders.

Hogan, D. (1999). Non-Hodgkin's lymphoma. In C. Miakowski & P. Buchsel, (Eds.). *Oncology nursing: Assessment and clinical care* (pp. 1453-1470). St. Louis: Mosby.

Jeha, S. (2001). Tumor lysis syndrome. *Seminars in Oncology, 38*(Suppl. 3), 6-11.

Jeha, S. (2006). Current and emerging treatment options for patients with tumor lysis syndrome. *Johns Hopkins Advanced Studies in Nursing, 4*, 49-57.

Krishnan, K., Urbanski, C., & Quillen, J. (2002). *Tumor lysis syndrome.* Retrieved July 4, 2005, from http://www.emedicine.com/med/topic2327.htm.

Lee, K. (2002). *Tumor lysis syndrome.* Retrieved July 4, 2005, from http://www.med.unc.edu/medicine/web/tumorlysissyn.pdf.

Lydon, J. (2005). Tumor lysis syndrome. In C. Yarbro, M. Frogge, & M. Goodman (Eds.). *Cancer nursing: Principles and practice* (6th ed., pp. 946-958). Sudbury, MA: Jones & Bartlett.

Oksenholt, N. & Seelig, F. (1999). Burkitt's lymphoma. In C. Miakowski & P. Buchsel (Eds.). *Oncology nursing: Assessment and clinical care* (pp. 1353-1372). St. Louis: Mosby.

Reedy, A. (2006). Targeting tumor lysis syndrome: New therapeutic options. *John Hopkins Advanced Studies in Nursing, 4*, 38-48.

Richerson, M. (2004). Electrolyte imbalances. In C. Yarbro, M. Frogge, & M. Goodman (Eds.). *Cancer symptom management* (3rd ed., pp. 440-460). Sudbury, MA: Jones & Bartlett.

Wossmann, W., Schrappe, M., Meyer, U., et al. (2003). Incidence of tumor lysis syndrome in children with advanced stage Burkitt's lymphoma/leukemia before and after introduction of prophylactic use of urate oxidase. *Annals of Hematology, 82*, 160-165.

Hematologic Emergencies   *Jeanene "Gigi" Robison*

Disseminated Intravascular Coagulation

DEFINITION

- A disorder in which there is a progressive and abnormal overstimulation of the normal coagulation system

- This results in varying degrees of concomitant systemic thrombosis and hemorrhage.

EPIDEMIOLOGY

- Risk increases when associated with:
  ○ Infections, sepsis
  ○ Leukemias, especially acute promyelocytic leukemia (APL), acute myelogenous leukemia (AML), acute lymphoblastic leukemia (ALL)

  ○ Lymphomas, especially immunoblastic lymphoma and Hodgkin disease
  ○ Cancers, including biliary, breast, colon, gastric, lung, ovarian, pancreas, and prostate and malignant melanoma
  ○ Massive tissue injury (e.g., major surgery, head trauma, burns, electrical shock)
  ○ Placement of prosthetic devices: intraperitoneal shunt;

LeVeen or Denver shunts; aortic balloon assist devices
- Transfusions: hemolytic transfusion reaction, multiple transfusions of whole blood
- Vascular disorders: aortic aneurysm, vasculitis, grafts, hemangiomas
- Acute liver disease: obstructive jaundice; acute hepatic failure
- Pregnancy and obstetrical complications
- Other: heat stroke, malignant hyperthermia, fat embolism, snakebite, acute pancreatitis, glomerulonephritis
- In persons with cancer, disseminated intravascular coagulation (DIC) is the most common serious thrombotic state that occurs.

CANCERS ASSOCIATED WITH DISORDER

- Leukemias, especially APL, and including AML, chronic myelogenous, and ALL
- Lymphomas, especially immunoblastic lymphoma and Hodgkin disease
- Cancers, including biliary, breast, colon, gastric, lung, ovarian, pancreas, prostate, gallbladder, and unknown primary; rarely, malignant melanoma

PATHOPHYSIOLOGY

- In the normal coagulation system, hemostasis is maintained through a balance between the processes of clot formation (thrombosis) and clot breakdown (fibrinolysis).
- One component of the DIC process is abnormal thrombus formation.
  - Triggered by an overwhelming thrombogenic stimulus, such as infection, malignancy, or trauma
  - Intrinsic or extrinsic pathway of the clotting cascade is triggered, which leads to excessive circulating thrombin.
  - Results in multiple fibrin clots circulating in the bloodstream
  - Platelets are trapped by the excess fibrin clots.

- Leads to formation of microvascular and macrovascular fibrin thrombi (stationary blood clots)
- When part of the thrombus is dislodged, then an embolus (or "thromboembolus") is formed. This traveling clot can lead to diffuse microvascular obstruction and result in ischemia, impaired organ perfusion, and end-organ damage.
- Second component is fibrinolysis.
  - Leads to bleeding and hemorrhaging
  - Normally, the fibrinolytic system is activated once a clot has been formed to control how large the clot becomes and to reopen the healed blood vessel over time.
  - During this process, plasminogen is converted to plasmin by tissue plasminogen activator.
  - The release of plasmin causes enzymatic lysis of the fibrin clot.
  - Breakdown of fibrin clot causes release of fibrin split, or degradation, products (FSPs, FDPs).
  - If fibrinolysis process becomes uncontrolled:
    - FDPs not effectively removed from circulation and accumulate in the bloodstream.
    - Accumulation contributes to the bleeding that is observed in patients with DIC.
  - Coagulation factors consumed at a rate greater than the body's ability to replace them during the thrombosis formation; also leads to the bleeding

SIGNS AND SYMPTOMS

- Signs of bleeding:
  - Skin
    - Pallor
    - Petechiae
    - Purpura
    - Ecchymosis
    - Hematomas
    - Epistaxis

- Scleral hemorrhage
- Gingival or mucosal bleeding from oral cavity
- Acral cyanosis (i.e., generalized sweating with cold, mottled fingers and toes)
- Bleeding (which can range from oozing to frank hemorrhaging) from any invasive site, including a wound, incision, injection site, intravenous (IV) or central line site
- Respiratory
  - Dyspnea
  - Tachypnea
  - Shortness of breath
  - Hypoxia
  - Hemoptysis
  - Cyanosis
  - Abnormal lung sounds
- Gastrointestinal
  - Tarry stools
  - Hematemesis
  - Abdominal tenderness, pain, or distention
  - Positive results with the guaiac stool test
- Genitourinary/gynecological
  - Hematuria (may be associated with burning), dysuria, frequency and pain on urination
  - Decreased urinary output
  - Renal failure
  - Heavily prolonged vaginal bleeding
- Cardiovascular
  - Hypotension
  - Tachycardia
  - Weak and thready pulse
  - Decreased peripheral pulses
  - Narrow pulse pressure
  - Sluggish capillary refill
  - Changes in color and temperature of extremities
  - Cool and clammy skin
- Neurological
  - Headache
  - Altered mental status
  - Changes in level of consciousness or pupil reaction
  - Restlessness
  - Confusion
  - Lethargy

- Seizures
- Coma
  - Musculoskeletal
    - Joint pain and stiffness

DIAGNOSTIC TESTS

- General laboratory tests to assist in the diagnosis of DIC:
  - Platelet count: usually decreased
  - Fibrinogen level: usually decreased
  - D-dimer assay (often done in combination with the FDP titer): increased
  - Fibrin degradation product (FDP) titer: increased
  - Prothrombin time/international normalized ratio (PT/INR): usually prolonged
  - Activated partial thromboplastin time (aPTT): may be prolonged
  - Thrombin time (TT): usually prolonged
- Laboratory tests to determine accelerated coagulation:
  - Antithrombin III level: decreased
  - Fibrinopeptide A: increased
  - Prothrombin activation peptides: increased
  - Thrombin-antithrombin complex: increased
- Laboratory tests to determine accelerated fibrinolysis:
  - Plasminogen level: decreased
  - Plasmin alpha 2-antiplasmin complex: decreased
- Other tests to assist in diagnosis of DIC:
  - Guaiac stool, urine, emesis, and nasogastric tube secretions
  - Radiology: chest x-ray film (PA and lateral): to rule out acute respiratory distress syndrome (ARDS)

DIFFERENTIAL DIAGNOSIS

- Infection, septicemia (bacteria, viruses)
- Intravascular hemolysis (transfusion reactions, thrombotic thrombocytopenic purpura [TTP], hemolytic uremic syndrome [HUS])
- Leukemia, metastatic malignancy
- Trauma
- Acute liver disease
- Vascular disorders
- Obstetrical accidents
- ARDS

TREATMENT

- Treatment of the underlying, predisposing condition(s) causing the DIC
- Supporting the patient's hemodynamic status
- Managing the signs/symptoms related to bleeding or thrombosis that are present

Pharmacologic Management

- Remove the trigger of the DIC by treating the underlying, predisposing condition.
  - For example, administer chemotherapy if malignancy is the cause; administer antibiotics if infection is the cause.
- Hemodynamic support
  - Administer fluid replacement to treat hypotension.
  - Provide oxygen therapy to treat hypoxia.
- IV vasopressor (i.e., dopamine)
  - Administer to maintain blood pressure
- Diuretics or IV fluids
  - Administer to maintain central venous pressure
- Platelet transfusions
  - Indicated if platelet count is less than 20,000/mm^3 or if patient is actively bleeding.
  - Indicated for use in patients with DIC and APL
- Washed, packed red blood cells (RBCs)
  - Indicated if hemoglobin is less than 8 g/dL or if patient is actively bleeding
- Blood components that contain fibrinogen (e.g., fresh-frozen plasma [FFP], cryoprecipitate, whole blood)
  - Use is controversial; the fibrinogen in these products may aggravate the DIC condition.
- Cryoprecipitate
  - May be indicated in cases of extreme hyperfibrinolysis

- Provides fibrinogen and factor VIII.
- Plasmapheresis
  - Removes triggers of coagulation
  - Replaces coagulation factors.
- Heparin (IV or subcutaneous)
  - Interferes with thrombin production
  - Use is controversial; primary side effect is bleeding
  - Do not administer to patients with APL because of increased risk of death related to hemorrhaging.
- All-transretinoic acid
  - Administer to patients with APL who have DIC.
  - Support their treatment with platelets and plasma.
  - Addition of retinoic acid may result in less hemorrhage and transfusion requirements for APL patients who are being treated for DIC.
- Fibrinolytic inhibitor medications
  - Used to manage excessive bleeding, in spite of other measures to control the DIC:
  - Epsilon-aminocaproic acid (EACA) (Amicar)
    - Use is controversial; EACA inhibits the fibrinolytic system
    - Primary side effect is clotting
    - Can lead to organ failure from large vessel thrombosis
- Antithrombin III
  - Inhibits procoagulants and fibrinolytic process
- Tranexamic acid (Cyklokapron)
  - Can lead to widespread fibrin deposits; usually given after heparin therapy

Nonpharmacologic Management

- Monitor hemodynamic signs and symptoms and vital signs often.
- Monitor intake and output every 1-2 hours during periods of acute DIC.
- Monitor all sites of bleeding often.
- Note amount of bleeding: count peripads, weigh affected dressings, measure bloody drainage.

- Measure abdominal girth every 4 hours if abdominal bleeding is suspected.
- Apply direct pressure or apply pressure dressings or sandbags to sites of active bleeding.
- Elevate sites of active bleeding, if possible

PATIENT TEACHING

- Goal of treatment is to reverse the hypercoagulable state and to maintain normal coagulation levels.
- Define DIC and describe the signs and symptoms.
- Explain the purpose of the laboratory tests, nursing care, and treatments for DIC.
- Teach patients self-care measures to maximize their safety: maintain bed in a low position with side rails up; clear pathways in room and hallway; minimize activities that trigger bleeding; take precautions against accidental bleeding because even minor scrapes or bumps could result in bleeding.
- Teach patients to minimize activities that contribute to clot formation, including avoid constrictive clothing or devices; do not dangle feet on side of bed; do not use pillows under knees or knee gatch; and move the toes, feet, and legs often.
- Teach patient and family to save urine, stool, and emesis for nurse to check for blood.
- Teach patient about critical signs and symptoms to report: any bruising, red rash, headache, black stools, blood in the urine or stools, and bleeding from the gums, nose, eyes, vagina, or rectum.

FOLLOW-UP

- Continue to monitor for signs and symptoms of DIC.
- Monitor laboratory findings as to the continuation or resolution of DIC.
- Provide additional resources, such as home equipment or assistance, as needed, as a result of severe

complications of DIC (e.g., organ dysfunction, activity limitations).

BIBLIOGRAPHY

Ezzone, S. (2000). Disseminated intravascular coagulation. In D. Camp-Sorrell & R. Hawkins (Eds.). *Clinical manual for the oncology advanced practice nurse* (pp. 683-688). Pittsburgh, PA: Oncology Nursing Press.
Gobel, B. (2005). Disseminated intravascular coagulation. In C. Yarbro, M. Hansen, & M. Goodman (Eds.). *Cancer nursing: Principles and practice* (6th ed., pp. 887-894). Sudbury, MA: Jones & Bartlett.
Gobel, B. (2005). Metabolic emergencies. In J. K. Itano & K. N. Taoka, (Eds.). *ONS core curriculum for oncology nursing* (4th ed., pp. 383-421). St. Louis: Elsevier Saunders.
Lin, E. (2001). Oncologic emergency: case 3. In E. Lin (Ed.). *ONS advanced practice in oncology nursing: Case studies and review* (pp. 312-319). Philadelphia: W. B. Saunders.
Miaskowski, C. (1999). Oncological emergencies. In C. Miaskowski & P. Buchsel (Eds.), *Oncology nursing: Assessment and clinical care* (pp. 221-223). St. Louis: Mosby.

Deep Vein Thrombosis

DEFINITION

- Deep vein thrombosis (DVT) is the partial or complete occlusion of blood flow in the deep veins caused by thrombus (clot) formation.

EPIDEMIOLOGY

- Third most common type of vascular disease
- The two most common presentations:
  - DVT of the lower extremities
  - Pulmonary embolus (PE); a life-threatening complication
- In persons with cancer, thrombosis is a common complication of malignancy.
- Potentially fatal complication that primarily affects hospitalized patients
  - Two million Americans are affected yearly.

- Approximately 200,000 hospital visits are due to DVT.
  - About 50% of persons with DVT have symptoms.
  - The other 50% are asymptomatic and therefore do not receive treatment, which increases the risk for a significant complication.

- Increased risk:
  - Surgery, especially lengthy surgical procedures
  - Active cancer (treatment or palliation within previous 6 months)
    - Can cause a hypercoagulable state
  - History of thrombotic events, especially DVT
  - Conditions in which local clotting takes place
    - Phlebitis
    - Trauma
    - Inflammation
  - Conditions that promote venous stasis
    - Prolonged bed rest
    - Prolonged immobility resulting from pain, trauma, surgery, or paralysis
    - Recent casting of a lower extremity (within 4 weeks)
    - General debility
    - Heart failure
  - Infections related to gram-negative or gram-positive bacteria
  - Hypercoagulable state (e.g., disseminated intravascular coagulation)
  - Peripheral vascular disease
  - Medications
    - Antiestrogens such as tamoxifen or raloxifene and estrogen
  - Medications that induce endothelial damage
    - Chemotherapy (especially adjuvant therapy for breast cancer)
    - Some vasopressor agents (i.e., dopamine)
    - Contrast medium
    - High-dose antibiotics.
  - Burns or fractures that cause damage to the vessel.
  - Use of central venous catheter

○ Antiphospholipid antibodies (associated with systemic lupus erythematosus)

CANCERS ASSOCIATED WITH DISORDER

- Mucin-secreting adenocarcinoma of the gastrointestinal (GI) tract
- Small cell lung carcinoma
- Non–small cell lung cancer
- Colon cancer
- Pancreatic tumors
- Ovarian carcinoma
- Endometrial carcinoma
- Intracranial carcinoma
- Acute promyelocytic leukemia
- Myeloproliferative disorders
- Breast carcinoma
- Prostate carcinoma
- Bladder carcinoma

PATHOPHYSIOLOGY

- Patients with cancer have a higher incidence of development of DVT because thrombi formation is a common complication of malignancy.
  ○ Formation of a thrombus occurs within the cardiovascular system.
  ○ Can lead to formation of an "embolus" (or "thromboembolus"), which is a traveling clot
    ■ Embolus may be formed when part of the thrombus is dislodged.
- Three factors predispose cancer patients to a higher risk of thrombus formation:
  ○ Cancer patients may have increased coagulability in their blood, which is induced by malignant cells.
    ■ Tumor cells often induce this hypercoagulable state directly through the secretion of procoagulant factors.
    ■ Tissue factor and cancer procoagulant can directly activate factor X, which results in the initiation of the clotting pathway.
  ○ Venous stasis predisposes a person to clot formation.
    ■ Pooling allows coagulation factors to accumulate and

increases the chance of platelet aggregation and clot formation.
    ■ Venous stasis often occurs in the lower extremities, especially in persons who are immobile or paralyzed.
    ■ Also occurs when tumors cause external pressure of the blood vessel and impede blood flow
    ■ Venous stasis is seen most commonly in persons with superior vena cava syndrome.
  ○ Damage to the blood vessel wall (endothelial) or abnormality causes platelets to adhere to the wall and activates clotting factors, which results in formation of a thrombus.
    ■ Direct invasion of blood vessels by tumors can affect the vascular endothelium and promote clot formation.
- A life-threatening complication of DVT is development of PE.
  ○ When the blood clot is detached from the original source, the embolus travels with the blood flow.
  ○ The embolism may migrate from the distal vein to the inferior vena cava, right atrium, right ventricle, and then may enter the pulmonary artery.
  ○ A very large embolus may lodge in the main pulmonary artery, and smaller emboli will pass to more distal branches of the pulmonary artery.
  ○ When the embolus lodges in the pulmonary artery or one of its branches, then it can cause partial or total occlusion of the vessel.

SIGNS AND SYMPTOMS

- Clinical manifestations
  ○ A dull ache, tight feeling or frank pain in the calf, which is made worse with standing or walking and is made better with elevation
  ○ Localized tenderness or pain over the involved vein

  ○ Tender, palpable venous cord of involved vein
  ○ Swollen calf or thigh by measurement
  ○ Calf swelling of more than 3 cm in circumference in the symptomatic leg
  ○ Unilateral pitting edema in involved extremity
  ○ Warmth and erythema of involved extremity
  ○ Dilated superficial venous collateral vessels (nonvaricose)
  ○ Low-grade fever is possible.
- Assessing for Homan's sign as part of the physical examination
  ○ Calf pain a positive sign
    ■ Produced by dorsiflexion of the foot, with the knee bent in about 30 degrees of flexion
  ○ Positive results seen in less than 50% of patients.
  ○ High incidence of false-positive results
  ○ Because Homan's sign test may cause embolism, the test should NOT be performed if DVT is suspected.
- Signs and symptoms of PE may be first indication of DVT.
  ○ May include dyspnea, chest pain, tachypnea, tachycardia, and fever

DIAGNOSTIC TESTS

- Laboratory
  ○ D-dimer
    ■ Blood assay detects blood clot fragments, which are produced by clot lysis
    ■ May be used with other diagnostic tests to rule out DVT
    ■ A negative result has shown a high negative predictive value for DVT in patients without cancer, but a negative result does not reliably rule out DVT in cancer patients.
- Radiology
  ○ Lower extremity venous ultrasonography is initial test of choice for diagnosis of DVT
    ■ Less accurate than venography

- Low cost, noninvasive test that is highly sensitive and specific for diagnosing symptomatic DVT
  - Less sensitive and specific for detecting proximal and calf DVT for the high risk postoperative patient who is without symptoms
  - Doppler ultrasonography
    - Uses both scanning and compression to detect the thrombus by direct visualization or by interference when the vein does not collapse during gentle compression
  - Impedance plethysmography
    - Detects changes in blood volume that can occur with obstruction
- Contrast venography (phlebography)
  - Determines the presence of DVT by infusing contrast material into the venous system by a catheter in the foot
  - A positive result would be any obstruction to the flow of dye within the vein, and this would indicate the presence of a thrombus.
  - Not the first choice of diagnostic tests for DVT because it is expensive, invasive, and carries significant side effects resulting from hypersensitivity reactions to contrast medium.
  - Gold standard for diagnosing DVT
  - Used when the diagnosis of DVT remains unclear after clinical evaluation and initial testing
- Magnetic resonance imaging (MRI)
  - May be alternative to venography
  - Especially useful for detecting thrombi in the pelvic vein.
- Computed tomography (CT)
  - Spiral CT and CT angiography have been used to diagnose DVT.

- Radionuclide scintigraphy
  - Uses a variety of radiopharmaceuticals to detect DVT
  - Less reliable in the calf
  - Results do not differentiate between intrinsic and extrinsic compression.
  - Expensive and not as reliable in recurrent DVT.

DIFFERENTIAL DIAGNOSIS

- Calf muscle strain or tear
- Intramuscular hematoma
- Cellulitis
- Superficial phlebitis
- Obstruction of lymphatics by tumor, from irradiation or lymph node dissection
- Acute arterial occlusion
- Ruptured Baker's cyst
- Chronic venous insufficiency
- Lymphangitis/fibrositis
- Kidney, liver, or heart disease: usually has bilateral edema
- Hypoalbuminemia

TREATMENT

- Medications
  - Anticoagulants
- Surgery
  - Placement of inferior vena cava filter to prevent PE in recurrent DVT has been advocated
    - Uses an endoluminal filter to interrupt the blood flow through the inferior cava vein
    - Filters may not be beneficial and may actually increase the risk of recurrent DVT.
  - Treatment of choice in patients with contraindications for anticoagulant therapy

Pharmacologic Management

- Prevention
  - Acetylsalicylic acid (aspirin, ASA) may be administered on a daily basis.
  - Low-dose subcutaneous heparin may be administered for lower abdominal, pelvic, and lower extremity.

- Low-molecular-weight heparin (LMWH) may be administered for lower abdominal, pelvic, and hip or knee replacement surgeries
  - Enoxaparin (Lovenox)
  - Ardeparin (Normiflo)
  - Danaparoid (Orgaran)
  - Dalteparin (Fragmin)
- Low-dose warfarin (Coumadin) may be administered to patients with long-term indwelling central venous catheters.
- Management
  - Anticoagulant therapy
    - To interrupt thrombosis
    - Allows the lytic system to dissolve the clot
    - Unfractionated heparin is the traditional standard for the initial treatment of DVT because of its rapid onset of action.
    - About 5 days of IV heparin is followed by a course of oral anticoagulants (warfarin).
    - LMWH drugs have been shown to be equally safe and effective in patients who are hemodynamically stable and effective in patients who are not candidates for warfarin therapy.
    - Enoxaparin and tinzaparin are approved in the United States for treatment of DVT, with or without PE.
    - Vitamin K antagonists (e.g., warfarin) are oral agents that are used for long-term anticoagulation after thromboembolism occurs and for secondary prophylaxis.
    - These agents may be initiated concurrently with heparin:
  - Thrombolytic therapy (e.g., streptokinase, rtPA)
    - Promotes rapid resolution of emboli
    - Commonly not recommended for persons with DVT
    - May be used in persons with extensive obstruction of venous outflow

Nonpharmacologic Management

- Bed rest is indicated for the first 5 to 7 days, with leg elevation, for acute DVT.
- Mild analgesics and warm compresses may be used for comfort for persons with acute DVT.
- Frequent leg exercises (range of motion [ROM] or isometric), if bedridden:
  - Every 1 to 2 hours while awake to improve venous flow
  - Heel pumping and ankle circles, for 10-12 repetitions
- Supplemental oxygen by nasal cannula may be administered to maintain a PaO_2 of higher than 80 mm Hg in persons with acute DVT.
- Frequent ambulation, if able to tolerate, after the 5-7 days of bed rest
- Antiembolitic stockings/hose should be applied before surgery.
- Pneumatic compression stockings/devices may be used postoperatively to stimulate circulation and prevent DVT.
- Elevation of foot of bed 15-20 inches, with slight knee flexion
  - Leg elevation should not exceed 45 degrees.
- Avoid popliteal pressure, which is produced by crossing the legs, placing pillows behind the knees, and elevation of the knee gatch.
- Do not massage the legs of persons with DVT.
- Regular position changes should be encouraged to prevent hypoventilation.
- Avoid smoking and caffeine to prevent vasoconstriction.
- Adequate hydration
- Do not perform Homan's test once DVT is diagnosed or test result is positive.

PATIENT TEACHING

- Goals:
  - Stimulate patient's circulation.
  - Prevent additional DVTs.
  - Minimize or prevent respiratory compromise.
  - Resolve the pulmonary embolism.
- Define DVT.
- Describe the signs and symptoms of DVT.
- Explain the purpose of the laboratory and diagnostic tests, nursing care, and treatments.
- Encourage patient to wear the pneumatic compression stockings/devices, as ordered.
- Teach patient the rationale for ambulating as soon as possible after surgery.
- Encourage patient to change position regularly, avoid sitting or standing for long periods, drink 8-10 glasses of fluid per day, avoid smoking and caffeine, and perform ROM or isometric exercises.
- Teach patients to avoid constrictive clothing or devices; to keep the legs elevated and straight; to move the toes, feet, and legs often; and to avoid pressure in the back of their knees (popliteal) to prevent a clot from forming in the arms or legs.
- Teach patient to take warfarin at the same time every day.
- Teach patient to avoid any contact sports that could lead to serious injury.
- Teach patient to use a soft toothbrush for oral care and use an electric razor, if there is a need to shave.
- Teach patient to maintain a diet consistent in the amount of vitamin K, if on warfarin.
  - Foods that are high in vitamin K: green leafy vegetables (spinach, kale) and liver
  - Foods that contain small amounts of vitamin K: milk, meats, eggs, cereal, fruits, and vegetables
  - Recommended Daily Allowances of vitamin K in adults: 80 mcg/day for men and 65 mcg/day for women.
  - Do not take vitamin K supplements; vitamin K improves blood clotting.
- Patient is to report any leg pain, bleeding, or signs of thrombophlebitis or PE.

FOLLOW-UP

- Continue to monitor for signs and symptoms of DVT.
- Monitor laboratory findings as to the continuation or resolution of DVT.
- Provide additional resources, such as home equipment or assistance, as needed, as a result of severe complications of DVT (e.g., PE).

BIBLIOGRAPHY

Anderson, J. (2004). Advances in anticoagulation therapy: the role of selective inhibitors of factor Xa and thrombin in thromboprophylaxis after major orthopedic surgery. *Seminars in Thrombosis and Hemostasis, 30,* 609-618.

Brant, J. (1999). Cervical cancer. In C. Miaskowski & P. Buchsel (Eds.). *Oncology nursing: assessment and clinical care* (pp. 657-688). St. Louis: Mosby.

Brophy, S., & George-Gay, B. (2002). Chapter 21: Musculoskeletal. In B. George-Gay & C. Chernecky (Eds.). *Clinical medical-surgical nursing: A decision-making reference* (pp. 720-763). Philadelphia: W. B. Saunders.

Burke, C. (1999). Surgical treatment. In C. Miaskowski & P. Buchsel (Eds.). *Oncology nursing: assessment and clinical care.* (pp. 29-58). St. Louis: Mosby.

DeSancho, M. T., & Rand, J. H. (2001). Bleeding and thrombotic complications in critically ill patients with cancer. *Critical Care Clinics, 17,* 599-622.

Friend, P., & Pruett, J. (2004). Bleeding and thrombotic complications. In C. Yarbro, M. Frogge, & M. Goodman (Eds.). *Cancer symptom management* (3rd ed., pp. 233-251). Sudbury, MA: Jones & Bartlett.

George-Gay, B. (2002). Deep vein thrombosis. In B. George-Gay & C. Chernecky (Eds.). *Clinical medical-surgical nursing: a decision-making reference* (pp. 500-509). Philadelphia: W. B. Saunders.

Hooper, V. (2002). Deep vein thrombosis. In B. George-Gay & C. Chernecky (Eds.), *Clinical medical-surgical nursing: a decision-making reference* (pp. 500-509). Philadelphia: W. B. Saunders.

Khushal, A., Quinlan, D., Alikhan, R., et al. (2002). Thromboembolitic disease in surgery for malignancy: rationale for prolonged thromboprophylaxis. *Seminars in Thrombosis and Hemostasis, 28,* 569-576.

Kwaan, H. C., & Gorgon, L. I. (2001). Thrombotic microangiopathy in the cancer patient. *Acta Haematologica, 106,* 52-56.

Larsen, J. *Vitamin K: ask the dietitian.* (1995-2003). Retrieved December 1,

2006, from http://www.dietitian.com/vitam ink.html.

Lee, A., Levine, M., Butler, G., et al. (2006). Incidence, risk factors, and outcomes of catheter-related thrombosis in adult patients with cancer. *Journal of Clinical Oncology, 24*, 1404-1408.

Levine, M. (2003). Low-molecular-weight heparin or oral anticoagulation for secondary prevention of deep vein thrombosis in cancer patients. *Seminars in Thrombosis and Hemostasis, 29*, 9-11.

Mousa, S. (2004). Low-molecular-weight heparin in thrombosis and cancer. *Seminars in Thrombosis and Hemostasis, 30*(suppl 1), 25-30.

Prandoni, P. (2003) Recurrent thromboembolism in cancer patients: incidence and risk factors. *Seminars in Thrombosis and Hemostatsis, 29*, 3-8.

Story, K. (2000). Deep vein thrombosis. In D. Camp-Sorrell & R. Hawkin (Eds.). *Clinical manual for the oncology practice nurse* (pp. 235-243). Pittsburgh: Oncology Nursing Press.

Story, K. (2005). Alterations in circulation. In J. Itano & K. Taoka (Eds.). *ONS core curriculum for oncology nursing* (pp. 364-379). St. Louis: Elsevier Saunders.

Turpie, A. (2002). State of the art: a journey through the world of antithrombotic therapy. *Seminars in Thrombosis and Hemostasis, 28*, 3-11.

Yarbro, C., Frogge, M., & Goodman, M. (Eds.). (2004). Cardiopulmonary function. In *Oncology nursing review* (3rd ed., pp. 147-167). Boston: Jones & Bartlett.

Hemolytic Uremic Syndrome

DEFINITION

- A potentially life-threatening disorder with a symptom complex characterized by microangiopathic hemolytic anemia, thrombocytopenia, and acute renal failure

EPIDEMIOLOGY

- Clinically rare complication
  - Incidence in cancer patients is estimated to be approximately 5%.
  - Delayed and potentially fatal complication after bone marrow transplantation (BMT)

- Risk increases when associated with:
  - Infections, particularly infections with the Shiga toxin-producing *Escherichia coli* (STEC)
  - Disorders of the complement system
  - Disorders interfering with the degradation of von Willebrand factor (VWF)
  - High-dose chemotherapy conditioning regimes (e.g., BMT)
  - Rejection after BMT
  - Chemotherapy regimens, especially with mitomycin C
  - Immunosuppressive drugs: cyclosporin A, tacrolimus
  - Immune disorders: systemic lupus erythematosus (SLE), human immunodeficiency virus (HIV) infection
  - Cobalamin metabolism
  - Pregnancy/hemolysis
  - Elevated liver enzymes
  - Syndrome of hemolysis, elevated liver enzymes, and low platelets (HELLP)

CANCERS ASSOCIATED WITH DISORDER

- Adenocarcinomas, including gastric cancer, lung cancer, and breast cancer
- Lymphoma

PATHOPHYSIOLOGY

- Two different forms of hemolytic uremic syndrome (HUS): typical (HUS) and atypical (aHUS)
  - HUS:
    - Occurs most often, primarily in children, and is usually epidemic
    - It is generally caused by infections with toxin-producing *E. coli* of the serotype 0157:H7.
    - The virulence of these microbes is associated with the Shiga toxin or Shiga-like toxins, which exert a direct effect on renal epithelial cells. This toxin has been shown to injure the endothelium, thereby

exposing the subendothelium.
    - Tissue factor is released, which renders the vessel wall prothrombotic.
    - The Shiga toxin also binds to and activates platelets.
    - Frequently associated with diarrhea
    - Most patients show acute renal failure.
    - Usually only one episode of HUS
    - Overall prognosis good
    - Renal function generally recovers.
  - aHUS:
    - Can be sporadic or familial
    - Not associated with the Shiga toxin or diarrhea
    - Sporadic form can be due to genetic defects. May be triggered by complement disorders, disorders interfering with the degradation of vWF, pregnancy, *Streptococcus pneumoniae*, drugs (cyclosporin A), diseases (SLE), or infection with HIV
    - Familial form rare; associated with a significant risk of morbidity and mortality.
    - Recurrent aHUS subgroup: strong relationship to diseases of the complement system; prognosis is often poor.
    - Patients often have end-stage renal disease; will require a kidney transplant.
    - Common for patients in this subgroup to have severe arterial hypertension and require multidrug therapy
  - Trigger is endothelial damage
    - Can be caused by defects in the complement system, which acts as a central defense of innate immunity
    - Endothelial damage leads to platelet aggregation, thrombocytopenia, and subsequent renal, neurological, and pulmonary dysfunction.

- Renal vasculature is primarily affected; result is often irreversible renal damage in aHUS.
  - No clear-cut distinction between cancer-associated thrombotic thrombocytopenic purpura (TTP) and aHUS
    - Many patients are diagnosed as having the TTP/HUS disorder on the basis of clinical and laboratory findings alone.
    - The patient's history can help distinguish between TTP and HUS. For example, a history of bone marrow transplant or Shiga toxin hemorrhagic colitis is suggestive of HUS. Also, renal impairment is the dominant feature in patients with HUS.

SIGNS AND SYMPTOMS

- In a person who has received a bone marrow transplant, the typical onset of HUS is 30 to 875 days post transplant. Patients have a triad of symptoms, including:
  - Microangiopathic hemolytic anemia: hematuria, fatigue
  - Renal insufficiency: increased creatinine levels, reduced creatinine clearance, fluid retention
  - Thrombocytopenia: increased bleeding, hemorrhaging

DIAGNOSTIC TESTS

- Complete blood cell count (CBC)—decreased platelets
- Red blood cell (RBC) morphology—increased schizocytes
- Blood: vWF assay, ADAMTS13 (vWF cleavage protein)
- Lactate dehydrogenase (LDH): elevated
- Haptoglobin levels: low or undetectable
- Reticulocyte counts: elevated
- Coombs' test: negative (nonautoimmune, non-drug-induced hemolytic anemia) or positive (autoimmune, drug-induced hemolytic anemia)

- Prothrombin times, activated partial thromboplastin times, factor V, factor VIII, and fibrinogen—usually normal
- Fibrinogen degradation products (FDP): may be elevated
- Thrombin times: may be prolonged
- Blood urea nitrogen (BUN), serum creatinine: may be elevated
- Electrolytes
- Blood cultures
- Urine: dipstick, urinalysis, 24-hour creatinine clearance, urine culture
- Radiology: renal sonogram, renal angiogram, intravenous pyelogram, computed tomographic (CT) scan of abdomen

DIFFERENTIAL DIAGNOSIS

- Thrombocytopenic purpura (TTP): classical or cancer associated
- Microangiopathic hemolytic anemia (MAHA)
- Disseminated intravascular coagulation (DIC)
- Hematuria related to other diseases (e.g., infection, intrinsic kidney disease, benign prostatic hypertrophy)
- Hematuria related to other medications (e.g., ifosfamide, high-dose cyclophosphamide, intravesicular chemotherapy)
- Hematuria related to radiation therapy (e.g., pelvic radiation, prostate seed implants)

TREATMENT

- Supportive care:
  - Plasma infusions
  - Plasma exchanges
  - Dialysis
  - Other supportive therapies

Pharmacologic Management

- Prevention:
  - Vigorous pretransplant hydration, parenterally or orally
  - Continuous bladder irrigations with normal saline solution
- Management:
  - Plasma exchange: less effective in TTP/HUS, with response

rates of 20%-30% compared with response rates of 80% in classical TTP
  - Plasma infusion
    - Pathogen-reduced fresh frozen plasma (FFP) is preferred.
    - Repetitive plasma infusions have increased risk of infection. Initially, the recommended volume is 60-65 mL/kg/week.
    - During maintenance, the recommended volume is 20 mL/kg/week.
  - Immunization program (including hepatitis A and B)
  - Discontinue drugs that are inducing the HUS. Discontinue administration of chemotherapy or immunosuppressive drugs, which may be inducing the HUS.
  - Avoid platelet transfusions: Contraindicated; can lead to worsening of the microvascular thrombi

Nonpharmacologic Management

- Nephrology consultation to determine the most appropriate renal therapy.
- Renal replacement therapy
  - May include peritoneal dialysis and hemodialysis
  - May be successful treatments for patients with recurrent aHUS
  - Renal transplantation is complicated by recurrence of the disease, and the failure rate is >70%.
  - No kidney transplant is recommended in patients with soluble complement disorders.
- Liver transplantation
  - Combined renal and liver transplant is a logical form of treatment because both factors H and I are synthesized in the liver.
  - Not recommended in persons with complement disorders

PATIENT TEACHING

- Goals:
  - Blood cell counts return to normal levels.
  - Symptoms (bleeding, renal symptoms) will subside.
- Define HUS.
- Describe the signs and symptoms of HUS.
- Explain the purpose of the laboratory tests, nursing care, and treatments for HUS.
- Encourage patient to drink at least 8-10 glasses of fluid each day.
- Patient is to report any increase in bleeding, blood in their urine, or the occurrence of renal symptoms.

FOLLOW-UP

- Continue to monitor for signs and symptoms of HUS.
- Monitor appropriate laboratory findings (especially platelet count and hemoglobin/hematocrit) as to the continuation or resolution of HUS.
- Provide additional resources, such as home equipment or assistance, as needed.
- Monitor bone marrow transplant patients treated with high-dose chemotherapy for potential long-term sequelae.

BIBLIOGRAPHY

Boyle, D. (2000). Hematuria. In D. Camp-Sorrell & R. Hawkins (Eds.). *Clinical manual for the oncology advanced practice nurse* (pp. 485-489). Pittsburgh, PA: Oncology Nursing Press.

Buchsel, P. (1999). Bone marrow transplantation. In C. Miaskowki & P. Buchsel (Eds.). *Oncology nursing: assessment and clinical care* (pp. 143-186). St. Louis: Mosby.

DeSancho, M., & Rand, J. (2001). Bleeding and thrombotic complications in critically ill patients with cancer. *Critical Care Clinics, 17,* 599-622.

Friend, P., & Pruett, J. (2004). Bleeding and thrombotic complications. In C. Yarbro, M. Frogge, & M. Goodman (Eds.). *Cancer symptom management* (3rd ed., pp. 233-251). Sudbury, MA: Jones & Bartlett.

Kavanagh, D., & Goodship, T. (2006). Membrane cofactor protein and factor I: mutations and transplantation. *Seminars in Thrombosis and Hemostasis, 32,* 155-159.

Kwaan, H. (2005). Thrombotic thrombocytopenic purpura: a diagnostic and therapeutic challenge. *Seminars in Thrombosis and Hemostasis, 31,* 615-624.

Kwaan, H., & Gorgon, L. (2001). Thrombotic microangiopathy in the cancer patient. *Acta Haematologica, 106,* 52-56.

Zimmerhackl, L. B., Besbas, N., Jungraithmayr, T., et al. (2006). Epidemiology, clinical presentation, and pathology of atypical and recurrent hemolytic uremic syndrome. *Seminars in Thrombosis and Hemostasis, 32,* 113-120.

Zipfel, P., Misselwitz, J., Licht, C., et al. (2006). The role of defective complement control in hemolytic uremic syndrome. *Seminars in Thrombosis and Hemostasis, 32,* 146-154.

Pulmonary Embolism

DEFINITION

- Partial or complete occlusion of blood flow in the pulmonary artery, or one of its branches, by an embolus, which migrates from the distal veins and lodges in the pulmonary blood vessel

EPIDEMIOLOGY

- Third most common type of vascular disease
  - Two most common presentations
    - Deep vein thrombosis (DVT) of the lower extremities
    - Pulmonary embolus (PE), a life-threatening complication of DVT
- In persons with cancer, thrombosis is a common complication of malignancy.
- The most common preventable cause of death in hospitalized patients
  - Estimates of 100,000 cases of fatal PE yearly
  - Contributing cause of death in a further 100,000 patients in the United States
- Up to 80% of PEs are small and clinically undetectable because the pulmonary circulation

has several sources of collateral flow.
- Pulmonary infarction occurs in 10%-15% of cases, usually in persons with cardiopulmonary disease.
- About 1% of persons with PE will have a fatal outcome.
  - High mortality rate associated with persons with PE who have large or multiple emboli.
- Increased risk from:
  - Surgery, especially lengthy surgical procedures
  - Active cancer (treatment or palliation within previous 6 months): can cause a hypercoagulable state
  - Hypercoagulable state (e.g., disseminated intravascular coagulation [DIC])
  - History of thrombotic events, especially DVT
  - Conditions in which local clotting takes place: phlebitis, trauma, inflammation
  - Conditions that promote venous stasis: prolonged bed rest; prolonged immobility resulting from pain, trauma, surgery, or paralysis; recent casting of a lower extremity (within 4 weeks); general debility; heart failure
  - Infections related to gram-negative or gram-positive bacteria
  - Peripheral vascular disease
  - Medications: antiestrogens (such as tamoxifen, raloxifene), estrogen
  - Medications that induce endothelial damage: chemotherapy (especially adjuvant therapy for breast cancer), some vasopressor agents (i.e., dopamine), contrast medium, high-dose antibiotics
  - Burns or fractures that cause damage to the vessel
  - Use of central venous catheter
  - Antiphospholipid antibodies (associated with systemic lupus erythematosus)

Oncologic Emergencies

CANCERS ASSOCIATED WITH DISORDER

- Mucin-secreting adenocarcinoma of the gastrointestinal (GI) tract
- Small cell lung carcinoma, non–small cell lung carcinoma
- Colon cancer
- Pancreatic tumors
- Ovarian carcinoma
- Endometrial carcinoma
- Intracranial carcinoma
- Acute promyelocytic leukemia
- Myeloproliferative disorders
- Breast carcinoma
- Prostate carcinoma
- Bladder carcinoma

PATHOPHYSIOLOGY

- Patients with cancer have a higher incidence of development of a PE as a complication of the existing DVT.
- Thrombus formation is a common complication of malignancy.
  - Formation of thrombi occurs within the cardiovascular system.
  - Can lead to formation of an "embolus" (or "thromboembolus"), which is a traveling clot
  - Embolus may be formed when part of the thrombus is dislodged.
- Three factors predispose cancer patients to a higher risk of thrombus formation in a blood vessel:
  - Increased coagulability of cancer patient's blood.
    - Tumor cells often induce this hypercoagulable state directly through the secretion of procoagulant factors.
    - Tissue factor and cancer procoagulant can directly activate factor X, which results in the initiation of the clotting pathway.
  - Venous stasis predisposes a person to clot formation.
    - Pooling allows coagulation factors to accumulate and increases the chance of platelet aggregation and clot formation.

- Venous stasis often occurs in the lower extremities, especially for persons who are immobile or paralyzed.
- It also occurs when tumors cause external pressure of the blood vessel and impede blood flow, such as in persons with superior vena cava syndrome.
  - Damage to the blood vessel wall (endothelial) damage or abnormality:
    - Causes platelets to adhere to the wall and activates clotting factors: results in formation of a thrombus
    - Direct invasion of the blood vessels by tumors can affect the vascular endothelium and promote clot formation.
- When the blood clot is detached from the original source, the embolus travels with the blood flow.
  - Embolism migrates from the distal vein to the inferior vena cava, right atrium, right ventricle, and enters the pulmonary artery.
  - Very large embolus may lodge in the main pulmonary artery
  - Smaller emboli will pass to more distal branches of the pulmonary artery.
- Pulmonary embolus is most commonly a blood clot.
- Embolus may also be a fat globule, air, tumor, amniotic fluid, other tissue fragment, bacterial emboli, or a foreign body.
- When the embolus lodges in the pulmonary artery or one of its branches, then it can cause partial or total occlusion of the vessel.
  - The result of mechanical occlusion of a regional pulmonary artery
    - Changes in perfusion and ventilation of the section of the lung that is supplied by that artery
  - Lung volumes and compliance are usually reduced.
  - Pulmonary shunting may cause hypoxia.

- Pulmonary artery pressure may become elevated.
- If massive PE, the right ventricle may be unable to generate a pressure that is high enough to maintain an adequate cardiac output.
- Right ventricular failure can cause right arterial pressure to rise and cardiogenic shock to ensue.

SIGNS AND SYMPTOMS

- Can be difficult to diagnose through tests; clinical presentation is important in guiding management approaches.
- May be few or no symptoms when the emboli are small
- Acute right ventricular failure, systemic hypotension, and sudden death may occur in patients with a massive PE.
- Clinical manifestations of PE may vary, depending on the size of the embolus and on the patient's preexisting cardiopulmonary status.
  - Dyspnea, usually with sudden onset (occurs in about 60% of patients with PE): can vary from mild to severe, and from intermittent to progressive
  - Tachypnea (respiratory rate >24/min)
  - Respiratory crackles/wheezing/rales
  - Diminished breath sounds
  - Tachycardia
  - Low-grade fever: occurs in about 40% of patients with PE
  - Chest pain: often anginal type at onset, and worsens with deep breathing; later, chest pain becomes pleuritic
  - Cough
  - Hemoptysis (usually a later symptom), bloody sputum
  - Diaphoresis
  - Syncope
  - Back or abdominal pain
  - Lower extremity pain, tenderness, or swelling
  - Thrombophlebitis symptoms: warmth, erythema, cord like
  - Anxiety, apprehension, restlessness

DIAGNOSTIC TESTS

- Radiology
  - Ventilation-perfusion (V/Q) lung scan
    - Normal perfusion scan result: definitively rules out clinical PE. Low or intermediate result: indicates a possible PE.
    - Venous thrombosis studies or pulmonary arteriogram is indicated. High probability result: indicates probable PE.
    - In conjunction with clinical signs, this test definitively indicates the need for immediate treatment of PE.
  - Chest x-ray film
    - Elevation of a hemidiaphragm and pulmonary infiltrates most commonly identified.
    - Findings often determined to be abnormal; however, these are frequently related to medical history of chronic obstructive pulmonary disease (COPD) or cardiac history and not due to PE.
  - Lower extremity venous ultrasonography
    - Noninvasive test that identifies any obstruction or reduced blood flow to a specific area
    - Intermediate result of the V/Q scan and a negative result of the lower extremity venous ultrasound does not exclude the presence of a PE.
  - Venography (phlebography)
    - Any obstruction to the flow of dye within the vein indicates the presence of a thrombus.
    - A positive result confirms the diagnosis of thrombophlebitis.
  - Pulmonary arteriography (angiography)
    - Although expensive, the high sensitivity makes this the definitive test for PE.
  - Electrocardiogram (ECG)
    - Tachycardia and nonspecific ST-T wave changes are most often observed but are not diagnostic for PE.
  - Magnetic resonance imaging (MRI)
    - May be an alternative to venography.
    - Especially useful for detecting thrombi in the pelvic vein.
  - Computed tomography (CT).
    - Spiral CT and CT angiography have been used to diagnose both DVT and PE.
- Laboratory tests:
  - D-dimer
    - Blood assay detects blood clot fragments, which are produced by clot lysis.
    - May be used with other diagnostic tests to rule out DVT.
    - Negative result has shown a high negative predictive value for DVT in patients without cancer.
    - A negative result does not reliably rule out DVT in cancer patients.
  - Arterial blood gas analysis
    - Results usually normal.
    - Hypoxia may be seen in massive PE.
    - Nondiagnostic test; hypoxia may be present in many medical conditions.

DIFFERENTIAL DIAGNOSIS

- Congestive heart failure
- Myocardial infarction
- Dissecting aortic aneurysm
- Pneumothorax
- Infection (e.g., pneumonia, pulmonary interstitial pneumonitis, pericarditis)
- Pleural effusions (PE can lead to pleural effusions)
- Pulmonary fibrosis
- Superior vena cava syndrome

TREATMENT

- Medications
  - Anticoagulants
- Surgery
  - Placement of inferior vena cava filter to prevent PE in recurrent DVT has been advocated.
    - Procedure uses an endoluminal filter to interrupt the blood flow through the inferior cava vein.
    - Filters may not be beneficial and may actually increase the risk of recurrent DVT.
    - Treatment of choice in patients with contraindications for anticoagulant therapy
  - Thrombectomy or embolectomy (rare):
    - Performed either as a surgical procedure or as a catheter technique under radiographic guidance.
    - Performed only in extreme cases

Pharmacologic Management

- Prevention
  - Goal is to prevent DVTs so pulmonary embolism does not occur.
  - Aspirin may be administered on a daily basis.
  - Low-dose subcutaneous heparin may be administered for lower abdominal, pelvic, and lower extremity surgeries.
  - Low-molecular-weight heparin (LMWH) may be administered for lower abdominal, pelvic, and hip or knee replacement surgeries:
    - Enoxaparin (Lovenox)
    - Ardeparin (Normiflo)
    - Danaparoid (Orgaran)
    - Dalteparin (Fragmin)
  - Low-dose warfarin (Coumadin) may be administered to patients with long-term indwelling central venous catheters.
- Management:
  - Anticoagulant therapy:
    - Interrupts thrombosis
    - Allows the lytic system to dissolve the clot
    - PE usually responds to treatment.
    - Unfractionated heparin is the traditional standard for the initial treatment of venous

thromboembolism, including PE, because of its rapid onset of action.

- LMWH drugs have been shown to be equally safe and effective in patients who are hemodynamically stable, and effective in patients who are not candidates for warfarin therapy. Enoxaparin and tinzaparin are approved in the United States for treatment of DVT, with or without PE.
- Vitamin K antagonists (e.g., warfarin) are oral agents that are used for long-term anticoagulation after thromboembolism occurs and for secondary prophylaxis. These agents may be initiated concurrently with heparin.
  - Thrombolytic therapy promotes rapid resolution of emboli; role of thrombolysis for acute PE is not established.
  - Novel anticoagulants
    - Synthetic, indirect factor Xa inhibitors (e.g., fondaparinux)
    - Direct thrombin inhibitors (e.g., ximelagatran)

Nonpharmacologic Management

- Bed rest is indicated for the first 5 to 7 days, with leg elevation, for acute DVT and acute PE.
- Frequent leg exercises (range of motion [ROM] or isometric), if bedridden
  - Every 1 to 2 hours while awake to improve venous flow
  - Includes heel pumping and ankle circles, for 10-12 repetitions.
- Mild analgesics and warm compresses may be used for comfort for persons with acute DVT and acute PE.
- Supplemental oxygen by nasal cannula may be administered to maintain a PaO_2 of higher than 80 mm Hg in persons with acute DVT and acute PE.
- Frequent ambulation, if able to tolerate, after 5-7 days of bed rest

- Antiembolitic stockings/hose should be applied before surgery.
- Pneumatic compression stockings/devices may be used postoperatively to stimulate circulation and prevent DVT and PE.
- Elevation of foot of bed 15-20 inches, with slight knee flexion. Leg elevation should not exceed 45 degrees.
- Avoid popliteal pressure, which is produced by crossing the legs, placing pillows behind the knees, and elevation of the knee gatch.
- Do not massage the legs of persons with DVT or PE.
- Regular position changes should be encouraged to prevent hypoventilation.
- Avoid smoking and caffeine to prevent vasoconstriction.
- Adequate hydration.
- Do not perform Homan's test once DVT is diagnosed or test result is positive.

PATIENT TEACHING

- Goals:
  - Stimulate patient's circulation.
  - Prevent additional DVTs.
  - Minimize or prevent respiratory compromise.
  - Resolve the PE.
- Define PE and describe the signs and symptoms.
- Explain the purpose of the laboratory and diagnostic tests, nursing care, and treatments.
- Encourage patient to wear the pneumatic compression stockings/devices, as ordered.
- Teach patient the rationale for ambulating as soon as possible after surgery.
- Encourage patient to change position regularly, to avoid sitting or standing for long periods, to drink 8-10 glasses of fluid per day, to avoid smoking and caffeine, and to perform ROM or isometric exercises.
- Teach patients to avoid constrictive clothing or devices; to keep the legs elevated and straight; to move the toes, feet, and legs often; and to avoid pressure in

the back of the knees (popliteal) to prevent a clot from forming in the arms or legs.
- Teach patient to take warfarin at the same time every day.
- Teach patient to maintain a diet consistent in the amount of vitamin K, if on warfarin.
  - Foods that are high in vitamin K: green leafy vegetables (spinach, kale) and liver
  - Foods that contain small amounts of vitamin K: milk, meats, eggs, cereal, fruits, and vegetables
  - Recommended Daily Allowances of vitamin K in adults: 80 mcg/day for men and 65 mcg/day for women
  - Do not take vitamin K supplements: vitamin K improves blood clotting.
- Teach patient to avoid any contact sports that could lead to serious injury.
- Teach patient to use a soft toothbrush for oral care and to use an electric razor, if there is a need to shave.
- Patient is to report any leg pain, bleeding, or signs of thrombophlebitis or PE.

FOLLOW-UP

- Continue to monitor for signs and symptoms of PE or DVT.
- Monitor laboratory findings as to the continuation or resolution of PE.
- Provide additional resources, such as home equipment or assistance, as needed.

BIBLIOGRAPHY

Anderson, J. (2004). Advances in anticoagulation therapy: The role of selective inhibitors of factor Xa and thrombin in thromboprophylaxis after major orthopedic surgery. *Seminars in Thrombosis and Hemostasis, 30,* 609-618.

Brant, J. (1999). Cervical cancer. In C. Miaskowski & P. Buchsel, (Eds.), *Oncology nursing: assessment and clinical care* (pp. 657-688). St. Louis: Mosby.

Burke, C. (1999). Surgical treatment. In C. Miaskowski & P. Buchsel (Eds.). *Oncology nursing: assessment and clinical care* (pp. 29-58). St. Louis: Mosby.

Friend, P., & Pruett, J. (2004). Bleeding and thrombotic complications. In C. Yarbro, M. Frogge, & M. Goodman, (Eds.). *Cancer symptom management* (3rd ed., p. 233-251). Sudbury, MA: Jones & Bartlett.

George-Gay, B. (2002). Deep vein thrombosis. In B. George-Gay & C. Chernecky (Eds.). *Clinical medical-surgical nursing: a decision-making reference* (pp. 500-509). Philadelphia: W. B. Saunders.

Henke, S. (2000). Pulmonary embolism. In D. Camp-Sorrell & R. Hawkin (Eds.), *Clinical manual for the oncology practice nurse* (pp. 183-188). Pittsburgh: Oncology Nursing Press.

Hooper, V. (2002). Deep vein thrombosis. In B. George-Gay & C. Chernecky (Eds.). *Clinical medical-surgical nursing: a decision-making reference* (pp. 500-509). Philadelphia: W. B. Saunders.

Khushal, A., Quinlan, D., Alikhan, R., et al. (2002). Thromboembolitic disease in surgery for malignancy? rationale for prolonged thromboprophylaxis. *Seminars in Thrombosis and Hemostasis, 28,* 569-576.

Larsen, J. *Vitamin K: ask the dietitian.* (1995-2003). Retrieved December 1, 2006, from http://www.dietitian.com/vitamink.html.

Lee, A., Levine, M., Butler, G., et al. (2006). Incidence, risk factors, and outcomes of catheter-related thrombosis in adult patients with cancer. *Journal of Clinical Oncology, 24,* 1404-1408.

Levine, M. (2003). Low-molecular-weight heparin or oral anticoagulation for secondary prevention of deep vein thrombosis in cancer patients. *Seminars in Thrombosis and Hemostasis, 29,* 9-11.

Lin, E. (2001). Oncologic emergency: case 10. In E. Lin (Ed.). *Advanced practice in oncology nursing,* (pp. 371-373). Philadelphia: W. B. Saunders.

Mousa, S. (2004). Low-molecular-weight heparin in thrombosis and cancer. *Seminars in Thrombosis and Hemostasis, 30*(suppl 1), 25-30.

Prandoni, P. (2003) Recurrent thromboembolism in cancer patients: incidence and risk factors. *Seminars in Thrombosis and Hemostatsis, 29,* 3-8.

Turpie, A. (2002). State of the art: a journey through the world of antithrombotic therapy. *Seminars in Thrombosis and Hemostasis, 28,* 3-11.

Yarbro, C., Frogge, M., & Goodman, M. (Eds.). (2004). Cardiopulmonary function. In *Oncology Nursing Review* (3rd ed., pp. 147-167). Sudbury, MA: Jones & Bartlett.

Sepsis

DEFINITION

- Systemic inflammatory response to pathogenic microorganisms in the bloodstream, which can lead to septic shock and multiple organ dysfunction syndrome (MODS)

EPIDEMIOLOGY

- Bacterial infection the most common cause of septic shock; responsible for 45%-50% of cases of septic shock
- Fungi, viruses, anaerobes, and protozoa are other organisms that also cause septic shock.
- In the United Stated, an estimated 750,000 cases of sepsis, which results in 210,000 deaths, occur annually. In noncoronary intensive care units, septic shock is the second leading cause of death, and mortality rates vary from 20%-50%.
- Highest risk for development of infection:
  - Neutropenia (absolute neutrophil count [ANC] <500/mm^3)
  - Chemotherapy: high dose, especially patients undergoing bone marrow transplantation
  - Radiation therapy: total body irradiation
  - Febrile neutropenia and one or more high risk factors (e.g., mucositis, diarrhea, clinical instability, advanced disease, or overt organ dysfunction)
- Moderate risk for development of infection:
  - Neutropenia (ANC between 500-1,000/mm^3)
  - Chemotherapy: standard doses
  - Radiation therapy: localized
  - Corticosteroids and immunosuppression therapy
  - Age >65 years old or <1 year old
  - Splenectomy
  - Breakdown of skin or mucous membranes
  - Invasive procedures/devices, including tunneled central venous catheters
  - Antibiotic use
  - Protein-calorie malnutrition
  - Comorbid conditions:
    - Diabetes
    - Organ-related disease (e.g., renal, hepatic, cardiovascular, gastrointestinal [GI], pulmonary)
- Lowest risk for development of infection:
  - Neutropenia (ANC between 1,000-1,500/mm^3)
  - Chemotherapy: low dose

CANCERS ASSOCIATED WITH DISORDER

- Leukemia, especially acute leukemia and chronic lymphocytic leukemia
- Lymphoma (e.g., Hodgkin disease, non-Hodgkin lymphoma)
- Multiple myeloma
- Disease with bone marrow metastasis

PATHOPHYSIOLOGY

- The greatest predictor of infection in persons with cancer is neutropenia.
  - The mature neutrophil is the first line of defense against bacterial infection.
- Infectious Disease Society of America (IDSA) definition
  - ANC of 500/mm^3, or
  - ANC of 500-1,000/mm^3 in patients in whom further decline is expected
- Sepsis is one stage in the continuum from infection to septic shock to MODS.
- Six phases of the septic shock cascade:
  - Infection
    - Inflammatory response to invasion of host tissue by microorganisms
  - Bacteremia/fungemia
  - Presence of viable bacteria (or fungus) in the bloodstream
  - Evidenced by positive blood cultures

Oncologic Emergencies

○ Systemic inflammatory response syndrome (SIRS)/sepsis
  ▪ The clinical, systemic inflammatory response to invasion by microorganisms
  ▪ Manifested by two or more of
    □ Temperature >38° C (100.4° F) or <36° C (96.8° F)
    □ Heart rate >90 beats/min
    □ Respiratory rate >20 breaths/min or $PaCO_2$ <32 mm Hg
    □ White blood cell count (WBC) >12,000 cells/mm^3, WBC <4,000 cells/mm^3, or >10% immature (band) cells
○ Severe sepsis
  ▪ Sepsis associated with hypotension (systolic blood pressure <90 mm Hg or reduction of >40 mm Hg from baseline)
  ▪ Organ dysfunction, hypoperfusion (e.g., dry, warm, and flushed skin; decreased breath sounds; decreased GI motility; oliguria; lactic acidosis; mental status changes)
○ Septic shock
  ▪ Severe sepsis with hypotension
  ▪ Presence of perfusion abnormalities such as acrocyanosis
  ▪ Cold, pale, and clammy skin
  ▪ Shortness of breath
  ▪ Pulmonary edema
  ▪ Acute respiratory distress syndrome (ARDS)
  ▪ Stress ulcers, GI bleeding
  ▪ Increased liver function test (LFT) results
  ▪ Jaundice
  ▪ Anuria
  ▪ Increased blood urea nitrogen (BUN)/creatinine
  ▪ Acute renal failure
  ▪ Anemia
  ▪ Decreased albumin, potassium, sodium, calcium, magnesium, and phosphate
  ▪ Obtundation
  ▪ Coma

○ MODS
  ▪ Alteration in organ function
  ▪ Homeostasis cannot be maintained without intervention
  ▪ Can lead to death

SIGNS AND SYMPTOMS

- Signs and symptoms may be subtle or absent.
- Initial clinical presentation of sepsis
  ○ Fever or hypothermia
  ○ Diaphoresis
  ○ Chills or shaking chills (e.g., rigors)
  ○ Hypotension
  ○ Tachycardia
  ○ Tachypnea
  ○ Purulent drainage from wound or central venous catheter (not present in neutropenic patients, who are unable to exhibit this sign of infection)
  ○ Mental status changes
- Later, as the infection and sepsis progresses, the clinical manifestations of organ dysfunction in severe sepsis includes:
  ○ Integument
    ▪ Dry, flushed skin
  ○ Metabolic
    ▪ Temperature >38° C or <36° C
  ○ Renal
  ○ Decreased urine output
  ○ Increased osmolality
  ○ Cardiovascular
    ▪ Sinus tachycardia, cardiac output normal or increased
    ▪ Systolic blood pressure <90 mm Hg or a reduction of >40 mm Hg from baseline
    ▪ Decreased systemic vascular resistance
  ○ Pulmonary
    ▪ Tachypnea
    ▪ Shallow breaths
    ▪ Hypoxic on room air
    ▪ Respiratory and metabolic acidosis
    ▪ Decreased breath sounds and crackles
  ○ GI
    ▪ Nausea and vomiting
    ▪ Decreased motility

○ Hematology
  ▪ Leukopenia or leukocytosis
  ▪ Thrombocytopenia
  ▪ Prolonged prothrombin time (PT)/partial thromboplastin time (PTT) prolonged
  ▪ Decreased fibrinogen
  ▪ Increased fibrin degradation products

DIAGNOSTIC TESTS

- Before initiation of chemotherapy, measure:
  ○ Temperature
  ○ Complete blood count (CBC), electrolytes, LFTs, renal function tests (RFTs)
- At the first suspicion of sepsis, obtain:
  ○ STAT blood cultures from two peripheral sites or from a peripheral site and a central venous access site. Always culture an invasive line in the febrile immunosuppressed patient.
  ○ Chest x-ray films: posteroanterior and lateral
  ○ Urine culture and sensitivity
  ○ Other cultures, as appropriate (e.g., sputum, drainage, stool, wound, central line site)
  ○ Laboratory tests: CBC, chemistry panel, uric acid, LFTs, coagulation studies, arterial blood gases (ABGs)
- Continuing evaluation:
  ○ Temperature
  ○ ABGs
  ○ Pulse oximetry
  ○ Antibiotic levels, as indicated
  ○ Laboratory tests: CBC, chemistry panel, electrolytes, LFTs, RFTs, serum lactate
  ○ Serologies and cultures for viral diseases

DIFFERENTIAL DIAGNOSIS

- Tumor-associated fever, especially in lymphoma, acute leukemia, chronic leukemia, multiple myeloma, solid tumors, and cancers with metastasis to liver or central nervous system (CNS)
- Febrile response related to drug administration may occur at the

start of therapy or 1 to 2 weeks later (e.g., amphotericin B, ganciclovir, interferons, interleukins)
- Allergic reaction to drug or blood products
- Nosocomial fever
- Early sign of septic shock

TREATMENT
- Treatment of the underlying, predisposing condition(s) causing the infection
- Supporting the patient's hemodynamic status
- Managing the clinical manifestations of infection/sepsis that are present

Pharmacologic Management
- Prevention
  - Prophylactic antibiotics may be administered to neutropenic patients.
  - WBC growth factors (e.g., granulocyte colony-stimulating factor [G-CSF] and granulocyte-macrophage colony-stimulating factor [GM-CSF]) may be administered to decrease the period of neutropenia and decrease the incidence of infection after chemotherapy administration.
- Management
  - Empirical antibiotics
    - Initiated at the first suspicion of sepsis and after blood cultures are obtained
    - Broad spectrum antibiotics, which cover against common gram-negative and gram-positive organisms, are given.
  - Empirical antifungal therapy
    - Initiated when the patient remains febrile for 5 to 7 days after the empirical antibiotic therapy is started
    - Amphotericin B has been the drug of choice for years
    - Antifungal agents are commonly administered prophylactically, including nystatin, clotrimazole, fluconazole, or amphotericin B.

- Antiviral agents (e.g., acyclovir, ganciclovir) and various formulations of immunoglobulin are used to prevent and treat viral infections.
  - Antipyretic therapy (primarily acetaminophen)
    - Administered for decreasing the patient's temperature and for minimizing the discomforts of fever (e.g., chills, seizures, delirium)
  - Fluid resuscitation
    - May be administered to manage hypotension or oliguria
    - Crystalloid solutions (e.g., normal saline solution, lactated Ringer's solution) are used most commonly during the early phases of sepsis
    - Colloid solutions (e.g., dextran, albumin, plasma protein fraction) are also used.
  - Vasopressors
    - Dopamine is first-line therapy for its vasopressor and inotropic effects
    - Norepinephrine may be added for increased vasopressor support
    - Dobutamine may be added for increased inotropic effects.

Nonpharmacologic Management
- Encourage hydration (drinking 8-10 glasses of fluid per day).
- Monitor vital signs every 4 hours or as clinically indicated.
- Monitor changes in laboratory values and report significant changes, including organism growth in cultures and increase in WBC count.
- Monitor signs/symptoms of infection and obtain an order for a culture for suspicious sites.
- Monitor signs/symptoms of fluid overload, including rales, edema, and weight gain.
- Monitor intake and output.

- Monitor pulse oximetry and patient's response to oxygen therapy.
- Physical methods of controlling body temperature: tepid baths, sponging, cool washcloths; ice packs; cooling blankets; air conditioning; fans; applying blankets during periods of chilling
- High-calorie, high-protein diet is important to provide proper nutrition.

PATIENT TEACHING
- Goal is to protect patient from infection and maintain normal temperature.
- Define sepsis and/or septic shock and describe the signs and symptoms.
- Explain the purpose of the laboratory tests (especially ANC), diagnostic tests, nursing care, and treatments for sepsis.
- Teach patient/family to prevent infection with frequent handwashing and to keep his or her body clean by bathing daily and washing hands after using the bathroom.
- Teach patient to brush the teeth at least twice a day and to floss once daily.
- Encourage patient to drink 8-10 glasses of fluid per day.
- Teach patient to avoid infection by avoiding large crowds, by avoiding people who are sick, and by avoiding infants, children, and adults who have been vaccinated within 3 weeks.
- Teach patient to not clean up cat litter or clean up excreta from animals.
- Verify that the patient and family understand how to take the patient's temperature and provide additional teaching, as needed.
- Teach patient to turn, cough, and deep breathe to maintain optimum respiratory functioning.
- Teach patient rationale and schedule for oral prophylactic antibiotics or WBC growth factors, if indicated.

Oncologic Emergencies

- Teach patient rationale and schedule for having blood drawn for CBC.
- Patient is to report any temperature greater than 100.5° F and any symptoms of infection, such as redness, swelling, warmth, pain, or drainage.

FOLLOW-UP

- Continue to monitor for signs and symptoms of infection or sepsis.
- Monitor laboratory findings, especially CBC, as to the continuation or resolution of sepsis.
- Provide additional resources, such as home equipment or assistance, as needed.

BIBLIOGRAPHY

Bone, R., Balk, R. A., Cerra, F. B., et al. (1992). The American College of Chest Physicians/ Society of Critical Care Medicine consensus conference: definitions for sepsis and organ failure and guidelines for use of innovative therapies in sepsis. *Chest, 101,* 1644-1655.

Ezzone, S. (2000). Fever. In D. Camp-Sorrell & R. Hawkin (Eds.). *Clinical manual for the oncology practice nurse* (pp. 813-824). Pittsburgh, PA: Oncology Nursing Press.

Gobel, B. (2005). Metabolic emergencies. In J. Itano & K. Taoka (Eds.). *ONS core curriculum for oncology nursing* (4th ed., pp. 383-421). St. Louis: Elsevier Saunders.

Lin, E. (2001). Oncologic emergency: case 6. In Lin, E. (Ed.). *ONS advanced practice in oncology nursing: case studies and review* (pp. 333-342). Philadelphia: W. B. Saunders.

Moore, S. (2005). Septic shock. In C. H. Yarbro, M. H. Hansen, & M. Goodman (Eds.). *Cancer nursing: principles and practice* (6th ed., pp. 895-909). Sudbury, MA: Jones & Bartlett.

Shelton, B. K. (2005). Infection. In C. H. Yarbro, M. H. Frogge, & M. Goodman (Eds.). *Cancer nursing: principles and practice* (6th ed., pp. 698-722). Sudbury, MA: Jones & Bartlett.

Wujcik, D. (2004). Infection. In C. H. Yarbro, M. H. Frogge, & M. Goodman (Eds.). *Cancer symptom management* (3rd ed., pp. 252-267). Sudbury, MA: Jones & Bartlett.

Thrombotic Thrombocytopenic Purpura

DEFINITION

- A potentially life-threatening disorder with a symptom complex of microangiopathic hemolytic anemia (MAHA), thrombocytopenia, and formation of microthrombi in several organs
- Associated with varying severity of neurologic, renal, cardiac, abdominal, and constitutional symptoms

EPIDEMIOLOGY

- Incidence is rare.
  - Estimated incidence of two to ten cases per million/year in all racial groups
  - Occurs more often in women, with a female/male ratio of 3:2.
  - Cases have been described in patients ranging from 1 to 90 years old, with the third decade being the time of peak incidence.
  - Incidence in adults is 90%-95%.
  - Incidence in children is 5%-10%.
  - Mortality rate was very high (80%-90%) before plasma exchange was introduced.
  - Mortality rate currently remains unacceptably high (10%-20%), despite the significant improvements from treating thrombotic thrombocytopenic purpura (TTP) with plasma exchange.
- Risk increases for idiopathic TTP.
  - Rheumatoid arthritis, polyarthritis
  - Systemic lupus erythematosus
  - Endocarditis
  - Drug induced (e.g., iodine, oral contraceptives, statin treatment, and some poisons)
  - Genetic basis (10%)
  - During pregnancy or in postpartum period
  - Sjögren's syndrome

- Risk increases for cancer-associated TTP.
  - Advanced cancer + MAHA
  - Chemotherapy or drug induced (e.g., cyclosporin, sulfonamides, zoledronic acid)
  - Bone marrow transplantation

CANCERS ASSOCIATED WITH DISORDER

- Lymphoma
- Cancers that are being treated by bone marrow transplant
- Advanced cancers

PATHOPHYSIOLOGY

- Endothelial cell injury is considered the central and most likely inciting factor that sustains the microangiogenic process in TTP.
  - The nature and extent of the endothelial damage is unclear.
  - Drug toxicity and autoimmune injury to endothelial cells is believed to be the cause in some subsets of TTP.
- Unusually large (UL) von Willebrand factor (vWF) multimers are synthesized in endothelial cells and megakaryocytes.
  - When endothelial cell injury occurs, ULvWF multimers are released into the blood.
  - In healthy persons, ULvWF multimers usually do not circulate because the normal proteolysis of ULvWF multimers will rapidly reduce them into smaller multimers after their release.
  - This reduction is due to cleavage by a plasma metalloprotease, ADAMTS13.
- In persons with TTP, accumulation of ULvWF multimers in the patient's plasma and deficiencies of ADAMTS13 have been reported consistently.
  - The absent or severely inhibited ADAMTS13 activity limits the cleavage of ULvWF multimers.
  - With the failure of proteolysis, these large VWF multimers will

accumulate and remain anchored to the endothelial cells in long strings.

○ These large multimers lead to excessive aggregation of circulating platelets with small amounts of fibrin.

○ Microthrombi formation is initiated in places where there is high shear stress (e.g., in arterioles and capillaries) throughout the body, and microangiopathic hemolytic anemia results.

• The pathophysiology of TTP has been clarified since 1998.

○ It was shown that TTP in adults was most often associated with an acquired deficiency of ADAMTS13, which is the VWF-cleaving protease, as a result of autoantibodies against ADAMTS13.

○ Also shown that TTP in children was most often associated with a hereditary autosomal recessive severe deficiency of ADAMTS13.

○ The disease name in children has changed from "congenital TTP" and "Upshaw-Schulman syndrome" to "hereditary ADAMTS13 deficiency."

• Conflicting research related to ULVWF multimer levels and ADAMTS13 activity exists.

○ Many patients with TTP have a severe deficiency of ADAMTS13 and did not have any ULVWF multimers in their circulation. Therefore, this research supports that the deficiency of ADAMTS13 is not the only determinant of ULVWF abnormalities in TTP.

• Cancer-associated TTP is distinct from the classic idiopathic form of TTP (Moschcowitz syndrome).

○ Main features in classic TTP are fever, hemolytic anemia, thrombocytopenia, and neurological and renal abnormalities.

○ The manifestations of cancer-associated TTP are less pronounced.

○ Many patients do not present with the full syndrome.

• There is no clear-cut distinction between cancer-associated TTP and hemolytic uremic syndrome (HUS).

○ Both diseases are characterized by localized microvascular thrombosis.

○ Difficulty in identifying the differential diagnosis arises because many of the findings are nonspecific and commonplace.

○ On the basis of clinical and laboratory findings alone, many patients are diagnosed as having the TTP/HUS disorder.

○ Clinical presentation one distinguishing factor

■ In patients with TTP, clinical presentation is dominated by hemorrhages and neurological symptoms.

■ In patients with HUS, renal impairment is the dominant feature.

■ Patient's history can also help distinguish between TTP and HUS.

□ For example, a history of Shiga toxin hemorrhagic colitis is suggestive of HUS.

SIGNS AND SYMPTOMS

• Patients who have been diagnosed with a classic case of TTP have the full syndrome of fever, hemolytic anemia, thrombocytopenia, and renal and neurological abnormalities as a result of the widespread formation of microvascular thrombi.

• Cancer patients who have been diagnosed with TTP have less pronounced symptoms. These signs and symptoms may include:

○ Anemia (average hemoglobin with TTP is between 7 and 9 gm/dL)

○ Hemorrhaging

■ Purpura (occurs in more than 90% of cases)

■ Retinal and choroidal hemorrhaging

■ Epistaxis

■ Gingival bleeding

■ Hematuria

■ Gastrointestinal hemorrhaging

■ Menorrhagia

■ Hemoptysis

○ Neurological symptoms

■ Confusion

■ Headache

■ Paresis

■ Aphasia

■ Dysarthria

■ Visual problems

■ Coma

○ Fever (usually is not seen at the onset; is almost always present during the illness)

○ Renal involvement is common.

■ Proteinuria and microhematuria are most constant findings.

■ Decreased renal function in 40%-80% of patients

• Abdominal pain (10%-30%)

• Pancreatitis

• Heart involvement: infrequent

• Lung involvement: rarely alveolar and interstitial infiltrates

DIAGNOSTIC TESTS

• Complete blood cell count (CBC): decreased platelets

• Red blood cell (RBC) morphology: increased schizocytes

• Blood: VWF assay, ADAMTS13 (VWF cleavage protein)

• Lactate dehydrogenase (LDH): elevated

• Haptoglobin levels: low or undetectable

• Reticulocyte counts: elevated

• Coombs' test: negative (nonautoimmune, non-drug induced hemolytic anemia) or positive (autoimmune, drug-induced hemolytic anemia)

• Prothrombin times, activated partial thromboplastin times, factor V, factor VIII, and fibrinogen: usually normal

• Fibrinogen degradation products (FDP): may be elevated

• Thrombin times: may be prolonged

• Electrolytes

• Urine: dipstick, urinalysis, 24-hour creatinine clearance, urine culture

- Radiology: renal sonogram, renal angiogram, intravenous pyelogram, computed tomographic (CT) scan of abdomen

DIFFERENTIAL DIAGNOSIS

- HUS
- MAHA
- Disseminated intravascular coagulation (DIC)
- Graft-versus-host disease (GVHD), venous occlusive disease (VOD), diffuse alveolar hemorrhage (DAH), or cytomegalic (CMV) viral infection in persons undergoing bone marrow transplant
- Hematuria related to other diseases (e.g., infection, intrinsic kidney disease, benign prostatic hypertrophy)
- Hematuria related to other medications (e.g., ifosfamide, high-dose cyclophosphamide, intravesicular chemotherapy)
- Hematuria related to radiation therapy (e.g., pelvic radiation, prostate seed implants)

TREATMENT

- Identify those with symptoms of TTP.
- Initiate plasma exchange as soon as possible.

Pharmacologic Management

- Prevention
  - Vigorous pretransplant hydration before bone marrow transplant, parenterally or orally
  - Continuous bladder irrigations with normal saline solution
- Management:
  - No consistently effective treatment is currently available.
  - Plasma exchange
    - Most effective; removes the circulating antibodies

- Fresh-frozen plasma or cryo-poor plasma more effective than albumin.
  - Immunosuppression therapy may be given in addition to plasma exchange. This might include the administration of corticosteroids or intravenous gamma globulin.
  - Potent immunosuppressive agents are usually administered for refractory TTP or chronic relapsing TTP. These agents include cyclophosphamide, azathioprine, rituximab, and cyclosporine.
  - Discontinue drugs that are inducing the TTP.
    - For a patient undergoing allogeneic bone marrow transplant in whom TTP develops while on cyclosporine, discontinuing cyclosporin A is reasonable.
    - May not reverse the complication and GVHD may worsen.
    - Switching to tacrolimus has been recommended.
  - Ineffective treatments
  - Antithrombotic measures (e.g., anticoagulants, urokinase, aspirin) have NOT been found to be effective.
  - Platelet transfusions should be avoided, if possible, in the management of cancer-associated TTP because this could lead to additional microthrombi formation.
  - Platelet transfusions may be required if major bleeding complications occur.

Nonpharmacologic Management

- Splenectomy
  - 50% success rate at best.
- Nephrology consultation
  - Needed to determine the most appropriate renal therapy.
- Renal replacement therapy

- May include peritoneal dialysis and hemodialysis
- May be successful treatments for patients with recurrent cancer-associated TTP.

PATIENT TEACHING

- Goal is that the patient's blood cell counts will return to normal levels and the symptoms (hemorrhaging, neurological) will subside.
- Define TTP and describe the signs and symptoms.
- Explain the purpose of the laboratory tests, nursing care, and treatments for TTP.
- Patient is to report any increase in hemorrhaging or the occurrence of neurological symptoms.

FOLLOW-UP

- Continue to monitor for signs and symptoms of TTP.
- Monitor appropriate laboratory findings (especially platelet count and hemoglobin/hematocrit) as to the continuation or resolution of TTP.
- Provide additional resources, such as home equipment or assistance, as needed.

BIBLIOGRAPHY

Buchsel, P. (1999). Bone marrow transplantation. In C. Miaskowki & P. Buchsel (Eds.). *Oncology nursing: assessment and clinical care* (pp. 143-186). St. Louis: Mosby.

Friend, P., & Pruett, J. (2004). Bleeding and thrombotic complications. In C. Yarbro, M. Frogge, & M. Goodman (Eds.). *Cancer symptom management* (3rd ed., pp. 233-251). Sudbury, MA: Jones & Bartlett.

Galbusera, M., Bresin, E., Noris, M., et al. (2005). Rituximab prevents recurrence of thrombotic thrombocytopenic purpura: a case report. *Blood, 106,* 925-928.

Galbusera, M., Noris, M., & Remuzzi, G. (2006). Thrombotic thrombocytopenic purpura? Then and now. *Seminars in Thrombosis and Hemostasis, 32,* 81-89.

Kwaan, H. (2005). Thrombotic thrombocytopenic purpura: a diagnostic and therapeutic challenge. *Seminars in*

Thrombosis and Hemostasis, 31, 615-624.

Loirat, C., Veyradier, A, Girma, J., et al. (2006). Thrombotic thrombocytopenic purpura associated with von Willebrand factor-cleaving protease (ADAMTS13) deficiency in children. *Seminars in Thrombosis and Hemostasis, 32,* 615-624.

Qu, L., & Kiss, J. (2005). Thrombotic microangiopathy in transplantation and malignancy. *Seminars in Thrombosis and Hemostasis, 31,* 691-699.

Ruggenenti, P., & Remuzzi, G. (1990). Thrombotic thrombocytopenic purpura and related disorders. *Hematology Oncology Clinics of North America, 4,* 219-241.

Yomtovian, R., Niklinski, W., Silver, B., et al. (2004). Rituximab for chronic recurring thrombotic thrombocytopenic purpura: a case report and review of the literature. *British Journal of Haematology, 124,* 787-795.

Palliative Care and End-of-Life Issues

Palliative and Hospice Care

Debra E. Heidrich

Health care professionals are generally not as comfortable dealing with issues related to death and dying as they are with supporting the patient through curative treatment. Knowledge and skill in providing physical and emotional comfort to dying patients and their families is essential to providing optimum care to persons with advanced, progressive diseases. Palliative care is a relatively new specialty that focuses on promoting the best possible quality of life for patients facing serious life-threatening illness through optimal management of physical, psychosocial, emotional, and spiritual symptoms. This specialty grew out of the hospice movement and is continuing to evolve as more palliative care teams are integrated into health care systems, more palliative care content is taught in schools of medicine and nursing, and more research is conducted to support an evidence base for palliative interventions.

DEFINITION

Palliative care is both a philosophy of care and an organized, highly structured system for delivering care. The goal of palliative care is to prevent and relieve suffering and to support the best possible quality of life for patients and their families, regardless of the stage of the disease or the need for other therapies (National Consensus Project for Quality Palliative Care [NCPQPC], 2004). Palliative care expands traditional disease-model medical treatments to include the goals of enhancing quality of life for the patient and family, optimizing function, helping with decision making, and providing opportunities for personal growth. It can be delivered concurrently with life-prolonging care or as the main focus of care.

Palliative care can and should be initiated at the diagnosis of a serious life-threatening or chronic, progressive illness and continued throughout the course of the illness across all care settings. As illustrated in the figure on page 438, palliative care is started along with life-prolonging therapies at the initial diagnosis of a life-threatening illness. As the disease progresses, there is a greater and greater emphasis on palliative interventions versus life-prolonging interventions. Hospice care is the part of the palliative care continuum when the emphasis is no longer on life prolongation, but primarily on comfort. In the United States, this is often defined as the last 6 months of life and is based on the eligibility requirements for hospice benefits under Medicare.

The NCPQPC defines palliative care as "medical care provided by an interdisciplinary team…focused on the relief of suffering and support for the best possible quality of life for patients facing serious life-threatening illness, and their families. It aims to identify and address the physical, psychological, spiritual, and practical burdens of illness" (NCPQPC, 2004). Palliative care is distinguished from routine symptom management by the following:

- The interdisciplinary approach
- Focus on physical, psychosocial, emotional, and spiritual symptoms
- Inclusion of the family in the unit of care

See the box on page 438 for a summary of the practice guidelines outlined by the NCPQCP.

PALLIATIVE CARE IN PERSONS WITH CANCER

Every patient diagnosed with cancer needs good symptom management from the time of diagnosis. Patients whose cancer is diagnosed at an advanced stage or whose cancer progresses during or after treatment are likely to have multiple physical, psychological, emotional, or spiritual concerns. The expertise of the palliative interdisciplinary team can be especially helpful at this time.

In general, the following patient populations are appropriate for palliative care:

- Persons diagnosed with large, poorly differentiated tumors
- Persons with distant metastasis at the time of diagnosis
- Persons whose diseases progress while on treatment or with short progression-free intervals after completing a course of treatment have a worse prognosis.
- Persons with a declining functional status
- Persons with multiple symptoms or those with one or more symptoms that are difficult to manage. Common symptoms include pain, dyspnea, nausea, vomiting, anorexia, constipation, fatigue, anxiety, and confusion.

MODELS OF PALLIATIVE CARE DELIVERY

Palliative care services are most effective when integrated into the care setting. Various models are used to facilitate access to the expertise of the palliative care team. These models include one or a combination of some of the following:

- Consultation service team, consisting of physician, nurse, or social work evaluations
- Dedicated inpatient unit in an acute or rehabilitation hospital, nursing home, or free-standing inpatient hospice
- Hospital- or private practice–based outpatient palliative care practice or clinic
- Hospice-based palliative care at home
- Hospice-based consultation in outpatient settings

HOSPICE PALLIATIVE CARE

The figure on page 438 illustrates that hospice care is the part of the palliative care continuum when life-prolonging therapies are no longer providing benefit. The focus of care is on comfort and quality of living by affirming life and viewing dying as a normal process. Services provided by the hospice interdisciplinary team include pain and symptom management, psychosocial and spiritual support, assistance and support with direct caregiving, and bereavement care for both the patient and family. The practice guidelines outlined by the NCPQPC (see box on

Palliative Care & End-of-Life Issues

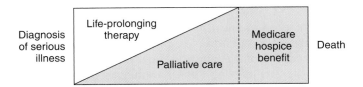

Palliative care's place in the course of illness. From National Consensus Project for Quality Palliative Care. (2004). Clinical practice guidelines for quality palliative care. Retrieved February 5, 2007, from http://www.nationalconsensusproject.org.

right) also apply to the organized, comprehensive services available through hospice programs.

Medicare, some state Medicaid programs, and some private insurance companies require that patients have a 6-month or less prognosis to be eligible for hospice services. However, the median length of stay in hospice programs in 2005 was only 26 days (National Hospice and Palliative Care Organization, 2006). Barriers that interfere with initial and timely referrals to hospice programs include the following (Friedman, Harwood, & Shields, 2002):

- Discomfort in discussing end-of-life care issues by patients, family members, and health care professionals
- Difficulty in determining a prognosis of 6 months or less
- Lack of information or misinformation about hospice care by patients, family members, and health care providers
- Real or perceived requirement to discontinue life-prolonging therapies to receive hospice services

Eligibility requirements and an outline of the services provided under the Medicare hospice benefit are listed in the table on page 439. Hospices receive a per diem rate from Medicare to pay for all services related to the terminal illness. Traditional Medicare coverage remains in place for services related to problems other than the identified terminal illness. Many private insurance companies have hospice benefits that are similar to those provided under Medicare.

The services from hospice programs are much more comprehensive than can be provided under a traditional home care insurance benefit, giving the patient and family more clinical, psychosocial, emotional, and spiritual support over a longer period of time than is available under other benefits. Patients whose residence is a long-term care facility receive these same benefits in addition to the services provided by the facility.

Services not paid for under the Medicare hospice benefit include treatment or medications intended to cure the terminal illness rather than for symptom control, care from any provider or in any facility that is not arranged by the hospice team, and room and board. Because Medicare does not pay for room and board at nursing homes, patients who qualify for skilled care in a long-term care facility may have less out-of-pocket expense by using their "skilled days" before enrolling in a hospice program. This is unfortunate because many of these patients and families

Clinical Practice Guidelines for Quality Palliative Care

1. STRUCTURE AND PROCESSES OF CARE
1.1. The plan of care is based on a comprehensive interdisciplinary assessment of the patient and family.
1.2. The care plan is based on the identified and expressed values, goals, and needs of patient and family and is developed with professional guidance and support for decision making.
1.3. An interdisciplinary team provides services to the patient and family, consistent with the care plan.
1.4. The interdisciplinary team may include appropriately trained and supervised volunteers.
1.5. Support for education and training is available to the interdisciplinary team.
1.6. The palliative care program is committed to quality improvement in clinical and management practices.
1.7. The palliative care program recognizes the emotional impact on the palliative care team of providing care to patients with life-threatening illnesses and their families.
1.8. Palliative care programs should have a relationship with one or more hospices and other community resources to ensure continuity of the highest-quality palliative care across the illness trajectory.
1.9. The physical environment in which care is provided should meet the preferences, needs, and circumstances of the patient and family to the extent possible.

2. PHYSICAL ASPECTS OF CARE
2.1. Pain, other symptoms, and side effects are managed on the basis of the best available evidence, which is skillfully and systematically applied.

3. PSYCHOLOGICAL AND PSYCHIATRIC ASPECTS OF CARE
3.1. Psychological and psychiatric issues are assessed and managed on the basis of the best available evidence, which is skillfully and systematically applied.
3.2. A grief and bereavement program is available to patients and families on the basis of the assessed need for services.

4. SOCIAL ASPECTS OF CARE
4.1. Comprehensive interdisciplinary assessment identifies the social needs of patients and their families, and a care plan is developed to respond to these needs as effectively as possible.

5. SPIRITUAL, RELIGIOUS, AND EXISTENTIAL ASPECTS OF CARE
5.1. Spiritual and existential dimensions are assessed and responded to on the basis of the best available evidence, which is skillfully and systematically applied.

6. CULTURAL ASPECTS OF CARE
6.1. The palliative care program assesses and attempts to meet the culture-specific needs of the patient and family.

7. CARE OF THE IMMINENTLY DYING PATIENT
7.1. Signs and symptoms of impending death are recognized and communicated, and care appropriate for this phase of illness is provided to patient and family.

8. ETHICAL AND LEGAL ASPECTS OF CARE
8.1. The patient's goals, preferences, and choices are respected within the limits of acceptable state and federal law and form the basis for the plan of care.
8.2. The palliative care program is aware of and addresses the complex ethical issues arising in the care of persons with life-threatening debilitating illness.
8.3. The palliative care program is knowledgeable about legal and regulatory aspects of palliative care.

From: National Consensus Project for Quality Palliative Care. (2004). *Clinical practice guidelines for quality palliative care.* Retrieved February 5, 2007, from http://www.nationalconsensusproject.org.

The Hospice Medicare Benefit

Eligibility criteria	The patient must: • Be eligible for Medicare Part A • Be certified as having a terminal diagnosis with a prognosis of 6 months or less by a physician • Agree to waive traditional Medicare coverage for the terminal illness • Enroll in a Medicare-approved hospice program
Services covered	All services for the terminal illness: • Physician care • Nursing care • Medical equipment • Medical supplies • Medications for symptom control and pain relief (there may be a small copayment) • Home health aide and homemaker services • Physical and occupational therapy • Speech therapy • Social work services • Dietary counseling • Grief and loss counseling for the patient and family • Short-term inpatient care • Short-term respite care • Volunteer services
Services not covered	• Treatment intended to cure the terminal illness • Prescription medications to cure the terminal illness rather than for symptom control • Care from any provider or in any facility that is not arranged by the hospice team • Room and board
Benefit periods	• There are two 90-day periods followed by an unlimited number of 60-day periods. • At the start of each period of care, the hospice medical director must recertify that the patient is terminally ill.

Payment for services	• Hospice programs are paid a per diem rate to provide all the services
	• The per diem rate is based on the level of care:
	  • Routine home care
	  • Must account for at least 80% of all care provided by a hospice program
	  • Includes private home, assisted living facility, boarding home, or long-term care facility
	  • Respite care—short-term inpatient care to relive caregivers
	  • General inpatient care for management of uncontrolled physical or psychosocial problems
	  • Continuous home care for management of uncontrolled physical or psychosocial problems in the home

From Centers for Medicare and Medicaid Services. (2005). *The hospice benefit*. CMS Publication No. 02154. Baltimore, MD: Author.

would benefit from the expertise and support of the hospice team during this time. Palliative care teams in long-term care facilities, when available, can address the symptom management and support needs of this population of patients.

REFERENCES

Friedman, B., Harwood, K., & Shields, M. (2002). Barriers and enablers to hospice referrals: an expert overview. *Journal of Palliative Medicine, 5*, 73-81.

Glare, P. (2005). Clinical predictors of survival in advanced cancer. *Journal of Supportive Oncology, 3*, 331-339.

National Consensus Project for Quality Palliative Care. (2004). *Clinical practice guidelines for quality palliative care*. Retrieved February 5, 2007, from http://www.nationalconsensusproject.org.

National Hospice and Palliative Care Organization. (2006). *Hospice facts and figures*. Retrieved February 5, 2007, from http://www.nhpco.org/files/public/2005-facts-and-figures.pdf.

ADDITIONAL RESOURCES

Doyle, D., Hanks, G., Cherney, H., et al. (Eds). (2004). *Oxford textbook of palliative medicine* (3rd ed.). New York: Oxford University Press.

Ferrell, B., & Coyle, N. (Eds.). (2005). *Textbook of palliative nursing* (2nd ed.). New York: Oxford University Press.

Communication in Palliative Care

Debra E. Heidrich

Good communication is essential for decision making throughout the course of an illness. As a disease progresses, new symptoms emerge, more specialists are consulted, and the emotional stresses of managing the illness mount. Adequate communication among the patient, family, primary care providers, multiple specialists, and health care professionals from various settings is necessary to coordinate care and decrease fragmentation. Information shared with patients and families must be honest, clear, and consistent to enhance understanding of the disease process and the patient's overall health status, to guide decision making, to assist in setting realistic goals, and to prepare for the end of life.

Health care professionals often do not receive adequate training in communication (Back et al., 2005). This is especially true when it comes to giving bad or sad news to patients and families. Health care professionals also avoid these conversations because of fears of provoking emotional distress, lack of knowledge on how to handle the emotional reactions of patients and family members, concern about how health care professionals will handle their own emotions, and a desire to avoid confronting one's own fear of death (Fallowfield, 2005).

Several factors interfere with good communication between persons living with advanced illnesses and their health care professionals:

- Use of medical terms that may be misinterpreted or not understood
- Concerns that discussing a poor prognosis will cause harm

- Difficulty in determining prognosis
- Attitudes held by both health care professionals and the public that death is a failure of medical interventions

These factors can lead to collusion to produce false optimism about recovery (The, Koeter, & van der Wal, 2000). This collusion is seen when, instead of clearly discussing the overall illness trajectory, both health care professionals and patients focus on available treatments and their associated side effects. Patients often interpret "treatment" as "can be cured," whereas health care professionals often use the term treatment to mean "can be controlled." The collusion of false optimism continues when prognosis is not discussed because both the health care professionals and the patients are waiting for the other person to bring up the subject.

KEYS FOR EFFECTIVE COMMUNICATION

Effective communication requires that the individuals trust, share information with, listen to, and respond to each other. People do not openly express their questions, fears, and concerns unless they trust the other. Establishing trust, then, is the basic foundation of good communication. In the health care system, patients are often not treated by a trusted primary care physician with whom they have established a trusting relationship over years. Instead, the health care professionals with whom these patients interact must work quickly to develop trusting relationships.

Establishing Trust

Trust develops when people feel that the other cares about them and will act to do what is best for them or their loved ones. Patients want to be treated as whole people, not as diseases. Trust can be threatened when patients and family members get inconsistent or conflicting information from health care providers. It is vitally important that all specialists and team members are in communication about the patient's overall condition and treatment plans.

The following strategies may assist health care providers to develop a trusting relationship with patients and family members (Back & Arnold, 2005; Tulsky, 2005):

- Let them know you are interested in knowing the *person* and the impact of the disease on the patient and family. Encourage patients and family members to talk so as to learn their understanding of the illness, what the patient's life was like before the illness or hospitalization, and how the patient and family are coping with the current situation. Open-ended questions help to initiate discussion (e.g., "What do you understand about your illness at this time?").
- Recognize the concerns of patients and family members. If these concerns involve not receiving adequate information or receiving conflicting information from other health care providers,

validate that you understand this is a concern without contradicting other health care providers. Commit to clarifying any conflicting information the patient or family has heard.
- Acknowledge any errors or misunderstandings that may have occurred and establish a plan to avoid them in the future. Denial and defensiveness interfere with trust.
- Demonstrate respect for the patient and family at all times. Frame the situation as a mutual issue of concern that the health care team wants to work in collaboration with the patient and family to address.
- Do not force decisions. When decisions are needed, ensure that the patient and family understand the risks and benefits of all options, give them time to think about the information that has been presented, and set up a time for follow-up.

SHARING INFORMATION

Health care professionals must provide information in straightforward language that patients and family members can understand. Avoid medical jargon that can be misinterpreted (see box below). Provide information in

---

Examples of Medical Language That Causes Confusion

TERMS OPEN TO MISINTERPRETATION
Disease progression
- Clinical meaning: deterioration
- Lay meaning: improvement

Disease regression
- Clinical meaning: improvement
- Lay meaning: deterioration

Advanced
- Clinical meaning: unfavorable prognosis
- Lay meaning: favorable prognosis

Positive biopsy
- Clinical meaning: presence of disease
- Lay meaning: absence of disease

Negative biopsy
- Clinical meaning: absence of disease
- Lay meaning: presence of disease

Terms With Unclear Meanings
- Tumor
- Growth
- Spot
- Lump
- Mass

MEDICAL JARGON
- Benign
- Malignancy
- Carcinoma
- Metastasis
- Hydration and nutrition
- Ventilation or intubation
- Full code
- CPR
- DNR

small chunks so that it can be understood one piece at a time. Verify that the information was heard correctly by asking the patient or family member to state in his or her own words the information that was shared (Ambuel & Weissman, 2005; Back et al., 2005).

It is helpful to have more than one person present when bad or sad news needs to be communicated. A family meeting is often very helpful to share the information with all concerned individuals at one time, to provide an opportunity for everyone to hear each other's questions, and to have questions answered.

Avoid any phrases that exacerbate fears and suffering. For example, statements such as "nothing more can be done" may lead to images of abandonment, symptoms out of control, and helplessness. Reassure patients, that although their disease is no longer responding to available treatments, there are many interventions available to ensure that they do not experience uncontrolled pain or other symptoms.

LISTENING AND RESPONDING

Listening is an active process requiring full attention to the speaker. Minimize distractions by holding meetings/conversations in as private an area as possible and silencing cell phones and pagers. Useful communication tools include the following:

- Using head nods or statements such as "Yes, go on…" to encourage the speaker to continue discussion of important issues
- Summarizing or paraphrasing to show that the listener understands the message, such as "It sounds like you are most concerned about…"
- Allowing silences so that the speaker has the time to think and respond. This is especially helpful when discussing issues that generate emotional responses.
- Empathizing with the speaker by reflecting the emotions, such as saying, "I can see that you are very worried" or "This must feel so overwhelming."

REFERENCES

Ambuel, B., & Weissman, D. E. (2005). *Fast facts and concepts #11: delivering bad news—part 2* (2nd ed). End-of-life Palliative Education Resource Center. Retrieved February 5, 2007, from http://www.eperc.mcw.edu/fastFact/ff_011.htm.

Back, A. L., & Arnold, R. M. (2005). Dealing with conflict in caring for the seriously ill. *Journal of the American Medical Association, 293*, 1374-1381.

Back, A. L., Arnold, R. M., Baile, W. F., et al. Approaching difficult communication tasks in oncology. *CA: A Cancer Journal for Clinicians, 55*, 164-177.

Fallowfield, L. (2005). Communication with the patient and family in palliative medicine. In D. Doyle, G. Hanks, N. I. Cherny, et al. (Eds.). *Oxford textbook of palliative medicine* (3rd ed, pp. 101-107). New York: Oxford University Press.

The, A., Hak, T., Koeter, G., et al. (2000). Collusion in doctor-patient communication about imminent death: an ethnographic study. *British Medical Journal, 321*, 1376-1381.

Tulsky, J. A. (2005). Beyond advance directives: importance of communication skills at the end of life. *Journal of the American Medical Association 294*, 359-365.

Cultural Issues in Cancer Care

Mary Murphy

DEFINITION OF CULTURE

A universal system of symbols and beliefs learned and shared among generations. Begins at birth, shared, adaptive and affects roles and responsibilities of the individual within the group

AFFECTS

- Language
- Food practices/rituals
- Symptom management
- Birth rituals
- Family relationship
- Illness beliefs
- Health practices
- Spiritual orientation
- Death rituals

CULTURAL COMPETENCE

- Awareness of one's own background and its influence on patient care
- Knowledge of how culture affects health care practices
- Accepting and respecting cultural difference and their impact on health care delivery.
- Awareness that health care providers and client beliefs may vary and may affect care
- Avoidance of judgmental acts and beliefs
- Openness to cultural encounters
- Adaptation of care to meet cultural needs
- Patient/caregiver education tools (Purnell & Paulanka, 2003)

STRATEGIES TO PROMOTE CULTURAL COMPETENCE

- Make it part of the organization's mission statement
- Facilitate cultural resources
  ○ Community (internal/external)
  ○ Religious affiliation
  ○ Interpreters
  ○ Volunteers
  ○ Internal staff
- Include in internal policy availability of internal resources references
  ○ Journals
  ○ Teleconference
  ○ Will sites
  ○ Books

ASSESSMENT TOOLS

The evaluation of cultural beliefs and practices must be part of the continuing clinical assessment as the client receives treatment; during treatment decisions and outcomes the impact of culture will have an impact on the decisions and care delivery practices.

ASSESSMENT

- Select a model of assessment with appropriate intervention related to area of care delivery.
- Use measurable outcomes to determine whether culturally sensitive care is being provided.
- Select model that staff can administer and understand.

SAMPLE ASSESSMENT MODEL—CONFHER

- **C:** Communication—how does the client communicate?
- **O:** Orientation—what are the values that influence the client? Length of time in country and resources
- **N:** Nutrition—food practices that may cause concerns with treatment. Food feeding issues if patient is unable to eat
- **F:** Family relationships—structure, roles, whose needs are nourished? Male/female roles. Who is the caregiver?
- **H:** Health and beliefs—health systems, values, beliefs. What does illness mean to the culture? What will interfere with delivery of care?
- **E:** Education—what is their education level? Occupation, competence to understand. Health care delivery process

- **R:** Religion—what is the religion? How does it affect care delivery and final outcomes? (see Fong, 1985)

BARRIERS TO CULTURAL COMPETENCE

- Ethnocentrism: using one's customs or values to judge others
- Common values of a dominant society reflected in the United States. A cookie cutter identity
- Youth, beauty
- Competition
- Achievement: financial, marital, and recognition
- Technology driven
- Financial success
- Conformity to rigid norms: clubs, organizations, sports, or those things that create an identity
- Stereotyping
  - Past values
  - Limited expense
  - Influence of media

DEALING WITH CULTURAL DILEMMAS

Dealing with cultural dilemmas can influence outcomes, compromise care, and result in staff/client/caregiver discomfort. Key components should be in place before the dilemma include the following (see table on pages 442-444):

- Identity cultural varies that may influence care issues.

Specific Cultural/Ethnic Population Cancer Profile

Ethnic Group	Cancer Problems	Lifestyle Risk Factors	Barriers to Prevention	Possible Approaches
African American	Highest overall cancer incidence rate Highest overall cancer mortality rate Survival 30% lower than whites Prostate cancer Breast cancer Lung cancer Colorectal cancer Pancreatic cancer Esophageal cancer	Poverty Diet Smoking Hazardous occupational exposures Obesity Alcohol consumption Urban living	Low education and literacy levels Lack of credible messengers with whom community can identify For the poor, survival, not prevention, is priority Decreased access to health care and prevention	Use African American professional for health care and as speaker Church-based information and speakers Forums at public housing sites Smoking cessation efforts directed to unique smoking habits of this group
Hispanic	Gallbladder cancer among New Mexico Hispanics of Native American ancestry Liver cancer among Mexican Americans Cervical cancer among women from Central and South America Pancreatic cancer among Mexican Americans	Genetic tendency Possibly diet Young age of first sexual encounter Poverty and possibly associated alcohol use	Low literacy, even in Spanish Fear of cancer General belief that cancer is God's will and only God can cure Modesty and sexuality issues associated with gynecological examinations Lack of Spanish-speaking caregivers	Public service advertisements, Hispanic media Speaker's bureau of Hispanic health professionals Outreach through neighborhood stores, restaurants Spanish videotapes Telenovelas Use Hispanic professionals for health care Use of friends (compadres) as role models

Specific Cultural/Ethnic Population Cancer Profile—cont'd

Ethnic Group	Cancer Problems	Lifestyle Risk Factors	Barriers to Prevention	Possible Approaches
		Dietary changes with associated acculturation		Advocate use of 1-800-4Cancer, number for Spanish translation and counseling
	Prostate cancer		Male reluctance to have examinations	
			Decreased access to health care prevention	
			Decreased awareness of cancer warning signs and screening tests	
Asian/Pacific Islander, Chinese	Nasopharyngeal cancer	Epstein-Barr virus Salt fish consumption Genetic predisposition	Low education and literacy in native languages	Include screening examinations and prevention education crisis care visits
	Liver cancer	Hepatitis B	"Prevention model" nonexistent	Outreach with messages through stores
	Esophageal cancer	Consumption of salted foods, hot tea, silica fiber, and contaminated grain Smoking Indoor pollutants	Lack of trust in Western health care Leaders lack health knowledge Decreased access to health care	Tie in with English as second language Integrate traditional healers, herbs, and practices
	Lung cancer	Smoking and passive smoke exposure Vitamin A deficiency		
	Stomach cancer	Loss of gastric acidity Salted food consumption Family history of gastric cancer		
Asian/Pacific Islander, Japanese	Stomach cancer	Age over 65 years Salted food consumption Low vitamin C intake Family history of gastric cancer Loss of gastric acidity		
	Esophageal cancer	Consumption of rice gruel cooked in hot tea Chronic esophagitis		
	Liver cancer	Hepatitis B		
	Gallbladder cancer	Gallstones High-fat diet		
Korean	Liver cancer	Hepatitis B		
	Biliary cancer	History of gallstones High-fat diet		
	Lymphoma	Unknown		
	Thyroid cancer	Unknown		
Filipino(a)	Liver cancer	Hepatitis B		
	Biliary cancer	History of gallstones High-fat diet		
	Lymphoma	Unknown		
Native American	Lowest overall cancer incidence and mortality of all U.S. populations Survival rates are uniformly low Tribal cancer rate differences are important		Inhospitable health care environment and insensitive personnel Lack of transportation to health clinic Low education and literacy levels Underfunded and overburdened health care system	Integrate cultural beliefs and practices Enlist support of key tribal leaders and organizations Perform examinations with strict attention and concern for modesty, tribal customs, and gender and dress differences
Ogalala women	Lung cancer Cervical cancer Stomach cancer	Smoking Lack of services	Generalized lack of financial resources	Integrate prevention and screening into other health care visits
Ogalala, Alaska,	Lung cancer	Smoking	Lack of integration of traditional practices with	

Continued

Specific Cultural/Ethnic Population Cancer Profile—cont'd

Ethnic Group	Cancer Problems	Lifestyle Risk Factors	Barriers to Prevention	Possible Approaches
Oklahoma, Northern Plains tribes			Western health care practice	
Oklahoma tribes and Alaska natives	Stomach cancer Colon cancer	Lack of dietary fiber		
Oklahoma, Navajo, and Aberdeen tribes	Breast cancer	Obesity		
Tribes of Rosebud, Sioux reservation, Ft.. McDowell community, North Carolina	Cervical cancer	Lack of adequate nutrition		
Alaska natives	Liver cancer	Hepatitis B Epstein-Barr virus		
	Nasopharyngeal cancer	Cigarette smoking Salted fish consumption		
Southwestern and Oklahoma tribes	Gallbladder cancer	Diet Genetic factors		
Navajo men	Lung cancer	Uranium mining		
Western, Washington tribes	Gallbladder cancer	Diet Possibly genetics		
	Cervical cancer	Access to health care issues		

From: Schulmeisten, L. K. (1999). Cultural issues in cancer care. In C. Miaskowski & P. Buchsels (Eds.). *Oncology Nursing: Assessment and Clinical Care* (pp. 387-399). St. Louis: M. Mosby.

- What is the durable power of attorney/do not resuscitate (DNR) status?
- What is the relationship with the physician, length of time, trust level, communication pattern?
- What are the resources?
- Who is the decision maker?
- What are the ethical dilemmas related to cultural diversity issues?
- What internal resources are available in the health care system?
- Have all barriers been removed?

EVALUATION OF CULTURAL PROGRAMS

- Evaluate at least yearly.
- Review current policies/procedures.
- Evaluate and update resources.
- Consider case conferences on specific cases.
- Review need for patient education material and need for updates.
- Consider yearly lecture or clinical update.

BIBLIOGRAPHY

Davis, M. (2000). The rules of ethnicity, race, religion and socioeconomic status in end-of-life care in icu. In J. R. Curtis & G. D. Rubenfeld (Eds.). *Managing death in the ICU* (pp. 215-229). New York: Oxford University Press.

Deshotells, J. M. (2002). Cultural awareness. In K. K. Kubher & P. Esper (Eds.). *Palliative care practices for the bedside clinician* (pp. 67-69). Pittsburgh, PA: Oncology Nursing Press.

Dhruva, A., Cheng, J., Kwong, M., et al. (2006). Contrasts, conflicts and change: a case in cultural oncology. *The Journal of Supportive Oncology, 4*, 301-304.

Fong, C. M. (1985.) Ethnicity in nursing practice. *Topics in Oncology Nursing, 7*, 1-10.

Itanko, J. K. (2005). Coping: cultural issues. In J. K. Itanko & K. N. Taoka (Eds.). *Core curriculum for oncology nursing* (4th ed., pp. 59-79). St. Louis: Elsevier Saunders.

Lipson, J. C., Dibble, S. L., & Minarik, P. A. (1996). *Culture & nursing care: a pocket guide*. San Francisco: UCSF Nursing Press.

Mazanec, P., & Tyler, M. K. (2003). Cultural considerations at end-of-life. *American Journal of Nursing, 103*, 50-59.

Oncology Nursing Society. (1999). *Oncology Nursing Society multicultural outcomes: guidelines for cultural competencies*. Pittsburgh, PA: Author.

Patten, C. W., & Kammer, R. M. (2006). Better communication with minority patients: seven strategies for achieving cultural competency. *Community Oncology, 3*, 295-295.

Purnell, L. D., & Paulanka, B. J. (2003). *Transcultural health care* (2nd ed.). Philadelphia: F. A. Davis.

Reese, D. J., Melton, E., & Ciavlino, K. (2004). Programmatic barriers to providing cultural competency at end-of-life care. *American Journal of Palliative Care, 21*, 357-364.

Schulmeisten, L. K. (1999). Cultural issues in cancer care. In C. Miaskowski & P. Buchsels (Eds.). *Oncology Nursing: Assessment and Clinical Care* (pp. 387-399). St. Louis: M. Mosby.

Taylor, E. J. (2001). Spirituality, culture, and cancer care. *Seminars in Oncology Nursing, 17*, 197-205.

Wood, S. A., Ersek, M., & Kraybill, B. M. (2004). Culture. In J. T. Panke & R. Coyle (Eds.). *Conversations in palliative care* (pp. 41-57). Pensacola, FL: Phol Publishing.

Ethical Considerations

Mary Murphy

Ethics plays a major role in oncology nursing practice and the delivery of care to patients. The American Nurses Association (ANA) Code of Ethics (2001) established the groundwork for practice, which includes the following:

1. Practices with compassion and respect
2. Commitment to the client
3. Promotes health and safety
4. Responsibility to individual nursing practice
5. Ownership of same duties to self as others
6. Establishes and maintains healthy environment
7. Advocates for professional practice, education, and administration
8. Collaborates to meet health care needs
9. Responsibility to maintain the nursing profession

Ethics is derived from the Greek term *ethos*, meaning customs, conduct, or character, and involves the study of how a person determines right and wrong, which involves principles of thinking, reasoning, and decision making when faced with choices of conflict.

ETHICAL THEORIES

- Utilitarian theory: Actions should produce the best consequences and produce happiness.
- Right approach: Respects and protects the rights of the individual
- Fairness and justice approach: Treats all patients as fair or in a just manner
- Common-good approach: Selective of the best alternative for the common good
- Care-based approach: The most responsive to individual needs

KEY PRINCIPLES OF ETHICS

- Autonomy: Self-determination
- Nonmaleficence: Avoids harm
- Beneficence: Promotes good
- Justice: Fairness
- Veracity: Truth telling

FRAMEWORK FOR ETHICAL DECISION-MAKING

- Identify the ethical issue
- Gather relevant data
- Determine values at stake
- Identify options
- Make choice(s)
- Support choice(s)
- Evaluate the preventable dilemma (Scanlon & Glover, 1995)

INFORMED CONSENT

An ethical and legal commitment to provide risk, benefit, and alternatives needed to make at decision

Requirements

- Adequate decision-making capacity
- Competence
- Comprehension
- Privacy and confidentiality
- Provision of advocacy if there is a lack of decisional capacity
- Provision of guardianship including:
  - Surrogate (next of kin)
  - Durable power of attorney (DPOA)
  - Living wills
  - Guardianships
  - Do not resuscitate (DNR) orders
- Accurate documentation
- Respect for individual differences
- Adequate support

Barriers to Ethical Decision-Making and Informed Consent

- Language
- Culture
- Time commitment
- Altered mental capacity (physical or emotional)
- Bias (previous preconceived ideas)
- Lack of family/caregiver support or documented wishes
- Age of patient
- Literacy
- Religious beliefs
- Suddenness of event
- Legal disputes for criminal involvement

TYPES OF ETHICAL DILEMMAS

- Prolongation of life
- Medical futility
- Mechanical ventilation
- Resuscitation
- Tube feedings
- Dialysis
- Sedation at end of life
- Assisted suicide and euthanasia research
- Clinical trials

Palliative Care & End-of-Life Issues

NURSE'S ROLE IN ETHICAL DECISION-MAKING

- Provide education
- Offer support
- Facilitate communication
- Serve as an advocate
- Serve as a witness
- Documentation of events

CONSIDERATIONS TO ASSIST THE NURSE IN ETHICAL SITUATIONS

- Administrative policies and support
- Ethics committee
- Nurse Practice Act
- Code of ethics for nurse's with interpretive guidelines
- Peer support

BIBLIOGRAPHY

American Nurses Association. (2001). *Code of ethics with interpretive statements.* Washington, DC: Author.

Beuchamp, T. L., & Childress, J. F. (2001). *Principles of biomedical ethics* (5th ed.) New York: Oxford University Press.

Calman, K. (2004) Ethical issues. In D. Doyle, G. Hanks, N. Cherry, et al. (Eds). *Oxford textbook of palliative medicine* (3rd ed., pp. 55-61). New York: Oxford Palliative Press.

Nelson-Martin, P., & Glover, J. (2005). Selected ethical issues in cancer care. In J. K. Itanko & K. N. Taoko (Eds.). *Core curriculum for oncology nursing* (pp. 909-920). St. Louis: Elsevier Saunders.

Scanlon, C., & Glover, J. J. (1995). A professional code of ethics: providing moral compass in turbulent times. *Oncology Nursing Forum 22,* 1515-1521.

Stanley, K. J., & Zoloth-Dorfman, L. (2001). Ethical considerations. In B. R. Ferrell & N. Coyle (Eds.). *Textbook of palliative nursing* (pp. 663-681). New York: Oxford University Press.

Taylor, C. (2002). Ethics. In K. K. Kuebler & P. Esper (Eds.). *Palliative practices from A-Z for the bedside clinician* (pp. 105-109). Pittsburgh, PA: Oncology Nursing Press.

Final Hours

Mary Murphy

Similar characteristics, both physical and psychosocial, are seen during the final hours of a patient's life. These are often divided into two major categories: the preactive phase and the active phase.

PREACTIVE PHASE (7-14 DAYS BEFORE DEATH)

- Increased weakness
- Need for assistance with activities of daily living
- Bed to chair or bed-bound status
- Increased sleeping
- Disorientation or episodes or near death awareness (talking to or seeing visions)
- Limited food and fluid intake
- Swallowing difficulty, including a need to discontinue or alter the route of medication
- Restless, agitated, withdrawal, loss of bowel and bladder control, withdrawal from family and

friends, fear of the dying process or asking when will it be
- Increased spiritual needs

ACTIVE PHASE (2-3 DAYS BEFORE DEATH)

- Altered vital signs, lowered blood pressure, temperature, abnormal respiratory pattern (apnea, Cheyne-Stokes breathing) present or increasing, rapid heart rate or faded muffled heart sounds
- Decreased level of consciousness
- Terminal congestion
- Cooling and mottling of skin
- Decreased responsiveness to external stimuli
- No or very limited oral intake
- Picking or reaching out
- Relaxed facial muscles
- Staring or disconnected viewing of environment
- Crying out, moaning, whimpering

NURSING CONSIDERATIONS BEFORE DEATH

- Discuss:
  - Review advance directives and durable power of attorney (DPOA) status, automatic implantable cardioverter defibrillator (AICD) deactivation.
  - Review wishes for dispensation of body or desire for autopsy; offer resources.
  - Need to be present at time of death; list of family members to call
  - Goals of care: palliation versus active treatment
  - Hydration/feeding concerns
  - Signs and symptoms of terminal phase
  - Treatment modalities to relieve symptoms
  - Provide supportive environment to deliver bad news
  - Rituals, traditions, rites that may be important to care, related to religious or cultural beliefs
  - Coaching families in distress to use four tasks (Byock, 1997):
    - Ask for forgiveness.
    - Say "Thank you."
    - "I love you."
    - "Good-bye."

PALLIATIVE THERAPY OPTIONS FOR END-OF-LIFE PATIENTS
Pain Management

- Use observation scales that are appropriate to level of alertness.
- Do not discontinue opioids or benzodiazepines.
- Seek alternative routes as needed.

Dyspnea

- Use oxygen for support.
- Elevate head of bed.
- Suction mildly as needed.

- Use of benzodiazepines and low-dose opioids

Dehydration
- Mouth/lip care
- Sips of fluids as appropriate
- Hypodermoclysis if appropriate
- Discuss food/fluid issues

Incontinence
- Skin care
- Foley catheter
  (assess for bladder distention)
- Incontinence barriers
- Manual impaction removal with use of suppository only if distention and discomfort present

Confusion and Agitation
- Use of benzodiazepines and phenothiazines

Death Rattle
- Suction only if necessary.
- Medication management:
  - Hyoscyamine (Levison)
  - Atropine
  - Scopolamine

Physical Care
- Mouth care
- Turning and positioning for comfort
- Skin care
- Provide safety.
- Emotional care
- Quiet environment or sounds that are comforting (tapes, voices)
- Story telling (past pleasant events)
- Call by name.
- Tell who is in the room.
- State who you are and what you are doing.

Special Considerations
- More preparation is needed if anticipated related to diagnosis.
  - Hemorrhage
  - Seizures
  - Severe and uncontrolled terminal agitation
  - Children or younger patient(s)

NURSING CARE AFTER DEATH
- Clarify who needs to be present or notified before body is removed.
- Determine whether any ritual needs to take place (poem, prayer).
- Removal of personal items (rings, hair, personal items)
- Offer support services (chaplain, bereavement)
- Preparation of the body

- Final good-byes
- Last-minute concerns

BIBLIOGRAPHY

Bayne, S., Farnham, C., & Fenick, P. (2006). Death bed phenomena and their effect on a palliative care team: a pilot study. *American Journal of Hospice and Palliative Care, 23,* 17-24.

Berry, P., & Griffie, J. (2001). Planning for the actual death. In B. R. Ferrell & N. Coyle (Eds.). *Textbook of palliative nursing* (pp. 382-394). New York: Oxford University Press.

Berry, P. H., Griffie, J., & Heidrich, D. (2002). The dying process. In K. K. Kuebler, P. H. Berry, & D. E. Heidrich (Eds.). *End of life care* (pp. 39-50). Philadelphia: W. B. Saunders.

Byock, I. (1997). *Dying well: the prospects for growth at end-of-life.* New York: Riverhead Books.

Callanan, M., & Kenny, P. (1992). *Final gifts: understanding the specific awareness needs, and communications of the dying.* New York: Bantam Books.

Ho, K. (2004). Changes as death approaches. In J. T. Panke & P. Coyne (Eds.). *Conversations in palliative care* (pp. 201-215). Pensacola, FL: Phol Publishing.

Nguyen, V. D., & Ash, M. J. (2002). The last days: the actively dying patient. In B. M. Kinzbrunner, N. J. Weinreb, & J. S. Policzer (Eds.). *20 Common problems in end-of-life care* (pp. 241-274). New York: McGraw-Hill.

Loss, Grief, and Bereavement

Mary Murphy

- Loss and its movement toward grief begin at the time the diagnosis of cancer is identified.
- Loss is defined by Guillaume (2004) as a loss of a possession or multiple possessions.
- Patients with cancer experience loss from both physical and emotional aspects, which includes roles, role identity, appearances, performance (job and personal), and relationships.
- Grief begins when losses become permanent or the reality of the situation overcomes the event.
- As situations change, continuing bereavement may be necessary to allow adjustment to losses that may be permanent or move to a serious outcome. They may also include altered or final losses for caregivers and spouses.

LOSS
Definition
- The absence of a possession or multiple possession(s) (Guillaume 2004)

GRIEF
Definition
- The emotional, mental, physical, behavioral, and spiritual response to loss (King, 2003)

BEREAVEMENT
Definition
- Includes grief and mourning and inner feelings and the outward reaction of survivorship (King, 2003)

Affected By

- Support systems (children, organizations, family)
- Previous experiences
- Suddenness of event
- Coping mechanisms
- Relationship and significances to person or event
- Knowledge and understanding
- Timing of event
- Life sequence of event
- Concurrent stresses
- Rituals and expectations
- Religious/spirituality, culture
- Boundaries
- Financial burden or support
- Events from diagnosis to death
- Role in family and community
- Personal value system (body image, self-concept)
- Role in family internal/external
- Perception of the loss, esteem, identity
- Future goals, "What will not be"

Characteristics

- Behavioral response
- Cannot be felt by others
- Decreased interest and motivation in usual tasks
- Withdrawal (social)
- Feelings of guilt
- Anger, withdrawal, anxiety
- Inability to concentrate or remember normal events
- Restlessness, agitation, mood changes
- Decreased ability to accomplish tasks
- Crying
- Avoiding thinking about or talking about the events, changes, or losses
- Apathy
- Increased in use of psychoactive substances
- Sleep disturbances
- Talking about event or loss repeatedly and to excess
- For caregivers, repeated need to revisit circumstances or illness and their outcomes

Physical Symptoms

- Weight loss/gain
- Fatigue (even without activity)
- Heart palpitations
- Headache
- Nausea/vomiting
- Constipation/diarrhea
- Muscle weakness
- Dry mouth
- Tightness of chest, jaw, or throat
- Difficulty swallowing
- Shortness of breath
- Sweating, chills, and hot flashes

TYPES OF GRIEF

- Anticipatory: fear of the unknown, based on losses experienced and fear of future loss
- Normal grief: a state loss and expected response; the ability to continue on with life and interact

Four Types of Complicated Grief

- Chronic: a normal grief cycle that continues for longer than expected
- Delayed: a postponed grief related to suicide, homicide, unexpected death, or unbearable losses. May be coping mechanism, a form of denial, and repression
- Exaggerated: the survivor uses self-destructive methods to cope with a loss such as suicide
- Masked: the survivor does not understand the behaviors he or she displays are elements of loss, such as substance abuse, mental illness, spiritual suffering, and physical focus on ongoing symptoms

Complicated grief may manifest itself in the forms of denial, shock, anger, feelings of hopelessness, panic attacks, numbness, or helplessness.

Other Forms of Grief

- Disenfranchised grief: a grief that cannot be expressed due to the nature of the loss such as the diagnosis of human immunodeficiency virus (HIV) infection, an affair, a crime that was committed, or information that cannot be shared with others. Nurses may experience this type of grief based on the inability to deal with the loss of a patient or an intense situation; there is an inability to talk to anyone or the thought that this is just part of the job
- Children's grief: is based on the developmental level and may affect sleep, bowel, eating patterns and is displayed by anger, nightmares, sexual promiscuity, compulsive behavior, accidents, deviant behavior, and focus on illness

Stages and Tasks of Grief

Stage I: Notification and Shock
- The task is to share acknowledgment of the reality of the loss and assist the survivor in coping with the initial impact of death.
- Survivors may feel numb, be in shock, or display poor daily functioning, isolation, and avoidance.

Stage II: Experience the Loss Emotionally and Cognitively
- Share in the process of working through the pain of the loss.
- Characteristics include:
  - Anger at the person who died and the health care system that failed them
  - Guilt
  - Sadness
  - Loneliness
  - Emptiness, and lack of interest in life
  - Insomnia

○ Appetite changes
○ Disorganization.

Stage III: Reintegration
- This stage allows for recognition and restructuring of family systems and reinvestment in relationships.
- Characteristics include:
  ○ Feelings of hope in the future
  ○ Increased energy
  ○ Participation in social events
  ○ Acceptance of the death.

TREATMENT

- Referral for identification of long-term and complication concerns
- Normal fear versus alteration in functioning
- Identification of risk factors that may cause increased distress
- Community referral(s), support groups
- Private referral counseling and independent counseling.
- Identification of pathology
- Counseling or psychiatric referral

RESPONSE AND SUPPORT

- Response to loss, grief, and bereavement issues include:
  ○ Identification
  ○ Validation of grief
  ○ Active listening, touch, silence
  ○ Normalize the grief process.
  ○ Explore healthy coping skills.
  ○ Offer emotional and spiritual support.
  ○ Mediation support as needed

SPOUSE/CAREGIVER AND FAMILY SUPPORT

- Spouses, caregivers, and families experience the similar affects to the diagnosis, treatments, and outcomes as the patients do, often forgetting that they can have both a positive and negative influence on the patient's treatment outcome.
- These individuals who are now expected to offer support may become a hindrance or compete with the patient on the basis of their own past experiences with loss, previous coping methods, role relationship to the patient, and their own support systems.
- Incorporation and understanding of these individuals at time of diagnosis will assist the health care team to understand and support the treatment and outcomes of the patient's disease.

BIBLIOGRAPHY

Bozeman, M. (2002). Bereavement. In B. M. Kinzbrunner, N. J. Weinreb, & J. S. Policzer (Eds.). *20 Common problems end-of-life care* (pp. 276-293). New York: McGraw-Hill.

Grimm, P. (2005). Coping: psychosocial issues. In J. K. Itano & K. N. Taoka (Eds.). *Core curriculum for oncology nursing* (4th ed., pp. 29-58). St. Louis: Elsevier Saunders.

Guillaume, C. (2004) Loss and grief. In C. Yarboro, M. Frugge, & M. Goodman (Eds.). *Cancer symptom management* (3rd ed., p 709). Boston: Jones & Bartlett.

King, S. (2003). Bereavement. In M. Finch & E. Burreura (Eds.). *Handbook of advanced cancer care* (pp. 126-136). New York: Cambridge University Press.

Pitorak, E. F. (2004). Bereavement. In J. Panke & P. Coyne (Eds.). *Conversations in palliative care* (pp. 241-250). Kingwood, TX: Pohl Publishing.

Roberts, K., & Berry, P. (2002). Grief and bereavement. In K. K. Kuebler, P. H. Berry, & D. E. Heidrich (Eds.). *End of life care clinical practice guidelines* (pp. 53-64). Philadelphia: W. B. Saunders.

Palliative Care & End-of-Life Issues

Patient Teaching

ALOPECIA (HAIR LOSS)

WHAT IS ALOPECIA?

- Alopecia is hair loss that can occur with certain cancer treatments such as chemotherapy and radiation therapy.
- Cancer treatments may not only kill cancer cells but also affect healthy cells in your body.
- Hair loss or thinning can occur on the head, face, and body with chemotherapy treatments. With radiation therapy, hair loss occurs only in the treated areas.
- Hair loss usually begins within 1 to 3 weeks after your first treatment.
- The amount of loss that you have will depend on the treatment you receive and the dose.

WILL MY HAIR GROW BACK?

- Hair will usually regrow after your treatment, except in cases of radiation given in doses greater than 6,000 cGY. You may notice some regrowth before the end of your treatment, but in almost all cases you will see regrowth by 3 months after the end of your treatments.
- Sometimes your hair may grow back a little different than it was before your treatments: it may be curly if it was straight, or gray if it was black, or thick if it was thin! Usually these changes are not permanent.
- It may take 6 to 12 months to grow back completely.

WHAT CAN I DO?

If your health care provider has told you to expect hair loss as part of your treatment's side effects, then you should be prepared:

- Consider purchasing a wig before your treatment begins so that you can match your color and style easily. Your insurance may cover the cost of a wig if a prescription is written for "scalp prosthesis." If your insurance doesn't help with the cost of a wig, contact the local American Cancer Society or other local cancer organization for help getting a wig free of charge. You can have your wig cut or professionally styled. Wear "stickies" to keep your wig on securely. The cost of wigs, scarves, false eyelashes, and so forth are considered tax-deductible medical expenses.
- You may want to consider wearing a turban, scarf, or hat instead of a wig.
- When outside, cover your head to protect it from the cold or the sun. Use a good sunscreen, applying it every 90 minutes or after getting wet.
- If you shave your head, be careful to avoid nicking or cutting your scalp.
- Use a mild soap or shampoo on your scalp. You may use a nonfragrant, mild lotion if your scalp is dry or sensitive. If itching or redness occurs, stop using anything on your scalp. Do not use anything on your head if you are receiving radiation therapy to the head, unless your radiation oncology doctor or nurse has approved it.
- If your hair is thinning, you may want to consider the following. However, these suggestions are only to protect fragile hair and might slow hair loss, but they will not prevent it from falling out if it has been severely damaged by your treatment:
  - Use a mild shampoo every 4 days and pay dry.
  - Avoid blow dryers, hot curling irons, hair rollers, barrettes and rubber bands.
  - Avoid hair dyes, rinses, bleaching, or permanents.
  - Use a soft-bristle brush.
  - Sleep on a satin pillowcase to decrease friction rubbing.
  - If you feel that getting your hair cut, colored, or permed is important to you and makes you feel better about yourself, then do it!

Losing your hair can be a very emotionally trying experience. It can affect how you feel about yourself or your self-image. Everyone's experience is different, so it is important to talk with your doctor or nurse about how you are dealing with your hair loss. You might want to join a support group or talk to a counselor. The American Cancer Society offers a class called "Look Good, Feel Better" (www.lookgoodfeelbetter.org) for persons who have hair loss during their cancer treatment.

Patient Teaching

ANOREXIA

WHAT IS ANOREXIA? WHAT CAUSES IT?

- Anorexia, or *loss of appetite* is a common problem in people with cancer.
- Certain types of cancer can affect your metabolism, especially ovarian, pancreatic, and stomach cancers.
- Side effects from your cancer treatment may also affect your appetite including mouth sores, dry mouth, nausea, constipation, pain and difficulty swallowing.
- Some medications can alter your appetite by affecting your metabolism too.

Make sure you tell your doctor if you are having any of these problems.

WHAT WILL ANOREXIA DO TO ME?

- Losing your appetite may cause you to eat less, not feel hungry at all, or feel full after eating small amounts.
- A persistently poor appetite can lead to weight loss and malnutrition, and this can affect your ability to tolerate your treatment.

WHAT CAN I DO ABOUT ANOREXIA?

- Weight loss in people with cancer is a combination of losing fat and lean muscle mass; therefore, it takes more than just eating to fix the problem.
- Your doctor may recommend nutritional supplements or other medications to stimulate your appetite.
- Here are some tips to help you eat better and gain weight during cancer treatment:
  - Add cold, sour, or acidic foods to diet.
  - Give yourself permission to eat less.
  - Use smaller dinner plates to avoid being overwhelmed.
  - Eat more at times during the day when you are most hungry.
  - Increase seasonings in food.
  - Take pain medications 30-60 minutes before meals if eating is painful.
  - Eat smaller, more frequent meals/snacks.
  - Try using plastic utensils.
  - Keep snacks available and take them with you when you go out.
  - Drink liquids 30-60 minutes before or after meals, to avoid getting full on fluids alone.
  - Use liquid meal replacements such as Boost, Ensure, and Carnation Instant Breakfast when it is hard to eat.
  - Rest before eating.
  - Try to eat something at bedtime.
  - Try softer, bland foods, but not tasteless ones.
  - Maintain good oral hygiene and rinse your mouth before and after meals.
  - Make sure teeth/dentures are in good condition.
  - Eat larger meals when feeling well.
  - Never force yourself to eat.
  - Plan meals with your favorite foods.
  - Let someone else cook/shop for you.
  - Plan music during meals and create a pleasant setting.
  - Keep mealtimes relaxed and unhurried.
  - Avoid empty calories; eat nutrient-rich foods.
  - Avoid tobacco products, which suppress appetite.
  - Add calories and protein to meals by adding sauces, gravy, butter, cheese, peanut butter, cream, and nuts.
  - Avoid eating a meal alone; when possible, have friends or family eat with you.
  - Try light exercise such as a 20-minute walk an hour before meals to stimulate your appetite. (Always check with your doctor before starting an exercise program.)
  - If okay with your doctor, drink a glass of sherry or wine before a meal to stimulate your appetite.

Submitted by Wendy H. Vogel.

Patient Teaching

CANCER PAIN MANAGEMENT

TEAMWORK IS THE KEY!

Not everyone with cancer has pain. Those who do know that pain can affect you in many ways. It can keep you from being active, sleeping, eating, and enjoying life. It can make you depressed. We will work with you as a **TEAM** to control your pain.

It is very important for you to talk to us about your pain. We will need to know things about your pain, such as:

- On scale of 1-10 (10 being the worst pain), how do you rate your pain?
- What are you taking for pain now?
- After taking your pain medications, how do you rate your pain?
- What makes it worse?
- What makes it better?
- Describe your pain.
- Where is it located? Does it travel anywhere else?
- Do you have any other symptoms?
- Are there certain times it is better or worse?
- Sometimes it is helpful to keep a pain journal. We will give you one to fill out if this would be helpful.

We need **YOU** to tell us about your fears or concerns you have about medication or your treatment. You are the biggest part of our **TEAM**!

WHAT IS CHRONIC PAIN?

Chronic pain is pain that lasts longer than 6 months. It doesn't have a purpose, like when you touch your hand on a hot stove and it hurts so that you will stop touching the stove. You may not have many physical symptoms of pain like raised blood pressure or elevated pulse, but you may see more symptoms like depression, trouble sleeping, or mood swings.

WHAT CAUSES MY PAIN?

There can be many causes of chronic pain. Most cancer pain comes when a tumor presses on a bone, nerve, or body organ. Cancer treatments sometimes can cause pain too. There are also other types of pain that have nothing to do with your illness. You can get headaches, muscle strains, arthritis pain, and other pains, just like anyone else.

HOW WILL YOU TREAT MY PAIN?

Chronic pain is usually treated with medicine. But sometimes surgery, radiation therapy, and other treatments may be used along with medicines to give better pain relief. There are many types of pain medicines. **Ask us if you have any questions about your particular medication.** Here are several types of pain medications:

Nonopiods: Acetaminophen and nonsteroidal anti-inflammatory drugs (NSAIDs), such as aspirin and ibuprofen. These are drugs such as Tylenol, aspirin, Motrin, Naprosyn, and others. Some of these you can buy without a prescription (over the counter).

Opioids: These include morphine, hydromorphone, oxycodone, codeine, Lortab, Tylenol #3, Percocet, Dilaudid, MS Contin, Darvocet, morphine sulfate, fentanyl, Avinza, Kadian, OxyContin and others. You must have a prescription for these medications, and most of these cannot be called into your drug store because they are federally regulated. If you are unable to pick up your prescriptions yourself, whoever picks up the prescription must present his or her driver's license for identification purposes and a copy will be made for our records.

Antidepressants: Amitriptyline, imipramine, doxepin, Trazone, Elavil, Desyrel, Sinequan, and others. A prescription will be required for these medications. If you are taking one of these medications, it does not necessarily mean that you are depressed or have a mental illness. These medications may be useful for tingling or burning pains (nerve pains).

Antiseizure medications: These might include Dilantin or Tegretol or others. You will need a prescription for these medications. Taking these medications does not mean that you could have a seizure. These medications work well for nerve pain also.

Steroids: Prednisone, Decadron, and others may be useful for controlling pain caused by swelling or infection. You will need a prescription for these medications.

WHAT ABOUT SIDE EFFECTS?

All medications have side effects. But, **not everyone gets side effects and you will *not* have all the side effects listed here!** You will not have the same side effects as someone else taking the same medicine. Every person is different. Most side effects of pain medications occur within the first few days and gradually go away. The most common side effects and what to do about them are listed below:

Constipation: Just about all pain medications can cause constipation. The best way to prevent constipation is to take a daily stool softener. **If you take pain medicine every day, you will likely need a stool softener every day.** There are many different kinds of stool softeners and laxatives. Ask us for more information on constipation.

Continued

Patient Teaching

CANCER PAIN MANAGEMENT—cont'd

Drink plenty of fluids (8-10 oz) per day. Exercise regularly. Increase fiber in your diet (such as eating cereal for breakfast and an apple a day).

Nausea and Vomiting: Just about any pain medication can cause some nausea. The key is not to take it on an empty stomach and to start at a smaller dose and gradually increase as needed. Usually if nausea or vomiting occurs, it should only last for the first few doses and then your body adjusts to the medication. **This does not mean you are allergic to the medication.** Keep taking the medicine unless you are vomiting severely or have a rash or shortness of breath. You may want to halve the dose for a short while until your body gets used to the medication. Please call us if you are having any trouble with this. Sometimes taking a medicine to prevent nausea about 30 minutes before you take your pain medication is helpful.

Sleepiness: Some people feel drowsy or sleepy after taking pain medications, especially short-acting medications. Your body will usually adjust to this after a few days and you will be less sleepy. Short-acting medications generally cause more sleepiness than long-acting medicines. **Do not drive or operate machinery if you experience this side effect.**

HOW WILL I BE TAKING MY PAIN MEDICATIONS?

Most pain medications are taken by mouth **(orally)**. Oral medicines are easy to take and usually cost less. Most are in tablet or capsules, but some come in liquid form as well. You can also take pain medications by:

Rectal suppository: medication that dissolves in the rectum and is absorbed by the body.

Patches: these are patches filled with medicine, placed on the skin and absorbed by the body.

Injections: this is given with a needle either subcutaneously (just under the skin) or intramuscularly (into a muscle). This type of route is not recommended for chronic pain.

Intravenous (through a vein): this is given with a needle inserted into a vein. This could be by an IV, central, Hickman catheter, PICC, or Groshong line.

Epidural or intrathecal: this is medication given into the back beside the spinal cord. This can give pain relief that can last a long time.

WHAT ELSE IS IMPORTANT TO KNOW?

1. **You are in charge of your pain control.** We will assist you in every way possible, **but you must take your medications as ordered.** We will work with you to find the right medication and the right dosage. We do not want you to hurt!

2. **Medications for chronic pain work better when taking regularly** (around the clock). **Long-acting medications must be taken regularly to work correctly. Long-acting medications are given to PREVENT pain. Do not skip a dose of these medications, even if you are not in pain at the time the medication is due.** Not being in pain means the medication is working! Long-acting medications (time-released) may include MS Contin, OxyContin, Duragesic, Kadian, Avinza, and others. **Do NOT break any long-acting medication in half.**

3. Sometimes, even when taking a long-acting medication like MS Contin, you may have what we call **"break-through" pain.** This is pain that occurs when you increase your activity, like coming to the doctor, riding in a car, etc. It could be any activity that makes your pain worse. You should have short-acting medication for this pain, such as Percocet, Lortab, or OxyIR. These medications work quickly (within 15-30 minutes) to **GET** you comfortable. Long-acting medications **KEEP** you comfortable! **If you find that you need a lot of "break-through" medication, please let us know, because we may need to increase the dose of your long-acting medication.**

4. **If you are taking pain medications only when needed (a short-acting medication), then take it before pain becomes bad!** Pain is much harder to stop once it begins to hurt badly. It is easier to control before it is bad.

5. **If you have followed our instructions and you are still in pain or if your pain increases or changes, call us! Call us if you are having other problems!** We want to help and we will work with you to make you comfortable.

CANCER PAIN MANAGEMENT—cont'd

6. **If you take pain medications every day, you will most likely need a stool softener every day.** See the section on constipation, under side effects.

7. **Call us early for refills (3-4 days before you run out). Don't wait until you run out.** We may not be able to refill pain medications over the weekends or holidays.

WHAT ABOUT GETTING ADDICTED?

Many people worry about getting addicted to or "hooked" on pain medications. Many studies have shown that when you have real, chronic pain, addiction to pain medication is rare. When your pain decreases, you will be able to decrease your pain medication as well. If you have had or have an addition to drugs or alcohol, please let us know. We still want to treat your pain. It is important that you be comfortable.

AREN'T DRUGS LIKE OXYCONTIN DANGEROUS?

If you take your medication as you are instructed, it should be safe for you to take. Many problems that you have heard about on TV or in the news come from persons who obtain these drugs illegally and use them in ways that are not intended. Do not share your medication with others, including family members. Do not sell or give away unused medications. Many times, it is better not to tell many people that you are taking pain medications.

I AM AFRAID IF I TAKE TOO MUCH NOW, IT MIGHT NOT WORK LATER.

Many people worry that pain medications might stop working if they take them now and they will be in severe pain later on in life. That is **not** true. The medicine will **not** stop working. Sometimes your body can get used to the medicine and that is called tolerance. Tolerance is not usually a problem with chronic pain because the amount of medicine or dose can be changed or other medications can be given. **Chronic pain can be relieved. Don't deny yourself pain relief now.**

WHERE CAN I GET MORE INFORMATION?

NCI: National Cancer Institute: 1-800-4-CANCER or www.nci.nih.gov
American Cancer Society: 1-800-ACS-2345 or www.cancer.org
Ask us for more information about pain control.

Submitted by Wendy H. Vogel.

Patient Teaching

CANCER PREVENTION AND DIET

DOES MY DIET AFFECT MY CHANCES OF GETTING CANCER?

Although the cause of cancer is not known, about 1 in 3 cancers may be related to what you eat and drink. For example, a diet that is high in fat may increase your risk for getting cancers of the breast, uterus (womb), prostate, colon, and rectum. Being overweight increases your risk of cancers of the uterus, gallbladder, kidney, stomach, colon, and breast. A fatty diet and being overweight also increase your risk for heart and circulation problems. Cancers of the stomach and esophagus have been linked to smoked and cured meats. Heavy use of alcohol may be related to cancers of the mouth, throat, esophagus, larynx (voice box), and liver.

DO ANY FOODS HELP PREVENT CANCER?

No foods are guaranteed to protect you from cancer, but fruits and vegetables contain fiber, vitamins, and phytochemicals that have a role in preventing cancer.

Fiber is the plant material in our diet that is not digested. It keeps food moving through our intestines. Fiber comes from whole-grain breads and cereals, as well as fruit and vegetables.

Vitamins C and E act as antioxidants. Antioxidants help prevent or repair damage to cells caused by pollution, sunlight, and normal body processes. Excellent sources of vitamin C are citrus fruits, brussels sprouts, peppers, and tomatoes. Vitamin E is found in vegetable oils, seeds and nuts, leafy green vegetables, and tomatoes.

Vitamin A and folate both help cells develop normally. Vitamin A is present in liver, fortified dairy products, eggs, and butter. Asparagus, leafy green vegetables, and fortified cereals are good sources of folate.

Vitamin C is present in some vegetables, such as potatoes, and in many fruits, especially tomatoes and citrus fruits.

Ask your health care provider about vitamin and mineral supplements.

Phytochemicals are natural chemicals that give plants their color, flavor, smell, and texture. Phytochemicals are only found in plants, so it is important to eat a variety of fruits, vegetables, and beans.

For a diet that helps protect you against cancer:
- Get more fiber in your diet. Foods that are rich in fiber help you to feel full and maintain your weight. Oat bran, fruits, and beans also help lower cholesterol.
- Eat more whole-grain breads, pastas, and cereals.
- Eat less fat. When you eat meat, trim off the fat and skin. Use nonfat or low-fat dairy products. Remember that desserts are usually high in both fats and calories.
- Eat more fish and white meat (chicken, turkey) and less red meat (beef, lamb, pork). Eat less smoked and processed meats and fish.
- Change how you cook. Grilling, broiling, and frying meat at high temperature creates chemicals that may increase cancer risk. The same meat cooked in a stew or steamed, poached, or microwaved is safer.
- Drink alcohol moderately if at all. Your risk of cancers of the mouth, pharynx, larynx, esophagus, and liver are increased if you drink more than 1 drink a day if you're a woman or 2 drinks a day if you're a man.
- Eat 5 to 13 servings a day of fruits and vegetables.
- Eat a variety of foods.
- If you are overweight, talk to your provider about losing weight.

Diet and lifestyle changes can help you take control of your health. Make healthy choices about regular physical activity, weight, consumption of alcohol, smoking, and the foods you eat. Talk your health care provider if you have questions or special concerns about your risk of cancer.

Patient Teaching

CANCER: SEVEN WARNING SIGNS

There usually are no signs or symptoms when cancer is in its very early stage. Sometimes early symptoms do not seem like anything serious. Learning what to look for can lead to early detection. Early detection of a cancer greatly increases the chances of curing cancer.

The American Cancer Society has identified **seven major warning signs** of cancer:
1. A change in bowel or bladder habits
2. A sore that does not heal
3. Unusual bleeding or discharge from any place
4. A lump in the breast or other parts of the body
5. Chronic indigestion or difficulty in swallowing
6. Obvious changes in a wart or mole
7. Persistent coughing or hoarseness.

You should have a check up soon if you have any of these warning signs. Having one of these warning signs does not mean you are sure to have cancer. However, if you are diagnosed with cancer, early treatment greatly increases your chances to be cured if a cancer is found.

To learn more about the warning signs of cancer, call your local chapter of the American Cancer Society, or call (800) ACS-2345 or the National Cancer Institute at (800) 4-CANCER.

Patient Teaching

CANCER TREATMENT TEAM

WHAT TYPES OF SPECIALISTS HELP TREAT CANCER?

The different members of your cancer team offer many kinds of help. They can help you deal with the physical and emotional effects of having cancer.

The treatment team may include:
- your primary health care provider
- medical oncologist
- radiation oncologist
- radiation technologist
- surgeon
- oncology nurses
- dieticians
- physical therapist
- pharmacist
- social worker, psychiatrist, or psychologist.

WHAT DO THESE SPECIALISTS DO?

Your primary health care provider will continue to provide your usual care. Your provider will also help you manage any other health problems you may have during your cancer treatment, such as high blood pressure or diabetes. Often the primary health care provider coordinates treatments and communication among the other specialists on the team.

A medical oncologist is a doctor who has had special training in the treatment of cancer. He or she sees patients after they have been diagnosed with cancer and prescribes chemotherapy and recommends other cancer treatments. Your oncologist may be a team leader, keeping a check on all treatments and making referrals to other specialists as needed.

Radiation oncologists are doctors who have special training in the use of radiation therapy. Radiation therapy is the use of high-energy rays to shrink or destroy tumors. These doctors determine the dosage and scheduling of radiation treatments and they manage side effects. Another type of specialist, the radiation technologist, performs the radiation treatment.

Surgeons are doctors who remove tissue for diagnosis, insert special tubes called catheters for giving chemotherapy, and do operations to remove cancerous tissue.

Oncology nurses provide nursing care to cancer patients. They give medicine and watch for side effects. They can give tips and advice for dealing with drug side effects and problems caused by the cancer. Nurses may care for you at the hospital, outpatient clinics, or home.

Dietitians design a diet to meet your particular needs. They can help you know how to get the calories and nutrients you need during your illness and treatment. The diet will help you maintain a healthy weight. Proper nutrition can make it easier for your body to fight the cancer. A healthy diet will also help fight the side effects of treatments and any infections that might develop. Dietitians can also give you tips about increasing your appetite if you have nausea, stomach upset, or tiredness from your illness or treatment.

A physical therapist designs an exercise program that is right for you. Proper exercise can help you maintain muscle tone and adapt to any physical changes that may result from your treatment. Physical therapists can provide exercise even if you are bedridden.

Pharmacists prepare the medicines used in cancer treatment. These medicines include the drugs used in chemotherapy and other prescription drugs.

Social workers or psychologists help you cope with the stress of the diagnosis and treatment of cancer. They can provide counseling for you and your family and help you find a support group. Social workers can help coordinate your hospital discharge. Psychiatrists are doctors who can prescribe medicine for depression or anxiety.

Finally, remember that you are the most important member of this team. Don't be afraid to ask questions and get any information you need. Let the other members of the team know when you need help and care.

For more information, contact:
- American Cancer Society (800-ACS-2345, http://www.cancer.org)
- National Cancer Institute (800-4-CANCER, http://www.cancer.gov).

CHEMO BRAIN (COGNITIVE DYSFUNCTION)

WHAT IS CHEMO BRAIN?

Sometimes after cancer treatments such as chemotherapy people have problems with memory or concentration. You may hear it called chemo fog or cognitive dysfunction. Some symptoms are as follows:
- Memory loss
- Trouble paying attention
- Trouble finding the right words
- Trouble learning something new
- Trouble managing daily things you have to do
- Trouble doing math
- Mood swings

WHAT CAUSES CHEMO BRAIN?

No one is sure of what causes chemo brain. There are some things that can make chemo brain worse, including low blood counts, stress, depression, anxiety, tiredness, not sleeping well, certain medications, and changes in hormones.

WHEN DOES IT START AND HOW LONG DOES IT LAST?

Some people say it can start around the time you were told you have cancer. Other people notice it during their chemotherapy treatments.

Submitted by Wendy H. Vogel.

Patient Teaching

CHEMOTHERAPY (DRUG THERAPY FOR CANCER)

WHAT IS CHEMOTHERAPY?

Chemotherapy is the use of medicines to control, slow, or cure medical conditions. The term chemotherapy is most often used to refer to the medicines given to slow or stop the growth of cancer cells. A problem with these medicines is that some of them also damage healthy cells.

The goals of chemotherapy are:
- To cure the cancer with the fewest or least harmful side effects.
- To control the cancer. This is done by keeping the cancer from spreading; slowing the cancer's growth; and killing cancer cells that may have spread to other parts of the body from the original tumor.
- To relieve symptoms that the cancer may cause. Relieving symptoms such as pain can help people who have cancer live more comfortably.

WHAT ARE THE DIFFERENT TYPES OF DRUG THERAPY FOR CANCER?

Chemotherapy uses many drugs. In general they fall into 3 categories:
- antimitotic drugs
- hormones and hormone inhibitors
- biological therapy.

Most of the chemotherapy drugs are antimitotics. This means that they stop cancer cell growth by stopping cells from dividing into more cells. There are many ways that scientists have found to do this, so there are now many different kinds of these drugs. They include names you may have heard: Adriamycin (doxorubicin), Cytoxan (cyclophosphamide), and 5FU (5-fluorouracil).

Hormone therapy plays a very important role in chemotherapy. Sex hormone inhibitors are used to treat tumors that grow better with the hormones estrogen and testosterone. (These are hormones that naturally occur in the body.) The inhibitors stop the hormones from helping the tumor grow. Two commonly used hormone inhibitors are tamoxifen, which blocks female hormones in breast cancer, and finasteride, which blocks testosterone in men with prostate cancer. Hormones, such as cortisone (prednisone), are also used to treat some tumors.

Biologic therapy, or immunotherapy, is a new name for a growing group of cancer drugs. They are medicines that help the immune system work better and fight the cancer. Interferon is an example of one of these drugs. Another example of biologic therapy is the use of antibodies. The goal is to identify or create antibodies that can bind to cancer cells. The antibodies can keep the cancer cells from multiplying, or they may destroy them. This type of therapy is also called biotherapy or biological response modifier therapy (BRM).

HOW IS CHEMOTHERAPY USED?

Chemotherapy is used in several ways:
- one drug alone
- a combination of drugs
- combined with surgery
- combined with radiation
- combined with both surgery and radiation.

The treatment depends on what type of tumor you have, where the tumor is, and how much it has spread. It can be given on many different schedules: daily, weekly, or monthly. The schedules are based on what research has found to work best for each type of cancer. The medicine can be given by mouth, by shot, or in a tube put in a vein (IV, or intravenous). If given by shot, it can be injected into a muscle or it may be given into the spinal cord area.

IV medicine may be given over a few minutes or a few hours. You may be able to give some treatments to yourself at home. Portable pumps are available for chemotherapy treatments that go into the vein. The pump makes sure the prescribed dose of medicine is given over the correct period of time.

WHAT SIDE EFFECTS SHOULD I EXPECT?

Common side effects of the antimitotics are fatigue, nausea, and hair loss. Other side effects depend on the drug, the dose, and your health. Examples of other possible side effects of these drugs are:
- sores in your mouth
- weight loss
- lowered blood counts that make you more likely to get an infection.

An otherwise healthy person receiving chemotherapy may tolerate it very well. Someone who has several other serious medical problems in addition to cancer may have a more difficult time with side effects.

Common side effects from hormone inhibitors are symptoms of menopause for women taking the estrogen-blocking tamoxifen and lowered sex drive for men taking testosterone-blocking finasteride.

Continued

CHEMOTHERAPY (DRUG THERAPY FOR CANCER)—cont'd

The biologic therapies (immunotherapies) often cause people to have flulike symptoms: fever, aches, chills, nausea, and loss of appetite.

Your health care provider will be watching closely for any side effects and help you manage them. If the side effects become severe, the dose of the drug may be lowered or the treatment may be postponed. Sometimes hospitalization is required for severe side effects. In extreme cases, treatment might be stopped.

WHAT ARE CLINICAL TRIALS?

Ask your health care provider about clinical trials. These are studies being done to test new treatments, new medicines, and new combinations of medicines. Research programs sometimes allow you to receive the latest treatments. Ask your provider where the closest clinical trials are (often at universities and participating doctors' offices) and how you can learn more about them. Making an appointment to talk about a clinical trial does not mean you have to take part in the trial. The options, the risks, the costs, and whether your insurance will pay will be explained to you. Then you can decide if you want to join the study.

HOW SHOULD I TAKE CARE OF MYSELF DURING TREATMENT?

- First, follow your health care provider's instructions for your treatment. Always ask questions to make sure you understand the directions. It is often helpful to have a friend or family member go with you to help you remember what is said at visits with your provider. You may want to take notes.
- Be sure to tell your provider about all medicines, vitamins, supplements, and any alternative or complementary therapies you are using. Some of these might interact with your chemotherapy and cause more side effects.

- Several doctors may be giving you care: your family health care provider, a cancer specialist (oncologist), a radiation oncologist (a doctor who specializes in the use of radiation for treatment), and a surgeon. Help your providers communicate with each other. Always take a list of your current medicines and chemotherapy drugs with you to ALL of your doctor visits, review the list with the doctor, and ask for the list to be included with your medical chart. Also share your test results from one provider's office with another by carrying copies of the results with you.
- Get specific instructions about what to eat and drink and what to avoid.
- Ask if you will need pain medicine and how to take it. If your cancer or your treatment is causing pain, it is usually best to take the pain medicine either on a regular basis or just when the pain is starting. There is usually no need to wait until the pain is severe.
- Let trusted family members and friends help you. Give them specific suggestions for what they can do to help and make your life easier. They want to help.
- Save your energy for important things and things you enjoy.
- Laughter is the best medicine. Humor helps the immune system work. Read funny books or watch funny movies— whatever makes you laugh.

For more information visit the following Web sites:
- American Cancer Society: http://www.cancer.org
- National Cancer Institute: http://www.cancer.gov

You can also call:
- American Cancer Society: 800-ACS-2345
- National Cancer Institute: 800-4-CANCER.

COMMON SKIN CONDITIONS CAUSED BY TARGETED TREATMENTS

Targeted treatments effectively manage many different kinds of cancer. These drugs are designed to block different mechanisms by which cancer cells are nourished, grow, divide, and possibly spread.

Targeted treatments differ from chemotherapy in that their focus is to prevent cancer cells from growing as well as kill the cancer cells themselves. Chemotherapy can harm healthy cells as it kills cancer cells.

Some of the targeted therapies may lead to skin problems. In particular, the type that inhibits epidermal growth factor receptors (EGFRs) sometimes causes rashes and other irritating skin conditions. Although it is not readily known why the rash occurs, recent research suggests that the rash may indicate that the EGFR inhibitor treatment is effective.

Targeted treatments, particularly those that block EGFRs, commonly cause four skin-related side effects: follicular eruption, nail toxicity, dry skin, and hair changes.

Follicular Eruption
- Refers to inflammation of the hair follicles.
- Rash appears on the face, scalp, chest, back, and areas behind and in front of the ears.
- Very rarely occurs on the buttocks, arms, or legs.
- Looks very similar to acne—some health care providers call it an acne-like rash.
- Tends to occur in many people who take EGFR-blocking drugs.
- Usually appears about 1 week to 10 days after starting treatment
- Can occur as late as 6 weeks after the first dose of medication

Treatment
- Rash may appear and disappear; mild forms may sometimes disappear without treatment.
- Rarely becomes so severe that targeted therapy is stopped.
- Mild cases
  ○ Steroid creams
    ▪ Help reduce inflammation, pain, and discomfort
    ▪ Tend to be more powerful than over-the-counter brands
    ▪ Available only with a doctor's prescription (e.g., hydrocortisone valerate [Westcort and others])
    ▪ Apply after cleaning the skin very gently with a mild, soap-free cleanser, such as Cetaphil.
    ▪ Use very carefully, particularly on the face.
    ▪ Side effects include thinning and whitening of the skin; the appearance of visible blood vessels; and a red, pimply, or acne-like rash.

  ○ Other topical treatments include
    ▪ Acne treatments such as benzoyl peroxide
    ▪ Retinoids (a class of drugs including Retin-A)
    ▪ Topical antibiotics (typically erythromycin, clindamycin, or metronidazole).
    ▪ All have been shown to help some people with follicular eruptions.
    ▪ Can irritate and dry the skin; use carefully
    ▪ It is advised to use these drugs every other day at first and then slowly increase to daily use.
  ○ Nontopical treatments include oral antibiotics, usually tetracyclines
    ▪ Help relieve inflammation.
    ▪ May take several weeks to start reducing symptoms.
    ▪ Increase the skin's sensitivity to the sun so use sunscreen daily or avoid exposure to the sun or tanning rays if possible.
- Severe eruptions
  ○ Can be treated with antibiotics and a stronger steroid cream
    ▪ Clobetasol (Temovate and others).
    ▪ If eruptions are persistent, isotretinoin (Accutane and others) might be useful.
- Treatment of pain symptoms
  ○ Can be treated with an over-the-counter pain reliever, such as acetaminophen (Tylenol and others).
  ○ If pain persists, a doctor may prescribe a more potent pain reliever.
- Treatment of pruritus (itching)
  ○ Over-the counter antihistamines (Benadryl, Claritin, Allegra, and other) may help.
  ○ Hydroxyzine (Atarax, Vistaril) is a prescription antihistamine you discuss with your health care provider.
- Infections
- Follicular eruptions may become infected, worsen despite treatment
- Your health care provider may test a sample of the rash for bacteria.
- If bacteria are present, your health care provider may prescribe an antibacterial cream or ointment such as mupirocin (Bactroban and others).

Nail Toxicity
- Changes that occur in the nails of the fingers or toes or in the skin around them.
- Skin around the nails becomes very dry and cracked and may even begin to peel away from the ends of the fingers or toes.
- The cuticle may swell, and some nails may become ingrown.
- Tends to occur weeks or months after beginning an EGFR-inhibiting targeted treatment,
- Often persists for weeks or months after a person stops taking the drug.

Continued

COMMON SKIN CONDITIONS CAUSED BY TARGETED TREATMENTS—cont'd

- Tends to affect the toes and thumbs more often than the fingers.
- Can improve or get worse during treatment or may even disappear without treatment.
- Nail conditions do not seem to indicate whether a medication is effective.

To help prevent nail problems if you are taking EGFR-inhibiting drugs:
- Try not to bite your nails.
- Avoid using fake nails or wraps.
- Consult your health care provider before having a manicure.
- Don't wear tight-fitting shoes.
- Don't push back your cuticles.

To prevent fingernails from drying out:
- Wear gloves while washing dishes, doing household chores, or when using chemical cleaning agents.
- Moisturize your hands and feet frequently.
  - Petroleum jelly (Vaseline) works best
  - Apply to skin around the nails throughout the day.
  - Apply a thick coat of petroleum jelly to your hands and feet at night and then cover them with white cotton gloves and socks.

Treatment
- Disinfecting or antibacterial soap (Lever 2000), as well as antibiotic and antifungal ointments, to prevent infection.
- Steroid ointment (clobetasol) may also help relieve inflammation.
  - Wrap the treated area with a bandage or clear plastic wrap to help the ointment penetrate the area completely.
- You can also apply a liquid bandage to the area at the first sign of any skin cracking.

Dry Skin
- One of the most common side effects of EGFR inhibitors.
- The skin can become very itchy and become infected without treatment
- To reduce irritation
  - Take short lukewarm showers (one each day, or less if possible)
  - Use a moisturizing fragrance-free cleanser designed for sensitive skin
  - After showering or bathing, apply a fragrance-free hypoallergenic body lotion to your damp skin to help your skin retain moisture and prevent dryness.
- Apply a moisturizer at least twice a day
- Petroleum jelly is the most effective, but it can be greasy.
- Good alternatives include Eucerin moisturizing creams and lotions, Aquaphor ointment, or Cetaphil moisturizing creams and lotions.
- Your health care provider may prescribe a steroid cream and an antihistamine drug for extreme itchiness

Gentle Cleansers for Sensitive Skin
- Cetaphil-brand cleansers and bars
- Neutrogena Extra Gentle Cleanser
- Dove Sensitive Skin Foaming Facial Cleanser
- Basis Sensitive Skin Bar
- Fragrance-free cleansers

Hair Changes
- Hair changes may occur about 2 to 3 months after starting EGFR-targeted treatments.
- Hair may become fine, brittle, or curly.
- There may be permanent hair loss in the front of the scalp or hair growth may slow down.

Treatment for Itchy Skin
- To relieve itchy skin, try the following:
  - Moisturize frequently.
  - Take short, lukewarm showers, using a moisturizing soap.
  - Bathe in lukewarm water plus 1 to 2 cups of baking soda or the contents of an Aveeno bath treatment packet.
  - After showering or bathing, be sure to moisturize your skin immediately while it's still damp, to prevent dryness.
  - Use an over-the-counter hydrocortisone cream or ointment.
- For severe or persistent itching ask about steroid cream or antihistamine
  - Available over the counter
  - Stronger doses available by prescription

Hirsutism (Facial Hair)
- Facial hair growth may increase.
- Upper lips may become a little hairier
- Eyelashes and eyebrows may get longer

Treatment
Problematic excess facial hair can be removed with electrolysis, laser treatment, or waxing.
- Long eyebrows and eyelashes can be trimmed to prevent eye irritation.

There are numerous changes in skin, nails, and hair that may occur in patients receiving EGFR inhibitor drugs for the treatment of cancer. Patients should be well informed of the potential complications, how to treat them, and what to report to their health care practitioners.

COMPLETE BLOOD COUNT TEST (CBC)

WHAT IS THE COMPLETE BLOOD COUNT TEST (CBC)?

Many blood tests measure the amount of a particular chemical or protein in your blood, but a complete blood count checks the blood cells themselves. It measures the numbers of different types of blood cells, their sizes, and their appearance. It is a very common and useful blood test.

In general, the test measures 3 main components of blood:
- **Red blood cells** (also called erythrocytes or RBCs). The test measures the number, size, shape, and appearance of the RBCs, and also the amount of hemoglobin in them. Hemoglobin carries oxygen from the lungs to the rest of the body. The part of the test called a hematocrit measures the percentage of your blood that is red blood cells.
- **White blood cells** (also called leukocytes or WBCs). The total count of white cells is measured. White blood cells help the body's immune system fight infection. When the amounts of each of the different types of white blood cells are also measured, the test is called a differential. The most common types are neutrophils (also called polymorphonuclear cells, PMNs, polys, or granulocytes) and lymphocytes.
- **Platelets** (also called thrombocytes). Platelets are not actually blood cells. They are fragments of large blood-forming cells. These fragments are essential for normal blood clotting.

WHY IS THIS TEST DONE?

This test is usually done to see if:
- You have anemia (too few red blood cells).
- You have a high level of white blood cells (also called leukocytosis). A high white-blood-cell count is often a sign of infection.
- This test may be done for other reasons as well, such as to:
  ○ Look for the cause of anemia.
  ○ Check for certain diseases.
  ○ Check the number of platelets.

HOW DO I PREPARE FOR THIS TEST?

- You may need to avoid taking certain medicines before the test because they might affect the test result. Make sure your health care provider knows about any medicines, herbs, or supplements that you are taking. Don't stop any of your regular medicines without first consulting with your health care provider.

HOW IS THE TEST DONE?

A small amount of blood is taken from your arm with a needle. The blood is collected in tubes and sent to a lab. A machine in the lab measures the amounts of the different components in the sample of blood. The blood sample may also be viewed with a microscope to double check the different kinds of white blood cells.

Having this test will take just a few minutes of your time. There is no risk of getting AIDS, hepatitis, or any other blood-borne disease from this test.

HOW WILL I GET THE TEST RESULT?

Ask your health care provider when and how you will get the result of your test.

WHAT DO THE TEST RESULTS MEAN?

The normal ranges in most labs are:
- red blood cells (RBC): 4 to 6 million cells per microliter
- white blood cells (WBC): 5,000 to 10,000 cells per microliter
- hematocrit: for women, 36% to 45%; for men 41% to 47%
- hemoglobin: for women, 12 to 15 grams per deciliter; for men, 14 to 16 grams per deciliter
- platelets: 150,000 to 450,000 per microliter

These ranges may vary from lab to lab. Normal ranges are usually shown next to your results in the lab report.

Some of the reasons your **red blood cell** count may be **higher than normal** are:
- You haven't had enough fluids.
- You are a smoker.

Continued

COMPLETE BLOOD COUNT TEST (CBC)—cont'd

- You have polycythemia vera, a disease that causes your blood to be too thick because you're making too many red blood cells.
- You have smoker's lung disease.

A red blood cell count or hemoglobin level **lower than normal** is called anemia. The size of the red blood cells gives an important clue to possible causes of anemia:
- Anemia with small red blood cells (called microcytic anemia) may be caused by:
  - a lack of iron
  - bleeding, such as from a stomach ulcer.
- Anemia with large red blood cells (called macrocytic anemia) may be caused by a lack of the vitamins:
  - B_{12}
  - folate.

Some of the reasons your **white blood cell** count may be **higher than normal** are:
- You have an infection.
- You have inflammation.
- You are taking certain medicines, such as prednisone.
- You have a type of cancer called leukemia.

Your white blood cell count may be **lower than normal** if you have a viral infection, including the common cold, or if you are receiving chemotherapy treatments.

Your **platelet count** may be **higher than normal** if you have an autoimmune disease, such as rheumatoid arthritis or Crohn's disease.

Some of the reasons your platelet count may be **lower than normal** are:
- You are receiving chemotherapy treatments.
- You are taking certain medicines, such as sulfa drugs, quinine, or heparin.
- You have sepsis (blood infection) or another serious illness.
- You have an autoimmune disease, such as lupus.

WHAT IF MY TEST RESULT IS NOT NORMAL?

Test results are only one part of a larger picture that takes into account your medical history and current health. Sometimes a test needs to be repeated to check the first result. Talk to your health care provider about your result and ask questions.

If your test results are not normal, ask your health care provider:
- if you need additional tests
- what you can do to work toward a normal value
- when you need to be tested again.

CONSTIPATION

WHAT IS CONSTIPATION?

Constipation is infrequent or uncomfortable bowel movements. Often the bowel movements are small, hard, or dry.

HOW DOES IT OCCUR?

You may have constipation because:
- You wait too long to have bowel movements.
- You do not drink enough fluids.
- You overuse some types of laxatives.
- You do not eat enough fiber.
- You don't have enough physical activity.
- You are taking iron pills or a medicine that has a side effect of constipation, such as narcotic pain medication.

Other possible causes are:
- pregnancy
- depression or stress
- some medical conditions and diseases.

WHAT ARE THE SYMPTOMS?

Symptoms may include having:
- small bowel movements
- hard, dry bowel movements
- uncomfortable or painful bowel movements that are hard to pass
- a longer time than usual between bowel movements.

Normal bowel movements vary from person to person. For some people, 3 times a day is normal. For others once every 3 days may be normal. What's important is whether there is a change in what has been normal for you.

HOW IS IT TREATED?

To ease your constipation:
- Drink more fluids.
- Add more fiber to your diet.
- Increase your physical activity.
- Do not delay bowel movements. Make sure that you go to the bathroom whenever you feel that you need to go.

Laxatives may be used for a short time, generally less than 1 week. Many people find fiber supplements, such as Metamucil, Citrucel, or other psyllium products, to be helpful, but in a few cases they make constipation worse.

Ask your health care provider if any medicines you are taking may be causing constipation.

Tell your health care provider if:
- You start having constipation after years of normal bowel movements.
- You have bouts of constipation alternating with bouts of diarrhea.
- You have pain during bowel movements or for some time afterward.
- Your bowel movements are dark or tar-colored or have blood in them.
- You are losing weight without trying.

HOW CAN I TAKE CARE OF MYSELF?

To help take care of yourself:
- Eat fresh vegetables and fruit every day.
- Exercise regularly. For example, walk for at least 20 minutes every day.
- Drink prune juice or eat stewed fruits at breakfast.
- Drink plenty of fluids.
- Increase the whole-grain fiber in your diet by eating cereals with 5 or more grams of fiber per bowl (for example, shredded wheat or bran flakes).
- Take a fiber product such as Metamucil or Citrucel once or twice a day for several days if you are constipated. If the problem continues, tell your health care provider.
- Avoid overusing other laxatives, such as cathartics, which are products that will cause a liquid bowel movement. Cathartics, including milk of magnesia or Epsom salt, irritate the lining of the intestines.
- Ask your health care provider about taking fiber products or laxatives or giving yourself an enema.
- Contact your provider if constipation lasts longer than 1 week.

Published by McKesson Provider Technologies. Developed by Phyllis G. Cooper, RN, MN, and McKesson Provider Technologies. Copyright © 2005 McKesson Corporation and/or one of its subsidiaries. All Rights Reserved.

Patient Teaching

CONTROLLING NAUSEA AND VOMITING

WHAT ARE THE CAUSES OF NAUSEA AND VOMITING?

There are many causes of nausea and vomiting. Chemotherapy is one reason, but the good news is: just because you are taking chemotherapy does not mean you have to be sick! Other causes of nausea and vomiting are medications such as pain medications or antibiotics, anesthesia, certain surgeries, certain types of cancers or diseases, constipation, riding in a car, liver disease, radiation to the stomach area, fluid in the abdomen (belly), brain metastases, and throat irritation.

HOW MANY TYPES OF NAUSEA AND VOMITING ARE THERE?

There are also several types of nausea and vomiting:
Anticipatory: occurs before the chemotherapy is given or just by the thought of chemotherapy or something that has made nausea and vomiting occur before. This type of nausea and vomiting may occur as a result of certain sights or smells.
Acute: occurs during the 24-48 hours after chemotherapy.
Delayed: occurs after the first 48 hours after chemotherapy.
Breakthrough: occurs when patient has already taken some medication to prevent nausea and vomiting.

WHAT MEDICATION CAN I TAKE TO HELP WITH MY NAUSEA AND VOMITING?

There are many different types of medications that can help control or prevent nausea and vomiting:

- **5-HT$_3$ receptor antagonists (such as Zofran, Kytril, Anzemet):** These work very well in patients taking chemotherapy or after surgery. They work best in the first 24-48 hours after chemotherapy. They are often given before chemotherapy or radiation therapy. They can be given by IV (through a vein) or by mouth. They may be taken:
  - **Zofran (ondansetron): 8 mg every 12 hours by mouth**
  - **Kytril (granisetron): 1 mg every 12 hours by mouth**
  - **Anzemet (dolasetron): 100 mg per day by mouth**
  - Side effects of these drugs might include headache, constipation, lightheadedness, and sedation. These side effects are usually mild if they occur. Constipation is more likely to occur if these are taken for several days in a row.
- **Dopamine receptor antagonists:** These work very well in patients taking chemotherapy or after surgery. They are often combined with 5-HT$_3$ antagonists. They work well for nausea caused by pain medications or other medicines and bowel obstructions. They make be taken:
  - **Reglan (metoclopramide): 10-40 mg two to four times per day by mouth**
  - **Compazine (prochlorperazine): 10-20 mg every 6 hours by mouth**
  - **Thorazine (chlorpromazine): 10-50 mg every 6 hours by mouth**
  - **Haldol (haloperidol): 1-4 mg every 6 hours by mouth.**
  - Side effects might include drowsiness, dizziness, dry mouth, constipation, nasal congestion, or restless legs.
- **Corticosteroids:** These work well for many types of nausea, alone or with other drugs. They may also be used to stimulate appetite, enhance mood, or to treat symptoms of brain metastases.
  - **Decadron (dexamethasone): 4-8 mg twice a day for delayed nausea (there are many other doses as well)**
  - **Medrol (methylprednisolone): 40-125 mg by mouth (there are many different doses)**

Continued

Patient Teaching

CONTROLLING NAUSEA AND VOMITING—cont'd

- Side effects might include difficulty sleeping, increased blood sugar, hiccups, and mood changes. Long-term use can cause more difficult problems.
- **Antihistamines/anticholinergics:** these are often useful in nausea caused by motion sickness, inner ear problems, liver disease, or nausea caused by pain medications.
  - **Phenergan (promethazine): 12.5-25 mg every 6 hours**
  - **Benedryl (diphenhydramine): 12.5-25 mg every 6 hours**
  - **Scopolamine (transderm Scop): 1-2 patches applied every 72 hours**
  - **Levsin (hyoscyamine): 0.125-0.25 mg up to four times a day**
  - Side effects could include drowsiness, confusion, dizziness, dry mouth, and constipation.
- **NK1 receptor antagonist:** this is a new class of drugs used to prevent delayed nausea and vomiting, in combination with other medications.
  - **Emend (aprepitant): 125 mg before chemotherapy and 80 mg each morning for 2 days**
  - Side effects could include fatigue, constipation, loss of appetite, hiccups.
- **Other medications for nausea and vomiting:** These might include benzodiazepines, antihistamines, and cannabinoids.
  - **Ativan (lorazepam): 0.5-2 mg every 6 hours**
  - **Marinol (dronabinol): 5 mg before chemotherapy, then 2.5-5 mg every 4 hours.**

WHAT YOU HAVE BEEN ORDERED AND HOW TO TAKE IT:

_____

_____

_____

_____

If your nausea and vomiting is not relieved by these medications, please call us. Have this paper nearby to refer to and to help your health care provider suggest the best possible treatment for you. You will probably be asked:

1. What kind of cancer or illness you have and other symptoms you may be having.
2. How you are being treated: what kind of chemotherapy, radiation therapy to what part of your body, or other treatment.
3. What kind of medications were ordered for your nausea and vomiting and how you have been taking them.

Submitted by Wendy H. Vogel.

COPING WITH CHEMOTHERAPY

WHAT IS CHEMOTHERAPY?

Chemotherapy is the use of natural and man-made drugs to treat cancer. These drugs attack cancer at the cellular level. Chemotherapy can be used by itself or in combination with surgery, radiation, or drugs that affect the immune system. Chemotherapy can prolong life, relieve pain, and sometimes cure certain types of cancer.

I'VE HEARD THAT CHEMOTHERAPY HAS SOME AWFUL SIDE EFFECTS. IS THIS TRUE?

Yes, there are some side effects in some patients. Everyone reacts differently, so you may not have any side effects, and if you do, these can be well controlled most of the time. You are going to hear a lot of "horror stories" from well-meaning friends and relatives in the next few weeks, but remember that most side effects can be controlled! Your health care providers and nurses will be working with you to keep side effects to a minimum.

WHAT ARE SOME OF THE SIDE EFFECTS OF CHEMOTHERAPY?

- *Nausea and vomiting* and **loss of appetite** can be a side effect of chemotherapy. The severity will depend on the drug, the amount that is given, how often you get it, and how you take the medications prescribed for nausea. It may start as soon as 2 hours after your treatment but should not last much more than 24-48 hours.
- *Hair loss (alopecia)* could be a side effect of chemotherapy. This will depend on the drug that is given to you. The extent can be just thinning of your hair to total loss of all body hair. Generally hair loss will begin 1-3 weeks following your first treatment. It will usually begin to grow back 2-3 weeks after your last treatment. Some insurance companies, including Medicare, will assist with the cost of a wig or hairpiece. Ask your health care team if you have any questions.
- *Low blood cell counts* could occur after chemotherapy. Blood cells that fight infection, clot your blood, and carry oxygen are made by the bone marrow. These cells can be sensitive to some chemotherapy drugs. If your white blood cell counts become low, you might not be able to fight off an infection very easily. If your platelet count becomes low, you might bruise and bleed more easily. If your red blood cell count becomes low, you might become "anemic," tiring easily and getting short of breath. Your health care team will be watching your blood cell counts carefully and will let you know if you need to take extra precautions because of low blood cell counts.
- *Diarrhea or constipation* can occur after chemotherapy. These are commonly treated just like diarrhea or constipation caused by an illness. If these are caused by chemotherapy, they will generally clear up quickly, but if they do not, you will need to contact your health care provider.
- *Fatigue* is quite common after chemotherapy. Unfortunately, there are no medications for fatigue. It will be important for you to get plenty of rest, eat well, and do some form of physical activity each day.
- *Mouth sores* can sometimes occur after chemotherapy. There is a special mouthwash that can be given to you to ease this discomfort. These generally do not last more than a few days.
- *Numbness or tingling in your arms or legs* can occur as a result of some chemotherapy's effects on certain nerves. These will generally go away when the chemotherapy is stopped.
- *Stopping of menstruation either partly or totally* can occur. This may or may not be permanent. Hot flashes may be experienced. Some chemotherapy can cause sterility (the inability to have children) in both men and women. Discuss this with your health care provider before your chemotherapy treatment if you have concerns over this.

Remember that not everyone has every side effect and that most can be controlled! Ask your health care team if you have any questions or concerns.

WHEN SHOULD I CALL MY HEALTH CARE PROVIDER ABOUT A SIDE EFFECT?

You should call the oncology office or the doctor on call if you:
- Have a fever of 100.5° F or greater or severe chilling.
- Develop any new rashes.

Continued

Patient Teaching

COPING WITH CHEMOTHERAPY—cont'd

- Have any unusual bruising or bleeding, bleeding gums, or blood in the urine or bowel movements.
- Have nausea and vomiting for more than 24 hours.
- Have any unusual weakness or shortness of breath.
- Have watery diarrhea for more than 24 hours.
- Have any redness, swelling, or a sore that develops where the chemotherapy drug entered the skin.
- Have any other unanticipated side effect.

HOW WILL CHEMOTHERAPY AFFECT MY DAILY LIFE?

Most patients can continue to live normal lives. Many patients continue to work, taking only a day or so off around their treatment schedule. Your diet does not have to change unless directed by your health care team. A well-rounded diet is important. Most prescribed medications can be taken with chemotherapy, but it is important that your health care team know every medication that you take, including those that are not prescription drugs (such as aspirin and cough syrup).

WHAT ARE SOME PRECAUTIONS I MIGHT NEED TO KNOW?

It is important that you keep your regular checkups with your health care providers. Before any surgery, emergency treatment, dental work, or medical tests, tell the physician that you have recently received chemotherapy.

Please ask us if you have any other questions or concerns.

Submitted by Wendy H. Vogel.

DIARRHEA ASSESSMENT

This assessment will help your health care providers advise you on the treatment for the diarrhea you are having. Please answer every question the best that you can.

1. How often do you NORMALLY have a bowel movement when not having diarrhea? _____ per day or _____ per week

2. How many times per day are you having bowel movements NOW? _____

3. Are you running a fever of 100.5° F or greater?
    _____ yes _____ no

4. Are you having any abdominal pain?
    _____ yes _____ no

    If yes, please describe: _____
    _____

5. Is there any blood in your bowel movements?
    _____ yes _____ no

    If yes, do you have any bleeding hemorrhoids?
    _____ yes _____ no

6. Have you recently taken any laxatives or stool softeners? _____ yes _____ no

7. Do any medicines seem to make the diarrhea worse?
    _____ yes _____ no

    If yes, please list _____

8. Does the diarrhea seem to be related to eating?
    _____ yes _____ no

    If yes, please describe _____
    _____

9. When did the diarrhea start?
    _____

10. Did the diarrhea start suddenly _____ or gradually _____?

11. Describe your bowel movements (check all that apply):

    _____ soft, formed   _____ hard
    _____ soft, not formed   _____ varies from hard to soft
    _____ mushy   _____ bloody
    _____ jellylike   _____ has undigested food in it
    _____ loose   _____ has mucus or pus in it
    _____ watery

12. How much diarrhea do you have each time you go?
    _____ small amount
    _____ moderate
    _____ large amount

13. Are you having any cramping?
    _____ a little
    _____ moderate
    _____ severe

14. Have you lost any weight since the diarrhea started?
    _____ yes _____ no

    If yes, how many pounds have you lost? _____

15. When does the diarrhea occur? (check all that apply)
    _____ day
    _____ night
    _____ after meals
    _____ after certain foods
    _____ after treatments

16. Are you having any incontinence (leaking of stool)?
    _____ yes _____ no

17. How is the diarrhea affecting your everyday life? (check all that apply)
    _____ getting up at night
    _____ avoiding going out of the house
    _____ embarrassment
    _____ extreme tiredness
    _____ can't participate in your normal activities
    _____ change in sexual activity

18. Are you having any of the following? (check all that apply)
    _____ fever
    _____ thirst
    _____ dry mouth
    _____ not urinating as much
    _____ feeling of weakness
    _____ dizzy or lightheaded
    _____ chills
    _____ skin breakdown in rectal area
    _____ back pain
    _____ nausea or vomiting
    _____ rectal pain

19. What have you tried to control the diarrhea?
    _____
    _____

20. Has this helped? _____ yes _____ no

Submitted by Wendy H. Vogel.

FATIGUE

WHAT IS FATIGUE?

Fatigue is a condition of tiredness or weakness that is physical or mental, or both.

HOW DOES IT OCCUR?

Fatigue can happen for many reasons, but it is especially likely when you are having a lot of physical or mental stress. Fatigue may be caused by:
- an illness
- hormone problems
- overexertion
- poor physical condition
- lack of exercise
- not enough sleep
- overweight
- poor diet
- stress
- emotional or psychological problems, especially depression
- some medicines.

Fatigue can also be a symptom of a heart attack, especially in women. It usually is new and severe fatigue that starts a day or two or just a few hours before a heart attack. Sometimes the fatigue starts a couple of weeks before a heart attack. Because new, unexplained fatigue can mean a heart attack is about to happen, it should be checked by your health care provider.

Overwhelming fatigue that lasts for at least 6 months and interferes with your daily life may be caused by a medical problem called chronic fatigue syndrome.

WHAT ARE THE SYMPTOMS?

Symptoms of fatigue are:
- weakness
- tiredness
- indifference
- lack of energy.

HOW IS IT DIAGNOSED?

Your health care provider will review your symptoms and ask about your daily routine, work habits, environment, and emotional well-being. Your provider will examine you. You may have blood tests to check for diseases that can cause fatigue, such as diabetes, hypothyroidism, heart disease, lung disease, and anemia.

HOW IS IT TREATED?

The treatment depends on the cause. If fatigue is a symptom of another condition or illness, that condition or disease will be the focus of treatment. If the cause is emotional or psychological, your health care provider may refer you to a therapist for counseling.

If new fatigue is caused by worsening heart health, prompt recognition and treatment of heart disease may prevent a heart attack.

HOW LONG DO THE EFFECTS LAST?

The effects will last as long as the cause of the symptoms exists.

HOW CAN I TAKE CARE OF MYSELF?

- Get enough rest and sleep.
- Eat a healthy diet. If you are overweight, begin a weight loss program after checking with your health care provider.
- Walk or exercise according to your health care provider's recommendations. Exercise can increase your energy and improve your mood.
- See a counselor if you are having emotional problems.
- Learn to use deep breathing techniques, visualization, and meditation to relieve stress.
- Allow yourself time to relax and do things you enjoy.
- Meet new people and develop new interests.

HOW CAN I PREVENT FATIGUE?

- If you are working longer hours or doing more physical work, allow yourself more time to sleep or rest.
- If your work activity has become more strenuous, take breaks during the day to sit and rest.
- Ask your provider about taking vitamin and mineral supplements.
- Consider eating smaller meals 4 to 6 times a day if that seems to help you maintain a higher energy level. Eat more complex carbohydrates such as rice and pasta, and eat less fat. Avoid foods that contain a lot of sugar. Avoid overeating.
- Stop smoking.
- Avoid caffeine, alcohol. and other drugs.

Published by McKesson Provider Technologies.Developed by Phyllis G. Cooper, RN, MN, and McKesson Provider Technologies. Copyright © 2005 McKesson Corporation and/or one of its subsidiaries. All Rights Reserved.

Patient Teaching

HOT FLASHES

Hot flashes may be a side effect of menopause, some diseases, or some medications. Hot flashes can occur in both women and men. Here are some things that may be effective for you in dealing with hot flashes. Not every measure will help every patient. You will need to see what works for you!

1. Vitamin E taken after meals with fat or with lecithin (this contains phosphorus) to aid absorption. Begin at 100 International Units, and may increase to 800 International Units or until symptoms are relieved. If you have high blood pressure, heart disease, or diabetes, check with your health care provider before trying. You may also obtain vitamin E from your diet in wheat germ, whole grains, vegetable oils, soybeans, peanuts, and spinach.

2. Vitamin B complex. Taken one or two per day after meals. You can also get vitamin B complex in your diet with whole grains, wheat germ, yogurt, brewer's yeast, and milk.

3. There are some prescription medications that may help with hot flashes. They include:
   - **Estrogen:** this is given to women going through menopause. There are both risks and benefits to estrogen. You will want to discuss this with your health care provider.
   - **Clonidine:** this is a topical patch used for high blood pressure. In low doses, it can be effective in controlling hot flashes.
   - **Effexor or Paxil:** these are antidepressants that have proven helpful in controlling hot flashes.
   - **Bellergal:** this is a combination of phenobarbital, belladonna, and ergotamine used to decrease hot flashes.

4. Wear layered, loose-fitting clothing. 100% cotton is best. Peel off a layer (or two) when you have a flash.

5. If you have a bed-mate, buy electric blankets with separate controls.

6. Keep track of what seems to trigger hot flashes for you: spicy foods, alcohol, stress, anger, embarrassment, fear, etc. Some people avoid these; others learn to adjust to them.

7. Be calm! A hot flash won't hurt you. It will be over in less than 2 minutes! Take deep breaths and exhale deeply. Laugh about these hot flashes! Keep your sense of humor! Consider them POWER SURGES!

Submitted by Wendy H. Vogel.

Patient Teaching

LOW PLATELET COUNTS

Although chemotherapy can kill cancer cells, it can affect normal cells, too, destroying some of your cells called *platelets* that help your blood form clots. Forming clots is the way your body controls bleeding. When you have too few of these cells, it is called having a *low platelet count*. Sometimes, a low platelet count does not cause problems. However, you will need to follow these precautions if your platelet count becomes extremely low, to prevent too much bleeding if you should injure yourself.

PRECAUTIONS

- Be very careful to prevent accidents. Sometimes an accident could injure the inside of your body, where you cannot see bleeding. Also, a bruise is a warning that you are bleeding inside your body.
- Ask a family member and someone you work closely with to read this sheet. Ask them to call your family doctor if you
  - Become easily confused
  - Act restless or irritable in ways that are not normal for you
  - Have constant headaches that are not normal
  - Have blackouts or feel dizzy
- Check your skin every few days for any small red or purple spots which may be tiny bruises.
- Do not use suppositories or take enemas. Do not take your temperature rectally. These could cause bleeding inside your body.
- Do not use toothpicks or dental floss. Use only a toothbrush with very soft bristles, if you can. If you use mouthwash, mix it half-and-half with water beforehand, or use ½ teaspoon soda in half a glass of water.
- Do not take aspirin or medicines containing aspirin. Instead take Tylenol or Datril.

- Do not use alcohol on cuts or scratches. Instead, apply firm, not hard, pressure to any bleeding or apply ice packs. Use an ice pack for a nosebleed. If your gums bleed, apply ice wrapped in clear wrap such as Saran wrap to prevent the ice from sticking to your gums.
- Use an electric razor for shaving, to prevent cuts.
- Do not clip your fingernails or toenails so closely that it could cause bleeding.
- Do not get injections, or shots, unless your doctor approves. Be sure to warn the doctor or nurse that you have low platelet count, and make sure firm pressure is applied to the spot for five minutes or until bleeding has stopped.
- Try to avoid blowing your nose forcefully.
- If you strain to have bowel movements, take a stool softener or laxative such as milk of magnesia to prevent straining.
- Avoid drinking alcohol while your platelet count is low.

CALL YOUR DOCTOR OR NURSE IF YOU HAVE...

- An increase in bruising.
- Blood in your urine.
- Blood in your stool or black, sticky stools that you have not had before. (If you take iron, you can expect black stool.)
- More menstrual flow or a longer flow than usual.
- Frequent nosebleeds or gum bleeding of more than a few drops that do not stop easily.
- Blood in vomit or sputum of more than a few drops.

Patient Teaching

LYMPHEDEMA: PREVENTION AND TREATMENT

WHAT IS IT?

- Lymphedema is an abnormal swelling of a body part, such as an arm or leg.
- Many times this can be treated or controlled.
- Lymphedema may cause a feeling of heaviness, difference in appearance, and mild discomfort and can make you more susceptible to an infection in that affected area.
- Lymphedema can interfere with wound healing and can cause a chronic inflammatory condition.

WHY DOES IT OCCUR?

- Some types can have no apparent cause, but many types of lymphedema are caused by the surgical removal of lymph nodes.
- It can also be caused by an injury, chronic infection of the lymph system, or by a parasite.
- It can occur right after surgery for the removal of lymph nodes, within a few months, a couple of years, or even 20 years after the surgery.
- It can be caused by radiation therapy as well.

HOW CAN I PREVENT IT?

Any person who has had surgical removal of lymph nodes is at risk. Below are some ways to prevent lymphedema from occurring:

- Avoid hot tubs, saunas, sunburn, insect bites, pet/animal bites, heavy lifting, obesity, needle sticks, or blood pressure cuffs on the affected limb.
- Do not ignore any slight increase of swelling in your body. If this occurs, talk with your health care provider.
- Keep the "at-risk" limb very clean. Be sure to gently dry well.
- Don't carry heavy handbags or bags with over the shoulder straps.
- Don't wear tight jewelry or elastic bands around affected fingers or arms.
- Avoid extreme temperature changes when bathing or washing dishes.
- Avoid any type of trauma.
- Wear gloves while doing housework, gardening, or any type of work that could result in even a minor injury.
- When manicuring your nails, avoid cutting your cuticles.
- Exercise is important, but do not overtire an arm at risk. If it starts to ache, lie down and elevate it (higher than your heart). Ideal exercises are walking, swimming, light aerobics, bike riding, and yoga. Do not lift more than 15 pounds.
- When traveling by air, wear a compression sleeve. Increase fluid intake while in the air.
- Wear a well-fitted bra: not too tight and with no wire support. Avoid heavy breast prostheses.

- Maintain your ideal weight with a well-balanced, low-sodium, high-fiber diet. Avoid smoking and alcoholic beverages.
- Use an insect repellent when outdoors. An insect bite may develop into cellulitis (infection of the skin).
- If you have lymphedema of the leg, use proper footwear, and avoid high-heeled or tight-fitting shoes. Never walk barefoot. Take extra precaution with foot care.
- Throughout the day, elevate the affected limb. Elevate it all night. Legs should be elevated higher than your hips; arms should be elevated higher than your heart.

WHEN TO CALL YOUR HEALTH CARE PROVIDER

Call your health care provide if:

- You have any signs of an infection: warmth, redness of the skin, fever, chills, or increased swelling.
- You develop a fungal infection of the fingernails or toenails or feet.
- You have any questions regarding lymphedema or its treatment.
- You have had congestive heart failure, venous or arterial obstruction, blood clots, or an infection.

IS THERE A TREATMENT FOR LYMPHEDEMA?

- There are treatments for lymphedema and most are covered by insurance. The treatment will depend on the cause of the lymphedema.
- If caused by an infection, you will be treated with antibiotics.
- If it is not caused by infection, there are other treatments including:
  - compression sleeves
  - manual lymph drainage (MLD) by specially trained therapists
  - special bandaging
  - sequential gradient pump
  - some medications, although diuretics may have little effect

FOR MORE INFORMATION

National Lymphedema network: 1-800-541-3259 or
  www.lymphnet.org
National Breast Cancer Coalition: www.ntalbcc.org
International Society of Lymphology: (520) 626-6118
Lymphedema International network:
  www.lymphedema.com

Submitted by Wendy H. Vogel.

Patient Teaching

MANAGING YOUR CANCER TREATMENT–RELATED FATIGUE

Factors that contribute to fatigue:
- Cancer itself
- Low blood cell counts
- Nutritional problems
- Sleep problems

SIGNS OF FATIGUE

- Feeling weary or exhausted. It may be physical, emotional, or mental exhaustion.
- Your body, especially your arms and legs, may feel heavy.
- Less desire to do normal activities such as eating or shopping.
- Difficulty concentrating or thinking clearly

WHAT YOU CAN DO TO MANAGE YOUR FATIGUE

Rest
Rest and sleep are important, but don't overdo it. Too much rest can decrease your energy level.

Activity
Stay as active as you can. Regular exercise, such as walking several times each week, may help. Set short-term goals for yourself (i.e., 10 minutes, two blocks), and then increase as you are able.

Nutrition
Drink plenty of liquids. Eat as well as you can, and eat nutritious foods. Carbohydrates and proteins are quick energy foods. Supplements, although nutritious, haven't been proven to directly reduce fatigue.

Energy Conservation
You can do more by spreading your activities throughout the day. Take rest breaks between activities. Do not force yourself to do more than you can manage.

Energy Restoration
Do activities that you enjoy and make you feel good. Many people enjoy nature activities such as bird watching or gardening. Try listening to music, or visiting with friends and family, or looking at pleasant pictures. Try to do these activities at least three times per week.

SUGGESTED STRATEGIES FOR ENERGY CONSERVATION

Activities of Daily Living
- Sit down to bathe and dry off. Wear a terry robe instead of drying off.
- Use a shower/bath organizer to decrease leaning and reaching.
- Install grab rails in the bathroom.
- Use extension handles on sponges and brushes.
- Use an elevated toilet seat.

Organize Time to Avoid Rushing
- Lay out clothes and toiletries before dressing.
- Minimize leaning over to put on clothes and shoes.
- Bring your foot to your knee to apply socks and shoes. Fast bra in front then turn to back.
- Modify the home environment to maximize efficient use of energy. For example, place chairs to allow rest stops (e.g., along a long hallway).
- Wear comfortable clothes and low-heeled, slip-on shoes. Wear button front shirts rather than pullovers.

Housekeeping
- Schedule household tasks throughout the week.
- Do housework sitting down when possible. Use long-handled dusters, dust mops, and so forth. Use a wheeled cart or carpenter's apron to carry supplies.
- Delegate heavy housework, shopping, laundry, and child care when possible.
- Drag or slide objects rather than lifting. Use proper body mechanics. Use your leg muscles, not your back, when working.
- Sit when ironing and take rest periods.
- Stop working before becoming tired.

Shopping
- Organize list by aisle.
- Use a grocery cart for support.
- Shop at less-busy times.
- Request assistance in getting to the car.
- Purchase clothing that doesn't require ironing.

Continued

Patient Teaching

MANAGING YOUR CANCER TREATMENT–RELATED FATIGUE—cont'd

Meal Preparation
- Use convenience foods/easy-to-prepare foods.
- Use small appliances (they take less effort to use).
- Arrange the preparation environment for easy access to frequently used items.
- Prepare meals sitting down.
- Soak dishes instead of scrubbing and let dishes air dry.
- Prepare double portions and freeze half.

Child Care
- Plan activities to allow for sitting down (e.g., drawing, pictures, playing games, reading, and computer games).
- Teach children to climb up on the lap or into the highchair instead of being lifted.
- Make a game of the household chores so that children will want to help.
- Delegate child care when possible.

Workplace
- Plan workload to take advantage of peak energy times. Alternate physically demanding tasks with sedentary tasks.
- Arrange work environment for easy access to commonly used equipment and supplies.

Leisure
- Do activities with a companion.
- Select activities that match energy level.
- Balance activity and rest (don't get overtired).

Fatigue Fighting Tips for Cancer Caregivers
- It is important to maintain your own health and well-being so that you can provide the best possible care to your loved one.
- Take some quality time for yourself—schedule a "day-off" or some quiet time at home.
- Watch for signs of stress, such as impatience, loss of appetite, or difficulty sleeping.
- Ask for or accept help from friends or family—suggest specific tasks or projects that they can do to help you.
- Make sure you are educated about your loved one's illness—knowledge is empowering.
- Use resources in your community that can help you. Take advantage of transportation agencies, home care services, support groups, and educational programs.
- Openly acknowledge your caregiving situation or discuss your feelings with family and friends. With proper support and education, caregiving can actually bring families closer together.
- Give yourself credit—the care you give does make a difference.

MUCOSITIS: PROBLEMS AND SOLUTIONS

Mucositis occurs when cancer treatments break down the rapidly divided epithelial cells lining the GI tract, particularly in the oral cavity, leaving the mucosal tissue open to ulceration and infection. Mucositis can occur anywhere along the digestive tract from the mouth to the anus. Oral mucositis is probably the most common, debilitating complication of cancer surgery, chemotherapy and radiation. It occurs in 20-40% of patients treated with chemotherapy alone and up to 50% of patients receiving combination radiation and chemotherapy. The consequences of mucositis can be mild, requiring little intervention, to severe (hypovolemia, electrolyte abnormalities, and malnutrition) that may result in fatal complications.

Taste loss tends to increase in proportion to the aggressiveness of treatment. Nausea, pain, vomiting, diarrhea, a sore or dry mouth may make eating difficult and a challenge to maintain adequate nutrition for cancer patients. Reduction of caloric intake can lead to weight loss, loss in muscle mass strength and other complications, including a decrease in immunity. Cancer patient education must include the risks and the underreporting of mucositis. Delayed or reduced medical treatment doses may limit chances for a cure. The potential impact of morbidity and mortality with oral mucositis should not be underestimated and requires active treatment.

Chemotherapy and radiation to the head and neck prevent cells in the mouth and GI tract from reproducing, which makes it hard for tissue to be repaired. The mouth has a delicate balance of natural bacteria and fungi, so if you receive any one or both of these therapies, it can lead to a decrease in salivation. This decrease in salivation upsets the natural balance of bacteria in the mouth causing infections, mouth sores and tooth decay.

It is important to know who is at risk of mucositis and to prevent complications to help improve quality of life and maximize your therapy. These risk factors include radiation to the head and neck, high dose chemotherapy, bone marrow transplantation, certain single agent anticancer drugs or a combination of these. Symptoms of mucositis should be treated as soon as they appear. It is important to be educated about proper nutrition and oral hygiene to help prevent or lessen these symptoms. Once you are aware of proper nutrition, you will be able to maintain adequate hydration, immunity and help prevent nausea, as well as protecting your teeth.

TOPICS TO DISCUSS WITH YOUR MEDICAL TEAM

1. Notify your doctor for any excessive bleeding, nausea, fever or pain associated with your mucositis.
2. Let your doctor know of all your medication allergies and a list of your current medications (including over-the-counter drugs, herbal products and vitamins).
3. Ask your medical team for dietary and nutritional needs tailored just for you.
4. Do not allow pain or nausea to get out of control. Take your medicine at the beginning of symptoms to prevent vomiting or excessive pain.
5. Make sure you have an emergency contact phone number from your medical team in case of any emergencies.
6. Keep your medical team well informed for any signs of infection. Also make sure you tell them of symptoms getting better or worse.
7. Keep a journal of your pain scale and when you have nausea so your medical team can make the best recommendations for you.

PREVENTION AND TREATMENT

Prevention will not stop mucositis from occurring, but it can help alleviate some pain and lessen some of the side effects and symptoms of mucositis. It is important to be educated about mucositis, how to take care of yourself and to have a good relationship with your physician and dentist.

The first step in prevention is to see if your doctor can recommend a dentist that deals with cancer patients. You will need to have your teeth and gums evaluated and if you wear dentures, you will need to make sure they fit properly. If any work is needed (teeth extractions or refitting of dentures), it should be completed at least one month prior to starting therapy to make sure your mouth has completely healed and prevent damage to your existing teeth, gums or jaw bones.

The next step to taking care of your mouth is proper brushing techniques and oral hygiene. If you smoke, it is extremely important that you stop smoking. Your doctor will be able to help you with smoking cessation programs. You should use a soft bristle toothbrush and brush your teeth 2 to 3 times daily (after eating). If necessary, due to sensitivity or mouth sores, you may need to use foam

Continued

MUCOSITIS: PROBLEMS AND SOLUTIONS—cont'd

toothbrushes with an antibacterial rinse. You should choose mild tasting toothpaste with fluoride: for example Prevident. Some flavorings in toothpaste may irritate the mouth. *If your toothpaste is still too irritating, you can use a solution made of 1 teaspoon of salt dissolved in 4 cups of water.* You should gently floss your teeth once daily.

If you develop mucositis or it worsens, you may need to increase brushing to every 4 hours and at bedtime. This will help keep the mouth moisturized and help prevent any infections. It is important to brush and floss very gently. You will want to rinse your mouth frequently to prevent cavities with antiseptic mouth rinses, for example: Peridex or Periogard. *You can make your own rinse by mixing 1 teaspoon of baking soda in 8 ounces of water or ½ teaspoon salt and 2 tablespoons baking soda dissolved in 4 cups of water.* If you are being treated with high dose chemotherapy or a bone marrow transplant, your doctor can give you some new medication that can prevent or shorten the duration of mucositis.

Your mouth may become dry and you will want to keep it moisturized. This can be due to a decrease in your saliva production or the mucositis directly. Some easy remedies include chewing ice chips, chewing sugarless gum, or sucking tart candy. If these do not work there are artificial saliva products that your physician can prescribe for you or some over-the-counter products are available such as Oral Balance. Since your saliva barrier is compromised you should avoid eating or drinking products containing sucrose to prevent cavities.

Pain is also a very serious complication of mucositis. Aspirin containing products and nonsteroidal anti-inflammory products like Motrin or Naprosyn should be avoided due to their effect on platelets, which can increase the risk of bleeding. You can also use topical products like Orajel or some prescription products like viscous lidocaine or a new product called Gelclair. If the pain becomes more severe you may need your doctor to prescribe you stronger pain medications, such as Vicodin, Percocet or Tyco #3. *To help clean oral sores you can rinse with a solution consisting of 1 part 3% hydrogen peroxide with 2 parts of saltwater (1 teaspoon of salt dissolved in 4 cups of water).*

Saliva helps protect the mouth and gums from infection. These infections can be bacterial, fungal or viral in nature. For mild fungal infections, topical oral suspensions or dissolving tablets can be prescribed. You will need to swish or dissolve the medicine in your mouth and depending on your doctor's directions, either swallow or spit out the medicine. It is important to not use any medicine containing alcohol because it will burn the mouth. For worsening fungal, bacterial and viral infections, your physician will need to prescribe oral medications, such as antibiotics, to eradicate them. You should also remove any dental appliances and soak them in antiseptic solutions (Listerine or Peridex).

NUTRITION TIPS

These nutrition tips will help if you are experiencing dehydration, taste changes, decreased appetite or pain with eating.

1. Eat small frequent meals throughout the day.
2. Try to have a balanced diet to maintain energy and your immunity.
3. Avoid spicy, hot or cold foods if it is painful to eat or you are having nausea. Eat food that is a little bland and at room temperature.
4. Drink lots of fluid, broth or drinks such as Gatorade. This will keep you hydrated.
5. Eat food high in calories and protein to maintain weight and nutrition. Take vitamins and minerals.
6. If your mouth is too sore, eat soft or blended foods such as ice cream, pudding, soup, and applesauce.
7. Zinc supplements may help with taste changes.
8. Some prescription medications are available to help increase appetite such as Megace or Marinol.
9. Avoid your favorite foods when you are receiving chemotherapy. You may develop a taste aversion to them by association.
10. Use spices or flavoring to make your food taste better. Eat whatever you can tolerate to maintain weight.

CancerSupportiveCare.com. *Fifth Dimension Therapy*™ www.cancersupportivecare.com © rev 2005 11/28/2005.

MUSCLE ACHES AND JOINT PAIN

Patient Name: _____

This guide will give you helpful hints to reduce muscle aches and pain in your joints.

SYMPTOM AND DESCRIPTION

Pain in your shoulders, hips, or knees can occur any time from 48-72 hours after you receive chemotherapy. When in your joints, this pain is called *arthralgia*; when it is located in your muscles, it is called *myalgia*. It is a side effect of your chemotherapy. The pain can range from a mild discomfort or ache to a severe pain. You may feel like you have the flu or you may have trouble moving around, for example, getting out of bed or a chair.

This muscle and joint pain may be more noticeable if colony-stimulating factors or growth factors (such as Neupogen) is a part of your treatment.

This side effect may not occur with every treatment; you may experience the pain after one treatment and not feel any aches the next treatment. You are at risk of having muscle aches and joint pain because of your cancer therapy. The drug you are taking called _____ is the cause.

You may also be at risk for this side effect:
• If you have diabetes
• If you have a history of alcohol use
• If you have a history of arthritis
• If you have neuromuscular disease

PREVENTION

The first thing to remember is that the symptoms do not appear until 48-72 hours after your treatment is given and that the aches can last for 4-7 days.

It is difficult to prevent muscle aches and joint pain because the drug you are getting for your cancer treatment causes it.

Some helpful hints to reduce the symptoms include:
• Medication can be taken if you experience this side effect. Your doctor has ordered the following to be taken after treatment:

_____

_____

MANAGEMENT

These are some ideas on how to manage these side effects at home:
• Take the medication prescribed by your doctor.

• Get plenty of rest and plan your activities to include rest periods.
• A heating pad or hot water bottle may give comfort to an achy area.
• Keep the pad or bottle covered with a towel when putting it next to your skin.
• Use the heat for short periods, 5-10 minutes several times a day.
• Keep your nutrition up by eating healthy, regular meals.
• Relaxation techniques, such as guided imagery or biofeedback, may be helpful.
• Taking a warm bath or whirlpool may be comforting.
• Massage therapy to the area may help.

Be sure to ask your doctor or nurse for more information if you are interested in trying any of these measures and you need additional information.

FOLLOW-UP

It may be helpful to keep a record of the muscle or joint pain, recording when it starts, what makes it better, and when it goes away.

Record the day and the degree of pain you feel by using a scale from 0-10. Also note what you did to relieve the pain (for example, took a warm bath, took Tylenol or ibuprofen, tried to rest, etc.).

The pain rating scale key:
0------1------2------3------4------5------6------7------8------9------10
0 = no pain; 10 = worst possible pain

Day/Time of Pain	Pain Rating	What made it better?
_____	_____	_____
_____	_____	_____
_____	_____	_____
_____	_____	_____

Bring this information with you when you visit the doctor or the nurse.

If at any time you are uncomfortable and the pain does not go away, please call the doctor or the nurse.

Telephone numbers to call: _____

Daytime _____

Evening or weekend _____

Patient Teaching

NEUTROPENIA

WHAT IS NEUTROPENIA?

Neutropenia is an abnormally low number of white blood cells (neutrophils). White blood cells protect the body from infection.

People with neutropenia tend to develop infections easily because their white blood cell count is too low to fight off germs, such as bacteria. Most of these infections occur in the lungs, mouth, throat, sinuses, and skin. Some people get gum infections, ear infections, or infections of the urinary tract, colon, rectum, or reproductive tract.

HOW DOES IT OCCUR?

Neutropenia has many possible causes. Some people are born with neutropenia. It can happen during or after a viral infection. In some cases the cause may be the side effect of a drug or exposure to certain poisons. Not having enough vitamin B-12 or folate (folic acid) in your diet can also cause neutropenia. It may result from diseases such as systemic lupus erythematosus (SLE). Having chemotherapy for cancer can also cause it.

WHAT ARE THE SYMPTOMS?

You may have not symptoms, or you may have symptoms of an infection, which may include:
• fever
• sore throat
• cough or shortness of breath
• diarrhea
• nasal congestion
• unusual vaginal discharge or itching
• burning during urination
• shaking chills
• redness, swelling, or warmth at the site of an injury.

HOW IS IT DIAGNOSED?

Your health care provider will do a test called a complete blood count (CBC) to measure white blood cells.

HOW IS IT TREATED?

Treatment for neutropenia depends on the cause and the severity. You may need to:
• Take antibiotics to prevent infections.
• Make changes in your diet or take vitamin supplements.
• Avoid chemicals or medicines that are known to cause neutropenia.

New medicines called colony-stimulating factors may also be used to stimulate the growth of neutrophils. These medicines help restore immune system function.

HOW LONG DO THE EFFECTS LAST?

How long neutropenia lasts depends on its cause. For example, neutropenia related to vitamin deficiency usually goes away after 2 weeks of treatment with vitamins. Other causes may take longer to clear up.

HOW CAN I HELP TAKE CARE OF MYSELF?

• Wash your hands often with an antibacterial soap, especially before eating and after using the bathroom.
• Avoid vaginal douches, bubble bath, and bath salts.
• Avoid cuts, scrapes, and burns.
• Use an electric razor instead of a blade.
• Don't squeeze or scratch pimples or sores on your skin.
• Avoid people with colds, flu, or any type of infection or open sores.
• Do not have vaccinations such as flu shots unless your health care provider approves.
• Never use rectal thermometers or suppositories.
• Avoid sunburn.
• Clean the furnace and heating ducts once or twice a year. Replace filters monthly.
• Eat a healthy diet. Make sure your food is completely cooked.
• Avoid constipation and consume plenty of fiber.
• Always use a soft toothbrush. Avoid dental floss.
• Tell your dentist you have neutropenia. You may need to take antibiotics before and after any dental work or cleaning.
• Get plenty of rest.

NUTRITION AND CANCER

The American Cancer Society states that approximately one third of the 500,000 cancer deaths each year in the United States are due to dietary factors. It is never too late to start practicing healthy eating to reduce your health and cancer risk.

Many dietary factors can affect your cancer risk, such as the types of food you eat, how they are prepared, portion sizes, food varieties, and calories. Cancer risk can be reduced by a diet with lots of plant foods and limited amounts of meat, dairy, and other high-fat foods, and by balancing calories and physical activity. Unfortunately, many Americans are eating more calories and high-fat foods and getting less physical activity.

The American Cancer Society recommends four steps to reduce cancer risk for people over the age of 2 years:
• Choose most of the foods you eat from plant sources.
• Eat five or more servings of vegetables each day.
• Eat other plant sources, such as bread, cereals, grain products, rice, pasta, or beans several times each day.

• Limit your intake of high-fat foods, especially from animal sources.
• Choose foods low in fat.
• Limit consumption of meats, especially high-fat (red) meats.
• Be physically active and keep at a healthy weight.
• Be at least moderately active for 30 minutes or more on most days of the week.
• Stay within your healthy weight range.
• Limit consumption of alcoholic beverages, if you drink at all. For women this is <1 drink/day on average. For men, <2 drinks/day.
• Stop smoking!

For more specific information on nutrition and cancer, you may contact the American Cancer Society or the National Cancer Institute.

Submitted by Wendy H. Vogel.

OSTEOPOROSIS

Osteoporosis is a condition in which the bones become so weakened that the slightest injury can cause a break in the bone.

- Hip and wrist fractures are the most common, with vertebrae following.
- Eight out of 10 people affected with osteoporosis are women.
- It is estimated that 50 out of 100 women will have an osteoporosis-related fracture after age 50 years. There are no warning signs of osteoporosis such as pain, stiffness, or joint swelling. You may not even know you have osteoporosis until you break a bone!

THE BONES

- Outside: cortical bone—hard and dense
- Inside: the marrow—makes blood cells
- 75%-80% of the bone is cortical bone
- The time of greatest bone density is between ages 25 and 35 years.
- As we age, more bone is broken down than is produced.

CALCIUM

- 9 out of 10 women don't get enough
- 99% of calcium is stored in the bone
- Needed for strong teeth and bones, for muscles, blood clotting, the heart, and the nervous system.
- Found in milk (300 mg in 1 cup of milk), yogurt, sardines, tofu, salmon (60 mg/cup), cheese (around 250 mg/ounce), collard/turnip greens and kale, and broccoli (150-250 mg/cup serving).
- Vitamin D (400-800 IU/day) needed to absorb calcium properly. We get vitamin D from sun exposure and supplements.
- The typical American diet does not have enough calcium or vitamin D.

RISK FACTORS FOR OSTEOPOROSIS

- Age
- Female sex
- Caucasian or Asian race
- Small-boned and thin
- Menopause
- Smoking or alcohol
- Too much salt or phosphorus in diet
- Not enough exercise or calcium
- Certain medicines and medical conditions

DIAGNOSIS

- Medical history
- DEXA scan (bone mineral density test) examines lower spine and hips

PREVENTION AND TREATMENT

- Exercise: Weight-bearing exercise (walking, jogging, tennis, aerobics, jump rope, etc.) for 30 minutes or more three to four times/week.
- Calcium: premenopausal: 1,500-1,800 mg/day; postmenopausal: 1,800-2,000 mg/day; take with meals; no more than 600 mg at a time
- Eat right. Phosphorus, such as in soft drinks, may keep you from absorbing enough calcium. Limit salt intake.
- Limit alcohol; stop smoking.
- Estrogen unless contraindicated
- Tamoxifen for women at high risk for breast cancer.
- DEXA scan as a baseline at menopause or around age 50 years
- Medications such as Actonel, Fosamax, Miacalcin, Evista

Submitted by Wendy H. Vogel.

PICC LINE CARE

WHAT IS A PICC LINE?

A **PICC** line is a type of long flexible tubing that is inserted into a vein in the arm and then threaded into a larger vein in the central part of the body. The end of the catheter that sticks out of the skin has a special cap. The **PICC** line can be used to get blood samples or to give medicines. **PICC** is the abbreviation for peripheral intravenous central catheter.

WHY DO I NEED A PICC LINE?

A **PICC** line may be used if you need intravenous (IV) medicine that may irritate the smaller veins usually used for IVs. A **PICC** line may also be used if you need many doses of IV medicines.

HOW IS THE PICC LINE PUT IN?

A **PICC** line is put in by your health care provider. First you will be given a local anesthetic so that the insertion of the line will not hurt. After the **PICC** line is put in, a transparent dressing will be put over the end of the catheter where it enters the skin. Then you will have an x-ray taken to make sure that the other end of the catheter is in the right place.

HOW DO I CARE FOR MY PICC LINE?

To keep the **PICC** line open and working properly:
- Flush the line with a small amount of fluid a couple of times a week. Your provider will show you how to do this and tell you how often to do it.
- Keep the area where the **PICC** line enters the skin clean and dry.
- Watch for signs of infection (redness, pus, tenderness). If you see these signs, tell your provider.
- Avoid catching the end of your catheter on your clothing or other things.

HOW IS THE PICC LINE REMOVED?

When you are done with your **PICC** line it will be removed by your health care provider. The line is pulled out of the vein and then pressure is applied over the spot where it entered the skin. Removing the **PICC** line is usually a painless procedure.

Patient Teaching

RESOURCE LIST: CANCER

AMC CANCER RESEARCH CENTER AND FOUNDATION
1600 Pierce Street
Denver, CO 80214
800-321-1557
Web site: http://www.amc.org
Educational materials, counselors to work through grief or discuss an individual case by phone

AMERICAN BRAIN TUMOR ASSOCIATION
2720 River Road
Des Plaines, IL 60018
800-886-2282
Educational materials, specialist referrals, support group listings

AMERICAN CANCER SOCIETY, INC.
National Headquarters
1599 Clifton Road NE
Atlanta, GA 30329
Web site: http://www.cancer.org
800-227-2345
Referrals to specialists and local chapters (local units sponsor services for patients and families including transportation programs and some supplies), educational materials

NATIONAL CANCER INSTITUTE CANCER INFORMATION SERVICE
31 Center Drive, MSC 2580
Building 31, Rm. 10A-03
Bethesda, MD 20892-2580
800-4CANCER (422-6237)
301-435-3848
TTY: 800-332-8615
Web site: http://www.cancer.gov
Spanish Web site: http://www.cancer.gov/espanol
English/Spanish educational materials, printed information, referrals to a local mammography center, cancer information specialists

NATIONAL COALITION FOR CANCER SURVIVORSHIP
1010 Wayne Avenue, Suite 770
Silver Spring, MD 20910
877-622-7937
Web site:http://www.cansearch.org/
Information and resources to support people after cancer diagnosis.

THE SKIN CANCER FOUNDATION
245 5th Avenue, Suite 1403
New York, NY 10016
800-SKIN-490 (754-6490)
Web site: http://www.skincancer.org
Public information services, printed and video information

UNITED OSTOMY ASSOCIATIONS OF AMERICA
19772 MacArthur Blvd., Suite 200
Irvine, CA 92612-2405
800-826-0826
Web site: http://www.uoaa.org
Educational materials, specialist referrals, local chapters, printed information, audio information, visual information

Y-ME NATIONAL BREAST CANCER ORGANIZATION
212 W. Van Buren
Chicago, IL 60607-3908
English: 800-221-2141
Spanish: 800-996-9505
Emergency Hotline (24 hours): 312-986-8228
Web site: http://www.y-me.org
Educational materials on treatment options, patient concerns, and questions; telephone peer counseling by breast cancer survivors

Your health care plan, local hospital, or regional cancer center are other sources for cancer information. Your health care plan may cover individual and family counseling. If not, speak to the health care plan social worker about mental health resources within your community.

Group counseling helps those faced with cancer to explore their feelings. People who have had cancer and who have been treated actively participate in these groups. They share their experiences of going through the process after a diagnosis of cancer is made. These people have experienced the psychological factors as well as the treatment factors for the diagnosis of cancer. Some groups meet only during the period of hospitalization, while others continue after the diagnosis is made and treatment is started. Some groups meet only with the patients, while others include spouses, family members, and other special people. These groups also provide an opportunity to exchange treatment tips and hints, as well as give support and information to help patients, families, and friends gain some control over their lives.

Faith is a source of strength for many people. Members of the clergy can provide comfort. Some are trained to minister to those coping with life-threatening illnesses. Contact the faith community of your choice. The chaplain of your local hospital will be able to guide you to clergy who are experienced in supporting people after a cancer diagnosis is made.

Patient Teaching

SEXUALITY AND CANCER

SEXUALITY

- Human sexuality is more than just sexual function. It is a combination of feelings and behaviors that are different for each person. Sexuality includes sexual response, intimacy, emotions, fertility, and hormonal function. Sexual function is a specific aspect of sexuality that includes gender and involves the mind and body.
- Sexuality is an important part of normal life for most people and is important to their quality of life.
- Many patients have some kind of sexual problems during or after cancer treatments and do not talk to their doctors or nurse practitioners about this.

WHAT CAUSES PROBLEMS WITH SEXUALITY IN CANCER PATIENTS?

- Cancer and/or cancer treatments (chemotherapy, biotherapy, surgery, or radiation therapy) may damage one of the body systems, such as hormonal, vascular, neurologic, or psychological systems, needed for healthy sexual responses.
- Certain medications may affect sexuality:
  - antihypertensives such as sympatholytics, alpha-adrenergic blockers, beta-adrenergic blockers, vasodilators, diuretics
  - psychotropic agents such as major tranquilizers, antidepressants, antianxiety agents
  - controlled substances such as alcohol, cocaine, narcotics, nicotine
  - other medications such as hormonal agents, anticholinergics, histamine H_2 receptor blockers, clofibrate, digoxin, and finasteride

WHAT ARE SOME SIGNS OF SEXUAL PROBLEMS?

- Females:
  - decreased libido (less desire for sex)
  - painful sex
  - difficulty reaching orgasm
  - changes in how you see yourself
  - amenorrhea (stopping of menstrual periods)
  - menopausal symptoms such as hot flashes, vaginal dryness, mood swings
  - infertility (unable to have children)
- Males:
  - decreased libido (less desire for sex)
  - erectile dysfunction (unable to have an erection or to maintain an erection)
  - premature ejaculation
  - difficulty reaching orgasm
  - changes in how you see yourself
  - infertility (unable to have children)

WHAT WILL MY DOCTOR OR NURSE PRACTITIONER DO?

- A physical examination

- Blood work may be done.
- You will be asked some personal questions that will help your health care provider know best how to treat you.
- Sometimes you may need to be referred to a specialist.

SUGGESTIONS TO HELP WITH SEXUAL PROBLEMS

It is important that you talk with us about your problem. We know this can be embarrassing or uncomfortable, but we want to help.

- For men:
  - Medications may be helpful
  - Vacuum devices
  - Testosterone therapy
  - Penis injections

- For women:
  - Stop any activity that causes pain or irritation.
  - For vaginal dryness, water-based lubricants, vaginal moisturizers, nonirritating lubricants (such as Replens) or a low-dose estrogen (vaginal ring or suppository) may be considered.
  - Consider position changes during sex, perhaps with the female on top.
  - Muscle exercises, relaxation techniques, and stress reduction techniques may be helpful.
  - For pain, topical lidocaine may be used. Mild oral analgesics such as Tylenol may be helpful.
  - Regular sexual activity will help prevent stiffening of the vaginal opening after surgery or radiation to the pelvic area.
  - Vaginal dilation may be used to prevent stiffening of the vagina after surgery or radiation to the pelvic area.

GENERAL SUGGESTIONS FOR EVERYONE

- Practice safe sex and talk to us about contraception during and after treatments.
- Avoid sexual relations during times of low blood counts.
- Exploration of other means of sexual expression besides intercourse.
- Control nausea and vomiting before sex:
  - Antiemetics 1 hour and light meal or crackers before sexual activity
  - Partner should avoid perfumes, colognes, or scented candles
- Control pain:
  - Take pain medication 1 hour before sexual activity.
  - Use relaxation techniques, massage, warm bath before sexual activity.
  - Support painful areas with cushions/pillows.
- For fatigue:
  - Take a 30-60 minute nap before sexual activity.
  - Avoid large meal before sexual activity.
- For shortness of breath:
  - Try sexual positions that take minimal effort on part of the patient.

Patient Teaching

SLEEP HYGIENE

Many cancer patients have difficulty with sleep, either being unable to sleep (insomnia) or sleeping too much (hypersomnia). If you are having trouble with sleep, please let your physician or nurses know. We want to help.

WHAT CAUSES SLEEP PROBLEMS?

- Active chemotherapy treatment
- Chronic medical illness
- Depression/anxiety
- Symptoms such as pain, nausea, diarrhea, itching, etc.
- Fatigue
- Older age
- Perimenopause
- Personal or family history of insomnia
- Recent life stressors
- Unpleasant environment
- Use of alcohol
- Withdrawal from certain medications
- Shortness of breath or difficulty breathing or lying down
- Having to urinate frequently
- Hormonal problems
- Hot flashes
- Restless legs
- Sleeping during the day (even as much as 15 minutes)
- Caffeine intake
- Change in environment
- Certain medications such as:
  - Amphetamines
  - Antiseizure medication
  - Biologicals such as interferons, interleukins, and tumor necrosis factor
  - Breathing treatments or medications
  - Caffeine
  - Chemotherapy
  - Steroids
  - Decongestants
  - Dieting agents
  - Hormonal agents
  - Illegal drugs
  - Long-term use of pain medications
  - Monoamine oxidase inhibitors (MAOIs)
  - Selective serotonin reuptake inhibitors (SSRIs)
  - Theophyllines

WHAT CAN YOU DO FOR MY SLEEP PROBLEMS?

- Sometimes a sleep study may be ordered to help decide what is causing the sleep problem.
- We will need to review your medications to make sure this isn't part of the problem. We may suggest changes in doses or timing of some medications.
- Certain medications may be given for a short period of time, usually no more than 2-3 weeks.
- After 2-3 weeks, you may want to try to taper off the sleep medication little by little and then take it only as needed.

WHAT CAN I DO TO HELP MY SLEEP PROBLEM?

- Keep a sleep journal to record information about your sleeping times, symptoms that keep you from sleeping, medications taken, food eaten, etc.
- Sometimes things such as counting, refocusing, meditation, or guided imagery may assist in controlling racing thoughts or worries.
  - Thought stopping is repeating the word "the" or "stop" every 3 seconds.
- Other types of relaxation training include progressive muscle relaxation, biofeedback, yoga, or hypnosis.
- Sleep hygiene

WHAT IS SLEEP HYGIENE?

- Sleep hygiene is a healthy way to go about sleeping. Here are some suggestions that may help:
  - Stay in the bed only during hours intended for sleep.
  - Establish a routine wake time and bedtime.
  - Avoid stimulants such as caffeine.
  - Refrain from exercising at least 6 hours before bedtime.
  - Decrease or eliminate nighttime use of tobacco products.
  - Determine the best sleep environment for you.
  - Do not nap during the day, or at least limit naps to 20 minutes, avoiding all napping after 3 PM.
  - Create a bedtime routine.
  - If not asleep within 15-20 minutes, get out of bed and do some nonstimulating activity until sleepy and then return to bed.
  - Avoid heavy foods at bedtime.
  - Consider keeping a sleep log.
  - Remove bedroom clock.

WEEDING THROUGH THE WEB

Many patients get information about their health from the Internet. But how do you know if you are getting accurate information? This educational sheet is designed to help you weed through the volumes of information that are on the Web.

Make sure the information is current. Check when the Web site was posted and when it was last updated. Many sites are made and not maintained. Old information may be worse than no information at all.

Who created the Web site? Was it a reputable institution (such as the American Cancer Society [ACS] or National Cancer institute [NCI])? Was it an individual with the health problem? Was it a pharmaceutical company trying to sell a particular drug? What are the credentials of the author of this Web site? Be sure that the author of the Web site is someone you would trust getting information from.

What is the goal of the Web site? Is the Web site trying to sell a product or service? Is the author trying to deliver a message? Are there a lot of advertisements or "pop-ups" on the site? You will want to know what the goal is because this can influence the information you are getting.

Where is the Web site getting its information? What sources or references are posted? Are they clearly identified? Are the sources from reputable studies? Remember that just because it is on the Internet does not mean it is true.

Can you understand the information you are getting? Most Web sites are written at a 12th grade level or above. This is difficult for the average American to understand. Ask a health care professional to help you understand the information if needed.

HELPFUL AND RELIABLE WEB SITES

General
National Institutes of Health: www.nih.gov
American Dietetic Association: www.eatright.com
Center for Patient Advocacy: www.patientadvocacy.org

Breast Cancer
Living with it.org: www.livingwithit.org
Share: www.sharecancersupport.org
American Breast Cancer Foundation: www.abcf.org
Susan G. Komen Breast Cancer Foundation:
  www.breastcancerinfo.com
Y-ME National Breast Cancer Organization: www.y-me.org
Breast Cancer Answers: www.medsch.wisc.edu/bca
National Lymphedema Network: www.lymphnet.org
Johns Hopkins Breast Center:
  www.med.jhu.edu/breastcenter
SusanLoveMD.com: www.susanlovemd.com

Lung Cancer
Living with it.org: www.livingwithit.org
Lung Cancer Profile—Know Your Risk:
  www.lungcancer.org

Ovarian Cancer
Conversations!: www.ovarian-news.org
FORCE: www.facingourrisk.org
Gilda Radner Familial Ovarian Cancer Registry:
  www.ovariancancer.com
Gilda's Club: www.gildasclub.org
Gynecologic Cancer Foundation: www.sgo.org/gcf
National Ovarian Cancer Coalition: www.ovarian.org
Ovarian Cancer National Alliance: www.ovariancancer.org
The Ovarian Cancer Research Fund: www.ocrf.org
Ovarian Plus: www.monitor.net/ovarian
Share: www.sharecancersupport.org

Prostate Cancer
American Foundation for Urologic Disease:
  www.prostatehealth.com

Cancer (all types)
National Cancer Institute: www.cancer.gov/
Gillette Women's Cancer Connection:
  www.gillettecancerconnect.org
Cancer Consultants Patient Resource Center:
  www.411cancer.com
American Cancer Society: www.cancer.org/
International Cancer Alliance: www.icare.org/

Continued

WEEDING THROUGH THE WEB—cont'd

CancerEducation.com:
www.cancereducation.com/cancersyspagesnb/
splash.cfm
Cancer News on the Net: www.cancernews.com
American Institute for Cancer Research: www.aier.org
Cancer Hope Network: www.cancerhopenetwork.org
National Coalition for Cancer survivorship:
www.cansearch.org
Cancer Care, Inc: www.cancercare.org
Oncology Nursing Society: www.ons.org
Association of Oncology Social Work: www.aosw.org
Association of Cancer Online Resources, Inc:
www.acor.org
Oncology.com: www.oncology.com

Clinical Trials (Research)
The National Foundation for Cancer Research:
www.nfcr.org
National Cancer Institute: www.cancer.gov/clinicaltrials/
CenterWatch, Inc: www.centerwatch.com

For Children Dealing With Family Member's Cancer
Kids Konnected: www.kidskonnected.org

Hospice
National Hospice and Palliative Care Organization:
www.nhpco.org

Palliative Care
National Institute on Aging: www.nia.nih.gov
National Hospice and Palliative Care Organization:
www.nhpco.org

General Links
Cancer Links: www.cancerlinks.net/

Submitted by Wendy H. Vogel.

Newly Released Oncology Drugs

During the time this book has been developed and published, several new medications have been approved for use by the Food and Drug Administration (FDA). Other medications currently in use for specifically approved cancers have earned additional indications. To remain up to date on oncology products, the United States FDA has a website that serves as a reference. Interested providers may sign up for free email updates. Access to information on new oncology drug products from the FDA Center for Drug Evaluation and Research is found at http://www.fda.gov/cder/Offices/OODP/whatsnew.htm.

There are new drugs in development that may be approved for general use in the future. To access information on drugs in development, go to Center Watch, a clinical trials service, at http://www.centerwatch.com/professional/cwpipeline.

The following monographs are for oncology drugs approved in 2007.

Dasatinib (Sprycel)

DRUG CLASS

- Inhibitor of multiple tyrosine kinases

ROUTE OF ADMINISTRATION

- Oral

PRETREATMENT GUIDELINES

- Measure potassium and magnesium levels prior to therapy. Correct abnormalities prior to starting therapy.

USE

- Treatment of adults with chronic, accelerated, or myeloid or lymphoid blast phase chronic myeloid leukemia resistant to or intolerant of prior therapy including imatinib.
- Treatment of adults with Philadelphia chromosome-positive acute lymphoblastic leukemia with resistance to or intolerant of prior therapy.

PHARMACOKINETICS

- Following oral administration, maximum plasma concentrations occur between 0.5 and 6 hours.
- Terminal half-life is 3-5 hours.

USUAL DOSE AND SCHEDULE

- Dose is 140 mg/day. Administer in two divided doses of 70 mg, take one in morning and one in evening.
- May be taken with or without food.
- Tablets should not be crushed, cut, or chewed.
- Dose escalation to 90-100 mg twice daily was allowed for patients that did not achieve a hematologic or cytogenetic response at recommended dose.
- Myelosuppression is managed by dose interruption, dose reduction, or discontinuation.

SIDE EFFECTS

- Myelosuppression
- Hemorrhage: CNS or gastrointestinal
- Fever
- Pleural effusion
- Pneumonia
- Thrombocytopenia
- Anemia
- Cardiac failure
- Fluid retention
- Diarrhea
- Nausea
- Abdominal pain
- Vomiting

DRUG INTERACTIONS

- Strong inducers of CYP3A4 may decrease level of dasatinib. Such drugs include: dexamethasone, carbamazepine, phenytoin, phenobarbital, rifampin, rifabutin, rifampicin, and St. John's Wort.
- Strong inhibitors of CYP3A4 may increase blood concentrations of dasatinib. Such drugs include: atazanavir, clarithromycin, erythromycin, indinavir, itraconazole, ketoconazole, nefazodone, nelfinavir, ritonavir, saquinavir, and telithromycin.

PREGNANCY

Category D

SPECIAL CONSIDERATIONS

- Drug may cause QT prolongation. Correct hypokalemia or hypomagnesemia and monitor during therapy.

PATIENT EDUCATION

- Patients should report symptoms of pleural effusion: dyspnea or dry cough.
- Patients should not take an antacid 2 hours before or after taking dasatinib.
- Avoid taking medications that lower acid levels in stomach such as cimetidine, ranitidine, omeprazole, lansoprazole, esomeprazole, or rabeprazole.
- Report any bleeding
- Avoid use of grapefruit or grapefruit juice while taking dasatinib.

BIBLIOGRAPHY

Bristol-Myers Squibb Company. (2007). *Sprycel® (dasatinib). Manufacturer package insert.* Princeton, NJ: Author.

Dexrazoxane hydrochloride (Totect)

DRUG CLASS

- Inhibits topoisomerase II reversibly, iron chelator

ROUTE OF ADMINISTRATION

- Intravenous (IV)

HOW TO ADMINISTER

- Totect is given IV for 3 days in a row starting as soon as possible, within six hours, following an anthracycline extravasation.
- Dose is administered over 1 to 2 hours through a large vein away from or in another extremity from the site of extravasation.

PRETREATMENT GUIDELINE

- Measure complete blood count (CBC), liver enzymes, and renal function.
- Patients with renal insufficiency will need a 50% dose reduction when creatinine clearance is less then 40 ml per minute.
- Monitor liver enzymes.

USE

- Treatment of anthracycline extravasation from daunorubicin, doxorubicin, epirubicin, or idarubicin.

PHARMACOKINETICS

- Pharmacokinetic studies following dosing for anthracycline extravasation have not been studied.
- When administered prior to doxorubicin, half-life was 2-2.5 hours.

USUAL DOSE AND SCHEDULE

- Administer 1000 mg/m^2 on Days 1 and 2 with 500 mg/m^2 on Day 3.
- Dose should not exceed a total of 2000 mg on days 1 and 2 with no more than 1000mg on day 3.

- Give Day 2 dose 24 hours after Day 1 dose with Day 3 dose 48 hours following Day 1 dose.

SIDE EFFECTS

- Neutropenia
- Thrombocytopenia
- Fever
- Nausea
- Vomiting
- Infusion site reactions
- Increased liver enzyme levels

NADIR

- Treatment is associated with leukopenia, neutropenia, and thrombocytopenia, specific time frame not identified.

STORAGE

- Store drug in carton at room temperature, protect from heat.

MIXING INSTRUCTIONS

- Reconstitute with supplied diluent to make a concentration of 10mg/mL. The solution will have a slight yellow color. The total dose is injected into a 1000 ml bag of normal saline.

PRODUCT STABILITY

- Reconstituted product should be used immediately after mixing, within 2 hours. Mixed, diluted product is stable for 4 hours below 25° C (77°F).

COMPATABILITY WITH OTHER DRUGS/IV FLUIDS

- Dimethylsulfoxide (DMSO) should not be used in patients receiving dexrazoxane for anthracycline-induced extravasation. DMSO may reduce the efficacy of dexrazoxane.
- Do not mix in infusion bag with other drugs.

DRUG INTERACTIONS

- None identified

PREGNANCY

Category D

SPECIAL CONSIDERATIONS

- Remove application of ice from site of extravasation at least

15 minutes prior to the administration of Totect.

PATIENT EDUCATION

- Women should be advised that drug may cause fetal harm.
- Instruct patient to remove ice at least 15 minutes prior to infusion.

BIBLIOGRAPHY

Schulmeister, L. (2007). Totect: A new agent for treating anthracycline extravasation. *Clinical Journal of Oncology Nursing, 11*(3), 387-395.

Totect™ (2007). *Package insert*. Manufactured for TopoTarget A/S, Copenhagen, Denmark: Author.

Ixabepilone (Ixempra)

DRUG CLASS

- Epothilone: Microtubular inhibitor

ROUTE OF ADMINISTRATION

- Intravenous (IV) infusion

HOW TO ADMINISTER

- Administer over 3 hours every 3 weeks using a non-DEHP infusion container and administration set. Use an in-line filter with a microporous membrane of 0.2 to 1.2 microns.

PRETREATMENT GUIDELINES

- Measure liver enzymes and complete blood count.
- Assess for degree of peripheral neuropathy, stomatitis, or diarrhea
- Administer an H$_1$ antagonist (e.g., diphenhydramine 50 mg orally or equivalent) and an H$_2$ antagonist (e.g., ranitidine 150 to 300 mg orally or equivalent) one hour prior to infusion to prevent hypersensitivity reaction. Should patient have a hypersensitivity reaction to ixabepilone or has a low grade hypersensitivity reaction to another cremophor-containing product, administer dexamethasone in addition to the H$_1$ and H$_2$ antagonists.

DOSE ADJUSTMENTS

- Reduce dose by 20% for febrile neutropenia, neutrophil count <500 cells/mm^3 lasting 7 days or longer, or thrombocytopenia (<25,000/mm^3 without bleeding or <50,000/mm≥ with bleeding).
- When used in combination with capecitabine, hold ixabepilone for concurrent stomatitis or diarrhea until platelet count >50,000/mm^3 or until neutrophil >1,000 cells/mm^3.

For patients receiving ixabepilone as monotherapy, reduce dose for hepatic impairment:

- Mild impairment: For AST or ALT ≤10 x upper limits of normal (ULN) and bilirubin ≤1.5 x ULN, dose reduced to 32mg/m^2
- Moderate impairment: For AST and ALT ≤10 x ULN and bilirubin between >1.5 - ≤3 x ULN, dose reduced to 20–30mg/m^2.
- Ixabepilone is contraindicated with the use of capecitabine when AST or ALT >2.5 x ULN or bilirubin >1 x ULN.

Dose reduction for neuropathy:

- Grade 2 lasting ≥7 days or grade 3 lasting <7days, reduce dose by 20%. Grade 3 lasting ≥7days or disabling neuropathy, discontinue ixabepilone.

CONTRAINDICATIONS

- Severe (grade 3/4) hypersensitivity to Cremophor® EL or its derivatives, such as polyoxyethylated castrol oil.
- Baseline neutrophil count <1500 cells/mm^3 or platelet count <100,000/mm^3 .
- Patients with AST or ALT >2.5 x ULN or bilirubin >1 x ULN when used in combination with capecitabine.

USE

- Metastatic or locally advanced breast cancer.
- When used in combination with capecitabine, must have a tumor that is resistant or refractory to prior anthracycline and taxane treatment.
- When used as monotherapy, must have a tumor that is resistant or refractory to prior anthracycline, taxane, and capecitabine therapy.

PHARMACOKINETICS

- Ixabepilone is metabolized in the liver.
- Terminal half-life is approximately 52 hours.

USUAL DOSE AND SCHEDULE

- Administer 40mg/m^2 IV over 3 hours every 3 weeks.
- Dose adjust per manufacturer guidelines.

SIDE EFFECTS

- Peripheral neuropathy: primarily sensory. Is cumulative, predictable, manageable, and generally reversible
- Myelosuppression: primarily neutropenia although leucopenia, thrombocytopenia, and anemia occur.
- Hypersensitivity reactions: premedicate with H$_1$ and H$_2$ antagonists to prevent. If patient has low-grade hypersensitivity to Cremphor, additional premedication with intravenous dexamethasone is suggested.
- Fatigue
- Myalgia/arthralgia
- Alopecia
- Nausea and vomiting
- Stomatitis/mucositis
- Diarrhea
- Musculoskeletal pain
- Additional side effects when administered with capecitabine include: hand-foot syndrome, anorexia, abdominal pain, nail changes, and constipation.

NADIR

- Not listed in package insert

STORAGE

- Ixabepilone is supplied as a kit containing one vial of drug for injection and one vial of diluent. Kit is refrigerated in original package at 2° to 8° C (36° to 46° F).

MIXING INSTRUCTIONS

- Constitute ixabepilone with supplied diluent. Remove from refrigerator and allow to stand at room temperature for 30 minutes prior to constitution.
- Further dilution is made using Lactated Ringer's injection to a final concentration of 0.2mg/ml to 0.6mg/ml

PRODUCT STABILITY

- Reconstituted ixabepilone should be further diluted in Lactated Ringer's solution as soon as possible. However, the constituted vial may be stored no longer than an hour at room temperature and room light before final dilution.
- Final solution of ixabepilone diluted in Lactated Ringer's solution must be used within 6 hours of mixture.

COMPATIBILITY WITH OTHER DRUGS/IV FLUIDS

- Lactated Ringer's for injection is indicated. Ixabepilone is stable in a pH between 6 to 7.5. Dilute only with supplied diluent and recommended solution for injection.

DRUG INTERACTIONS

- The use of CYP3A4 inhibitors may increase the concentration of ixabepilone. Avoid concurrent use with ketoconazole, itraconazole, clarithromycin, atazanavir, nefazodone, saquinavir, telithromycin, ritonavir, amprenavir, indinavir, nelfinavir, delavirdine, or voriconazole. Avoid use of grapefruit juice.
- The use of CYP3A4 inducers may decrease the concentration of ixabepilone. The drugs that may interact in this manner include: dexamethasone, phenytoin, carbamazepine, rifampin, rifampicin, rifabutin, phenobarbital, and St. John's wort.

PREGNANCY

Category D

- Ixabepilone is excreted in human milk.

SPECIAL CONSIDERATIONS

- Use caution when used with patients with a history of cardiac disease. Should patient develop impaired cardiac function or develop cardiac ischemia, consider discontinuation of drug.
- Drug contains dehydrated alcohol, cognitive impairment may occur.
- If patient has a hypersensitivity reaction, add dexamethasone to the premedications and infuse at a slower rate.

PATIENT EDUCATION

- Avoid grapefruit juice while receiving ixabepilone.
- Report symptoms of numbness, tingling, or burning in hands or feet.
- Report any itching, flushing; chest tightness; trouble breathing; sudden swelling of face, throat or tongue; heart palpitations; feeling dizzy; or unusual weight gain.

BIBLIOGRAPHY

Bristol-Myers Squibb. (2007). Ixabepilone *Full prescribing information*. Princeton, NJ: Author.

Nilotinib (Tasigna)

DRUG CLASS

- Tyrosine kinase inhibitor: Targets BCR-ABL and c-KIT

ROUTE OF ADMINISTRATION

- Oral

PRETREATMENT GUIDELINES

- Measure potassium and magnesium levels prior to therapy. Correct abnormalities prior to starting therapy.
- Due to potential for prolonged QT interval, obtain electrocardiogram (ECG) at baseline, seven days after starting drug, and periodically thereafter.
- Measure complete blood count (CBC), liver functions, and electrolytes prior to initiating therapy and thereafter. CBC should be checked every two weeks for the first two months and then monthly.

USE

- Treatment of adult patients with chronic phase or accelerated phase of Philadelphia chromosome positive chronic myelogenous leukemia (CML) resistant to or intolerant to therapy with imatinib.

PHARMACOKINETICS

- Half-life is approximately 17 hours.
- Steady state is achieved by day 8.

USUAL DOSE AND SCHEDULE

- Dose is 400 mg twice a day.
- Swallow capsule whole with water on an empty stomach.
- Food increases the blood levels of nilotinib. Do not eat for at least 2 hours prior and one hour after taking medication.

SIDE EFFECTS

- Neutropenia
- Febrile neutropenia
- Thrombocytopenia
- Bleeding including intracranial hemorrhage
- Pneumonia
- Fever
- Elevated lipase
- Rash
- Pruritus
- Nausea
- Fatigue
- Nausea
- Headache
- Constipation
- Diarrhea
- Vomiting

DRUG INTERACTIONS

- Nilotinib is metabolized by the CYP3A4 route.
- Strong inducers of CYP3A4 may decrease level of nilotinib. Such drugs include: dexamethasone, carbamazepine, phenytoin, phenobarbital, rifampin, rifabutin, rifampicin, and St. John's Wort.
- Strong inhibitors of CYP3A4 may increase blood concentrations of nilotinib. Such drugs include: atazanavir, clarithromycin, erythromycin, indinavir, itraconazole, ketoconazole, nefazodone, nelfinavir, ritonavir, saquinavir, and telithromycin.
- Nilotinib is a substrate of P-glycoprotein (Pgp). Drugs that inhibit Pgp may result in an increased concentration of nilotinib.

PREGNANCY

Category D

SPECIAL CONSIDERATIONS

- Nilotinib may increase bilirubin levels, monitor levels.
- Food will affect absorption. Take on an empty stomach.

PATIENT EDUCATION

- Patients and caregivers may find further information about nilotinib or CML at www.CMLALLIANCE. com or www.LivingwithCML.com
- If patient misses a dose, take the next dose as scheduled. Do not take a double dose to make up for the missed dose.
- Avoid grapefruit juice, grapefruit, or supplements that contain grapefruit extract.
- Provide your healthcare worker with an updated list of medications, vitamins, and supplements.
- Report any problems with lactose. Nilotinib capsules contain lactose.
- Do not become pregnant or breastfeed while on nilotinib.
- Take medication on an empty stomach.

BIBLIOGRAPHY

Burger, V. (2007). Pharmacy corner: Drug provides alternative for Imatinib resistance. *Oncology Nursing Forum, 34*(3), 737.

Novartis. (2007). Tasigna® *(nilotinib) prescribing information*. East Hanover, NJ: Author.

Raloxifene Hydrochloride (Evista)

DRUG CLASS
- Estrogen agonist/antagonist

ROUTE OF ADMINISTRATION
- Oral

HOW TO ADMINISTER
- Oral agent administered once daily

PRETREATMENT GUIDELINES
- Evaluate for presence of or history of deep vein thrombosis or pulmonary embolism.
- Evaluate for presence of coronary artery disease.
- Evaluate for menopausal status.

USE
- Treatment and prevention of osteoporosis in postmenopausal women
- Reduction in risk of invasive breast cancer in postmenopausal women with osteoporosis
- Reduction in risk of invasive breast cancer in postmenopausal women at high risk for invasive breast cancer.

PHARMACOKINETICS
- Drug is absorbed rapidly following oral administration.
- Half-life is 27.7 hours after oral dosing.

USUAL DOSE AND SCHEDULE
- 60 mg tablet taken orally once daily

SIDE EFFECTS
- Deep vein thrombosis (DVT)
- Pulmonary embolism (PE)
- Retinal vein thrombosis
- Hot flashes
- Leg cramps
- Peripheral edema
- Flu syndrome
- Arthralgia
- Sweating

DRUG INTERACTIONS
- Cholestyramine reduces the absorption of raloxifene.
- Prothrombin time may be decreased by 10% when coumadin is given with raloxifene.

PREGNANCY
Category X

SPECIAL CONSIDERATIONS
- Not recommended to be taken at the same time as estrogen supplement.
- Monitor triglyceride level if triglyceride level was previously elevated while on estrogen supplement.
- Hold drug at least 3 days prior to and during prolonged immobilization due to DVT/PE risk.

PATIENT EDUCATION
- When administered for osteoporosis treatment or prevention, patient should be advised to take supplemental calcium and vitamin D.
- Patients should be instructed to participate in regular weight-bearing exercises, quit smoking, and limit alcohol intake.
- Patients should perform monthly self breast exam, have regular breast exam and have regular mammograms.

BIBLIOGRAPHY
Eli Lilly and Company. (2007). Raloxifene. *Manufacturer package insert.* Indianapolis, IN: Author.

Temsirolimus (Torisel)

DRUG CLASS
- Targeted Therapy: mammalian target of rapamycin (mTOR) inhibitor

ROUTE OF ADMINISTRATION
- Intravenous (IV)

HOW TO ADMINISTER
- Given as a weekly infusion over 30 to 60 minutes.

PRETREATMENT GUIDELINES
- Obtain baseline glucose and lipid profiles and measure every 2 weeks.
- Measure baseline renal function and throughout treatment.
- Administer antihistamine, such as diphenhydramine 25 to 50 mg, 30 minutes prior to treatment.

USE
- First line therapy for advanced renal cell carcinoma

PHARMACOKINETICS
- The half-life of sirolimus, the active metabolite of temsirolimus, was 54.6 hours.

USUAL DOSE AND SCHEDULE
- Dose is 25 mg administered weekly using a non-DEHP infusion bag and administration set with an in-line filter no larger than 5 microns.
- Hold dose for absolute neutrophil count (ANC) <1,000 cells/mm^3, platelet count <75,000 cells/mm^3, or any grade 3 or greater toxicity.
- When toxicities resolved to a grade 2 or less, may resume at a reduced dose. Dose is reduced by 5mg/week to a dose no lower than 15 mg/week.

SIDE EFFECTS
- Hyperlipidemia
- Hyperglycemia

- Interstitial lung disease: report cough, dyspnea, hypoxia, and fever
- Bowel perforation
- Intracranial hemorrhage
- Renal failure
- Rash
- Nausea
- Edema
- Fatigue
- Mouth sores
- Loss of appetite

NADIR

- None noted in package insert

STORAGE

- Drug must be refrigerated and protected from light. Store at 2° to 8° C (36° to 46° F).

MIXING INSTRUCTIONS

- Mix with 1.8 ml of diluent provided. Total volume will be 3 ml and drug concentration is 10 mg/ml.
- Withdraw required amount of constituted solution and inject into a 250 ml bag of normal saline.

PRODUCT STABILITY

- Product constituted with diluent is stable for up to 24 hours at room temperature.
- Once final concentration of drug is mixed with saline infusion solution, administration should be completed within 6 hours.

COMPATIBILITY WITH OTHER DRUGS/IV FLUIDS

- Use non-DEHP infusion bags and administration sets. The use of an in-line filter with a pore size of not greater than 5 microns is recommended.
- Drug should not be mixed with other medications in the IV solution.

DRUG INTERACTIONS

- Strong inducers of CYP3A4/5 may decrease level of temsirolimus. Such drugs include: dexamethasone, carbamazepine, phenytoin, phenobarbital, rifampin, rifabutin, rifampicin, and St. John's Wort.
- Strong inhibitors of CYP3A4 may increase blood concentrations of temsirolimus. Such drugs include: atazanavir, clarithromycin, indinavir, itraconazole, ketoconazole, nefazodone, nelfinavir, ritonavir, saquinavir, and telithromycin.

PREGNANCY

Category D

SPECIAL CONSIDERATIONS

- Monitor glucose, blood lipids and triglyceride levels every two weeks.
- Monitor renal function.

- Patients with central nervous system tumors and/or on anticoagulation therapy may have an increased risk for intracranial hemorrhage.
- Patients should not receive or be around anyone that has received a live vaccination while on temsirolimus.
- CBC should be monitored weekly and chemistry panel every 2 weeks.

PATIENT EDUCATION

- Patients should report any new or worsening respiratory symptoms.
- Patients should report any abdominal pain, fever, bloody stools, or diarrhea.
- Patients should not take St. John's Wort while on temsirolimus.
- Avoid use of grapefruit or grapefruit juice while on temsirolimus.

BIBLIOGRAPHY

Burger, V. (2007). Pharmacy corner: Treatment for kidney cancer with Torisel can prolong survival. *Oncology Nursing Forum, 34*(6), 1222.

Roethke, S. (2007). Abstract 2539: Safety consideration for temsirolimus (Torisel™, a novel inhibitor of mammalian target of rapamycin, in treatment of patients with advanced renal cell carcinoma. *Oncology Nursing Forum, 34*(6), 1245-1246.

Wyeth Pharmaceuticals. (2007). Torisel *(temsirolimus) package insert.* Philadelphia, PA: Author

Index